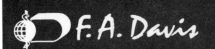
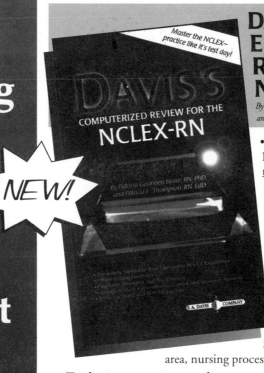
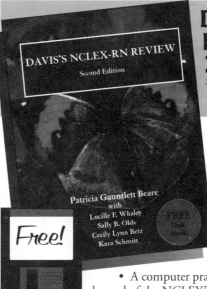

Davis's Q & A for the NCLEX-RN

Patricia Gauntlett Beare, RN, PhD

Professor
Louisiana State University
School of Nursing
New Orleans, Louisiana

Patricia E. Thompson, RN, EdD

Associate Professor
Chair, Parent-Child Department
College of Nursing
University of Arkansas for Medical Sciences
Little Rock, Arkansas

 F. A. DAVIS COMPANY • Philadelphia

F. A. Davis Company
1915 Arch Street
Philadelphia, PA 19103

Printed in the United States of America

Last digit indicates print number: 10 9 8 7 6 5 4 3 2 1

Publisher, Nursing: Robert G. Martone
Nursing Editor: Alan Sorkowitz
Production Editor: Stephen D. Johnson
Cover Designer: Louis J. Forgione

As new scientific information becomes available through basic and clinical research, recommended treatments and drug therapies undergo changes. The author and publisher have done everything possible to make this book accurate, up to date, and in accord with accepted standards at the time of publication. The authors, editors, and publisher are not responsible for errors or omissions or for consequences from application of the book, and make no warranty, expressed or implied, in regard to the contents of the book. Any practice described in this book should be applied by the reader in accordance with professional standards of care used in regard to the unique circumstances that may apply in each situation. The reader is advised always to check product information (package inserts) for changes and new information regarding dose and contraindications before administering any drug. Caution is especially urged when using new or infrequently ordered drugs.

Library of Congress Cataloging–in–Publication Data

Beare, Patricia Gauntlett.
    Davis's Q & A for the NCLEX-RN / Patricia Gauntlett Beare.
    Patricia E. Thompson.
        p.   cm.
    ISBN 0-8036-0282-0 (alk. paper)
    1. Nursing–Examination, questions, etc.   I. Thompson, Patricia
E.   II. Title.
    [DNLM: 1. Nursing Care–examination questions.   2. Nursing–
examination questions. Not acquired]
RT55.B428 1998
610.73′076—dc2
DNLM/DLC
for Library of Congress   97-29247
                                                                CIP

Preface

You are about to take one of the most important tests of your life. The authors of these textbook questions recognize this and have done their best to prepare test questions that will help you to review your nursing knowledge and skills and apply these in clinical situations.

These practice tests will help you think about different situations in which nurses must take correct nursing actions. Every question is written according to the NCLEX-RN format and provides a rationale for the correct as well as incorrect options.

We hope this book will help you build confidence in your nursing knowledge and skill as well as your test-taking skills.

We hope soon to welcome you as a member of a very special group of people—a registered nurse!

Acknowledgments

Many people, too numerous to mention, have helped make this book a reality.

To Alan Sorkowitz, Nursing Editor for F. A. Davis, who supervised the production of the text, special thanks for his patience.

To the many special contributors who shared their expertise and generated many new ideas for student preparation for the NCLEX-RN licensure examination.

To Danielle Trepagnier, who typed and modified the manuscript several times.

To Herb Powell, Director of Production for F. A. Davis, who adroitly guided this book through the production process, special thanks and gratitude.

To the reviewers, who, through their constructive critiques, greatly enhanced the quality of this unique NCLEX-RN review book.

A very special acknowledgment to all our students, personal friends, and colleagues for their support.

Contributors

Golden Tradewell, RN, MA, MSN, PhD$_c$
Assistant Professor
McNeese University
Lake Charles, Louisiana

Susan R. Pryor, RN, MN, DNS$_c$
Assistant Professor
Southeastern University
Hammond, Louisiana

Kathy A. Viator, RN, MN, DNS$_c$
Assist Professor
Southeastern University
Hammond, Louisiana

Pauline F. Bohannon, RN, MN, CS
Faculty
Baton Rouge General School
  of Nursing
Baton Rouge, Louisiana

Ola Burns Allen, RNC, DNS
University of Mississippi
  Medical Center
School of Nursing
Jackson, Mississippi

Bonnie Juvé Meeker, RN, MN, DNS
Southeastern Louisiana
  University
Hammond, Louisiana

Eileen W. Keefe, RN, C, MS
Assistant Professor
Louisiana State University
School of Nursing
New Orleans, Louisiana

Alexandra Weis, RN, MN
Instructor
Louisiana State University
School of Nursing
New Orleans, Louisiana

Rebecca Hall Cagle, RN, C, DSN, FNP
Access Family Health Services, Inc.
Family Nurse Practitioner
Assistant Professor of Nursing
Mississippi University for Women

Mary Taylor Martoff, RN, EdD
Associate Professor
Louisiana State University
Medical Center
New Orleans, Louisiana

Lizabeth Carlson, RN, C, MSN
Maternal Child Coordinator
Copiah-Lincoln Community College
Wesson, Mississippi

Louise Plaisance, RN, C, DNS
Education Coordinator
King Faisal Specialist Hospital and
  Research Center
Riyadh, Saudi Arabia

Jane S. Savage, RN, MS, ACCE
Assistant Professor
Louisiana State University
  Medical Center
School of Nursing
New Orleans, Louisiana

Lola J. Case, RN, DNS, FNP
Pediatric and Adolescent Clinic
Natchez, Mississippi

Lynn Ryan, RN, MN
Instructor
Louisiana State Univesity
    Medical Center
School of Nursing
New Orleans, Louisiana

Susan I. Ray RN, MS
Instructor in Nursing
Copiah-Lincoln Community College
Wesson, Mississippi

Linda K. Calhoun, MNSc, NNP, RN
Instructor
Henderson State University
Department of Nursing
Arkadelphia, Arkansas

Carla Hester, RNC, MNSc
Instructor
University of Arkansas for Medical
    Sciences
College of Nursing
Little Rock, Arkansas

Donna J. Middaugh, MSN, RN
Clinical Assistant Professor
University of Arkansas for Medical
    Sciences
College of Nursing
Little Rock, Arkansas

CONTENTS

unit**three**
INTEGRATED PRACTICE TESTS 541

appendix**a**
STATE BOARDS OF NURSING...................................647

unitone

WHAT YOU NEED TO KNOW ABOUT THE NCLEX-RN

chapter 1

Development, Administration, and Scoring of the NCLEX-RN*

by Kara Schmitt, PhD

The National Council Licensure Examination for Registered Nurses (NCLEX-RN), developed by the National Council of State Boards of Nursing (NCSBN), is designed to measure a licensing candidate's knowledge of the nursing process and client health needs. Using the test plan, "each assembled NCLEX-RN examination reflects the knowledge, skills and abilities essential for application of the phases of the nursing process to meet the needs of clients with commonly occurring health problems."[1] It is used to determine whether a candidate can appropriately react and respond to various problems commonly associated with a registered nurse's (RN's) responsibilities in typical clinical settings. The examination content is structured in such a manner that jurisdictional Boards of Nursing can be reasonably assured that individuals who pass the examination are *minimally competent* to practice entry-level RN nursing and to protect the health, safety, and welfare of its citizens.

APPLYING TO TAKE THE NCLEX-RN

Effective April 1994, the NCLEX-RN changed from a paper-and-pencil administered examination to a computerized adaptive examination. The examination is offered daily in at least one location in each of the states and U.S. territories that require passing the NCLEX-RN

prior to licensure. In order to sit for the examination, you have to submit certain documentation and fees to both the Board of Nursing in the jurisdiction where you wish to be licensed and to The Chauncey Group. Generally, two separate submissions of documents and fees are required, although some jurisdictions may ask that both the licensure application and fee and examination application and fee be sent directly to them.

The Board of Nursing requires a licensure application along with verification of education such as a certificate of completion or an official transcript from an approved school of nursing. Depending on the jurisdiction, you also have to submit a licensure fee, application fee, and/or temporary license fee. All relevant documents and fees must be submitted to the appropriate Board office prior to being allowed to take the examination.

Because each jurisdiction has different requirements, it is essential that you be thoroughly familiar with the specifications associated with the jurisdiction in which you wish licensure. In most instances, faculty from the nursing program that you attended can instruct you as to the necessary forms and fees to submit. Typically, your program also has the necessary licensure and examination applications for you to complete. If your program does not furnish you with these instructions and forms, or you wish to be licensed in a jurisdiction other

---

*NCLEX, NCLEX-RN, and NCLEX-PN are trademarks of the National Council of State Boards of Nursing, Inc.

than where you received your education, it is your responsibility to contact the specific Board office for these forms and/or information, including the *NCLEX Candidate Bulletin*, which contains the registration form and instructions for registering. Appendix A includes a listing of all Boards, their addresses, and phone numbers.

It is essential that you complete the licensure application accurately, enclose the correct fee, and ensure that all additional documentation is forwarded to the Board as soon as possible. Remember, you will *not* be allowed to take the examination until the appropriate Board has determined that you are eligible.

Candidates with a physical disability should contact the licensing jurisdiction as early as possible to arrange for special accommodations. Information will be provided as to how to request the required accommodations as well as what type of documentation is necessary to initiate the process.

Foreign-educated candidates should recognize that additional documentation of education and proof of English-language competency may be required when submitting the licensure application. For this reason, if you were educated outside of the United States, you should contact the appropriate Board to ascertain what specific documentation and/or examination results are required. Additionally, you may want to contact the Commission on Graduates of Foreign Nursing Schools (CGFNS) for various requirements that you may have to fulfill. The address and phone number for CGFNS is:

Commission on Graduates
of Foreign Nursing Schools
3624 Market Street
Philadelphia, PA 19104
(215) 349-8767

In addition to applying for a license, you need to apply to sit for the examination either through The Chauncey Group or through the jurisdiction where you wish to be licensed. Examination applications can be obtained through your school of nursing or the desired licensing jurisdiction. The examination application, along with the fee, may be submitted to The Chauncey Group at any time, even prior to completing your education or being deemed eligible to take the test. Candidates seeking licensure from Florida, Illinois, Massachusetts, and New York do not register with The Chauncey Group. Follow instructions from your Board of Nursing.

If you have a credit card, you can call The Chauncey Group using its toll-free number (1-800-551-1912, Monday through Friday, 8 A.M. to 8 P.M. Eastern Time) to register for the examination. An additional fee is charged for this service. Should you wish to phone in your registration, you will be asked for your credit card number, its expiration date, and the exact name that appears on your card, in addition to the examination application information. The money placed on credit card registration is not refundable.

The information included on the application, or given over the phone, is entered into the computer system. Your registration is considered inactive, however, until your licensing jurisdiction indicates that you are eligible to take the examination. Remember, it will take your jurisdiction time to determine your eligibility, and if you sent your licensure application prior to graduation, no action can be taken until *all* required documents have been received and approved. The quicker your educational program submits the necessary graduation information, the quicker the jurisdiction can determine your eligibility.

Once the jurisdiction in which you wish to be licensed has determined your eligibility, you are sent an *Authorization To Test (ATT)*. This document is required to schedule an appointment and *must* be presented at the test site in order for you to take the exam. As soon as you receive this document, verify that the spelling of your name is correct and that it matches *exactly* the name included on the official signed photographic identification you will be using for admission to the examination. If the two names do not match, call 1-800-551-1912 immediately. If your *ATT* and identification do not match, you may be denied admission to the examination.

In addition to an *ATT,* you also will receive a brochure explaining computerized adaptive testing (CAT), a list of the testing centers, and a toll-free number to call for any new sites. Be sure to read the brochure carefully and follow the instructions provided. You will receive the booklet *Scheduling and Taking Your NCLEX* and a list of centers with the cities and phone numbers of the centers.

Scheduling an Appointment

Once you receive the *ATT,* you may call any of the testing centers where you wish to be tested or the toll-free number (1-800-800-1123) to schedule an appointment. Be sure to have your *ATT* available when you call because you will be asked for your authorization number, identification number, expiration date for testing (determined by the appropriate Board of Nursing), as well as your name and phone number. You cannot make an appointment without your authorization number. The site personnel will verify your name and address as shown in the computer.

You will be asked if the first available date and time are convenient for you; if they are not, you will be asked for your preferred testing date and time. If the site, date, or time you have requested is not available, you will be provided with alternatives. If you are calling the toll-free number, you will first be asked for your preferred testing location.

If you are a first-time candidate, you will be scheduled within 30 days of calling, if you desire. If you are a repeat candidate, you will be scheduled within 45 days, if you desire. You do not need to call for an appointment as soon as you receive the *ATT.* Even if you do call immediately, you do not need to schedule an appointment within the 30 or 45 days. You may schedule your examination appointment at a time convenient for you, provided that it is before the expiration date shown on the

ATT. If you call for an appointment after the expiration date, you will be told to contact the nursing jurisdiction to obtain information as to what you must do. ONLY after you have received this document can you schedule your examination.

Because you have the opportunity to make a specific appointment, be sure to select a time that is convenient for you. Do not schedule your test at the same time as another critical event. Plan for a full 5 hours plus transportation and check-in time. Be sure *not* to schedule your test immediately prior to or after the delivery date for your or your spouse's baby, immediately before a wedding (your own or that of someone close to you), prior to a change in jobs or living arrangements, and so forth. Schedule the examination when you will be able to devote 100 percent to the examination and not be worrying about something else. If, however, you have scheduled your examination and later learn that it will not be convenient, you can reschedule the appointment by calling the testing center where you are scheduled or the central toll-free number at least 3 days prior to the appointment date. You will first have to cancel the original appointment and then make another one. You are limited as to the number of times you can cancel and reschedule without an additional fee. If you are applying for licensure in Florida, Illinois, Massachusetts, or New York, you must register through your jurisdiction. Do not send your registration material or fee to The Chauncey Group.

An important feature of CAT is that testing is conducted at least 5 days a week, typically in at least one site in every jurisdiction. During peak administration times (June and July), some sites may be open for up to 15 hours a day and may offer examinations up to 7 days a week. The number of daily administrations, as well as the number of days each site is open, is contingent on the number of candidates requesting a site. In some instances, the demand at a particular site might be so low that it is only open a few days per month. Specifics regarding each site and available testing times will be conveyed to you when you call for an appointment.

Another significant change relating to CAT is that you do not have to take your examination in the same state in which you have applied for licensure. Perhaps you attended school in Iowa but want to be licensed in Hawaii. You can apply directly to the Hawaiian Board of Nursing. Once Hawaii determines you are eligible, you can schedule your examination administration in Iowa. The results of the examination will be submitted automatically to Hawaii even though you sat in Iowa.

Once you have called for an appointment, be sure to write the location, date, and time somewhere so that you will remember the information. You will also be given directions for finding the site. You might want to put all of this on your *ATT* because you will need to bring it with you to the examination.

If you lose your *ATT,* call The Chauncey Group to request another. If you discover it missing immediately prior to your examination, you should still call The Chauncey Group so that the testing center can be alerted that you do not have the document. You will probably still be allowed to test provided you have sufficient identification.

BASIS FOR THE EXAMINATION CONTENT

The purpose of the NCLEX-RN is to help Boards of Nursing determine whether licensure candidates are *minimally competent* to practice entry-level nursing, thus protecting the public. In order to accomplish this purpose, it is necessary for the NCSBN to know what an entering nurse actually does *on the job.* Once this is known (based on a job analysis), an accurate evaluation instrument (examination) can be created to measure a candidate's knowledge, skills, and abilities relative to these activities.

The first step in a job analysis involves the determination of tasks that are likely to be performed by new licensees. After these tasks have been agreed on by a committee of nurse supervisors, faculty, and new nurses, a survey is prepared and sent to a random sample of more than 3000 newly licensed RNs whose characteristics (i.e., age, sex, race) represent the total population. After the surveys are returned, the data are analyzed so that an accurate picture of the tasks performed by entering nurses can be obtained.

The primary purpose of a job analysis is to ascertain the frequency with which certain tasks are performed by entering nurses as well as the criticality of these tasks (which tasks, if performed incorrectly, could do serious or critical harm to the patient). Some tasks, such as performing cardiopulmonary resuscitation, may not be done on a regular or daily basis; however, if they are not done immediately and correctly, the patient could die. While it is important to know both the frequency of performance and the criticality of incorrect performance, the criticality is the more important factor. Accordingly, the criticality of a task is given greater weight in the development of a test plan (which determines the examination content) than the frequency of performance.

The July 1988 NCLEX-RN was the first administration of the examination using the results of a job analysis completed in 1986.[2] Another RN job analysis was completed in 1993,[3] and the results of this analysis were implemented in 1995.

EXAMINATION CONTENT (TEST PLAN)

The examination is *not* designed to merely measure a candidate's ability to recall or recognize certain facts. Its primary purpose is to assess how well an individual can apply the facts learned in school to common nursing situations. Accordingly, most items in the examination relate to a candidate's ability to (1) apply information or knowledge acquired in one situation and correctly transfer that knowledge to a similar situation; or (2) an-

TABLE 1–1. NCLEX-RN Test Plan Matrix (1996)

	Phases of the Nursing Process				
Client Health Needs	Assessment (17–23%)	Analysis (17–23%)	Planning (17–23%)	Implementation (17–23%)	Evaluation (17–23%)
Safe, effective care environment (15–21%)					
Physiological integrity (46–54%)					
Psychosocial integrity (8–16%)					
Health promotion and maintenance (17–23%)					

alyze a complex relationship by breaking it into simpler components, making comparisons or identifying the relationships between or among certain pieces of information. Remember, the examination is designed to measure how well you will respond in typical, real-life clinical settings and not necessarily whether you know the exact number of bones or muscles in the arm. The examination content is based on the following premise:

> Upon entry into nursing practice, the registered nurse is expected to care for the client and/or to assist the client's significant others in the provision of care. The registered nurse is expected to identify the health needs/problems of clients throughout their life cycle and in a variety of settings, to plan and to initiate appropriate action based upon nursing diagnoses derived from these assessments and to evaluate the extent to which expected outcomes of the plan of care are achieved.[1]

Based on this premise and the results of the job analysis, the test plan,[4] or specifications for constructing each form of the examination, consists of five phases of the nursing process. Each of these phases is weighted approximately the same; that is, an approximately equal number of items measures each phase of the nursing process (17–23%) of the total number of items covering each phase. The test plan also includes four general categories of client health needs. Accordingly, the test plan is a 5 × 4 matrix (Table 1–1), and all items in an examination must fit into one of the corresponding 20 cells.

In order to better understand the nursing process and client health needs, a brief description of each is provided below.

Phases of the Nursing Process

Assessment is the establishment of a database from which a decision can be made. This phase includes (1) gathering both objective and subjective information re-

lating to the client, (2) confirming the data, and (3) communicating the information acquired to the relevant parties.

Analysis involves the identification of actual or potential health-care needs as a result of the assessment phase. This stage includes (1) interpreting data, (2) formulating the client's nursing diagnoses, and (3) communicating results of the analysis.

Planning means the establishment of goals to meet the client's needs and the design of strategies to reach these goals. In order to plan, the nurse must (1) prioritize the nursing diagnoses, (2) determine the goals of care, (3) formulate the outcome criteria for each goal, (4) develop a plan of care and modify as necessary, (5) collaborate with other health team members to plan delivery of care, and (6) communicate the plan of care.

Implementation is the initiation and completion of actions necessary to accomplish goals. To implement a plan, one must (1) organize and manage the care of a client, (2) counsel and teach client and others, (3) provide care to achieve established care goals, (4) supervise and coordinate the delivery of care, and (5) communicate nursing intervention.

Evaluation is the final phase in the process and involves the extent to which the client's goals have been met. Aspects of a nurse's work in this phase include (1) comparing the actual outcomes with the expected outcome of care, (2) evaluating the client's ability to implement self-care, (3) evaluating the health-care team's ability to implement care, and (4) communicating the evaluation findings.

Client Needs

There are four broad categories associated with the health needs of clients. A brief description of these needs, together with the percentage of items covering each, is as follows:

Safe, effective care environment (15–21%) is achieved by providing and directing nursing care that promotes the achievement of the client's needs through (1) coordinated care, (2) environmental safety, and (3) safe and effective treatment and procedures.

Physiological integrity (46–54%) is provided by the nurse giving care that achieves the client's needs of (1) physiological adaptation, (2) reduction of risk potential, and (3) provision of basic care.

Psychosocial integrity (8–16%) in stress and crisis-related situations is obtained by the client when the nurse promotes achievement in (1) psychosocial adaptation and (2) coping skills.

Health promotion and maintenance (17–23%) of the client is obtained when the nurse provides care that assists in (1) continued growth and development, (2) self-care and support systems, and (3) prevention and early treatment of disease.

COMPUTERIZED ADAPTIVE TESTING

In April 1994, the NCLEX-RN examination underwent a significant change. No longer would RN candidates take a paper-and-pencil examination; no longer would candidates have to take the examination only in February or July; no longer would hundreds or even thousands of candidates have to take a 2-day examination in one large conference hall; no longer would candidates have to wait several months for results.

Instead, the examination is administered by computer at a convenient location on a day convenient for the candidate, and only a small number of candidates are tested at the same time. In most instances, 10 or fewer candidates are in a room, and the maximum number of candidates is 15. Results are available to the candidate's licensure jurisdiction within 48 hours of taking the test.

When the examination was administered via paper and pencil, there was a predetermined number of items asked of *every* candidate and a maximum amount of time allocated to answer all of the questions. Candidates were finished with the exam either when they had answered all of the items or when they had been told to stop writing.

With computerized adaptive testing (CAT) there is still a maximum amount of time allowed (5 hours) and a maximum number of items presented (265), but each candidate receives an examination that is tailor-made to fit ability levels. It is very unlikely that any two candidates will receive exactly the same items, because no two candidates have exactly the same ability. The selection of items presented, as well as the number of items, is based on how well a candidate answers the preceding items (a determination of his or her ability).

A *minimum* of 75 items, of which 15 are experimental items (unscored items used solely to determine how well they work and their difficulty), are presented. Because the experimental items are not identified, candidates should answer *all* items as if they were scored. The *maximum* number of items presented is 265, including the 15 experimental items. The number of items presented does not, however, automatically indicate whether a candidate has passed or failed.

All items have a known difficulty level; that is, an item is either easy or difficult for the candidate population to answer correctly. This information is obtained by analyzing the experimental items given to a large number of candidates. If every candidate answers an item correctly, it would be considered easy. If only a few candidates answer an item correctly, it would be considered difficult. Based on this information, items are placed on a scale such as the following one with a (−3) used to indicate the easiest items and a (+3) to indicate the most difficult items.

$$\underline{\quad -3 \quad -2 \quad -1 \quad 0 \quad +1 \quad +2 \quad +3 \quad}$$
$$\text{Easiest} \hspace{4.5cm} \text{Hardest}$$

At the start of the examination, you will be given an item that has a low or moderate difficulty level (a value of between −2 and 0). If you answer the item correctly, you will be given a slightly more difficult item. If you answer the initial item incorrectly, you will be given a slightly easier item. The computer will continue selecting items based on how well you responded to previous items. If you miss an item, the next item will be slightly easier. If you answer the next item correctly, the following item will be slightly more difficult. Throughout the examination, you will be presented with items that are targeted to your ability level; they will be neither too easy nor too difficult for *you*. The computer is programmed to stop presenting items when one of the following conditions has occurred:

1. Your measure of competence is known to be *above* or *below* the passing standard and at least 75 items have been answered
2. You have taken the maximum number of items (265)
3. You have tested for the maximum number of hours (5)

Before the computer stops the test, all candidates are presented with a sufficient number of items covering the test plan to determine accurately whether they possess the necessary knowledge, skills, and abilities to practice competently. Regardless of your level of competence, you will be tested on *every* aspect of the test plan.

Perhaps the most confusing aspect of CAT for candidates is how accurate pass-fail decisions can be reached if some candidates take only 75 items and others take 265 items. The following illustration may assist you in understanding this phenomenon:

Suppose a track coach is trying to decide who on the team should participate in the high jump event. The coach knows that individuals need to jump a minimum of 4 ft in order to be competitive (passing score).

Ten students decide to try out for this event. The coach sets the bar at 4 ft and asks the 10 students to jump over it. Two students "sail over" the bar with no difficulty; two students hit the bar with their stomachs; and the other six students either just make it over or their foot strikes the bar.

For the two students who had no problem with the jump, the coach raises the bar to 4.5 ft, and the two students are able to jump without problems. The bar is then raised to 5 ft; the students are able to meet this standard. Based on these three jumps, the coach is confident that these two students have more than adequately demonstrated their competence to meet the minimum level of 4 ft (passing score).

For the two students who had considerable difficulty with the bar at 4 ft, the coach lowers the bar to 3.7 ft. If the students are unable to get over that height, the bar is lowered again to 3.5 ft. Based on these three jumps, the coach is confident that these two students are not capable of meeting the minimum level of 4 ft (passing score).

Finally, the coach has to determine the competence of the remaining six students. In order to make a decision about the ability of these students, the coach has to keep raising and lowering the bar. Sometimes the students complete the jumps with no problems; other times they hit the bar. Only after 8 to 10 attempts is the coach able to feel confident whether a particular student is or is not capable of meeting the minimum level of 4 ft.

The same principle applies in the CAT. The computer can determine more quickly that a candidate is competent if he or she consistently answers the more difficult items correctly. At the other extreme, a quick decision can be made that a candidate is not minimally competent if the candidate is only able to answer items in the very easy range. The computer requires more time to determine a candidate's competence when he or she is responding to items in the -1 to $+1$ range.

The minimum passing level was determined by the National Council's Board of Directors, based on input from a panel of nurses who evaluated a typical examination and other sources. The panel was instructed thoroughly in the definition of "minimally competent" and what this term means in real life. After there was consensus as to the meaning of this term, the members were asked to individually evaluate each item in terms of "the percentage of 100 minimally competent RN candidates who would answer the item correctly." If an item was considered relatively easy, a greater percentage of candidates would be likely to answer the item correctly. If an item was considered more difficult, a smaller percentage of candidates would answer the item correctly. Individual decision making was done for each of the items presented. After every member of the panel provided an estimate of the percentage of minimally competent candidates who would answer each item correctly, the values obtained for each item for each panel member were averaged. The end numerical value was provided to the Board of Directors to assist them in making a decision about the minimum passing score required on an examination.

Item Format

The examination consists of a number of multiple-choice items involving a clinical setting (situation) on which a question is based or an individual statement or question relating to a client and/or family members. Following each situation or introductory statement, you are required to select which of four choices *best* responds to the question being asked. Because the examination is designed to measure an individual's competence to practice safely in the work setting, the items generally relate to various "real-life" situations in which nursing intervention and decision making are required. Although you must possess basic nursing knowledge (i.e., facts about the human body and the way it operates), the primary focus is on whether you are able to correctly apply these concepts in a variety of typical clinical settings.

Whether the item includes an introductory scenario or not, each item includes a question (*stem*) to which the candidate must respond. Following the stem are four choices (*options*). Only one of these options is correct (*key*); the other three are known as *distractors*. Distractors are created in such a way that they may seem correct to someone who is unfamiliar with or uncertain about nursing terminology, procedures, or general practice. The items are not designed to "trick" candidates. Rather, they are constructed in such a manner that it is possible to discriminate between candidates who are minimally competent (qualified to enter the profession) and those who are not.

Each item is presented on a single computer screen in one of two formats.

Situational or Scenario Item. The situation is presented on the left half of the screen, and the stem and four options are shown on the right half of the screen.

An 83-year-old male client is scheduled for the removal of a cataract from his left eye. His operative prescriptions include the instillation of mydriatic eye drops.	*When administering eye drops to the client, the nurse should instill them into which of the following parts of the eye?* a. Inner canthus b. Sclera c. Conjunctival sac d. Cornea

Individual or Stand-Alone Question. With this format the stem is presented on the left half of the screen, and the four options are shown on the right half of the screen.

Which of the following would be most *important for the nurse to consider in the home management of a young child who is mentally retarded?*	a. Having the same person teach him all new activities b. Limiting the amount of stimulation he receives from his environment

c. Maintaining a consistent routine for the performance of his activities of daily living
d. Teaching him amenities that will help him be accepted by others

Examination Administration

On the day of your examination, you should plan on arriving at the site a half-hour before your appointment. After you arrive, you will be shown to another area for identification verification and initial instructions.

You will need to present your *Authorization To Test* (*ATT*) and two pieces of identification, one which must be an official identification that includes your photograph and signature. The name shown on your official signed photographic identification must match *exactly* with the information stored in the computer as well as that printed on your *ATT*. If your name does not match, you may not be allowed to take the examination. Because of the necessity to have your identification match the name on your *ATT,* you should call ETS as soon as you receive the admission document if there is a discrepancy between the *ATT* and your photographic identification. The name on your second piece of identification should be very similar to the name on your *ATT,* although it does not have to be exact (e.g., Mary Jones versus Mary C. Jones). The identifying information in the computer will be verified, you will be photographed and fingerprinted, and you will be asked to sign an examination administration log. These security procedures are in place to protect the fairness and integrity of the examination. Although they may appear excessive, each of the steps is important to guaranteeing that the examination is not compromised and that you are really the person scheduled to take the examination.

At this time, you will also be given basic instructions on the operations of the computer and the manner in which you are to select answers and move on to the next item. Should you have any questions about the information presented, be sure to ask for clarification.

Before entering the testing room, you will be required to place *all* of your personal belongings in a locked cabinet to which you will have a key. Your individual storage facility is very small and cannot accommodate large books, briefcases, or large purses (no, you cannot even bring a purse into the testing room). Furthermore, the testing center will not assume any responsibility for personal property brought to the center. You will *not* be allowed to bring anything, except your two pieces of identification, into the testing room. Even a pencil will be furnished for you at your workstation.

Each testing room consists of a small number of computer workstations with partitions between them. Each station's padded chair is designed so that you can change its position to one that is comfortable for you. The computer screen can also be adjusted to match your personal requirements. When you enter the room, you will notice at least one viewing window from which a proctor can observe all activity in the room. A camera is also installed and will be taping both activity and sound in the room. These two features are incorporated into the testing room in order to maintain the security of the examination. If you need assistance during the course of the examination, raise your hand and the proctor will come into the room.

You will be shown to a specific computer that will be identified with your picture—a copy of the one taken during check-in. All personal identifying information has been fed into a specific computer so that it "knows" who is taking the examination. At the start of the examination, you will be given a practice session to help you become familiar with the keys required to take the examination.

The mechanics involved in using the computer are quite *simple*. There are only *two* keys that you use to answer the questions, and you do not have to have any computer experience in order to take the examination. The two required keys are the *space bar* and the *enter key*. All other keys will be inoperable during the administration of the examination. This means that you do not have to worry about what will happen if you hit the wrong key—nothing will happen. The space bar is used to move the cursor (a small line on the computer screen) from one option to another. Once you decide which option is correct, you need to hit the enter key. This will highlight the option you have selected. If you are confident of your response, hit the enter key again; your answer will be recorded and you will be shown another item. You must respond to every item presented before being allowed to go on to the next item.

Based on your response, the computer will select an appropriate item for you in the same or different area of the test plan. Because the correctness of each answer you give determines the difficulty of the next item, you will not be allowed to return to a previously shown item, nor will you be able to skip an item. You must respond to every item presented and continue to move forward.

Do not worry about the possibility that you selected the wrong answer several items previously. If you make a mistake, the computer's estimate of your competence will not be permanently affected. Once you give a correct answer, the computer will recalculate your competence level and will present a more difficult item. Keep in mind that even when the NCLEX-RN was presented as a paper-and-pencil test, you were not expected to get every item correct. The same is true with CAT. A wrong response on the CAT does not mean you are incompetent; it simply means that you do not know everything associated with the field of nursing.

As stated previously, you will have a maximum of 5 hours in which to complete the test. During the first year of testing, almost 90 percent of the candidates were presented with fewer than the maximum number of items. In fact, approximately one-half of the candidates had their examination terminated after the minimum number of items. Although most candidates finish with their examination in less than the allocated 5 hours, you should not be worried if you take the entire time. Just as was true with the paper-and-pencil NCLEX, some candidates will finish their CAT examination more quickly than others. Your examination result does not depend on how quickly you answer the questions.

After 2 hours of testing, the computer will automatically stop, and you will be required to take a 10-minute break. You must leave the computer room, but you do not have to leave the testing center. After 10 minutes, you can resume testing. An optional break will be permitted after an additional 1½ hours of testing. During either of these two breaks, your computer screen will indicate a break and no item will be shown until the test administrator releases the "break" from your screen. You may also take "unscheduled" breaks anytime during the 5 hours by raising your hand and requesting permission to leave the room. The item on which you were working will remain on the computer screen while you are on break. Before you consider taking a break, remember that if you take the optional break or any unscheduled break, you will be given no additional time to complete the examination. The computer is set for 5 hours, and the time will continue to elapse whether you are out of the room or answering items.

Your examination will end when (1) the computer can accurately determine your level of competency, (2) the maximum number of items has been answered, or (3) 5 hours have elapsed. Once you have "completed" the examination, the computer automatically retains the exact items presented to you as well as your responses to each of the items. Your level of competency (pass versus fail) is also retained.

At the conclusion of the examination, you will be given the opportunity to respond to a number of questions about your testing experience. It is not mandatory that you respond, but your comments, both positive and negative, will help to improve the testing experience for others.

Immediately following your examination, the items you responded to as well as the responses given are transmitted to a central location for processing. Within 48 hours, your results are electronically transmitted to the jurisdiction in which you wish to be licensed. A paper copy of your results is also mailed to the jurisdiction at the same time.

Each jurisdiction must complete its own processing of the results. The processing involved determines how quickly results are submitted to candidates. In general, you should receive your results 4 to 6 weeks after taking the examination.

Candidates who pass the examination will receive a notification of pass; no score will be provided. Depending on the jurisdiction's procedures, you may or may not receive your license with your test results.

Candidates who do not pass the examination will receive a notice of fail. No numeric score will be provided. You will, however, be sent a Diagnostic Profile, similar to the one shown in Table 1–2, that indicates your personal areas of strength and weakness on the NCLEX test plan and an Interactive Diagnostic Profile Progam designed to assist NCLEX examination candidates in understanding the information on the Diagnostic Profile and in preparing a course of study. The following information will appear at the top of the Diagnostic Profile: your name, date of birth, Social Security number, program code, and program name. For most jurisdictions (Michigan candidates will not have a photograph shown), a copy of the photograph taken of you at the examination site will also be included.

In this example, the candidate was close to passing and performed fairly well in the areas of Analysis; Planning; Safe, Effective Care Environment; and Psychosocial Integrity. The area of greatest weakness was Evaluation. The candidate should focus his or her studying not only on Evaluation, but also on the other four areas in which performance was weak.

A failing notice will also include information on how often you can repeat the examination and how soon you can reapply for a re-examination. The NCSBN has established a retake policy of no more than four administrations per year and no more frequently than once in any 3 months. Jurisdictions have the authority to impose other restrictions, provided that their retake policy is no more lenient than the one established by the NCSBN.

You cannot overcome these restrictions by applying to another state for licensure, changing your name, or applying to take the examination in another state. The computerized registration system continues to track candidates after they have first applied to take the examination. Once you register, you are assigned a permanent, unique identification number that is used every time you apply to take the examination.

If you fail the examination, you can request an examination review, but hand scoring will not be available. The reason is that there is nothing to hand score. The answers you selected were automatically entered into the computer and stored. Accordingly, there is no possibility that your answers were "misread."

An examination review is feasible because the exact items presented to you, along with your responses, were retained by the computer. Should you wish to review your test and your licensing jurisdiction permits it, you will need to submit a written request and fee to the jurisdiction. Once your request is approved, your test and answers will be transmitted to the testing center chosen by the jurisdiction. This location may not necessarily be the one in which you took the examination. Although you can take the examination outside of the licensing jurisdiction, you will be required to review the examination within the licensing jurisdiction at the specified site.

You will be shown only the items you answered incorrectly. The answer you selected as well as the correct answer will be presented. If you wish to challenge an item, you will be asked to prepare documentation as to why you should be given credit for the item.

TABLE 1–2. Sample of an Actual Diagnostic Profile (Candidate identifiers deleted)

NCLEX-RN™ CANDIDATE DIAGNOSTIC PROFILE
National Council Licensure Examination for Registered Nurses

Test Date:	MM/DD/YY
Test Center:	X9999
Candidate Number:	123-45-678
Date of Birth:	12/31/58
Social Security Number:	123-45-6789
Program Code:	99-999
Program Name:	Smalltown College of Nursing
	Smalltown, OH

CANDIDATE'S
PHOTOGRAPH HERE

WALTER P SMITH
123 MAPLE ST.
SMALLTOWN, OH 12345

WALTER P SMITH, an applicant for licensure by the
OHIO BOARD OF NURSING,
HAS NOT PASSED the National Council Licensure Examination for Registered Nurses.

The scale below, titled "Overall Performance" Assessment," shows how well you did on the NCLEX-RN. The "X" shows how far below passing your performance fell. Passing is indicated by the "I" shown in the box.

On the NCLEX-RN, no candidate is administered more than 265 questions. The box titled "Number of Items Taken" shows that the computer reached a decision after you had answered 164 questions.

Due to the adaptive nature of the test, the closer your number of questions answered is to the maximum number of 265, the closer you are to the passing level.

The back of this form lists the nine test plan content areas. The "X"s in the nine boxes at the bottom of this page show how well you did in those content areas. This will help you know which areas to study before you take the test again.

PERCENTAGE OF THE TEST PLAN MASTERED

NUMBER OF QUESTIONS TAKEN

PHASES OF THE NURSING PROCESS
Assessment (17–23% of the test)

CATEGORIES OF CLIENT NEEDS
Safe, Effective Care Environment (15–21% of the test)

low performance	high performance	low performance	high performance

Analysis (17–23% of the test)

Physiological Integrity (46–54% of the test)

low performance	high performance	low performance	high performance

Planning (17–23% of the test)

Psychosocial Integrity (8–16% of the test)

low performance	high performance	low performance	high performance

Implementation (17–23% of the test)

Health Promotion/Maintenance (17–23% of the test)

low performance	high performance	low performance	high performance

Evaluation (17–23% of the test)

low performance	high performance

TABLE 1–3. CAT Questions and Answers

What is the exam application deadline?	None
Where is the exam application submitted?	State Board, ETS, or the Board's Testing Service
Where is the licensure application submitted?	State Board or State's Testing Service
What is the exam fee?	The exam fee is $88 plus any additional exam administration fee charged by your Board.
What are the exam administration dates?	Whenever convenient for the candidate after being deemed eligible.
What types of items are used in the exam?	Multiple choice
How long does the exam take?	Maximum of 5 hr in 1 day. Most candidates will be finished sooner.
How many items are on the exam?	A *minimum* of 60 scored and 15 try-out; a *maximum* of 250 scored and 15 try-out.
Do all candidates answer the same items?	No, each candidate is presented with items specific to his or her competency level.
Where are the exams administered?	There is at least one site in each jurisdiction.
Must I take the exam in the jurisdiction in which I want to be licensed?	No, candidates can take the exam in any jurisdiction, and results will be transmitted to the licensure jurisdiction.
How is the passing score determined?	A criterion-referenced procedure is used.
When will I receive my results?	Results are sent to the jurisdiction within 48 hr; results should be sent to candidates within a few weeks.
If I fail, can I retake the exam?	Yes
How many times can I retake the exam?	That depends on the rules of each jurisdiction but no more than 4 times a year.
Can I have my answers hand scored?	No, there is nothing to hand score.
Can I review my exam?	Yes, depending on the rules of the licensing jurisdiction.
During a review, will I be shown all items included in the test?	No, you will only be shown the items that you missed, the answer that you selected, and the correct answer.
Can I challenge an item I missed?	Yes

In all of the years that the NCLEX-RN has been administered, there have been very few challenges to the examination items, and none of the challenges has resulted in a score change. The reason for this is that prior to including an item on an examination, it has been reviewed numerous times by many individuals involved in the nursing profession, and it has been placed on an examination as a try-out item so that adequate statistics have been obtained. All items have been scrutinized thoroughly before they are actually presented to candidates and scored.

2. Taking the examination whenever and wherever you want
3. Taking the examination in pleasant, noncrowded conditions
4. Answering 265 or fewer items
5. Completing the examination in 5 hours or less
6. Receiving results in less time
7. Being able to start work as a licensed RN sooner

Some of the similarities and differences between CAT and paper-and-pencil testing are shown in Table 1–3. After you have reviewed the information in this table, you will quickly see that CAT is the preferred method of testing.

SUMMARY

Although CAT may be a new experience for you, you should not be unduly worried or anxious about the format of the examination. It is still a multiple-choice test. The main differences are that the items are displayed on a computer screen instead of on paper and you use two computer keys instead of a pencil. These are minor differences compared with the many advantages associated with the CAT:

1. Quicker administration of the examination after you have been determined eligible by the licensing jurisdiction

REFERENCES

1. National Council of State Boards of Nursing: Test Plan for the National Council of Licensure Examination for Registered Nurses. NCSBN, Chicago, 1989.
2. Kane, M, et al: A Study of Nursing Practice and Role Delineation, and Job Analysis of Entry-Level Performance of Registered Nurses. National Council of State Boards of Nursing, Chicago, 1986.
3. Chornick, N, et al: 1992–1993 Job Analysis Study of Newly Licensed, Entry-Level Registered Nurses. National Council of State Boards of Nursing, Chicago, 1993.
4. National Council of State Boards of Nursing: Test Plan for the National Council Licensure Examination for Registered Nurses. NCSBN, Chicago, 1987.

chapter 2

Computerized Adaptive Testing Questions and Answers

by Kara Schmitt, PhD

This chapter briefly answers some of the most frequently asked questions about computerized adaptive testing (CAT). More detailed information can be found in Chapter 1 or by speaking with the staff at the National Council of State Boards of Nursing (NCSBN), The Chauncey Group, or your Board of Nursing.

1. What is CAT?

Computerized adaptive testing is a method of presenting multiple-choice items to candidates in such a manner that each examination is tailor-made to match the individual candidate's competence level. No two candidates are likely to receive the exact set of items, because no two candidates are exactly alike in their level of competence. All candidates are tested on the same content (test specifications), but the actual items vary.

2. Why did the NCSBN decide to implement CAT?

There are a variety of reasons why the NCSBN decided that CAT, as compared with the traditional paper-and-pencil method, was a more appropriate manner in which to test candidates. Some of these reasons are as follows:

a. CAT can provide a more accurate measure of a candidate's competency.

b. Examination security is enhanced because examination forms do not have to be transported to all jurisdictions, they do not have to be stored at an examination site, and the same items are not seen by all candidates at one time.

c. Candidates are able to take the examination throughout the year. Depending on candidate volume in the individual jurisdictions, the examinations are typically offered twice a day, 6 days a week, every week in the year. During peak testing times, the examinations may be offered even more frequently.

d. The testing environment is more conducive to test taking. The number of candidates tested at a single time is small (no more than 15 candidates in a room), and the examination is offered in more pleasant surroundings.

e. Results are available more quickly. Results are sent to the individual jurisdictions within 48 hours after a candidate has tested. Depending on the policy and practice of each jurisdiction, candidates probably receive their results within a few weeks after the examination administration.

f. Candidates are able to enter the workforce more quickly because of a faster turnaround time for receiving results.

g. Candidates can schedule the examination at their convenience, not at predetermined times. If desired by the candidate, first-time candidates can be scheduled within 30 days after calling for an appointment; re-examination candidates are scheduled within 45 days.

h. Candidates who need to be re-examined can be tested up to four times a year but no more frequently than once in a 3-month period. The actual retake policy is determined by the individual boards.

i. Testing time is reduced. Registered nurse candidates have their examination administered in 1 day with no more than 5 hours of testing. During the 1993 field testing of CAT, approximately 50 percent of the candidates completed the examination in about 2 hours.

j. The examination can be administered in any approved testing center regardless of the jurisdiction in which a candidate wishes to be licensed.

3. What are the minimum and maximum number of items that must be answered?

All candidates are required to answer *at least* 60 scored items and 15 try-out items (a total of 75 items) before the computer will terminate the examination. This minimum number ensures that each candidate has been tested in each of the areas of the NCLEX-RN test plan. The maximum number of items given to a candidate is 250 scored items plus the 15 try-out items for a total of 265 items.

4. What are the minimum and maximum testing times?

There is no minimum testing time, but the maximum time allowed a candidate is 5 hours. Candidates can go at their own pace. Some candidates are able to respond to the minimum number of items in less than an hour; others may take 2 hours to respond to the same number of items. Provided that at least 75 items have been administered, the examination will be terminated once a decision can be reached about the candidate's level of competence.

5. Can I change my answer to a previously asked question, and can I leave an item unanswered?

The answer to both these questions is *no.* Your response to each item, whether you are right or wrong, determines the difficulty of the next item presented. If you answer an item incorrectly, either because you do not know the correct response or because of a careless error, you will receive an easier item. If this item is answered correctly, you will receive a more difficult item. The CAT methodology enables you to demonstrate your true competence. Research has shown that the inability to change an answer to a previous question or leave a question blank does not make a significant difference in a candidate's performance.

6. If each candidate receives a "different" test, how can CAT determine accurately my level of competency?

Although each candidate receives different items, all candidates are tested on the same material. That is, all candidates receive items measuring each of the areas included in the NCLEX-RN test plan as shown in Chapter 1. All candidates also have to demonstrate competency at the same passing point. Finally, all candidates have sufficient opportunity to demonstrate their true level of competency because the test will not stop until an accurate pass-fail decision can be made. The only exception to this is if 5 hours have elapsed or the maximum number of items have been presented. If a candidate's competency level is not above the passing point, the candidate fails the examination.

7. How does the computer decide when a candidate's test is finished?

Basically, the examination ends when an accurate decision can be made that the candidate is reliably above or below the minimum level of required competency *or* after 5 hours of testing. Candidates whose competence level is close to the passing point need to answer more items in order for the computer to determine whether they are competent. Candidates whose competency level is farther away, either positively or negatively, from the required passing point need to answer fewer items.

8. Is the number of candidates passing the CAT examination any different from those passing the paper-and-pencil test?

There should be no difference in the pass-fail rate of candidates taking the CAT compared with that for the traditional method of examination administration. The requirement for passing the examination, the passing standard, remains the same as it was with the paper-and-pencil examination. The only time this requirement would change is if a new NCLEX-RN test plan was implemented.

9. Am I allowed to take a break during the testing?

All candidates are required to take a 10-minute break after 2 hours of testing. An optional break is available after 3½ hours of testing. If necessary, you can request an "unscheduled" break by raising your hand and asking the proctor for permission to leave the testing room. As was true with the paper-and-pencil testings, you are not given additional testing time should you decide to take a break.

10. How much does the examination cost?

The current fee for CAT is $88 in cashier's check, money order, or certified check payable to the National Council of State Boards of Nursing. If you decide to register by phone, you will be charged an additional fee on your credit card. This does not, however, include any additional fee charged by your jurisdiction for application processing, temporary license, and/or initial license. Each jurisdiction institutes its own fees for these items. Your licensure application should indicate the fee required by the jurisdiction.

11. What are the steps involved in taking the NCLEX-RN?

In order to take the NCLEX examination, candidates must generally go through the following steps listed in chronological order:

A. Apply to the Board of Nursing for a license following instructions from that board.

B. Candidate gets an *NCLEX Candidate Bulletin* from the Board of Nursing.

C. Candidate submits a registration form to The Chauncey Group (the National Council's contracted testing service) or registers by phone. The Chauncey Group will acknowledge the candidate's registration by mail.

Note: Candidate seeking licensure from Florida, Illinois, Massachusetts, and New York do not register directly with The Chauncey Group. Follow registration instructions provided by those Boards of Nursing.

D. The Board of Nursing will communicate the candidate's eligibility to test to The Chauncey Group.

E. The Chauncey Group will send the candidate an Authorization To Test (ATT) with a booklet called *Scheduling and Taking your NCLEX* and a list of testing centers.

F. The candidate will call a testing center and schedule an appointment to test.

G. On the appointed day, the candidate will take the test at a testing center.

H. The testing center transmits the test results to The Chauncey Group. After verifying the accuracy of the results, The Chauncey Group transmits them to the designated Board of Nursing.

I. The Board of Nursing sends the results to the candidate.

The answer to this question is reprinted with permission from "Overview of the NCLEX Examination Testing Process," National Council of State Boards of Nursing, Inc., http://www.ncsbn.org/pfiles/nclex/testproc.html, accessed 6/2/97. Copyright 1997 by the National Council of State Boards of Nursing, Inc.

12. How do I register for the NCLEX?

There are two methods for registering for the NCLEX. The method you use depends on the jurisdiction in which you are applying for a license.

METHOD 1:

If you are applying for licensure in one of the following jurisdictions, Florida, Illinois, Massachusetts, or New York, you must follow the registration procedures established by the jurisdiction. You must register through your jurisdiction. Do not send your registration materials or fee to The Chauncey Group. You also must not call The Chauncey Group Quick Registration telephone number.

METHOD 2:

If you are applying for licensure in a jurisdiction not listed in Method 1, you may register with The Chauncey Group for the examination either by mail or telephone.

If you are registering by mail,

- you must enclose a certified check, cashier's check, or money order for $88 in U.S. currency drawn on a bank in the United States with your registration. Use the enclosed envelope to return your registration form and payment. Personal checks, cash, foreign currency, stamps, receipts, or proofs of payment will not be accepted. Credit cards cannot by used when registering by mail. There will be no refund of the registration fee for any reason.

- the check or money order must be made payable to the National Council of State Boards of Nursing.

- registrations that are not properly completed and/or are not accompanied by the proper payment will be returned to you and will delay your testing.

Registering by telephone is a quicker way to register for the NCLEX. If you are registering by telephone,

- you must pay by using a valid VISA, MasterCard, or American Express credit card.

- have your credit card ready when you make your telephone call. You must supply the name shown on the credit card, the credit card number, and the expiration date.

- credit cards will be verified before registrations are processed.

- there is a $9.25 service fee charged for telephone registration. Therefore, the total amount that will be charged to your credit card is $97.25.

13. Can I really take the examination at any time and at any location?

Basically, *yes*. Prior to being scheduled, however, you must first be deemed eligible by the appropriate licensing jurisdiction. You do not, however, have to take the examination in the jurisdiction in which you have applied for licensure. You may take the examination in any jurisdiction that recognizes the NCLEX-RN for licensure. The only other limiting factor would be if the site that you are requesting is full on the desired day; in that case, you may need to be tested on an alternative date or go to another site if one is nearby. Even if you have to select another day for testing, if you are taking the examination for the first time you can be scheduled within 30 days after calling, if you so desire.

14. Can I be scheduled to take my examination at the same time that friends are taking theirs?

Certainly, provided there is space available and you have all been determined to be eligible by the jurisdiction in which you wish to be licensed.

15. Should I learn about computers and the keyboard configuration before taking the CAT?

That is not necessary. There are only *two* keys you will need to use in order to select an answer and move to the next item. The space bar moves the cursor (line on the screen that indicates where you are) among the options. The enter key is used to highlight and select an answer and must be struck twice in order to actually record the choice and move to the next item. These keys will be identified on the keyboard so that you will know which ones are needed for taking the test. All other keys are "turned off" once the examination actually begins; that is, even if you strike another key, nothing will happen.

You will also have an opportunity to practice using the computer and keys at the start of the examination. This will enable you to become familiar with the general format of the examination as well as with the layout of the keys needed for taking the test.

16. What will the computer screen look like?

All items are presented in one of two layouts, and all the information you need to answer an item is shown on the computer screen. This is true regardless of whether you are presented with a short situation first and then the question (stem) and possible answers (options) or whether you are shown merely a stem and options.

The question (stem) will appear here.	a. Option #1 b. Option #2 c. Option #3 d. Option #4
The background information (situation) will appear here.	The question (stem) will appear here. a. Option #1 b. Option #2 c. Option #3 d. Option #4

17. What happens to my examination and the answers I've made if there is a power failure?

All computers have surge protection devices to minimize the potential for loss of data. Each center is equipped with an uninterruptible power supply that provides continuous processing in the case of a short-term power failure. All answers are automatically saved so that in the case of a long power failure, your answers and performance on the examination up to that time will not be lost.

18. If I fail the examination, can I still ask for hand scoring or examination review?

The Interactive Diagnostic Profile Program is an interactive version of the NCLEX Examination Candidate Diagnostic Profile. The Diagnostic Profile is an individualized document sent to candidates who fail the NCLEX-RN or NCLEX-PN examination. This interactive program is designed to assist NCLEX examination candidates in understanding the information on the diagnostic profile and in preparing a course of study to improve performance in retakes of the examination.

Because your answers are automatically entered into the computer system, there is no need to hand score any examination. Hand scoring was feasible under the old administration mode because you were marking your answers on paper and then a computer was reading these answers. If you marked too lightly or went outside the circle, there was a slight possibility that the computer might have misread your response. In CAT, there is no possibility of your responses being misread because you entered them directly into the computer.

Examination reviews by candidates are feasible. As indicated previously, the items presented to you and the answers you made are automatically recorded. If you wish to review your examination, this will be conducted at a testing center selected by your jurisdiction. The items you missed, your response to each item, and the correct answer to each item missed will be transmitted to the testing center at a mutually agreed on date and time. The transmittal will indicate which items you answered incorrectly as well as what the correct answer should have been. A separate fee is charged for examination reviews.

19. How often can I retake the examination if I fail?

The current NCSBN recommendation is that candidates be allowed to take the examination once every 91 days. The retake policy may be changed at a later date as the item bank is expanded. Each jurisdiction, however, determines its own retake policy, which can be no more frequently than the policy of the NCSBN. Because the computer system tracks each candidate based on a unique identification number, the retake policy will be in effect even if you decide to apply to another jurisdiction for licensure.

20. If I have to repeat the examination, will I be given the same items that I answered the first time?

No. All the items shown you during one administration are "locked" so that they cannot be used on any subsequent administration. This means that you will still be tested on each of the areas of the test specifications *and* you will be given items that match your ability level but each item will be different from any given you previously.

21. Are special accommodations provided for candidates with a disability?

Yes. Near the completion of your education, you should contact your licensing jurisdiction for specific information regarding the procedures. In general, you need to submit a written letter documenting the disability and describing the accommodations requested. You also need to have a health professional qualified to make the particular diagnosis write a letter to the jurisdiction. Each jurisdiction determines whether your request can be honored or whether some modifications are necessary.

All sites, including the testing room and rest rooms, are wheelchair accessible. At least one computer table at each site can be repositioned to accommodate a wheelchair. Additional modifications, such as timing or size of the letters on the screen, can be made as required.

chapter 3

Preparing for and Taking the NCLEX-RN

by Kara Schmitt, PhD

While preparing for and taking the NCLEX- RN, you must constantly remember that you have the ability to pass the examination. Although the manner in which you will be responding to items may be different (computer instead of paper and pencil) and there may be more items than included in previous tests, the examination is still just an examination. As you study for the examination, remember that *confidence, like success, is a result of hard work and preparation*. In order to do well, you must be both psychologically and intellectually prepared.

TEST ANXIETY

Although stress and anxiety do *not* have exactly the same definition, these terms are used interchangeably in this chapter. Stress and anxiety are normal reactions to situations such as preparing for and taking a major test like the NCLEX-RN. If you were to ask friends who have already passed the examination if they were anxious before and during the examination, their answer would certainly be *yes*. In fact, some amount of anxiety is actually *good* and has been found to improve test-taking ability. On the other hand, uncontrollable anxiety will hurt your ability to do well. It has been said that stress is "the spice of life or the kiss of death—depending on how we cope with it."[1] By learning how to recognize and deal with stress effectively, you can use it to your advantage.

The ability to recognize and respond to stress or anxiety varies from person to person. There is no one method that will work for everyone; therefore, the information included in this chapter is presented merely to give you some ideas of ways in which you might be able to reduce seemingly uncontrollable and perhaps incapacitating stress.

The best way to deal with stress is to take specific steps to cope with and reduce the stress-producing situation. Proper study behaviors and a thorough preparation for an examination are the *best* ways to reduce the stress experienced prior to and during an examination.

An inappropriate approach, which in the end will increase the stress, is to deny the importance of the task (examination) that you must accomplish. Statements such as "The exam is filled with trick questions anyway, so why bother studying" or "If I don't do well, I just wasn't lucky" are inappropriate and will not help you. You need to concentrate your efforts on studying properly and thinking positively.

Some of the characteristics frequently associated with test anxiety include:

1. Feeling insecure about your performance
2. Worrying a great deal about things not under your control
3. Thinking about how much brighter or better others are
4. Thinking about what will happen should you fail
5. Feeling that you are not as prepared as you could or should be (assuming that you really did prepare)
6. Worrying about not having enough time to finish the test
7. Feeling that you will be letting yourself and others down
8. Feeling that you could and should have done better[2]

These eight feelings can be categorized into four major symptoms of anxiety,[3] which can and must be handled in order to overcome the anxiety-producing situation. Each of these four symptoms is discussed briefly.

Anxiety-Producing Mental Activities. Worrying about nonspecific problems or situations and fretting over everything that *could* go wrong are associated with this symptom. Self-criticism, self-blame, and generally negative self-talk lead to low self-confidence and disorganized problem solving. Telling yourself that you cannot do something or that you are stupid will lead to failure. Another trait associated with this symptom is false thinking about yourself and the world around you—the "everyone is so much better than I am" syndrome.

Misdirected Attention. Instead of focusing on the task at hand, such as studying for or taking an examination, you focus on internal and external distractors. These could include watching other people study, looking at the clock, or daydreaming. If you focus on the wrong thing, you will be less efficient and more likely to become emotionally upset.

Physiological Distress. When you are anxious, your body reacts both physiologically and psychologically. Some of the physiological symptoms include sweating, increased heart rate, nervous stomach, or headache. If you focus on the physiological symptoms to a significant degree, you will be less able to focus on your studies or the examination.

Inappropriate Behavior. This symptom is exhibited by avoiding the task that needs to be done (procrastination), by withdrawing prematurely from the task, or by doing something else when you should be focusing on the task at hand (talking to your neighbor instead of studying). Other aspects of inappropriate behavior include rushing through the examination or study material without focusing on the information or, at the opposite extreme, being excessively compulsive and rereading everything more than is necessary. A final element is trying to push yourself to keep going when you are tense rather than taking the time to relax.

In order to reduce stress to a manageable level, you need to determine what symptoms or behaviors you are exhibiting. One way to learn more about your individual expressions of stress is to find a comfortable, relaxing environment; close your eyes; and really imagine and concentrate on how you feel or what you do when you study. How are you going to feel when it is 1 week before the examination? When it is 1 day before the examination? When it is the day of the examination? When you are sitting at the computer taking the examination? Try to think carefully about these events and how you *really* will feel. If you are honest in the evaluation of these situations and your feelings, you will be better able to change the way you handle stress.

Another activity you can do to learn more about your own coping ability is to reflect on and make note of what you actually do while studying. Do you watch other people? Do you daydream? Do you begin worrying about the test? Do you stop studying because you think it will do no good? You will probably need to keep a log of your behaviors following several study periods in order to obtain an accurate picture of your behaviors.

After you have recorded all of your distractors, make a list of what you could do to reduce your level of anxiety. For instance, telling yourself that you can never learn the material is self-defeating. Instead, remind yourself that you learned the material in the past and did well in school. After all, you are ready to graduate or have graduated, so you must have learned what was necessary to reach this stage in your pursuit of a nursing career.

Another aid to learning more about yourself and your reaction to stress is to respond *true* or *false* to each of the following statements in terms of what you do or how you respond during periods of stress.

	True	False
1. I bite my nails, fidget with my hair, tap my fingers, or perform other similar behaviors constantly.		
2. I smoke or drink more frequently.		
3. I tend to eat more or eat less, or I eat less healthy foods.		
4. I avoid doing what I should be doing.		
5. I feel like there is too much to do in too short a time.		
6. I worry about everything—the examination, my health, my family, my work, etc.		
7. I seem to have more physical or health-related problems.		
8. I become irritated or lose my temper more quickly over trivial matters.		
9. I seem to have less energy and seem to want to sleep more.		
10. I have trouble falling asleep or sleeping my normal amount of time.		
11. I am more critical of myself or think of myself as worthless.		
12. I seem to forget more day-to-day activities or responsibilities, such as forgetting to get groceries, forgetting an appointment, or forgetting to return a phone call.		
13. I have trouble relaxing and enjoying myself even when at a social event or with people I like.		
14. I tend to daydream more.		

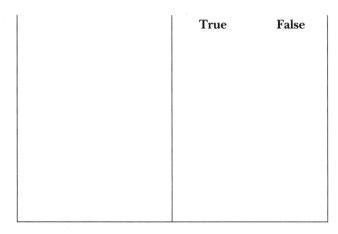

True	False

Items 1 through 3 may be viewed as bad habits, which simply become more prevalent during times of stress or anxiety. The key to deciding whether these three behaviors are detrimental to successful completion of the required task is to determine whether you are doing them *more than usual* during times of stress. If the answer is *yes* they could be negatively influencing your effectiveness while preparing for and taking the examination. At the same time, if you try to become "perfect" and eliminate normal bad habits during a stressful situation, you may actually increase your level of stress. It is not necessary for you to eliminate all bad habits at this time, but you should keep them under control.

The other items (4 through 14) focus more on symptoms of anxiety. If you responded *true* to most of these items, it is time for you to re-evaluate your thoughts about yourself and the future examination. You need to focus less on what is going on around you or inside you and more on understanding and solving the problem that is causing the anxiety. Begin to view the examination as a problem to be solved or a challenge you must meet. Do not view it as something that is a punishment or an imaginary catastrophic event.

Begin to view the test realistically. It is not a measure of your self-worth, your ability to be successful, or your future happiness. It is merely a single measure of what you know.

Develop a positive attitude toward the test. Eliminate the negative thoughts and feelings you have about it, and do not think about how poorly you might perform on the examination.

Choose to take the test. The examination is not being forced on you; rather, you elected to take it. By viewing the examination as something you want to do, you are in control and the examination is no longer controlling you. Because you have chosen to take the test, you must also choose to study for it.

Concentrate on what you can and must do *now*. Do not think about what you should have studied yesterday (the past) or what your NCLEX-RN results will be (the future). Rather, direct your attention to the present and expend your energy on the current task. Right now, you need to concentrate on studying for the examination. On the day of the examination, your energy must be fo-

cused on understanding the questions and responding correctly.

As stated previously, *some* test anxiety is actually good for you. Too much, however, will hinder your performance, and you will not be able to demonstrate adequately the knowledge you actually possess. Some ways in which test-anxious persons can be helped are by:

1. Learning to be less demanding of themselves
2. Revising their expectations about the consequences of failure and viewing the task as less alarming
3. Strengthening their study skills
4. Gaining more self-control over their worry and emotionality[4]

If anxiety is handled in a positive manner, it can assist in "promoting survival, healthy adaptation and development. In its nonadaptive modes, it can promote incompetence and extreme and lasting misery."[5]

In any situation, if you convince yourself that you are going to fail, you will. Instead of being negative about yourself, trying to decide what others will think of you if you fail, or deciding that you will do poorly on the examination, think *positively*. Negative statements made to yourself or others can reduce significantly the effectiveness of the preparation you do. Think positively and you will feel positive.

Read the examples of typical negative and positive statements shown in Table 3–1. Are you guilty of making any of the negative statements? If so, begin using and believing in the statements shown in the right (positive) column.

Avoid *why*, *if only*, and *what if* types of questions or statements, such as "Why did I ever think I could be a nurse?" or "If only I had more time, I could do better," or "What if I don't do well on the examination?" These expressions tend to reinforce feelings of helplessness, frustration, and anger. Eliminate them from your internal thoughts and external statements.

Stress and anxiety can and will be reduced if you take *positive* action and think *positive* thoughts about yourself and your abilities. At the same time, recognize that it is natural for you to feel some anxiety about the examination. The statement "don't worry" is ridiculous advice because all of us worry about the unknown to some extent. You must, however, worry in a constructive manner and must be prepared for the examination.

STUDY ENVIRONMENT

Not only is what you study important, but the conditions under which you study also are important in your ability to learn and remember. Both internal (daydreaming) and external (noise) distractions will interfere with your ability to concentrate and learn.

Think about where and how you generally study. Are you studying in an optimal place and manner? You want to be comfortable and relaxed while studying, yet at the

TABLE 3–1. Changing Negative Self-talk to Positive

Negative Statements	Positive Statements
"I have to get a perfect score."	"I want to do well, but I don't have to get every item correct."
"I always get upset during a test."	"If I feel myself getting tense during the test, I know how to relax."
"I'm a failure because I didn't remember . . . "	"Just because I forgot about . . . doesn't mean that I'm a failure. I remembered lots of the other material."
"If the test has questions on . . . topic, I'll just die."	"Since I'm not real comfortable with . . . topic, I had better study it more."
"What if I fail the exam?"	"I don't expect to fail, but if I do, I'll just have to study harder and do better the next time."
"I'll let my family down if I don't pass this test."	"Sure, my family wants me to do well, but they'll still accept me if I don't pass."
"I'm too stupid to be a nurse."	"I made it through school, and I can make it through the exam."
"The test is designed to trick candidates, so it doesn't matter if I study."	"If I study, I can do well; it's my responsibility to prepare."
"I'll never be able to understand all of this material."	"Just relax and try rereading this section. I know I can figure it out."
"Thank heavens I made it through this study session!"	"Wow, I really learned a lot while studying today. Hope tomorrow goes as well."
"I just know I'll be scared during the exam."	"I know I'll do well on the exam because I'm capable and I studied."
"Everyone expects me to do poorly, so why bother trying to do otherwise?"	"I don't care what others think about my chance of passing the exam; I know I can do it."
"I don't know why I have to take this test. I got good grades in in school and that should be good enough."	"I want to take this test simply because it will confirm that I really did learn while I was in school."

same time you need to be able to focus all of your attention and energy on the material you are reading, reviewing, and learning.

The following series of questions should assist you in your evaluation of whether the location and manner in which you study are the most conducive to learning.

1. When I begin studying, do I have all necessary books, paper, pencils and pens, and study materials with me so that I do not waste time finding them?
2. Do I schedule a block of time (1 to 2 hours) for studying?
3. Do I take short breaks (10 to 15 minutes) while studying for long periods of time and then return to work immediately?
4. Do I spread out my studying over a period of time rather than trying to do all of it at the last minute?
5. If I study with friends, do they have good study habits and do we really study?
6. Do I have a plan for studying and stick to it?
7. Do I feel rested when I study?
8. If I begin to feel tense or tired, do I stop studying for a while and try to relax?
9. If I begin to daydream or worry, do I take a few minutes to permit myself to daydream or worry rather than let these activities interfere with my studying?
10. Do I concentrate on the material that I am studying rather than think about other things?
11. Have I included some time in my schedule for social activities and exercise?
12. When I am done studying for the day, do I feel I have accomplished something?
13. Am I able to remove myself mentally from my environment; that is, can I block out potential distractions?
14. Is the area in which I study relaxing and comfortable, but not to such an extent that I fall asleep?
15. Is the area in which I study quiet and basically free from interruptions?
16. Is my desk (study area) neat and well organized so that I have enough room to study effectively?
17. Is the lighting sufficient and nonglaring?
18. When it is time to study, do I do so immediately and eagerly?
19. Do I reward myself when I feel I have done an exceptionally good job of studying?

Each of these questions should have been answered *yes* if you are studying in an appropriate atmosphere and with the proper frame of mind. If there were some questions to which you answered *no*, try to determine what you need to do to improve the conditions. Remember, how, when, and where you study does make a difference in your ability to concentrate and learn.

PREPARING FOR THE NCLEX-RN

One of your first tasks is to learn all you can about the actual examination—how it is constructed, the type of questions included, how long you have to complete the test, and so on. The information provided in Chapter 1 serves as a good starting point, but you should also read the material provided by the National Council of State Boards of Nursing and ask your instructors about the test. The better informed you are about the examination, the better you can prepare for it in a positive manner.

You also need to keep in mind that everything you did during your education to become a nurse—attending classes, applying good listening skills, taking clear and concise notes, doing your homework, reading all assignments, and taking course examinations—have helped you to prepare for the NCLEX-RN. Draw on these experiences as you prepare to take the final step in the learning process.

The suggestions in this section are provided to help you learn to study more aggressively and actively. Underlining or highlighting key words or passages is a good start, but that is passive learning and is not as effective for long-term memory. You need to develop active learning skills to improve your chances for remembering the material.[6,7]

Relate the material you have just read to information you learned in the past. Does knowledge of the new material relate to something else? Does this knowledge help you understand how to deal with any specific nursing situation? Is there a relationship among various facts that you have already learned? If so, what is that relationship? **Think, do not just memorize!**

Ask yourself questions about the material you have just read. Predict how the material might be worded in the examination.

Form study groups to review information and ask each other questions. This is an excellent way, if done correctly, to share your knowledge while you benefit from the knowledge of others. When you form a study group, keep the following points in mind.[8]

1. Study with others who are at your ability level or slightly above. If you were an average student in school, do not study with those who always got As. They may skip over material that is necessary for you to review. On the other hand, if you consistently got As, do not study with students who received Cs. They will want to study and review material that you don't need to study. Remember, the members of the study group should assist each other.

2. Keep sufficient time available for you to study on your own. Do not plan on all of the allocated study time to be spent with the group.

3. Keep the group serious. While there will be times when you "get off the subject," you should keep this to a minimum. Always keep in mind the real purpose for being together, and do not become distracted with trivial matters.

4. Keep the group small. If there are more than five people working together, there is a greater tendency to become distracted.

5. Do not meet too often. A few short meetings will provide the intensity and seriousness needed to accomplish the task. Also, you need time between meetings to prepare on your own.

6. Come to the meetings prepared with questions on areas you do not understand. Prepare mock test items to share with the others.

Above all, all members of the study group need to be actively involved in the process and willing to devote sufficient time to prepare for the meetings and to interact in a beneficial manner during the meetings.

Make notes of key concepts that are important to remember. Also, take notes on areas in which you feel less certain and use them as a reminder that you need to continue learning more about those topics.

Develop flash cards to help you remember dates, facts, formulas, and other factual material. Use 3×5 index cards to write short, factual questions on one side (What is the normal blood pressure for an adult?) and the answer on the reverse side. Add to the set of cards as you continue studying; review the cards on a weekly basis. At first you may want to read the questions and answers together to help you learn. Later you should ask yourself the questions and respond aloud. Check to see if you are correct. You can also have someone else read the questions to you. If you do not know the answer to a question, put that card back into the stack and ask the question again. If you know the material, you should be able to answer each question in a few seconds.

Be interested in the material. Just because you have wanted to be a registered nurse (RN) for a number of years, this does not mean everything you studied in school was personally of interest to you. Regardless of your interest in a subject or the profession, there were undoubtedly some topics that you found boring, uninteresting, or irrelevant. As you prepare, however, you need to become interested in the total field in order to learn better. Convince yourself that the boring topics are really critical, and try to determine how they can be related to topics that are of interest to you.

Use prepared test questions such as those in this book to help you study. Take a general, comprehensive RN-related examination as a practice test to help you determine your strengths and weaknesses. Use this information as a basis for preparing your study schedule. The better you do on the practice test, the less time you may need to devote to studying. Be sure to be honest with your appraisal of your performance and the areas you need to study. Start with the areas of weakness first so that you can devote more time to studying these. After you have reviewed the weak areas, take the same test or another one to see what improvements have been made. Use various sources of test items to become familiar with different ways in which the same information can be asked.

As you respond to each item, read the stem and options carefully, select the option you think is correct, and go on to the next item. Do not leave items blank, and do not return to items after you have made your selection. Because you answer each item presented in computerized adaptive testing (CAT) before going on to the next, now is the time to get into the habit of, and feel comfortable with, responding to a single item and moving forward.

Set specific goals for yourself. A goal of "I need to learn about nursing" or "I need to know enough to pass the test" will not be of assistance to you. Rather, you need to decide which nursing components you will learn during the week and then during each day. Have specific, concrete goals for each study period.

Establish a schedule for each day's studying and reviewing. Remain flexible, however, so that should you wish to go to an unplanned party or go out to dinner when you have scheduled a study period, you can do so without feeling guilty. At the same time, too much flexibility (procrastination) can cause you to become tense and stressed as you realize that instead of studying 10 hours during the week, you have only studied 2 hours. When you establish a weekly schedule, plan for the "unplanned" event to occur. If you do this, you will not feel guilty or stressed when something you want to do becomes available. Also, remember that if you do forfeit some study time on one day, you need to make up that time on another day.

Write summaries of what you have read. Rephrase information so that you can understand it better. Use mnemonics or silly phrases to remember certain facts. Use word associations. In other words, writing out the information either in your own words or with the help of a clever saying can help you remember the material better.

If information is not clear in one book, read another to see if the same material is explained any better. Although the same material may be included in a number of books, the manner in which it is explained and the way it is presented (with or without drawings, charts, and so forth) can make a difference in how well you understand the information. You should also rely on your instructors and peers for clarification of material that may be difficult for you to grasp.

Visualize the information you have just read. Mentally try to see how what you have read would actually look or work. Try to visualize a patient with certain conditions or symptoms. What would you be observing? Try to visualize yourself performing a certain procedure. How would you perform it?

Overlearn the material. Everyone forgets information regardless of how much studying was done. You should not expect to remember all of the material you were taught during your nursing education. You can, however, improve the likelihood of remembering more if you continue to review and relearn the material even after you think you know it. The more active (visualizing, rephrasing, verbalizing) your learning, the greater the probability of remembering.

At the conclusion of each study period, take a few minutes to **outline the key material you have just studied and learned.** These outlines can then serve as future review materials. Some key elements of a good outline include:

1. Using underlining or symbols to identify key points
2. Using sufficient space to allow for clarification or expansion based on later studying
3. Recording all formulas, equations, and rules exactly
4. Writing legibly on one side of the paper
5. Writing your own ideas or questions as well as facts
6. Using your own words to help reinforce a concept
7. Using personal nursing care experiences to clarify points

Now that you have learned what you should be doing to become a more active learner, you need to put these activities into place. During the next few study periods, do not try to study any differently than you would normally. Instead, at the end of each study period, take the assessment test shown in Table 3–2. Use the questions to evaluate how you need to change your studying behavior.

Whenever you answered *no*, keep those points in mind the next time you study. Do not feel frustrated if you find that you have not included all of the steps in your studying; just keep trying to improve. The overused phrase "Rome wasn't built in a day" is applicable in this instance as well as in your overall preparation for the examination. It might take you some time and effort to learn how to study more effectively and actively.

HOW TO TAKE MULTIPLE-CHOICE TESTS

There is a right way and a wrong way to answer multiple-choice items. Although you have probably answered thousands of them during your course of study, you may find it advantageous to review the suggestions given in this section of the chapter. Part of doing well on any examination is being *test wise*, that is, knowing how to figure out the correct answer even if you are not 100 percent certain. You may have a wealth of knowledge and be one of the smartest in your class, but if you do not know how to respond to multiple-choice questions, you will be unable to prove this knowledge. For better or worse, part of the score you receive on any examination depends on your test-taking ability.

Budget your time and pace yourself accordingly. Even with the CAT, in which the number of questions and actual time spent will vary, you know that you will have a maximum of 5 hours and a maximum of 265 items. This works out to slightly over **1 minute per item.** You should keep this time frame in mind as you are presented with each item. Although you might need to spend more than 1 minute for certain items, your overall goal should be 1 minute per item.

TABLE 3–2. Study Approach Checklist

Questions	Yes	No
1. Did you make a note of the material you were unsure of in order to restudy it later?		
2. Did you look over the topic headings as well as any study questions at the end of the chapter before beginning to read the entire section?		
3. When you finished the initial reading, reciting, and reviewing, did you look over your notes and check your memory of the major headings and subpoints under each heading?		
4. Did you carefully determine the most important topics to be learned (or the topics with which you are least knowledgeable) and determine your time frame for learning them?		
5. Did you take clear and concise notes while you studied?		
6. Did you read the material and try to answer questions you developed that covered the key information?		
7. After reading a section or chapter, did you answer correctly the questions included at the end, and did you try to develop examples of nursing situations in which this knowledge might be useful?		
8. Did you vary your speed of reading according to the difficulty and familiarity of the material as well as according to your purpose for reviewing the material?		
9. Did you pause after reading each section to underline or jot down the important points, and did you make notes on material you did not understand completely?		
10. Did you go back to the material that you were unsure of and review it again (in the same book or in a different book)?		

Keep moving at a steady pace. If a question is difficult and you are spending too much time on it, make an educated guess and move on to the next item. Remember, in CAT, if you select an incorrect option you will be given the opportunity to demonstrate your competence with a slightly easier item. If you get the next one correct, you will be given a slightly more difficult item. One or two incorrect responses will not fail you!

Read each question thoroughly, but quickly. Do not keep reading the same question over and over. Select your response and move on. In general, your first reaction to a question is the correct one. Do not try to second-guess what might be intended or try to figure out if there is a "trick" to the question. As a rule, the items are straightforward, basic, and designed to determine if you are *minimally* competent. Read each of the stems and all of the options carefully and then make your selection.

Concentrate on one item at a time. Do not worry about how many more items will be presented to you, how many of the candidates have already left the testing room, or how much time remains. Focus only on the item on the screen in front of you at that time (you should already be pacing yourself so that you answer one item approximately every minute).

Do not stop trying. Even if there are several items in a row that seem unfamiliar to you, do not start worrying about the examination as a whole. Just answer the items to the best of your ability and move forward.

Focus on key words in the stem. Mentally highlight these words or phrases and keep them in mind as you read the options. You might even want to jot down some key words on scratch paper to help you remember them as you read the options.

Focus on whether the item is asking for a positive or negative response. Negative words (*not, except*) are usually emphasized in the stem to help you recognize that you must reverse your thought process. When you respond to a negatively worded item, read each of the options and decide whether it is a true or false statement. If the item asks you to select the procedure that you would *not* follow, the false option is the correct response.

If a question requires calculations, **talk yourself through each step of the process.** At the same time, do not try to do the calculations in your head. Use the scratch paper provided at your workstation. Double-check your computations to make certain you have not made some minor arithmetical error. Generally, the incorrect options included in computational questions are based on mistakes typically made in the calculations (for instance, dividing instead of multiplying). This means that you may find the answer as you worked the problem and still be wrong.

Break down complex stems into smaller, more manageable sections. Make certain that the response you select is correct for each of the separate components within the stem. If an option works for one segment of the question, but not another, then the option is probably incorrect.

Reword a difficult stem and see if that helps you to better understand the intent of the item. Use your own words to ask the question included in the stem.

Try answering the question before you have read the options provided. The stem should provide sufficient information so that you know the direction of the question and the general response being sought. Start thinking about what you should be looking for as you read the options. This process will help you save time even if the answer you initially think is correct is not one of the options provided. At least you will be thinking about what to look for.

Read all options before selecting the one you think is correct. A well-constructed test will have four plausible responses, and it is your responsibility to select the *best*. Too often candidates read the first few options and decide that one of them is correct without reading all of the options. While one of those options may be *good*, it may not be the *best*.

Eliminate the distractors that are obviously wrong, and then pick between the remaining ones by using a rational thought process. At the same time, do not eliminate an option unless you are absolutely certain you understand every word in the phrase or sentence.

Use logic and common sense to figure out the correct response. The items are based on situations that an entering nurse would encounter. The items do not include exotic or unique situations or problems that only an experienced nurse would be able to understand. If the situation presented is one that you have not personally experienced, try to recall a similar situation and how you handled it. Then look at the options to see if you can apply any of them to a situation with which you are familiar.

Relate each option to the stem. Make sure that the answer you selected fits the intent of the stem and is grammatically correct.

Try to figure out the meaning of unfamiliar words in the stem and options in terms of the context of the sentences. You might also be able to figure out the meaning of words by dividing them into prefixes and suffixes that you know.

Use cues in the stem and distractors to help you figure out the correct response.

If you must guess, do so logically. After you have eliminated the options that you know are wrong, see if there are any test construction flaws that might help you figure out the intended answer. Given the extensive editing done prior to assembling the NCLEX-RN, it is doubtful that these "errors" will be found, but you might as well look for them. Some of the more common test constructions flaws are:

Length: Select the longest response if all other options are approximately equal in length.

Location: The correct response is more likely to be in the middle unless the options are ordered in terms of length.

Grammar: Incorrect options may not always fit the stem grammatically.

Language: Unusual or highly technical language typically indicates that the particular option is not correct.

Qualification: If one option includes qualifiers such as "generally," "tends to," or "usually," and the other options do not, select the option that includes the qualification.

Generalizability: The correct option will tend to have greater applicability and flexibility.

Specifics: Options that include the words "always" or "never" are typically not correct. There are very few instances in life that "always" occur.

SCHEDULING YOUR STUDY TIME EFFECTIVELY

The following schedule will help you prepare for the NCLEX-RN without trying to learn and remember everything at the last minute. Keep in mind that cram-

ming has no long-term benefit. You may remember the material for a few hours after you have studied, but probably not for the duration of the examination. Not only should the studying you do prepare you for the examination, but it should also provide an additional benefit—help you become a better nurse as you start your career.

At some point during your education, you probably stayed up all night studying for an examination, took the examination, and returned to your room and slept. How much of the material did you remember later that day? Probably not much! Therefore, if you want to do well on the examination and in your career, you have to begin preparing early and *not* try to cram all the information into a few nights or hours of studying.

Even though you do not know the exact day on which you will take the examination, you should be able to make a reasonable estimate that it will take place 4 to 6 weeks after you graduate, assuming that all of the required applications and fees have been submitted on time. You can certainly schedule the examination later if a different time would fit your work and personal schedule better. With an estimate of when you will likely take the test in mind, count backward from that date *2 to 3 months* and start doing the following activities:

1. Begin organizing your textbooks and class notes in a meaningful manner.
2. Begin making notes of the nursing subjects with which you feel least comfortable.
3. Begin learning more about the format and content of the examination as well as what will be expected of you. Review the first two chapters in this book as well as other material that describes the test; look at the format of items presented in this book and others; and talk to your instructors or friends who may have already taken the examination. Thoroughly understand all facets of the NCLEX-RN.
4. Take a practice test that includes items similar to those likely to be on the actual NCLEX-RN to see how well you do and to assess your strengths and weaknesses.
5. Establish a study schedule that includes adequate time to prepare but also recognizes the need for flexibility, social activities, family or personal responsibilities, and so forth. You might consider developing a 3-month calendar on which you write down all known events or activities as well as reasonable study times (4 to 5 days per week with 1 to 3 hours of study per day). The number of times you study per week as well as the amount of time spent each day should be based on how well you did on the practice test, how confident you feel, and the number of weeks prior to the test that you start studying.

Starting *4 to 8 weeks before the examination,* you should:
1. Begin reviewing the areas of weakness *first* so that you have time to review these areas again before the exam.
2. Develop, organize, and maintain your own notes

in each subject for a final review prior to the examination.

3. Form a study group that meets once a week. Prepare specific topics and questions for discussion prior to each meeting.

4. Take at least one review test every few weeks to help you become more familiar with the type of items that might be asked as well as to reassess your performance.

5. After a month of studying, take the original pretest to see how well you are now doing. Have you improved in those areas in which you were initially weak? Have you maintained your knowledge in those areas in which you were initially strong? Review the results and adjust your study schedule accordingly.

6. Develop your own situational questions as a technique for reviewing.

7. As soon as you know your test date, make reservations at a hotel or motel close to the site, preferably within walking distance, for the night before the examination. This should be done particularly if you live more than 1 hour from the site and your examination is scheduled for the morning. Even if you have an afternoon administration, you should consider staying close to the site so that you are not rushed in the morning. Car problems, traffic, road repairs, and so forth can and do occur. Even if these events do not make you late for the examination, they will definitely increase your anxiety level.

8. Maintain sufficient time for eating, sleeping, exercising, socializing, and working. Do *not* become a study hermit!

One week before the examination, you need to:

1. Begin a concentrated *review* of the material.

2. Take the pretest for the last time and evaluate your performance.

3. Recite key ideas to yourself. Make sure you have memorized and understand all essential formulas, equations, or procedural steps.

4. Rest, eat well, and do not dwell on the test during the nonstudy times.

5. Make certain you have all documents required for admission to the examination. If you have any questions, call the testing center where you will be taking the examination, The Chauncey Group, or your Board of Nursing office (see Appendix A). If you have doubts, take the time to obtain the correct information.

On the *day before the examinations:*

1. Whether you are staying at a hotel or your own home, drive to the site to make certain you know exactly how to get there, how long the drive will take, and whether there is any road construction that might delay your travel.

2. Do something you enjoy during the day. Have a nice quiet dinner and relax that evening. Do not keep thinking about the test and whether or not you will do well.

3. If you are with colleagues who are taking the test, refrain from discussing it with them.

4. If you feel you absolutely have to review your notes, do so once and then not again. Do *not* keep returning to them.

5. Get sufficient sleep. You need to be both physically and mentally alert the next day.

6. Double-check to make certain you have all required documents for the next day.

COPING WITH THE ACTUAL EXAMINATION ADMINISTRATION

The examination day has finally arrived, and although you may be anxious or worried, you know you have prepared adequately as well as how to maintain a helpful level of anxiety. Be confident as you start the day.

1. Get up early enough so that you are not rushed and can have a good breakfast. As a nurse, you have studied enough nutrition to know that breakfast is the most important meal of the day.

2. Wear comfortable clothes, preferably layered so that you can be comfortable regardless of the room temperature.

3. Make certain you have everything you need—*Authorization To Test,* an official signed photographic identification as well as another piece of identification, money, directions to the site, something to do while waiting for the start of the examination, and so on.

4. Arrive at the examination site on time and preferably early. If you are driving, start at least one-half to 1 hour *earlier* than you think is necessary in case an unexpected problem occurs. It is better to arrive early than late! If you are early, do not just sit and wait. Do something that will take your mind off the examination—read a book, work on a crossword puzzle, work on a craft.

5. Avoid discussing the examination with others who are waiting to take the examination. Leave your review notes and books at home or the hotel.

6. Listen carefully to the instructions given prior to entering the testing room. If you have any questions, ask them at this time.

Most researchers have found that the greatest level of anxiety in a testing situation occurs while you wait for the test to begin or during the first few minutes of the examination. If you find this happening to you at the start of the test, or anytime during the test, some rapid relaxation may be helpful. You should use this technique as soon as you are aware of feelings of anxiety. If you wait, these feelings may become heightened and more difficult to reduce.

One recommended procedure[9] is as follows:

1. Close your eyes. As you sit in your chair, tense all your muscles. Really try to "scrunch up" as many muscles as you can.

2. Once you have tensed the muscles, take a deep breath (inhale through your nostrils) and hold your breath for a count of five, keeping your muscles tensed all the time.

3. After reaching the count of five, simultaneously exhale rapidly through your lips and quickly let go of your muscle tightness by silently telling yourself to *relax*.

4. With your eyes still closed, go as limp in the chair as you possibly can after relaxing.

5. Now, with your muscles relaxed, take a second deep breath through your nostrils. Hold your breath for a couple of seconds. Then *slowly* exhale through your lips.

6. As you exhale, repeat the word "calm" to yourself. You will probably repeat the word 7 to 10 times while slowly exhaling.

7. Repeat these steps once or twice to achieve greater relaxation. Each time through the steps will take approximately 30 seconds.

In addition to the above relaxation technique, there are a number of other steps you should take to remain calm during the examination.

1. As soon as the examination starts, jot down formulas or ideas that you think you might forget during the examination on the scratch paper provided.

2. Develop an *assertive* yet realistic attitude. Approach the test determined that you will do your best, but also accept the limits of what you know. Use everything you know to do well, but do not get angry with yourself if you are uncertain about the answer to a particular item.

3. Remember the guidelines on how to take multiple-choice tests.

4. Do not spend too much time thinking about alternative responses once you have selected the one you think is correct. At the same time, before striking the enter key a second time, quickly double-check your answer and the other options just to make certain you do not make a careless mistake.

5. Concentrate on the critical task—doing well on the examination—and give it your complete attention. Do not waste time worrying, doubting yourself, or wondering how others are doing. Do not become concerned if one or more candidates leave the testing room before you do. Do not worry about what you should have done; instead, concentrate on what you are doing now. Your only concern should be how well one person is doing and that person is *you*.

6. Budget your time. Although sufficient time has been allocated for the examination, you need to be aware of the time constraints. Wear a watch (turn off the alarm if you have one on your watch) and refer to it periodically, but do not be ruled by it. The watch should not become a distraction to your ability to concentrate. The computer screen will also display the time, but a watch is a better way to keep track of the time.

7. Do not permit lapses of memory to create unhealthy anxiety or fear; you are not expected to remember everything you learned in school.

8. Do not waste time with emotional reactions to the items. If you do not know the answer to an item, that's fine. Select an option that seems the most reasonable and proceed to the next item.

9. Above all, *remain confident* and resolve to work at top efficiency throughout the entire examination. Remain positive and convinced that you will do well.

At the conclusion of the examination, you should be pleased with your performance. Whether you took 1 hour or 5 hours to complete the examination is unimportant and not an indicator of how well you did. If you did well in school and prepared for the examination, you should have had no major problems with the questions asked. Now is not the time to worry about your performance, because there is nothing you can do about the results except wait. Fortunately, the wait should not be very long, and within a few weeks you will know the actual outcome of your performance.

REFERENCES

1. Fiore, N, and Pescar, SC: Conquering Test Anxiety. Werner Books, New York, 1987.
2. Sarason, IG (ed): Test Anxiety: Theory, Research and Application. Laurence Erlbaum Associates, Hillsdale, NJ, 1980.
3. Ottens, AJ: Coping with Academic Anxiety. The Rosen Publishing Group, New York, 1984.
4. Sarason, op cit.
5. Sarason, op cit.
6. Sherman, TM, and Wildman, TM: Proven Strategies for Successful Test Taking. Charles E. Merrill Publishing, Columbus, Ohio 1982.
7. Kesselman-Turkel, J, and Peterson, F: Test Taking Strategies. Contemporary Books, Chicago, 1981.
8. Fry, Ron: "Ace" Any Test. Career House, Hawthorne, NJ, 1992.
9. Ottens, op cit.

unittwo
CONTENT AREAS Q & A

chapter 4

Maternity Nursing Q & A

*by Linda Calhoun, Lizabeth L. Carlson,
Carla Hester, Jane Staton Savage, and
Golden Tradewell*

1. A normal gynecoid pelvis is described as:
   A. A well-hollowed sacrum, blunt spines, and wide pubic arch
   B. Flat sacrum, prominent spines, and a wide pubic arch
   C. Deeply hollowed sacrum, narrow pubic arch, and blunt spines
   D. Flat sacrum, narrow pubic arch, and prominent spines

2. Ovulation usually occurs:
   A. At varying, irregular intervals
   B. Fourteen days before the end of the menstrual cycle
   C. Two days after menstrual flow has ceased
   D. When the ovary is stimulated by sexual intercourse

3. In which period of gestation is the embryo/fetus most likely to be damaged by teratogens?
   A. First trimester
   B. Second trimester
   C. Third trimester
   D. Equally throughout pregnancy

4. The sex of the developing fetus is externally identifiable at which month of gestation?
   A. First
   B. Third
   C. Fifth
   D. Seventh

5. Which laboratory tests are usually repeated at each prenatal visit?
   A. Hematocrit
   B. Urinalysis for glucose and albumin
   C. Syphilis and GC screening
   D. Blood typing and antibody titers

6. In most pregnant women, urinary frequency is most problematic:
   A. At 20 weeks' gestation
   B. Following "lightening"
   C. Following "quickening"
   D. During the second trimester

7. Heartburn during pregnancy is commonly attributed to the normal physiological changes of:
   A. Increased output and work load of the heart
   B. Increased peristalsis and increased gastric acidity
   C. Increased peristalsis and decreased food intake
   D. Decreased gastric motility with reflux of stomach contents

8. The vaginal discharge during pregnancy is characteristically:
   A. Whitish and thick
   B. Yellow and frothy
   C. Thin and blood-tinged
   D. No different than nonpregnant state

9. Your patient is being prepared for an amniocentesis. Before the procedure is performed, it is most important for the nurse to obtain:
   A. The heart rate of the fetus
   B. The mother's body temperature
   C. A urine specimen from the mother
   D. A blood specimen from the mother

10. The underlying cause of variable decelerations in the fetal heart rate is:
    A. Head compression
    B. Cord compression
    C. Placental insufficiency
    D. Medications

11. One of the main objectives of a childbirth preparation program is to:
    A. Strengthen the couple's marital relationship
    B. Enhance the pregnant woman's self-esteem
    C. Provide practical tools for the labor process
    D. Educate the mother about the changes in childbirth practices

12. Of the following assessment findings, which would be the most concerning to the nurse during a postpartum examination?
    A. A temperature of 99.8°F
    B. A positive Homans' sign
    C. Edema of the perineal area
    D. Uterine contractions during breastfeeding

13. The nurse explains to a woman that a diaphragm is an excellent method of contraception, providing she:
    A. Does not use any contraceptive cream, jelly, or foam that might make it slip out of place
    B. Removes it promptly following intercourse
    C. Leaves it in place for 6 to 8 hours following intercourse
    D. Inserts it at least 4 to 6 hours prior to intercourse to ensure a protective seal

14. The *main* purpose of relaxation during labor is to:
    A. Allow the woman to conserve energy and allow the uterine muscles to work more efficiently
    B. Promote resting and control
    C. Replace unfavorable with controlled, favorable behaviors
    D. Provide a quiet birthing environment

15. Vitamin K is administered to a newborn in order to:
    A. Stimulate the growth of intestinal flora
    B. Improve the conjugation of bilirubin
    C. Prevent potential bleeding problems
    D. Improve the production of RBCs

16. Which of the following physical characteristics serves to decrease the loss of heat from the newborn?
    A. Larger body surface relative to the adult's
    B. Limited subcutaneous fat
    C. Blood vessel dilatation
    D. Flexed posture

17. Your client is scheduled for a nonstress test (NST). After 20 minutes, you have noted four fetal movements accompanied by accelerations of the fetal heart rate 15 or more beats per minute, each lasting 15 seconds. You interpret this test to be:
    A. Nonreactive
    B. Reactive
    C. Negative
    D. Positive

18. When an epidural is given during the first stage of labor, an important nursing intervention in monitoring this client is to:

A. Position the laboring woman flat in bed to avoid a postanesthesia headache.
B. Monitor the client's blood pressure for hypertension.
C. Monitor the client's blood pressure for hypotension.
D. Ensure that the client voids frequently.

19. Descent, flexion, and internal rotation are the cardinal movements of labor. These movements are designed to:
    A. Allow the fetus to progress rapidly through the birth canal.
    B. Allow the smallest presenting diameter of the fetus to pass through the birth canal first.
    C. Shorten the second stage of labor.
    D. Allow engagement of the presenting part of the fetus.

20. A neonate is delivered at 27 weeks' gestation weighing 1400 grams. Based on this weight and gestation age, how would you classify this neonate?
    A. Low birth weight
    B. Small for gestational age
    C. Large for gestational age
    D. Preterm

21. The embryonic period of pregnancy is critical because:
    A. Genetic information is duplicated at this time.
    B. All organ systems are developed.
    C. Urine is secreted by the kidneys.
    D. Subcutaneous fat is deposited.

22. When conducting a urine pregnancy test, what specific hormone will produce a positive test for pregnancy?
    A. Estrogen
    B. Prolactin
    C. Alpha-fetoprotein
    D. Human chorionic gonadotropin

23. At a client's first prenatal visit you obtain a pregnancy history. She has two living children, has experienced two spontaneous abortions, and currently has a positive pregnancy test. Which of the following best describes your client's status?
    A. Gravida V para II AB II
    B. Gravida IV para IV AB II
    C. Gravida III para II AB II
    D. Gravida II para II AB II

24. Your client is 25 weeks' pregnant. Her glucose screening test shows a blood sugar level of 180 mg/dl. What follow-up care, if any, would be indicated for this client?
    A. No follow-up is required because the blood sugar is within normal limits.
    B. A glucose tolerance test is indicated.
    C. She should be placed on insulin injections to maintain her glucose within normal levels.
    D. She will need weekly nonstress tests to validate fetal well-being.

25. Your client is a gravida III para I. Her first child weighed 4100 gms at birth. She had a spontaneous abortion early in her second pregnancy. With her current pregnancy, her GTT shows elevated blood sugar levels. Because this client has no history of diabetes except during her pregnancies, she is classified as having:
    A. Insulin-dependent diabetes
    B. Type II diabetes mellitus
    C. Type I diabetes mellitus
    D. Gestational diabetes mellitus

26. A fetal ultrasound is done prior to an amniocentesis in order to:
    A. Ensure the fetus is mature enough to withstand the amniocentesis
    B. Evaluate the amount of amniotic fluid
    C. Locate the fetus and implantation site of the placenta
    D. Evaluate fetal lung maturity

27. Your client is a 16-year-old gravida I para 0 who is 37 weeks' gestation by dates. Based upon your knowledge of the maternal physiological changes that normally occur in pregnancy, which of the following assessment findings concern you?
    A. Complaints of dyspnea
    B. Facial and upper body edema
    C. Pulse of 64 beats per minute at 8 weeks, 74 beats per minute at 37 weeks
    D. Hematocrit 39 percent

28. Based on your knowledge of genetic inheritance, which of these statements is true for an autosomal recessive genetic disorder?
    A. Heterozygotes are affected.
    B. The disorder is always carried only on the X chromosome.
    C. Only female offspring are affected.
    D. If both parents are affected they will always have affected offspring.

29. What is the causative agent of syphilis?
    A. *Chlamydia trachomatis*
    B. *Neisseria gonorrhoeae*
    C. *Treponema pallidum*
    D. *Trichomonas vaginalis*

30. Chorioamnionitis is a maternal infection usually associated with:
    A. Post-term deliveries
    B. Maternal dehydration
    C. Prolonged rupture of membranes
    D. Maternal pyelonephritis

31. A positive Babinski's reflex in a newborn would indicate:
    A. The infant has a neurological dysfunction.
    B. The infant has normal, intact neurological function.
    C. The infant has experienced perinatal asphyxia.
    D. The infant has most likely experienced a spinal cord injury during the birthing process.

32. Molding of the fetal head during birth would result in:
    A. Widely spaced suture lines
    B. A collection of fluid across the scalp
    C. Overriding suture lines or a small space between the cranial bones
    D. Depressed fontanelles

33. Your client is 1-day postpartum following a vaginal birth with a second-degree episiotomy. She is complaining that her bottom is sore and it is very uncomfortable for her to sit. She states that she won't have a bowel movement for a few days until the soreness is gone. Which nursing diagnosis would be most accurate for your patient's plan of care?
    A. Ineffective individual coping related to pain of episiotomy
    B. Activity intolerance related to postpartal status
    C. Constipation related to episiotomy pain
    D. Pain related to effects of episiotomy

34. Maternal adaptation to pregnancy causes many changes to occur in the cardiovascular system. Which statement reflects normal changes that occur in the hematologic system of a pregnant woman?
    A. Increased total blood volume, decreased total RBCs, and decreased WBCs
    B. Decreased hemoglobin and hematocrit early in pregnancy with an increase occurring after the second trimester
    C. Increased RBCs, increased WBCs, and decreased hemoglobin and hematocrit
    D. Decreased total blood volume, increased systemic blood pressure, and decreased cardiac output

35. Your client is 10 weeks' pregnant and you are providing her with nutritional education that will be important throughout her pregnancy. She is of average weight for her height. Based on the recommended weight gain during pregnancy, you will advise her that she should gain:
    A. 10 to 20 pounds
    B. 15 to 22 pounds
    C. 25 to 35 pounds
    D. 38 to 50 pounds

36. To improve iron absorption, you should instruct your client at her prenatal visit to take the supplement:
    A. At bedtime with citrus juice, and avoid coffee or tea
    B. Between meals when her stomach is empty
    C. When she takes her prenatal vitamins
    D. Only when she does not eat foods rich in iron daily

37. Your client states she is experiencing gastrointestinal discomforts. Your recommended intervention should be:
    A. Lie down for a short time after each meal.

B. Always include coffee or tea as a beverage with meals.

C. Eat six to eight small meals per day instead of three large ones.

D. Take over-the-counter antacids whenever these episodes occur.

38. In order to accurately measure the duration of contractions, the nurse should measure the time interval between:

A. The beginning of the contraction and the peak of that same contraction

B. The beginning of the contraction and the end of the same contraction

C. The beginning of one contraction and the beginning of the next contraction

D. The peak of one contraction to the peak of the next contraction

39. Effacement is a term used to describe the process by which the cervix:

A. Opens to its widest diameter

B. Lengthens during a normal pregnancy

C. Becomes hypotonic to prepare for dilation

D. Softens and thins with contractions

40. A laboring client who is pregnant for the second time becomes very anxious as transition progresses. She begins to cry and hyperventilate, which upsets her husband. Your best intervention at this point would be:

A. Have the client explain what happened in her previous labor and delivery.

B. Scold her for losing control and assist her in controlling her breathing.

C. See if she is ready for her epidural.

D. Explain to both of them that she is making good progress and assure them that you will remain there to assist them both.

41. During the descent phase of labor, the fetal monitor begins to indicate variable decelerations with each contraction. As the nurse, your best intervention would be to:

A. Notify the physician or nurse midwife immediately.

B. Assist the client in more effective pushing techniques.

C. Move the client to a side-lying position.

D. Continue to assist the client with each contraction because variable decelerations are not worrisome.

42. The cardinal movements of an ROA labor and delivery are descent, flexion, internal rotation, and extension. The main purpose of these movements is to:

A. Shorten the birth process.

B. Allow the largest fetal part to pass through the largest portion of the birth canal first.

C. Provide the most comfortable birth for the mother.

D. Provide the safest outcome for the fetus.

43. To ensure a safe outcome for a client who has been placed an oxytocin for induction of labor, the nurse should assess the client for:

A. Nausea, hyperstimulation of the uterus, and poor urine output

B. Hypertension, headache, and arrhythmias

C. Nervousness, diarrhea, and hypertonic contractions

D. Fluid overload, hypertension, and elevated temperature

44. Kegal exercises are important for mothers following birth because they:

A. Assist in relieving perineal pain

B. Tone the abdominal muscles.

C. Assist in preventing postpartal hemorrhage.

D. Tone the perineal muscles and promote healing.

45. Your client explains that her menstrual period is 2 weeks late and she believes she is pregnant. You respond based on your knowledge that the positive signs of pregnancy are:

A. Amenorrhea, nausea, breast changes, and urinary frequency

B. Uterine enlargement and a positive pregnancy test

C. Demonstration of fetal heart tones and verification of fetal movement by someone other than the mother

D. Braxton Hicks contraction, urinary frequency, and a positive pregnancy test

46. Your client, who is 24 weeks' gestation, asks you to tell her about her baby. Your description includes the following:

A. Twelve inches in length, profuse vernix, and external sexual characteristics that are not clearly discernible

B. Ten inches in length, weight about 2 pounds, with nails to tips of fingers and toes

C. Eye complete, lanugo present, viable, and hearing present

D. Testes in scrotum, strong suck reflex, good tone, and large amount of head hair

47. Which of the following statements by your client would indicate concerns that would cause you to further evaluate her learning needs?

A. At 22 weeks' gestation: "My husband and I have enrolled in some parenting education classes."

B. At 16 weeks' gestation: "I know it's about time for me to feel the baby moving and I can hardly wait."

C. At 26 weeks' gestation: "I can still get by with my regular clothes and I don't think I'm going to have to buy any maternity clothes."

D. At 20 weeks' gestation: "My husband came with me for my check-up today. He wants to hear the baby's heartbeat."

48. In assessment of a postpartum client, you discover a boggy uterus with increased lochia flow. Your first nursing intervention should be to:
 A. Increase her oxytocin (Pitocin) flow rate.
 B. Encourage her to ambulate to the bathroom to empty her bladder.
 C. Gently massage the fundus.
 D. Examine her cervix for lacerations.

49. As you enter the room of a third-day postpartum client, you discover her crying. She tells you that she doesn't know why she is crying but she can't seem to stop. Her behavior would indicate:
 A. Disappointment in the gender of her new baby
 B. Dissatisfaction with the care she is receiving in the hospital
 C. Postpartum psychosis
 D. Postpartum blues

50. At the first prenatal visit, the client says that she has been a one-pack-a-day smoker for 3 years and knows it is not good for her baby, so she plans to quit. However, at her subsequent visits she tells you she has not been able to quit. Her fundal height measurements are suggestive of intrauterine growth retardation (IUGR) of her fetus. What fetal assessment tool would give an accurate diagnosis of IUGR?
 A. Amniocentesis
 B. Doppler blood flow analysis
 C. Contraction stress test
 D. Chorionic villi sampling

51. A client is scheduled for an amniocentesis in her 36th week of pregnancy. She has had several episodes of preterm labor and is being evaluated to determine the L/S ratio. This would reveal which of the following?
 A. Amount of amniotic fluid
 B. Fetal lung maturity
 C. Fetal weight
 D. Position of the placenta

52. Upon rupture of membranes during labor, the amniotic fluid is noted to be meconium stained. What preparations for the nurse midwife to respond to this event will the nurse need to make?
 A. Explain to the client the need for an immediate cesarean section and begin to prepare the environment.
 B. Anticipate and begin your client on oxytocin (Pitocin) to speed her labor.
 C. Prepare the equipment so that the nurse midwife can provide early suctioning of the infant as soon as the head delivers. *done 2nd*
 D. Increase your monitoring of the fetus to ensure fetal well-being during the remainder of the mother's labor.

53. You receive a phone call from a client who is 36 weeks' gestation. She complains of painless vaginal bleeding that started suddenly without any spe-

cific precipitating event. You advise her to come to the hospital immediately because you are concerned that she may have a/an:
 A. Placenta previa
 B. Placenta accreta
 C. Abruptio placentae
 D. Ectopic pregnancy

54. A client with late third trimester bleeding would not receive a digital vaginal examination due to an increased risk of:
 A. Initiating undesired labor
 B. Separating a low-lying placenta
 C. Infection for the mother and fetus
 D. Fetal distress prior to labor

55. Most pregnancy tests evaluate the presence of hCG, which is produced by the:
 A. Trophoblastic layer of the blastocyst
 B. Chorionic villi
 C. Anterior pituitary gland
 D. Corpus luteum

56. The fetal structures that allow blood to be shunted to the placenta with very little flowing through the lungs are the:
 A. Ductus arteriosus and foramen ovale
 B. Ductus venosus and ductus arteriosus
 C. Foramen ovale and ductus venosus
 D. Umbilical vein and ductus venosus

57. A woman who suffered a spontaneous abortion at 8 weeks' gestation, delivered one infant at 40 weeks, and is now pregnant would be classified as:
 A. Gravida II para II
 B. Gravida III para III
 C. Gravida III para I
 D. Gravida III para II

58. Betty R. is worried that her newborn will not sleep once she takes him home because they live so close to a railroad track. As her nurse, you explain to her that newborns can decrease their response to annoying stimuli after repeated exposure. This response is known as:
 A. Level of comfort
 B. Habituation
 C. Responsibility
 D. Consolability

59. You are teaching a childbirth and parenting class to a group of expectant mothers. As you describe the different states of an infant, you tell the participants that the characteristics of the quiet alert state of an infant are:
 A. Minimal body activity, widening of eyes, and a regular breathing pattern
 B. Variable activity levels, heavy lidded eyes, and an irregular breathing pattern
 C. Nearly still body activity, no eye movements, and a smooth, regular breathing pattern
 D. Minimal body activity, rapid eye movements, and an irregular breathing pattern

60. Stacy M. states that she is very disappointed that she cannot breastfeed her infant since her breasts are too small and would not provide enough milk. The nurse's best response would be:
   A. "You are probably right. It would be very difficult for you to produce enough milk. Commercial formula is just as healthy for your baby."
   B. "I understand your concern. Perhaps you could provide some breast milk occasionally and provide formula for all the other feedings to ensure that he receives enough calories."
   C. "The size of your breasts really don't have anything to do with it. However, formula is much easier and less stressful for you."
   D. "The size and shape of your breast are related to the amount of fatty tissue and are not what influence your milk production. The amount of glandular tissue is what is important. You should be successful with breastfeeding."

61. Marge W. tells you she would like to use the measurement of basal body temperature to control pregnancy. You explain the rationale for determining the time of ovulation by this method. During ovulation you know that the basal body temperature:
   A. Drops sharply, remaining low
   B. Rises sharply, remaining high
   C. Drops slightly and then rises
   D. Rises slightly and remains high for 72 hours

62. Clara M. has come to the clinic in which you work to have an intrauterine device (IUD) inserted. In explaining this contraceptive method you tell Clara a common problem is:
   A. Painful intercourse
   B. Repeated vaginal and uterine infections
   C. Spontaneous expulsion of the IUD
   D. Cessation of menstrual flow

63. Doris L. is admitted to the ER complaining of a sharp lower right abdominal pain. During the nursing history, she reports that her last menstrual period was 7 weeks ago. A question the nurse would ask is:
   A. "Are you experiencing any shoulder pain?"
   B. "Have you ever been pregnant before?"
   C. "How many children do you have?"
   D. "Can you feel a hard mass on your right side?"

64. Faye M. has just had her 6-week pregnancy confirmed at the clinic. She is a gravida I, and she asks the nurse how long it will be before she will be able to feel her baby moving. The nurse's best response would be:
   A. "It won't be for several weeks. You need to focus on how you can best take care of yourself and your baby now instead of things that won't happen for quite some time."
   B. "Most first-time mothers don't experience that feeling for several weeks. Sometimes as late as 18 to 20 weeks."

   C. "You should be able to feel the baby begin to move within the next month or so. It really just depends on the size of your baby and his or her activity level."
   D. "Sometimes first-time mothers don't even realize they are feeling their baby move, because they think it is gas pains. Let's focus on your diet and some other things that are important for you to learn during your first trimester."

65. During her prenatal physical assessment, Ginny P, overhears the physician tell the nurse that Ginny has a positive Chadwick's sign. Following the exam Ginny asks the nurse to explain the comment. The nurse knows that a positive Chadwick's sign means that:
   A. Cervical softening with an increase in vascularity has taken place.
   B. Softening of the lower uterine segment has occurred.
   C. Softening of the cervix has started.
   D. The vaginal mucosa has a purplish color.

66. Hillary A. has come in for her first prenatal visit. The results of her blood work show a physiologic anemia. The nurse knows that:
   A. Her diet is poor without enough iron intake.
   B. Her liver is dysfunctional and not able to keep up with the increased demands of pregnancy.
   C. Her blood volume has increased, causing hemodilution.
   D. Her blood work needs to be repeated because of a probable laboratory error.

67. The nurse is discussing the labor process with a client who is pregnant for the first time. The nurse explains that the client should come to the hospital when:
   A. She loses her mucus plug and has a bloody show.
   B. She is having regular contractions that are very uncomfortable.
   C. Her membranes rupture or her contractions are regular at 5 to 7 minutes apart.
   D. Her contractions are 10 to 15 minutes apart.

68. The nurse is teaching her primigravida client about the difference between true and false labor. She knows that true labor will:
   A. Cause contractions that are felt in the abdomen and spread to the lower back and cause cervical changes to occur
   B. Produce contractions that are somewhat irregular and may disappear with activity
   C. Be more tolerable for the client if she is lying down
   D. Occur only after the membranes have ruptured and contractions are regular

69. The labor-and-delivery nurse monitoring a client discovers on examination that the membranes

have ruptured. She notes that the amniotic fluid is greenish-yellow. She knows that this:
A. Is a normal appearance for amniotic fluid
B. May be an ominous sign that indicates the presence of bilirubin
C. May indicate the presence of meconium and is indicative of fetal distress
D. May indicate chorioamnionitis, an infection of the membranes

70. A client is admitted to the labor-and-delivery room with contractions that are regular, lasting 50 seconds and 3 to 5 minutes apart. She reports that she had a bloody show early this morning. Vaginal examination reveals that her cervix is 100 percent effaced and 8 cm dilated. The nurse knows that this information indicates that Margaret is in which phase of labor?
A. Active phase
B. Latent phase
C. Retention phase
D. The fourth stage

71. A client is admitted to the labor-and-delivery suite at 42.5 weeks' gestation following her report of loss of her mucous plug with a bloody show, slow leak of what she believes to be amniotic fluid, and low back pain. She denies experiencing any contractions. As the nurse, you know that you should prepare:
A. For an emergency cesarean section
B. For possible augmentation of labor
C. For an amnioinfusion
D. To send her home until she is in true labor

72. A client comes into the labor-and-delivery suite stating that her membranes ruptured about 5 hours ago, but that she is not having contractions. She wants to be examined to see if she is dilating. She states that her baby has stopped moving, but she wants to return to work if she is not in labor. The nurse knows that:
A. Following a vaginal examination to check for dilation, the client will most likely be allowed to return to work until her contractions are in a regular pattern.
B. The client should be sent home to rest in a familiar environment until she is in true labor.
C. She should evaluate for fetal heart rate and check for a prolapsed cord.
D. The client will be routinely admitted because she will most likely develop a regular contraction pattern soon.

73. Penny Y., who is 41 weeks' gestation, is undergoing induction of labor with IV oxytocin. As the nurse monitoring this client, you should routinely assess for:
A. Uterine tetany
B. Deep tendon reflexes
C. Hyperglycemia
D. Tearing of the perineum

74. Rita M. is laboring at 39 weeks' gestation. Upon vaginal examination the nurse records her assessment of 100 percent effaced, 9 cm dilated, and +1 station. The nurse knows that the presenting part is:
A. Still high in the pelvis
B. Level with the ischial spines
C. Slightly below the ischial spines
D. Slightly above the ischial spines

75. The previous shift's nurses' notes on a client indicated that the client had a third-degree laceration on delivery. The nurse knows that this means:
A. The perineal laceration extends through the skin.
B. An extensive cervical laceration has occurred.
C. The perineal laceration extend through the perineal body and anal sphincter and involves the rectal wall.
D. The perineal laceration extends through the perineal body to the anal sphincter.

76. Sally H. is now 4 hours' postpartum following the vaginal birth of a term infant weighing 7 lb 6 oz. The nurse has encouraged her to try to void, although she does not feel the urge. The nurse knows that urinary retention can cause:
A. Postpartal urinary tract infection (UTI)
B. Uterine atony
C. Postpartal uterine infection
D. Uterine tetany

77. The nurse realizes that Terri, who is 12 hours' postpartum and successfully breastfeeding her new son, needs additional breastfeeding instruction when she states:
A. "I must remember to keep lotion handy for my breasts so they won't dry out."
B. "I must remember to wash my hands real good each time before I put the baby to breast."
C. "I plan to put a large safety pin on my bra after each feeding so that I can remember which breast the baby nursed from at each feeding."
D. "I know how important it is to drink lots of fluids now."

78. At her first postpartal visit to the clinic at 4 weeks, the client tells the nurse that she has been experiencing a lot of leg cramps at night. The best advice the nurse can give is to:
A. Be sure that she exercises on a regular basis and drinks plenty of water
B. Increase her milk intake since she most likely has hypocalcemia
C. Increase her intake of bananas and dark yellow vegetables since she most likely has hypokalemia
D. Take a long relaxing bath each evening to relieve the stress common with new mothers

79. Wanda R. tells the nurse that a friend told her that newborns cannot get sick since they get immunity

from their mothers before they are born. The nurse knows that Wanda is probably referring to:

A. Active immunity
B. Latent immunity
C. Passive immunity
D. Natural immunity

80. The nurse knows that the client needs additional teaching when the client asks how she can get rid of the pimples on her baby's face. The nurse's best response is:

A. "Those spots are called milia and are very common in newborn babies. you should not try to open them. They will disappear on their own over a short period of time."
B. "Those spots are called vernix and will disappear on their own very soon."
C. "I'll be glad to get you a basin of warm water and a wash cloth so that you can bath the baby. Those spots should come off easily enough when you clean his face."
D. "Don't worry about them. When we bathe him in the nursery, we'll take care of spots. Lots of babies have them."

81. Following the birth of her newborn, your client is afraid when she notices her baby jumping and throwing out his arms when his bed is bumped. She is sure that her baby has some kind of brain damage. The nurse knows that his action by the baby is called the:

A. Tonic neck reflex
B. Babinski reflex
C. Moro reflex
D. Galant's reflex

82. A client is very concerned about the purplish spots on her baby's buttocks. She feels sure the baby was dropped while in the nursery. In developing a nursing plan of care for this mother, an appropriate nursing diagnosis would be:

A. Knowledge deficit related to normal newborn characteristics and variations
B. Altered thought processes related to lack of understanding of newborns
C. Ineffective individual coping related to new family member
D. Anxiety related to inadequate information

83. Your client is concerned when she discovers that she is 7 weeks' pregnant because she had spent a weekend with her friends that was filled with alcohol and drug use. It was the first weekend following her menstrual period, and she is sure this is when she got pregnant because she has not had intercourse since that time. She is certain that her infant will be badly deformed because of her drug and alcohol use that weekend. Your knowledge of the occurrence of teratogenic effects of drugs:

A. Leads you to believe that she does have a great deal to worry about

B. Helps you to explain that she has little to be concerned about since substances used prior to implantation will have an all-or-nothing effect
C. Leads you to recommend that this mother might want to consider terminating this pregnancy since there will likely be major deformities
D. Helps you to explain that fetal and maternal circulations are separate and what she ingested during the weekend will not harm her fetus

84. Your client at 41 weeks' gestation is scheduled for a test to determine how her infant will withstand the stress of labor and delivery. You know this is describing a:

A. Transvaginal ultrasound
B. Nonstress test
C. Amniocentesis
D. Contraction stress test

85. During a routine ultrasound in the sixth month of gestation, it is discovered that a client has a low-lying placenta. It would be important to teach this client the danger signs of:

A. Placenta previa
B. Placenta accreta
C. Abruptio placentae
D. Placental infarction

86. A client delivered a 36-week-gestation male infant following diagnosis of Hemolysis Elevated Liver enzymes Low Platelets (HELLP) syndrome. In the postpartum recovery room she is receiving IV magnesium sulfate (MgSO$_4$) and hydralazine (Apresoline). You take her vital signs every 15 minutes and you are checking DTRs and urinary output. You know that the client continues to be at risk for seizure activity for how long after delivery?

A. 12 hours
B. 24 hours
C. 48 hours
D. 1 week

87. The most appropriate nursing diagnosis for a client in postpartal recovery who is being managed for HELLP syndrome is:

A. High risk for infection related to changes in RBC morphology
B. High risk for injury related to possible seizure activity
C. Risk for hemorrhage related to HELLP syndrome
D. Anxiety related to unknown outcome of disease process

88. Baby boy J. was born at 28 weeks' gestation. As his nurse you know that one of the most common immediate problems of preterm infants is:

A. Central nervous system edema
B. Biliary atresia

C. Respiratory distress
D. Hyperglycemia

89. The nurse working with premature neonates knows that the gastrointestinal system of the infant:
    A. Is no different from that of a term infant
    B. Has a smaller capacity stomach, slower emptying time, and low gastric acidity
    C. Has faster motility and therefore absorbs fewer nutrients as foods pass through
    D. Has a higher gastric acidity and therefore reflux is more common

90. Judith A. is recovering from a hysterectomy as a result of uncontrollable bleeding following placenta previa. One of the top priority teaching needs prior to discharge would be:
    A. Explanation of the rationale for the immediate onset of menopause
    B. Explanation of resumption of a normal menstrual cycle
    C. Discussion of the type of birth control most suited for posthysterectomy clients
    D. Discussion of expected feelings of grief and loss

91. The nurse should explain to the client that the most common side effect of the contraceptive Depo-Provera is:
    A. Irregular and unpredictable menstrual bleeding
    B. Weight loss
    C. Hyperactivity
    D. Hypertension

92. Your client is concerned because her 34-week-gestation newborn has undescended testicles. Your explanation to her should be based on the knowledge that:
    A. The testes do not normally descend into the scrotal sac until 1 year of age.
    B. The testes normally descend into the scrotal sac at about 36 weeks' gestation.
    C. It is not important for the testes to descend until puberty.
    D. The baby will require immediate surgery in order to move the testes into the scrotal sac.

93. The characteristic signs and symptoms of pregnancy-induced hypertension (PIH) include:
    A. Trace of proteinuria, BP increase greater than 15 mm Hg above the systolic baseline, and lower extremity edema.
    B. Epigastric pain, diastolic pressure of 90 mm Hg, dizziness
    C. BP increase of 30 mm Hg systolic, 15 mm Hg diastolic above the baseline, greater than 1+ proteinuria, and edema greater than 1+
    D. Hypertension, glucosuria, and upper body edema

94. Your client is concerned that she does not have breast milk the second day following delivery of her newborn. She complains that the yellow stuff will not be enough for her baby. Your explanation to this client should include the following:
    A. She will need to supplement with commercial infant formula.
    B. The yellowish secretion is colostrum, which is important for her newborn because it is contains antibodies and is high in nutritional value.
    C. She will have an ample amount of breast milk by the end of the first month.
    D. Many women with small breasts do not have an adequate early production of breast milk.

95. The diagnosis of pregnancy-induced hypertension (PIH) is suspected if the following are found:
    A. Ankle edema and hyporeflexia
    B. Ankle edema and glucosuria
    C. Hypertension and glucosuria
    D. Hypertension and proteinuria

96. A major complication of eclampsia is:
    A. Infection
    B. Aspiration
    C. Polyuria
    D. Extremity injuries

97. The most common cause of early postpartal hemorrhage is:
    A. Uterine atony
    B. Retained placental fragments
    C. Cervical lacerations
    D. Infection

98. The nursing diagnosis of highest priority for a client who has experienced a postpartal hemorrhage is:
    A. Alteration in comfort
    B. Anxiety
    C. Altered tissue perfusion
    D. High risk for infection

99. When administering $MgSO_4$ for treatment of pregnancy-induced-hypertension (PIH), which of the following findings are of concern?
    A. Sixteen respirations per minute
    B. Reflexes of 2+
    C. Irritability and nervousness
    D. Urinary output less than 20 ml/hr

100. Magnesium sulfate ($MgSO_4$) is used in the treatment of pre-eclampsia to:
    A. Prevent seizures
    B. Decrease blood pressure
    C. Increase urine output
    D. Decrease edema

101. A client arrives at the clinic for her first prenatal visit. She states that her last menstrual period was May 12 to 16. Using Naegele's rule, determine her EDC:

A. February 23
B. August 15
C. February 19
D. March 3

102. Physiological anemia is a result of:
    A. Increased erythropoiesis in the first 2 weeks of pregnancy
    B. Decreased dietary intake of iron
    C. A plasma volume increase that is greater than the RBC increase
    D. Increased demand on the maternal liver

103. Your client is 12 hours' postpartum. On assessment you note her fundus is one fingerbreadth above the umbilicus and deviated to the right. What is your understanding of this finding?
    A. This is a normal fundal position for this stage of recovery.
    B. This position indicates a lazy uterus.
    C. This position indicates that the clients bladder is distended.
    D. This position is an early sign of postpartal hemorrhage.

104. A client with three prior cesarean sections is in active labor and scheduled for a repeat cesarean delivery. The nurse's primary concern for the client would be:
    A. Tetanic contractions
    B. Precipitous labor
    C. Uterine rupture
    D. Abruptio placentae

105. Following an amniocentesis, the client should be monitored for an hour for:
    A. Breast tenderness
    B. Increased fetal activity
    C. Temperature elevation
    D. Rupture of membranes

106. In order to decrease complaints of frequent indigestion, the nurse suggests the client should:
    A. Use an antacid as needed.
    B. Decrease intake of spicy foods.
    C. Increase amount of fruit eaten.
    D. Discontinue the use of sugar substitutes.

107. A client reports a weight gain of 1 pound a week during her eighth month of pregnancy. Which of the following actions should be taken?
    A. None, because this is a normal weight increase.
    B. Make an appointment with the nutritionist.
    C. Suggest a weight-loss program.
    D. Check for proteinuria and hypertension.

108. The client reports concern about alternating periods of fetal activity and inactivity. The nurse recognizes the need for further teaching and replies:
    A. "Inactivity may be a signal that something is wrong."
    B. "The fetus goes through wake/sleep cycles just like a baby."

C. "This type of activity pattern usually indicates a male fetus."
D. "Your baby is responding to changes in temperature and barometric pressure."

109. A pregnant client has been taking tetracycline during her pregnancy. Fetal damage resulting from tetracycline is:
    A. Deafness
    B. Webbed fingers
    C. Discolored teeth
    D. Mental retardation

110. The nurse would suspect placenta previa when her pregnant client experienced which of the following?
    A. Painless bleeding
    B. Painful bleeding
    C. No bleeding
    D. Intermittent bleeding

111. An internal fetal-monitor lead is applied after the amniotic membrane ruptures. The nurse observes the tracing for which of the following, indicating severe fetal distress?
    A. Hiccups
    B. Late decelerations
    C. Early decelerations
    D. Beat-to-beat variability

112. A client's husband plans to accompany his wife (G4P3) into the delivery room. When should the nurse plan to have him change into scrub attire?
    A. During the latent phase of labor.
    B. Once active labor is established.
    C. When complete dilation occurs.
    D. When the fetal head is visible.

113. The best position for a client, 28 weeks' gestation, receiving ritodrine for premature labor is:
    A. Prone
    B. Trendelenburg's
    C. Supine
    D. Side-lying

114. A client has a history of pelvic inflammatory disease (PID). This would increase the risk of:
    A. Ectopic pregnancy
    B. Placenta previa
    C. Abruptio placentae
    D. Molar pregnancy

115. A pregnant client with anemia is prescribed ferrous gluconate. In addition, the nurse would expect the physician to order:
    A. Folic acid
    B. Riboflavin
    C. Thiamine
    D. Calcium

116. A client asks about a safe level of physical activity while she is pregnant. The nurse's best teaching is that she should:

A. "Maintain your normal level of activity if there are no problems."
B. "Gradually increase your activity to improve endurance."
C. "Gradually decrease your activity because there is a potential for premature labor."
D. "Decrease activities in the second trimester because your increased oxygen demands will endanger your baby."

117. A client, G2P1, is expecting twins. An important goal for her care is to:
A. Limit weight gain.
B. Promote physical endurance.
C. Equalize size of the twins.
D. Prevent premature delivery.

118. Baby boy J. has just been born prematurely at 35 weeks, weighing 4 lb 4 oz. His Apgar scores are 7 and 8. His respiratory status is stable. You are the nurse providing care for him and his mother in the Labor Delivery Recovery Postpartum (LDRP) room. Your most immediate major concern is to:
A. Obtain his footprints and place a name band on his arm
B. Administer blowby oxygen as you assess him
C. Provide body temperature support with a warmer or warmed blankets
D. Assess vital signs q 15 minutes

119. While you are performing your admission assessment of a term newborn female infant born in the frank breech position, you note asymmetrical gluteal and thigh folds. She has a positive Ortolani's maneuver. You know that these assessment findings are indicative of:
A. Femoral nerve palsy
B. CNS nerve damage
C. Acetabulum atresia
D. Congenital hip dislocation

120. Angela Y. brings her baby in for his first newborn appointment. She tells you that the baby has some funny white patches and sores in his mouth and he has been having a little diarrhea. You know that these signs and symptoms most likely indicate that the baby has:
A. Herpes simplex
B. Thrush
C. *Staphylococcus aureus*
D. Epstein pearls

121. You are admitting a newborn into the nursery whose mother had a rupture of membranes (ROM) 23 hours prior to delivery. You know that one of the complications for which you must carefully monitor is:
A. Respiratory distress syndrome
B. Retinopathy of prematurity
C. Meconium aspiration syndrome
D. Neonatal sepsis

122. Kandy W., who has insulin-dependent diabetes mellitus and is 9 weeks' pregnant, has come into the ER with signs of insulin overdose. She has not adjusted her insulin dosage. What change has likely taken place?
A. Because she is in her first trimester of pregnancy, she has been hungry and has added a lot of foods containing simple sugars to her diet.
B. She has had some nausea and vomiting and a subsequent loss of appetite caused by morning sickness.
C. She has been concerned about the baby and has stopped her exercise routine.
D. Because of her increased sleep requirements, she has not checked her blood glucose levels on a regular basis.

123. You are providing care for a client who has been hospitalized for internal radiation therapy following a diagnosis of cervical cancer. One of your main nursing interventions will be to:
A. Maintain a close bedside vigil to closely assess the client for signs and symptoms of radiation sickness
B. Closely monitor how frequently the client is voiding because the implants sometimes cause difficulty voiding
C. Monitor liquid and subsequent low-residue diet
D. Ensure that the client remains in a high Fowler's position to prevent the implants from migrating upward

124. A 38-weeks'-pregnant client was admitted to the labor-and-delivery suite with contractions 15 minutes apart. As she is being assisted into bed by the nurse, her membranes rupture and the nurse notes the umbilical cord has prolapsed. The best position for the nurse to place the client in the bed is:
A. Supine
B. Trendelenburg
C. Fowler's
D. Lithotomy

125. Upon admission to the labor-and-delivery suite, a client who is 37 weeks' pregnant is experiencing vaginal bleeding and complains of severe abdominal pain. On assessment, the nurse discovers a woodlike fundus and signs of shock. The client states she has not felt the baby move "in a long time." The nurse knows that she has most likely experienced:
A. A placenta previa
B. An incomplete abortion
C. An abruptio placentae
D. An intrauterine fetal death

126. A client has experienced an early postpartal hemorrhage due to uterine atony following a vaginal

birth 48 hours ago. Her bleeding has finally been controlled. A pertinent priority nursing diagnosis would be:

A. Pain related to traumatic events
B. High risk for infection related to decreased immunity.
C. High risk for altered parenting related to forced separation of mother and infant.
D. Altered maternal tissue perfusion related to hypovolemia.

127. A client at 32 weeks' gestation presents in the ER with an asthma attack that she has not been able to control with her usual medications. Her husband states that she has been very stressed at work lately since the company for which she works has discussed layoffs. The client is diagnosed as experiencing status asthmaticus and is admitted to the ICU. You know that the major physiological concern for her and her infant is:

A. Related to the effects of medications and hypoxia
B. Related to hypoxia and required bed rest
C. Related to the risk of nosocomial infections because of the lengthy hospital stay
D. Related to fluid overload from required intravenous fluids and medications

128. Julie Y.'s last menstrual period began August 23. Using Naegele's rule, her estimated date of confinement is:

A. June 23
B. May 30
C. April 25
D. November 23

129. During the client's first prenatal examination the certified nurse midwife (CNM) determines that the client is approximately 11 weeks' gestation. Which of the following signs of pregnancy would the CNM be able to assess at this gestational age?

A. Fetal movements
B. Fetal heart rate with a stethoscope
C. Chadwick's sign
D. Presence of breast milk

130. You receive a phone call from your client, who is in her first trimester of pregnancy, telling you that she has had trouble keeping her breakfast down each morning. Her early morning symptoms have bothered her for about 2 weeks. Your best nursing advice to this client is:

A. Skip an early morning breakfast and wait until about midmorning before eating.
B. Sip black coffee with her breakfast because the caffeine seems to settle the stomach.
C. Eat only fruit in the morning in order to avoid foods containing fats, which increase the nausea.
D. Eat dry crackers before getting out of bed in the morning.

131. At her first prenatal visit, Ms. Anderson tells you that she has an occasional alcoholic drink when she and her husband go out to dinner. Your best nursing advice to Ms. Anderson in regard to drinking alcoholic beverages during pregnancy is:

A. An occasional drink should not hurt her or her baby throughout her pregnancy.
B. Abstinence from alcohol during pregnancy is recommended.
C. Drinking only wine or beer is suggested since their alcohol content is lower than other alcoholic beverages.
D. Mixed drinks tend to cause less stomach upset and are therefore preferred over wine or beer.

132. You are discussing weight gain during pregnancy with a client who is in the clinic for her prenatal visit. She is of average height and within her recommended weight range for her age and height prior to pregnancy. Based on your knowledge of nutritional needs of pregnancy and appropriate weight gain, your best advice to her would be:

A. She should not be so concerned with how much weight she gains as the types of foods she is eating.
B. She should control her weight gain to within 15 lb so that she will have less weight to lose after the birth of the baby.
C. A weight gain of about 2 lb per month will ensure an adequate growth curve for her baby.
D. A weight gain of 25 to 35 lb over the prepregnancy weight will allow for normal growth of the fetus and the maternal organs.

133. A client is complaining that she has continued to have problems with constipation throughout her first trimester of pregnancy. The nurse should teach that a good way to help relieve constipation is:

A. Purchase a good over-the-counter laxative to use on occasion.
B. Decrease the amount of unrefined sugars in the diet.
C. Increase fluid intake and exercise.
D. Decrease the amount of fat in the diet.

134. The nurse is assisting a client in her 34th week of pregnancy onto the examination table in order to check the heart rate of her fetus. She is lying supine and complains to the nurse that she is feeling dizzy. The nurse notes that she is pale. The best nursing action at this time is:

A. Immediately check her blood pressure because she is likely hypotensive.
B. Request that the client lean forward and place her head between her knees.
C. Check for vaginal bleeding because she may be hemorrhaging.
D. Place a pillow under either side to get the client into a side-lying position.

135. During Ms. Carter's monthly prenatal visit, the nurse will be performing Leopold's maneuvers.

The nurse should provide instruction to Ms. Carter prior to the examination. She will instruct her to:

A. Empty her bladder prior to the examination
B. Remain NPO for 8 hours prior to her appointment time
C. Lie on her left side during the entire examination
D. Drink plenty of fluids so that the full bladder will make visualization better

136. Ms. Surtane has called the client for advice regarding the diarrhea she has been experiencing for the past 36 hours. The nurse knows that her best advice to this client is to:

A. Take an over-the-counter medication specific for diarrhea
B. Increase the bulk in her diet
C. Come into the clinic to be evaluated and examined
D. Increase her fluid intake to avoid dehydration

137. During her prenatal visit at 18 weeks, Ms. Lennom asks about wearing her seat belt when she is riding in her car. She tells the nurse that she has heard that the belt can crush her baby if she is in an accident. The nurse's best response should be:

A. "You are right. During pregnancy, only the shoulder belt should be worn. The lap belt can cause an injury to your baby if you are involved in an accident."
B. "You should only wear the lap belt. It is difficult to position the shoulder belt over your enlarging abdomen."
C. "Since you really shouldn't be traveling any long distances during your pregnancy, you needn't worry about using seat belts. They can do more harm than good."
D. "You should wear the lap belt as low as possible over the pelvic bones and below your enlarging abdomen and the shoulder belt should be firm but comfortable. You can put a pad on the shoulder belt if it touches the side of your neck."

138. Sara H., a 15-year-old primigravida who has been admitted to the labor-and-delivery unit with regular contractions, tells the nurse that she is very frightened because she is already having painful contractions. Sara states that she did not think having a baby really hurt until just before the baby is born. The nurse correctly explains to Sara that the pain she is experiencing in the first stage of labor is caused primarily by:

A. The dilatation and effacement of the cervix
B. The pressure of the baby on the spine
C. The tightening of the uterine muscles
D. Her pain threshold

139. A term, small for gestational age (SGA) infant is admitted to the newborn nursery at 1 hour of age. As the nurse assigned to the nursery, you know

that it is essential to evaluate this infant for signs of hypoglycemia. The main signs and symptoms of hypoglycemia in a newborn are:

A. Hyperthermia, cyanosis, and lethargy
B. High-pitched cry, respiratory distress, and doll's eyes
C. Hypothermia, absent Babinski, and tremors
D. Hypothermia, high-pitched cry, respiratory distress, and tremors

140. During a birth preparation class, the nurse is teaching parents about the anatomy and physiology of the placenta and umbilical cord. She correctly describes the cord as containing:

A. One artery and one vein
B. One artery and two veins
C. Two arteries and one vein
D. Two arteries and two veins

141. Judy B. has been discussing her varicose veins in her legs with the nurse. The nurse accurately teaches Judy that she should avoid certain items of clothing because of her varicosities. These include:

A. Flat shoes without adequate support
B. Clothing with elastic waistbands
C. Girdles or panty hose
D. Knee-high or thigh-high hose

142. Kegel exercises are important for the pregnant mother in order to:

A. Strengthen the perineal muscles
B. Strengthen the abdominal wall muscles
C. Prevent varicose veins
D. Strengthen the lower back

143. A client has come to the prenatal clinic because her menstrual period is 5 weeks late. She is quite certain that she is pregnant since her periods are usually very regular. The nurse knows that the following symptom would be identified as a presumptive sign of pregnancy.

A. Constipation
B. Breast tenderness
C. Shortness of breath
D. Headaches

144. A pregnant client is concerned that the splotches on her face will not go away. The nurse correctly explains to her that:

A. "Chloasma or melasma—blotchy, irregular hyperpigmentation of the forehead, cheeks, nose, and upper lip—is caused by hormonal changes that occur during pregnancy. This condition generally fades after delivery, but in some women never disappears completely."
B. "Linea nigra is common in pregnancy in darker-skinned women and will disappear completely after delivery."
C. "Striae frequently occur during pregnancy. Unfortunately, they do not usually go away following pregnancy."

D. "There are many vascular changes that occur during pregnancy. There is no way to know for sure which will remain after delivery. You really don't need to worry about these things so early in your pregnancy."

145. You are providing preconception counseling for birth control to a client in the clinic. She is interested in oral contraceptives. You know that if she indicates she has experienced any of the following problems in her past medical, it will *not* be advisable for her to use that type of birth control.
A. Amenorrhea
B. Hyperglycemia
C. Breast cancer
D. Premenstrual syndrome

146. The nurse is counseling her client on the use of her new diaphragm for contraception. She advises her client that the minimum length of time following intercourse that the diaphragm must be left in place in the vagina is:
A. 30 minutes
B. 1 hour
C. 6 hours
D. 24 hours

147. Mr. and Ms. Tosh have just experienced a perinatal loss. Ms. Tosh delivered a stillborn term infant just 3 hours ago. When the nurse enters the room to evaluate the client's postpartal status, she discovers Ms. Tosh alone and crying. Which statement would be the most therapeutic?
A. "Your husband should be here with you during this time. You will both need a lot of support and you should be helping each other."
B. "I am so sorry you lost your baby. I know this is a very difficult time for you right now."
C. "You really shouldn't be alone now. Would you like for me to call someone to come and stay with you?"
D. "I'll get you a sleeping pill to help you rest. It will make everything all better."

148. Your client is classified as a high risk in need of a definite diagnosis of pregnancy. Ultrasound will be used to determine if she is pregnant. Confirmation of pregnancy during the first trimester using ultrasound is based on:
A. Laboratory analysis of a sample of amniotic fluid
B. Measurement of femur length of the fetus
C. Visualization of the yolk sac
D. Level of HCG in the urine sample

149. Your client is scheduled for chorionic villus sampling (CVS) during her first trimester of pregnancy. During your patient teaching you explain to her that the purpose of this test is to:
A. Obtain a sample of fetal cells on which to perform genetic analysis

B. Measure the length of the fetus to establish gestational age
C. Evaluate the volume of amniotic fluid to ensure adequate volume
D. Evaluate placenta perfusion

150. A client is in the clinic for her prenatal visit at 31 weeks. You have measured her fundal height and find it is within normal limits for her gestational age. What would you expect her fundal height to be at this time?
A. 27 cm
B. 31 cm
C. 33 cm
D. 40 cm

151. A client has just had an amniocentesis to determine fetal lung development. If the lungs were considered mature, you would expect the lecithin-sphingomyelin ratio (L/S) to be equal to or greater than:
A. 3 : 1
B. 1 : 2
C. 2 : 1
D. 5 : 2

152. A client is admitted to the labor-and-delivery unit. As she is placed on the electronic fetal monitor, she asks the nurse to explain her baby's heart beat. You know that the normal range for a term fetal heart rate per minute would be:
A. 80 to 100
B. 100 to 160
C. 120 to 160
D. 130 to 180

153. You are monitoring a client in the labor-and-delivery unit. Her electronic fetal monitor is indicating early decelerations of 40 beats per minute below baseline. Your first nursing action would be to:
A. Immediately move her to her left side to improve fetal perfusion.
B. Continue to monitor her because this is not a concerning pattern.
C. Increase the rate of the maintenance IV fluids to correct maternal hypotension.
D. Administer O_2 per facial mask at 10 to 12 L/min.

154. A client is laboring with her first child. She reports to the nurse that she has had a cold for the past few days prior to her admission. The electronic fetal monitor shows a baseline fetal heart rate (FHR) of 175 to 185 beats per minute with good beat-to-beat variability (BTBV) and no decelerations. The most likely cause of the FHR is:
A. Maternal anxiety caused by her primigravida status
B. Elevated maternal temperature related to her cold
C. Fetal distress related to maternal hypotension
D. Fetal distress related to maternal dehydration

155. As you are caring for a client in the labor-and-delivery unit, you notice a fall in the fetal heart rate that begins at the peak of each contraction and ends several seconds after the end of the contraction. This type of pattern is known as:
    A. A variable deceleration
    B. An early deceleration
    C. A late deceleration
    D. A mixed deceleration

156. A client asks the nurse why vaginal examinations are done during her laboring process and what she is feeling for. The nurse's best response is:
    A. "It is important for us to be able to assess the fetus as he moves down through the birth canal. I am feeling for the baby's head."
    B. "This helps us to know how the baby is tolerating the labor. I am checking the baby's heart rate."
    C. "We can determine if the baby is progressing through the birth canal correctly. I am feeling for the edge of your cervix."
    D. "It is important for us to identify the baby's position and to assess how your cervix is dilating. I am feeling the baby's fontanelle and the edge of your cervix."

157. Early adolescents whose parents are expecting a new baby often have a difficult time accepting the infant as a part of the family unit because:
    A. They feel they have lost the attention and therefore the love of their parents.
    B. This is an age when peers have more influence than family and they fear rejection.
    C. They are in the middle of developing their own sexual identity and believe their parents are no longer sexually active because of their age.
    D. Many parents place additional expectations on teenage children when a new baby arrives and adolescents are resentful.

158. You know that pregnancy is considered a maturational crisis. Which one of your clients would most likely have difficulty adjusting to this crisis and be most concerning to you?
    A. Helen, 17 years old, who is single and lives alone. She no longer has contact with the infant's father.
    B. Sue, a 30-year-old who is married and has recently moved into a new community.
    C. Lou, 22 years old, who lives at home with her parents and is engaged to be married in 3 months.
    D. Judy, a 26-year-old interior designer who is married to her high school sweetheart and came to your office for preconceptual counseling 8 months ago.

159. A client delivered her fourth child vaginally 18 hours ago and is now complaining of a sore bottom and what she thinks are hemorrhoids. As the nurse providing care for her, you inspect her perineum and anus. You observe an edematous perineum and several protruding hemorrhoids during your inspection. What step of the nursing process are you using?
    A. Assessment
    B. Diagnosis
    C. Planning
    D. Evaluation

160. A client is in the clinic for her second prenatal visit. She asks the nurse to tell her what they test in her urine sample at each of her visits. The nurse's best response would be:
    A. "We check the hematocrit to see if you are anemic."
    B. "The urine is tested for antibody titers."
    C. "We check the urine for glucose and albumin."
    D. "We make sure there are no bacteria to cause infection."

161. A client asks the nurse to explain what will be done to her during each of her prenatal visits. The nurse's best response would be:
    A. "We will check your weight and urine and do a pelvic exam to see if you are having cervical changes."
    B. "You will be weighed, your blood will be drawn, and we will do an ultrasound."
    C. "Your weight will be checked, and we will talk with you about your nutrition."
    D. "We will check your vital signs, weight gain, and urine and measure your fundal height."

162. Your breastfeeding client questions you about providing cereal to her newborn at age 6 weeks to 2 months. She asks if this will affect her milk production. Based on your knowledge of breastfeeding, you know that:
    A. Most infants are ready for solids at about 2 months of age and should be started on rice cereal even if they are breastfed.
    B. This will greatly decrease her milk supply because it will decrease the infant's sucking and consequently the milk production.
    C. This will increase her milk supply because it will strengthen the infant's sucking musculature.
    D. Introduction of solids will not affect milk production and should be started whenever the infant is no longer sleeping through the night.

163. Your laboring client overhears your statement that the baby's head is engaged. She is concerned about this statement and frightened that something is wrong with her baby. Your best explanation of engagement is:
    A. "I'm sorry you were frightened. Engagement means that the largest part of your baby's head has passed into the pelvic inlet. She is moving into position to be born."
    B. "I didn't mean to frighten you, but you need to know that you still have a long way to go before the baby will be born."

C. "Please don't worry. We are taking care of everything to ensure your baby's safety. Just relax since you have a lot of work ahead of you."

D. "Engagement means that your baby's head is pressing against your cervix. This is necessary to help you dilate so the baby can be born."

164. A client, a gravida I para 0, comes into the labor-and-delivery suite with her husband. She is crying and very agitated in the early stages of labor. She tells you that her contractions are extremely painful, and she appears frightened and anxious. As you reassure her, your examination shows that she is 50 percent effaced, fingertip dilated, −2 station, with contractions 8 to 10 minutes apart. Your best nursing intervention at this time would be:
A. Quickly obtain an order for IV meperidine (Demerol) to calm her.
B. Provide a quiet, reassuring environment for her with her husband in the room with her.
C. Begin teaching her relaxation and rhythmic breathing with her contractions.
D. Explain that she needs to get a grip on her emotions and grow up.

165. You are providing care for a newborn who has been diagnosed with congenital heart disease. It is imperative that the ductus arteriosus remain open in order to provide oxygenated blood to his circulation. The medication used for this purpose is:
A. Dopamine
B. Pancuronium (Pavulon)
C. Phenytoin (Dilantin)
D. Prostaglandin

166. You are working in the delivery suite in the role of newborn stabilization. One of the most important points of neonatal stabilization immediately following birth in the delivery room is:
A. Quickly drying the infant to decrease the chance of iatrogenic hypothermia.
B. Checking a rectal temperature to ensure the infant does not become hypothermic.
C. Providing humidified blowby O_2 to ensure adequate oxygenation during transition
D. Evaluating the presence of any physical deformities that the parents will need to know about before viewing their infant.

167. Baby girl Smith presents at birth with cyanosis, respiratory distress, and a scaphoid abdomen. Based on your knowledge of this triad of symptoms, you know she most likely has:
A. Respiratory distress syndrome (RDS)
B. Diaphragmatic hernia
C. Pneumothorax
D. Congenital heart disease

168. Following a difficult vaginal birth, Baby boy Thompson is diagnosed with Erb-Duchenne paralysis. You know that this is a result of trauma to the:

A. Facial nerves with resulting facial muscle paralysis
B. Brachial nerve with resulting lower arm paralysis
C. Fifth or sixth cervical nerve resulting in paralysis of the upper portion of the arm
D. Clavicle with resulting paralysis in the arm on the affected side

169. You are providing care for a preterm infant requiring gavage feedings. The infant's mother is concerned that her baby is not getting fed like other newborns. Your best explanation to her for this type of feeding would be:
A. "Infants who are compromised by respiratory distress or are too immature to have coordinated suck and swallow reflexes will be fed this way until they are able to take in their food by sucking."
B. "Babies who are little are fed this way because they are too small to be held outside of the incubator for a long enough period of time to take in all they need."
C. "Premature babies have very small stomachs and need to be gavage fed to control their intake."
D. "Premature babies don't know how to suck yet, and so we will feed your baby this way until her sucking reflex is mature."

170. A client is assisting you while her preterm newborn is being fed by oral gavage (OG) feeding. You have placed a pacifier in the infant's mouth during the feeding. The client questions you about the reason for the pacifier since the baby is on OG feedings. Based on your knowledge of preterm newborn feedings, you explain that this is called:
A. Parenteral nutrition
B. Non-nutritive sucking
C. Rhythmic sucking
D. Nutritive sucking

171. You are providing care in the labor-and-delivery suite for a primigravida who is being inducted for postdates. In which situation would it be safe to *continue* the administration of oxytocin for the induction of labor?
A. Decreased BTBV with periodic late decelerations
B. Uterine contractions q 1 minute lasting 90 seconds
C. Absent BTBV following an IV dose of meperidine (Demerol)
D. Maternal urine output of 150 ml in the past 4 hours

172. A client, a gravida I para 0, is 100 percent effaced and dilated to 3 cm. Her uterine contractions have decreased in frequency and intensity, but her fetus has a good tracing and is not demonstrating any signs of fetal distress. You can expect to prepare her for:

A. A cesarean section delivery
B. A fetal scalp pH sampling
C. Augmentation of labor with oxytocin
D. Cervical softening with prostaglandin gel

173. As you monitor a client during her progress of labor, you notice that the contraction pattern on the monitor strip has changed from an intermittent wave form to a flat line pattern. Your first nursing action should be:
A. Immediately turn the client to her left side to increase fetal oxygenation.
B. Increase her IV fluid rate to prevent hypotension.
C. Adjust the position of the electronic fetal monitor transducer.
D. Provide oxygen to the client per nasal cannula.

174. Your laboring client complains of severe low back pain. Her first stage of labor has been much longer than normal. Based on your knowledge of fetal positioning, in what position would you suspect her fetus to be?
A. Breech presentation
B. Posterior presentation
C. Transverse presentation
D. Anterior presentation

175. You are providing care in the labor-and-delivery suite for a client who is now in the active phase of labor. Which statement would she most likely make at this stage of her labor?
A. "Why don't you turn the TV up just a little, it's hard for me to hear with everything that's going on."
B. "Get out of my face! I have to push now!"
C. "My breathing exercises really paid off. I hope I can keep this up."
D. "I just can't do this any more! Please make it be over now!"

176. A client received meperidine (Demerol) and promethazine (Phenergan) approximately 1 hour prior to delivery of her term infant. The baby did not experience any delay in respiratory effort at birth, however, the nursery nurse was not surprised that the infant experienced:
A. An early passage of meconium
B. A slow and diminished suck reflex
C. Cyanosis during the first hour after birth
D. A weak shrill cry

177. A client questions you about the red mark on her baby's forehead and between his eyes. She states that it becomes brighter when he cries and goes away when she presses on it. Based on your knowledge of normal newborn variations, your best explanation is:
A. "That is probably an abrasion he got during birth. I think they may have used forceps to help get him out."
B. "That is called a port wine stain and will get bigger as he gets older. You'll just have to learn to live with it."
C. "Those are called mongolian spots and lots of babies have them. They will go away over the next few months."
D. "Some people call those 'stork bites.' They are nevi and usually disappear during the first 2 years, although some people have them into adulthood. They usually fade a bit. Many babies have them and there isn't a need to worry."

178. A client is concerned that her baby must be under the phototherapy light for hyperbilirubinemia. During your patient teaching you will explain to the mother that it is important to:
A. Ensure that the baby's head is covered while under the light.
B. Hold all of the baby's feedings while under the light.
C. Keep the baby's eyes covered while under phototherapy.
D. Keep the baby still and quiet while under phototherapy.

179. Mr. and Ms. Lawson have a preterm newborn in the newborn intensive care unit. It is important for them to be able to openly discuss their feelings about their critically ill newborn. What nursing statement would most likely provide them with the opportunity to discuss their feelings?
A. "You guys look really depressed. What's on your mind?"
B. "I know you are glad to be here to visit your baby. It must really be exciting to have such a beautiful new baby daughter."
C. "I know you probably need a little help right now, so I have made up a list of phone numbers for you to reach the social worker here in the hospital."
D. "Most parents understandably feel pretty overwhelmed when they have a premature baby. Would you like to sit down with me, so we can talk over things and you can ask all the questions you like. I'll be glad to help you sort through things."

180. Baby boy O'Hare has been diagnosed with neonatal sepsis. As the nurse providing care for him, you will expect to.
A. Place him in reverse isolation.
B. Administer antibiotics.
C. Restrict parental visits.
D. Prepare him for an exchange transfusion.

181. As you prepare the nursing care plan for a client who vaginally delivered her third child 18 hours ago, you know that a nursing diagnosis for her should include:
A. Objective data
B. Subjective data
C. A nursing clinical judgment statement
D. Both objective and subjective data

182. You are educating your client who has experienced a molar pregnancy. You will encourage her to be consistent in follow-up care because:
    A. She will likely be infertile following the molar pregnancy.
    B. The risk of choriocarcinoma increases following a molar pregnancy.
    C. The risk of spontaneous abortion is high should a normal pregnancy occur.
    D. She is at risk for uterine rupture following a molar pregnancy.

183. Following a very complicated delivery, you suspect your client is experiencing disseminated vascular coagulation (DIC) because you observe:
    A. Hypertension and increased WBC
    B. Increased bleeding from a venipuncture site
    C. Uncontrollable shaking of the extremities
    D. Pitting edema in the lower extremities

184. You are educating your client concerning breast self-examinations. You instruct her in the appropriate technique for the examination and tell her that she should perform this:
    A. Each month right after her period
    B. Monthly just before her period starts
    C. Every other month during her period
    D. Every other month on the same date

185. During the physical assessment of a newborn, the finding that would be most concerning to you would be:
    A. Dark gray-blue pigmented lesions over the lumbosacral region
    B. Overriding cranial sutures
    C. A soft, flat anterior fontenelle
    D. A head circumference that is 5 cm less than the chest circumference

186. Judy T. requests to breastfeed her newborn in the delivery room. As the nurse providing care for Judy and her newborn, your best response is:
    A. Tell the mother that she and her newborn will need to rest first.
    B. Assist the mother in placing the infant to the breast.
    C. Tell the mother that the infant will need a first feeding of sterile water.
    D. Reassure the mother that the infant will not be hungry for a few hours.

187. Baby girl Newton is a postmature newborn. As the nurse providing care for this infant, you know that she is at risk for cold stress as a result of:
    A. Dry, peeling skin
    B. Decreased birth weight
    C. Decreased subcutaneous fat
    D. Increased coating of vernix caseosa

188. A client is being discharged home 24 hours following the vaginal delivery of her first child. Since late-onset group B hemolytic infection may appear after the immediate newborn period and up to 4 months following birth, you will want to teach her about the signs and symptoms of infection in her newborn. The symptoms it is important for you to teach her are:
    A. Spitting up and fever
    B. Extremely high fever and difficulty sleeping
    C. Feeding intolerance and diarrhea
    D. Irritablity, poor appetite, and fever

189. A client has delivered her first infant by scheduled cesarean section 8 hours earlier. She is 28 years old, 5 ft 1 inch tall, and weighs 280 lb. Which of the following factors would predispose her to thrombophlebitis?
    A. Placement of a Foley catheter prior to delivery
    B. Epidural anesthesia
    C. Maternal obesity
    D. Infusion of lactated Ringer's during surgery

190. A term primigravida tells you that she is concerned that she might need to have a cesarean section. She states that several of her friends have required surgery and that she is worried. She asks you to explain the reasons she might need to have a cesarean section. You explain one common reason cesarean section is required would be:
    A. A history of chronic hypertension
    B. Ruptured membranes greater than 18 hours
    C. A low maternal pain threshold
    D. Cephalopelvic disproportion

191. You are the nurse providing care for a multigravida with a history of several spontaneous abortions. She has been admitted for placement of a cerclage. Based on your knowledge of this procedure, you know it is necessary because of:
    A. An incompetent cervix
    B. A cervical infection
    C. Vaginal bleeding
    D. Repeated prolapsed umbilical cords

192. A client has had increasing blood pressure and is suspected of having mild pre-eclampsia. She is started on magnesium sulfate ($MgSO_4$) intravenously. Based on your knowledge of this drug, you know it is given as a(n):
    A. Antihypertensive to lower blood pressure
    B. Central nervous system stimulant to maintain a stable blood pressure
    C. Smooth-muscle relaxant that decreases uterine contractions
    D. Central nervous system depressant that prevents seizures

193. Baby boy Richards is 45 minutes old in the term nursery. You know that the two anatomic systems that undergo the most profound changes are the:
    A. Gastrointestinal and hematologic
    B. Cardiovascular and respiratory
    C. Hepatic and renal
    D. Neurological and immunological

194. You are conducting a physical assessment on a 1-

hour-old newborn female infant. The physical finding that would be the most concerning would be:
  A. Mottled skin over the trunk and extremities
  B. Small, white nodules over the chin and bridge of nose
  C. An imperforate anus
  D. Blood-tinged vaginal discharge

195. A 20-year-old single mother who will be living alone in a town without close family is being prepared for discharge at 24 hours' postpartum. Her term male newborn is her first child. The most appropriate nursing diagnosis is:
  A. Knowledge deficit related to self and newborn care secondary to lack of childbirth and parenting experience
  B. Alteration in urinary elimination related to perineal edema secondary to trauma of childbirth
  C. Potential for infection related to multiple vaginal examinations and vaginal delivery
  D. Alteration in comfort: pain related to perineal trauma secondary to vaginal delivery

196. You have spent time teaching your prenatal client about breastfeeding. The statement that would indicate to you her understanding of the prevention of sore nipples would be:
  A. "I really shouldn't let the baby suck longer than 5 to 10 minutes per breast at each feeding."
  B. "I guess I had better find a shopping day so that I can buy some lotion for my breasts so they don't get sore."
  C. "In the beginning I'll supplement with formula so that my baby doesn't have to nurse so often. I don't want my breasts to be sore."
  D. "I think we should review the positioning of the baby again. I don't want my breasts to get sore because I didn't get the baby attached right."

197. During the labor process, a high-risk antepartal client is attached to an electronic fetal monitor. She complains of being restricted to the bed during this time. An appropriate nursing diagnosis would be:
  A. Alteration in comfort related to imposed bedrest
  B. Anxiety related to restriction of movement
  C. Impaired physical mobility related to restrictions secondary to monitor cords
  D. Activity intolerance related to imposed immobility secondary to labor process

198. A high-risk antenatal patient asks the nurse to explain why the electronic fetal monitor (EFM) is necessary. She wants to know why the nurse cannot just listen to the baby every few minutes to be sure everything is going OK. As the nurse providing care, your best response would be:
  A. "Listening with the fetoscope takes up too

much of my time. I have other things that I need to be doing for you."
  B. "I know the cords are in your way, but we are required by law to have these attached since you are a high-risk patient."
  C. "Sometimes we just have to tolerate things we don't like very much when we understand that they are the best thing for us."
  D. "Electronic fetal monitoring provides a continuous recording of the baby's heart rate and your contractions. Listening only intermittently wouldn't give us a complete picture of the condition of your baby."

199. A client pregnant at 10 weeks' gestation is being treated for an upper respiratory tract infection. The nurse recognizes that which of the following treatments is inappropriate for this stage of pregnancy?
  A. Drink eight cups of fluid a day.
  B. Acetaminophen, 500 mg PO, every 4 to 6 hours for elevated temperature
  C. Rest at frequent intervals during the day
  D. Erythromycin, 500 mg PO tid, for infection

200. A 24-year-old primipara in the 28th week of gestation reports that she has been diagnosed with a vaginal yeast infection. She asks if this is a common occurrence in pregnancy and, if so, why. Which of the following explanations by the nurse is most accurate?
  A. Vaginal yeast infections are common in pregnancy because of increased blood sugar levels.
  B. Vaginal yeast infections are uncommon in pregnancy because of decreased blood sugar levels.
  C. Vaginal yeast infections are common in pregnancy because of decreased vaginal acidity.
  D. Vaginal yeast infections are uncommon in pregnancy because of increased vaginal acidity.

201. An 18-year-old client at 36 weeks' gestation has been diagnosed with a vaginal yeast infection. She asks you how to help prevent recurrence of vaginal yeast infections. In assessing the effectiveness of your teaching, which of the following client responses indicate a need for further teaching?
  A. "I should eat some live culture yogurt every day."
  B. "I should douche with vinegar and water daily."
  C. "I should wear cotton underwear."
  D. "I should wear loose clothing."

202. A 24-year-old multigravida in the 32nd week of pregnancy comes into the clinic with complaints of nasal stuffiness, epistaxis, and right-sided hearing loss. Which of the following statements by the nurse is most accurate in explaining the symptoms?
  A. "This sounds like a bad cold. You need to take a decongestant."

B. "These symptoms are highly unusual. You need to be seen by an ear, nose, and throat specialist."

C. "These symptoms are common in pregnancy because of increased blood flow caused by a pregnancy hormone."

D. "It sounds like you have a sinus infection. They are caused by cold drafts and sleeping on your right side. Avoid drafts and change your position from side to side at night.

203. A client in the second trimester of pregnancy has blood drawn for routine 18-week laboratory work. Which of the following results would be considered normal for this stage of pregnancy?
A. Decreased hemoglobin
B. Increased hemoglobin
C. Decreased blood glucose
D. Decreased coagulation time

204. A nurse educator teaching a first trimester prenatal class discusses breast changes. Which of the following breast changes would be expected during the first trimester?
A. Lightening of the areola, increased breast size, and striae
B. Breast tenderness, vein prominence, and Montgomery's tubercles
C. Inverted nipples, lightening of the areola, and decreased breast size
D. Nodularity, darkened areola, and colostrum

205. A 32-year-old company executive in the first trimester of her pregnancy tells the nurse that her pregnancy was planned, but that "I'm feeling like maybe this wasn't such a good idea." Which of the following responses by the nurse would best indicate an understanding of the emotional tasks of this stage of pregnancy?
A. "You should be happy to be pregnant at your age. Here is the name of our social worker, she can help you overcome these unnatural feelings."
B. "It's OK to feel ambivalence at this stage—you'll love your baby once it is born."
C. "Many women who feel like you do have an abortion. Have you considered one?"
D. "Many women have mixed emotions during the early stages of pregnancy. They don't mean you won't be a loving parent."

206. Paternal support and adaptation to pregnancy assist the woman in accomplishing her own developmental tasks. Which of the following actions by the nurse would be most appropriate in assisting a father to attach to the fetus and validate the reality of the pregnancy?
A. Allow the father to listen to fetal heart tones.
B. Show the father a model of a fetus at the developmental stage of the pregnancy.
C. Give the father a typed handout on fetal development.

D. Encourage the father to attend an ultrasound of his fetus.

207. An 18-year-old woman comes in for her first prenatal appointment. Some blood is drawn for ABO typing, Rh testing, and antibody screening. The purpose of these tests is to determine the potential for which fetal condition?
A. Erythroblastosis fetalis
B. Down syndrome
C. Erythemia neonatorum
D. Caudal regression

208. A 38-year-old client in the 28th week of her pregnancy has been admitted to the obstetric unit with a blood pressure of 160/90, swollen hands, 3+ proteinuria, and complaints of persistent headache. These signs and symptoms are most likely due to which of the following pregnancy complications?
A. Preterm labor
B. Preterm premature rupture of the membranes
C. Hyperemesis gravidarum
D. Pregnancy-induced hypertension

209. A 31-year-old woman at term has been in active labor for 5 hours. A vaginal examination reveals −1 station, 4 to 5 cm dilation, and 90 percent effacement of the cervix. The fetal heart rate baseline is in the 140s to 150s. Three variable decelerations were observed within the last hour with a quick return to baseline. What is the most appropriate nursing action?
A. Place the client on her back so the fetal heart rate strip is more accurate.
B. Prepare for a stat cesarean section.
C. Turn the client to her left side.
D. Prepare for augmentation of labor with oxytocin (Pitocin).

210. A client at 32 weeks' gestation is admitted for possible preterm labor. The health-care provider performs an amniocentesis. Which nursing actions should occur immediately following the procedure?
A. Monitor the needle entry site for signs and symptoms of infection.
B. Monitor fetal heart tones and for uterine contractions.
C. Explain the purpose of the amniocentesis to the client.
D. Encourage the client to verbalize her concerns regarding the procedure.

211. Analysis of amniotic fluid obtained from a client at 36 weeks' gestation reveals a lecithin-sphingomyelin (L/S) ratio of 3:1 and the presence of phosphatidylglycerol (PG). The nurse correctly identifies this result as indicating which of the following fetal conditions?
A. Fetal distress
B. Erythroblastosis fetalis

C. Down syndrome

D. Pulmonary maturity

212. A 24-year-old primipara at 32 weeks' gestation asks if she would be able to successfully breastfeed since, "My breasts are so small." Which of the following explanations by the nurse would be most accurate?

A. "The size of the breast is related to the amount of fatty tissue present and has nothing to do with the ability to produce milk. All women have the ability to produce adequate amounts of breast milk."

B. "You are probably right. Breasts as small as yours have fewer lactiferous ducts than women with larger breasts."

C. "You do have small breasts, but you can probably breastfeed your baby if you also supplement with formula."

D. "You should talk to a representative from La Leche. She can give you important information on how women with small breasts can successfully breastfeed."

213. Several pregnant women are attending a class on prenatal nutrition. A 16-year-old client at 8 weeks' gestation reports that she is a semivegetarian and asks if there are any diet modifications she will need to make for protein intake since she is now pregnant. Which of the following explanations by the nurse would be the most accurate?

A. "You will need to be referred to the dietitian for nutritional counseling because your protein needs cannot be met by fruits and nuts alone."

B. "No special considerations are needed with this type of diet."

C. "You need to increase your intake of milk and cheese to get the protein needed for the pregnancy."

D. "If you drink soy milk and add tofu to your diet, and combine legumes with grains, you can meet your protein requirements."

214. A 32-year-old G3P2 client, with a history of postpartum deep vein thrombosis, has been on prophylactic heparin therapy for 2 weeks. The nurse should monitor the results of which of the following laboratory tests?

A. H&H

B. CBC

C. PTT

D. HCV

215. A postpartum Vietnamese client received discharge teaching about nutrition and breastfeeding just before lunch. When the nurse picked up the client's lunch tray, she noticed that the sandwiches, fruit, and salad had not been touched. The client then asked the nurse to heat up some soup brought by her family. She then handed the nurse a container of a dark green liquid with what looked like seaweed floating in it. Which of the following actions should the nurse take?

A. Try to talk the client into eating the balanced diet that she was served.

B. Offer the client chicken noodle soup.

C. Ask, "What is this stuff, anyway?"

D. Heat up the soup.

216. A 17-year-old primigravida comes in for her 32-week prenatal appointment. The nurse asks her about her plans after delivery. Which of the following information would indicate that this family may be at high risk for ineffective family functioning?

A. "I plan to live at home with my parents. My mom will take care of the baby while I go to school for half a day and then work the other half. We have a nursery fixed up in a corner of my room. It'll be hard, but I think we can make it."

B. "I'm going to get an apartment in a few weeks. That way I can keep AFDC and Medicaid. I don't have a job."

C. "My boyfriend and I are getting married after the baby is born. He's older—20, and in the Army. They pay pretty good and have good benefits. He'll be going to Germany pretty soon, so I'll move back home with my parents. I plan to get my GED later, when the baby is older."

D. "I'm giving the baby up for adoption. I'm just not ready to be a parent yet. It'll be an open adoption and I'll get to see the baby and stuff."

217. A 24-year-old breastfeeding client on the first day postpartum calls the nurse to her room. She reports that she can't get the baby to "stay on the breast." She exclaims in tears, "All he does is turn red and scream!" The nurse asks the client to put the baby to the breast. The nurse observes that the mother holds the infant in the cradle position with the infant's head turned to the side. Which of the following nursing diagnoses would be most appropriate?

A. Ineffective breastfeeding, related to lack of knowledge of correct positioning of infant

B. Altered nutrition (infant), less than body requirements, related to the infant's refusal to nurse

C. Body image disturbance, related to client's discomfort with breastfeeding

D. Anxiety, related to infant's refusal to nurse

218. A 27-year-old client at 22 weeks' gestation comes into the clinic and has a CBC drawn. Results include a WBC of $10^3/mm^3$, RBCs of $5.0 \times 10^6/mm^3$, hemoglobin 9 gm/dl, hematocrit 32 percent. Which of the following explanations by the nurse would be most accurate?

A. "Your laboratory results are normal for this stage of pregnancy. At your next visit, we'll need to check your blood sugar levels."

B. "It looks like you have an infection. I'll notify the health-care provider of these results and get you a prescription for an antibiotic."

C. "The H&H are low, but still in the normal range for pregnancy. We'll check it again at your next visit."

D. "It looks like you are slightly anemic. Take the iron pills your health-care provider ordered, twice a day. And take them with some orange juice."

219. A 36-year-old client at 32 weeks' gestation has been admitted to the obstetric unit for pregnancy-induced hypertension. Her blood pressures have been ranging from 142/100 to 160/110. She has 3+ proteinuria, generalized edema, and has been complaining of an unrelenting headache. Which care environment would be most appropriate for this client?

A. Semiprivate room, up ad lib., vital signs every shift with fetal heart tones, fetal stress testing daily, and 2 gm sodium diet

B. Private room, bedrest with bathroom privileges, vital signs with fetal heart tones every 4 hours, fetal nonstress testing daily, and regular diet

C. Three-bed ward, ambulate tid, vital signs bid with fetal heart tones, fetal nonstress testing twice a week, and low protein diet

D. Labor room, strict bedrest, vital signs every 15 minutes with continuous fetal heart monitoring, and NPO except for ice chips

220. A 32-year-old breastfeeding G5P5 client delivered a 10-pound baby boy 36 hours ago. Which of the following medications would the nurse anticipate administering?

A. Bromocriptine (Parlodel)

B. Medroxyprogesterone (Depo-Provera)

C. Insulin

D. Methylergonovine (Methergine)

221. A 26-year-old G2P1 at term gestation has had a normal progression of labor and is now pushing. The fetal presentation is vertex with the presenting part occiput posterior (OP) and between 0 and 1+ station. Which of the following procedures would the nurse expect to prepare the client for?

A. The fetal presenting part is in the desired position; the nurse should continue to coach the client to push.

B. A mediolateral episiotomy and Simpson's forceps delivery

C. A second-degree midline episiotomy and fundal pressure administered by the nurse

D. A third-degree midline episiotomy and a Piper forceps delivery

222. A 23-year-old client in the 34th week of gestation has just been admitted to the labor-and-delivery observation room. She calls the nurse and says, "I felt a gush. I think my water broke." Which of the following nursing actions has priority?

A. Prepare for a sterile vaginal examination.

B. Check the vital signs of the client.

C. Prepare for a sterile speculum examination.

D. Check the fetal heart tones.

223. A 28-year-old client was admitted 24 hours ago in preterm labor. She has received IV terbutaline at 8 mg/min for the last 10 hours. She received three 500 cc boluses of IV fluids since admission. The IV of normal saline has been infusing at 125 cc/hr since the last bolus of IV fluids. Which of the following symptoms should the nurse monitor for that would indicate a complication of therapy?

A. Palpitations, nervousness, tremors, and tachycardia

B. Drowsiness, lethargy, slurred speech, and blurred vision

C. Decreased fetal heart rate variability, neonatal hypotonia, and drowsiness

D. Decreased urine output, fluid retention, and rales

224. A breastfeeding client is being discharged home with her 24-hour-old infant. Which of the following statements would indicate the client needs further instruction about nipple care?

A. "I should wash my nipples with soap and water and then let them air dry."

B. "I should leave the flaps of my bra down between feedings."

C. "I should rub a little breast milk on my nipples after nursing and let it dry."

D. "I should hold the baby in a different position each time we breastfeed."

225. A bottle-feeding mother who was discharged home with her term infant calls the obstetrical clinic when the infant is 3 days old. She is concerned because the infant is taking only ½ ounce at each feeding. Which of the following explanations by the nurse would be most accurate?

A. "Your baby needs to take at least 1 ounce at every feeding. If you squeeze the nipple while it's in the baby's mouth and then stroke his/her throat, it'll get down."

B. "Maybe the baby is allergic to the formula. You should try a soy formula."

C. "If the baby has four wet diapers a day, (s)he is getting enough."

D. "A newborn's stomach can't hold much at first, but your baby should be taking an ounce or more in a few days."

226. A healthy term infant was admitted to the well-baby nursery 3 hours ago. Which of the following symptoms would indicate cold stress in the infant?

A. An increased respiratory rate and a decreased blood glucose level

B. Cool, clammy skin and decreased blood glucose levels

C. Acrocyanosis and flexion of the extremities

D. Bluish lips and an increased respiratory rate

227. A 28-week-old newborn had a septic work-up performed at 6 hours of age. Blood cultures came back positive. A peripheral heparin lock was then inserted for intravenous antibiotic therapy. The infant has now been on antibiotic therapy for 72 hours. At the time of antibiotic therapy, an attempt is made to make the routine heparin flush. Resistance is met and blood is observed at the hub of the catheter. To ensure the best outcome for the infant, which of the following actions is most desirable for the nurse to use?

A. Clear the catheter using pressure and a small amount of sterile saline. Administer the antibiotics.

B. Clear the catheter by removing the cap of the lock and attempting to aspirate any clots. Replace the cap and administer the antibiotics.

C. Discontinue the catheter and insert an intravenous needle at a new site. Administer the antibiotics.

D. Discontinue the catheter. Hold the antibiotics until the physician can be contacted for an order to discontinue them.

228. A 22-year-old client in the 34th week of gestation attended a natural childbirth class offered at the local hospital. Which of the following statements by the client would indicate the client needs further instruction?

A. "If I practice these techniques, I won't have any labor pain."

B. "My husband will be my coach and help me to relax during the contractions."

C. "When a labor pain starts, I'll imagine I'm floating on a cloud in the sun."

D. "I should practice my Kegel exercises several times a day."

229. A 28-year-old client with Hemolysis Elevated Liver enzymes, Low Platelets (HELLP) syndrome prenatally delivered a small-for-gestational-age term male infant 2 hours ago. Because of the client's history, which of the following nursing measures are most important in her postpartum care?

A. Careful monitoring for headaches, visual changes, epigastric discomfort, or elevated blood pressure

B. Postpartum checks of fundus, lochia, and vital signs every 15 minutes, and assessment of maternal-infant attachment processes

C. Monitoring of blood glucose levels hourly for 12 hours; then finger-stick glucose levels every morning and after every meal

D. Assessment of self and infant care abilities, instruction and return demonstrations of infant bathing and feeding techniques

230. A breastfeeding client who is 1-week postpartum calls the obstetric clinic with a report of a hard lump and localized tenderness in the upper outer quadrant of the left breast. She also reports a temperature of 102°F, headache, and malaise. Considering these symptoms, which of the following instructions by the nurse would be most appropriate?

A. "You should come into the clinic for a breast examination and maybe a biopsy. A painful lump could indicate cancer."

B. "You should be admitted to the hospital right away. You have a serious breast infection and need to be started on IV antibiotics."

C. "It is normal to have tender, lumpy breasts when you are breastfeeding. It will go away when you wean the baby."

D. "Go to bed with your baby. Nurse every chance you get. Take acetaminophen (Tylenol) and drink lots of water."

231. A breastfeeding client has put the infant to the breast for the first time. To facilitate latching on, the nurse should teach the mother which position for the infant?

A. Using a finger to depress the breast tissue so the infant can breathe while nursing.

B. Placing the forefinger and middle finger around the breast tissue in a "scissors" position to help the infant grasp the nipple and areola.

C. Ensuring that only the nipple is taken into the infant's mouth.

D. Placing the infant level with the nipple with the infant's whole body in a straight line with the head.

232. The nurse discussed the milk ejection reflex with a first-time breastfeeding client. Which of the following statements would reflect client understanding of the etiology of the milk ejection reflex?

A. "I should wear a firm-fitting bra 24 hours a day."

B. "I should drink lots of fluids without caffeine."

C. "I should use cold packs on my breasts several times a day."

D. "I should put my baby to the breast."

233. A primipara at 8 weeks' gestation has just attended a prenatal class that discussed precautions to take during pregnancy. Which of the following statements would indicate the client needs further instruction?

A. "I will have my husband empty the cat box until after the baby is born."

B. "I will take my iron pills twice a day with a citrus food."

C. "I can use my electric blanket since the weather has turned cold."

D. "I can eat or drink products with Nutrasweet in them."

234. A 37-year-old Rh negative client who is pregnant at 10 weeks' gestation is scheduled to undergo chorionic villus sampling. Considering the procedure,

the nurse should anticipate having which of the following medications available?

A. Oxytocin (Pitocin)
B. Methylergonovine maleate (Methergine)
C. Morphine
D. Anti-D globulin

235. A first-time mother is preparing for discharge with her term female infant. In discussing infant safety concerns, which of the following statements would indicate the client needs further instruction?

A. "We put the infant car seat in the back seat facing backward."
B. "We bought a backpack to carry the baby in."
C. "We stripped the crib and repainted it with lead-free paint."
D. "We will put the baby to sleep on her side or back."

236. A 38-year-old client has been trying to conceive for the last 2 years without success. She makes the following statement, "I wanted a career first. I thought I could get pregnant anytime. Why am I having problems?" Which of the following explanations by the nurse would be most accurate regarding achieving pregnancy after age 35?

A. Women who have used birth control pills for many years can have trouble conceiving.
B. Men older than 35 produce fewer sperm. how old is your partner?
C. Metrorrhagia is common in women around age 35. It is associated with infertility.
D. The ovaries may be producing fewer eggs because of aging.

237. A 16-year-old client pregnant at 16 weeks' gestation tells the school nurse that she has decided to put her baby up for adoption. Which of the following responses by the nurse would be the most appropriate?

A. Tell her that it is too soon to make such an important decision.
B. Support her decision and acknowledge her maturity in making it.
C. Ask her if she is being pressured by anyone into making this decision.
D. Question her reasons for giving up her baby for adoption.

238. A primipara delivered twins at 32 weeks' gestation. One infant died shortly after birth. The second infant is in the neonate intensive care unit (NICU) for respiratory distress but is responding well to treatment. The client is crying and states, "I wish both my babies had lived." Which response by the nurse would be most therapeutic?

A. "Many women would be happy for just one baby. You should be thankful, not sad."
B. "Many women who have lost a twin recover very well."
C. "It's a good thing your baby died before you became attached."

D. "I'm sorry your baby died. I'm here if you would like to talk."

239. A 24-year-old primipara at 6 weeks' gestation tells the clinic nurse that she does not understand why she should quit smoking just because she is pregnant. Which of the following explanations by the nurse would be most accurate?

A. Tobacco smoking causes fetal anomalies.
B. Tobacco smoking causes central nervous system damage.
C. Tobacco smoking causes low-birth-weight infants.
D. Tobacco smoking causes fetal addiction to nicotine.

240. A 24-year-old gravida II para I, who is pregnant at 10 weeks' gestation, has a hemoglobin of 10 and a hematocrit of 32 percent. She tells the nurse that she cannot take iron supplements because they make her too sick. The nurse should suggest which of the following menus to the client?

A. Turkey, cantaloupe, iceberg lettuce, green peas, rice, milk
B. Duck, dried apricots, kale, baked potatoes, pumpkin, lemonade
C. Chicken, baked apples, broccoli, navy beans, mashed potatoes, tea
D. Canned salmon, bananas, asparagus, egg noodles, apple juice

241. A gravida IV para III is admitted to the labor unit in early labor with contractions every 10 minutes, mild to moderate in intensity, cervix 4 cm, and 80 percent effaced. Membranes are intact with the presenting part at −2 station. Which of the following changes would indicate imminent delivery?

A. Cervical dilation of 8 cm, presenting part at +1 station
B. Client report of feeling like she has to have a bowel movement
C. Contractions every 5 minutes, hard intensity
D. Client starts to vomit and states, "I can't do this anymore!"

242. A 28-year-old client admitted with preterm labor (PTL) was treated with subcutaneous terbutaline and has had several boluses of IV fluids over the last 36 hours. The IV is now infusing at 125 cc hr. Which of the following symptoms would indicate fluid overload?

A. Pulse 118, heart palpitations
B. Intake of 1100 cc, output of 1400 cc
C. Fine crackles in the lower bases of the lungs
D. Pitting pedal edema of 2+

243. A 24-year-old multigravida abused cocaine while pregnant. The newborn male is rigid when held and is difficult to soothe. The nurse discusses appropriate play techniques for the infant with the mother. Which of the following statements would indicate the client understands?

A. "I'll get a musical mobile for his crib for him to see and hear."
B. "I've got a wind-up swing that I'll use when he cries."
C. "I'll tell my friends to get rattles for the baby to play with."
D. "I'll get a tape player and play soft music in his room."

244. A female infant born to a narcotic-addicted mother exhibits rigidity, tremors, and frantic crying. Which of the following approaches by the nurse would best console the infant?
A. Place the infant on her back and loosely cover her with a blanket.
B. Rock the infant back and forth while humming a lullaby.
C. Place the infant in the en face position and coo to her.
D. Place the infant over the shoulder and gently stroke her back.

245. The nurse suspects that a newly delivered infant was born to a mother with a narcotic addiction. Which of the following physical manifestations would the nurse expect to find in a narcotic-exposed newborn?
A. Rigid muscle tone, seizures, and a poorly coordinated suck-and-swallow reflex
B. Flat midface, lowset ears, small for gestational age
C. Small for gestational age, decreased head circumference, developmental delays
D. Poor muscle tone, flat face, epicanthal folds near the bridge of the nose

246. A 27-year-old primigravida is admitted to the labor unit at 36 weeks' gestation in active labor. She has a runny nose and is diaphoretic and restless. Needle tracks are observed on both forearms. On taking an obstetrical history, the nurse notes that the client has a history of heroin abuse. The client is nauseated and vomiting. Which of the following nursing actions would be most appropriate for this client?
A. Obtain an order for administration of intramuscular (IM) methadone.
B. Obtain vital signs on admission and every 4 hours thereafter.
C. Obtain an order for administration of IV butorphanol tartrate (Stadol).
D. Place the client in a dimly lit room on a quiet corridor.

247. A client who admits to recent cocaine usage is admitted to the labor unit in active labor. She has dilated pupils and is hostile and diaphoretic. Her vital signs are pulse 86, respirations 22, temperature 100.2°F, and blood pressure 158/92. She is complaining of extremely painful contractions. Which of the following nursing actions would be most appropriate?

A. Position the client in a semi-Fowler's position.
B. Place the bed in the lowest locked position and pad the side rails.
C. Place the client in a brightly lit room next to the nurses' station.
D. Offer narcotic analgesics PRN as ordered.

248. A well-dressed client who is 5 months' pregnant presents to the obstetrical unit with facial and abdominal bruises. She states that she walked into a door. Physical assessment reveals other wounds in various stages of healing. The nurse suspects intimate partner abuse. Which of the following approaches by the nurse would be best in this situation?
A. Ask the client, "Did someone hurt you?"
B. Accept the story. Abuse occurs only in the lower classes.
C. Encourage the client to leave her partner.
D. Refer the client to psychiatric counseling.

249. A pregnant woman reveals to the clinic nurse that she is a victim of partner abuse. She also reports that she deserved to be beaten up because, "I didn't have dinner on the table on time." She also reports that her partner was extremely remorseful after the incident and promises it will never happen again. The best response by the nurse would be which of the following?
A. "You're right, you shouldn't do things you know provoke him to anger."
B. "You need to leave this relationship right now. Here is the address of a shelter."
C. "If he's very sorry, I'm sure this won't happen again."
D. "No one deserves to be beaten up. How can I help you?"

250. A client is admitted to the obstetrical unit at 36 weeks' gestation. Which of the following symptoms would indicate a concealed abruptio placentae?
A. Painless, bright red vaginal bleeding
B. Decreased fundal height
C. A hard, boardlike abdomen
D. A fetal heart rate of 180

251. A woman on IV magnesium sulfate for PIH has respirations of 10 and depressed deep tendon reflexes. Besides discontinuing the medication, which of the following nursing actions would be most appropriate?
A. Stimulate the client to take deep breaths.
B. Administer calcium gluconate.
C. Monitor for increased uterine contractions.
D. Administer naloxone (Narcan).

252. A client who just delivered at term has tested positive for hepatitis B. Mother and baby were immunized with hepatitis B immunoglobulin and hepatitis B vaccine. Which of the following actions by the nurse would be appropriate.
A. Discuss the need for the mother to bottle feed.

B. Place the mother and baby in respiratory isolation.

C. Place the mother and baby in reverse isolation.

D. Discuss breastfeeding techniques with the mother.

253. A client whose newborn infant tested positive for phenylketonuria (PKU) has received teaching regarding the special needs of her infant with the clinic nurse. Which of the following statements would indicate the client understands the dietary needs of the infant with PKU?
    A. "I'll be able to continue breastfeeding."
    B. "I'll have to give my baby formula instead of breast milk."
    C. "I'll have to use a low-phenylalanine formula."
    D. "A soy formula will be best for my baby."

254. A client is getting ready for discharge to her home with her new infant. In preparing to teach the client about infant skin care, the nurse would include which of the following in the plan of care?
    A. A newborn needs a complete bath and shampoo every day.
    B. Baby lotion is necessary to keep the infant's skin from drying out.
    C. Shaking talcum powder on the infant's buttocks keeps the diaper area dry.
    D. Once the cord clamp is off, the area needs to be kept clean and dry.

255. A term female infant has just been born. To prevent cold stress, which of the following nursing actions have priority?
    A. Place the infant under the radiant warmer.
    B. Dry the infant and place dry blankets under her.
    C. Wrap the infant in a prewarmed blanket.
    D. Check the rectal temperature.

256. A first-time breastfeeding mother who delivered a term male infant 2 days ago is reviewing discharge instructions with the nurse. The nurse knows breastfeeding instruction has been effective when the client makes which of the following statements?
    A. "I know the baby is getting enough milk if he falls asleep while nursing."
    B. "If he has a firm bowel movement every other day, he is getting enough milk."
    C. "If he has six wet diapers a day, he is getting enough milk."
    D. "If he wants to nurse more than every 4 hours, I'll have to supplement."

257. A 15-year-old primipara at 14 weeks' gestation is discussing nutrition with the school nurse. She reports that "I don't like those foods. I only eat at fast-food restaurants." The nurse identifies which of the following fast foods maintain adequate nutrition?
    A. Cheeseburger, sausage and green pepper pizza, roast beef sandwich, baked potato with broccoli and cheese, orange juice, mixed salad with wine vinegar dressing
    B. A fully dressed hamburger, double cheese pizza, chicken nuggets, baked potato with sour cream, milkshake
    C. Chicken-fried steak, chili dog, french fries, lettuce salad with ranch dressing, diet cola
    D. Chili cheese dog, black olive pizza, onion rings, whole milk, salad bar

258. A client at term is admitted to the labor unit in active labor. She is 6 cm dilated with the fetal station at −1. An external fetal heart and contraction monitor is applied. Which of the following fetal tracings would indicate a non-reassuring pattern?
    A. Variable decelerations with a quick return to the baseline rate in the 140s. Short-term variability of 6 to 10 beats per minute.
    B. Late decelerations to 120 with a gradual return to the baseline rate in the 140s. Short-term variability of 3 to 4 beats per minute.
    C. Early decelerations, baseline rate in the 120s with a short-term variability of 8 to 12 beats per minute.
    D. Accelerations to 120 with contractions. A baseline rate of 110. Short-term variability is 8 to 10 beats per minute.

259. A client has been admitted to the labor unit with contractions every 5 minutes, strong in intensity, and duration of 45 to 60 seconds. Membranes are intact, dilation is 4 to 5 cm, and the presenting part is at 0 station. The fetal heart tracing is unreadable, but auscultation of the fetal heart rate for a full minute by fetoscope revealed a rate in the 150s. No decelerations were heard. Which of the following actions by the nurse is best.
    A. Place the client on her back to obtain a better fetal heart tracing.
    B. Turn the client to the left lateral position and start oxygen per nasal cannula.
    C. Place the client in knee-chest position and prepare for an emergency cesarean.
    D. Change the location of the external doppler.

260. A primipara with gestational diabetes at 36 weeks' gestation asks the nurse about indications for induction of labor. In evaluation of her teaching, which of the following statements would indicate the client needs further instruction?
    A. "If I go more than 2 weeks past my due date, the doctor might consider inducing labor."
    B. "If the nonstress tests show my baby isn't doing well, labor might be induced."
    C. "I can arrange with the doctor to induce labor any time now that I am at 36 weeks."
    D. "The doctor will probably induce labor at 38 weeks if the tests show the lungs are developed."

261. A client at 16 weeks' gestation has just discovered that she is HIV positive. The clinic nurse has offered counseling to the client and outlined her op-

tions. Which of the following statements would indicate that the client understands the implications of pregnancy and this disease?
A. "Breastfeeding will protect my baby from HIV."
B. "It's possible my baby won't be affected."
C. "I'm going to die before my baby can be born."
D. "My baby is going to die within 6 months of birth."

262. A 34-year-old client pregnant at 30 weeks' gestation has a prior pregnancy history that includes the cesarean delivery of a stillborn fetus at 20 weeks' gestation. Which of the following pregnancy complications is this client likely to develop?
A. Pregnancy-induced hypertension
B. An incompetent cervix
C. Preterm labor
D. Uterine rupture

263. The basal body temperature (BBT) method for testing for ovulation is based on the findings that body temperature:
A. Dips dramatically just prior to ovulation
B. Rises dramatically just prior to menstruation
C. Rises sharply within 24 hours of ovulation
D. Decreases significantly after the menstrual cycle

264. The identifiable signs that mark the end of the "unsafe" time when using the rhythm method for birth control include:
A. Three days of elevated basal body temperature (BBT) plus sticky cervical mucus
B. A return to preovulatory basal body temperature (BBT) and disappearance of minor discomforts
C. Breast tenderness and drop in basal body temperature (BBT)
D. A rise in basal body temperature (BBT) 1°F above the lowest temperature in the cycle

265. Which of the following is the main advantage to the use of levonorgestrel (Norplant) as a contraceptive?
A. Relatively inexpensive method of birth control
B. Client can discontinue the method on her own
C. Provides a low dosage of hormone, which means effective coverage with fewer side effects
D. Provides the most effective means of pregnancy prevention of all birth control methods on the market today

266. A client, 16 years old, presents to the local health department for information on birth control. She selects medroxyprogesterone (Depo-Provera) because of its convenience. Information that is of highest priority for her to receive would include:
A. She needs to return for an injection on a monthly basis.
B. This method does not protect her from sexually transmitted diseases (STDs).

C. If she should skip a menstrual period, she needs to report it to her health-care provider immediately.
D. She may experience mild tenderness at the site of the injection.

267. An increase in blood volume is one of the earliest adaptations to pregnancy. Which physiological process allows the body to accommodate this change?
A. Relaxation of smooth vascular tissue
B. An increase in collateral system
C. A decrease in red blood cell size and volume
D. A rise in the mean arterial pressure

268. A client, 36 weeks' twin gestation, has arrived for her ultrasound. After placing her supine on the exam table, she complains of nausea and dizziness. Your priority nursing action is:
A. Check the client's blood pressure.
B. Leave the room to get assistance.
C. Turn or wedge the client to her left side.
D. Assist the client to a sitting position.

269. The physiological basis for pseudoanemia in pregnancy is:
A. A decrease in red blood cells, resulting in a decreased oxygen-carrying capacity
B. An increase in plasma volume while red blood cells decrease
C. An increase in plasma volume while red blood cell count remains unchanged
D. An increase in both red blood cells and plasma, with plasma increasing in greater proportion

270. A client arrives in the prenatal clinic for her regular visit. She is 38 weeks' gestation. She is complaining of back pain and urinary frequency. The health-care provider orders a UA and a CBC. The UA results showed a trace of protein, negative in all other areas. The CBC showed a WBC of 16,000. What is your conclusion of these findings?
A. The UA is within normal limits, but the WBCs are elevated.
B. Both findings are within normal limits for the client's gestational age.
C. The WBC is within normal limits, but the UA findings are abnormal.
D. Both findings are abnormal and follow-up is required.

271. A client, 32 weeks' gestation, has arrived for her prenatal visit. When assessing her vital signs, you note her heart rate is 100 bpm. When you check her prenatal record, her baseline heart rate was 68 bpm. What is your nursing response?
A. Consider this a normal finding for this gestational age.
B. Ask the client if she has been having any difficulty breathing or chest pain with exertion.

C. Ask the client if heart disease runs in her family.

D. Have the client return to the clinic in 2 weeks instead of waiting a full month.

272. Your client is 22 weeks' gestation and complaining of urinary frequency, requiring her to get up at least every 2 hours at night. What further information would you obtain?

A. No further information is needed, because this is a normal finding for this gestational age.

B. The nurse would need to determine if the client also had burning or pain on urination or back pain.

C. The nurse would order a urinalysis and culture.

D. The nurse would instruct the client to limit fluids throughout the day to decrease urine output at night.

273. Which of the following changes in vital signs would be considered within normal limits for the client in the first trimester of pregnancy?

A. An increase in the resting heart rate of about 8 beats per minute

B. A rise in blood pressure of 5 to 10 mm Hg

C. A 20 percent increase in the respiratory rate

D. A drop in the basal body temperature

274. A client who is 12 weeks' pregnant complains about an increased amount of vaginal secretions. She describes the discharge as thin and white with no odor or discomfort. The nurse should advise the client to:

A. Wear tampons when the discharge gets very heavy.

B. Use over-the-counter medication to treat the yeast infection.

C. Keep her perineal area clean.

D. Douche with a weak vinegar and water solution.

275. When providing education for a client on her first prenatal visit, 8 weeks' gestation, which of the following would be considered danger signs that the client should be taught to report?

A. Excessive white vaginal discharge

B. Occasional malaise and lethargy

C. Bleeding and cramping

D. Gain of 2 to 3 pounds over a 6-week period

276. When counseling a client in regard to weight gain in pregnancy, what factors are most important to consider?

A. What was the client's prepregnancy weight?

B. How much weight does the client expect to gain?

C. What is the client's age?

D. What cultural influences may affect the client's dietary pattern?

277. A client, 28 weeks' gestation, complains of frequent heartburn. Nursing interventions should be based on the knowledge that:

A. In pregnancy, food is digested and moves through the digestive system more quickly than in the nonpregnant state.

B. This condition occurs because of an increased secretion of hydrochloric acid and pepsin.

C. Eating frequent, large meals will decrease the incidence of heartburn.

D. The cardiac sphincter is more relaxed, resulting in reflux of stomach content.

278. A client comes in for her prenatal visit. She is 20 weeks' gestation. You would expect to find the fundus:

A. At the umbilicus

B. Midway between the symphysis and the umbilicus

C. One to two fingerbreadths below the umbilicus

D. At the xiphoid process

279. Subjective changes that occur in pregnancy include which of the following?

A. The cervix and vagina become bluish purple in color.

B. The isthmus of uterus softens.

C. Darkening of areola of nipples

D. Breast tenderness

280. A client and her husband have been trying to get pregnant for 5 years. When pregnancy is confirmed, the client feels conflicting emotions, stating that she feels they have made a mistake. The nurse's best response would be to:

A. Encourage the client to seek abortion counseling.

B. Reassure the client that when she feels the baby move, the ambivalence will disappear completely.

C. Reassure the client that most women experience ambivalence in early pregnancy, even when the pregnancies are planned.

D. Express your concern and arrange psychological counseling for the client and her husband.

281. A client arrives for her 28-week prenatal visit. She confides that she has been on a strict diet and has lost 25 pounds. She was approximately 50 pounds overweight at her first prenatal visit. What would be the appropriate nursing response?

A. "As long as you supplement your diet with vitamins and minerals, the amount of weight gain in pregnancy is not important."

B. "Dieting in pregnancy will hurt your unborn baby."

C. "I understand how excited you must be to be losing weight. However, adequate weight gain in pregnancy is important for a healthy baby."

D. "I can see how excited you are with the success of your diet. Keep up the good work!"

282. You are caring for a pregnant client who was diagnosed with diabetes mellitus 2 years prior to this

pregnancy. Her physician told her that her insulin needs will increase during pregnancy. You know this information is based on the fact that:

A. The placenta produces a hormone that increases maternal glucose levels.

B. The placenta produces a hormone that decreases the effectiveness of maternal insulin.

C. Her diabetic condition is becoming more severe.

D. Maternal insulin has to cross the placenta to support the fetus.

283. A client who is diagnosed with gestational diabetes may be treated with:

A. Diet only

B. A combination of diet and oral hypoglycemics

C. A combination of exercise and oral hypoglycemics

D. A combination of diet, exercise, and insulin

284. A client is admitted to labor and delivery with a diagnosis of pre-eclampsia and is started on magnesium sulfate. The nurse evaluating the client's response knows the primary purpose for this medication is to:

A. Lower blood pressure

B. Prevent seizures

C. Decrease peripheral edema

D. Decrease protein lost in the urine by decreasing urine output

285. When caring for a client in labor, the nurse takes the client's blood pressure between contractions. The rationale for this nursing action is:

A. It is more comfortable for the client.

B. Diastolic blood pressure lowers during uterine contractions.

C. Systolic blood pressure increases during uterine contractions.

D. Blood pressure does not change during contractions.

286. The nurse is caring for a client in labor. A deceleration pattern is noted that mirrors the contractions pattern, but begins at the peak of the contraction and returns to baseline 20 seconds after the end of the contraction. The nurse knows that the most likely cause of this pattern is:

A. Fetal head compression

B. Uteroplacental insufficiency

C. Umbilical cord compression

D. Fetal activity

287. In caring for a gravida I in labor, it is noted that her fetus is in LOP position. Which of the following statements about this position will most likely be true of this client's labor?

A. Will have no effect on the average length of labor

B. Will facilitate the labor and allow it to progress more rapidly

C. Will prolong the client's second stage of labor

D. Will prolong the client's third stage of labor

288. You are caring for a client who is 36 weeks' gestation. Her recent laboratory work shows a hematocrit of 34. Her baseline hematocrit was 38. Your nursing action would be:

A. Advise the client that her laboratory work is abnormal and she needs to increase her iron supplement.

B. Assess the client for symptoms of occult bleeding.

C. Assure the client this is a normal finding, called pseudoanemia.

D. Assess the client's clotting factors.

289. Pregnant clients are at increased risk for urinary tract infections (UTIs) due to:

A. The relaxing effect of progesterone on smooth muscle

B. Engorgement of the ureters

C. Increased excretion of protein in the urine

D. Increased urine output that occurs in pregnancy

290. A client, G1P0, 39 weeks' gestation, presents to labor and delivery, complaining of contractions.

A. Encourage the client to ambulate.

B. Suggest the client return home until she is in active labor.

C. Anticipate that the client is at risk for a prolapsed cord.

D. Give the client an enema in preparation for labor induction.

291. A client, 25 weeks' gestation, has a 1-hour glucose test. The results are 150 mg/dl. The nurse should:

A. Review the client's exercise plan.

B. Schedule the client for a glucose tolerance test.

C. Have a hemoglobin A_{1c} drawn.

D. Understand this is a normal finding for this gestational age.

292. You are caring for a client on terbutaline (Brethine) for preterm labor. On assessment, you note that her respiratory rate has increased from a baseline rate of 20 to a current rate of 26. What is your nursing action?

A. Apply O_2 at 10 L/min to increase oxygenation.

B. Consider this a normal finding when this medication is used.

C. Assess breath sounds and notify physician.

D. Medicate the patient for pain.

293. The most common sexually transmitted disease seen in pregnant women is:

A. HIV

B. Syphilis

C. Gonorrhea

D. Chlamydia

294. You are caring for a client who is 40 weeks' gestation with ruptured membranes for 20 hours. Compared to the normal protocol for frequency of assessments, which of the following would the nurse assess *more* frequently?

A. Fetal heart rate
B. Maternal blood pressure
C. Maternal temperature
D. Uterine contractions

295. A client who is 6 hours' post-vaginal delivery, is complaining of severe perineal pain. On assessment, the nurse does not see anything out of normal range in the perineal area. What complication is this client most likely experiencing?
A. An unrepaired vaginal laceration
B. A hematoma of the vaginal wall
C. Excessive edema at the episiotomy site
D. Acute anxiety over the labor and delivery experience

296. The degree of glycemic control for a pregnant diabetic can be determined by:
A. Comparing weights from one visit to the next
B. Measuring the blood glucose at each visit
C. Reviewing the daily home monitoring of glucose levels
D. Measuring the glycosylated hemoglobin A_{1c}

297. You are caring for a client who is 34 weeks' gestation and has been diagnosed with gestational diabetes. When educating the client, the nurse should include the following information:
A. "You will be placed on oral hypoglycemics if your blood sugars are too high."
B. "I will teach you how to do urine dipsticks to check for sugar in your urine, because this is the most effective way to measure control at home."
C. "You will be placed on insulin if your glucose screening test (GST) is positive."
D. "Insulin is the drug of choice to control diabetes in pregnancy when medication is required."

298. The diagnosis of pregnancy-induced hypertension (PIH) is based on:
A. A BP elevation greater than 140/90
B. Severe headaches and right upper quadrant pain
C. Edema above the waist, 2+ protein in the urine, and a BP increase of 30 mm Hg systolic, 15 mm Hg diastolic above the baseline
D. BP increase of greater than 140/90, significant lower extremity edema, and glycosuria

299. During a routine OB visit, the physician orders an ultrasound for a client who is 12 weeks' gestation. The nurse understands the purpose of the ultrasound is to:
A. Determine chromosomal disorders
B. Confirm the gestational age
C. Assess the need for a cesarean delivery
D. Screen for gestational diabetes

300. When assessing a client in labor, it is determined that the fetus is a face presentation, LMA position. The M stands for:

A. Mouth
B. Maxilla
C. Mandible
D. Mentum

301. When assessing a client in labor, it is determined that the fetus is in an RSA position. Which of the following presentations does this represent?
A. Breech
B. Vertex
C. Occipital
D. Face

302. When assessing fetal heart tones on a client, the nurse first determines that the fetus is LOA. Based on this information, where should fetal heart tones be located?
A. Upper left
B. Upper right
C. Lower left
D. Lower right

303. The nurse determines that the client is in labor when:
A. Contractions are 5 minutes apart and lasting 30 seconds.
B. Effacement and dilatation of the cervix occur.
C. The client complains of pain mostly in the upper abdomen.
D. Contractions do not change with ambulation.

304. A client at her first prenatal visit asks what laboratory tests will be *routinely* done at her visits. The nurse's best response would be:
A. Blood for hemoglobin and hematocrit
B. Urinalysis
C. Blood sugar
D. Urine for protein and glucose

305. The nurse should explain that the most common side effect of the contraceptive Depo-Provera is:
A. Irregular and unpredictable menstrual bleeding
B. Weight loss
C. Hyperactivity
D. Hypertension

306. Your client is concerned because her 34-week gestation newborn has undescended testicles. Your explanation to her should be based on the knowledge that:
A. The testes do not normally descend into the scrotal sac until 1 year of age.
B. The testes normally descend into the scrotal sac at about 36 weeks' gestation.
C. It is not important for the testes to descend until puberty.
D. The baby will require immediate surgery in order to move the testes into the scrotal sac.

307. The characteristic signs and symptoms of pregnancy-induced hypertension (PIH) include:

A. A trace of proteinuria, BP increase greater than 15 mm Hg above the systolic baseline, and lower extremity edema
B. Epigastric pain, diastolic pressure of 90 mm Hg, dizziness
C. BP increase of 30 mm Hg systolic, 15 mm Hg diastolic above the baseline, greater than 1+ proteinuria, and edema greater than 1+
D. Hypertension, glucosuria, and upper body edema

308. A postpartum client is concerned that she does not have breast milk the second day following delivery of her newborn. She complains that the "yellow stuff" will not be enough for her baby. The nurse's explanation to the client should include:
A. She will need to supplement with commercial infant formula.
B. The yellowish secretion is colostrum, which is important for her newborn because it is contains antibodies and is high in nutritional value.
C. She will have an ample amount of breast milk by the end of the first month.
D. Many women with small breasts do not have an adequate production of breast milk early.

309. The diagnosis of PIH is suspected if the following are found:
A. Ankle edema and hyporeflexia
B. Ankle edema and glucosuria
C. Hypertension and glucosuria
D. Hypertension and proteinuria

310. A major complication of eclampsia is:
A. Infection
B. Aspiration
C. Polyuria
D. Extremity injuries

311. The most common cause of early postpartum hemorrhage is:
A. Uterine atony
B. Retained placental fragments
C. Cervical lacerations
D. Infection

312. Magnesium sulfate (MgSO$_4$) is used in the treatment of pre-eclampsia to:
A. Prevent seizures
B. Decrease BP
C. Increase urine output
D. Decrease edema

313. Physiological anemia is a result of:
A. Increased erythropoiesis in the first 2 weeks of pregnancy
B. Decreased dietary intake of iron
C. Plasma volume increase being greater than RBC increase
D. Increased demand on the maternal liver

314. A client is 12 hours' postpartum. On assessment you note her fundus is one fingerbreadth above the umbilicus and deviated to the right. What is your understanding of this finding?
A. This is a normal fundal position for this stage of recovery.
B. This position indicates a lazy uterus.
C. This position indicates that the client's bladder is distended.
D. This position is an early sign of postpartum hemorrhage.

315. A client diagnosed with mild pre-eclampsia should be encouraged to:
A. Restrict her sodium intake.
B. Plan for an early birth.
C. Ambulate at least once daily.
D. Bedrest in a left lateral position.

316. The nurse is caring for a client whose baseline blood pressure was 110/60. Her blood pressure in the latent stage of labor is 146/76. What is the appropriate nursing action?
A. The client's BP is still within an acceptable range. The nurse should continue routine monitoring of the BP.
B. The client's BP is expected to increase in this stage of labor. The nurse should consider this a normal finding.
C. If the client has no other complaints, the nurse should continue to observe her.
D. The nurse should consider this reason for concern and notify the primary health-care provider.

317. The nurse admits a 13-year-old in labor. The client is a gravida IV para 0 AB III, 40 weeks' gestation. On assessment the nurse notes that the fundal height is 40 cm, and the cervix is 100 percent effaced, 3 cm dilated and at −4 station. Based on these findings, what is the priority area of concern that should be considered?
A. Because the client has already had three babies, she will be at risk for hemorrhage.
B. The client will be emotionally upset because she has "lost" three other babies.
C. Because she is so young, her pelvis may be underdeveloped and not adequate for the fetus to pass through.
D. The fetus may be too small to survive the delivery.

318. The normal amount of amniotic fluid at 38 weeks' gestation is:
A. 200 to 300 cc
B. 500 to 600 cc
C. 800 to 1000 cc
D. 1500 to 2000 cc

319. A normal pH for the fetus would be:
A. 6.25
B. 7.00
C. 7.19
D. 7.28

320. The most common fetal trauma that occurs with the use of vacuum extraction (VE) is:
    A. Perineal lacerations
    B. Cephalohematomas
    C. Caput succedaneum
    D. Facial palsy

321. Descent, flexion, internal rotation, and extension allow for the normal birth process. These movements are designed to:
    A. Shorten the second stage of labor
    B. Ease the passage of the infant through the false pelvis
    C. Allow the smallest presenting diameter to pass through first
    D. Allow the infant to be born in an occiput anterior position

322. When labor is prolonged and the fetus does not descend past the ischial spines, which of the following complications may be suspected?
    A. Prolapsed cord
    B. Hydramnios
    C. Cephalopelvic disproportion
    D. Shoulder dystocia

323. You are caring for a client with intense contractions occurring every 2 minutes. She delivers less than 3 hours after her labor began. Based on your knowledge of the normal labor process, which of the following labor patterns did the client experience?
    A. Hypotonic
    B. Precipitous
    C. Prolonged
    D. Normal

324. A surgical incision to enlarge the perineal opening during a vaginal delivery is called what?
    A. AROM
    B. Cerclage
    C. Episiotomy
    D. Cesarean section

325. Afterpains during the postpartum period are caused by:
    A. Constipation
    B. Trauma during delivery
    C. Uterine contractions after birth
    D. A prolapsed uterus

326. Fertilization of the human ovum occurs in the:
    A. Uterus
    B. Vagina
    C. Fallopian tube
    D. Isthmus

327. Your client, who is 16 weeks' pregnant, asks if it is possible to tell on ultrasound if the baby is a boy or girl yet. Based on your knowledge of fetal development, what is your best response?
    A. "Yes, we can tell as early as 9 weeks what the sex of the baby is."
    B. "Yes, by 12 weeks, sex organs are developed so we should be able to get a good picture now."
    C. "No, sex is not determined until closer to 20 weeks' gestation."
    D. "No, an ultrasound is totally unreliable in determining the sex of the baby."

328. Nausea and vomiting that continues past the first trimester and is severe in nature is termed:
    A. Morning sickness
    B. Toxoplasmosis
    C. Hyperemesis gravidarum
    D. Toxemia of pregnancy

329. One of the common characteristics of placenta previa is:
    A. Separation of the normally implanted placenta
    B. Painless bleeding during the last trimester of pregnancy
    C. Sudden sharp pain not associated with vaginal bleeding
    D. A rigid abdomen and dark red vaginal bleeding

330. Narcotic analgesics are generally contraindicated in labor when the fetus:
    A. Has a congenital deformity
    B. Has macrosomia
    C. Is in a persistent posterior position
    D. Is premature

331. As a nurse for the prenatal clinic, you have been asked to set up a special educational program for teens, ages 15 to 18 years. Based on your knowledge of this age group, which of the following would be the most appropriate?
    A. One-on-one teaching sessions
    B. Group activities with their peer group
    C. Group activities with a mix of age groups
    D. Written materials that are age-appropriate

332. In the last 10 years, first-time pregnancies to women over age 35 have increased by 50 percent. Which of the following is the major reason for this increase?
    A. Women are becoming less involved in the work force.
    B. There has been a drop in teen pregnancy in recent years.
    C. Advances in reproductive technology have allowed timing of conception.
    D. Poverty and low educational levels of women in this decade have increased unplanned pregnancies after 35.

333. You are giving prenatal information to a 24-year-old gravida I para 0. She asks what the "mucus plug" is. Your best response would be:
    A. "The mucus plug seals the amniotic bag closed so none of the fluid leaks out."
    B. "The mucus plug prevents the cervix from opening up too early."
    C. "The mucus plug protects the fetus by acting as a barrier against bacteria."

D. "The mucus plug occurs when there is infection in the uterus."

334. At 20 weeks' gestation, the fundus of the uterus should be palpated:
A. Below the symphysis
B. At the symphysis
C. At the umbilicus
D. At the xiphoid process

335. During pregnancy, the vaginal walls become dark red or violet in color. The nurse knows this change occurs because of:
A. Increased blood flow to the area
B. Decreased blood flow to the area
C. Decreased estrogen production
D. Pressure from the products of conception

336. Anticipatory guidance surrounding the changes in posture that are occurring because of pregnancy for a primigravida at 38 weeks' gestation should include instructing the client to:
A. Lie flat with the feet elevated to prevent swelling of ankles and feet.
B. Keep the feet close together when lifting or ambulating.
C. Avoid leaning forward to lift objects.
D. Avoid back supporters during this stage of pregnancy.

337. When assessing a client, a gravida I at 28 weeks' gestation, you hear a systolic murmur. The client states that she has never had any heart problems before. Based on your knowledge of normal cardiovascular changes in pregnancy, you would:
A. Refer the client to a cardiologist, since heart murmurs are not a normal finding in pregnancy.
B. Instruct the client that she will have to be treated with antibiotics before surgery or dental work, but otherwise she should have no problems.
C. Assure the client that systolic murmurs occur very commonly in pregnancy, and inform the primary health-care provider of your findings.
D. Assure the client that there is no need for concern since all pregnant women develop a murmur in pregnancy.

338. You are evaluating a client who is 32 weeks' gestation. You note that she has had BP increase from her baseline of 110/60 to 124/76. Your further assessment of this client is based on the knowledge that:
A. An increase in BP at this gestational age is normal.
B. Unless the diastolic BP is greater than 90, there is no reason for concern.
C. It is a concern anytime there is an elevation in BP since BP normally drops slightly in pregnancy.
D. As long as the client is not symptomatic, there is no reason for concern.

339. You are caring for a client who is 32 weeks' pregnant. She asks why she is bothered so much with heartburn. Your response is based on the knowledge that:
A. Indigestion at this stage in pregnancy is abnormal and always indicates a severe disorder.
B. The increase in hydrochloric acid during pregnancy causes heartburn.
C. A combination of increased intragastric pressure and decreased esophageal tone causes heartburn.
D. Increased gastric motility causes an increased reflux of food and the symptoms of heartburn.

340. Your client, a 24-year-old female at 22 weeks' gestation, complains of reddened, swollen areas on her gums. She asks what they are and why she has them. What is your best response?
A. "These are called epulides, and though we are not sure of the cause, we believe it is connected with high levels of estrogen during pregnancy."
B. "You have gingivitis, a gum condition exclusive to pregnancy caused by not brushing your teeth well enough."
C. "These are called pica and are found in women who suffer from eating disorders."
D. "This is called ptyalism and is caused by excessive salivation."

341. Your pregnant client asks why the palms of her hands are red. Based on your knowledge of pregnancy, how would you respond?
A. "Red palms are common in pregnancy and occur because of an increase in circulating estogens."
B. "Red palms occur when your hematocrit is higher than the normal range."
C. "Red palms occur only with liver disorders; we need to have you see your physician immediately."
D. "I don't know why they occur; let's ask your physician."

342. Your client complains of right upper quadrant discomfort, noting that it is worse after eating fatty or spicy foods. Your concerns are based on which of the following facts related to pregnancy?
A. There is an increase in gastric motility that occurs in pregnancy.
B. The gallbladder becomes sluggish and more prone to the development of stones during pregnancy.
C. The liver becomes engorged with blood, causing stress on the capsule.
D. The increase in hydrochloric acid and pepsid predisposes the pregnant woman to peptic ulcer disease.

343. When your client, who is 18 weeks' pregnant, comes in for her routine check-up, you notice a brownish discoloration over the bridge of her nose,

fanning across both cheeks. It resembles a butterfly pattern. Based on your knowledge of changes in pregnancy, how would you explain this finding?

A. This is a condition called striae, a tearing of the connective tissue under the skin, causing a change in skin color.

B. This is caused by an increased blood flow to the face, a normal finding in pregnancy.

C. This is a pigmentation change that can occur in pregnancy and is called chloasma gravidarum.

D. This is a skin change that is only seen in lupus.

344. The hormone that causes a positive result in most over-the-counter pregnancy tests is:

A. Estrogen
B. Progesterone
C. FSH
D. hCG

345. Your client, whose menstrual cycle is about 2 months late, complains of nausea in the morning and breast tenderness. Based on your knowledge of pregnancy, these are considered:

A. Presumptive signs of pregnancy
B. Probable signs of pregnancy
C. Positive signs of pregnancy
D. Diagnostic signs of pregnancy

346. Your client, pregnant with her first baby, asks when she will be able to hear the baby's heartbeat with the "special stethoscope" (Doppler stethoscope). Based on your knowledge of fetal development, what is your best response?

A. "The baby's heartbeat can first be heard at about 20 weeks' gestation."

B. "The baby's heartbeat can first be heard by about 12 weeks."

C. "The baby's heartbeat can be heard with the Doppler stethoscope before it is picked up on ultrasound, at about 6 weeks' gestation."

D. "With a trained ear, the baby's heartbeat can be heard by 8 weeks; you probably won't be able to hear it until much later."

347. Your client, who is 10 weeks' gestation, is not immune to rubella. Based on your knowledge of the immunization, what information would you give the client?

A. "I need to give you a rubella vaccine now, because if you get rubella during your pregnancy, it could have detrimental effects on the fetus."

B. "It's too late to do anything for this baby; you should stay up to date on your vaccinations!"

C. "You will need a rubella vaccine as soon after delivery of this baby as possible. Have you been in contact with anyone with rubella?"

D. "We will immunize your baby for rubella as soon as possible to protect it from rubella."

348. You are caring for a client who is 23 weeks' gestation. She is Rh negative, and the father of the baby is Rh positive. She asks if she has to have a shot because of her blood type. Based on your knowledge of Rh compatibilities, how would you counsel your client?

A. "No, you won't need a shot until after the baby is born and we determine the baby's blood type."

B. "Yes, we give everyone a shot so we are sure we don't miss anyone."

C. "No, since your husband is Rh positive, the baby will be positive, and there is no reason for concern."

D. "Yes, because you are Rh negative, we will give you a shot now and you may need another one after the baby is born."

349. You are counseling a client on her prenatal care. What laboratory work would you expect a pregnant client to have drawn at 16 to 18 weeks' gestation?

A. Serum glucose
B. Rubella screen
C. Serum alpha-fetoprotein
D. Group B strep screen

350. A client arrives for her second prenatal visit. She asks why she has to give a urine specimen at every visit. What is your best response?

A. "We test your urine at every visit to see if there is protein, sugar, or ketones present. If any of those are present, the physician may order additional tests."

B. "We don't test your urine every time, just the first few visits."

C. "We have to test your urine every visit to make sure you don't have an infection."

D. "You don't need to worry about it. It's just part of our routine care."

351. You are performing a dipstick urine test on a client who is 14 weeks' pregnant. You note a large amount of ketones in her urine. What question would be appropriate to ask this client?

A. "Does it hurt or sting when you go to the bathroom?"

B. "Are you still having a lot of nausea and vomiting?"

C. "Are you eating a lot of sugar?"

D. "Are you having any right upper quadrant discomfort?"

352. You are caring for a client who is 32 weeks' pregnant. She is admitted with vague complaints of headache, sleeplessness, and inability to concentrate. On physical examination, you note several bruised areas over her abdominal and chest areas and immediately suspect abuse. How would you question the client?

A. "Do you sometimes fall and injure yourself?"

B. "How can you stay with someone who beats you up?"

C. "How did you get these bruises?"

D. "I notice you have several bruised areas. Has someone kicked, slapped, hit, or otherwise hurt you?"

353. When caring for a client that you suspect is suffering chronic physical abuse, what signs and symptoms would you expect to see? A client who:
   A. Is anxious to report her abuser
   B. Has obvious injuries to her face and extremities
   C. Has a very hostile, abusive attitude
   D. Is evasive and depressed

354. You are caring for a client during her first prenatal visit. Prior to the pelvic examination, why is it important to have the client void?
   A. The client may expel urine during the examination and contaminate the specimens.
   B. A full bladder will displace the cervix, making it difficult to obtain the specimens.
   C. The client will have increased discomfort during the examination.
   D. The client could experience bladder damage from the speculum during the examination.

355. At what gestational age should fundal height measurements begin?
   A. 12 weeks
   B. 16 weeks
   C. 20 weeks
   D. 26 weeks

356. You are caring for a client who is 14 weeks' pregnant with her first baby. She asks when she will feel her baby move. Based on your knowledge, what would be your best response?
   A. "I'm surprised you haven't felt the baby move by now."
   B. "Most women feel the baby by 16 weeks."
   C. "At around 18 to 20 weeks, you should begin to feel a fluttery feeling—that's the baby."
   D. "At about 28 weeks, you will begin to feel sharp punches—that will be baby's first movements."

357. Your client is 36 weeks' gestation and a gestational diabetic. Her physician has recommended that she have an amniocentesis prior to her planned cesarean section this week. Based on your knowledge, the amniocentesis is being done to determine:
   A. Fetal lung maturity
   B. Genetic deformities
   C. Meconium in the amniotic fluid
   D. Volume of amniotic fluid

358. You are performing a contraction stress test on a client who is 38 weeks' gestation. You note that the fetal heart rate averages in the 140s with no decelerations noted. How would you document these findings?
   A. A positive test
   B. A negative test
   C. A reactive test
   D. A nonreactive test

359. Your client, who is in the first trimester of pregnancy, is complaining of nausea and vomiting every morning. You suggest that she should:
   A. Limit her eating to regular mealtimes
   B. Drink plenty of fluids with her meals
   C. Eat dry crackers before arising in the morning
   D. Eat a high carbohydrate meal before bedtime

360. Your client, who is in the first trimester of pregnancy, is complaining of urinary frequency. She denies burning or discomfort with urination. Based on your knowledge, what instructions would you give her? She should:
   A. Limit her intake of oral fluids
   B. Have a UA done to check for infection
   C. Expect this until the second trimester
   D. Attempt to hold the urine for a while after the urge hits

361. You instruct a client who is beginning her second trimester of pregnancy and complains of a vaginal discharge that smells bad and is itching that she should:
   A. Wear cotton panties and change frequently
   B. Wear tampons to prevent the odor and irritation to her perineum
   C. Keep her perineum clean and dry and wear a minipad
   D. Come in and have an examination

362. Your client, who is in the last trimester of pregnancy, complains of constipation. What instructions would be most appropriate?
   A. "Increase the fiber in your diet and drink plenty of fluids."
   B. "Take a mild laxative each day with plenty of fluids."
   C. "Take 2 tablespoons of mineral oil after each meal."
   D. "Use a Fleet enema whenever you feel pressure in the rectum."

363. You are talking with a client who is in her third trimester of pregnancy. She comments that her feet are so swollen she cannot get her shoes on. Her blood pressure is within normal limits and her urine is negative for protein. How would you counsel in regard to her lower extremity edema?
   A. Lie flat with her feet elevated
   B. Limit her intake of salt
   C. Rest in a left lateral position
   D. Limit her intake of fluids

364. A student nurse asks why having an adequate hemoglobin is so important during pregnancy. What is the nurses' best response?
   A. "If the hemoglobin is low, there is not enough circulating blood volume to maintain blood pressure."
   B. "The biggest concern is that there are not enough red blood cells to carry oxygen to the tissue."

C. "Red blood cells help with the clotting process after delivery."

D. "The hemoglobin is stored in the white cells, which help fight infection."

365. You are counseling a client on the use of iron supplements during pregnancy. What information would assist the client to achieve maximum benefit from the supplement?

A. Only take the iron supplement on an empty stomach.

B. Only take the iron supplement with food.

C. Take the iron supplement with orange juice between meals.

D. Take the iron supplement with milk.

366. You are counseling a client who is 22 weeks' gestation, regarding her low hemoglobin. What foods would you recommend that she include in her diet to help build her iron stores?

A. Red meat and dark green vegetables

B. Poultry and yellow vegetables

C. Lima beans and cooked carrots

D. Whole milk and whole wheat bread

367. In reviewing a client's history, you note that she does low-impact aerobics twice a week, drinks one cup of coffee daily, has an indoor cat, and works as a nurse. What area of her history is most concerning and requires prenatal teaching?

A. The fact that she does low-impact aerobics.

B. The fact that she has a habit of drinking coffee each day.

C. The fact that she has a cat as an indoor pet.

D. The fact that her occupation is as a nurse.

368. Your client is 23 years old and planning her first pregnancy. She works in a daycare setting with preschool-age children. What information should you provide her regarding her job with regard to pregnancy?

A. Daycare workers are at increased risk of certain teratogenic infections because of contact with children.

B. Daycare workers are at low risk for illnesses because of the natural immunity they acquire from the children.

C. Daycare workers have the highest injury rate of all health-care providers.

D. Daycare workers require additional immunizations to protect against cytomegalovirus, a herpes type virus found frequently in children.

369. You are caring for a client in labor. She has a documented streptococcus B vaginal culture. Based on your knowledge of this infectious disease, what nursing actions would be priority for this client?

A. Monitor BP since there may be a precipitous rise during the perinatal period with this disease.

B. Order CBCs q 4 hours to monitor WBCs.

C. Monitor temperature every hour after rupture of membranes.

D. Monitor fetal heart rate for decelerations or bradycardia.

370. You are caring for a client who is 32 weeks' pregnant. She presents to labor and delivery with complaints of sudden onset of fever, chills, malaise, and loss of appetite. What priority nursing assessment would you perform to assist the physician in diagnosis?

A. Assess for Homans' sign

B. Assess costovertebral angle for pain

C. Assess breath sounds for wheezing and crackles

D. Assess fundus for contractions

371. What changes occur in pregnancy that increase the risk of a urinary tract infection?

A. Significant increase of protein in the urine

B. Increased bladder capacity

C. Presence of sugar in the urine

D. Shortening of the ureters

372. Based on your knowledge of normal pregnancy changes, what information can you provide to the pregnant client that will decrease her risk of developing a urinary tract infection?

A. Eat large amounts of carbohydrates daily.

B. Attempt to hold urine when the urge to void occurs in order to slowly increase bladder capacity.

C. Limit fluid intake to avoid having to void frequently.

D. Void before and after intercourse.

373. The most common form of sexually transmitted disease in the United States today is:

A. HIV

B. Gonorrhea

C. Syphilis

D. Chlamydia

374. Nutritional needs increase during pregnancy because of the needs of the growing fetus. How would you counsel a women in her second trimester about her caloric needs?

A. "You will need an additional 1000 calories per day to meet the needs of your body and the pregnancy."

B. "An additional 800 calories per day will provide adequate calories without excessive weight gain during the pregnancy."

C. "Most women need about 300 calories per day to meet the additional needs of pregnancy, depending on weight prior to pregnancy."

D. "Most women do not need to increase their caloric intake because they already exceed the recommended daily amount of calories."

375. You are counseling a teenager who is 16 weeks' pregnant on the recommended foods in pregnancy. She states, "But I don't like any of that

stuff!" Based on your knowledge of nutritional needs in pregnancy and the adolescent, what is your response?

A. "I am sorry you don't like any of that stuff, but you're going to have to eat it if you want a healthy baby."

B. "Let's look at the foods you do like. I bet we can get everything you need for a healthy pregnancy and still eat things you like."

C. "I can see this pregnancy is going to be hard on you."

D. "As long as you take your vitamins and mineral supplements, you can eat whatever you want."

376. You are discussing a client's 24-hour food recall with her when you note that she has written down "1 tablespoon of clay" twice on her list. What risk does this intake have on the nutritional status of the pregnancy?

A. This a fairly common practice with pregnant women called pica. The concern is that it may interfere with the absorption of her regular foods.

B. Research has shown that pregnant women eat nonfood items to make up for something lacking in their diet.

C. There is no concern with this practice as long as she bakes it prior to consuming it.

D. This a common practice and not of concern.

377. When counseling a woman on expected weight gain in pregnancy, what factors most influence the expected gain?

A. Age and diet preferences

B. Pre-pregnancy height and weight

C. Previous eating disorders

D. Economic status and ability to buy food

378. You are counseling a client about nutrition and weight gain in pregnancy. She is 60 lb over her normal weight at conception. Based on your knowledge, how would you counsel this client?

A. She still needs to gain the average amount of weight for pregnancy, which is 25 to 35 lb.

B. She does not need to gain any weight; the pregnancy will pull what it needs from her fat stores.

C. She needs to gain 15 to 25 lb to meet the needs of a healthy pregnancy.

D. Weight gain does not matter as long as she eats a nutritious diet.

379. You are counseling a client regarding her nutritional needs in pregnancy. She states that she is an aerobics instructor and does two to three classes per day, 4 days per week. Based on this information, you would advise her to:

A. Supplement her diet with complex carbohydrates to supply needed energy and maintain expected weight gain

B. Eat a regular diet and maintain her weight with this activity level

C. Decrease her activity level to promote a healthy pregnancy

D. Double the amount of calories to make up for the calories burned with exercise

380. You are caring for a client in the latent phase of labor. What position would most likely promote contractions and progress labor most effectively at this stage?

A. Lateral recumbent

B. Supine

C. Upright

D. Prone

381. The shortest anteroposterior distance between the sacral promontory and the symphysis pubis is called the:

A. Diagonal conjugate

B. Obstetrical conjugate

C. Pelvic inlet

D. Pelvic outlet

382. The physician has described the client's fetal attitude as military. So that the client understands, you explain that a military attitude means:

A. "That the head is flexed with the chin down on the chest"

B. "That the baby is coming head down just as he should"

C. "That the head is extended, with the face presenting first"

D. "That the head is slightly extended with the baby's brow presenting first"

383. Your client's fetus is in a left occipital posterior position. In terms of nursing interventions, what comfort measures would you expect to provide for this client in addition to regular nursing interventions?

A. Frequent adjustment of the fetal monitor

B. Ice chips as needed

C. Application of counter pressure to the low back

D. Change her position every 2 hours

384. You are caring for a client in labor. She has been in complete control of her labor up until this point, when suddenly she slaps her husband and screams at him to get out. Based on your knowledge of behavioral changes in labor, what phase or stage of labor is this client in?

A. The latent phase

B. The active phase

C. The transition phase

D. The second stage

385. A client calls and reports that she is due tomorrow. She complains of backache and diarrhea. Based on this information, what instructions will you give the client?

A. "It sounds like you are in labor. You better come on into the hospital."

B. "You may have a viral infection. Have you been around anyone who is sick?"

C. "It sounds like you may be getting ready to go into labor. Watch for other signs like contractions, leakage of fluid, or bloody discharge."

D. "This is not uncommon this late in pregnancy. You have probably overdone your activities."

386. A client calls to ask how she will know when she is having real contractions. The nurse's response should include:

A. "Contractions will be intense when you are lying down but may stop if you walk."

B. "Contractions will be felt in your back and upper fundus."

C. "Contractions will be felt in the low back and come around to the low abdomen."

D. "Contractions vary with individuals. You'll just know when it is time."

387. You have admitted a client to the labor-and-delivery unit. She is 38 weeks' gestation, has ruptured membranes, and is in the active phase of labor. On assessment, you note her heart rate to be 124. Based on your knowledge of the normal response to labor, what is the most likely cause of this elevation?

A. The client probably is infected secondary to the ruptured membranes.

B. The client may be anxious or in pain from the labor process.

C. An increased heart rate is a normal finding in the last trimester of pregnancy.

D. The client's heart rate may be increased because of pregnancy-induced hypertension.

388. You are caring for a client in the first hour postpartum after a vaginal delivery. You note that her heart rate has increased slightly with each set of vital signs and is now 118. Her BP is within normal limits. What is your concern based on these findings?

A. An elevated heart rate is the first indicator of maternal hemorrhage, and the client's vaginal flow needs to be evaluated carefully.

B. There is normally an elevation in heart rate during the postpartum period and this is nothing to worry about.

C. As long as the BP is within normal limits, the heart rate is not a concern.

D. The client may have an infection, causing an increase in heart rate.

389. You have admitted a client to the birthing unit in the latent phase of labor. She is term and considered low risk. After the initial fetal heart evaluation, how often should fetal heart tones be monitored?

A. Every hour in the latent phase of labor

B. Every 30 minutes in the latent phase of labor

C. Every 15 minutes, regardless of the phase of labor

D. Every 5 minutes, regardless of the phase of labor

390. When evaluating fetal heart tones, the baseline fetal heart rate is determined:

A. During contractions, over a 5-minute period

B. During a contraction and for 30 seconds after the contraction ends

C. Between contractions, over a 1-minute period

D. For a 5-minute period, both during and between contractions

391. You are caring for a client in the latent phase of labor. She is a gravida II para I, 2 cm dilated, and has been having regular contractions for 20 hours. What is the concern with regard to this client's labor pattern?

A. There is no concern with this client. She is within the expected time frame for the latent phase of labor.

B. The client is experiencing a prolonged latent phase of labor. The concern is the intensity of contractions will cause extreme discomfort for the client.

C. The client is experiencing a prolonged latent phase of labor. The concern is that the client may experience exhaustion, sleep deprivation, and frustration.

D. The client is experiencing a prolonged latent phase of labor. The concern is that the fetus may experience distress because of the prolonged labor.

392. You are caring for a client in the active phase of labor. She is 6 cm dilated and at −2 station. On vaginal examination, the midwife states the fetus has a caput forming. You know this is an indication of:

A. Too rapid progression through the birth canal

B. A normal finding at this fetal station

C. Possible cepholopelvic disproportion

D. Trauma to the fetal head, causing blood to accumulate under the scalp

393. You are caring for a client who is having labor induced with an oxytocin drip. You note that her last three contractions have lasted 120 seconds with 20 seconds between contractions. What is your priority nursing action?

A. Continue to observe the contraction pattern and the fetal response.

B. Notify the midwife caring for the client and report this pattern.

C. Assess the maternal blood pressure and heart rate.

D. Turn off the oxytocin and assess the FHR.

394. You are caring for a client in the latent phase of labor. From Leopold examination and visualization of abdominal shape, you suspect the fetus is in an occiput posterior (OP) position. In what position should you place the client for maximum comfort and to assist in rotation of the fetus?

A. Have the client maintain a left lateral position.

B. Have the client kneel, leaning forward for support.

C. Place the client in a semisitting position.

D. Have the client ambulate, resting as needed by leaning against the wall.

395. You are caring for a client in the early stages of labor. She is 2 cm dilated and at 0 station, membranes intact. What position will most likely facilitate progression of labor for this client?
    A. A left lateral position
    B. A right lateral position
    C. Ambulating or standing position
    D. Hands-and-knees position

396. You are caring for a client in the active phase of labor. She has been thrashing about and huffing and puffing with contractions. She suddenly becomes very frightened and complains of a feeling of dizziness and numbness around her lips and fingers. What is your nursing action?
    A. Have the client cup her hands together, place them over her face, and breathe into them.
    B. Place a paper bag over the client's face.
    C. Perform a vaginal examination to determine dilation.
    D. Have the client turn to her left side.

397. When assisting a client in the second stage of labor, which of the following behavioral signs indicate that the client is ready to commit to pushing?
    A. Restraint of vocalizations during pushing efforts
    B. Rectum retracts during pushing effort
    C. Verbalizes embarrassment over incontinence
    D. Client looks to her partner for support

398. A client who is 16 weeks' gestation asks what over-the-counter medications she can take for a headache. What is your best response?
    A. "Any nonnarcotic medication is acceptable for occasional use."
    B. "Acetaminophen is the only analgesic medication recommended during pregnancy and lactation."
    C. "Ibuprofen or acetaminophen are both acceptable choices."
    D. "Acetylsalicylic acid is one of the oldest and safest drugs on the market today."

399. A client who is 26 weeks' pregnant asks if she can safely continue her job as a computer programmer. Based on your knowledge of normal pregnancy, what is your best response?
    A. "Most pregnant women can continue to work but find it very hard to focus on their work."
    B. "As long as you get up and move around every few hours, there shouldn't be any reason why you can't continue your current position."
    C. "Because of the high risk of radiation from the computer screen, this is not recommended."
    D. "If you can, it would be better to take time off to adapt to the pregnancy."

400. You are caring for a client who is 32 weeks' pregnant. She asks the proper way to wear her car safety belt. You respond:
    A. "Place the shoulder strap behind your back so you won't have pressure across your abdomen."
    B. "Place the shoulder strap loosely across the chest and the lap belt low on the hips."
    C. "Place the lap belt below the abdominal bulge snug across the pelvic bones. The shoulder strap should be snug across the chest and shoulder."
    D. "It is better not to wear a seat belt when pregnant because of the risk of abdominal injury and possible fetal injury from the belt."

401. You are working in the emergency department. A client who is 36 weeks' pregnant arrives in full cardiac arrest. Which intervention is unique for a pregnant woman during cardiopulmonary resuscitation (CPR)?
    A. Slightly elevate the legs to increase central circulation.
    B. Use a ratio of 10 chest compressions to 1 breath.
    C. Listen for fetal heart tones before using heroic measures.
    D. Position the client so that vena cava compression does not occur.

402. You are caring for a client in the postpartum phase of pregnancy. She asks when she and her husband can resume sexual intercourse. You would respond:
    A. "As soon as you feel physically ready."
    B. "You should wait a minimum of 6 weeks, until the physician gives you the OK."
    C. "You should wait until the flow of lochia stops, which usually takes 3 to 4 weeks."
    D. "I can't believe you can even think about that now!"

403. You are caring for a client in early pregnancy. She asks if there is any reason why she cannot continue sexual relations with her husband. Your response should be based on the knowledge that:
    A. Pregnancy is a normal, natural occurrence and does not affect sexual relations.
    B. During pregnancy, because of the enlarging maternal abdomen, sexual intercourse may become very awkward. When this occurs, relations should be suspended.
    C. Most couples lose interest in intercourse early in pregnancy, so this will not be an issue.
    D. Unless the client is considered high risk, she and her husband should be able to continue intercourse.

404. You are caring for a client who delivered vaginally 12 hours ago. She had no problems during the intrapartal period but now has a temperature of 100.2°F. Based on your knowledge of the normal postpartal period, what would be the priority nursing intervention?

A. Notify the physician of the client's fever.
B. Assess for breast engorgement.
C. Encourage oral fluids and rest.
D. Assess vaginal bleeding and fundal position.

405. You are caring for a client who delivered 30 hours ago and is preparing for discharge. When you assess her vital signs, you note a temperature of 100.6°F. What is your priority nursing action?
A. Notify the client's primary health-care provider.
B. Instruct the client to drink large amounts of fluid when she gets home.
C. Order a CBC to rule our infection.
D. Discharge the client per orders with instructions to call her physician if the temperature does not go down in 2 to 3 days.

406. You are assessing a client who is 12 hours' postpartum. You note a heart rate of 130 beats per minute. Based on your knowledge of the normal postpartal range, your priority would be to assess the client's:
A. Respiratory status
B. Blood pressure
C. Excessive vaginal bleeding
D. Laboratory findings

407. You have arrived for a home visit with a client who delivered vaginally 5 days ago. When you assess her lochia flow, you note that it is pinkish brown, serosanguinous, and has a fleshy odor. What is your priority nursing action related to this finding?
A. Assess the client's temperature and heart rate.
B. Ask the client if she has any abdominal discomfort.
C. Ask the client if she has been exposed to any STDs.
D. Assure the client this is a normal finding for this stage postpartum.

408. A student nurse is caring for a client who delivered vaginally 3 hours ago and is being admitted from the recovery room. She asks how often she should assess this client's fundus. Based on the standard practice, your response would be:
A. "Every 15 minutes for the first 24 hours"
B. "Every 1 hour for the first 12 hours"
C. "Every 4 hours for the first 24 hours"
D. "Every 8 hours, at the beginning of each shift"

409. A mnemonic used to remember the assessment for an episiotomy is:
A. PERRL
B. BUBBLE-HE
C. REEDA
D. GTPAL

410. You are caring for a client who is 4 hours' postpartum. Her past assessments have been within normal limits. She now complains of pain and pressure in the perineal and rectal area, and she

appears to be restless and anxious. What nursing assessment is priority based on this information?
A. Assess the blood pressure to rule out shock.
B. Visualize perineum to assess for hematoma.
C. Do a vaginal examination to assess for an undetected second fetus.
D. Look for Homans' sign to assess for thrombus in the calf.

411. In caring for postpartum clients, the primary nursing intervention that prevents postpartum thromboembolic disease is:
A. Implementation of acetylsalicylic acid (ASA) therapy
B. Placement of TED hose
C. Early postpartum ambulation
D. Placement of a blanket behind the knees when sitting

412. The drug of choice for treatment of thromboembolic disease during pregnancy is:
A. Warfarin (Coumadin)
B. Protamine sulfate
C. Heparin
D. Streptokinase

413. You are caring for a client postpartum who is being treated with heparin therapy for thromboembolic disease. The client voices her concerns over the safety of breastfeeding while on this drug. Based on your knowledge of this medication, how would you advise this client?
A. "Because research has shown that heparin passes freely through breast milk, I would advise that you discontinue breastfeeding until this therapy is completed."
B. "Because we are unsure of the effect of heparin on the baby, I would encourage you to pump your breasts and discard the milk, and feed the baby by bottle."
C. "I would encourage you to continue breastfeeding. You only get one chance to provide these nutrients to your newborn baby."
D. "Research has shown that heparin is unlikely to pass through breast milk, and even if it does, it cannot be absorbed through the baby's gastrointestinal tract. Therefore, it is safe to breastfeed."

414. You are assessing a newborn who is 2 hours old. You note a mild murmur on auscultation. Previously documented assessments do not indicate a murmur. You also noted that the baby did not do well on its initial feeding, turning a little dusky during the feeding. What is your nursing action?
A. Listen again. Maybe you did not really hear a murmur.
B. Explain to the mother that her baby has a heart murmur, but it is probably nothing to worry about.
C. Document your findings on the baby's chart, along with the rest of the assessment findings.

D. Notify the physician of your findings, fully aware that murmurs are usually a normal finding in the neonatal period.

415. You are caring for a newborn who is 4 hours old, 38 weeks by examination, and weighs 5 lb 12 oz. After a visit to her mom, she has returned to the nursery. On assessment you note that her temperature is 96.8°F axillary; heart rate, 168, respiratory rate, 66. Based on your knowledge of the normal newborn, what is this baby most at risk for?
    A. Hyperbilirubinemia
    B. Hypoglycemia
    C. Prematurity
    D. Macrosomia

416. You are caring for a client who is in preterm labor, 28 weeks' gestation. Her labor progressed rapidly and delivery is imminent. The client asks why everyone is so concerned about the baby being born early. Your best response would be:
    A. "Because the baby is going to be so small, he won't have enough fat to keep himself warm."
    B. "At 28 weeks the lungs are immature. We will have to give a special medication to the baby after he is born to help the lungs work properly."
    C. "All of the baby's organs are nonfunctional. We will have to use all kinds of machines to do the jobs the organs normally would."
    D. "We aren't really concerned, we have babies this small all the time. I am sure your baby will be fine."

417. A gravida I para I is feeding her newborn baby her first feeding. She is concerned because the baby only took 30 cc from the bottle before falling asleep. Based on your knowledge of the newborn's gastrointestinal tract, how would you intervene with this mother?
    A. Take the baby from her and try to feed her a little more.
    B. Assure her that she and the baby will improve with practice.
    C. Assure her that 30 cc is a good amount for the first feeding.
    D. Ask the client to show her the position she was using.

418. You are caring for a client who just had an uncomplicated vaginal delivery. She asks when she can breastfeed her baby. Based on your knowledge of the first period of reactivity, when should this mother be encouraged to breastfeed?
    A. After the first hour of recovery, when vital signs and bleeding are determined to be within normal limits, the baby should go to breast.
    B. Within 2 hours of delivery to prevent the initial blood sugar drop that can occur
    C. Within 4 hours of delivery to assure establishment of a breastfeeding pattern
    D. The baby should go to breast immediately after delivery, if the mother and baby are stable.

419. You are orienting a new nurse to the newborn nursery. As she begins to assess a baby, you note that she listens to the apical heart rate for a full minute. How should you intervene in this situation?
    A. Tell her that it is a lot quicker if she listens for 15 seconds and multiplies that by four to get the heart rate.
    B. Instruct her to do a brachial pulse instead of listening to the apical heart rate.
    C. Give her positive feedback for performing this skill appropriately.
    D. Tell her that as she gets more experience, this skill will become easier.

420. You are assessing a newborn after a forcep-assisted vaginal birth. You note edema of the right side of the scalp that does not cross the suture line. This edema was not present when the baby first arrived in the nursery 2 hours ago. What condition of the newborn is most likely present?
    A. Cephalohematoma
    B. Caput succedaneum
    C. *Candida albicans*
    D. Hydrocephaly

421. You are assessing a newborn infant. You note that the baby has dry, leathery, peeling skin and deep creases that cover the entire sole of both feet. How would you interpret this finding?
    A. Normal for a preterm newborn
    B. Normal for a term newborn
    C. Normal for a post-term newborn
    D. Not a normal finding for any newborn

422. The purpose of the Ballard scale is to:
    A. Compare height to weight of the newborn
    B. Convert weight in kilograms to pounds and ounces
    C. Determine if the baby has a normal head size
    D. Estimate gestational age of the newborn

423. You are caring for a client during an uncomplicated vaginal delivery. She has complained of being extremely hot during the labor process, furthermore, the room temperature is set at 71°F, and you have a fan blowing directly on her. What is your first nursing action after delivery of the baby to prevent thermoregulation problems with the newborn?
    A. Turn up the heat in the room.
    B. Turn off the fan.
    C. Wrap the mother and baby in warm blankets.
    D. Take the baby to the radiant warmer.

424. You are preparing to give a newborn his vitamin K injection. Based on your knowledge of this drug and the newborn, what site should be used?
    A. Anterior deltoid
    B. Vastus lateralis
    C. Gluteus maximus
    D. Medial plantar

425. You are doing a follow-up visit for a newborn who is not 6 days old. The mother states that he is a "good baby." She says he sleeps all night without waking, and only cries to eat about three times in the daytime. On assessment, you note that the baby is lethargic, the tongue is dry, and the fontanelles are sunken. What is your first nursing action?
A. Call the physician and report your findings.
B. Try to feed the baby to determine ability to feed by mouth.
C. Discuss with the mother the need to feed the baby more frequently.
D. Place an oral-gastric (OG) tube and give sterile water.

426. You are the nurse in the delivery room. You receive the neonate, and despite resuscitation measures, at 1 minute the respirations are absent; heart rate, 80; muscle tone, flaccid; reflexes, grimace noted; color, blue. What Apgar score would this baby receive at 1 minute?
A. 0
B. 1
C. 2
D. 3

427. A 26-year-old female client is trying to conceive. She took the medication isotretinoin (Accutane) for a year as a 13-year-old. The nurse should include which of the following in her teaching? Isotretinoin _____
A. Is a mutagen that will affect embryonic development
B. Is a teratogen that will affect the future of her baby's embryonic development
C. Does not impact on fetal development
D. Will not influence fetal development because she stopped the medication at age 13

428. A 22-year-old female believes she is pregnant. Because she started spotting 9 days after the day of conception, the nurse should explain that
A. Seven to ten days after conception, some women experience mild implantation bleeding.
B. She has already had a spontaneous abortion. Early bleeding is a warning sign.
C. The bleeding is related to an increase of estrogen.
D. This is evidence of blastocyst formation.

429. Which of the following statements by an expectant client suggests to the nurse that more teaching is needed?
A. "My pregnancy should be about 40 weeks long."
B. "My baby should be born at the end of my third trimester."
C. "My pregnancy should last 11 lunar months."
D. "My pregnancy should last about 280 days."

430. Using Naegele's rule, calculate a nullipara's due date. Her last period started on August 1 (8/1) and it lasted 5 days.

A. November 8 (11/8)
B. May 8 (5/8)
C. November 27 (11/27)
D. May 27 (5/27)

431. A term multigravida is in early labor. Her membranes are ruptured. After 1 hour of oxytocin induction, she is in the left lateral position. The nurse determines her status: bladder, palpable; contractions, 8 to 10 minutes apart, 90 to 120 seconds long; dilation: 3 cm; effacement: 50 percent; station: −4; FHT: 120-130. The nurse should next:
A. Increase the rate of the oxytocin infusion and reposition the client to her right side.
B. Decrease the rate of oxytocin infusion and catheterize the client.
C. Stop the infusion and allow the client to ambulate to the bathroom.
D. Stop the oxytocin infusion; change over the primary infusion; and administer oxygen to the client.

432. The nurse assesses a laboring client. The fetal heart rate range is 60 to 80. Which of the following is the best explanation for this situation?
A. Early fetal hypoxia
B. Late profound fetal hypoxia
C. Maternal fever
D. Amnionitis

433. A client in labor is 7 cm dilated with membranes intact. She is having twins. The nurse positions her on her left side. The fetal heart rates are consistently within the 120 to 140 range. Twin A has had early decelerations in the previous hour and a series of three more have recurred. The best action would be to:
A. Wait and watch.
B. Assist the client to the right lateral position.
C. Prepare the client for a cesarean birth.
D. Prepare the client for an amnioinfusion.

434. A new mother takes a photograph of her newborn with a flash camera. The newborn responds by throwing out his arms and legs and crying. Identification of which of the following reflexes suggests accurate understanding by the mother?
A. Tonic neck
B. Babinski's
C. Doll's eye
D. Moro

435. A 21-year-old multigravida, 7 months' pregnant, comes with her husband to the emergency unit for treatment. Multiple cuts and bruises are visible on her face and arms. After the husband returns to the waiting area, the client says that her arm is hurting, "I think it is broken, but please quickly check the baby's heart rate." To establish trust with this client the nurse:
A. Sits next to her to take her history

B. Asks the husband if he would like to hear the baby's heart sounds
C. Alerts security that a crisis may arise
D. Checks her records to see if a pattern of ER visits has developed

436. For the client in labor, the nurse has identified the position that provides the least amount of oxygen to the fetus to be:
A. Left lateral
B. Hand and knees
C. Semisitting
D. Dorsal recumbent

437. A client in her first trimester is experiencing nausea and vomiting almost every morning. Which of the following statements by the nurse would be most beneficial to the client?
A. Skip breakfast on those morning sickness days.
B. Keep crackers at your bedside to eat before arising.
C. Brush your teeth first thing in the morning before breakfast.
D. Drink two 8-ounce glasses of ginger ale before going to sleep each night.

438. A client is at the beginning of her second trimester. She is concerned about having an adequate intake of iron. Which of the following statements indicates that clarification by the nurse is needed?
A. "I eat a serving of strawberries or melon every day."
B. "I take my iron tablet every morning with my breakfast of milk and a bran muffin."
C. "I avoid tea and caffeine when I take my iron tablet."
D. "I put a tomato slice on my hamburger patty."

439. A primipara is 8 cm dilated, 100 percent effaced, 0 station. She is trembling and saying that her hands are tingling. The best nursing action is to:
A. Transfer her to delivery.
B. Administer a prescribed narcotic analgesic.
C. Slow her rate of breathing.
D. Check capillary refill.

440. During an initial postpartal assessment of a client, the nurse notes a 10 cm bluish green discoloration over the sacral area and similar smaller discolorations under her right rib cage. The next priority is to
A. Share the observation and ask for an explanation.
B. Carefully document the assessment in the nurses' notes.
C. Alert social services.
D. Ask who hit her.

441. In reviewing guidelines for intimacy with expectant couples, which of the following situations is considered unsafe for expectant couples to have penile-vaginal intercourse?
A. Four weeks before the due date

B. Ruptured membranes
C. Multiple gestation
D. Presence of vaginal discharge

442. A postpartal client is HIV positive. Her infant was born at term via vaginal delivery. The newborn is asymptomatic for HIV and is low birth weight. Which of the following discharge goals have greatest priority?
A. Be free of opportunistic or nosocomial infection
B. Maintain physiological homeostasis via nutrition.
C. Identify effects of birth trauma.
D. Promote comfort.

443. A client is in her second trimester and has come to the clinic for her first prenatal visit. She has a history of urinary tract infections. The nurse implements a teaching plan specific to prevention of urinary tract infections. Which statement by the client signifies a need for clarification?
A. "I should wipe from front to back each time I use the bathroom."
B. "Bathing in warm soapy water will help cleanse the perineum."
C. "Wearing cotton underwear will help prevent an infection."
D. "Urinating after intercourse will help to flush out the bacteria."

444. The nurse completes the first expectant parent class on fetal development. Which of the following statements by an expectant mother is accurate regarding fetal development?
A. "At 16 weeks, my baby will receive antibodies from me."
B. "By 20 weeks, I should feel my baby move."
C. "When my baby is 4 weeks old, she can breathe."
D. "My baby can open and close her eyes at 24 weeks."

445. A client is in her first trimester. During a prenatal assessment, the nurse notes which one of the following clinical findings that relates specifically to the first trimester?
A. Increased flatulence
B. Backache
C. Diastasis recti
D. Nasal stuffiness

446. A 36-year-old primipara has just seen her healthcare provider. She is attending an early pregnancy class. Which one of the following statements implies that clarification by the nurse is needed?
A. "I must have a cesarean birth because my pelvis is too small."
B. "I am at risk for preterm labor because of my age."
C. "I need to drink more water when I walk four blocks in the afternoon."
D. "I should see the dentist regularly."

447. A 40-year-old attorney has just received the news that she is pregnant. She states, "I just do not know if I can do this . . . it is not the best time." The nurse's best response is:
    A. "Of course you can; women have babies every day!"
    B. "You have several options. Why don't you review this brochure and give me a call to discuss them in a few days?"
    C. "You sound overwhelmed. Would you like to talk about it?"
    D. "You will have 9 months to get ready, so don't worry."

448. A 30-year-old multipara is 5 cm dilated, zero station, and membranes intact. While in labor, she is changing upright positions every 30 minutes. The nurse recognizes that changing position will:
    A. Intensify the contraction
    B. Increase the risk of cord prolapse
    C. Slow the progress of labor
    D. Increase the need for catheterization

449. After spontaneous rupture of membranes, a laboring client has received an epidural anesthetic to help control her discomfort in labor. Thirty minutes later, the nurse notes the balls of her feet are warm and dry to the touch. The client is concerned about not being able to detect the sensation of the contraction anymore; it is most important for the nurse to:
    A. Verify catheter placement.
    B. Reassure the client.
    C. Reposition the client to the dorsal recumbent position.
    D. Perform vaginal exams every hour to verify progress.

450. A postpartal client is breastfeeding her 1-week-old infant. She is asking how she can decide if the baby is getting enough breast milk?
    A. Encourage her to pump the breast that the baby does not nurse from and measure it.
    B. The newborn will be satisfied with nursing every 4 hours.
    C. Give formula, one feeding per day, and measure amount of intake.
    D. The number of diapers the baby uses daily should be 10 or more.

451. A new mother is planning to return to work next week after her 4-week maternity leave. She wants to reduce the number of breastfeeding sessions and use supplements to feed her newborn while at work. Which comment indicates to the nurse that additional teaching is needed?
    A. "I will introduce the bottle by increasing the number of bottles one per day."
    B. "I will use fruit and cereal as a supplement for my baby."

    C. "My husband will feed her a bottle while I take a walk."
    D. "I will need to pump my breasts at work."

452. A gravida 2 para 1 is to receive epidural anesthesia. The nurse administers to the client a preload of 1000 cc lactated Ringer's IV because the fluid will:
    A. Prevent a postanesthesia headache
    B. Alleviate maternal hypotension
    C. Prevent dehydration
    D. Prevent pruritus

453. A client in labor is 7 cm dilated. She is experiencing low back pain between, as well as during, labor contractions. To increase the client's comfort, the nurse positions the client on her left side. The nurse is aware that the discomfort is related to the:
    A. Presentation of the fetus
    B. Phase of labor
    C. Urinary tract infection
    D. Maternal position

454. A nullipara has been in latent labor over 21 hours. She looks tired. Which of the following approaches by the nurse is best?
    A. Reassure her that her baby will be born soon.
    B. Prepare her for a cesarean birth.
    C. Discourage maternal movement.
    D. Encourage maternal mobility.

455. For a client scheduled to undergo labor induction, the nurse understands that which of the following is a contraindication for oxytocin induction of labor?
    A. Prolonged rupture of membranes
    B. Prolonged pregnancy
    C. Placenta previa
    D. Multipara with a history of rapid deliveries

456. During a home visit, the nurse assesses the uterine height of a primipara client on her third day after delivery. Where should the nurse expect to find it relative to the umbilicus?
    A. 1 cm above
    B. 1 cm below
    C. 4 cm below
    D. 3 cm below

457. Three days' postdelivery, a client calls the clinic to report night sweats and increased urinary output. The nurse should suggest that the client:
    A. Increase her breastfeeding time and increase her fluid intake
    B. Shower as needed and continue with normal fluid intake.
    C. Increase her intake of cranberry juice and try a sitz bath once a day
    D. Take her temperature and take acetaminophen if indicated

458. As the nurse prepares to perform an initial vaginal exam on a client in active labor, a thick, white substance is noted at the introitus. This substance is most likely to be:

A. The mucus plug
B. A portion of the amniotic sac
C. *Candida albicans* exudate
D. Trichomoniasis exudate

459. A client is transferred to the postpartum floor 2 hours after delivering a 7 lb 14 oz healthy male. Her first stage of labor was 26 hours. Her initial postpartum assessment yields a firm fundus, midline, 1 cm above the umbilicus; lochia heavy; and midline, second-degree laceration/episiotomy approximated, with ice pack applied. She states, "I am so tired and my bottom is sore." Which of the following is the most immediate nursing diagnosis for this client?
A. Pain, acute, related to mechanical trauma
B. Risk for infection related to tissue trauma
C. Alteration in urinary elimination related to tissue edema
D. Constipation related to perineal pain

460. The first postpartum assessment for a client is 20 minutes after the delivery of a viable female, 8 lb 2 oz. Vital signs are T 97.6°F; P 100; R 20; BP 110/70; fundus relaxed, 2 cm above the umbilicus; lochia: rubra, moderate to heavy; and bladder is not palpable. The nurse should first:
A. Increase her IV rate to hydrate her.
B. Massage the fundus.
C. Offer the client the bedpan.
D. Carefully reinspect the perineum.

461. A client is 6 cm dilated, 100 percent effaced, −4 station, FHR 130–140. Fifteen minutes after her physician ruptured her membranes, the nurse's assessment is 8 cm, 100 percent effaced, −4 station, FHR 80–100, cord protruding from the vagina. The nurse should first:
A. Call for assistance and prepare for a vaginal delivery.
B. With a gloved hand, carefully exert pressure on the presenting part to relieve cord compression.
C. Place the client in reverse Trendelenburg.
D. Sit her upright to bring the baby down into the pelvis.

462. A 30-year-old G1P1, just spontaneously delivered a viable 7 lb female. After the placenta is delivered, she states she is glad the baby is healthy, although she wanted a boy. Which of the following is the nurse's highest priority at this time?
A. Encouragement of relaxation
B. Promotion of bonding
C. Maintaining comfort
D. Discharge teaching

463. On postpartum day two, a 28-year-old multipara complains of pain in her lower left leg. Which of the following nursing interventions is most pertinent?
A. Massage the affected part.
B. Administer an analgesic and encourage walking.
C. Assess for Homans' sign.
D. Apply an ice pack to minimize the discomfort.

464. A client, gravida III, para II, is 8 months' pregnant. She has been vomiting for 36 hours. Currently, she complains of a headache, blurred vision, and some facial swelling. Vital signs include: T 98.6°F, P 78, R 20, and B/P 150/90 mm Hg. Her urine is 3+ protein. The nurse inserts an indwelling urinary catheter. Which of the following is the best rationale for this intervention?
A. To maintain bedrest
B. To reduce bladder fullness
C. To monitor renal functioning
D. To prevent bladder atony

465. A client is in active labor, 6 cm dilated, when she complains of extreme abdominal pain. The nurse notes a hard abdomen, tender to touch; bright red vaginal bleeding; and FHT of 80 to 90. The nurse knows that which of the following conditions is most conclusive?
A. Complete placenta previa
B. Pregnancy-induced hypertension
C. HELLP syndrome
D. Abruptio placentae

466. A 7 months' pregnant client with pregnancy-induced hypertension is admitted to the unit. She seems quiet and reluctant to talk. When she does talk, she is preoccupied with the well-being of her baby. The nurse knows that which of the following client responses suggests psychological well-being?
A. "I have to watch my diet to control my blood pressure."
B. "I need some time alone to think. I would prefer that my family not visit."
C. "I wonder if something else has happened that the doctor should investigate?'"
D. "I am afraid. I don't know how to help my baby."

467. In an emergency cesarean birth, which of the following nursing actions will facilitate lowering the mother's anxiety?
A. Give the client ample time to be alone.
B. Provide information in explicit detail.
C. Describe the cesarean as an alternate birthing option.
D. Reassure her that her baby will be fine.

468. A client with pregnancy-induced hypertension is in her 33rd week of pregnancy. The drug of choice for treatment of the preterm pre-eclamptic patient is:
A. IV hydralazine
B. IV magnesium sulfate
C. IV labetalol
D. PO diazoxide

469. After breastfeeding instruction, which of the following statements by the client would indicate the need for additional teaching by the nurse?
  A. "I can breastfeed my baby in the delivery room."
  B. "My breasts make colostrum before they make milk."
  C. "The more my baby nurses, the more milk I will produce."
  D. "My first milk, witch's milk, has antibodies to protect my baby."

470. The nurse is making a home visit to a client who was discharged within 24 hours after vaginal delivery with an episiotomy. The client is now 36 hours' postdelivery. The best intervention to promote perineal comfort and healing is to:
  A. Use clean technique when changing the daily peri-pad.
  B. Apply an ice pack for 15 minutes three times a day.
  C. Soak in a warm sitz bath for 15 minutes three times a day.
  D. Use tampons to keep the area clean and dry.

471. After her morning bath, a 1-week postpartum client calls the clinic to report she has experienced a gush of bright red bleeding with large clots. The best explanation for this situation is:
  A. Lochia rubra
  B. Endometritis
  C. Postpartum haemorrhagia
  D. Delayed healing of the episiotomy

472. Which of the following statements indicates additional teaching is needed for the low-risk mother-to-be?
  A. "I cannot have intercourse 2 weeks prior to my due date because it will rupture my membranes."
  B. "Although I have orgasms, it is not harmful to my baby."
  C. "I am not supposed to have intercourse if my membranes rupture."
  D. "I have noticed I am more interested in making love since I have reached my second trimester."

473. A nullipara, 36 weeks' pregnant, calls the clinic to tell the nurse that she is having contractions. Which of the following descriptions indicate false labor?
  A. When changing from resting to activity the contractions persist.
  B. When decreasing activity to resting, the contractions subside.
  C. The contractions progressively increase in strength.
  D. The contractions start in the back and radiate to the lower abdomen.

474. A 33 weeks' pregnant client has uncontrolled pregnancy-induced hypertension. The nurse knows the purpose of giving the client an injection of glucocorticoid 48 hours prior to her scheduled cesarean section is:
  A. To reduce inflammation
  B. To induce fetal lung maturity
  C. To increase placental perfusion
  D. To lower her blood pressure

475. A client in labor has diabetes mellitus. During active labor, the nurse should anticipate which of the following responses?
  A. Stabilization of blood sugar levels
  B. Hyperglycemia
  C. Hypoglycemia
  D. Ketoacidosis

476. A gravida IV, para IV client has given birth to a viable male infant weighing 8 lb 10 oz. The infant was delivered vaginally without complications. The client had a local anesthetic for episiotomy repair. As the placenta is delivered SD, the client begins to shake uncontrollably. The nurse knows that which of the following best explains the client's response?
  A. The client is having a toxic reaction to the anesthetic.
  B. The client is experiencing cerebral edema.
  C. The client is experiencing a sudden release of pressure on the pelvic nerves.
  D. The client is reacting to the anesthesia leaking into a blood vessel.

477. A multigravida client has HELLP syndrome. Which of the following laboratory reports indicates the client's condition has improved?
  A. Hemoglobin: 10 gm/dl
  B. Hematocrit: 40 percent
  C. LDH: 350 ImU/ml
  D. Serum platelets: 90,000/mm^3

478. A couple in their early 30s have been trying to conceive over 5 years with the help of a fertility expert. The couple has just been informed that her recent pregnancy test is negative. Which of the following nursing goals is the most immediate for the couple?
  A. The couple will state that they will continue with infertility treatment.
  B. The couple will verbalize comfort with the negative pregnancy test.
  C. The couple will verbalize their feelings.
  D. The couple will identify factors contributing to the situation.

479. A multipara is transported into the recovery area. The nurse notes that the client's whole body is shaking. Which of the following is the most effective independent intervention for the client?
  A. Ask her to describe how she is feeling.
  B. Cover her with warm blankets.
  C. Administer an ordered IM analgesic.
  D. Administer ordered IM diazepam (Valium).

480. A client is admitted with pregnancy-induced hypertension. Which of the following is an indicator for the nurse to discontinue magnesium sulfate in the client with intrapartal hypertension?
A. The client develops spontaneous bruising.
B. The client develops a warm sensation over her body.
C. The client's last 4 hours of urinary output is 100 cc greater than the previous 4 hours.
D. The client's deep tendon reflexes are 1+.

481. Which of the following behaviors should the nurse expect from the laboring mother during the second stage?
A. The client is walking during her contractions.
B. The client is anxious to see and hold her baby.
C. The client is expressing doubt about her ability to cope with her contractions.
D. The client is irritable and unable to concentrate.

482. A client is now pregnant for the fourth time. She has had one preterm, living baby, and two spontaneous abortions. Using the five-digit system, G-TPAL, which best describes the client's current status?
A. 3-1021
B. 4-0121
C. 4-3121
D. 2-2310

483. During a prenatal clinic visit, it is important for the nurse to initiate a discussion of a birth plan for which of the following reasons?
A. The birth plan will familiarize the expectant mother with how the hospital staff anticipates providing her with health care.
B. The birth plan is often an unrealistic prescription specifying an overall birth goal.
C. The introduction of birth planning provides a tool for parents to explore their childbirth options and identify those that are most important to them.
D. If the parents want any input in their birth experience, a formalized birth plan is developed.

484. A client is 20 weeks' pregnant. The nurse should locate uterine fundal height at the level of the:
A. Symphysis pubis
B. Umbilicus
C. Xiphoid process
D. Ischial spines

485. During a pelvic examination of a primipara in her first trimester, which of the following probable signs are visible?
A. Chadwick's sign
B. Goodell's sign
C. McDonald's sign
D. Piskacek's sign

486. To assess evidence of maternal role acquisition, which behavior should the nurse anticipate finding in the expectant mother?

A. An aversion to certain foods
B. Offering to baby-sit
C. Wearing her regular clothes as long as possible
D. Delaying the reporting of the news to significant others

487. In planning early pregnancy class topics, which of the following should the nurse include?
A. Minor discomforts
B. Distinguishing true labor from false labor
C. Menstrual cycle
D. Labor variations
D. Reassure her that her baby will be fine.

488. During a clinic phone call, a multipara in her last trimester shares that when she awoke this morning her ankles were so swollen that she could not wear her shoes. Her hands and face are puffy. The nurse should next:
A. Assess her intake of water and sodium-rich foods.
B. Review her compliance with taking prescribed diuretics.
C. Determine whether she has had dizzy spells or blackouts.
D. Assess her urinary output.

489. An expectant mother, 28 weeks' pregnant, expresses concern about the birth of her baby. She tells the nurse at the prenatal clinic that she and her partner have herpes simplex, type II (HSV-II). The nurse should
A. Advise her that she will not be able to deliver vaginally.
B. Advise her that her pregnancy will lessen the severity of the disease if it reoccurs.
C. Reassure the client that avoiding public restrooms will prevent disease transmission.
D. Reassure her that a vaginal delivery is possible if the herpes is inactive.

490. A 22-year-old primipara calls the labor unit stating that she is in labor. After reviewing true labor versus false labor with her, it is decided that she will stay home for a while. Which statement reflects that additional teaching is needed?
A. I will come to the hospital when my contractions are 60 seconds long and 3 to 5 minutes apart for 1 hour.
B. I will call the labor unit if I have any questions or concerns.
C. I may take a warm shower if my membranes are intact.
D. If I have a bloody show, I should come to the hospital right away.

491. A 35-year-old primigravida and her husband have been laboring together all night. After a spontaneous rupture of membranes, the nurse notes thick meconium staining in the amniotic fluid. With the couple's consent, a decision is made by the physician to perform a cesarean section.

Which of the following nursing interventions is specific to the diagnosis of anxiety?
A. Promote fetal and maternal well-being
B. Describe the perioperative procedure
C. Discuss feelings about previous childbirth expectations
D. Administer sedatives or perioperative narcotics

492. A 15-year-old primipara, 38 weeks' pregnant, is concerned about how often she should feel the baby move. The nurse's best response is:
A. "The baby slows down toward the end of your pregnancy. Do not be surprised if you do not feel any movement at all."
B. "You should feel at least 10 fetal movements for 2 days in a row."
C. "Has anything happened that could affect the baby?"
D. "When was the last time you remember the baby moving?"

493. The nurse plans to review nutrition in pregnancy with a multipara. Additional teaching is needed if the client states:
A. "My daily requirement of vitamins will come from the prenatal vitamins, so basically I can eat what I like."
B. "The greener the leafy vegetable and the redder the meat, the greater the iron content."
C. "Fresh fruits and vegetables are better than canned."
D. "I should not eat a bran muffin after I take my iron tablet."

494. A 35-year-old multigravida is in her first trimester. During a routine prenatal visit, she expresses concern about her baby because she has a couple glasses of wine to help her sleep every night. The nurse should respond:
A. "Difficulty sleeping is usually associated with the first trimester. A glass of wine every now and then is OK."
B. "You are addicted to alcohol and are threatening the life of your unborn child."
C. "Have you thought about taking rest periods throughout the day?"
D. "It took courage for you to share that with me today."

495. A multigravida has been in labor for 3 hours. She is 3 cm dilated, at −4 station, contractions are regular and strong, and fetal heart rate range is 130 to 150. The physician ruptures the membranes. The most likely outcome is:
A. Labor progression
B. Prolapsed umbilical cord
C. Vaginal delivery
D. Amniotic fluid embolism

496. The nursing assessment of a laboring client reveals: dilation, 5 cm; effacement, 80 percent; station, 0; presentation, vertex; membranes, ruptured; contractions, 3 to 5 minutes apart, 60 seconds long. The client is uncomfortable during her contractions but relaxing well in between. She wants to walk to the nursery to see the newborns. The nurse's best response is:
A. "Walking will stimulate the uterus to contract and a change of scenery will help."
B. "Because your membranes are ruptured, you cannot walk around because of the risk of cord prolapse."
C. "I know you are getting tired, why don't you get in the whirlpool?"
D. "Would you like me to call for your epidural now before it is too late?"

497. A nullipara, 18 years' old, is in labor. Her pelvis is determined to be gynecoid in shape. The nurse identifies what effect this pelvis shape will have on her labor?
A. Transverse arrest is common.
B. There may be delay at the inlet.
C. There will be good uterine function with spontaneous delivery.
D. The fetus is often in occiput posterior position.

498. A 30-year-old multipara with a normal pregnancy comes to the clinic in her ninth month with the following symptoms: decreased epigastric pressure, low backache, increased pelvic pressure, constipation, and urinary frequency. The most important nursing action is to:
A. Determine if dilation and effacement have occurred.
B. Encourage increased fluid intake.
C. Determine her current vital signs.
D. Explain that the sensation she describes is lightening.

499. During an initial vaginal examination of a multigravida at term, the nurse assesses that the fetal presenting part is at the level of the ischial spines. The nurse knows that which of the following has occurred?
A. Engagement
B. Lightening
C. Floating
D. Dipping

500. A nullipara client is in labor. The nursing assessment yields the following: contractions, 3 to 5 minutes apart; fetal heart tones (FHT), 130 to 140; dilation, 2 cm; effacement, 50 percent; station, −4. Which of the following outcomes is most consistent with the data assessed?
A. Dysfunctional labor is more common with a low station.
B. Rapid descent of a high fetal head is dangerous and abnormal.
C. Clients who start labor with high fetal station usually have lesser degrees of cervical dilation.
D. The incidence of pelvic disproportion is greater when the head is low at the beginning of labor.

501. After the nurse teaches a client about the use of a diaphragm with a spermicide, which of the following comments by the client would indicate understanding?

A. "I can use a petroleum-based lubricant to insert my diaphragym."

B. "The diaphragm combined with the spermicide increases my risk of pelvic inflammatory disease."

C. "The diaphragm and spermicide provide some protection against cervicitis and reduce my risk for cervical cancer."

D. "I must remove the diaphragm immediately after intercourse."

502. To determine the teaching effectiveness of a class on human reproduction, the nurse identifies which of the following statements by the client indicates additional teaching is needed?

A. "The ovaries produce estrogen."

B. "The fallopian tubes facilitate the movement of the fertilized ovum to the uterus."

C. "Only one sperm can fertilize an egg."

D. "The female clitoris is comparable to the male testes."

503. A multigravida is in second-stage labor. Which of the following nursing interventions is most effective at this time?

A. Wake the client at the beginning of her contractions.

B. Keep the client informed as she dilates and effaces.

C. Encourage the client to assume a position of comfort to bear down.

D. Encourage the client to void every 1 to 2 hours.

504. An Rh-negative nullipara has just spontaneously aborted after 10 weeks' gestation. Her partner is Rh-positive. Which of the following nursing actions is most relevant?

A. Observe the client for jaundice and fever.

B. Administer ordered Rh immunoglobulin to client.

C. Administer ordered Rh immunoglobulin to her partner.

D. Monitor the development of maternal antibody development.

505. A client's newborn is diagnosed with phenylketonuria (PKU), an inborn error of metabolism. The best explanation by the nurse is that:

A. Both genes of each parent are abnormal for this disorder to be expressed.

B. The abnormal gene is expressed even though it is linked with a normal gene.

C. The disorder is related to X-linked recessive inheritance.

D. The disorder is related to multifactor inheritance.

506. A postpartum client is asking for the specific rationale for doing pelvic floor (Kegel) exercises. The best response by the nurse is:

A. To increase emotional well-being

B. To strengthen the muscles of the pelvic floor

C. To increase intestinal peristalsis

D. To reduce the amount of lochia formation

507. A 30-year-old multigravida is in the clinic for prenatal care. She has a history of urinary tract infections. After the nurse determines that the client has a sufficient fluid intake, the nurse should next:

A. Review pelvic floor exercises and stress her ability to suppress urinary frequency.

B. Encourage fluid restriction before intercourse.

C. Review the importance of urinating before going to sleep at night.

D. Encourage the client to gradually hold her urine for longer time periods.

508. To determine if client teaching was effective for healthy urinary practices, which of the following outcomes would be reached?

A. The client drinks 1 quart of fluid a day.

B. The client wears cotton panties.

C. The client bathes every day.

D. The client is free from urinary tract infections.

509. An expectant mother, a 25-year-old nullipara, is a musician. She states during a routine, last trimester, prenatal visit that her hands tingle and she has been dropping things at home and work. The client believes her condition is worsening because she has experienced numbness in her hands over the past week. Which of the following is the best nursing diagnosis?

A. Impaired gas exchange

B. Risk for injury

C. Risk for decompensation of cardiac output

D. Risk for activity intolerance.

510. A 40-year-old primipara gave birth to a healthy baby girl 3 days ago. The nurse recognizes which of the following mother-infant interactions as the most positive?

A. The mother refers to the infant as "he."

B. The mother rooms in with her, pumps her breasts, and asks the nurse to bottle-feed her infant.

C. The mother allows relatives and friends to hold the baby.

D. The mother seeks out the source of the infant's discomfort when she cries.

511. To assess newborn behaviors that positively impact parental attachment, the nurse should observe for:

A. A sleepy infant with eyes closed most of the time

B. An infant who seeks attention from anyone in the room

C. An infant with an unpredicatable sleep-wake schedule

D. An infant with differential crying and vocalizing

512. A 30-year-old multigravida is breastfeeding for the first time. The client alerts the nurse to the small

gush of lochia she experienced during abdominal cramping. The best action by the nurse is to
A. Explain that breastfeeding facilitates uterine involution.
B. Return the infant to the nursery to allow the client to rest.
C. Assess the client's vital signs.
D. Administer a prescribed, mild analgesic.

513. After teaching a breastfeeding class, the nurse recognizes which of the following statements indicate that the client has a satisfactory understanding of basic breastfeeding?
A. "Breastfed infants require sugar water supplements until the mother's milk comes in."
B. "I should carefully cleanse the breasts and nipples with warm, soapy water."
C. "To prevent sore nipples, I should position my infant on her side facing my breast."
D. "Breastfeeding mothers lose weight more slowly because of their increased caloric intake."

514. A client has had a vaginal delivery with an epidural anesthetic. Which of the following symptoms would the nurse identify as a risk for hypovolemic shock?
A. A blood loss of 350 cc
B. A placenta that is delivered 30 minutes after the infant
C. Hypertension and headache
D. Tachycardia and hypotension

515. During a postpartum examination of a client 3 days' post vaginal delivery, the nurse would expect the lochia to be:
A. Rubra with clots
B. Serosa
C. Alba
D. Absent

516. Six hours after a vaginal delivery, a client expresses the desire to void for the first time. What nursing action will ascertain that the client is adequately emptying her bladder?
A. Ambulate her to the bathroom.
B. Palpate the suprapubic area for bladder fullness.
C. Catheterize the bladder.
D. Measure the volume of voided urine.

517. A primipara delivered a healthy newborn 1 hour ago. She wants to breastfeed her infant. The nurse should encourage her to:
A. Wait several hours until the infant has physiologically stabilized.
B. Express her milk into a bottle for feeding.
C. Put the infant to breast and support her efforts.
D. Determine if her let-down reflex is present.

518. Which of the following is accurate when identifying content to teach the postpartum client self-care?

A. Wash the perineum at least once a day with mild soap and water.
B. Avoid using soap and water on the perineum.
C. Tampons will provide the greatest absorption and comfort.
D. Change the pad only when it is completely saturated.

519. A 6-week postpartum client reports to the clinic on her scheduled first postpartum clinic appointment. During the examination, the nurse notes that the client's lochia is red with numerous clots and has a strong odor. Which of the following approaches by the nurse is best?
A. Provide her with perineal care.
B. Assess the amount of lochia.
C. Assess the status of uterine involution.
D. Instruct the client in perineal care.

520. A gravida II para II is 4 days' postdelivery. She has received IV antibiotics since the first postpartum day for an initial temperature of 101.8°F. Her present vital signs are temperature, 99.9°F; pulse, 100; respirations, 20; blood pressure, 110/70. The client denies anorexia and malaise. The uterus is 4 cm below the umbilicus. Her lochia is serosal with clots and has a fleshy odor. The nurse identifies the most likely source of her temperature elevation to be:
A. Endometritis
B. Pelvic thrombophlebitis
C. Toxic shock syndrome
D. Chorioamnionitis

521. A postpartum client is diagnosed with endometritis. Which of the following nursing actions will enhance the drainage of the uterine cavity?
A. Placing the client in a semi-Fowler's position
B. Placing the client in a modified Sims' position
C. Administering a vaginal irrigation
D. Assessing fundal contractibility

522. To ensure that the postpartal client does not develop an infection, the nurse plans for the best prenatal treatment modality to:
A. Administer a prescribed prophylactic round of antibiotic therapy.
B. Ensure good prenatal nutrition.
C. Encourage adequate fluid intake.
D. Ultrasound the uterus once per trimester.

523. A client calls to report that she has missed one of her daily doses of oral contraceptives. The best response by the nurse is to instruct the client to:
A. Take the missed dose immediately and take the next dose at the regularly scheduled time.
B. Take the missed dose at the regularly scheduled time and use a condom during intercourse until the end of her cycle.
C. Stop taking the pills and restart the cycle 5 days after bleeding begins.
D. Take two pills now and take one at the next scheduled time.

524. When the nurse is providing client education about family planning, which of the following client statements regarding oral contraceptives indicates that additional teaching is needed?
    A. "I have a greater risk for cardiovascular problems if I am over 35 or smoke."
    B. "Even though I have had liver damage from hepatitis, I can safely take the pill."
    C. "I should see my clinician immediately if I develop chest pain or shortness of breath."
    D. "I should expect to have less menstrual cramping and decreased pain at the time of ovulation."

525. When counseling clients for family planning, the nurse knows that for which of the following clients is an intrauterine device (IUD) contraindicated?
    A. A multigravida with a history of thrombophlebitis
    B. A 26-year-old gravida I para I with irregular menses
    C. A 35-year-old gravida II para II who smokes
    D. A 17-year-old nullipara with multiple sex partners

526. In reviewing a 24-hour nutrition diary, the nurse should check that which of the following foods is present for evidence of folic acid (folacin) intake in the expectant mother?
    A. Citrus fruits, green peppers, and strawberries
    B. Egg yolk, fish oil, and liver
    C. Skim milk, dried beans, and cheese
    D. Green leafy vegetables, whole wheat bread, and kidney beans

527. While reviewing data from the prenatal client's nutritional assessment, which of the following will alert the nurse to a maternal risk factor?
    A. A client who has had three or more pregnancies within 3 years
    B. A client with a maternal age of 30 years
    C. A client who exercises 30 minutes three times a week
    D. A client with a hemoglobin of 12 gms/dl

528. When reviewing the differing types of anemia, the nurse knows that the pregnant client is at greatest risk for:
    A. Iron deficiency anemia
    B. Folic acid deficiency anemia
    C. Thalassemia
    D. Hemoglobin C disease

529. In planning nursing care for the client with pregnancy-induced hypertension (PIH), which of the following is true?
    A. The majority of fetal deaths are related to nutritional deficits found in the mother.
    B. The PIH client is susceptible to blood loss at delivery.
    C. The epigastric pain associated with the PIH client is related to increased acid reflux.
    D. Vascular changes are limited to the placenta.

530. The nurse's assessment of a prenatal client's edema is 3+. This indicates that the client has
    A. Minimal edema at pedal and pretibial sites
    B. Marked edema of the lower extremities
    C. Evident edema in her face, hands, lower abdominal wall, and sacrum
    D. Generalized edema and massive with ascites

531. Which of the following laboratory values indicates a positive change in the client with PIH? *proteinuria HTN*
    A. An increase in blood urea nitrogen (BUN)
    B. An increase in hematocrit
    C. An increase in serum glutamic-oxaloacetic transaminase (SGOT)
    D. An increase in platelets

532. The nurse should observe the client receiving magnesium sulfate for magnesium toxicity, which would include:
    A. Respirations below 12 per minute
    B. Hyperreflexia
    C. Urinary output greater than 50 cc/hr
    D. CNS stimulation

533. A gravida II para I calls the unit to report that she is in active labor. The nurse should expect her contraction pattern to be:
    A. 15 to 30 minutes apart, lasting 30 seconds
    B. 3 to 5 minutes apart, lasting 60 seconds
    C. 2 to 3 minutes apart, lasting 90 seconds
    D. 2 to 3 minutes apart, lasting 60 seconds

534. A prenatal client, 32 weeks' gestation, has uncontrolled premature labor. A regimen of antenatal corticosteroids is recommended by her physician. After the physician leaves the room, the client asks the nurse to clarify how corticosteroids work. The best response by the nurse is:
    A. "Let met get your physician to answer that question for you."
    B. "The mechanism of action is unknown but produces consistently good results."
    C. "At this time in your baby's development, she does not have surfactant in her lungs. Without surfactant the air sacs collapse and cause lung damage. This medication stimulates the lungs to produce the needed surfactant."
    D. "Corticosteroids suppress the inflammatory response mechanism of the immune system. This suppression activates the trigger for surfactant production in the fetal lung."

535. A nullipara in her third trimester expresses concern about the dreams she has been having about her unborn baby. Which of the following responses by the nurse is best?
    A. "These dreams are normal. All expectant mothers have them."
    B. "I would not worry about the dreams. Have you investigated child care for your baby when you return to work?"
    C. "Tell me more about your dreams."

D. "Have you monitored what you eat before you go to sleep at night?"

536. The nurse is preparing a gravida II para II for discharge. Which one of the following is most important for the client to know before she returns home?
A. Signs and symptoms of postpartum blues
B. Community support for new parents
C. Immunization schedule for the newborn
D. Warning signs for hemorrhage, infection, and dehydration

537. A third-trimester client and her partner are undergoing an ultrasound examination on the antenatal unit of a community hospital. The desired outcome is that the client will:
A. Verbalize an independent decision regarding diagnoses.
B. Verbalize fears and concerns related to the outcome of the ultrasound.
C. Identify signs requiring medical evaluation.
D. Participate in screening procedures.

538. A gravida II para I client, at term, is admitted to the unit with vaginal bleeding. The best nursing action is to:
A. Assess dilation, effacement, and station.
B. Assess the amount, duration, and onset of vaginal bleeding
C. Determine if membranes are intact.
D. Determine if labor is in progress.

539. In discussing outcomes with a client with a low-lying placenta previa at 20 weeks, the nurse should inform the client to expect:
A. A cesarean birth
B. The placenta to migrate upward, away from the cervical os
C. A placenta abruptio to develop
D. A spontaneous abortion

540. A gravida III para III has delivered a healthy newborn. In recovery, the nurse notes that the client's placenta was diagnosed as low lying. Because of the client's history, which of the following nursing measures is most important in her immediate postpartum care?
A. Assess nature and degree of discomfort.
B. Assess for uncontrollable shaking.
C. Assess blood pressure and pulse every 15 minutes.
D. Assess location and consistency of fundus every 15 minutes.

541. A laboring client who has an IV solution of lactated Ringer's infusing at 125 cc/hr is complaining of sharp abdominal pain. During the assessment, the nurse notes the following information: profuse, bright red vaginal bleeding; fundus, firm and rounded; fetal heart rate, 60; contractions, absent. Which one of the following nursing interventions is most important?

A. Increase IV rate and start another IV of normal saline.
B. Determine effacement and dilation.
C. Perform Leopold's maneuvers.
D. Reposition the client on her left side.

542. A client presents in the labor unit with profuse, bright red bleeding. The fundus is firm and rounded, contractions are absent, and the fetal heart rate (FHR) is 80. The first nursing intervention is to:
A. Notify the family members.
B. Prepare the client for an emergency cesarean birth.
C. Determine the source of the bleeding.
D. Reassess the status of the FHR and contractions using an external fetal monitor for at least 20 minutes.

543. A client, gravida VIII para VII, is admitted to the labor unit. Her contractions are irregular; dilation, 4 cm; effacement, 50 percent. The nurse should anticipate which of the following?
A. Cesarean birth to control the delivery
B. Postpartum hemorrhage
C. Labor induction
D. Retained placenta

544. A laboring client is noted to have meconium staining when her membranes spontaneously rupture. The nurse accurately identifies that which of the following is a major factor in meconium-stained amniotic fluid?
A. Multiple gestation
B. Maternal upright position
C. Placenta anomalies
D. Fetal hypoxia

545. A client is experiencing labor dystocia. Which of the following is least likely to be associated with labor dystocia?
A. Ineffective uterine contractions
B. Pelvic diameters
C. Fetal bradycardia
D. Maternal psyche

546. After teaching human reproduction, which of the following client statements indicates a clear understanding of sex determination of the newborn?
A. "My diet during my pregnancy will determine the baby's sex."
B. "My husband's chromosomes determine the baby's sex."
C. "The way I carry my baby determines the sex of the child."
D. "If I dream about girls, the baby will be a girl."

547. A 21-year-old primipara has given birth to a fair-haired baby boy. She expresses to the nurse that she is disappointed. She thought her baby would be dark-haired, like herself, and that her family was expecting a girl. Which of the following nursing interventions conveys the nurse's understanding of the mother's immediate need?

A. Give the mother time alone with her infant.
B. Restrict family visitation.
C. Reassure her that her response is normal.
D. Ask another new mother to come and talk with her prior to discharge.

548. A couple is talking to the nurse about family planning. The primary task of the nurse as it relates to family planning is to:
A. Assess the couple's needs and suggest a limited number of alternatives from which they can choose.
B. Present an objective evaluation of options from which the couple can select.
C. Determine who will have the primary responsibility and assign decision making to that person.
D. Suggest use of the method with the highest rate of effectiveness.

549. During an early prenatal check-up, the nurse is reviewing the nutritional requirements with the expectant mother. Her diet assessment reveals a well-balanced intake. The nurse should reinforce additional intake of which of the following?
A. Vitamins A and D
B. Sodium
C. Vitamin C
D. Iron and folic acid

550. A nullipara, 40 years' old, is scheduled to have a diagnostic procedure to determine if any fetal anomalies are present. The nurse knows that which of the following tests screens for fetal neural tube defects?
A. Amniocentesis
B. Chorionic villi sampling
C. Alpha-fetoprotein
D. Coombs' test

551. Which of the following client statements indicates a clear understanding of the guidelines for exercise during pregnancy?
A. "My center of gravity is offset, and I have an increased risk of falling when I play tennis."
B. "To strengthen my abdominal muscles, I will do a set of 10 double leg lifts."
C. "I only need to drink water before my workout."
D. "If I get hip pain while walking, I should continue; no pain—no gain."

552. A client prepared by the Dick-Read method is in labor. Which of the following behaviors should the nurse expect from the client?
A. The use of a variety of paced breathing and relaxation techniques with labor support
B. The primary use of abdominal breathing during uterine contractions
C. Low lights in delivery
D. Positive affirmations and self-hypnosis

553. A prepared couple in early labor asks their nurse if they should call their family to come to the hospital while they labor. The best response by the nurse is:
A. "Often family members do not understand what is going on and they get in the way."
B. "It is advisable to only have two family members in your room at a time."
C. "How will your family be supportive of your efforts?"
D. "Have you considered asking them to come after the baby is born?"

554. A term client is admitted to the labor unit with severe, unstable PIH. After assessing the client's CNS involvement, the nurse minimizes the client's risk for injury by:
A. Providing a quiet environment with limited visitors
B. Monitoring oral intake
C. Assessing the client's level of knowledge
D. Providing information on the effect of bedrest on protein requirements

555. After the nurse reviews activity limitations with a high-risk pregnancy client, which of the following statements indicates additional teaching is necessary?
A. "I can travel by car in my last trimester if I get up and walk around every 4 hours or so."
B. "I should avoid sexual activity if I have low back pain."
C. "I should avoid traveling by plane."
D. "I will ask my family to do my Christmas shopping for me."

556. While interviewing a 15-year-old nullipara, the nurse realizes that the client used several words that were unclear and ambiguous. The nurse should:
A. Ask the client for clarification.
B. Ask the client to use words that the nurse understands.
C. Use the words while interacting with the client to gain credibility.
D. Make a note of the words and ask staff for clarification.

557. A prenatal client with a class II level of cardiac functioning is receiving digitalis glycosides. The nurse should monitor her for
A. PIH
B. Premature labor
C. Fetal tachycardia
D. Placental insufficiency

558. The nurse recognizes which of the following drugs should be used with caution in the third stage of labor in a client with cardiac disease?
A. Digitalis glycoside
B. Aminophylline
C. Nitroglycerine
D. Oxytocin

559. In a client with PIH receiving magnesium sulfate therapy, which of the following medications should the nurse have on hand?
A. Calcium gluconate
B. Methylergonovine
C. Morphine sulfate
D. Ergonovine

560. In the prenatal client with PIH, which of the following signs alerts the nurse to CNS involvement?
A. Decreased urinary output
B. Increased urinary output
C. Dyspnea
D. Headache

561. In the client with gestational diabetes mellitus, which of the following is a teaching priority for the nurse whose client is in the first trimester?
A. Discuss the signs and symptoms of hypoglycemia.
B. Discuss the client's risk for hyperglycemia.
C. Review the cause of ketoacidosis.
D. Discuss the need to limit physical activity.

562. Which of the following laboratory values should the nurse monitor in a client with gestational diabetes?
A. Fibrinogen levels
B. Hemoglobin and hematocrit
C. Estrogen levels
D. Lactic acid dehydrogenase (LDH)

563. The normal blood pressure range for a prepregnant client is 120/80. During this client's second trimester, the nurse anticipates her blood pressure to approximate which of the following?
A. 100/60
B. 80/40
C. 140/100
D. 120/80

564. In the third-trimester prenatal client with a nursing diagnosis of high risk for infection, urinary tract, which of the following is the most accurate rationale for urine testing?
A. Proteinuria suggests an increase in white blood cells.
B. Often, pregnant clients have asymptomatic bacteriuria.
C. Inadequate output concentrates the bacteria content of the urine.
D. Verification of diabetes.

565. In planning care for the prenatal client with bacteriuria, the nurse recognizes that the client is at risk for which of the following?
A. Protracted active labor
B. Cesarean birth
C. Preterm labor
D. Relaxation of the pelvic floor

566. To which of the following nursing diagnosis should the nurse assign highest priority for the client with hyperemesis gravidarum?

A. Altered health maintenance
B. Potential fluid volume deficit
C. Risk for fatigue
D. Risk for infection

567. The nurse is interacting with a couple seeking genetic counseling for the first time. Which of the following nursing actions has highest priority?
A. Review diagnostic procedures.
B. Refer to counseling.
C. Provide information about their specific genetic disorder.
D. Assess the nature, origin, and symptoms of their anxiety.

568. Once the couple seeking genetic counseling has been provided with information about diagnostic procedures, the next nursing intervention is to:
A. Refer them to community support groups.
B. Permit the couple to arrive at their own decision about testing.
C. Schedule the tests that will yield the best results.
D. Encourage the couple to make their decision as timely as possible.

569. Which of the following should the nurse suggest that the prenatal client experiencing urinary frequency omit from her diet?
A. 8 to 10 glasses of water per day
B. Cola beverages
C. Acidic fruit juices
D. Dairy products

570. Which of the following self-care practices for hemorrhoids and constipation should the nurse suggest that the client in her first trimester eliminate?
A. Eating a diet high in fiber
B. Elevating her buttocks on a pillow
C. Drinking coffee in the morning
D. Using ice packs for comfort

571. A client at 24 weeks' gestation is questioning the need for a glucose tolerance test (GTT). The best response by the nurse is:
A. "This test will indicate if your baby will have diabetes."
B. "GTT indicates the adequacy of your body to maintain this pregnancy."
C. "The GTT screens for gestational diabetes mellitus. This condition is associated with large babies and difficult labors."
D. "The outcome of the GTT will tell us the amount of your unique caloric need."

572. A client in her second trimester has varicosities of the legs and vulva. Which of the following measures would make the problem worse?
A. Wearing knee-high stockings
B. Wearing loose clothing
C. Elevating her hips and legs for 20 minutes three times a day
D. Dorisflexing her feet while sitting long periods at work

573. While weighing a second-trimester client, she states, "I do not understand why I must get weighed every time I come for a check-up. I just hate it." Which of the following is the best response by the nurse?
    A. "I have never met an expectant mother who enjoyed getting weighed."
    B. "I know it is not pleasant seeing yourself put on this weight, but it comes with the pregnancy."
    C. "Are you feeling guilty about not taking care of yourself?"
    D. "Our concern at this point in your pregnancy is detection of a sudden increase in weight."

574. While discussing discomforts of pregnancy with a primigravida, she asks when should she have Braxton Hicks contractions. The best response by the nurse is:
    A. "Women who are having babies for the first time generally note Braxton Hicks contractions in the first trimester."
    B. "Most women note second-trimester Braxton Hicks contractions."
    C. "The majority of primigravidas notice Braxton Hicks contractions in their third trimester."
    D. "Primigravidas do not experience Braxton Hicks contractions."

575. Which of the following positions should the nurse recommend to the third-trimester client experiencing altered urinary elimination?
    A. Supine
    B. Sitting upright
    C. Standing
    D. Left lateral

576. Which of the following types of exercise should the nurse suggest for the client in her third trimester?
    A. Swimming
    B. Race-walking
    C. Tennis
    D. Horseback riding

577. The nurse should anticipate that the multigravida who is dehydrated will evidence this by:
    A. A decrease in blood urea nitrogen (BUN)
    B. An increase in hematocrit
    C. A decrease in hematocrit
    D. Oligohydramnios

578. A multigravida shares that she is an alcoholic and her husband validates this. She wants to stop drinking now that she is pregnant and requests a referral to a clinic for disulfiram (Antabuse). The best action by the nurse is to:
    A. Support her decision to stop drinking and refer her the alcohol treatment center for her disulfiram.
    B. Determine the couple's need for family therapy.
    C. Describe the outcome of fetal alcohol syndrome.
    D. Explain that the safety of disulfiram has not been established for pregnancy.

579. When selecting a position for the prenatal client with vaginal bleeding, which of the following positions is contraindicated?
    A. Semi-Fowler's
    B. Supine with elevated hips
    C. Trendelenburg
    D. Left lateral

580. In the prenatal client with a positive gonorrhea infection, the nurse knows which of the following is true?
    A. Up to 30 percent of infants will contract gonorrhea during the passage through the birth canal.
    B. The majority of woman are symptomatic.
    C. Gonorrhea causes few problems for the postpartal client.
    D. Once a female has had gonorrhea and recovered, she will not become reinfected.

581. What is the purpose of giving the multigravida client who is a carrier of group B β-hemolytic streptococcus (GBS) antibiotics in her 39th week of pregnancy?
    A. To minimize the teratogenic effect on the fetus
    B. To maintain a peak drug level in the newborn
    C. To prevent recolonization of the bacteria (GBS)
    D. To prevent the development of a secondary, opportunistic viral infection in the mother

582. After teaching a client who had a McDonald's procedure, which of the following statements suggests to the nurse the need for further instruction?
    A. "If I feel contractions, I should limit my activity."
    B. "I will have a contraction stress test in my third trimester."
    C. "Immediately after the procedure, I should stay on bedrest for 48 hours."
    D. "I will report any fluid leaking to my healthcare provider."

583. A 25-year-old nullipara in the first trimester has been diagnosed with fetal demise. The products of conception have not been expelled for 6 weeks. Her laboratory values are: prothrombin time, elevated; fibrinogen levels, decreased; estrogen and progesterone levels, low. Because of the client's health status, which of the following indicates to the nurse that the client is at risk?
    A. Infertility
    B. HELLP syndrome
    C. Disseminated intravascular disease (DIC)
    D. Pre-eclampsia

584. To evaluate client teaching, which of the following statements by the client to the nurse indicates the best understanding of self-care to prevent a postabortion infection?
    A. "I may use tampons to absorb any vaginal bleeding."

B. "I should not have vaginal intercourse, but oral-vaginal sex is permissible."
C. "I may take baths as long as they are not too hot."
D. "I should call the clinic if my temperature is over 100.4°F."

585. A client who is 32 weeks' gestation is admitted to the labor unit for observation. She has been experiencing irregular contractions. The client's vital signs are: blood pressure, 128/80; pulse, 90; respirations, 20. The nurse recognizes which of the following as the best rationale for administering IV fluids to this client?
A. Hydration may decrease uterine irritability.
B. An IV line will provide access for medication in case of an emergency.
C. Hydration will promote renal clearance.
D. Hydration will reduce hypotension.

586. A client in preterm labor has been receiving terbutaline sulfate via an infusion pump for 8 hours. During an assessment, the nurse notes the following: contractions: mild, irregular, diminishing in number; blood pressure, 140/90; pulse, 100; respirations, 24, labored; breath sounds, rales. Which of the following nursing actions is indicated?
A. Increase the IV rate of infusion.
B. Stop the IV.
C. Monitor deep tendon reflexes.
D. Continue assessment of uterine contractions.

587. The nurse understands that which of the following conditions in a client experiencing preterm labor would likely prohibit steroid therapy to promote fetal lung maturity?
A. Multiple gestation
B. PIH
C. Placenta previa
D. Hyperemesis gravidarum

588. A client in early labor is admitted to the unit with ruptured membranes, irregular contractions, and diarrhea. The client reports that her bag of waters broke 5 hours ago and describes her amniotic fluid as straw-tinged with a noticeable odor. Which of the following nursing measures is most important?
A. Provide perineal care every 4 hours or as needed.
B. Monitor temperature, pulse, respirations, and white blood count.
C. Provide a bolus of oral fluids.
D. Monitor intake and output.

589. A laboring client is 5 cm dilated, 75 percent effaced, and at 0 station. Membranes have spontaneously ruptured. Her contractions are 3 to 5 minutes part, lasting 60 seconds. Her vital signs are: blood pressure, 120/84; temperature, 101.4°F; pulse, 88; respirations, 20. The fetal heart rate (FHR) ranges between 170 and 190. The nurse understands that which of the following factors best explains the increase in FHR?

A. Active labor
B. Maternal anxiety
C. Maternal fever
D. Cord prolapse

590. The results of fetal scalp blood test indicate a pH of 7.2. These results indicate which of the following?
A. A cesarean birth is indicated.
B. Routine fetal monitoring is appropriate and a repeat test should be done when fetal heart rate drops.
C. Constant fetal monitoring is necessary and a repeat test should be done within 30 minutes.
D. Fetal monitoring as needed is correct protocol.

591. A nullipara client in late active labor has an increased vaginal bloody show. The nurse knows that the change is indicate of:
A. Fetal descent
B. Placenta previa
C. Rupture of membranes
D. Crowning

592. A nullipara client and her partner are practicing prepared childbirth techniques. The client is in late active labor. They are in the process of deciding if the client should get an epidural. They have asked the nurse for an opinion. The best response by the nurse is:
A. "Most of our laboring mothers do receive some medication or anesthesia."
B. "This is your first baby, you have no idea how intense the pain will become."
C. "You both have worked so hard. Enjoy your labor; get the epidural."
D. "Why don't I find out your progress at this point, and then you can make a decision."

593. After examining a primigravida who is 8 cm dilated, 100 percent effaced, and at 0 station, she tells the nurse that she needs to push. The best response by the nurse is to:
A. Assist the client to the lithotomy position.
B. Encourage her to take a deep breath, hold it, and bear down.
C. Reposition her to a lateral position and encourage her to pant.
D. Re-examine her.

594. A client in the transitional phase of labor is "sleeping" between contractions. She tells the nurse she is having difficulty remembering who just spoke to her. The best action by the nurse is to:
A. Inform her when the contractions begin.
B. Decrease the environmental stimuli and encourage her to sleep.
C. Administer oxygen per nasal cannula.
D. Increase her IV Infusion rate.

595. The multigravida in transition announces to the nurse and her husband that "she is tired and wants to go home." The best response by the nurse is to:

A. Ask the husband to step outside and ask the client what is wrong.

B. After informing the client of her current progress, encourage her to deal with one contraction at a time.

C. Inform her that there is no turning back at this point.

D. Encourage her husband to distract her by discussing names for the baby.

596. A multigravida, completely dilated and at 0 station, begins to push. What type of behavior should the nurse anticipate from the client?
A. Relieved, eager to push
B. Withdrawn, internally focused
C. Anxious and uncertain
D. Passive and easily directed

597. During labor contractions, the nurse notes that the client is exhibiting clenched fists and jaw. The best action by the nurse is to:
A. Remind the client that pain and tension are cyclic.
B. Ambulate the client to distract her.
C. Assess the client's level of discomfort.
D. Massage the areas of tension and verbally remind her to release the tension.

598. A multigravida client delivered her baby after a prolonged second stage. After some difficulty with placenta removal, the uterus inverted. Which of the following nursing interventions is critical?
A. Place the client in Trendelenburg.
B. Administer volume replacement.
C. Administer ergonovine (Ergotrate) IM.
D. Aggressive fundal massage.

599. A term nullipara is having frequent mild contractions. Her contractions have shorter intervals. The fetal monitor shows a uterine resting tone of 20 mm Hg. She is 2 cm dilated and 20 percent effaced with intact membranes. Which of the following nursing measures is indicated?
A. Ambulate the client.
B. Position the client in semi-Fowler's.
C. Administer prescribed oxytocin.
D. Administer a prescribed narcotic analgesic.

600. After examining a labor client, the nurse determines that the fetal head is left occiput posterior. The next nursing intervention should be to:
A. Prepare the client for a cesarean birth.
B. Have the client assume hands-and-knees position.
C. Observe for occult cord prolapse.
D. Assess fetal heart rate.

601. A gravida III para II, 28 years' old, has vaginally delivered a healthy newborn after a 12-hour labor with an epidural. Which of the following factors places the client at high risk for fluid volume deficit?
A. The length of labor

B. The client's gravity and parity
C. The client's age
D. The epidural anesthesia

602. In the postpartum client with altered tissue perfusion, which of the following nursing measures would be least effective?
A. Gently massaging a soft uterus
B. Applying firm downward pressure on the fundus
C. Encouraging the client to void
D. Positioning the client in lateral recumbent

603. A multigravida with a midline episiotomy is admitted to recovery following the birth of her infant. She verbalizes perianal discomfort. Which of the following nursing measures will best enhance the client's comfort?
A. Apply a warm, moist compress to the episiotomy site.
B. Spray her perineum with a topical analgesic-antiseptic.
C. Apply an ice pack to the perineal area.
D. Apply dry heat to the perineal site.

604. During the first postpartum assessment of a gravida II para II, the nurse should note which of the following to be within normal limits?
A. Breasts firm
B. Breasts soft without tenderness
C. Fundus firm, 2 cm below the umbilicus
D. Lochia alba, scant, and odorless

605. A client, gravida I para I, 12 hours' postdelivery is verbalizing headache discomfort. After determining that the client's vital signs are within normal limits, which of the following nursing measures is best?
A. Administer an oral analgesic.
B. Determine if the headache is relieved after reclining.
C. Apply a cold compress to the forehead.
D. Minimize the environmental stimuli and retake the client's blood pressure in 15 minutes.

606. The postpartum client is breastfeeding her newborn for the first time. She calls the nurse for assistance after being unsuccessful in getting her newborn to latch on. The nurse learns the client has inverted nipples. The best nursing intervention is to:
A. Encourage the client to bottlefeed.
B. Administer an analgesic 30 minutes before breastfeeding.
C. Encourage the client to apply ice to her nipples before breastfeeding.
D. Apply a tea solution after breastfeeding.

607. A client with PIH is 3 days' postpartum after a vaginal delivery. Which of the following nursing diagnoses is applicable?
A. High risk for injury
B. High risk for fluid volume deficit

C. Alteration in bowel elimination: diarrhea
D. Self-care deficit

608. A gravida III para III vaginally delivered a stable newborn 4 hours ago. During labor the client experienced a significant increase in blood pressure that responded to magnesium sulfate. She received an epidural for pain management. After delivery of the placenta, an IV infusion of lactated Ringer's with 10 units of oxytocin was started. The blood loss from delivery was estimated to be 300 cc. The current nursing assessment reveals an examination within normal limits except for a soft uterus. The nurse knows that the most probable cause is what?
    A. The amount of blood loss in delivery
    B. A rebound effect of the oxytocin
    C. The administration of magnesium sulfate
    D. Vasoconstriction of the uterine musculature

609. During a postpartum assessment, the nurse notes that the client, a gravida II para II, has a severe diastasis recti. The nurse knows that the most probable outcome of this finding is that the client will be at risk for a(n):
    A. Alteration in comfort
    B. Alteration in bowel elimination: constipation
    C. Impaired physical mobility
    D. Injury

610. In providing discharge teaching for the early-discharge client, which of the following methods will best reinforce the nurse's teaching program?
    A. Openly discuss with the client and her family the need for a car safety seat.
    B. Administer a true-false quiz about breastfeeding and structure the discussion around the missed answers.
    C. Ask the client to identify the signs and symptoms of infection.
    D. Have the client show how to bathe her newborn.

611. A gravida I para I is 2 days' postpartum after a cesarean delivery. Which of the following nursing interventions will be the least effective in reducing the client's discomfort from gas pain?
    A. Encourage ambulation.
    B. Position the client in left lateral recumbent and support her extremities with pillows.
    C. Administer a prescribed, oral narcotic analgesic with ice water.
    D. Encourage use of the bedside rocking chair.

612. Before ambulating the gravida I para I client, who has had a cesarean delivery, for the first time, the nurse should:
    A. Encourage oral fluid intake.
    B. Splint the client's abdomen with pillows.
    C. Administer a prescribed narcotic analgesic.
    D. Allow her to sit on the bedside and dangle her feet.

613. The client is a gravida I para I who delivered her viable female infant via cesarean. After the sixth postpartal hour, which of the following laboratory reports shows to the nurse that the client is at risk for infection?
    A. Fasting plasma glucose of 136 mg/dl
    B. Mild proteinuria
    C. Leukocytes: 20,000/mm³
    D. Hemoglobin: 11 gms/dl

614. On postcesarean day 3, determining hypoactive bowel sounds in the client would lead the nurse to which of the following interventions?
    A. Encouragement of a regular dietary intake.
    B. Palpation of the abdomen with notation of distention or discomfort.
    C. Administration of a prescribed soap suds enema.
    D. Insertion of a nasogastric tube.

615. A client has given birth via cesarean delivery 24 hours ago. The nurse is ready to discontinue her IV. Which of the following data would alert the nurse to continue IV infusions?
    A. A urinary output of 25 cc/hr
    B. Fundal height at the umbilicus
    C. Peripad with moderate saturation of lochia rubra
    D. Verbalization of discomfort at the incision site

616. On receiving a postcesarean client from delivery, the nurse notes a scant amount of drainage on the lower abdominal dressing. The nurse should:
    A. Increase the IV rate of infusion.
    B. Outline and indicate the date and time on the dressing.
    C. Notify the physician.
    D. Change the dressing.

617. The nurse is teaching self-care to a multigravida client who will be discharged within 24 hours after a vaginal delivery. Which of the following client statements suggests the need for clarification by the nurse?
    A. "I should tighten my gluteal muscles before I sit down."
    B. "I can reinsert a hemorrhoid while wearing a rubber glove."
    C. "Afterpains should diminish after 24 hours."
    D. "Walking around my house a little more each day will help me to get stronger."

618. A 2-week postpartum client calls the clinic to talk with the nurse about a breastfeeding concern. During the conversation, the client tells the nurse she is experiencing bouts of unstoppable crying and feelings of being overwhelmed. The best response by the nurse is to:
    A. Encourage her to make an appointment at her earliest convenience.
    B. Assess the client's alteration in sleep pattern.
    C. Refer her to a mother support group.

D. Reassure the client that these feelings will leave as quickly as they have come.

619. Which of the following findings in a client who is 1-week postpartum suggests to the nurse the need for further assessment?
A. Fundal height approximately 7 cm below the umbilicus
B. Lochia serosa scant and odorless
C. Episiotomy edges approximated
D. Breast engorgement

620. After reviewing the nutritional needs for the lactating client, which of the following client statements indicates the need for additional teaching by the nurse?
A. "I should drink about 1000 to 1500 ml per day."
B. "To make sure that my milk supply is adequate, I need to take in an extra 500 to 800 kcal per day."
C. "I needed more protein when I was pregnant than I do now."
D. "I now need to increase my intake of foods rich in niacin."

621. A client returning to the clinic for her 6-week postpartum check-up reports that breastfeeding her son is going well. The client also tells the nurse that when she resumed intercourse with her husband it hurt. The best approach by the nurse is to:
A. Remind her that she was instructed to maintain pelvic rest for this reason.
B. Encourage her to wait 3 more weeks before attempting intercourse again.
C. Ensure that her episiotomy has healed and everything is fine.
D. Suggest the use of a water-soluble lubricant.

622. After ambulating to the bathroom for the first time, a primigravida complains to the nurse about a feeling of fullness at the vaginal outlet. The nurse knows that this sensation is most likely related to:
A. A full bladder
B. Prolapsed rectum
C. Pooled lochia draining from the uterus
D. Hematon formation

623. The nurse is concerned about preventing hypothermia in a newborn. The nurse should first:
A. Place the infant in well-heated isolette.
B. Wipe the newborn dry.
C. Wash the newborn with warm water.
D. Place the infant on an examination table open to room air.

624. After placing a newborn who was cool to touch in the heated isolette (38°C), the nurse notes that the infant has perspiration on his face and neck. The nurse knows that the perspiration is most likely related to:
A. The temperature of the incubator

B. Narcotic analgesics taken by the mother in labor
C. Hyperglycemia
D. Cold stress

625. A term infant is born. At 1 minute the nurse determines the crying infant's respiratory rate to be 40 and regular; heart rate, 120; muscle tone, arms and legs moving; color, body pink, extremities gray. Based on this data, the nurse should assess the Apgar score to be:
A. 3
B. 5
C. 7
D. 9

626. The client notes that her newborn has cold hands even though his head and body are covered. The best response by the nurse is:
A. "The newborn's hands and feet should remain covered to maintain a constant body temperature."
B. "Cold hands are the true indicator of the baby's temperature. Leave them exposed for a quick check."
C. "Cold hands are indicative of thermal heat loss, which results from inadequate clothing."
D. "The baby's hands are often cool to touch even though her body temperature is fine."

627. In providing nursing care for the prenatal client, which of the following parameters should the nurse use to accurately describe anemia in pregnancy?
A. At 16 weeks' gestation, the client has a hemoglobin of 12 gms/dl.
B. During the third trimester, the client has a hematocrit of 38 percent.
C. At any time during pregnancy, the client has a hemoglobin of less than 11 gms/dl.
D. If the pregnant client's hematocrit is 40 percent, she is anemic.

628. Which of the following signs and symptoms of iron deficiency anemia should the nurse observe for in the pregnant client?
A. Fatigue
B. Insomnia
C. Shortness of breath
D. Headache

629. In developing a plan of care for a gravida III para II client with hyperemesis gravidarum, which of the following nursing interventions would be most effective?
A. Provide diversional activities.
B. Monitor laboratory values.
C. Provide diet high in protein, fat, and carbohydrates.
D. Initiate hyperalimentation.

630. In providing care for the newborn of a mother with active syphilis, the nurse should assess the infant for which of the following?

A. Skin rash
B. Pneumonitis
C. Microcephaly
D. Cardiomyopathy

631. In counseling the postpartum gravida III para III client with diabetes mellitus about contraceptive choices, the nurse understands that which of the following is contraindicated?
A. Diaphragm
B. Condoms
C. Oral contraceptives
D. Tubal ligation

632. While assessing a postpartal client's complaint of coldness and pain in her lower left leg, the nurse notes that the client's left calf seems to be edematous. The next action by the nurse should be to:
A. Encourage ambulation.
B. Massage the left leg.
C. Encourage the client to wear knee socks.
D. Measure and record calf circumference of both legs.

633. During instructions for baby care, the parents voice concern to the nurse about caring for their premature newborn: "We have no idea how to take care of a baby; much less one so small." The best response by the nurse is:
A. "If you let me finish with my teaching, you will be better prepared."
B. "This baby will not stay this small forever, and you will get used to him."
C. "You sound overwhelmed. What frightens you the most about caring for your baby?"
D. "Your baby has grown 3 oz since birth; you have to measure progress in small increments."

634. A client, who has experienced perinatal loss, is talking with her nurse for a few hours after the infant was born. The client asks the nurse, "How could this have happened to me? I went to all the classes, ate all the right foods, and the baby was fine at my last check-up." The most supportive response is:
A. "You are feeling powerlessness and looking for a logical explanation for your loss."
B. "This experience will make you a stronger person."
C. "What did the doctor tell you at your last prenatal visit?"
D. "God never gives us more than we can handle."

635. After determining the first Apgar score, the nurse notes that the newborn has a wide-eyed stare. The nurse correctly attributes this to:
A. Alertness
B. Hypoxia
C. Hypoglycemia
D. Hypothermia

636. In providing care for a prenatal client with pulmonary tuberculosis, the nurse recognizes which of the following to be a probable outcome?

A. Cesarean birth
B. Therapeutic abortion
C. Congenital tuberculosis
D. Isolation from newborn

637. For the infant with hyperbilirubinemia, which of the following nursing interventions should be indicated?
A. Introduce early oral feedings.
B. Delay oral feedings.
C. Prolong time in nursery.
D. Maintain infant in left lateral position.

638. A laboring client has received an epidural for pain management. She is presently positioned on her left side. Which of the following will alert the nurse as an impending sign of hypotension?
A. Nausea and vomiting
B. Headache
C. Fainting
D. Nosebleed

639. While providing care to a newborn directly after birth, which of the following nursing interventions has the highest priority?
A. Assessing initial respiratory effort and rate
B. Placing the newborn in a prewarmed environment
C. Placing the infant in the parent's arms
D. Administering vitamin K

640. A newborn, 24 hours old, is diagnosed with neonatal withdrawal syndrome. Which of the following nursing measures is most important?
A. Observing infant for twitching, nystagmus, or tongue thrusting
B. Providing small, frequent feedings
C. Observing the quality of parent-infant interactions
D. Repositioning the infant every 2 hours

641. The nurse is providing prenatal care to a 15-year-old nullipara. Which of the following interventions is least effective for a nursing diagnosis of altered nutrition, less than body requirements?
A. Assess dietary intake using 24-hour recall.
B. Determine the client's protein requirement.
C. Give client pamphlets to read.
D. Assist client in choosing favorite foods to satisfy requirements.

642. An Rh-negative nullipara and her Rh-positive partner are present for the second prenatal health-care visit. The expectant mother is 12 weeks' pregnant. Which of the following nursing actions to reduce the risk of fetal injury will the nurse want to discuss?
A. The administration of Rh immunoglobulin (Rh IgG) at 28 weeks' gestation to the expectant mother to suppress the development of maternal antibodies.
B. To consider their options in carrying this pregnancy to term

C. To prepare for the immediate possibility of a fetal blood transfusion

D. The administration of Rh IgG to the expectant mother at 12 weeks' gestation

Focus on Obstetric-Gynecological Drug Dosage Calculation

643. A 38-year-old was diagnosed with endometriosis. The physician ordered danazol 400 mg bid. On stock were 200 mg tablets. How many tablets will the client receive?
A. 1 tablet
B. 1.5 tablets
C. 2 tablets
D. 2.5 tablets

644. The client, 42 weeks' pregnant, was admitted to have her labor induced. The physician ordered 10 units of oxytocin (Pitocin) to be added to 1 liter of 5% dextrose in lactated Ringer's solution. The physician wanted the client to receive 1 mU/min. How fast would the nurse set the rate to be delivered over 1 hour?
A. 4 ml/hr
B. 5 ml/hr
C. 6 ml/hr
D. 7 ml/hr

645. The 58-year-old client was demonstrating signs and symptoms of menopause. The physician ordered conjugated estrogens (Premarin) 0.6 mg daily. On hand were 1.25 mg tablets. The nurse instructed the client to take _____ tablets.
A. ½ tablet
B. 1 tablet
C. 1½ tablets
D. 2 tablets

646. A 45-year-old was seen by her gynecologist with complaints of abnormal uterine bleeding. The physician ordered conjugated estrogens (Premarin) for this breakthrough bleeding. He ordered the nurse to give the client 10 mg IM. On hand was a 25 mg/cc vial. How many milliliters did the nurse draw up?
A. 0.1 cc
B. 0.2 cc
C. 0.3 cc
D. 0.4 cc

647. A 68-year-old client was diagnosed with post-menopausal osteoporosis. The physician ordered 0.4 mg of estrone IM. On hand was a 2 mg/cc vial. The nurse drew up _____ ml.
A. 0.1 ml
B. 0.2 ml

C. 0.3 ml
D. 0.4 ml

648. A 25-year-old client was being seen at the physician's office with breast cancer. The physician ordered tamoxifen 10 mg PO tid for 3 months. The client received 2.5 mg tabs from the local pharmacist. How many tablets should the nurse instruct the client to take?
A. 1 tablet
B. 2 tablets
C. 3 tablets
D. 4 tablets

649. A 23-year-old was having difficulty getting pregnant. The physician's diagnosis was primary ovarian failure. He ordered estradiol 1 mg daily. On hand were 2 mg tablets. How many tablets should be taken?
A. ½ tablet
B. 1 tablet
C. 1½ tablets
D. 2 tablets

650. A 22-year-old postpartal client was experiencing severe breast engorgement. She decided not to breastfeed. The physician ordered 25 mg estradiol valerate (Delestrogen) IM. The nurse had on hand 40 mg/ml. How many milliliters would the nurse administer?
A. 0.2 ml
B. 0.4 ml
C. 0.6 ml
D. 0.8 ml

651. A 25-year-old was admitted with the complaint of bleeding during her second trimester. She later passed the fetus in a spontaneous abortion. The physician ordered dinoprostone 25 mg every 3 hours. On hand was 20 mg/ml. How many milliliters are needed?
A. 0.5 ml
B. 1 ml
C. 1.25 ml
D. 1.50 ml

652. A 25-year-old delivered a 6 lb 7 oz baby girl. During the postpartal assessment, the nurse noticed that the client had developed uterine atony. The physician ordered methylergonovine (Methergine) 0.2 mg IV over 1 minute. On hand was a 0.2 mg/ml vial. How many milliliters did the nurse use?
A. 0.5 ml
B. 1.0 ml
C. 1.5 ml
D. 2.0 ml

653. A young woman was admitted in premature labor. The physician ordered ritodrine 150 mg/500 ml of 5% dextrose in water. How many milligrams are delivered per milliliters of solution?
A. 0.1 mg

B. 0.2 mg
C. 0.3 mg
D. 0.4 mg

654. The physician ordered 0.25 mg terbutaline every hour subcutaneously for a young woman in premature labor. The nurse had 0.2 mg/ml on hand. How many milliliters did the nurse administer?
   A. 0.5 ml
   B. 1.0 ml
   C. 1.25 ml
   D. 1.50 ml

$0.25 \times \dfrac{1\,ml}{0.2}$

655. A 65-year-old was being treated for breast cancer. The physician ordered ethinyl estradiol (Estinyl) 1 mg tid PO. The client had 0.5 mg tabs on hand. The nurse instructed the client to take _____ tablets.
   A. 0.5 tablet
   B. 1.0 tablet
   C. 1.5 tablets
   D. 2.0 tablets

656. A 25-year-old was experiencing postpartal breast engorgement after she returned home from the hospital. The physician ordered ethinyl estradiol (Feminone) 1 mg every day times 3 days. The pharmacist sent 0.5 mg tablets. How many tablets should the client take?
   A. 0.5 tablet
   B. 1.0 tablet
   C. 1.5 tablets
   D. 2 tablets

657. A 67-year-old was being treated with megestrol-acetate (Megace) 320 mg/day for endometrial cancer. How many 40 mg tablets are required per day to deliver 320 mg?
   A. 2 tablets
   B. 4 tablets
   C. 6 tablets
   D. 8 tablets

658. A young woman was treated for AIDS. The physician ordered 400 mg of megestrol (Megace) IM. Using a 200 mg/5 ml vial, how many milliliters did the nurse administer?
   A. 4 ml
   B. 6 ml
   C. 8 ml
   D. 10 ml

659. An 18-year-old complained of amenorrhea. The physician ordered progestin 375 mg IM. Using a 400 mg/5 ml vial, how many milliliters did the nurse administer?
   A. 5.0 ml
   B. 6.0 ml
   C. 7.0 ml
   D. 8.0 ml

660. A 30-year-old was being treated with norethindrone (Micronor) 20 mg for endometriosis. The pharmacist dispensed 5 mg tablets with the instruction to take _____ tablets.

A. 2 tablets
B. 4 tablets
C. 6 tablets
D. 8 tablets

661. A young woman was seeking contraception without the use of birth control pills. The physician ordered medroxyprogesterone (Depo-Provera) 400 mg every 3 months. On hand was 400 mg/ml. How many milliliters did the nurse administer?
   A. 0.5 ml
   B. 1.0 ml
   C. 1.5 ml
   D. 2.0 ml

662. The physician ordered medroxyprogesterone (Provera) 500 mg IM to a young woman with endometrial cancer. Using a 400 mg/ml vial, the nurse administered how milliliters to the client?
   A. 0.5 ml
   B. 1.0 ml
   C. 1.25 ml
   D. 1.50 ml

663. A young woman was having a difficult time becoming pregnant. The physician ordered clomiphene citrate (Clomid) 75 mg every day times 5 days. The nurse instructed the client to take how many 50 mg tablets?
   A. 1 tablet
   B. 1.5 tablets
   C. 2 tablets
   D. 2.5 tablets

664. A young woman with irregular menses was diagnosed with decreased follicular growth. The physician ordered menotropins (Pergonal) 75 IU. How many milliliters will be needed if each vial reconstituted delivers 17 IU/ml?
   A. 2 ml
   B. 3 ml
   C. 4 ml
   D. 5 ml

665. Preoperatively, the physician ordered fentanyl 2 mg IM as a sedative for a 55-year-old undergoing a hysterectomy. Using a 2.5 mg/ml vial, the nurse administered how many milliliters?
   A. 0.5 ml
   B. 0.6 ml
   C. 0.7 ml
   D. 0.8 ml

666. A 15-year-old was found to have a lesion on the anterior pituitary gland. After removal of the lesion, the physician ordered gonadorelin hydrochloride (Factrel) 100 μg IM to stimulate the anterior pituitary gland to initiate menses. Once reconstituted, the vial will contain 500 μg/2 ml. How many milliliters did the nurse administer?
   A. 0.1 ml
   B. 0.2 ml

C. 0.3 ml
D. 0.4 ml

667. A 29-year-old was seen in the ER with severe asthma. The client was in her second trimester. The physician ordered dexamethasone (Decadron) 4 mg IV. The nurse administered how many milliliters from a 16 mg/ml vial?
A. 0.1 ml
B. 0.15 ml
C. 0.2 ml
D. 0.25 ml

668. A 32-year-old was diagnosed with fibrocystic breast disease. The physician ordered danazol (Danocrine) 300 mg PO. The nurse instructed the client to take how many 200 mg tablets?
A. 0.5 tablet
B. 1.0 tablet
C. 1.5 tablets
D. 2.0 tablets

669. A 29-year-old was experiencing breast engorgement postpartally secondary to a stillborn birth. The physician ordered 50 mg testosterone IM to reduce the symptoms. The nurse drew up how many milliliters from a 100 mg/ml vial?
A. 0.5 ml
B. 1.0 ml
C. 1.5 ml
D. 2.0 ml

670. A 16-year-old rape victim was given diethylstilbestrol 25 mg twice a day times 5 days to prevent conception. The nurse instructed the client to take how many 5 mg tablets?
A. 2 tablets
B. 3 tablets
C. 4 tablets
D. 5 tablets

671. A 17-year-old was diagnosed with herpes genitalis. The physician ordered acycolovir (Zovirax) 200 mg every 4 hours while awake (8 AM, noon, 4 PM, and 8 PM) times 5 days. The nurse instructed the client to have on hand how many 200 mg tablets?
A. 10 tablets
B. 15 tablets
C. 20 tablets
D. 25 tablets

672. A young woman was complaining of burning on urination. The physician diagnosed cystitis and ordered ampicillin 250 mg IM every 6 hours. After reconstitution, the vial contained 500 mg/5 ml. How many milliliters will the nurse administer?
A. 1 ml
B. 1.5 ml
C. 2.0 ml
D. 2.5 ml

673. A 33-year-old was diagnosed with monilial vaginitis. The physician ordered nystatin 400,000 units

qid. The suspension contained 100,000 unit/ml. The nurse instructed the client to take _____ ml.
A. 1 ml
B. 3 ml
C. 4 ml
D. 5 ml

674. A 22-year-old pregnant woman was diagnosed with chlamydia. Because of the pregnancy, the physician ordered erythromycin 250 mg qid times 2 weeks. The nurse instructed the client to take how many milliliters of a 100 mg/2.5 ml suspension?
A. 4.25 ml
B. 5.0 ml
C. 5.25 ml
D. 6.25 ml

675. A 15-year-old was seen in the ER with symptoms of burning on urination and a foul vaginal discharge. The physician diagnosed acute syphilis. He ordered 2.4 million units of penicillin G IM. The reconstituted vial contains 600,000 unit/ml. How many milliliters must the nurse administer?
A. 2 ml
B. 4 ml
C. 6 ml
D. 8 ml

676. A 23-year-old AIDS client received zidovudine 200 mg every 4 hours. The client had 100 mg tablets. How many tablets must be administered?
A. 1 tablets
B. 2 tablets
C. 3 tablets
D. 4 tablets

677. A 23-year-old was in premature labor. The physician ordered betamethasone (Celestone) 12 mg prior to the delivery to help with fetal lung maturation and prevent hyaline membrane disease. The nurse using a 4 mg/ml vial withdrew how many milliliters?
A. 1 ml
B. 2 ml
C. 3 ml
D. 4 ml

678. A 16-year-old was diagnosed with *Candida albicans.* The physician ordered 1200 mg miconazole (Monistat) in 50 cc 5% dextrose in water IV. The tubing delivers 10 gtt/min/mil. What rate should the nurse set?
A. 15 gtt/min
B. 16 gtt/min
C. 18 gtt/min
D. 19 gtt/min

679. A 31-year-old was diagnosed with bacterial vaginosis. The physician ordered clindamycin 450 mg every 6 hr IM. Using a 300 mg/ml vial, the nurse administered how many milliliters?
A. 0.5 ml
B. 1.0 ml

C. 1.5 ml
D. 2.0 ml

680. A 38-year-old woman in her second trimester was admitted for congestive heart failure. The physician ordered digoxin 0.5 mg as an initial dose. The nurse administers how many milliliters from a 0.25 mg/ml vial?
A. 1.0 ml
B. 1.5 ml
C. 2.0 ml
D. 2.5 ml

681. A 27-year-old was admitted for pre-eclampsia. The physician ordered 4 gms of magnesium sulfate IV as a loading dose. On hand was 50% magnesium sulfate (50 gms in 100 ml). How many milliliters will the nurse administer?
A. 2.0 ml
B. 4.0 ml
C. 6.0 ml
D. 8.0 ml

682. Routinely after delivery, a newborn receives vitamin K IM to treat hemorrhagic disease. The physician ordered 0.5 mg after birth. Using a 2 mg/ml vial, the nurse administered how many milliliters?
A. 0.15 ml
B. 0.25 ml
C. 0.35 ml
D. 0.45 ml

683. An obese 40-year-old delivered an 8 lb 10 oz baby boy. Within 24 hours postpartal, she began complaining of leg pain. The physician was notified and ordered 7,500 units of heparin IV immediately for possible deep vein thrombosis. Using a 10,000 unit/ml vial, the nurse administered how many milliliters?
A. 0.25 ml
B. 0.50 ml
C. 0.75 ml
D. 1.0 ml

684. The obese client with the deep vein thrombosis began experiencing severe respiratory distress. The physician suspected a pulmonary embolus. He added warfarin (Coumadin) 15 mg PO daily to the medical regimen. The nurse had 10 mg tablets on hand. How many tablets did the nurse administer?
A. 0.5 tablet
B. 1.0 tablet
C. 1.5 tablets
D. 2.0 tablets

685. A 19-year-old was experiencing gestational diabetes during her second trimester of pregnancy. The physician ordered 10 units of Humulin regular insulin for a blood sugar of 150 mg/dl. Using a tuberculin syringe, how many milliliters would the nurse administer?
A. 0.1 ml

B. 0.2 ml
C. 0.3 ml
D. 0.4 ml

686. A 32-year-old pregnant woman was exposed to hepatitis B during a recent blood transfusion prior to pregnancy. The physician ordered 1 ml of the hepatitis B vaccine. Using a 10 mg/0.5 ml vial, how many milliliters of the vaccine would the nurse administer?
A. 10 mg
B. 15 mg
C. 20 mg
D. 25 mg

687. A 16-year-old pregnant teen was diagnosed with iron deficiency anemia. The physician ordered Femiron 600 mg daily PO. The pharmacist dispensed 300-mg tablets. The nurse instructed the teen to take _____ tablets.
A. 1 tablet
B. 2 tablets
C. 3 tablets
D. 4 tablets

688. A 30-year-old woman in her third trimester began experiencing congestive heart failure symptoms. The physician ordered furosemide 40 mg IV push. Using an 80 mg/ml vial, how many milliliters did the nurse administer?
A. 0.2 ml
B. 0.3 ml
C. 0.4 ml
D. 0.5 ml

689. During her annual physical, a 31-year-old woman complained of burning on urination. The urine specimen revealed that she had a urinary tract infection. The physician ordered nitrofurantoin (Macrodantin) 100 mg PO. On hand was a 25 mg/5 ml suspension. How many milliliters did the nurse administer?
A. 10 ml
B. 20 ml
C. 30 ml
D. 40 ml

690. An 18-year-old was experiencing severe labor pains. The physician ordered butorphanol tartrate (Stadol) 2 mg IM. Using a 1 mg/ml vial, how many milliliters did the nurse administer?
A. 0.5 ml
B. 1.0 ml
C. 1.5 ml
D. 2.0 ml

691. After administering butorphanol tartrate (Stadol) to a postoperative client, she developed severe respiratory depression. The physician ordered naloxone (Narcan) 0.4 mg IV immediately. Using a 1 mg/ml vial, how many milliliters did the nurse administer IV?
A. 0.2 ml

B. 0.4 ml
C. 0.6 ml
D. 0.8 ml

692. A 17-year-old was experiencing severe pain during labor. The physician ordered nalbuphine hydrochloride (Nubain) 0.5 mg subcutaneously. Using a 10 mg/ml vial, how many milliliters did the nurse administer?
   A. 0.5 ml
   B. 1.0 ml
   C. 1.5 ml
   D. 2.0 ml

693. A 40-year-old woman was experiencing pain after a vaginal hysterectomy. The physician ordered 0.5 mg oxymorphone subcutaneously. Using a 1.5 mg/ml vial, how many milliliters did the nurse administer?
   A. 0.1 ml
   B. 0.2 ml
   C. 0.3 ml
   D. 0.4 ml

694. A 15-year-old pregnant teen was diagnosed with thiamine deficiency. The physician ordered thiamine hydrochloride (Biamine) 100 mg IM. Using a 250 mg/ml vial, how many milliliters did the nurse administer?
   A. 0.2 ml
   B. 0.4 ml
   C. 0.6 ml
   D. 0.8 ml

695. A 35-year-old female executive was experiencing premenstrual symptoms. Because of her severe agitation and restlessness, the physician ordered alprazolam (Xanax) 0.5 mg PO at the hour of sleep. The pharmacist dispensed 1-mg tablets and instructed the client to take _____ tablet(s).
   A. ½ tablet
   B. 1 tablet
   C. 1½ tablets
   D. 2 tablets

Answers

1. **(A)** Nursing process phase: assessment; client need: health promotion and maintenance; content area: maternity nursing

Rationale
(A) This is the description of a pelvis that is ideal for the birthing process. It will allow movement of the fetus through this passage for a safe birth. (B) Prominent spines and a flat or shallow sacrum will not be adequate for a normal birth. The interspinous diameter is the smallest diameter that the fetus must accommodate and prominence of these spines will likely prevent normal descent through the birth canal. (C) A narrow pubic arch would likely not allow passage of the fetal head as it ex-

tends during birth. (D) A narrow pubic arch and prominent spines would impede the normal descent of the fetus during the birthing process. A flat sacrum would also prevent the fetus from making the cardinal movements necessary for birth.

2. **(B)** Nursing process phase: assessment; client need: health promotion and maintenance; content area: maternity nursing

Rationale
(A) Ovulation may vary for some individuals; however, the term "cycle," referring to the menstrual cycle, implies regularity and predictability. Generally speaking, each woman's body establishes a routine reproductive cycle with ovulation occurring at a regular interval for her. (B) Ovulation generally occurs at the end of the proliferative phase, beginning the secretory phase of the menstrual cycle. This usually occurs at about the 14th day of the cycle based on a 28-day menstrual cycle. (C) As the ischemic phase of the cycle takes place and the endometrial tissue is sloughed off, blood begins to escape with the tissue and mucus marking the menstrual flow. Ovulation does not occur until the estrogen and progesterone levels have risen and the endometrium has begun to prepare for implantation of the fertilized ova. About 2 weeks are required for the follicle to develop adequately with the increase of FSH. (D) Intercourse does not play a part in the stimulation or maturation of the ovum.

3. **(A)** Nursing process phase: assessment; client need: health promotion and maintenance; content area: maternity nursing

Rationale
(A) The period following fertilization until the implantation of the zygote is thought to be relatively free of teratogenic influences. However, the embryonic period is one of the most highly susceptible to the influence of teratogenic effects due to the organogenesis that occurs at this time. (B & C) The second and third trimesters, though critical periods of development, are not as likely to result in major morphologic abnormalities if teratogens are present. Physiological defects and minor morphologic abnormalities may occur during this time frame. (D) Teratogenic effects are not equal throughout pregnancy. Once the organ systems are developed they are not as susceptible to the damage of teratogens.

4. **(B)** Nursing process phase: assessment; client need: health promotion and maintenance; content area: maternity nursing

Rationale
(A) At conception, chromosomal or genetic sex is determined. During the first month, primordial germ cells are internally visible. (B) Reproductive development occurs in conjunction with the urinary system. Testes develop in the fetal abdomen as early as 7 weeks. However, external genitalia are not well developed and identifiable until after the ninth week. By the 16th week, oogenesis has been established. (C) By the 20th week, the external genitalia are well defined though they continue to refine until close to term. (D) The seventh month finds the fetal external genitalia continuing to be more clearly defined. The sexual characteristics of the external genitalia are easily distinguished at this time.

5. **(B)** Nursing process phase: assessment; client need: health promotion and maintenance; content area: maternity nursing

Rationale

(A) The hematocrit is done at the first prenatal visit and generally not repeated until the 32nd to 36th week. If the reading is low, a complete work-up is done to screen for anemia. (B) A urine specimen is obtained and a urine dipstick test is done during each prenatal visit. Screening is done for glucose and protein. Glucose may identify hyperglycemia and diabetic problems. Protein may indicate pre-eclampsia if other signs and symptoms are present. (C) STD screenings are done at an early prenatal visit but are not routinely repeated throughout pregnancy unless the client is symptomatic. (D) Blood typing is done early in pregnancy. Coombs' test should be repeated at 28 weeks in Rh-negative women. Antibody titers for rubella are drawn early and will be repeated later in pregnancy if the titer is more than 1:128.

6. **(B)** Nursing process phase: assessment; client need: health promotion and maintenance; content area: maternity nursing

Rationale

(A) Urinary frequency usually occurs in the first trimester as a result of the enlarging uterus and the resulting pressure on the bladder. During the second trimester the uterus rises out of the pelvic cavity, reducing the weight on the bladder. (B) During the third trimester, with descent of the presenting part the enlarged uterus compresses the bladder, causing urinary frequency. (C) Quickening, the time when the mother may feel fetal movement, will not have any influence on urinary frequency. (D) During the second trimester, when the uterus rises out of the pelvic cavity, the woman's feeling of urinary urgency usually disappears.

7. **(D)** Nursing process phase: assessment; client need: health promotion and maintenance; content area: maternity nursing

Rationale

(A) The cardiac output and workload of the heart are not related to the incidence of heartburn during pregnancy. (B) Though gastric acidity does change during pregnancy, peristalsis decreases rather than increases. (C) Peristalsis decreases during pregnancy by about 50 percent. These women have increased nonpropulsive esophageal motor activity with a decrease in wave amplitude and slower spread of peristaltic waves. Food intake amount may or may not change; however, this is not a primary factor in the occurrence of heartburn. (D) The common complaint of heartburn in pregnancy is a result of the diminished gastric emptying time and acid reflux into the esophagus. The amount of gastric secretions is somewhat lower in the first and second trimesters but increases dramatically in the third trimester. Acid indigestion may include burping and an acidic taste in the mouth.

8. **(A)** Nursing process phase: assessment; client need: health promotion and maintenance; content area: maternity nursing

Rationale

(A) Due to the hormonal changes that occur during pregnancy, there is an increased sloughing of cells from the cervical and vaginal walls, causing an increase in the amount of vaginal mucus or leukorrhea. The discharge may be thin and milky or thick and sticky but should not cause irritation to tissues. (B) Yellow discharge may indicate the presence of an infection. (C) Blood-tinged mucus would be of concern because this may indicate preterm labor. (D) There is a definite difference in the vaginal discharge during pregnancy. The degree of change varies from woman to woman.

9. **(A)** Nursing process phase: implementation; client need: safe, effective care environment; content area: maternity nursing

Rationale

(A) Prior to an amniocentesis, the fetal heart tones are monitored for a baseline. (B) Maternal vital signs are monitored prior to and following this procedure. The mother's vital signs will be monitored during the procedure with the major concern being her blood pressure. Maternal and fetal vital signs are monitored for approximately 30 minutes to 1 hour following the procedure. (C) The woman will need to empty her bladder in order to avoid the possibility of nicking the bladder during the procedure. There is no connection between a urine specimen and an amniocentesis. (D) There is no need for a maternal blood specimen. The amniocentesis is used to evaluate the amniotic fluid and its cellular components for identification of birth defects and genetic diseases. It may be used later in pregnancy to check fetal lung maturity.

10. **(B)** Nursing process phase: analysis; client need: safe, effective care environment; content area: maternity nursing

Rationale

(A) Early decelerations of the fetal heart rate are due to a gallop response to head compression during a contraction. These are usually seen in the second stage of labor following rupture of membranes. (B) Variable decelerations are caused by cord compression. The decelerations may occur with contractions but are not of major concern, though they do indicate a need to follow the infant's response closely. (C) Late decelerations are a result of fetal distress from uteroplacental insufficiency. (D) Infants may respond to maternal medications given during labor by a slightly lower or higher baseline heart rate. However, decelerations with contractions generally are not related to maternal medication admnistration.

11. **(C)** Nursing process phase: implentation; client need: health promotion and maintenance; content area: maternity nursing

Rationale

(A & B) Many expectant mothers may not have a supportive partner. Although childbirth education may indeed strengthen a couple's relationship and increase a woman's self-esteem, these are not the primary focuses of the class. (C) Educating the mother in order to provide her with practical tools that will equip her to cope effectively with the stress brought about by the last weeks of pregnancy, the birth of her baby, and the early postpartal period are the main objectives in childbirth programs. (D) Many childbirth preparation classes do include this type of information; however, it is not the primary focus of the class.

12. **(B)** Nursing process phase: implementation; client need: safe, effective care environment; content area: maternity nursing

Rationale

(A) A slightly elevated temperature during the first hours after birth is common due to dehydration. A temperature above 100.4°F would be concerning due to the possibility of infection. (B) A positive Homans' sign would be of great concern to the nurse. Postpartal clients are predisposed to the formation of phlebitis and thromboembolisms due to the decreased venous return, increased viscosity from fluid loss, and the temporary elevation in clotting factors that occur in the time following delivery. (C) Edema of the perineal area is common following a vaginal delivery and would not be of unusual concern. (D) During breastfeeding, uterine contractions are normal as a result of the release of oxytocin.

13. **(C)** Nursing process phase: implementation; client need: health promotion and maintenance; content area: maternity nursing

Rationale
(A) A diaphragm, which is a curved rubber dome enclosed by a flexible metal ring, is used as a mechanical barrier for contraception. Spermicidal cream or jelly is placed in the cup portion and on the rim of the diaphragm before insertion. (B & C) The diaphragm should be left covering the cervix at least 6 hours but no longer than 24 hours following intercourse. (D) It is effective for contraception as soon as it is in place. It should be placed just prior to intercourse.

14. **(A)** Nursing process phase: assessment; client need: physiological integrity; content area: maternity nursing

Rationale
(A) The discomforts that normally occur in the later part of pregnancy may cause many women to experience fatigue during this time. The application of skills of controlled relaxation will enhance her ability to withstand the stress of labor. It will teach her body awareness and will improve her ability to conserve energy between contractions and provide relaxation of the uterine muscles. This will improve the work of each contraction to more effectively move the fetus through the birth canal. (B) Resting between contractions is important and a woman is more able to remain in control when she is not overly fatigued; however, in addition, movement of the infant through the birth canal is an important reason for relaxation. (C) Although this is a hoped-for result of remaining relaxed, it is not the main focus. (D) A quiet environment is ideal and may be a factor that will assist the mother to be more in control and relaxed.

15. **(C)** Nursing process phase: implementation; client need: safe, effective care environment; content area: maternity nursing

Rationale
(A & B) This vitamin does not increase the growth of the intestinal flora nor does it assist in the conjugation of bilirubin. (C) Hemorrhagic disease of the newborn results from a deficiency of prothrombin and other clotting factors. Vitamin K, which is produced in the bowel, is low in the newborn due to the decreased bacterial flora. (D) Healthy full-term infants have sufficient iron stores for synthesis of red blood cells until the third to fourth month after birth. Anemia may result if supplemental iron is not given beyond that time. Most commercial formulas contain supplemental iron.

16. **(D)** Nursing process phase: analysis; client need: safe, effective care environment; content area: maternity nursing

Rationale
(A) The increased ratio of body surface area can cause an increased heat loss. (B) Term newborns have an increased amount of subcutaneous and brown fat to improve their ability to conserve heat. (C) Blood vessel dilatation should not be an issue in the normal term newborn. (D) Thermoregulation is important in the newborn. The flexed position of the newborn assists in decreasing the amount of heat lost. However, drying with warmed blankets or towels, placing on a prewarmed bed or mother's abdomen, and preventing drafts following birth will decrease heat loss in the newborn.

17. **(B)** Nursing process phase: evaluation; client need: safe, effective care environment; content area: maternity nursing

Rationale
(A) A nonreactive nonstress test is one in which the fetus does not meet these criteria. This test is considered non-reassuring and further evaluation of fetal well-being would be done. (B) The NST is used to identify the fetus who may not be adapting well to the intrauterine environment. The FHR is monitored for accelerations in relation to fetal movements. These increases are a sign of an intact central and autonomic nervous system. A reactive nonstress test is one in which in a 20-minute time frame there are two FHR accelerations, each of at least 15 beats per minute, lasting at least 15 seconds in conjunction with fetal movements. (C & D) Positive and negative are not terms that are appropriately used to describe the results of a nonstress test.

18. **(C)** Nursing process phase: implementation; client need: safe, effective care environment; content area: maternity nursing

Rationale
(A) Vena caval compression may result if the client is placed in a flat position. Headache is not common after epidural administration, though it may occur as a result of poor technique. (B) Elevated blood pressure is not a common side effect of epidural anesthesia. (C) Epidural anesthesia is very effective for a labor and vaginal and operative births. Major complications are uncommon; however, because of initial vasodilation following administration, hypotension is always expected due to pooling of blood in the legs. (D) There is no relationship between frequent voiding and epidural anesthesia.

19. **(B)** Nursing process phase: analysis; client need: safe, effective care environment; content area: maternity nursing

Rationale
(A) The cardinal movements are essential for normal progression but do not influence the speed of labor. (B) The female pelvis is varied in contour and diameter. The fetal presenting part must adapt to the birth canal by a series of turns and adjustments that are termed the cardinal movements of labor. These include engagement, descent, flexion, internal rotation, extension, external rotation, and expulsion. (C) These cardinal movements of labor are completed prior to the second stage. (D) Engagement of the fetal presenting part occurs prior to descent, flexion, and internal rotation.

20. **(D)** Nursing process phase: analysis; client need: physiological integrity; content area: maternity nursing

Rationale
(A) The average weight for an infant at 27 weeks' gestation is approximately 1100 gms. This infant exceeds the average weight. (B & C) In order to determine whether an infant is SGA or LGA, the length, as well as the weight, is required for

calculation. (D) An infant of less than 37 weeks' gestation is classified as preterm.

21. (B) Nursing process phase: analysis; client need: physiological integrity; content area: maternity nursing

Rationale

(A) Duplication of genetic material occurs during the pre-embryonic period (weeks 1 to 3) following conception. The exact duplication of genetic material is essential for cell differentiation, growth, and biologic maintenance of the embryo. (B) Weeks 4 through 8, known as the embryonic period, is the period when organogenesis occurs. All major organs and systems are formed. During this period of growth and development the greatest potential for major congenital malformations exists. (C) Kidneys do not secrete urine until the 13th to 16th weeks of gestation. (D) Subcutaneous fat is not deposited until the final week prior to delivery at term.

22. (D) Nursing process phase: assessment; client need: physiological integrity; content area: maternity nursing

Rationale

(A) Though estrogen levels do change during pregnancy, it is not used as the main hormone of evaluation in pregnancy tests. (B) Maternal serum levels of prolactin rise throughout pregnancy in preparation for breastfeeding but there is no evidence of increased urine levels that could be used to determine pregnancy. (C) Alpha-fetoprotein is the major protein in the serum of the embryo produced initially by the yolk sac. Increased levels may indicate neural tube defects, abdominal wall malformations, fetal demise, or renal anomalies. Low levels are associated with chromosomal trisomies and gestational trophoblastic disease. (D) Human chorionic gonadotropin is the biochemical basis for pregnancy tests. Produced by the placenta, it helps to maintain the corpus luteum. Levels increase rapidly following conception, peaking at about 8 weeks and gradually decreasing to low levels at about 16 weeks.

23. (A) Nursing process phase: analysis; client need: health promotion and maintenance; content area: maternity nursing

Rationale

(A) This client has been pregnant five times, delivered two infants, has had two abortions, and is currently pregnant. (B) This client has been pregnant four times, delivered four infants, and has had two abortions. (C) This client has been pregnant three times, delivered two infants, and has had two abortions. (D) This client has been pregnant two times, delivered two infants, and has had two abortions.

24. (B) Nursing process phase: evaluation; client need: safe, effective care environment; content area: maternity nursing

Rationale

(A) A normal blood sugar level would be less than 140 mg/dl. (B) A glucose tolerance test is indicated for any glucose screening result of 140 mg/dl or greater. (C) The need for insulin control cannot be determined based on a glucose screening test. (D) Although nonstress tests may be indicated later in pregnancy to determine the well-being of the fetus, the priority at this gestational age is to achieve euglycemia.

25. (D) Nursing process phase: analysis; client need: physiological integrity; content area: maternity nursing

Rationale

(A & C) Insulin-dependent diabetes mellitus, also known as type I diabetes, usually appears before 30 years of age with an abrupt onset of symptoms requiring insulin for management. It is not related to onset during pregnancy, though maintenance of a steady state may be more difficult if a diabetic woman becomes pregnant. (B) Type II diabetes, also known as non–insulin-dependent diabetes mellitus, usually appears in older adults. It is characterized by a slow onset and progression of symptoms. It may be managed by diet, exercise, oral hypoglycemic medications (not recommended during pregnancy), or insulin. (D) Gestational diabetes mellitus develops during pregnancy and typically resolves following delivery. Symptoms are usually mild and not life threatening to the mother but pose increased risks of fetal morbidity and other fetal complications. Individuals who are diagnosed with gestational diabetes are at an increased risk for the development of diabetes in later years.

26. (C) Nursing process phase: assessment; client need: safe, effective care environment; content area: maternity nursing

Rationale

(A) Amniocentesis can be safely performed as early as 15 to 17 weeks. (B) Ultrasound can evaluate amniotic fluid volume, which may be used to determine congenital anomalies. That is not the purpose prior to an amniocentesis. (C) Amniocentesis involves aspiration of a small amount of amniotic fluid for evaluation. The needle inserted through the abdominal wall is guided by ultrasound to evaluate the position of the placenta and the fetus to avoid needle injuries. (D) Amniocentesis can be performed to assess for lung maturity. Fetal ultrasound can be used for gestational dating through measurements of the femur and biparietal diameter. Ultrasound does not determine fetal lung maturity.

27. (B) Nursing process phase: analysis; client need: safe, effective care environment; content area: maternity nursing

Rationale

(A) Dyspnea is a common complaint in the third trimester of pregnancy due to the increasing size of the uterus resulting in pressure against the diaphragm. (B) Facial/upper body edema may be indicative of pre-eclampsia and would be very concerning to the nurse. Further evaluation of the BP and a urine dipstick to check for proteinuria would be in order. (C) A heart rate increase of 10 to 15 beats per minute is a normal physiological change of pregnancy due to the multiple hemodynamic changes that occur. (D) This hematocrit is within the normal range. Less than 35 percent would warrant follow-up.

28. (D) Nursing process phase: assessment; client need: health promotion and maintenance; content area: maternity nursing

Rationale

(A) The term "heterozygote" refers to an individual with one mutant allele and one normal or unaffected allele at a given locus on a pair of homologous chromosomes. An individual who is heterozygous for the abnormal gene does not manifest obvious symptoms. (B) Disorders carried on the sex chromosome, either the X or Y chromosome, are referred to as sex-linked recessive. (C) Both males and females may be affected by the autosomal recessive genetic disorders because the responsible allele can be found on any one of the 46 chromosomes. (D) If both parents are affected by the disorder and not just carriers, then all of their children will manifest the same disorder.

29. (C) Nursing process phase: assessment; client need: physiological integrity; content area: maternity nursing

Rationale
(A) *Chlamydia trachomatis* is the bacteria causing chlamydia. (B) *Neisseria gonorrhoeae* is the bacteria causing gonorrhea. (C) *Treponema pallidum* is the spirochete that causes syphilis. (D) *Trichomonas vaginalis* is the protozoan causing trichomonas.

30. (C) Nursing process phase: assessment; client need: physiological integrity; content area: maternity nursing

Rationale
(A) Post-term deliveries have not been shown to increase the incidence of chorioamnionitis unless there has been prolonged rupture of membranes. (B) Though extremely concerning, maternal dehydration is not related to chorioamnionitis. (C) Chorioamnionitis is an inflammation of the amnion and chorion surrounding the fetus. It is generally associated with premature or prolonged rupture of membranes. (D) Pyelonephritis, a kidney infection that develops as a result of an untreated UTI, is the most common nonobstetric cause for hospitalization during pregnancy.

31. (B) Nursing process phase: assessment; client need: physiological integrity; content area: maternity nursing

Rationale
(A) The absence of Babinski's reflex in a newborn would indicate neurological dysfunction. (B) Stroking the lateral aspect of an infant's sole from heel to toe should elicit a positive Babinski's reflex with dorsiflexion of the great toe and extension of the other toes. This normal developmental reflex disappears before 2 years of age. (C) The absence of a palmar grasp reflex can indicate an infant has suffered hypotonia or perinatal asphyxia. (D) The absence of a plantar grasp reflex is seen in infants with hypotonia or spinal cord injuries.

32. (C) Nursing process phase: assessment; client need: physiological integrity; content area: maternity nursing

Rationale
(A) Widely spaced suture lines in a newborn may be an indication of hydrocephaly. (B) Caput succedaneum is an easily identifiable edematous area of the scalp of a newborn. The sustained pressure of the presenting fetal scalp during a vaginal delivery may result in compression of local vessels, slowing venous return and causing a edematous swelling. This swelling extends over the suture lines of the skull and disappears spontaneously within 3 to 4 days. (C) Molding is a normal occurrence from the pressure on the fetal head during the birthing process. The cranial bones are not fused, allowing the movement necessary for the fetal head to pass through the birth canal. There may be a small space between the cranial bones or overriding may occur. (D) Depressed fontanelles may possibly indicate dehydration. Fontanelles should feel soft and flat.

33. (D) Nursing process phase: planning; client need: health promotion and maintenance; content area: maternity nursing

Rationale
(A) Carpenito defines this ND as a state in which individuals experience the inability to adequately manage internal or environmental stressors because of inadequate resources. (B) Activity intolerance indicates an individual with compromised physical conditioning. Though this is true for this client this ND does not adequately address the issue of bowel retention. (C) Though the client will likely become constipated if she does avoid a bowel movement for several days, this ND does not address the issue that is currently causing the problem. (D) This ND addresses the cause of this client's problem in which the nurse can intervene in order to prevent further complications from developing.

34. (C) Nursing process phase: analysis; client need: physiological integrity; content area: maternity nursing

Rationale
(A) Total blood volume increases by approximately 1500 ml. Red blood cell production increases but at a slower rate than total blood volume. Total white blood cell volume increases primarily in granulocytes. (B) Hemoglobin and hematocrit values decrease even though there is an increase in red blood cell production. The decrease is more noticeable during the second trimester. (C) Red blood cell and white blood cell production increases. The decreased hemoglobin and hematocrit are related to the rapid expansion of blood volume, which occurs at a faster rate than the increase in cell production. This condition is known as physiological anemia. (D) There is an increase in total blood volume and an increase in cardiac output of 30 to 50 percent by the 32nd week of pregnancy. Many factors influence maternal blood pressure such as anxiety, maternal position, maternal age, activity level, and chronic health problems.

35. (C) Nursing process phase: implementation; client need: health promotion and maintenance; content area: maternity nursing

Rationale
(A & B) This amount of weight gain would not allow for an adequate growth of the fetus and the maternal organs. Inadequate weight gain may lead to low-birth-weight infants. (C) This is the recommended amount of weight a woman should gain during pregnancy if she is of average weight prior to pregnancy. The rate or gain should not be linear but should begin slowly in the first trimester while the embryo is small, increasing to about 1 pound per week during the second and third trimesters. This will allow for adequate growth of the fetus and the maternal organs. (D) This amount of weight gain is above the recommended amount.

36. (A) Nursing process phase: implementation; client need: health promotion and maintenance; content area: maternity nursing

Rationale
(A) Absorption of iron is best when the supplement is taken at bedtime with a citrus juice. However, if gastrointestinal upset is experienced, it may need to be taken with a meal. Coffee, tea, milk, and calcium supplements decrease absorption of iron. (B) Taking an iron supplement between meals on an empty stomach will likely cause gastrointestinal upset. (C) Though taking these two supplements together might assist the client in establishing a routine to avoid forgetting her supplements, taking them together does not increase or improve iron absorption. In fact, the calcium that is included in pre-

natal vitamins impedes iron absorption. (D) An increased intake of iron is needed during pregnancy because of the increase in maternal blood volume, fetal blood formation, fetal iron stores for early infancy, and blood loss that occurs during delivery. Iron absorption from the diet does increase during pregnancy; however, it is almost impossible for a client to meet her iron requirements from food intake without overeating. Therefore, iron supplements of 30 to 60 mg/day are recommended.

37. **(C)** Nursing process phase: implementation; client need: health promotion and maintenance; content area: maternity nursing

Rationale
(A) Sitting up for an hour after meals is recommended to assist in decreasing the incidence of heartburn. This will decrease the amount of reflux of stomach contents into the esophagus. (B) Coffee, tea, alcohol, chocolate, and acidic juices should be avoided because they are gastric irritants that increase GI discomforts. (C) Eating several small meals per day, separating solid foods from liquids, not overfilling the stomach, decreasing gastric irritants, and limiting gas-producing foods will assist the client in reducing GI discomforts. (D) Antiemetics are not recommended unless prescribed by a physician or other healthcare provider. Nonpharmacological methods should be implemented first.

38. **(B)** Nursing process phase: implementation; client need: physiological integrity; content area: maternity nursing

Rationale
(A) The duration of a contraction is the amount of time of the entire contraction, not just a portion of it. (B) This is the accurate definition of the duration of a contraction. It is measured from the beginning to the end of the same contraction and is usually recorded in seconds. (C) This describes the frequency of contractions. Frequency is usually recorded in minutes. (D) There is no measurement done from the peak of one contraction to the peak of another.

39. **(D)** Nursing process phase: assessment; client need: physiological integrity; content area: maternity nursing

Rationale
(A) Opening of the cervix is called dilation. (B) The cervix does not lengthen during pregnancy. (C) Hypotonic is not a term used to describe the cervix. (D) Effective contractions lead to cervical changes. The cervix softens and thins with each contraction, drawing slowly and progressively up into the lower uterine segment.

40. **(D)** Nursing process phase: implementation; client need: psychosocial integrity; content area: maternity nursing

Rationale
(A) Because each labor experience is different, knowing what happened in previous experiences would not be helpful at this time. (B) During transition, it is important that the woman receive a great deal of encouragement from her caregivers. Assisting her with each contraction and giving specific directions is important. Monitoring her breathing will help to decrease the incidence of hyperventilation. (C) If an epidural will be used it is administered earlier in the laboring process, generally after the cervix has dilated to at least 4 cm.

It is generally not placed this late in the laboring process. (D) Transition is a time when the laboring client requires a great deal of support. Reminding her that her baby is almost here, giving specific directions, and encouraging her are important. The woman's need for reassurance intensifies. The nurse should interpret the progress and labor to both members of the couple and affirm their coping abilities.

41. **(C)** Nursing process phase: evaluation; client need: safe, effective care environment; content area: maternity nursing

Rationale
(A) Variable decelerations are a result of cord compression. Although an occasional variable deceleration is not terribly worrisome, repetitive decels are serious and could indicate serious fetal distress. There are interventions that should reduce their occurrence prior to notification of the physician or nurse midwife. (B) Variables are often seen toward the end of labor following rupture of membranes with accompanying cord compression. More effective pushing techniques will not change their occurrence. (C) Using the lateral Sims' position as the first intervention may relieve pressure on the cord. The knee-chest position may help to move the fetus off the cervix if the Sim's position is not effective. (D) Variable decelerations resulting from cord compression may be a result of nuchal cord, presence of the cord between the fetus and uterine wall, a knot in the cord, cord prolapse, or pressure on the cord as a result of oligohydramnios. This is a potentially serious condition.

42. **(B)** Nursing process phase: analysis; client need: physiological integrity; content area: maternity nursing

Rationale
(A) These cardinal movements may indeed shorten the birth process but this is not the main purpose for the movements. (B) The main purpose of the cardinal movements of birth is to allow the largest diameter of the fetal head to pass through the largest diameter of the pelvis. (C) This birth presentation and the cardinal movements may be the most comfortable for the mother because they will tend to shorten the birth process; however, this is not the main purpose. (D) These cardinal movements do not ensure safe passage of the fetus.

43. **(A)** Nursing process phase: assessment; client need: safe, effective care environment; content area: maternity nursing

Rationale
(A) Nausea, hyperstimulation of the uterus, and poor urine output are common side effects of oxytocin. (B) Hypotension, not hypertension, plus headache, and arrhythmias are common side effects of oxytocin. (C) Hypertonic contractions are a common side effect of oxytocin. It does not cause nervousness or diarrhea. (D) Because of the antidiuretic effect of oxytocin it may cause fluid overload. Hypertension and elevated temperature are not common side effects.

44. **(D)** Nursing process phase: analysis; client need: health promotion and maintenance; content area: maternity nursing

Rationale
(A) Kegel exercises themselves do not relieve perineal pain, but because they promote healing they may result in less pain

overall. (B) Kegels do not assist in toning the abdominal muscles. (C) Postpartal hemorrhage is not prevented by the toning of the pelvic floor muscles. (D) Toning of the pelvic floor muscles around the reproductive organs by performing Kegel exercises will assist in preventing stress incontinence and prolapsed uterus later in life. Because Kegels increase the flow of circulation to the episiotomy area, they will assist in the healing process.

45. **(C)** Nursing process phase: assessment; client need: health promotion and maintenance; content area: maternity nursing

Rationale
(A) These signs are considered presumptive signs of pregnancy because they may be caused by conditions other than pregnancy. (B) These are considered probable signs of pregnancy. These signs strongly suggest pregnancy but do not confirm it. (C) Fetal heart tones and fetal movement documented by someone other than the mother as well as visualization of the fetus with ultrasound are considered positive signs of pregnancy. (D) Frequency of urination may be caused by infection and the accuracy of a pregnancy test may vary depending on the time it is done. Other signs of pregnancy such as Braxton Hicks contraction may occur with pseudocyesis, or pseudopregnancy, when a woman believes very strongly that she is pregnant.

46. **(C)** Nursing process phase: implementation; client need: health promotion and maintenance; content area: maternity nursing

Rationale
(A) A 24-week fetus is about 9 inches in length, has thick vernix caseosa, and clearly identifiable external sexual characteristics. (B) At 24 weeks, the fetus is about 9 to 10 inches in length, and weighs about 2 pounds, but fingernails are just beginning to be clearly defined. They will not be complete until 32 weeks and will not be over the tips of fingers and toes until about 38 weeks. (C) Lanugo does not begin to disappear until about 28 weeks, eye formation is complete, hearing is present, and the fetus weighs about 700 to 800 gms. If born at this time, the infant would be considered viable. (D) Testes will not begin to descend into the scrotum until around 28 weeks and will not be fully descended until closer to term. The suck reflex is not well developed until after 34 weeks. The head hair may be quite long but muscle tone is not well developed at this time.

47. **(C)** Nursing process phase: evaluation; client need: health promotion and maintenance; content area: maternity nursing

Rationale
(A) This is a good time for couples to begin to evaluate their parenting skills. A midpregnancy parent education class would be an excellent idea at this time. (B) Quickening occurs at about the 16th to 18th weeks of pregnancy. This is a significant point in pregnancy for many women. Primiparas may not be able to discern fetal movement as early as multiparas. (C) A woman's uterus should have enlarged enough by 26 weeks' gestation that she should be requiring maternity clothes. If she continues to attempt to wear her prepregnancy clothes, it may indicate a denial of the pregnancy or a financial hardship. This statement would be concerning and would require further evaluation by the nurse. (D) Toward the end of the first trimester, before the uterus is an abdominal organ, the fetal heart tones can be heard with an ultrasound or Doppler. Anytime after this is a good time for the woman and her family to be offered the opportunity to hear the fetal heart beat.

48. **(C)** Nursing process phase: implementation; client need: safe, effective care environment; content area: maternity nursing

Rationale
(A) Changes in the flow rate of a medication require a physician's order. This is not an independent nursing judgment unless you are operating under standing protocol orders. Even so, uterine atony generally responds to fundal massage. (B) Uterine tone must be maintained. Ambulating to the bathroom will not increase the tone. Lack of tone may be a result of a full bladder, in which case your assessment would reveal a uterus that was deviated to the side. (C) Gently massaging the fundus will usually increase the uterine tone. This would be your first action. Failure to respond to the massage might indicate more serious problems and would require further evaluation. (D) Cervical tears or lacerations generally present as a firm uterus with persistent, moderate bright red flow.

49. **(D)** Nursing process phase: analysis; client need: psychosocial integrity; content area: maternity nursing

Rationale
(A) Some women may indeed think that they will feel disappointed if the gender of their child is not what they have anticipated. However, research shows that this is usually not the case. Bonding and attachment begin prior to the infant's birth and, usually, discovering that they have a healthy infant removes any doubts that they may feel about the gender. (B) Her expression that she doesn't know why she is crying and is unable to stop does not indicate that she is dissatisfied with the care she is receiving. (C) Postpartum psychosis is characterized by acute psychotic behavior generally characteristic of other disorders such as schizophrenic, affective, or organic disorders. The actions of the clients are exaggerated. Quiet crying is not a sign of postpartum psychosis. (D) Postpartum blues, or postpartum depression, is common in the first few days following delivery. This is considered to be a normal mild, transient mood disturbance lasting a few days or more. Some research indicates there is a connection between this mood disturbance and the drop in estrogen and progesterone that normally occurs during this period.

50. **(B)** Nursing process phase: assessment; client need: safe, effective care environment; content area: maternity nursing

Rationale
(A) An amniocentesis is done to obtain a sample of amniotic fluid containing fetal cells. It is used to evaluate for genetic disorders, assessment of pulmonary maturity, and diagnosis of fetal hemolytic disease. (B) Doppler blood flow analysis provides a noninvasive evaluation of the fetus and placenta. It is used in at-risk pregnancies to evaluate for IUGR, multifetal gestation, and preterm labor as well as many other high-risk problems. (C) A contraction stress test is performed near term to evaluate the fetus's ability to withstand the stress of labor and delivery. It will not give you an accurate diagnosis of IUGR. (D) Chorionic villa sampling is used early in preg-

nancy for genetic studies. The procedure is done between 10 and 12 weeks' gestation. About 90 percent are done to evaluate for genetic disorders in situations of advanced maternal age.

51. **(B)** Nursing process phase: evaluation; client need: safe, effective care environment; content area: maternity nursing

Rationale

(A) The amount of amniotic fluid could be evaluated during this procedure as a real-time ultrasound would be done in conjunction to determine the position of the fetus and placenta to avoid injury to either. However, this is not the main reason for an amniocentesis at this time. (B) Analysis of the lung profile will reveal the lecithin-sphingomyelin ratio (L/S). The ratio of these phospholipids produced by the type II alveolar cells increases with gestation and a ratio of 2:1 indicates lung maturity. (C) A sample of amniotic fluid will not provide information indicating fetal weight. (D) Position of the placenta and fetus would be determined during the ultrasound that would be performed at the same time. The main reason this test would be done on this client now would be to determine lung maturity.

52. **(C)** Nursing process phase: implementation; client need: safe, effective care environment; content area: maternity nursing

Rationale

(A) An emergency cesarean section is not necessary in this situation. The fetus has responded to some stressful event and close monitoring is required. (B) Increasing the speed of your client's labor is not necessary and in fact may increase the stress on the fetus. (C) Early suctioning while the infant's head is on the perineum will be necessary. The nares and oral cavity will be cleaned to prevent the aspiration of meconium-stained fluid by the infant with the initial breath. (D) Good fetal monitoring is the best practice throughout the labor process. You should continue to be vigilant of the condition of the fetus throughout the entire labor and delivery.

53. **(A)** Nursing process phase: implementation; client need: safe, effective care environment; content area: maternity nursing

Rationale

(A) Placenta previa occurs when the placenta is implanted in the lower segment of the uterus rather than in the body of the uterus. A portion or all of the placenta may cover the cervical os. During the latter part of pregnancy when the cervix begins to efface, the placenta may pull away from the wall of the uterus and bleeding begins. Bleeding is not related to activity level and the uterus is relaxed and nontender. (B) Placenta accreta is defined as an anomaly in which the placenta trophoblastic tissue entered the myometrium when the placenta was first formed. When separation occurs at delivery, parts of the placenta continue to adhere to the wall and prevent uterine contracture. (C) Abruptio placentae is a premature separation of the normally implanted placenta. Signs of vaginal bleeding often occur as labor begins. Pain may occur with increasing pain indicating concealed bleeding. (D) Ectopic pregnancy occurs when the fertilized ovum implants in the fallopian tube or a foreign site other than the normal implantation site of the uterus. It would not be likely that a woman

could progress to 36 weeks' gestation without major problems becoming obvious prior to that time.

54. **(B)** Nursing process phase: analysis; client need: safe, effective care environment; content area: maternity nursing

Rationale

(A) Labor occurring late in the third trimester is not of great concern because this is close to term for the pregnancy. (B) Painless bleeding late in the third trimester might indicate a placenta previa where the implantation site of the placenta occurs over the cervical os. As the cervix begins to efface late in pregnancy the placenta begins to separate and bleeding begins. A digital vaginal exam might dislodge more of the placenta. Therefore, after the first speculum exam to evaluate for the presence of a placenta previa, no vaginal exams would be done. (C) When done correctly, the examination should not result in an infection. (D) A vaginal exam could lead to increased fetal distress prior to labor if the exam caused the low-lying placenta to separate further.

55. **(A)** Nursing process phase: analysis; client need: physiological integrity; content area: maternity nursing

Rationale

(A) Human chorionic gonadotropin (hCG) is secreted by the trophoblastic layer of the blastocyst. Its function is to maintain the corpus luteum until the placenta can produce adequate amounts of pregnancy hormones. The levels of hCG in urine or serum provide the basis for pregnancy tests. (B) These villi are structures forming the fetal side of the placenta. They do not play a part in urine or serum evaluation of pregnancy. (C) The anterior pituitary gland ceases its release of follicle-stimulating hormone (FSH) and luteinizing hormone (LH) during pregnancy. It does not play a part in urine or serum evaluation of pregnancy. (D) Following ovulation, luteinizing hormone (LH) induces changes in the ruptured follicle from which the egg has been released. The empty follicle is now known as the corpus luteum. It does not play a part in urine or serum evaluation of pregnancy.

56. **(A)** Nursing process phase: analysis; client need: physiological integrity; content area: maternity nursing

Rationale

(A) Most of the highly oxygenated blood from the inferior vena cava is diverted to the left atrium through the foramen ovale. Increased pressure caused by fetal pulmonary constriction directs a great deal of blood away from the pulmonary vessels and to the aorta through the ductus arteriosus. (B) Highly oxygenated blood comes to the fetus from the placenta through the umbilical vein and is shunted past the liver by the ductus venosus, continuing through the inferior vena cava to the right atrium. (C) The foramen ovale is a flap that allows blood to flow only from the right to the left sides of the heart. The ductus venosus does not play a part in directing the blood away from the fetal lungs. (D) The umbilical vein brings highly oxygenated blood to the fetus from the placenta. It does not play a part in directing the blood away from the fetal lungs.

57. **(C)** Nursing process phase: analysis; client need: health promotion and maintenance; content area: maternity nursing

Rationale

(A) A gravida II para II has been pregnant two times and delivered two babies beyond 20 weeks' gestation. (B) A gravida III para III has been pregnant three times and delivered three babies beyond 20 weeks' gestation. (C) A gravida III para I has been pregnant three times, delivered one baby beyond 20 weeks' gestation, and is currently pregnant. We cannot tell from this description whether the other pregnancy was a spontaneous or induced abortion. (D) A gravida III para II has been pregnant three times, has delivered two babies, and is currently pregnant.

58. **(B)** Nursing process phase: implementation; client need: health promotion and maintenance; content area: maternity nursing

Rationale

(A) This is an incorrect response. The level of comfort of the infant may have some influence on the length of sleep; however, this phrase does not describe the infants' response. (B) Habituation refers to an infant's ability to decrease responses to repeated environmental stimuli. (C) This is not a correct description of the newborn's response. (D) Consolability refers to the infant's ability to bring itself, or to be brought by others, to a lower state.

59. **(A)** Nursing process phase: implementation; client need: health promotion and maintenance; content area: maternity nursing

Rationale

(A) This is a correct description of a quiet alert state in an infant. Infants react to sensory stimuli because this is the most optimum state of arousal. (B) This describes an infant in a drowsy awake state. (C) This describes an infant in a deep sleep state. (D) This describes an infant in a light sleep state.

60. **(D)** Nursing process phase: implementation; client needs: health promotion and maintenance; content area: maternity nursing

Rationale

(A) This statement is incorrect. The size of Stacy's breasts does not influence her ability to produce enough milk. (B) This is not a correct statement. This again indicates that breast size influences milk production. Providing some breast milk in addition to formula would not be necessary. (C) This statement is also incorrect. Although it indicates that breast size does not influence milk production, it infers that formula is a better choice for infants and more convenient for mother. (D) This is a correct statement. If there are no other complications that influence this mother's ability to breastfeed, she should not be unsuccessful based on the size of her breasts.

61. **(C)** Nursing process phase: implementation; client needs: physiological integrity; content area: maternity nursing

Rationale

(A) At the approach of ovulation, the drop is slight and not sharp and it does not remain low. (B) At ovulation the temperature does not rise sharply and does not remain high. (C) Just prior to ovulation, there is a slight drop in the basal temperature with the increase in estrogen. At the time of ovulation, the basal body temperature rises with an increase in progesterone. (D) The temperature does not remain high for an extended time.

62. **(C)** Nursing process phase: implementation; client need: health promotion and maintenance; content area: maternity nursing

Rationale

(A) Women with IUDs do not report painful intercourse as a result of the IUD. (B) There is no evidence that IUDs increase the occurrence of these infections. (C) The IUD may cause contraction of the uterus because of an increased irritability. These contractions may cause spontaneous expulsion of the IUD. (D) The opposite may be true. Following insertion, many women report an excessive menstrual flow for several months.

63. **(A)** Nursing process phase: evaluation; client need: safe, effective care environment; content area: maternity nursing

Rationale

(A) Because of the rupture of the fallopian tube during an ectopic pregnancy and the subsequent blood loss, pressure on the diaphragm may cause referred shoulder pain. (B) Ectopic pregnancy results from abnormalities that prevent the movement of the fertilized ovum through the tube and into the uterus. It is not related to the number of times a woman has been pregnant. (C) Again, this is not relevant to an ectopic pregnancy. (D) This would be difficult for the woman to evaluate on her own. It would be a part of the physical assessment by the nurse or other health-care provider.

64. **(B)** Nursing process phase: implementation; client need: health promotion and maintenance; content area: maternity nursing

Rationale

(A) This is not a therapeutic response. Even though Faye may not experience quickening for several weeks, it is an important event in her pregnancy and her question should be addressed more directly. (B) This is a correct as well as a therapeutic statement. (C) This statement is not accurate. Most pregnant women recognize quickening somewhere between 16 to 20 weeks. The baby's size and activity level are not pertinent factors. (D) Some first-time mothers do mistake quickening for gas pains early on; however, this statement is not therapeutic since it really does not answer Faye's question. Also, putting her off by changing the subject is not a therapeutic teaching technique.

65. **(D)** Nursing process phase: implementation; client need: health promotion and maintenance; content area: maternity nursing

Rationale

(A) This is known as Ladin's sign. (B) This describes Hegar's sign. (C) Goodell's sign refers to cervical softening. (D) Increased vaginal vascularity with blood vessel engorgement results in the vaginal mucosa taking on a purplish color known as Chadwick's sign.

66. **(C)** Nursing process phase: analysis; client need: safe, effective care environment; content area: maternity nursing

Rationale

(A) Maternal dietary iron intake is not related to physiological anemia. (B) There is nothing to indicate that the client's liver is dysfunctional. This does not explain physiological anemia of pregnancy. (C) During the first trimester of pregnancy, maternal blood volume increases approximately 50 percent, causing a decrease in the concentration of hemoglobin and erythrocytes. This is known as physiological anemia of pregnancy. (D) Physiological anemia of pregnancy is common, and these results do not indicate any laboratory error. Hillary's laboratory work does not need to be repeated at this time.

67. **(C)** Nursing process phase: implementation; client need: health promotion and maintenance; content area: maternity nursing

Rationale
(A) This could occur several hours prior to delivery. This would indicate the very early stages of labor and would be much to soon for a primigravida to come to the hospital. (B) The nurse needs to be much more specific about the frequency of contractions. (C) Ruptured membranes can increase the mothers' chance of infection or possibly a prolapsed cord. Regular contractions that are 5 to 7 minutes apart would indicate a need for the mother to come to the hospital. She is in true labor and cervical changes are probably occurring. (D) With intact membranes, contractions of 10 to 15 minutes' frequency would be too early for a primigravida to come to the hospital. She will be more comfortable at home in a familiar environment.

68. **(A)** Nursing progress phase: implementation; client need: health promotion and maintenance; content area: maternity nursing

Rationale
(A) Although the client will not be able to judge whether or not cervical changes are occurring, she should be told to come to the hospital when she has a bloody show; her contractions are regular, between 5 and 7 minutes apart, or irregular with increasing intensity that does not decrease with activity; or her membranes rupture. Cervical dilation and effacement are palpable on sterile vaginal examination by the health-care provider. (B) True labor contractions do not decrease or disappear with activity. (C) True labor contractions persist regardless of the position of the mother. Although this may be a true statement for some women, this will not help her identify the difference between true and false labor. (D) Membranes may remain intact throughout most of the labor process. Contractions may continue to be of an irregular pattern well in the active phase.

69. **(C)** Nursing process phase: analysis; client need: safe, effective care environment; content area: maternity nursing

Rationale
(A) At term, the amniotic fluid should be colorless with small particles of vernix caseosa present. (B) Amber-colored amniotic fluid indicates the presence of bilirubin. Rh isoimmunization causing destruction of RBCs releases bilirubin into the amniotic fluid. (C) Amniotic fluid that is greenish-yellow in color indicates the presence of meconium and suggests fetal distress. With a decrease in oxygen supply to the fetus, the anal sphincter relaxes, causing the release of meconium into the fluid. (D) Cloudy amniotic fluid with purulent material and usually a foul odor indicates infection.

70. **(A)** Nursing process phase: analysis; client needs: safe, effective care environment; content area: maternity nursing

Rationale
(A) The first stage of labor including the active phase is from 3 cm to full cervical dilation. Contractions are strong, closer together, and usually last 30 to 60 seconds. Additionally, the deceleration phase includes a change in behavior such as irritability, and nausea and vomiting. (B) The latent phase begins with the onset of true labor and continues to a cervical dilation of 3 cm. Contractions are 15 to 30 minutes in frequency and mild to moderate in intensity. (C) This terminology does not refer to a phase of labor. (D) The fourth stage of labor occurs up to and through 4 hours after the delivery of the fetus and placenta. It is considered a stabilization phase of the mother.

71. **(B)** Nursing process phase: analysis; client need: safe, effective care environment; content area: maternity nursing

Rationale
(A) There is no indication that she or her fetus are in distress. There would not be an indication for an emergency cesarean section at this time. (B) Since she is postdates and not contracting, she will most likely receive oxytocin as an augmentation to labor unless she begins to experience a regular progressive pattern of labor right away. (C) There is no indication for an amnioinfusion, a procedure that infuses sterile saline into the uterus and is used in cases of oligohydramnios accompanied by variable decelerations to relieve the compression on the umbilical cord. (D) It is unlikely that she would be sent home. She is postdates and has signs of early labor.

72. **(C)** Nursing process phase: analysis; client need: safe, effective care environment; content area: maternity nursing

Rationale
(A) Once membranes have ruptured, women should be admitted to the labor-and-delivery suite for monitoring. There is an increased risk for infection once the membranes are no longer intact. (B) This client would not be sent home with ruptured membranes. (C) The first nursing action should be to evaluate the status of the fetus. The description this client has given indicates the possibility of a prolapsed cord that has compromised the oxygen supply to the fetus. (D) The client would be admitted and will most likely develop a regular contraction pattern soon; however, it is obvious from the mother's description that the nurse needs to investigate the situation further to ensure the well-being of the fetus.

73. **(A)** Nursing process phase: analysis; client need: safe, effective care environment; content area: maternity nursing

Rationale
(A) Oxytocin is a neurohyopohyseal hormone that stimulates contraction of the uterine smooth muscle. It is used for induction and augmentation of labor. One of the main adverse reactions is uterine tetany. The nurse should assess for contractions that occur at less than 2-minute intervals or last longer than 90 seconds. These hypertonic contractions can lead to impaired fetal blood flow or in some cases uterine rupture. (B) It is not necessary to monitor deep tendon reflexes when a patient is receiving oxytocin. (C) Hyperglycemia is

not a side effect of oxytocin. (D) This is not a side effect of oxytocin.

74. **(C)** Nursing process phase: assessment; client need: safe, effective care environment; content area: maternity nursing

Rationale
(A) When the presenting part is high in the pelvis above the ischial spines, the station is recorded with negative numbers. (B) A station of 0 indicates the presenting part is at the level of the ischial spines. (C) This is a correct statement. +1 station indicates the presenting part is slightly below the ischial spines. (D) A station of −1 would indicate the presenting part is slightly above the ischial spines.

75. **(D)** Nursing process phase: analysis; client need: safe, effective care environment; content area: maternity nursing

Rationale
(A) This describes a first-degree perineal laceration. (B) Cervical lacerations are not documented by degrees. (C) This describes a fourth-degree perineal laceration. (D) This is a correct description of a third-degree laceration of the perineum. Lacerations of the perineum, vagina, or cervix may occur as a result of forceps delivery, precipitous or rapid delivery, delivery of a large infant or multiple infants. They may also occur following a normal spontaneous vaginal delivery.

76. **(B)** Nursing process phase: analysis; client need: safe, effective care environment; content area: maternity nursing

Rationale
(A) Though urinary stasis may lead to an increase risk of UTI, this is not the most immediate concern. (B) Urinary retention postpartally may lead to lack of uterine tone as a result of the pressure of the distended bladder on the uterus. This pressure and subsequent displacement prevents the uterus from clamping down adequately, leading to postpartal hemorrhage. (C) Urinary retention is not related to an increased risk of uterine infection postpartally. (D) Uterine tetany is not a postpartal concern. Clamping down of the uterus is desirable following delivery.

77. **(A)** Nursing process phase: assessment; client need: health promotion and maintenance; content area: maternity nursing

Rationale
(A) Washing the breast prior to each feeding or applying lotions or creams to the breast are not recommended. (B) Good handwashing prior to each feeding is encouraged. There is no need to wash the nipple prior to each feeding, though good hygiene is encouraged. (C) Mothers are encouraged to either alternate breasts at each feeding or alternate the breast that is used first at each feeding. Placing some type of reminder on the bra, such as a safety pin or ribbon, is a good way for mothers to remember which breast was used first at the previous feeding. (D) Lactating women should have approximately 2500 to 3000 ccs of fluid daily to produce a sufficient amount of breast milk.

78. **(B)** Nursing process phase: implementation; client need: health promotion and maintenance; content area: maternity nursing

Rationale
(A) Exercise and good fluid intake are highly recommended for new mothers; however, this is probably not the cause of her leg cramps. (B) Leg cramps are generally a result of low calcium levels. Milk and dark green vegetables are a good source of calcium. (C) Low potassium levels are not usually related to leg cramps. (D) Though this may indeed be a good stress reliever for new mothers, the cause of the leg cramps has still not been addressed. They are most likely a result of inadequate nutrition.

79. **(C)** Nursing process phase: assessment; client need: health promotion and maintenance; content area: maternity nursing

Rationale
(A) Active artificial immunity is acquired through vaccinations, active natural immunity refers to immunity acquired following the occurrence of a disease in an individual. (B) This is not correct terminology used to describe immunity. (C) Passive natural immunity occurs when immunity develops in the fetus from an antigen-antibody response in the mother. (D) This does not correctly describe immunity acquired transplacentally.

80. **(A)** Nursing process phase: implementation; client need: health promotion and maintenance; content area: maternity nursing

Rationale
(A) Milia are a very common finding in newborns. They are blocked sebaceous glands commonly found on the face, nose, forehead, and upper torso of newborns. They will disappear in a short time without intervention. (B) Vernix caseosa is a white, unctuous substance covering the body of infants. It is present for protection of the skin in utero. (C) This is not an appropriate response for the nurse, since milia are common findings and should not be disturbed. Encouraging the mother to attempt to remove them with washing is not an appropriate nursing intervention. (D) It is true that lots of babies have milia; however, they should not be removed with bathing. It is important to teach new mothers about milia and encourage them to wait patiently for them to disappear on their own.

81. **(C)** Nursing process phase: implementation; client need: psychological integrity; content area: maternity nursing

Rationale
(A) The tonic neck reflex, or fencing reflex, is elicited by turning the infant's head to one side while he or she is lying supine. The extremities on the same side extend and those on the opposite flex. The position gives the appearance of a fencing position. (B) The Babinski reflex is elicited when the baby's foot is stroked along the lateral aspect of the sole from heal up and across. The infant responds by hyperextending the toes and dorsiflexing the great toe. This reflex is intact until about 1 year of age. (C) The Moro or startle reflex is normal and is elicited when the infant is startled. The response is an abduction and extension of the arms in a symmetrical pattern. This reflex is intact until about 4 to 5 months of age. (D) Galant's reflex, or trunk incurvation, is elicited when the infant is prone. When the infant's back is stroked firmly about 2 inches from the spine in a downward motion, the body curves to the side of the stimulus. This reflex is present until approximately 3 months of age.

82. **(A)** Nursing process phase: implementation; client need: psychosocial integrity; content area: maternity nursing

Rationale

(A) This is an appropriate nursing diagnosis for this mother. She is not knowledgeable concerning mongolian spots in newborns and does not realize that this is a normal variation. (B) Her lack of understanding of normal variations in the newborn is not related to any altered thought process. (C) This is not an appropriate nursing diagnosis in relation to her lack of knowledge. She may have some alteration in her coping strategies related to a new family member, but this does not refer to her need for additional information. (D) Anxiety is common in new mothers; however, this nursing diagnosis does not adequately address the reason for her anxiety, which, of course, is her lack of knowledge of newborns.

83. **(B)** Nursing process phase: implementation; client need: psychosocial integrity; content area: maternity nursing

Rationale

(A) If this weekend was an isolated event and this young woman has not used substances since that time, it is unlikely that her fetus will be affected. (B) Teratogens used in the first 2 weeks after conception usually have an all-or-nothing effect; that is, it either prevents implantation, resulting in a spontaneous abortion, or leaves the fetus unharmed. (C) Again, if this was an isolated event, major deformities are unlikely. Other fetal well-being studies could be done if there continued to be concerns. (D) Maternal and fetal circulations are separate; however, this will not prevent teratogenic effects of substances that can cross this barrier.

84. **(D)** Nursing process phase: assessment; client need: health promotion and maintenance; content area: maternity nursing

Rationale

(A) Transvaginal ultrasounds allow the deep small organs of the pelvis, such as the ovaries and fallopian tubes, to be visualized clearly. These ultrasounds may be used to detect such things as ectopic pregnancies or to evaluate the fetus very early in pregnancy. (B) The nonstress test (NST) is used widely to assess fetal well-being. The NST uses Doppler ultrasound to obtain a baseline fetal heart rate and fetal movement as well as to evaluate uterine activity. It will not be used to evaluate the ability of the fetus to withstand the trials and stress of labor. (C) An amniocentesis is the removal of amniotic fluid during ultrasound. This test of fetal well-being is done to evaluate fetal lung maturity or to determine the presence of chromosomal abnormalities. It would not be used to determine the ability of the fetus to tolerate labor. (D) The contraction stress test (CST) is a third-trimester test of fetal well-being. This test subjects the fetus to uterine contractions and observing the FHR pattern to determine if the fetus will be able to withstand the stress of labor.

85. **(A)** Nursing process phase: implementation; client need: safe, effective care environment; content area: maternity nursing

Rationale

(A) This is a correct statement. A placenta that is implanted close to, or overlying, the cervical os is referred to as a placenta previa. (B) Placenta accreta refers to a placenta that has invaded the myometrium and cannot easily be separated at delivery. (C) A placenta that separates from the wall of the uterus prior to delivery of the fetus is referred to as abruptio placentae. (D) Placental infarction occurs when blood supply to the placenta is blocked and tissue necrosis occurs.

86. **(C)** Nursing process phase: implementation; client need: safe, effective care environment; content area: maternity nursing

Rationale

(A) Women with HELLP syndrome and severe pre-eclampsia continue to be at risk at 12 hours' postpartum. (B) Women with HELLP syndrome and severe pre-eclampsia continue to be at risk at 24 hours' postpartum. (C) Women with HELLP syndrome and severe pre-eclampsia usually stabilize and are no longer at risk for seizure activity following postpartum diuresis, which usually occurs by 48 hours. (D) Women with HELLP syndrome and severe pre-eclampsia are no longer at risk for seizures at 1 week postpartum. Postpartum diuresis has usually occurred by 48 hours.

87. **(B)** Nursing process phase: planning; client need: safe, effective care environment; content area: maternity nursing

Rationale

(A) Clients with HELLP syndrome are not at greater risk for infection than other postpartum clients. RBC morphology is not changed. (B) Women diagnosed with HELLP syndrome continue to be at risk for seizure activity for approximately 48 hours following delivery. Postpartum diuresis has usually occurred by this time. (C) This is not an appropriately stated nursing diagnosis. Women with HELLP syndrome are at risk for hemorrhage because of their low platelet count, which is one of the triad of symptoms of the syndrome. (D) Anxiety may be a problem for these clients though they are generally sedated. This, however, is not the priority nursing diagnosis for this client.

88. **(C)** Nursing process phase: analysis; client need: safe, effective care environment; content area: maternity nursing

Rationale

(A) This is not a common immediate problem of preterm infants. (B) Biliary atresia does not occur more commonly in preterm infants than in term infants. It is not a condition related to prematurity. (C) Respiratory distress syndrome is a common problem in preterm newborns. The lungs are not sufficiently developed in infants at 28 weeks because of the decreased numbers of alveoli and insufficient amounts of surfactant. (D) Hypoglycemia is more likely to be the problem in preterm newborns. Infants at 28 weeks' gestation have a decreased production and store of glucose.

89. **(B)** Nursing process phase: assessment; client need: physiological integrity; content area: maternity nursing

Rationale

(A) Nutrition in the preterm newborn is quite challenging. It differs a great deal from the term neonate. (B) The preterm newborn has a smaller capacity stomach, slower motility, limited store of nutrients, decreased ability to digest proteins, and decreased ability to absorb nutrients as well as an immature enzyme system. (C) This is not an accurate statement. Motility and emptying time are slower in the preterm neonate. (D) Reflux is a common problem in preterm newborns because of an immature sphincter, which allows stomach contents to reflux into the esophagus. It is not caused by a higher gastric acidity.

90. (D) Nursing process phase: implementation; client needs: safe, effective care environment; content area: maternity nursing

Rationale
(A) Since only the uterus is removed during a hysterectomy and not the ovaries, the secretion of ovarian hormones is not effected and, consequently, menopause does not occur as a result. (B) With removal of the uterus, menstruation will no longer occur. (C) The posthysterectomy client will no longer need birth control. However, she should know that she will continue to need protection from sexually transmitted diseases if she is not in a mutually monogamous relationship. (D) Feelings of grief and loss may result following an unplanned hysterectomy because the client suffers the structural loss and subsequently the ability to conceive and bear a child. Clients should be taught that feelings of loss or depression are normal and should be provided with emotional support.

91. (A) Nursing process phase: implementation; client need: safe, effective care environment; content area: maternity nursing

Rationale
(A) Depo-Provera prevents the regular release of ova, inhibiting normal changes in the endometrial lining of the uterus. (B) More commonly, women report weight gain rather than loss. (C) Women may experience fatigue rather than increased metabolic activity. (D) Hypertension has not been reported in the literature as a side effect of Depo-Provera.

92. (B) Nursing process phase: implementation; client need: pychosocial integrity; content area: maternity nursing

Rationale
(A) By 1 year of age, the incidence of undescended testes in all boys is less than 1 percent. (B) The testes descend into the scrotum in 90 percent of newborns by 36 to 40 weeks' gestation. (C) Although spermatogenesis does not occur until puberty, the higher temperature of the abdominal cavity causes deterioration of the sperm cells. (D) The ideal time frame for surgery for undescended testicles is 2 to 3 years of age.

93. (C) Nursing process phase: assessment; client need: physiological integrity; content area: maternity nursing

Rationale
(A) Traces of proteinuria and lower extremity edema are normal findings in pregnancy. A BP increase of this level would need to be followed closely but is not indicative of PIH. (B) Epigastric pain may be seen in PIH; however, dizziness is not a common symptom. (C) This is the classic triad of symptoms of PIH. (D) Mild glucose in the urine is a common finding in pregnancy. The hypertension is not specifically defined to meet the PIH criteria.

94. (B) Nursing process phase: implementation; client need: health promotion and integrity; content area: maternity nursing

Rationale
(A) Formula supplementation is not recommended until the breast milk supply is well established. (B) Colostrum is uniquely suited to the needs of the newborn, providing vital antibodies and concentrated nutrition in the small volume typical of early feedings. (C) Colostrum gradually changes to breast milk between the third to fifth postpartum day. (D) Breast size is related to the amount of fatty tissue and gives no indication of the functional capacity of the breast.

95. (D) Nursing process phase: assessment, client need: physiological integrity; content area: maternity nursing

Rationale
(A) Hyperreflexia is commonly seen with PIH. (B & C) Glucosuria is not a common finding with PIH. (D) Hypertension and proteinuria are two of the classic triad of symptoms found in PIH. The other symptom of this triad is greater than 1+ edema.

96. (B) Nursing process phase: assessment; client need: physiological integrity; content area: maternity nursing

Rationale
(A) Infection is not associated with eclampsia. (B) Eclampsia is characterized by seizure activity, which often results in aspiration as a common complication. (C) Renal perfusion is decreased with hypertension, resulting in decreased urine output (D) Extremity injuries may occur with seizure activity but are not considered a major complication.

97. (A) Nursing process phase: assessment; client need: physiological integrity; content area: maternity nursing

Rationale
(A) Uterine atony, failure of the uterine muscle to contract firmly, is the most common cause of excessive bleeding following childbirth. It occurs in 75 to 85 percent of postpartum clients. (B) Retained placental fragments commonly cause late postpartal hemorrhage. (C) Cervical lacerations are seen less often and are characterized by slow, continuous bleeding with a contracted uterus. (D) Postpartal infection is not necessarily associated with postpartal hemorrhage. It occurs in only about 6 percent of postpartum women.

98. (C) Nursing process phase: planning; client need: safe, effective care environment; content area: maternity nursing

Rationale
(A) Though clients may experience postpartal pain, this is not usually associated with hemorrhage. (B) Clients may be anxious; however, the priority focus in this situation should be adequate organ perfusion. (C) Altered tissue perfusion results from hemorrhage and should be the nurse's highest priority to maintain the client's physiological well-being. (D) Though postpartal patients are at increased risk for infection, this diagnosis is not related to hemorrhage.

99. (D) Nursing process phase: evaluation; client need: physiological integrity; content area: maternity nursing

Rationale
(A) This is a normal respiratory rate. (B) 2+ reflexes are expected with PIH. (C) $MgSO_4$ more typically results in mild sedation because of the CNS effects. (D) Urinary output of less than 30 ml/hr is considered an abnormal amount. Magnesium sulfate is excreted by the kidneys. Toxicity may result

when the kidney function is decreased as a result of reabsorption of the drug. Decreased urine output is a common side effect of $MgSO_4$ toxicity.

100. (A) Nursing process phase: analysis; client need: physiological integrity; content area: maternity nursing

Rationale
(A) $MgSO_4$ prevents seizures by blocking neuromuscular transmission. (B) With the administration of $MgSO_4$, a slight drop in blood pressure may be seen as a result of the relaxation of smooth muscles. However, $MgSO_4$ is not an antihypertensive drug. (C) $MgSO_4$ treatment does not result in an increased urine output but may actually cause a decrease with toxicity. (D) Decreasing edema as a result of diuresis caused by the increased perfusion of the kidney is a positive sign. However, decreasing edema is not the primary purpose of $MgSO_4$ administration.

101. (C) Nursing process phase: assessment; client need: health promotion and maintenance; content area: maternity nursing

Rationale
Nägele's rule, the most common method of determining a delivery date, is obtained by subtracting 3 months from the first day of the last menstrual period and then adding 1 year and 7 days to that date. The correct answer is: May minus 3 months is February. Adding 1 year and 7 days to the 12th results in an EDC of February 19.

102. (C) Nursing process phase: assessment; client need: physiological integrity; content area: maternity nursing

Rationale
(A) Erythropoiesis normally increases after the first trimester but is unrelated to physiological anemia. (B) Dietary intake of iron is unrelated to the development of physiological anemia. (C) There is a 30 to 50 percent increase in maternal blood volume by the end of the first trimester. Although RBCs do increase at this time, plasma volume increases more rapidly, resulting in hemodilution. (D) The liver changes in size, structure, and form during pregnancy, but these changes have no impact on physiological anemia.

103. (C) Nursing process phase: assessment; client need: physiological integrity; content area: maternity nursing

Rationale
(A) At 12 hours postpartum the fundus should be midline and at the umbilicus. (B) At 12 hours postpartum a lazy uterus will generally be deviated to the left side but should be firm and at the umbilicus. (C) Bladder distention pushes the uterus up and generally to the right side. This may cause poor contraction of the uterine muscle increasing the risk for postpartal hemorrhage. (D) Though postpartal hemorrhage may result from a boggy uterus caused by a distended bladder, this assessment does not necessarily indicate the presence of a hemorrhage.

104 (C) Nursing process phase: evaluation; client need: physiological integrity; content area: maternity nursing

Rationale
(A, B, & D) These conditions are not associated with repeat cesarean sections. (C) Uterine rupture along the previous scar is a primary concern for clients who previously have had cesarean deliveries.

105. (D) Nursing process phase: evaluation; client need: physiological integrity; content area: maternity nursing

Rationale
(A) Breast tenderness is not associated with an amniocentesis. (B) Increased fetal activity may occur but would not present a problem. (C) Signs of infection would not be evident in the first hour after the procedure. (D) Rupture of the membranes is a potential complication of amniocentesis.

106. (B) Nursing process phase: implementation; client need: physiological integrity; content area: maternity nursing

Rationale
(A) Antacids should not be used unless prescribed by the primary health-care provider. (B) Reducing or eliminating spicy foods during pregnancy usually eliminates or decreases indigestion. (C & D) These are not related to indigestion during pregnancy.

107. (A) Nursing process phase: evaluation; client need: physiological integrity; content area: maternity nursing

Rationale
(A) This weight gain is normal during the third trimester. (B–D) These actions are not necessary because the weight gain is normal.

108. (B) Nursing process phase: assessment; client need: health promotion and maintenance; content area: maternity nursing

Rationale
(A) As long as there are periods of activity mixed with the inactivity, this would not be an indication that something is wrong. (B) Periods of fetal activity and inactivity are normal during pregnancy. (C) Fetal activity patterns are not associated with gender. (D) This statement is not true.

109. (C) Nursing process phase: evaluation; client need: physiological integrity; content area: maternity nursing

Rationale
(A, B, & D) These conditions are not associated with tetracycline use during pregnancy. (C) Permanent, brown coloration of tooth enamel occurs in the fetus following maternal ingestion of tetracycline during pregnancy.

110. (A) Nursing process phase: assessment; client need: physiological integrity; content area: maternity nursing

Rationale
(A) Painless or silent bleeding is a classic indication of placenta previa. (B–D) These are not indications of placenta previa.

111. (B) Nursing process phase: evaluation; client need: physiological integrity; content area: maternity nursing

Rationale
(A) Hiccups are normal occurrence. (B) Late decelerations are usually indicative of fetal distress. (C & D) These are normal occurrences.

112. (B) Nursing process phase: planning; client need: safe, effective care environment; content area: maternity nursing

Rationale
(A–D) Multiparas may progress rapidly once labor is established. To avoid a last-minute rush and to ensure the husband's presence, an early change to scrub attire is recommended.

113. (D) Nursing process phase: implementation; client need: safe, effective care environment; content area: maternity nursing

Rationale
(A) A prone position is usually uncomfortable at this stage of pregnancy and has no relationship to the drug the client is receiving. (B) A head-down position would place pressure on the diaphragm and has no relationship to ritodrine. (C) This position places pressure on the abdominal aorta and is not related to ritodrine. (D) The side-lying position reduces the risk for supine hypotensive syndrome while administering a drug with a common side effect of hypotension.

114. (A) Nursing process phase: assessment; client need: physiological integrity; content area: maternity nursing

Rationale
(A) PID often causes strictures of the fallopian tubes that increase the risk of ectopic pregnancy. (B–D) These conditions are not associated with PID.

115. (A) Nursing process phase: implementation; client need: safe, effective care environment; content area: maternity nursing

Rationale
(A) Folic acid supplements improve the absorption of iron. (B–D) These supplements are not related to iron absorption.

116. (A) Nursing process phase: planning; client need: health promotion and maintenance; content area: maternity nursing

Rationale
(A) Normal activity patterns during a normal pregnancy are encouraged. New, strenous, or hazardous activities (i.e., sky diving or scuba diving) are discouraged. (B) Maintaining normal activity is the goal. There is no need to improve endurance during pregnancy. (C) Normal activity during a normal pregnancy will not cause premature labor. (D) This statement is not true.

117. (D) Nursing process phase: planning; client need: safe, effective care environment; content area: maternity nursing

Rationale
(A) Weight gain is necessary during pregnancy. (B) Physical endurance is not a goal of pregnancy. (C) This is an unrealistic goal and not possible to accomplish. (D) Premature delivery is a primary risk of multiple gestation. Term delivery is the desired goal.

118. (C) Nursing process phase: implementation; client need: safe, effective care environment; content area: maternity nursing

Rationale
(A) Although these interventions are important and must be accomplished, they are not your most immediate concern with a preterm infant who is small. (B) If the infant is stable respiratorily, there is no need to provide O₂ indiscriminately. (C) At birth the newborn moves into an environment that is 20 to 30 degrees cooler than his core body temperature. If appropriate heat loss prevention is not provided, his body temperature can drop up to 2 degrees within 5 to 10 minutes. Drying the infant thoroughly following birth, using radiant overhead warmers, or wrapping in heated blankets are all top priorites in preventing cold stress in the newborn. Infants who are born prematurely and are small are at an even greater risk of cold stress than a term infant. (D) Institution protocols vary on timing of vital signs. However, in general, an initial set is done soon after birth followed by a second set in 15 minutes. If the vital signs are stable, hourly measurements are done for the first 3 to 4 hours and then changed to q 4 to 8 hours. Unless there is an identified problem, q 15 minute vital signs are usually not necessary.

119. (D) Nursing process phase: analysis; client need: physiological integrity; content area: maternity nursing

Rationale
(A) Brachial nerve palsy sometimes occurs with damage to the nerves of the brachial plexus following shoulder dystocia if there is excessive traction on the infant's head and neck, which pulls at the cervical nerve roots. Femoral nerve palsy is not an appropriate term. (B) Central nervous system damage would not produce these types of gluteal folds or a positive Ortolani's maneuver. (C) Acetabulum atresia would be a major congenital structural defect. It would not, however, produce these signs and symptoms. (D) Infants who have been in the frank breech position in utero are at high risk for congenital dislocation of the hip. Common signs and symptoms of this condition are appearance of a shortened femur on the affected side, thigh and gluteal fold creases that are deeper on the affected side. An Ortolani's test or maneuver is done to evaluate for hip dislocation. With the infant supine, the nurse places the middle fingers on the outside of the femur and the thumb on the inside and flexes the infant's legs so that the hips and knees are at right angles. The knees are then abducted. If the hip is dislocated, the nurse will be able to hear and/or feel a click.

120. (B) Nursing process phase: analysis; client need: physiological integrity; content area: maternity nursing

Rationale
(A) Herpes simplex virus, a member of the herpes virus group including those that cause herpes simplex, herpes zoster, and varicella, produces symptoms such as fever blisters or cold sores. Herpes simplex virus does not produce white patches inside the mouth. (B) Thrush, an infection of the mouth caused by *Candida albicans*, is characterized by formation of white patches and ulcers. Infants often have a low-grade fever and gastrointestinal inflammation with this infection. (C) *Staph. aureus* infection does not present with these signs and symptoms. (D) Epstein pearls are epidermal inclusion cysts that are found on the palate or gums of the newborn. They disappear early in infancy.

121. **(D)** Nursing process phase: planning; client need: physiological integrity; content area: maternity nursing

Rationale

(A) Respiratory distress syndrome (RDS) is caused by a decreased number of alveoli and a lack of lung surfactant. ROM will not cause RDS. (B) Retinopathy of prematurity is thought to be a result of oxygen administration causing vasoconstriction of retinal blood vessels. It is not related to ROM. (C) Meconium aspiration syndrome occurs when the infant aspirates meconium-stained amniotic fluid that has been passed in utero. It is not related to lengthy ROM. (D) Infants born of mothers who had prolonged rupture of membranes are at high risk for infection with organisms that normally inhabit the vaginal tract. Early-onset sepsis causes severe illness in the newborn with mortality rates as high as 50 percent.

122. **(B)** Nursing process phase: analysis; client need: safe, effective care environment; content area: maternity nursing

Rationale

(A) An intake of more sugars would require an increased insulin need to maintain good glycemic control. (B) Morning sickness that normally occurs in the first trimester can complicate glycemic control. During the first trimester there is a lowering of the plasma glucose level, which is related to the action of estrogen. This can compound the problem that results from the nausea that may accompany pregnancy. Insulin requirements change periodically throughout pregnancy, and the woman needs appropriate teaching to maintain glycemic control. (C) Exercise lowers blood glucose levels and decreases the risks of cardiovascular complications such as hypertension and hyperlipidemia. Exercise lowers insulin requirements. If she had stopped her exercise routine, she would likely require more insulin. (D) Sleep requirements do change some in the first trimester; however, it is unlikely that they would reach a point where a woman would not be able to check her glucose levels because of sleep demands.

123. **(C)** Nursing process phase: implementation; client need: physiological integrity; content area: maternity nursing

Rationale

(A) Lengthy periods of exposure to the client should be avoided because of the potential for overexposure to the radiation. Clients should be taught that children and woman who are pregnant will not be allowed to visit. (B) The client will have a urinary catheter in place in order to keep the bladder decompressed to avoid distention and potential displacement of the radiation implants. (C) Clients with internal radiation will be placed on a liquid diet and progressed to a low-residue diet. Antidiarrheal agents that reduce peristalsis and prevent pressure from bowel movements will be given. (D) Clients with internal radiation will remain supine with the head of the bed no higher than 20 degrees to prevent displacement of the implants. She will not be permitted to move from side to side and will require active range-of-motion (ROM) exercises and deep breathing exercises.

124. **(B)** Nursing process phase: implementation; client need: safe, effective care environment; content area: maternity nursing

Rationale

(A) The pressure of the infant against the cord is not reduced in this position. (B) It is imperative that the pressure of the infant's head be reduced against the cord to facilitate a good blood supply to the infant. Placing the mother in the Trendelenburg position will help to relieve some of this pressure. (C) A Fowler's position will increase the force of the infant's head against the cord, decreasing the blood supply to the infant. (D) The pressure of the infant against the cord is not reduced in this position.

125. **(C)** Nursing process phase: analysis; client need: safe, effective care environment; content area: maternity nursing

Rationale

(A) Placenta previa is the attachment of the placenta in the lower uterine segment rather than in the body of the uterus. The presentation signs of this problem are painless vaginal bleeding. (B) These are not the signs and symptoms of an incomplete abortion, which involves heavy bleeding with severe uterine cramping, with some tissue already partially out of the uterus and into the vagina. If loss occurred at 37 weeks, this would not be classified as an abortion. (C) Premature separation of the normally implanted placenta is referred to as an abruptio placentae. Separation often occurs at the onset of labor. Hemorrhage may be internally or externally visible with pain in varying degrees. The woman has a rigid abdomen and signs and symptoms of shock are common with large amounts of bleeding. (D) If more than half of the placenta is involved, intrauterine fetal death will likely occur. However, though there are many other reasons for fetal death in utero, the signs and symptoms this woman is experiencing indicate more has occurred than the death of the fetus.

126. **(D)** Nursing process phase: planning; client need: physiological integrity; content area: maternity nursing

Rationale

(A) This woman should no longer be experiencing any pain as a result of the blood loss. Though pain would be a postpartal nursing diagnosis, it would not be the greatest priority for this client at this time. (B) Infection is certainly a concern postpartally, however this would not be the priority diagnosis in relation to the blood loss. (C) There may have been a period of time that mother and infant could not be together, however this is not the priority diagnosis at this time. (D) With large volume blood loss, tissues become hypoxic as preload falls, cardiac output falls, pulse rises and blood pressure drops. Blood may pool in the peripheral circulation as metabolic acidosis with tissue damage occurs, platelet consumption takes place, and vasodilation reverses the protective vasoconstriction. This will cause further hypoxemia. This is a priority nursing diagnosis for this client.

127. **(A)** Nursing process phase: analysis; client need: physiological integrity; content area: maternity nursing

Rationale

(A) The major risk to a pregnant woman who suffers an asthma attack is the development of status asthmaticus, a lengthy period of reduced gas exchange, which in turn will lead to hypoxia in the fetus. The risk to the fetus is also related to the effects of the medication that may be used to reverse the bronchospasms in the mother. (B) Many high-risk pregnancies require periods of bedrest. This would not be the most concerning risk for the mother and fetus. (C) Although this is certainly a concern for anyone who must experience lengthy hospitalization, it is not the primary concern for this woman and her fetus. (D) IV fluids should be monitored very carefully, as they would be with any client. This will not be the major risk factor for this mother and her fetus.

128. **(B)** Nursing process phase: implementation; client need: health promotion and maintenance; content area: maternity nursing

Rationale
(A) This is not an accurate estimate using Naegele's rule. (B) To use Naegele's rule, count back 3 months from the first day of the last menstrual period, add 7 days and 1 year. August minus 3 months = May, 23 + 7 = 30. (C) This is not an accurate estimate using Naegele's rule. (D) This is not an accurate estimate using Naegele's rule.

129. **(C)** Nursing process phase: assessment; client need: physiological integrity; content area: maternity nursing

Rationale
(A) Fetal movement will not be felt by the mother until approximately 16 to 20 weeks in multigravida clients and as late as 24 weeks in primigravidas. (B) Auscultation of the fetal heart rate with a stethoscope is not possible until about 18 to 20 weeks. (C) Circulation to the vaginal and cervical tissues increases, causing the vaginal mucosa and cervix to take on a bluish-purple hue. This is known as Chadwick's sign. (D) Colostrum, the first breast milk, which is very rich in nutrients and antibodies, may be secreted in very small amounts as early as the second trimester. However, this is generally not noted as early as 11 weeks.

130. **(D)** Nursing process phase: implementation; client need: health promotion and maintenance; content area: maternity nursing

Rationale
(A) Skipping meals is not a good idea. Breakfast is a very important meal after being without intake for several hours during sleep. (B) Many women find that caffeine actually increases their nausea because of its acidity. In addition, many studies indicate that heavy caffeine use appears to affect fetal weight. The higher the caffeine intake, the smaller the fetus. (C) Fats do tend to increase nausea; however, fruits do not seem to be the answer to controlling morning sickness. Additionally, restricting the diet to one type of food is not the best choice. (D) Research shows that dry carbohydrate intake in the morning helps to decrease nausea. Also, reducing the intake of fats, spicy foods, and sweets and spacing meals closer together in smaller amounts is helpful.

131. **(B)** Nursing process phase: implementation; client need: health promotion and maintenance; content area: maternity nursing

Rationale
(A) Even small amounts of alcohol have been linked to fetal alcohol syndrome or other neurological abnormalities in fetuses. (B) Abstinence from alcohol use during pregnancy has been recommended by the surgeon general since 1981. Since the early weeks of pregnancy are the times that are most crucial, it is important that preventive education begin prior to pregnancy. (C) Abstinence is recommended during

pregnancy. (D) Abstinence is recommended during pregnancy.

132. **(D)** Nursing process phase: implementation; client need: health promotion and maintenance; content area: maternity nursing

Rationale
(A) Good nutrition is of vital importance to the health of a woman and her fetus during the course of the pregnancy; however, it is also important to maintain good weight control. (B) It is now recognized that inadequate weight during the course of a pregnancy poses a higher risk to the pregnant woman and her fetus than does excessive weight gain. An inadequate weight gain may lead to low-birth-weight infants, placing them at risk for continuing complications. (C) Weight gain during pregnancy should not follow a linear pattern but should start gradually in the first trimester (about 1 lb per month) and then rise to about 1 lb per week in the second and third trimesters. (D) A gain of 25 to 35 lb over the prepregnancy level allows for adequate growth of the fetus and the maternal organs. Women with multiple gestations should be encouraged to gain 35 to 45 lb, and adolescents within 2 years of menarche should gain about 5 lb more than mature women.

133. **(C)** Nursing process phase: implementation; client need: physiological integrity; content area: maternity nursing

Rationale
(A) The use of habit-forming over-the-counter laxatives should be discouraged. Stimulants or lubricants such as mineral oil should also be avoided. (B) Increasing fiber and complex carbohydrates in the diet will assist in relieving constipation. (C) Increasing fluid intake to at least eight glasses per day and increasing regular exercise will assist in relieving constipation during pregnancy. (D) Although this is a good overall suggestion to improve the diet, it generally will do little to change the elimination pattern of a pregnant woman unless other suggested changes are also made.

134. **(D)** Nursing process phase: implementation; client need: physiological integrity; content area: maternity nursing

Rationale
(A) The client is likely experiencing supine hypotension because of compression of the inferior vena cava. It is not necessary to obtain a blood pressure reading immediately until the situation has been resolved by changing the client's position. (B) This would be a difficult position for a client who is 34 weeks' gestation. It would also not be safe to place a client in this position on an examination table. (C) This is not the most common reason for pregnant clients to experience these symptoms when in the supine position. If changing positions of the client did not relieve the symptoms, further evaluation would be needed. (D) This client is likely experiencing supine hypotension because she is impeding venous return and decreasing the cardiac output since the gravid uterus is placing pressure on the inferior vena cava. The problem is most often relieved when the patient turns onto either side.

135. **(A)** Nursing process phase: implementation; client need: safe, effective care environment; content area: maternity nursing

Rationale

(A) The nurse should allow the client to empty her bladder prior to the performance of Leopold's maneuver, which is palpation of the fetal outline abdominally. This allows the examiner to feel for parts of the fetus in order to assess the position of the fetus in utero. (B) It is not necessary for the woman to remain NPO for any length of time prior to this assessment. (C) It is not recommended that the pregnant woman lie completely supine since this may cause supine hypotension; however, it is not necessary for her to be on her side during this examination. (D) There is no visualization of the fetus during this fetal assessment. It is uncomfortable for the client to have a full bladder during the examination.

136. **(C)** Nursing process phase: implementation; client need: physiological integrity; content area: maternity nursing

Rationale

(A) Over-the-counter medications should not be taken by pregnant women. Diarrhea in pregnancy is usually related to a food source or a viral infection. (B) Increasing the bulk in her diet will not relieve her diarrhea. She should be evaluated further. (C) Diarrhea that does not subside within a 24-hour time frame should be further evaluated. It would be important for this client to come into the clinic. She may be experiencing a viral infection or responding to a food source. In any case, dehydration is dangerous and can often precipitate preterm labor. (D) She will likely need fluid volume support, but it may need to be administered intravenously. She should be advised to come into the clinic for evaluation.

137. **(D)** Nursing process phase: implementation; client need: health promotion and maintenance; content area: maternity nursing

Rationale

(A) Wearing the shoulder belt alone can injure the ribs, spine, neck, or sternum. This is not appropriate information. (B) Lap belts worn alone or not fastened below the abdominal bulge may cause injury from the pressure of the buckle or injury to the intestines, spleen, kidneys, pancreas, stomach, bladder, or uterus may occur as a result of sudden flexion. This is not appropriate advice. (C) Automobile accidents are the leading cause of maternal mortality that is unrelated to pregnancy. Correct positioning for seat belts should be taught, and consistent use should be encouraged even for short trips. (D) This is appropriate information and guidance for seat belt use during pregnancy. During the discussion of proper seat belt use for the mother, the nurse should take the opportunity to introduce the guidelines for infant car seat use as well.

138. **(A)** Nursing process phase: implementation; client need: psychosocial integrity; content area: maternity nursing

Rationale

(A) Pain experienced in the first stage of labor is primarily a result of the dilatation and effacement of the cervix. During the first stage of labor, nerve impulses enter the sympathetic chain and travel to the posterior roots of the thoracic nerves and up the spinal cord to the thalamus. (B) Back pain during labor or "back labor," occurs primarily when the fetus is in an occiput posterior (OP) position because of the pressure of the occiput on the lower spine. (C) Pain is usually felt when the contraction intensity rises 15 to 20 mm Hg above the resting tonus of the uterus. (D) Pain threshold is intrauterine pressure above which contractions are painful. A high pain threshold may be explained by increased endorphin levels. Illness, fear, and fatigue will lower a person's pain threshold. Cultural expectations also affect a person's perception of pain and pain behaviors.

139. **(D)** Nursing process phase: assessment; client need: physiological integrity; content area: maternity nursing

Rationale

(A) Infants with hypoglycemia may be cyanotic; however, hyperthermia and lethargy are not signs and symptoms of this problem. (B) A high-pitched cry and respiratory distress are common signs of hypoglycemia. Doll's eyes are a common sign of a neurological problem and are not related to hypoglycemia. (C) Babinski's reflex is one sign of an intact neurological system and is not related to hypoglycemia. Hypothermia and tremors are commonly seen in an infant with hypoglycemia. (D) These are all appropriate signs and symptoms of hypoglycemia in the newborn.

140. **(C)** Nursing process phase: implementation; client need: physiological integrity; content area: maternity nursing

Rationale

(A) This is not accurate information. One umbilical artery is sometimes associated with congenital anomalies. (B) This is not accurate information. (C) The umbilical cord is made up of two arteries and one vein. Oxygenated blood and nutrients are transported to the fetus by one umbilical vein. The oxygen-depleted blood moves back to the placenta by the two umbilical arteries. (D) This is not accurate information. There are only three vessels in the cord.

141. **(D)** Nursing process phase: implementation; client need: health promotion and maintenance; content area: maternity nursing

Rationale

(A) Flat shoes that do not provide good support may increase leg aches; however, research does not indicate an increase in varicosities. (B) Many clothes that are designed specifically for pregnant clients have elastic waistbands in order to provide a comfortable stretch and fit. There is no reason to avoid these clothes. They are not related to an increase in varicosities. (C) There is no reason for a pregnant client to avoid a stretch girdle or panty hose. (D) Knee-high or thigh-high hose inhibit circulatory functioning in the lower extremities. This may cause or increase the presence of varicosities.

142. **(A)** Nursing process phase: analysis; client need: health promotion and maintenance; content area: maternity nursing

Rationale

(A) Alternately contracting and relaxing the pubococcygeal muscles, known as Kegel exercises, helps to strengthen these perineal muscles, which aids in preventing stress incontinence following delivery. Additionally, these exercises assist the women during the labor process. (B) Kegel exercises do not help to strengthen the abdominal muscles. (C) Kegels do not assist in preventing varicose veins. (D) Kegels do not assist in strengthening the muscles of the lower back.

143. **(B)** Nursing process phase: analysis; client need: physiological integrity; content area: maternity nursing

Rationale
(A) Constipation may occur during pregnancy; however, this is a symptom that may occur for a variety of reasons that do not involve pregnancy. (B) Breast tingling or tenderness and breast enlargement are considered possible or presumptive signs of pregnancy. (C) Shortness of breath should not occur early in pregnancy. This may be a complaint during the latter stages of pregnancy, when the gravid uterus is placing pressure on the diaphragm. (D) Headaches are common occurrences that do not necessarily relate to pregnancy.

144. **(A)** Nursing process phase: implementation; client need: pyschosocial integrity; content area: maternity nursing

Rationale
(A) This is a correct description of melasma, formally referred to as chloasma. It occurs more frequently in darker skinned women. (B) Linea nigra is a line that forms between the symphysis and the umbilicus as a result of hormonal changes. It generally disappears following pregnancy. (C) Striae gravidarum, commonly referred to as stretch marks, appear as pink or purple lines on the breasts, lower abdomen, or thighs. As pregnancy progresses and following delivery they become brown or silvery but never completely disappear. (D) This is not a therapeutic statement, even though it is accurate to state that there are many vascular changes that occur during pregnancy. If a client attempts to discuss an issue or question some event in her pregnancy, it is the responsibility of the nurse to provide accurate information in a therapeutic manner.

145. **(C)** Nursing process phase: analysis; client need: health promotion and maintenance; content area: maternity nursing

Rationale
(A) In and of itself, amenorrhea is not a condition that would prevent a woman from using oral contraceptives. If a condition existed that caused the amenorrhea, then that condition might prevent the use of oral contraceptives. (B) Women with a history of diabetes mellitus are not advised to use oral contraceptives; however, hyperglycemia alone would not be a reason to advise against the use of oral contraceptives. (C) A history of breast cancer as well as malignancies of the reproductive system would prevent a woman from being a good candidate for oral contraceptive use. In addition, women with a history of cystic breast disorder or vaginal bleeding of unknown causes should also not use oral contraceptives. (D) Symptoms of premenstrual syndrome would not prevent a woman from using oral contraceptives.

146. **(C)** Nursing process phase: implementation; client need: health promotion and maintenance; content area: maternity nursing

Rationale
(A & B) This would not be enough time to ensure that sperm are prevented from migrating into the fallopian tubes. (C)

The diaphragm must be left in place for at least 6 hours (but no longer than 24 hours) to ensure that the sperm cannot migrate up the fallopian tubes and initiate conception. An additional application of spermicidal foam or jelly should be used. Douching may dislodge the diaphragm and force sperm into the cervix. (D) Twenty-four hours is the maximum amount of time the diaphragm should be left in place, since research has shown an increased incidence of toxic shock syndrome when the diaphragm or other barrier methods are not removed.

147. **(B)** Nursing process phase: implementation; client need: psychosocial integrity; content area: maternity nursing

Rationale
(A) Giving the client instructions about her husband's presence will not be beneficial to the client at this time. Men and women grieve differently, and this is a judgmental statement. (B) Generally, a statement that conveys your sympathy concerning the loss is very beneficial to the client. Stating your sorrow at her loss and validating her feelings are therapeutic statements. (C) The client may have requested time alone. The nurse should not convey that being alone is bad or that having someone with her would diminish her pain. (D) Medications that delay the grieving process are not beneficial to parents who have experienced a perinatal loss. Even if the mother slept for a time, the pain of her loss would remain when she awakens. Grief must be lived.

148. **(C)** Nursing process phase: assessment; client need: physiological integrity; content area: maternity nursing

Rationale
(A) Sampling of the amniotic fluid requires an amniocentesis to obtain fluid. This is not a first trimester test. (B) The fetal skeleton is not developed during the first trimester. (C) During the first trimester, a real-time ultrasound can visualize and identify the developing yolk sac to confirm pregnancy. (D) A urine sample is not obtained during an ultrasound.

149. **(A)** Nursing process phase: implementation; client need: safe, effective care environment; content area: maternity nursing

Rationale
(A) During CVS a sample of chorionic villi are obtained to perform genetic analysis. Some birth defects can be identified in the early weeks of pregnancy in order to provide adequate time to determine the outcome of the pregnancy. (B) A CVS would not allow you to measure the length of the fetus. (C) Volume of amniotic fluid is not measured during a CVS. (D) This test does not evaluate the functioning level of the placenta.

150. **(B)** Nursing process phase: evaluation; client need: physiological integrity; content area: maternity nursing

Rationale
(A) At 31 weeks' gestation, a fundal height measurement of 27 cm would cause concern that the fetus was not growing appropriately or that the expected date of confinement (EDC) had been miscalculated. (B) At this time the fundal height should correspond to the number of weeks of gestation. This client should measure 31 cm. (C) At 31 weeks' gestation, you would be concerned that a fundal height of 33 cm would in-

dicate an LGA infant, multiple gestation, or inaccurate EDC. (D) Again, this measurement is much too large for a 31-week pregnancy. You would be concerned about the above complications.

151. (C) Nursing process phase: assessment; client need: physiological integrity; content area: maternity nursing

Rationale

(A) This is not an appropriate ratio for L/S. (B) These lungs would not be considered mature. (C) The presence of pulmonary surfactants in amniotic fluid is used to determine the degree of fetal lung maturity. Lecithin is the most critical alveolar surfactant required for lung expansion following birth. After the 24th week of pregnancy, lecithin increases. Sphingomyelin remains constant, and therefore a measurement of the ratio of the two pulmonary surfactants will give an accurate measurement of feta lung maturity, which occurs at about 35 weeks' gestation. The ratio should be 2:1. (D) This is not an accurate ratio for fetal lung maturity.

152. (C) Nursing process phase: assessment; client need: physiological integrity; content area: maternity nursing

Rationale

(A) This heart rate would be considered bradycardia and would be concerning. (B) The lower number of 100 beats per minute would be too low. (C) This is the normal heart rate per minute for a term infant. (D) This upper level would be considered tachycardia and might be concerning.

153. (B) Nursing process phase: evaluation; client need: physiological integrity; content area: maternity nursing

Rationale

(A) Changing the maternal position to a side-lying position will improve fetal perfusion; however, it is not a necessary nursing intervention for early decelerations. (B) Early decelerations are a result of fetal head compression and are considered a benign heart rate pattern. No nursing intervention is necessary. These usually occur during the first stage of labor as the cervix is dilating from 4 to 7 cm. Early decelerations are sometimes seen during the second stage of labor as the woman is pushing. (C) There is no indication of maternal hypotension with early decelerations. (D) This is not necessary since early decelerations are a benign fetal heart rate pattern.

154. (B) Nursing process phase: evaluation; client need: physiological integrity; content area: maternity nursing

Rationale

(A) This would not likely cause a high baseline in the fetus. (B) An elevated maternal temperature would increase the heart rate in response to the increased metabolic rate. The nurse should attempt to reduce the maternal fever with antipyretics as ordered and cooling measures. (C) Early fetal hypoxia will sometimes cause an increase in FHR above 160 beats per minute. Good beat-to-beat variability would be an encouraging sign. (D) There is no indication that this client is dehydrated. Maternal dehydration does not usually cause an elevated baseline FHR unless there is fetal distress. Good BTBV would be encouraging.

155. (C) Nursing process phase: analysis; client need: physiological integrity; content area: maternity nursing

Rationale

(A) Variable decelerations are those that occur any time during the contraction and are caused by umbilical cord compression. They are often U- or V-shaped with a rapid descent and ascent to and from the nadir of the deceleration. (B) Early decelerations are in response to fetal head compression and usually do not indicate fetal distress. Early decelerations are uniform in shape and correspond to the rise in intrauterine pressure as the uterus contracts. (C) Late decelerations are a result of uteroplacental insufficiency and are smoother, uniform patterns that mirror the intrauterine pressure during a contraction. They begin after the contraction has been established and last after the uterus has returned to the resting state. They usually indicate fetal distress and hypoxia and should be considered an ominous sign. (D) This is not an appropriate term.

156. (D) Nursing process phase: implementation; client need: safe, effective care environment; content area: maternity nursing

Rationale

(A) This statement is partially true but does not give a comprehensive explanation of what the nurse is assessing. (B) The fetal heart rate is monitored electronically or with a Doppler. Cervical examinations do not evaluate the fetal heart rate. (C) This statement is partially true but, again, does not give a comprehensive explanation of the examination. (D) Vaginal examinations are done to correctly identify the fetal position and presenting part as well as to evaluate the effacement and dilatation of the cervix. This is an accurate statement and a good explanation of the importance of vaginal checks.

157. (C) Nursing process phase: analysis; client need: psychosocial integrity; content area: maternity nursing

Rationale

(A) Though they may feel that parents no longer have as much time to devote to the relationship between the teen and the parents, this is not the primary reason for the lack of acceptance of the infant. (B) Peers have a tremendous impact on adolescents as they attempt to develop their own identity. However, they do not necessarily fear rejection as a result of the presence of a new infant in the family unit. (C) Preteen and early adolescent years are an important time for the development of a strong sexual identity. Early adolescents rationalize that their parents are too old to be sexually active and therefore may have a difficult time accepting the new infant into the family unit. (D) This may be a true statement but does not adequately describe the developmental issues surrounding the arrival of a new infant into a family of an adolescent.

158. (A) Nursing process phase: analysis; client need: health promotion and maintenance; content area: maternity nursing

Rationale

(A) Helen has no apparent social support system. At 17 years of age she has limited educational preparation to provide financial support for herself and infant. (B) Although Sue has made a recent move to a new community, she has the social and emotional support of her spouse. She would need good nursing support but would not likely be your most concerning client. (C) Even though Lou is unmarried and pregnant, it is apparent that she has a good support system available to her. She would need good nursing support but would likely do well in adjusting to the maturational crisis of pregnancy. (D) Judy would also need good nursing care, but because of her social and emotional support system as well as her obvious desire to be pregnant, she should adjust to her maturational crisis well. Her financial situation should be stable.

159. (A) Nursing process phase: assessment; client need: physiological integrity; content area: maternity nursing

Rationale
(A) During your observation of the client's perineum and anal area, you are using the assessment portion of the nursing process. You are using observation to collect data. (B) The diagnosis step of the nursing process includes a statement of the nursing diagnosis that can be made following a thorough assessment of the client. (C) Nursing interventions are prepared to guide the care to be provided to the client. This is the planning phase of the nursing process. (D) Following implementation of nursing intervention, care is evaluated and plans are revised.

160. (C) Nursing process phase: implementation; client need: health promotion and maintenance; content area: maternity nursing

Rationale
(A) Urine will not provide a hematocrit level. A sample of blood is the source of this test. (B) Again, a blood sample is needed for this test. (C) Urine is checked at each prenatal visit to screen for protein and glucose. These tests would be an early indicator of pre-eclampsia and gestational diabetes. (D) Urine can be screened for infection if a urinalysis is done. This is not a part of routine screening unless the urine is cloudy or blood-tinged or the woman is symptomatic.

161. (D) Nursing process phase: implementation; client need: health promotion and maintenance; content area: maternity nursing

Rationale
(A) Weight and urine will be checked, but cervical checks will not be done until close to the due date. (B) Blood tests are done early in the pregnancy at the first visit, and an ultrasound may be done during the second trimester if the client is high risk. They are not done routinely at each visit. (C) This is a true statement but is not a comprehensive explanation of all screenings done at a prenatal visit. (D) These are routine checks that are done at each prenatal visit. Blood pressure is monitored for signs of pregnancy-induced hypertension. Weight gain is monitored, and urine is checked for protein and albumin. Fundal height is measured to ensure that the fetus is developing appropriately.

162. (B) Nursing process phase: analysis; client need: health promotion and maintenance; content area: maternity nursing

Rationale
(A) Infants do not need solids this early and may be more prone to allergies if solids are begun so early. Breastfed infants receive adequate nutrition from breast milk alone. (B) Milk production is stimulated by the infant's sucking. Adding solids will interrupt the milk supply. (C) This is not a true statement. The infant will not increase sucking since her stomach will be full of solids and will not nurse as long. (D) Introduction of solids has not been shown to increase the amount of sleep time for most infants. Early introduction of solids to infants increases allergy responses. Breastfed infants do not need supplements if the mother is well nourished and has a good milk supply.

163. (A) Nursing process phase: implementation; client need: psychosocial integrity; content area: maternity nursing

Rationale
(A) Reassuring your client is important. A simple explanation is appropriate. This is an accurate definition of engagement. (B) Reassurance is important, but this statement does not give the client any information or explanation about engagement. This is a demeaning statement. (C) Again, this is a demeaning and condescending statement. It did not answer the client's question. (D) This is not an accurate explanation of engagement.

164. (C) Nursing process phase: implementation; client need: psychosocial integrity; content area: maternity nursing

Rationale
(A) Pain medications given so early in labor will slow or halt the progression. Opioid analgesics such as meperidine (Demerol) can cause respiratory depression in the woman and decreased fetal movements with resulting poor beat-to-beat variability. Protocols vary from institution to institution, but generally speaking, these analgesics are not given before labor is well established. (B) This would be a positive nursing action; however, it will not assist the woman in managing her pain. (C) Teaching this patient the elements of better pain management and control will assist her in taking charge of her labor process. Fear is probably playing a large role in her response to the pain. Nonpharmacological pain management can often work very well in the early stage of labor. (D) A condescending attitude and approach to this patient will not assist her in becoming more in control. Education and good emotional support are the keys.

165. (D) Nursing process phase: assessment; client need: physiological integrity; content area: maternity nursing

Rationale
(A) Dopamine is a pressor used to maintain blood pressure. (B) Pavulon is a paralytic agent. (C) Dilantin is used for seizure control. (D) Prostaglandin E_2 causes the smooth muscle of the ductus to remain relaxed. This is necessary in many forms of cyanotic heart disease so that the patent ductus arteriosus (PDA) can provide for the necessary mixing of oxygenated and unoxygenated blood.

166. (A) Nursing process phase: implementation; client need: physiological integrity; content area: maternity nursing

Rationale
(A) Newborn infants have a large surface area in proportion to mass, less subcutaneous fat, and lower vasomotor control and are therefore prone to hypothermia. Providing a warmed area and quickly drying the infant are critical immediately following birth to prevent heat loss. Severe consequences may result if the newborn is exposed to an environmental temperature above or below the neutral temperature zone. (B) The flexure of the sigmoid colon is at a depth of 3 cm in the infant. Insertion of a rectal probe to a depth of less than 5 cm will not provide an accurate core temperature,

and perforation of the rectum is likely at this depth. Therefore, routine use of rectal temperatures is not recommended for the neonate. (C) Infants who are not in respiratory distress do not routinely require supplemental oxygen. Supplemental oxygen should be viewed as a medication and should not be given indiscriminately. (D) Although good physical assessment to evaluate for physical deformities of the newborn is important, it is not the priority nursing intervention at the time of delivery.

167. (B) Nursing process phase: analysis; client need: physiological integrity; content area: maternity nursing

Rationale
(A) RDS usually presents with respiratory distress and quickly progresses to cyanosis. The infant may be grunting and may have nasal flaring and retractions. A scaphoid abdomen is not a symptom of RDS. (B) Diaphragmatic hernia, one of the most urgent emergencies in the newborn, is a defect in the diaphragm with herniation of the abdominal contents into the thoracic cavity. These are the classic symptoms of this defect. These infants should not be resuscitated with bag and mask ventilation but should be intubated immediately. (C) Symptoms of a spontaneous pneumothorax are decreased breath sounds on the affected side, respiratory distress, and cyanosis. A scaphoid abdomen is not a symptom of this disorder. (D) Congenital heart disease may present with respiratory distress and cyanosis; however, a scaphoid abdomen is not a symptom.

168. (C) Nursing process phase: analysis; client needs: physiological integrity; content area: maternity nursing

Rationale
(A) Facial paralysis is usually caused by pressure on the facial nerve during birth. Forceps are generally the cause. Often the condition is transitory and will resolve within hours or days following birth. (B) This is not an accurate description of the resulting injury to the brachial nerve. (C) Brachial paralysis, or Erb-Duchenne paralysis, is the most common type of paralysis associated with a difficult vaginal birth. This results from injury to the upper plexus when stretching or pulling on the shoulder occurs. Generally symptoms are a flaccid arm with the elbow extended and the hand rotated inward. The grasp reflex is intact. (D) Trauma to the clavicle will not cause paralysis in the arm unless the nerve tract has been damaged.

169. (A) Nursing process phase: implementation; client need: psychosocial integrity; content area: maternity nursing

Rationale
(A) Gavage feeding is used for infants who are respiratorily compromised, do not have a mature suck or swallow reflex, or who fatigue so easily that they are not able to take in the amount of calories they need for growth and development. (B) Preterm infants may be held outside of the incubator, depending on their weight and ability to maintain their body temperature. However, they may still be too small to take in the amount of formula they need for growth because of their immature suck and swallow reflex. (C) Stomach capacity in the preterm infant may be small, but this is not the reason for providing gavage feedings. (D) Preterm infants can suck, though their suck-swallow-breathe reflex may not be well developed. They will fatigue before they are able to take in the appropriate amount of formula for growth.

170. (B) Nursing process phase: implementation; client need: physiological integrity; content area: maternity nursing

Rationale
(A) Parenteral nutrition indicates nourishment that is obtained by any route other than the alimentary canal, such as IV, IM, mucosal, and so on. (B) Nonnutritive sucking is encouraged to allow the infant to suckle during gavage feedings, which results in improved oxygenation and decreased energy expenditure and increases attachment to the nipple when oral feedings are initiated. (C) This is not an appropriate term. (D) This is not an appropriate term as the infant is not receiving nutrition from the pacifier.

171. (D) Nursing process phase: evaluation; client need: physiological integrity; content area: maternity nursing

Rationale
(A) Oxytocin should be discontinued immediately if any nonreassuring FHR pattern occurs. (B) Oxytocin should be discontinued immediately if uterine hyperstimulation occurs. (C) Oxytocin should be discontinued immediately if any nonreassuring FHR pattern occurs. (D) Urine output should be at least 120 ml or more over a 4-hour period when a client is receiving oxytocin for an induction of labor.

172. (C) Nursing process phase: evaluation; client need: safe, effective care environment; content area: maternity nursing

Rationale
(A) There is no indication for a cesarean delivery at this time. (B) As long as the electronic fetal monitor tracings are indicating that the infant is experiencing no fetal distress, there is no indication for a fetal scalp pH sampling. (C) The client will likely be a candidate for augmentation of labor to stimulate her contractions. If labor has started spontaneously, yet is not progressing satisfactorily, contractions can be augmented with the administration of oxytocin. (D) Since the client has already dilated to 3 cm, there is no indication that cervical ripening is needed.

173. (C) Nursing process phase: implementation; client need: safe, effective care environment; content area: maternity nursing

Rationale
(A) There is no indication that the fetus is in distress. (B) There is no indication of maternal hypotension (C) Since the client has been progressing well through her labor, the sudden change in the contraction pattern to a flat line would most likely mean that the transducer has slipped off the fundus of the uterus and was not picking up the uterine activity. Repositioning the transducer would be the best nursing action. (D) There is nothing to indicate that the client is in need of additional oxygen.

174. (B) Nursing process phase: analysis; client need: physiological integrity; content area: maternity nursing

Rationale
(A) A breech presentation does not cause severe low back pain. (B) A posterior presentation causes low back pain because of the pressure of the bony occiput on the low spine. This presentation frequently slows the progress of the first stage of labor as the fetus attempts to make the first cardinal movements of birth. (C) A transverse presentation will cer-

tainly slow the progress of labor, but severe low back pain is not a complaint. (D) An anterior presentation is the most desirable presentation, because this allows the fetus to move easily through the birth canal. Some clients may complain of back pain, but it is not usually of a severe nature.

175. (C) Nursing process phase: assessment; client need: physiological integrity; content area: maternity nursing

Rationale

(A) During the latent first stage of labor, clients may still be focused outside themselves. They may be able to ambulate and talk through most contractions. (B) The urge to push does not come until the second stage of labor, when clients are near or completely dilated. (C) During the active phase of the first stage of labor, clients begin to work at maintaining control during contractions. They are quieter and accept coaching more readily. (D) Clients are irritable and agitated during transition. They frequently feel that they are not able to go on.

176. (B) Nursing process phase: evaluation; client need: physiological integrity; content area: maternity nursing

Rationale

(A) Pain medications may slow intestinal motility of newborns. (B) Meperidine (Demerol), a narcotic, may diminish the ability of the newborn to suck effectively if given too close to birth. The ability of the infant to clear the narcotic from his or her own system is slow. (C) There should not be any central cyanosis unless the infant is in respiratory distress or has delayed respiratory effort. In this case the infant should be given a narcotic antagonist such as naloxone (Narcan). (D) This should not be a response seen in a newborn as a result of narcotic medication in the mother prior to delivery.

177. (D) Nursing process phase: analysis, client need: physiological integrity; content area: maternity nursing

Rationale

(A) A nurse providing care for a newborn should know whether or not forceps were used during a delivery. Although skin abrasions and bruising may occur with forceps use, they appear different than telangiectatic nevi. (B) Port-wine stain, or nevus flammeus, is a red to purple macular lesion resulting from dilated capillaries under the epidermis. The lesions are permanent and do not blanch with pressure. (C) Mongolian spots are purplish spots on the trunk and buttocks or sacral area. They are most common in darker skinned individuals. They fade and disappear in early childhood. (D) Telangiectatic nevi are pink, macular lesions that blanch with pressure and become darker when the infant cries. These lesions may last as long as 1 to 2 years or may persist into adulthood. They appear most often on the forehead, eyelids, bridge of the nose, neck, and over the base of the occipital bones. They are a normal variation of the newborn and are not concerning.

178. (C) Nursing process phase: implementation; client need: safe, effective care environment; content area: maternity nursing

Rationale

(A) There is no need to cover the infant's head during phototherapy. As much of the skin as is possible needs to be exposed to the light for the maximum benefit. (B) Phototherapy increases the infant's insensible water loss. The feedings will not be held. On the contrary, fluids will be encouraged to increase intestinal motility to maximize bilirubin excretion through the bowel. (C) The infant's eyes are covered at all times while undergoing phototherapy to prevent retinal damage. Eye patches should be removed during feedings or every 4 hours to assess the eyes for signs and symptoms of infection and to promote visual stimulation. Eye patches should be firmly in place but should not cause undo pressure on the eyes because abrasions can result. (D) It is not necessary for the infant to remain still and quiet during phototherapy. This does not increase the effectiveness of the light.

179. (D) Nursing process phase: implementation; client need: psychosocial integrity; content area: maternity nursing

Rationale

(A) These parents are most likely depressed and overwhelmed by the events of the birth of their preterm newborn. This statement is flippant and does not show professional judgment. (B) This statement puts your feelings into play in the minds of these parents. They may not be excited at the thoughts of the events surrounding the birth of their daughter. This is a very frightening experience. (C) Though talking with a social worker or other professional may be helpful to these parents, you are the care provider who knows and understands the events of this infant. You will be the most convenient person to interact with these parents and will be most available to them. You should take every opportunity to reassure them and to answer their questions so that they can feel a part of the care of their new child. (D) This is an open-ended statement that will allow them to discuss any aspect of their feelings regarding the birth of their preterm child. You are not being judgmental or imposing your thoughts on them. You are giving them the opportunity to discuss their feelings and to ask direct questions about the status of their infant.

180. (B) Nursing process phase: planning; client need: safe, effective care environment; content area: maternity nursing

Rationale

(A) Infants with neonatal sepsis are not necessarily in isolation. It will depend on the responsible microorganism. The most common early-onset newborn infections are a result of group B hemolytic streptococci, *Escherichia coli*, and *Haemophilus influenzae*. Late-onset organisms are nosocomial and result from *Staphylococcus aureus*, *S. epidermidis*, and *Pseudomonas*. Compliance with universal precautions is essential. (B) Prevention is the best cure; however, when sepsis does occur, therapies are chosen carefully because side effects are common. Broad-spectrum antibiotics will be administered until microorganism-specific antibiotics can be selected following culture and sensitivity tests. (C) Parental visitation is encouraged. However, good hand washing and parent education is vital. (D) Exchange transfusions are not the treatment of choice for neonatal sepsis.

181. (C) Nursing process phase: planning; client need: health promotion and maintenance; content area: maternity nursing

Rationale

(A) The first part of the nursing process is assessment which includes objective data. (B) The first part of the nursing process is assessment which includes subjective data. (C) A nursing diagnosis is a three part statement that reflects a nursing clinical judgment statement about an individual, family, or community. Nursing diagnosis provide the basis for nursing interventions that will assist the client in achieving optimal health. (D) The first part of the nursing process is assessment which includes both objective andd subjective data.

182. **(B)** Nursing process phase: implementation; client need: safe, effective care environment; content area: maternity nursing

Rationale
(A) If diagnosis is made in the first trimester, the medical treatment is to remove the molar tissue by dilation and curettage. Later diagnosis may lead to a hysterotomy. The woman's desire for future pregnancy is considered when making treatment choices. Future pregnancies are possible following a molar pregnancy. (B) Without treatment, choriocarcinoma of the endometrium will develop in approximately 20 to 50 percent of cases of hydatidiform mole. A partial mole less frequently leads to malignancy. (C) Her risks for a spontaneous abortion in future normal pregnancies are not necessarily increased. (D) There is not an increased risk for uterine rupture during a normal pregnancy following a molar pregnancy.

183. **(B)** Nursing process phase: assessment; client need: physiological integrity; content area: maternity nursing

Rationale
(A) DIC does not necessarily produce hypertension or cause an increase in the WBC count. (B) Prolonged bleeding time from venipuncture sites or other areas of skin integrity interruption are common with DIC. (C) Shaking of the lower extremities is a very common occurrence following delivery. Several theories exist in regard to the causes including exhaustion, sudden decrease in intra-abdominal pressure, withdrawal of placental hormones, and reactions to fetal blood or amniotic fluid that may have entered the maternal circulation during placental separation. This shaking is not associated with elevated temperature. (D) Pitting edema in the lower extremities is not necessarily associated with DIC.

184. **(A)** Nursing process phase: implementation; client need: health promotion and maintenance; content area: maternity nursing

Rationale
(A) The best time for a woman to do breast self-examination is immediately after her period. At this time her breasts are not tender or swollen. If her periods are irregular, she should do it each month on the same day of the month unless it falls just before or during her period. (B) Just before a woman's period, her breasts are usually tender and may be swollen from retained fluid. This is not the ideal time to do breast self-examinations. (C) Many changes take place in a woman's breasts prior to and during her period. This is not the ideal time to do breast self-examination. (D) This is the best time to do breast self-examinations only if a woman's periods are very irregular or if she frequently skips periods. Her examination should not take place prior to or during her period.

185. **(D)** Nursing process phase: analysis; client need: physiological integrity; content area: maternity nursing

Rationale
(A) These are mongolian spots resulting from the deep dermal infiltration of melanocytes seen most frequently in Black,

Asian, or Latin infants. This is a normal variation. (B) Overriding cranial sutures are a normal variation that occur as the infant moves down through the birth canal. This molding allows for a normal descent of the infant. (C) The anterior and posterior fontanelles should feel soft and flat. This is a normal finding. (D) The chest circumference should always be 1 to 2 cm less than the head. The infant should be evaluated for microcephaly if the chest circumference is larger than the head circumference.

186. **(B)** Nursing process phrase: implementation; client need: health promotion and maintenance; content area: maternity nursing

Rationale
(A) The newborn will be in the first period of reactivity during the first 15 to 30 minutes after birth and alert and eager to suck. (B) This is an ideal time for maternal-infant bonding to begin. Even if the mother feels prepared to breastfeed her infant, assisting and encouraging her at this time is very important. (C) It is no longer felt to be necessary to initiate breastfeeding with sterile water. (D) Even if the infant is not hungry, this is an ideal time for the first breastfeeding. The infant will consume only a small amount of colostrum at the initial feeding.

187. **(C)** Nursing process phase: analysis; client need: physiological integrity; content area: maternity nursing

Rationale
(A) Postmature infants frequently have dry, peeling skin. This does not place them at an increased risk of cold stress. (B) Postmature infants will have normal length and head circumference but may have lost weight in utero as a result of decreased placental function after the 42nd week of gestation. This, however, does not necessarily place them at risk for cold stress. (C) There is a loss of subcutaneous tissue, which makes legs and arms look wasted. This also increases the risk of hypothermia in postmature infants. (D) There is a decrease in vernix coating as infants become more postmature.

188. **(D)** Nursing process phase: implementation; client need: health promotion and maintenance; content area: maternity nursing

Rationale
(A) Fever is never to be ignored. Parents should be told to notify their health-care provider if the fever is greater than 99°F. It is important for parents to distinguish between vomiting and spitting up. It is common for infants to have a small amount of spitting up. This is not a sign of infection. (B) Again, fever should never be ignored. Many infants "spike" a high fever with an illness. Motor behavior disturbances would be a better indicator of severity of illness. Many infants have difficulty accommodating to the family's schedule. This can be very disturbing to new parents, but generally it does not indicate severe illness. (C) An increase in the fluid consistency, frequency, and volume of stool can be a result of allergies or overintake of food. It is not necessarily an indication of severe illness. Health-care providers should be notified if dehydration is a concern. (D) Unexplained irritability, poor appetite, and fever are early indications of infections. Parents should be taught the signs of symptoms of newborn infection.

189. (C) Nursing process phase: analysis; client need: physiological integrity; content area: maternity nursing

Rationale
(A) There is no evidence that urinary catheters place a patient at an increased risk for thrombophlebitis. (B) There is no evidence that epidural anesthesia places a patient at an increased risk for thrombophlebitis. (C) Women who have pre-existing varicose veins or prior episodes are at increased risks of thrombophlebitis. Other factors that place women at risk are obesity, high parity, advanced maternal age, and previous heart disease. Bedrest associated with surgery and general anesthesia can also increase the risk. (D) Fluid replacement during surgery does not place a patient at increased risk for thrombophlebitis.

190. (D) Nursing process phase: implementation; client need: safe, effective care environment; content area: maternity nursing

Rationale
(A) Chronic hypertension is not associated with pregnancy but may be aggravated by it. Pregnancy can be very stressful for women who have chronic hypertension. However, these women do not necessarily require a cesarean section. (B) When amniotic membranes are ruptured for greater than 18 hours, the woman and fetus are at a greater risk of infection. However, if the labor is progressing normally, there is no reason a cesarean section is required based simply on the length of time of ruptured membranes. (C) The pain of a woman with low pain threshold will be treated and controlled as much as possible but does not require a cesarean section. (D) An arrest of descent of the fetus during the labor process will lead to an operative birth.

191. (A) Nursing process phase: analysis; client need: safe, effective care environment; content area: maternity nursing

Rationale
(A) Habitual spontaneous abortions as a result of loss of muscular integrity of the cervix may be caused by genetic, structural, immunologic, or hormonal problems. The placement of a cerclage or Skirodkar-Barter procedure is a common treatment for this problem. (B) Infections may lead to spontaneous abortions, however, the placement of a cerclage is not required. Treatment of the infection with antibiotics and limitations of activities are the common medical treatments. (C) Vaginal bleeding would be a symptom of a threatened spontaneous abortion. (D) Prolapsed cords are not an indication for a cerclage.

192. (D) Nursing process phase: analysis; client need: physiological integrity; content area: maternity nursing

Rationale
(A) A decrease in blood pressure is a positive side effect of magnesium sulfate. (B) Magnesium sulfate is not a CNS stimulant. It provides a neuromuscular blockade at the myoneural junction. (C) Magnesium sulfate inhibits muscle function, thereby decreasing uterine contractions. This patient is not being given $MgSO_4$ as a muscle relaxant. (D) Magnesium sulfate is the treatment of choice for prevention of eclamptic convulsions.

193. (B) Nursing process phase: analysis; client need: physiological integrity; content area: maternity nursing

Rationale
(A) For the first 15 to 30 minutes following birth, the term infant will be alert and eager to suck with a gastric capacity of 10 to 20 ml. Bowel sounds can be heard following the first period of reactivity. At birth the hematologic system is quickly infused with oxygen. Assessments of the hematologic system include the ability of this system to carry oxygen. These changes are vital but are not the systems undergoing the most profound changes. (B) These two systems are considered together. They are vital to survival. The first breath, establishment of respirations, and transitional circulation are the most important anatomic changes that must occur following birth. (C) The loss of placenta circulation at birth ends the newborn's dependence on the maternal renal system. Several changes take place over the first few months of life. The newborn liver is immature and continues to develop following birth; however, this system does not undergo the most profound changes following birth. (D) Thorough assessment of the neurological system is important in the early hours following birth. The newborn is subjected to temperature changes, lights, and other environmental stimuli. It is imperative that the newborn are able to transition normally. The immune system functions somewhat sluggishly at birth. This places the infant at increased risk for colonization and subsequently infection. However, these systems do not undergo the most profound changes following birth.

194. (C) Nursing process phase: analysis; client need: physiological integrity; content area: maternity nursing

Rationale
(A) Cutis marmorata, or mottling, is sometimes a result of chilling. It is caused by dilation of the small blood vessels. It is commonly seen in early infancy. (B) Milia, which are epidermal inclusion cysts, are common in newborns. These small, white papules may be seen on the chin, nose, and forehead. They usually disappear early in infancy. (C) An imperforate anus is worrisome and can be associated with tracheoesophageal fistula or esophageal atresia. (D) A blood-tinged vaginal discharge, or pseudomenses, is a result of withdrawal of maternal hormones following birth. It is a common variation of the newborn female.

195. (A) Nursing process phase: implementation; client need: health promotion and maintenance; content area: maternity nursing

Rationale
(A) This nursing diagnosis would be appropriate since she is a first-time mother with a limited support system available. (B) This nursing diagnosis would have been pertinent immediately following delivery but should have been resolved by 24 hours' postpartum. She would not be released from the birthing center if this diagnosis remained active. (C) This nursing diagnosis would also have been of primary concern soon after delivery and would continue to be an issue for this client for several weeks' postpartum. However, this could fall under the umbrella of knowledge deficit related to self-care. (D) This diagnosis could also be included in the knowledge deficit of self-care.

196. (D) Nursing process phase: evaluation; client need: physiological integrity; content area: maternity nursing

Rationale
(A) Limiting the time the baby breastfeeds contributes to engorgement. This can cause difficulty in latching on and actually increases the chances of sore nipples. (B) Prenatal preparation of the breasts for lactation is of little benefit. Rolling of nipples, lotions or creams, and manual expression of milk do

not decrease nipple trauma during lactation. Breasts should be cleaned with warm water and should be free of creams and lotions prior to placing the baby to breast. (C) Supplemental feedings of water or formula should be discouraged because they interrupt the establishment of an adequate milk supply. Supplements do not decrease the occurrence of sore nipples. (D) Substantial damage from poor positioning can result after only one feeding. It is imperative that infants latch on correctly and are positioned appropriately to decrease trauma to the nipple.

197. (C) Nursing process phase: planning; client need: psychosocial integrity; content area: maternity nursing

Rationale
(A) Altered comfort is a state in which an individual experiences an uncomfortable sensation in response to a noxious stimulus. Although she complains of being restricted to the bed during the labor process, this nursing diagnosis is not the most comprehensive. (B) Anxiety is a state in which an individual experiences feelings of uneasiness with activation of the autonomic nervous system in response to a vague, nonspecific threat. The monitor is not imposing a nonspecific threat. (C) This nursing diagnosis adequately defines the problem that is specific to her complaints. (D) Activity intolerance refers to a reduction in an individual's physiological capacity to endure activities. She is not impaired physiologically by the monitor.

198. (D) Nursing process phase: implementation; client need: safe, effective care environment; content area: maternity nursing

Rationale
(A) Some institutions prefer intermittent EFM. Guidelines for each perinatal center should be developed based on the Association of Women's Health, Obstetric and Neonatal Nursing (AWHONN) standards of practice. This statement is not appropriate since it is not therapeutic. (B) There is no law that requires continuous EFM. However, recommendations for care are based on AWHONN standards. Continuous monitoring is recommended for high-risk clients. (C) This is not therapeutic communication. (D) This statement provides the client with information so that she is able to understand the rationale for the nursing intervention. It is professional and therapeutic.

199. (D) Nursing process phase: analysis; client need: safe, effective care environment; content area: maternity nursing

Rationale
(A) Pregnant women need at least 2000 cc of fluid daily. (B) Tylenol is a nonteratogenic antipyretic and is safe for use in pregnancy. (C) Oxygen requirements increase during pregnancy; some women may experience dyspnea even at rest. (D) All antimicrobials cross the placenta. Erythromycin can cause fetal liver damage.

200. (C) Nursing process phase: implementation; client need: health promotion and maintenance; content area: maternity nursing

Rationale
(A) Maternal blood sugar increases slightly during the second trimester of pregnancy. However, this increase is not normally sufficient to contribute to the incidence of vaginal yeast infections. (B) Maternal blood sugar decreases during the first trimester of pregnancy. Lower blood sugar levels are associated with decreased incidence of vaginal yeast infections. (C) Vaginal pH increases from 4 to 6.5 during pregnancy, which leads to decreased acidity, a proliferation of yeast cells, and an increased incidence of vaginal yeast infections. (D) Vaginal yeast infections are common during pregnancy due to the increased vaginal pH.

201. (B) Nursing process phase: evaluation; client need: health promotion and maintenance; content area: maternity nursing

Rationale
(A) Evidence indicates that ingestion of live culture yogurt decreases the incidence of vaginal yeast infections. (B) Although vinegar and water douches do decrease vaginal pH, douching is not recommended during pregnancy. (C) Moisture in the perineal area contributes to the development of vaginal yeast infections. Cotton fabrics are more absorbent than synthetic or silk fabrics. (D) Tight-fitting clothing holds in moisture and heat. These conditions contribute to the incidence of vaginal yeast infections.

202. (C) Nursing process phase: implementation; client need: health promotion and maintenance; content area: maternity nursing

Rationale
(A) Increased estrogen levels cause engorgement, edema, and hyperemia of the capillaries in the upper respiratory tract. They will not be relieved by decongestants. (B) Referral to a specialist is not necessary because these are normal pregnancy symptoms. (C) The elevated levels of estrogen during pregnancy caused increased vascularization in the upper respiratory tract. Nasal stuffiness, earaches, hearing loss, and a tendency to nosebleeds are commonplace. (D) Cold drafts do not cause respiratory infections. Lying on one side or the other will not cause hearing loss.

203. (A) Nursing process phase: evaluation; client need: physiological integrity; content area: maternity nursing

Rationale
(A) Blood volume increases by 30 to 50 percent in pregnancy. This increase in blood volume causes hemodilution of red blood cells and a corresponding physiological anemia. (B) Hemoglobin normally decreases in pregnancy due to the increase in blood volume. (C) Blood glucose increases in the second trimester of pregnancy. (D) Increased production of factors VII, VIII, IX, X, and fibrinogen, plus depression of fibrinolytic activity during pregnancy, leads to hypercoagulability in pregnancy.

204. (B) Nursing process phase: implementation; client need: health promotion and maintenance; content area: maternity nursing

Rationale
(A) The areola darkens during pregnancy, breasts are swollen because of the influence of progesterone and estrogen, and striae are generally not seen until the third trimester. (B) Breast tenderness is an almost universal complaint during the first trimester of pregnancy, the increased blood supply to breast tissue results in veins becoming more visible, and the sebaceous glands (Montgomery's tubercles) enlarge. (C) Inverted nipples are not a pregnancy finding, the areola and nipple become more pigmented, and breast size increases. (D) Nodularity is caused by an increase in the size of the mammary

glands during the second trimester. The areola and nipples darken; colostrum is not secreted until the third trimester.

205. (D) Nursing process phase: implementation; client need; psychosocial integrity; content area; maternity nursing

Rationale

(A) Ambivalent feelings about pregnancy are common and do not require special intervention. In addition, this response is a block to therapeutic communication. The nurse is telling the client how she "should" feel. (B) "Mother love" does not necessarily appear right after birth, especially in a primipara. It may take time for such love to grow. (C) Even women with a desired pregnancy have occasional ambivalent feelings. Such feelings do not necessarily mean the woman desires an abortion. (D) Ambivalence is a normal response experienced by any individual preparing for a new role.

206. (D) Nursing process phase: implementation; client need: psychosocial integrity; content area: maternity nursing

Rationale

(A) Listening to FHT helps validate the reality of the pregnancy but does not help the father visualize the new family member, which best facilitates father-fetal attachment. (B) Fetal models are good teaching tools for explaining physical development and size of the fetus, but are not the best way of encouraging paternal attachment to his fetus. (C) Typed handouts are too abstract to be of help in encouraging paternal-fetal attachment. (D) Having a father present at the ultrasound of his fetus promotes paternal-fetal bonding by allowing him to see the features of his fetus. This visualization makes the pregnancy and new role more real.

207. (A) Nursing process phase: assessment; client need: physiological integrity; content area: maternity nursing

Rationale

(A) Erythroblastosis fetalis is caused by antibodies formed by a mother who has formed antibodies in her blood because of an ABO or Rh incompatibility. Blood and Rh typing and antibody screening can alert the health-care provider to the possible development of this condition so steps can be taken to ensure a healthy neonate. (B) Down syndrome is caused by an extra chromosome 21 and is diagnosed through analysis of amniotic fluid obtained by amniocentesis. (C) Erythemia neonatorum is a transient epidermal rash. It is found only in term infants during the first 3 weeks after birth. It has no clinical significance and requires no treatment. (D) Caudal regression syndrome is caused by uncontrolled and high maternal blood glucose levels. It can be diagnosed before delivery only by ultrasound.

208. (D) Nursing process phase: assessment; client need: physiological integrity; content area: maternity nursing

Rationale

(A) Preterm labor is characterized by repetitive uterine contractions lasting more than an hour that result in cervical changes. These contractions may or may not be painful. (B) Premature rupture of the membranes is characterized by uncontrolled leakage of clear fluid from the vagina. The fluid is nitrazine positive and demonstrates a characteristic "ferning" pattern when dried on a glass slide. (C) Hyperemesis is characterized by severe, persistent maternal vomiting that results in dehydration and a catabolic state. (D) Pregnancy-induced hypertension is characterized by blood pressures of 140/90 or above, > 2+ proteinuria, persistent or severe headache, visual disturbances, and edema of the face or fingers or over the sacrum.

209. (C) Nursing process phase, implementation; client need: safe, effective care environment; content area: maternity nursing

Rationale

(A) Compression of the major vessels of the pelvis occurs with a supine position. This will cause postural hypotension and compromise placental perfusion. (B) Fetal reserves are still present as evidenced by normal variability of 8 to 10 beats and a quick return to baseline after the decelerations. A cesarean section is not yet warranted. (C) Positioning a woman on her left side promotes fetal well-being by increasing placental perfusion and subsequent fetal oxygenation. This position change may very well stop the occurrence of the variable decelerations. (D) Oxytocin (Pitocin) causes or increases the intensity of uterine contractions. Increasing the intensity of the contractions can inhibit placental perfusion and compromise the fetus. In addition, labor is progressing normally in this client and no augmentation of labor is needed to speed up the process.

210. (B) Nursing process phase: implementation; client need: physiological integrity; content area: maternity nursing

Rationale

(A) Amniocentesis is done under sterile conditions. In addition, signs and symptoms of infection usually take 12 to 24 hours to manifest after an invasive procedure. (B) This invasive procedure involves inserting a long needle through the uterus and into the amniotic sac. There is a real risk for precipitation of uterine contractions and compromised fetal well-being. (C) Informed consent is required before this invasive procedure. Any explanations should occur before the amniocentesis is performed. (D) Although encouraging the client to verbalize concerns is always appropriate, physiological needs have priority over psychological needs.

211. (D) Nursing process phase: assessment; client need: physiological integrity; content area: maternity nursing

Rationale

(A) Fetal distress is evidenced by a fetal heart rate less than 110, poor variability, multiple decelerations, and a scalp pH indicating fetal acidosis. (B) Erythroblastosis fetalis is a hemolytic condition of the newborn caused by isoimmunization, which results from ABO or Rh incompatibility. (C) Down syndrome is caused by an extra chromosome 21 and is determined by chromosomal analysis of the amniotic fluid. (D) Mature fetal lungs have an L/S ratio of greater than 2:1. In addition, the presence of phosphatidylglycerol is a predictable indicator of lung maturity.

212. (A) Nursing process phase: implementation; client need: health promotion and maintenance; content area: maternity nursing

Rationale

(A) All women have approximately the same amount of milk-producing glandular tissue (mammary glands). The amount of fatty tissue present determines breast size. (B) Milk (lactiferous) ducts are the lumina that carry the breast milk to the nipple. They are not associated with either breast size or milk production. (C) Milk production is determined by how often the breasts are emptied of milk. Supplementation with formula can lead to less frequent emptying of the breasts and a decrease in milk production. (D) La Leche is a group support organization with the purpose of helping women successfully breastfeed. However, breast size (large or small) does not constitute any type of special need.

213. (B) Nursing process phase: implementation; client need: health promotion and maintenance; content area: maternity nursing

Rationale
(A) This diet is fruitarian. It consists of raw or dried fruits, nuts, honey, and olive oil. (B) The semivegetarian includes fish, poultry, eggs, and dairy products. Red meat and pork are avoided. There are no nutritional problems with this type of vegetarian diet. (C) The lactovegetarian supplements a vegetable diet with milk and cheese. Iron is the only deficiency in this diet. (D) The strict vegetarian follows an all-vegetable diet, which includes fruits, nuts, legumes, and grains. Special combinations of legumes and grains provide adequate amounts of vegetable protein for pregnancy.

214. (C) Nursing process phase: assessment; client need: physiological integrity; content area: maternity nursing

Rationale
(A) An H&H determines if a state of anemia exists by measuring the hemoglobin and hematocrit. (B) A complete blood count measures red and white blood cells. It does not include clotting factors. (C) Heparin affects the blood's clotting ability. Careful monitoring of the partial thromboplastin time is essential to achieve effective anticoagulation. (d) HCV measures the presence of antibodies to hepatitis C virus.

215. (D) Nursing process phase, implementation; client need: psychosocial integrity; content area: maternity nursing

Rationale
(A) According to cultural beliefs of the Vietnamese, the postpartum state is "cold" and "hot" foods are necessary to maintain the balance of the body. "Hot" foods are also thought to stimulate the flow of breast milk. Fruits, vegetables, and sandwiches are considered to be "cold" foods and therefore avoided. (B) Noodle soup is a better substitute because it is a "hot" food. However, seaweed soup is traditionally served to Vietnamese women during the postpartum state. Offering a substitute would not be culturally sensitive behavior. (C) This statement is neither culturally sensitive nor professional. (D) Heating up the soup as asked indicates respect for the cultural beliefs of the client.

216. (B) Nursing process phase: assessment; client need: psychosocial integrity; content area: maternity nursing

Rationale
(A) Financial resources and adequate family support are essential in ensuring effective family functioning. This client has a workable plan for the future and a good support system in her parents. (B) High-risk families include those below the poverty level, those headed by a single teenage parent, and those with unanticipated stress. This family has few financial resources and is headed by a single, teenaged parent. The family is at high risk for ineffective functioning. (C) This family is at some risk because of the age of the client and the pending separation of the couple. However, finances are secure and family support is available. (D) This client has the ability

to make mature decisions. She recognized her limitations and developed a plan to ensure the best environment for her baby. Her decision would not constitute a risk factor for ineffective family functioning.

217. (A) Nursing process phase: analysis and planning; client need: physiological integrity; content area: maternity nursing

Rationale
(A) The infant needs to be held belly to belly with his mother. Having the head turned to one side does not allow the infant to swallow, thus increasing the frustration of both mother and baby. (B) Newborn infants can utilize their stores of brown fat for energy for up to 72 hours after birth. This infant is not at risk for a lack of nutrition. (C) Evidence of body image disturbance would include expressions of distaste for the breast-feeding process and a refusal to demonstrate putting the baby on the breast. (D) While there is certainly anxiety, this is not the priority diagnosis. Physiological needs come before psychosocial needs.

218. (D) Nursing process phase: implementation; client need: health promotion and maintenance; content area: maternity nursing

Rationale
(A) Normal laboratory values for pregnancy are WBCs = 5,000 to 10,000/mm^3; RBCs = 4.2 to 5.4 × 10^6/mm^3, Hemoglobin = 12 to 16 gm/dl, and Hematocrit = 37 to 47%. This client is anemic. (B) The WBC count is within the normal range for pregnancy. (C) The hemoglobin and hematocrit are below the normal ranges for pregnancy. (D) Most cases of iron deficiency develop after the 20th week of pregnancy because of expanding blood volume and fetal demands. Any hemoglobin value below 10 gm/dl and/or hematocrit below 35 percent is generally considered to constitute a true anemia. Iron supplements are necessary. Vitamin C helps the body to more easily absorb iron.

219. (B) Nursing process phase: implementation; client need: safe, effective care environment; content area: maternity nursing

Rationale
(A) A semiprivate room would not afford the client the quiet environment she needs. Routine vital signs are not frequent enough to detect early changes in maternal or fetal condition. Stress testing is done to determine fetal reaction to uterine contractions and is inappropriate at this time. Salt restriction has no effect on the edema and is unnecessary. (B) Loud noises and bright lights can trigger seizures in a client with severe PIH; these stimuli can be minimized in a private room. The client needs to rest as much as possible and avoid stress. Vital signs and fetal heart tones should be monitored a minimum of every 4 hours. PIH can result in fetal intrauterine growth retardation. Twice daily fetal nonstress testing can help determine fetal well-being. There are no dietary restrictions for a client with PIH. (C) This client needs to be in a quiet environment and on bedrest. The VS and fetal heart tones are not frequent enough to detect early changes in maternal or fetal condition. Fetal nonstress testing is also too infrequent. A low protein diet is prescribed for clients with renal conditions. Pregnant clients need adequate amounts of protein to support the pregnancy. (D) Unless the condition of the client suddenly worsens or she starts to labor, there is no reason for her to be in a labor room. Continuous fetal

monitoring, VS every 15 minutes, and no NPO status are also not necessary.

220. (D) Nursing process phase: analysis and planning; client need: safe, effective, care environment; content area: maternity nursing

Rationale

(A) Parlodel is a (rarely used) medication for suppression of lactation. (B) Depo-Provera is a long-lasting (3 months), injectable form of birth control. It should not be given to nursing mothers until at least 6 weeks' postpartum. (C) The size of the infant could indicate the mother had undiagnosed gestational diabetes. However, once an infant is delivered, maternal blood glucose returns to normal within 24 hours. Insulin would not be needed. (D) A grandmultiperous woman is at risk of uterine atony and postpartum hemorrhage. Women who deliver an unusually large infant are also at risk for uterine atony. Methergine is an oxytocin that directly stimulates contractions of the uterus and is used to prevent and treat postpartum hemorrhage caused by uterine atony.

221. (B) Nursing process phase: implementation; client need: safe, effective care environment; content area: maternity nursing

Rationale

(A) A vertex OP position is not desired because it results in a larger diameter presenting to the pelvis and birth canal. The nurse should expect to prepare the client for an episiotomy and manual rotation of the presenting part to OA (occiput anterior). (B) OA (or face down) is the desired fetal position. The occiput has the smallest fetal diameter and makes passing through the birth canal easier. A mediolateral episiotomy gives more room for application of the forceps without the danger of the episiotomy extending into the rectum. Simpson's forceps are generally used to perform a midforceps (0 to <2+ station) delivery. (C) In a face presentation, a second-degree midline episiotomy would very likely tear the perineum into the rectum. Fundal pressure is contraindicated. Any assisted pressure administered by the nurse should be suprapubic to avoid prolapse of the uterus after delivery of the fetus. (D) A third-degree midline episiotomy would give the health-care provider more room to apply forceps, but would have the same risks of extending into the rectum as a second-degree midline episiotomy. Piper forceps are used for breech presentations to deliver the aftercoming head.

222. (C) Nursing process phase: implementation; client need: safe, effective care environment; content area: maternity nursing

Rationale

(A) A vaginal examination on a woman with ruptured membranes who is not in labor will increase her risk for infection. (B) It is important to obtain baseline vital signs and a temperature every hour after membranes have ruptured. The vital signs should be obtained after the sterile speculum examination. (C) A sterile speculum examination is done to confirm membrane status, to rule out cord prolapse, and to visualize the cervix for dilatation and effacement. A sample of any fluid can also be obtained with a sterile swab and checked for ferning. (D) Fetal heart tones should be monitored with an external fetal monitor to determine that the fetal heart rate is normal. The fetal monitor is placed in position after the sterile speculum examination has been completed.

223. (D) Nursing process phase: assessment; client need: physiological integrity; content area: maternity nursing

Rationale

(A) Terbutaline is a β-adrenergic agonist. Palpitations, nervousness, tremors, and tachycardia are normal maternal side effects. (B) Drowsiness, lethargy, slurred speech, and blurred vision are maternal side effects of magnesium sulfate therapy. (C) Decreased fetal heart rate variability, neonatal hypotonia, and drowsiness are fetal/neonatal side effects of magnesium sulfate therapy. (D) 8 mg/min of terbutaline for 10 hours is considered to be a high dose. The client also has received excessive amounts of IV fluids. β-adrenergic agonists increase plasma renin and arginine vasopressin, which is associated with sodium and water retention. This predisposes to pulmonary edema. In addition, excessive intravenous fluids combined with the antidiuretic effect of high doses of β-adrenergic agonists can result in fluid overload.

224. (A) Nursing process phase: evaluation; client need: health promotion and maintenance; content area: maternity nursing

Rationale

(A) Do not use soap on the nipples. It removes protective oils and causes drying. (B) Increased air circulation promotes drying and prevents maceration. (C) Colostrum or breast milk should be applied to the nipples after feedings because it has lysozymes and other healing properties. (D) The area of the nipple directly in line with the infant's nose and chin is most stressed during feedings. Varying the position of the infant during nursing can prevent any one area from overstress.

225. (D) Nursing process phase: implementation; client need: physiological integrity; content area: maternity nursing

Rationale

(A) A newborn's stomach capacity is approximately 15 ml. This lasts for the first few days of life. (B) Cow's milk allergy is manifested in a newborn by vomiting up each feeding. (C) A 3-day-old infant with adequate intake should have 6 to 10 wet diapers a day. (D) The average capacity of a newborn's stomach is 15 ml. However, the capacity increases to 75 to 90 ml by the end of the first week.

226. (A) Nursing process phase: assessment; client need: physiological integrity; content area: maternity nursing

Rationale

(A) Cold stress increases an infant's need for oxygen and can upset the acid-base balance. The infant reacts by increasing its respiratory rate. Cold stress also increases the metabolic rate and glucose stores are rapidly used up. (B) Hypoglycemia is manifested in a newborn by diaphoresis and a blood glucose level below 35 mg/dl. (C) Acrocyanosis is peripheral cyanosis and refers to the blue color of the hands and feet in most newborns. This peripheral cyanosis is normal and disappears in 7 to 10 days. Flexion of the extremities is the normal position for a healthy term newborn. (D) Cyanosis noted around the lips (central cyanosis) and an increased respiratory rate are indicators of a congenital cardiac defect, not cold stress.

227. (C) Nursing process phase: implementation; client need: safe, effective care environment; content area: maternity nursing

Rationale

(A) Infiltration of an intravenous line can have devastating effects on the fragile tissue of a preterm infant. Severe pain, necrosis, and tissue sloughing are common. (B) This technique involves breaking a sterile line and should not be attempted on any client. Preterm infants are especially vulnerable to the bacteria that gather during breaks in sterile technique. (C) It is appropriate to discontinue the catheter. Insertion of a new catheter into a different site minimizes the risk of infiltration of the medication and ensures that serum levels of the antibiotic remain therapeutic. (D) It is appropriate to discontinue the catheter; however, a neonate with sepsis is kept on antibiotics for a minimum of 10 days. Three days of intravenous antibiotics is not enough.

228. **(A)** Nursing process phase: evaluation; client need: health promotion and maintenance; content area: maternity nursing

Rationale
(A) Teachers of the Lamaze method recognize that labor is painful and do not promise a pain-free labor or birth. The techniques are used to increase the ability of the woman to cope with pain through conditioning and relaxation. (B) In the Lamaze technique, the labor coach assists the woman by providing feedback during labor. It is the responsibility of the coach to recognize when the woman is experiencing stress and helping her to relax. (C) Lamaze techniques typically use imagery in combination with relaxation exercises. (D) In the Lamaze technique, women learn exercises to condition and tone muscles to prepare for childbirth. Exercises include the pelvic tilt, tailor sit, and Kegel exercises.

229. **(A)** Nursing process phase: analysis and planning; client need: safe, effective care environment; content area: maternity nursing

Rationale
(A) HELLP syndrome often presents in late second or early third trimester but might not present until after delivery. The presence of HELLP syndrome is a risk factor for developing postpartum eclampsia. (B) Vital signs and postpartum checks are essential every 15 minutes in the first postpartum hour only. Assessment of the maternal-infant attachment process is important throughout the 6-week postpartum period. (C) Blood glucose levels need to be monitored only in the postpartum diabetic woman. The blood glucose level is not a concern for HELLP syndrome or eclampsia. (D) According to the theory of puerperal adaptation, the postpartum woman is most ready to start to care for herself and her infant about 24 hours postpartum. Assessment of these abilities and return demonstrations by the client are most logically assessed on the first or second postpartum day prior to discharge.

230. **(D)** Nursing process phase: implementation; client need: physiological integrity; content area: maternity nursing

Rationale
(A) Cancerous lumps are usually not painful or tender. These are the symptoms of early mastitis. A biopsy is not indicated. (B) These are the symptoms of early mastitis. Hospitalization and IV antibiotics are reserved for severe cases of breast infection. (C) As lactation is established, a lump may be felt. However, a filled milk duct will shift position from one day to the next. After the milk comes in on about the third postpartum day, breasts may be tender for about 48 hours. It is not normal for pain to persist for as long as a week postpartum. (D) Mastitis is an infection of a milk duct. Early mastitis can be effectively treated with rest, fluid, acetaminophen, and through emptying of the plugged milk duct. Some health-care providers recommend emptying the breasts with a pump; however, pumps are less effective than a breastfeeding infant and the organisms that cause mastitis are not present in breast milk.

231. **(D)** Nursing process phase: implementation; client need: health promotion and maintenance; content area: maternity nursing

Rationale
(A) Infant noses are made so they can breathe while nursing. It is not necessary to depress breast tissue to facilitate breathing. Depressing breast tissue at the nose can pull the nipple and areola out of the correct position in the infant's mouth. (B) Using the "scissors" position of the fingers can prevent the infant from taking in enough of the areola for effective breastfeeding. It can also lead to sore nipples and early termination of breastfeeding. (C) The lactiferous ducts are found underneath the areola. Proper latching on includes the nipple and as much of the areola as can be gotten into the infant's mouth. (D) Positioning the infant at nipple level prevents nipple trauma from pulling of the nipple. Keeping the body of the infant in a straight line with the head allows the infant to swallow when nursing.

232. **(D)** Nursing process phase: evaluation; client need: health promotion and maintenance; content area: maternity nursing

Rationale
(A) A firm-fitting bra is necessary for support of the breast tissue but also reduces stimulation to the breasts and will suppress the milk ejection reflex. (B) Breastfeeding mothers need noncaffeinated fluids to maintain their fluid needs and milk supply. This is not related to the milk ejection reflex. (C) Cold packs reduce inflammation and engorgement. They will also suppress milk production. (D) Nipple stimulation causes the release of oxytocin. Oxytocin is the hormone responsible for the milk ejection reflex.

233. **(C)** Nursing process phase: evaluation; client need: health promotion and maintenance; content area: maternity nursing

Rationale
(A) Cats can carry an organism called *Toxoplasma* in their stool. The organism can be picked up on the hands, or through inhalation of cat litter dust. Toxoplasmosis, the disease caused by this organism, can cause fetal damage. (B) Vitamin C enhances the absorption of iron. (C) Electric blankets can raise the body temperature to greater than 102°F. Temperatures this high or higher have been associated with fetal anomalies. (D) No studies have shown any harmful effects from moderate ingestion of aspartame (Nutrasweet) by most women during pregnancy. However, women with phenylketonuria (PKU) should avoid aspartame since it contains the amino acid phenylalanine.

234. **(D)** Nursing process phase: analysis and planning; client need: safe, effective care environment; content area: maternity nursing

Rationale
(A) Oxytocin is given to stimulate contraction of the uterus. It is used for induction of labor or immediately postpartum to control bleeding. It is contraindicated for this stage of pregnancy and procedure. (B) Methylergonovine maleate is an oral medication used to control postpartum hemorrhage

caused by subinvolution of the uterus. It is contraindicated in this instance. (C) Morphine is a schedule II narcotic in pregnancy risk category C. Animal studies have shown an adverse effect on the fetus. Maternal discomfort experienced during the procedure range from mild to severe. Nonnarcotic analgesics may be administered. (D) Since there is potential for leakage of fetal red blood cells into the mother's circulation, some studies recommend that all Rh negative women should be given an immunoglobulin.

235. (B) Nursing process phase: evaluation; client need: health promotion and maintenance; content area: maternity nursing

Rationale
(A) The back seat is the safest place in a car. The car seat should face the back of the seat until the infant weighs at least 20 lb. (B) Backpacks should only be used for infants old enough to be able to hold their heads up well alone. (C) An infant may chew the paint on a crib when teething starts. Lead paint causes brain damage. (D) Sudden infant death syndrome (SIDS) is associated with the abdominal position in young infants. Until the infant can turn over alone, the recommended position is on the back or side.

236. (D) Nursing process phase: implementation; client need: psychosocial integrity; content area: maternity nursing

Rationale
(A) Studies have shown that there is no connection between the use of birth control pills and difficulty conceiving, especially when the low-dose pills are used. (B) Men retain their ability to impregnate women into their eighties. Spermatogenesis is generally not affected by the aging process. (C) Metrorrhagia is abnormally heavy menses. It is normally associated with perimenopause. Perimenopause generally does not start until the forties or fifties. (D) After age 35 the ovaries are adversely affected by the normal aging process.

237. (B) Nursing process phase: implementation; client need: psychosocial integrity; content area: maternity nursing

Rationale
(A) An adolescent who becomes pregnant must decide what course of action she is going to take. Relinquishing an infant by adoption can be painful for the expectant teen. Making a decision earlier in the pregnancy allows feelings to be worked through before the birth of the baby. (B) The autonomous decision by an adolescent to relinquish her baby for adoption can be considered an important step toward maturity. (C) Teenagers who place their infant for adoption because of external pressure frequently feel anger at those who put the pressure on them, and painful feelings of grief. (D) The choice of adoption leaves the teenager with mixed messages from society regarding her pregnancy. The teenager needs both affirmation that this decision is a significant event and assistance in dealing with her feelings.

238. (D) Nursing process phase: implementation; client need: psychosocial integrity; content area: maternity nursing

Rationale
(A) Women who experience the loss of one child and the survival of another experience complex feelings of joy and grief. Parents do not grieve less for one child because of the joy in the survival of another. (B) This is an example of a blocking statement. The woman is not being allowed to express her feelings. (C) Parents who have experienced the loss of an infant often feel alone in their grief because society places less value on the loss of a newborn as compared to that of an older child or adult. (D) Recognition of the client's grief and offering her a chance to express her feelings validates her feelings of loss.

239. (C) Nursing process phase: implementation; client need: health promotion and maintenance; content area: maternity nursing

Rationale
(A) Fetal anomalies are caused by genetic changes, or alterations in physical development. Tobacco smoking does not alter the genetic makeup of infants, nor does it alter physical development. (B) Central nervous system damage is usually associated with inadequate intake of folic acid. Tobacco smoking does not hinder folic acid absorption. (C) Nicotine causes vasoconstriction and reduced placental blood flow. Carbon monoxide inactivate maternal and fetal hemoglobin and further decrease the oxygen carrying capacity of the blood. Other toxic elements of tobacco smoke cause abnormalities of the placenta. The major fetal consequences of smoking during pregnancy are intrauterine growth retardation, prematurity, and increased perinatal loss. (D) There is little evidence to associate maternal smoking and fetal nicotine addiction. The adverse fetal effects of nicotine and other tobacco byproducts are related to decreased oxygen delivery to the fetus.

240. (B) Nursing process phase: implementation; client need: health promotion and maintenance; content area: maternity nursing

Rationale
(A) Turkey is high in protein; cantaloupe high in vitamin C; iceberg lettuce high in fiber; green peas high in iron; rice high in carbohydrates; milk high in calcium (B) Duck, dried apricots, kale, baked potatoes, and pumpkin are high iron foods. Lemonade is high in vitamin C, which facilitates the absorption of iron. (C) Chicken is a high protein food; apples have soluble fiber; broccoli is high iron; navy beans have calcium; mashed potatoes have vitamin C; tea should be avoided. (D) Canned salmon is high in calcium; bananas are high in potassium; asparagus is high fiber; egg noodles have some iron; apple juice is high in simple sugars.

241. (B) Nursing process phase: assessment; client need: safe, effective care environment; content area: maternity nursing

Rationale
(A) The client is in transition, which is cervical dilation from 7 to 10 cm. Delivery will probably take place in approximately 2 hours. (B) Pressure of the presenting part as it progresses through the birth canal stimulates the sensation of needing to have a bowel movement. A vaginal examination needs to be done stat because delivery may occur very quickly. (C) Contractions can increase in frequency and intensity without much cervical change. A judgment about delivery time cannot be made from this information. (D) Vomiting and a sense of "having enough" are signs of transition. Transition is the shortest part of labor, lasting approximately 2 hours.

242. (C) Nursing process phase: assessment; client need: physiological integrity; content area: maternity nursing

Rationale
(A) A rapid pulse rate (up to 120) and palpitations are normal side effects of terbutaline. They do not indicate fluid overload. (B) This output exceeds the intake, which would lower the risk

of fluid overload. (C) Fluid overload results in pulmonary edema. The lower bases of the lungs are the first to fill with fluid. Rales would be auscultated. (D) Pitting pedal edema is not uncommon in pregnant women. 3+ pitting edema and edema of the hands or face could indicate PIH, not pulmonary edema.

243. (D) Nursing process phase: evaluation; client need: health promotion and maintenance; content area: maternity nursing

Rationale

(A) Visual and auditory stimulation should not be presented to the infant at the same time. Drug-exposed infants are easily stressed. (B) Wind-up swings have a clicking noise and also stimulate the infant visually. (C) Rattles stimulate the infant's vision and hearing. (D) Drug-exposed infants need physical contact and soft auditory stimulation. Playing soft music is appropriate for this infant.

244. (D) Nursing process phase: implementation: client need: physiological integrity; content area: maternity nursing

Rationale

(A) Bringing the arms to the midline and securing them helps console the infant. Leaving the arms loose contributes to frantic behaviors. (B) This technique includes both visual and auditory stimulation, which is to be avoided in drug-exposed infants. (C) This technique includes both visual and auditory stimulation, which is to be avoided in drug-exposed infants. (D) Placing the infant over a shoulder and gently stroking the back is a proven technique for preventing frantic crying in a drug-exposed newborn.

245. (A) Nursing process phase: assessment; client need: safe, effective care environment; content area: maternity nursing

Rationale

(A) Hypertonicity and poor coordination of the suck-and-swallow reflex are characteristic of the narcotic-exposed infant. Seizures may also be present in these newborns. (B) These features are typical of fetal alcohol syndrome. (C) These characteristics are typical of the tobacco-exposed infant. (D) These are the typical features of Down syndrome.

246. (A) Nursing process phase: intervention; client need: safe, effective care environment; content area: maternity nursing

Rationale

(A) Methadone should be given to the heroin-addicted client to prevent or stabilize heroin withdrawal during labor. When nausea and vomiting are present, it should be administered IM. (B) Heroin is a central nervous system depressant. It is essential to monitor the respiratory rate, pulse, and blood pressure at least every hour. (C) Butorphanol tartrate is a narcotic agonist that can cause acute maternal and fetal abstinence syndrome. (D) The heroin-addicted woman may leave the obstetrical unit well into her labor to avoid withdrawal. Close observation is necessary.

247. (B) Nursing process phase: implementation; client need: safe, effective care environment; content area: maternity nursing

Rationale

(A) Cocaine causes vasoconstriction of the placental vessels. The client should be positioned on her left side to maximize placental blood flow. (B) The laboring woman who has recently used cocaine is at risk for a hypertensive crisis and seizures. She must be protected from injury. (C) The client who has recently used cocaine is at risk for seizures. Environmental stimuli must be reduced as much as possible. (D) Narcotic analgesics can cause central nervous system depression in cocaine-using clients. Nonpharmacological comfort measures are preferred.

248. (A) Nursing process phase: implementation; client need: psychosocial integrity; content area: maternity nursing

Rationale

(A) The most significant intervention for partner abuse is just being asked about being hurt or frightened by a partner. Studies show that victims of partner abuse have frequently gone to a health-care provider with obvious injuries and waited for someone to ask about them because they were too ashamed to volunteer the information. (B) One in three women is a victim of partner abuse, regardless of socioeconomic status. Pregnancy in particular can precipitate abuse because the partner may perceive a loss of power in the relationship and resort to abuse as a way to restore power. (C) Many women fear that disclosure of abuse will result in being told they must leave their partner in order to receive treatment. Women who are pregnant or with a newborn are least likely to leave a relationship. (D) The client does not have a psychiatric problem. What is most needed is sensitivity, acceptance, and guidance regarding where she can obtain additional help when she is ready.

249. (D) Nursing process phase: implementation; client need: psychosocial integrity; content area: maternity nursing

Rationale

(A) Physical abuse concerns power. The abusive partner often does not perceive his violent behavior as a problem. The victim may not know what will provoke the abuse, but the abuser blames the woman for the violence. (B) Victims of abuse often remain in these relationships because they are financially dependent on the partner, especially if they are pregnant. They may feel that they have no options. It typically takes a victim three times to leave an abusive partner and three times before she succeeds. (C) Partner abuse occurs in a cycle that has three phases: (a) tension building, (b) an explosion, and (c) a honeymoon phase where the abuser expresses remorse and tries to "make it up" to the victim. This cycle continually repeats itself. (D) The abused woman often believes she is responsible for the violence against her. It is essential that the nurse let her know that no one deserves to be hurt for any reason. The person who hurt her is the one responsible for his action. The nurse should also teach the victim that violence is not normal, that it is usually repeated, that it is against the law, and that she has alternatives to staying in the relationship.

250. (C) Nursing process phase: assessment; client need: physiological integrity; content area: maternity nursing

Rationale

(A) Painless, bright red vaginal bleeding indicates a placenta previa. (B) A decreased fundal height is associated with "lightening," or the engagement of the fetal presenting part in the pelvic girdle. (C) Abruptio placentae is the separation of the placenta from the uterus. It can separate around the margins of the placenta, in which case there would be painful, dark red bleeding. Or it can separate in the middle of the placenta, in which case bleeding would be concealed. (D) Fetal tachycardia in the absence of tocolysis indicates maternal infection.

251. **(B)** Nursing process phase: implementation; client need: safe, effective care environment; content area: maternity nursing

Rationale

(A) Magnesium sulfate is a central nervous system depressant. Stimulating the client will have no effect on increasing respirations. (B) Calcium gluconate reverses the effects of magnesium sulfate. (C) Magnesium sulfate is also a tocolytic. It prevents uterine contractions by blocking the release of acetylcholine by motor nerve impulses. (D) Naloxone reverses the effects of narcotic analgesics. It is not effective for magnesium sulfate overdose.

252. **(D)** Nursing process phase: implementation; client need: health promotion and maintenance; content area: maternity nursing

Rationale

(A) Hepatitis B virus is excreted in breast milk. However, once the infant has been given immunoglobulin, bottle feeding is not required. (B) Hepatitis B is transmitted through blood and body fluids. It is not transmitted by the respiratory route. (C) Reverse isolation is used to protect immunocompromised individuals from nosocomial infections. It is not used to protect others from hepatitis B. (D) Breastfeeding is considered safe once the infant has been given immunoglobulin and hepatitis B vaccine.

253. **(C)** Nursing process phase: evaluation; client need: health promotion and maintenance; content area: maternity nursing

Rationale

(A) Breast milk contains the amino acid phenylalanine, which cannot be metabolized by the infant with PKU. Moderate to high levels of phenylalanine can result in mental retardation. (B) Formula is modified cow's milk, which also contains phenylalanine. (C) PKU is treated with a special low-phenylalanine diet. A special formula is used for infants. (D) Soy-based formulas also contain phenylalanine.

254. **(D)** Nursing process phase: analysis and planning; client need: health promotion and maintenance; content area: maternity nursing

Rationale

(A) A newborn does not need a full bath every day as long as the diaper area is kept clean and regurgitated milk is removed. Clear water only or a mild soap solution should be used. (B) Newborns have very dry skin that peels during the first weeks of life. This is because they were surrounded by fluid for 9 months and the outer layers of skin were not shed. The use of lotions or creams on the skin is unnecessary and may cause skin irritation. (C) Powders do not help keep the diaper area dry. They can cause chafing and skin irritation. In addition, shaking talc-based powders creates a dust cloud that can be inhaled by the infant, causing respiratory problems. (D) The cord should be cleaned three times a day with cotton swabs and peroxide or alcohol. The area should be kept dry by folding the diaper below the cord.

255. **(B)** Nursing process phase: implementation; client need: safe, effective care environment; content area: maternity nursing

Rationale

(A) The radiant warmer provides heat according to the infant's skin temperature. However, this is not the priority nursing action. (B) The infant should be dried before any other nursing or medical action. Heat loss from evaporation occurs when the infant's skin is wet. (C) Warming blankets will help prevent heat loss through conduction. However, the infant is not wrapped in a blanket until she is ready to be taken to the nursery. (D) Temperatures are usually obtained by the axillary route in newborns because of the risk of injury to the rectal area. An initial temperature is not obtained until the infant is taken to the nursery.

256. **(C)** Nursing process phase: evaluation; client need: physiological integrity (of infant); content area: maternity nursing

Rationale

(A) Infants get warm and comfortable against the mother's body and fall asleep. This may occur before enough milk has been ingested. (B) The stool of the breastfed baby is very soft. If the stool is hard, the infant many be becoming dehydrated. (C) The breastfed infant should have six to ten wet diapers daily. If there are fewer than six wet diapers, or if the infant has not voided for 12 hours, the health-care provider needs to be notified immediately. (D) Breast milk is more easily digested than formula. The breastfed infant will need to nurse every 1½ to 3 hours. In addition, the more often the baby empties the breasts, the more milk will be produced.

257. **(A)** Nursing process phase: analysis and planning; client need: health promotion and maintenance; content area: maternity nursing

Rationale

(A) The addition of cheese to hamburgers increases calcium and protein; adding vegetables to pizza increases vitamins; roast beef sandwiches are lower in fat and a good source of protein; adding broccoli and cheese to a baked potato increases calcium and vitamins; orange juice is high in vitamin C. A mixed salad with vinegar dressing increases fiber and vitamins with a minimum of added fat. (B) Dressings on hamburgers should be avoided because they are high in fat. Adding cheese increases calcium but also increases fat. Breaded foods are high in fat, as are potatoes with sour cream. A milkshake is preferable to carbonated drinks but is high in fat. (C) Breaded, fried foods are too high in fat, as are hot dogs and french fries. Iceberg lettuce is high in fiber but not in vitamins. Ranch dressing is too high in fat. Diet colas are high in sodium, caffeine, and phosphorus. (D) Chili cheese dogs are very high in fat and calories; olives are high in sodium; breaded fried foods are high in fat; whole milk is higher in fat and lower in calcium than skim milk. Salad bars typically have high fat and sodium choices such as cheese, bacon bits, pickles, and salad dressings.

258. **(B)** Nursing process phase: assessment; client need: physiological integrity (fetal); content area: maternity nursing

Rationale

(A) Variable decelerations are usually caused by cord compression. A quick return to baseline is reassuring. The baseline rate is within the normal fetal heart rate range of 110 to 160. A healthy fetus should exhibit short-term variability of at least 6 to 10 beats per minute. (B) Late decelerations indicate uteroplacental insufficiency. A gradual return to the baseline rate indicates exhaustion of fetal reserves. Short-term variability is non-reassuring. (C) Early decelerations are a normal reflexive response of the fetus to pressure on the fetal head. The fetal baseline should range from 110 to 160. Short-term variability is excellent. (D) Accelerations with contractions is one of the most reassuring signs of fetal well-being. The baseline rate is within normal limits. Short-term variability is excellent.

259. (D) Nursing process phase: implementation; client need: safe, effective care environment; content area: maternity nursing

Rationale

(A) The prone position will usually result in a better fetal heart tracing. However, this position causes compression of the aorta and inferior vena cava and compromises placental blood flow. (B) Positioning the client on the left side is the best position for placental blood flow, however there is currently no evidence of fetal compromise. Oxygen is not indicated. (C) Clients should be positioned in the knee-chest position and prepared for a cesarean when there is evidence of a prolapsed cord. Membranes must be ruptured for this event to occur. The membranes are intact in this client. (D) A monitor tracing that is not readable has little value in determining fetal status. The appropriate nursing action is to change the location of the external doppler to obtain a better reading.

260. (C) Nursing process phase: evaluation; client need: health promotion and maintenance; content area: maternity nursing

Rationale

(A) Fetal compromise is more likely when pregnancy is prolonged 2 weeks or more past a well-established expected date of birth (EDB). A post-term pregnancy is an indicator for induction of labor. (B) Non-reassuring nonstress testing can be an indicator of fetal compromise and is an indicator for induction of labor. (C) The FDA and American College of Obstetrics and Gynecology (ACOG) state that induction of labor is not an elective procedure. (D) Fetal-neonatal morbidity and mortality rates are decreased when gestational diabetics are delivered by the 38th week of gestation.

261. (B) Nursing process phase: evaluation; client need: health promotion and maintenance; content area: maternity nursing

Rationale

(A) Breastfeeding is contraindicated for the HIV positive mother as the virus is excreted in breastmilk. (B) HIV is diagnosed by the presence of antibodies in the blood. The infant will probably test positive for HIV for at least six months until the antibodies from the mother are exhausted. Many babies who tested HIV positive at birth will convert to negative within 12 months. (C) The average time from HIV diagnosis to the development of full blown AIDS is two or more years. It is unlikely with the use of AZT and other AIDS drugs that the client will die within six months. (D) HIV diagnosis of the mother does not necessarily condemn the infant to death. HIV is diagnosed by the presence of antibodies in the blood. The infant will probably test positive for HIV for at least six months until the antibodies from the mother are exhausted. Many babies who tested HIV positive at birth will convert to negative within 12 months.

262. (D) Nursing process phase: assessment; client need: physiological integrity; content area: maternity nursing

Rationale

(A) Pregnancy-induced hypertension is more common in primiparas, women under the age of 20 or over the age of 35,

pregnant diabetics, and clients with a history of chronic hypertension. (B) Incompetent cervix is associated with cervical surgeries and/or the ingestion of diethylstilbestrol (DES) by the mother of the client when pregnant. (C) Preterm labor is associated with urinary tract infections, illicit drug usage, dehydration, and multiple fetal gestations. (D) At 20 weeks, the lower uterine segment is not developed enough for a low segment transverse incision. A classical cesarean incision is necessary. Classical uterine incisions are associated with a high risk for uterine rupture.

263. (C) Nursing process phase: assessment; client need: health promotion and maintenance; content area: maternity nursing

Rationale

(A) The body temperature dips slightly 24 hours prior to ovulation. (B) The body temperature decreases slightly prior to menstruation. (C) The body temperature rises sharply within 24 hours of ovulation and the increase is maintained for the life of the corpus luteum. This is the basis of the BBT method of determining ovulation. (D) The body temperature does decrease slightly after the menstrual cycle, but has no significance to the BBT test for ovulation.

264. (A) Nursing process phase: assessment; client need: health promotion and maintenance; content area: maternity nursing

Rationale

(A) Progesterone is excreted in higher levels after ovulation and has a thermogenic effect. An initial BBT increase will occur approximately 24 hours prior to ovulation. Because the ovum is viable for only 1 day after ovulation, by the third day of BBT increase and with the change from clear and slippery to sticky cervical mucus, the client using this method can assume she is "safe." (B) The BBT remains elevated after ovulation until the day before the menstrual cycle. Minor discomforts may have little relation to ovulation. (C) Breast tenderness is usually seen prior to the menstrual cycle as in the drop in BBT. This is not the mark of the safe period. (D) A rise in BBT of approximately 1°F is indicative of ovulation and would not indicate a safe zone.

265. (C) Nursing process phase: analysis; client need: health promotion and maintenance; content area: maternity nursing

Rationale

(A) Norplant is more expensive than the birth control pill and other short-term methods. (B) Norplants have to be removed by a skilled health-care provider. (C) Norplants provide a slow release of synthetic progestin levonorgestrel. Because of the small amounts of hormone in the body, side effects are usually mild. (D) Although Norplant has an accidental pregnancy rate of 0.6 to 1.5 per 100 women, forms of the combined-regime pills are nearly 100 percent effective, with failure rates of only 0.1 to 0.5 percent.

266. (B) Nursing process phase: planning, client need: health promotion and maintenance; content area: maternity nursing

Rationale

(A) Depo-Provera is given every 3 months. (B) Many teens have the misconception that birth control methods protect from STDs as well as pregnancy. The client should be instructed to have her partner use a condom to protect against

STDs and HIV. (C) Skipping a menstrual period is a common side effect of this method and does not warrant immediate attention. (D) Clients may experience mild tenderness at the injection site, but this is not a priority for this client.

267. (A) Nursing process phase: analysis; client need: physiological integrity; content area: maternity nursing

Rationale
(A) Progesterone causes relaxation of the smooth vascular tissue, increasing the intravascular space. (B) Collaterals form when normal processes do not allow for normal blood flow patterns. The collateral system is not associated with normal pregnancy changes. (C) Red blood cells change very little in size and should increase in volume. (D) A rise in the mean arterial pressure is indicative of hypertension, a complication of pregnancy.

268. (C) Nursing process phase: implementation; client need: physiological integrity; content area: maternity nursing

Rationale
(A) The situation describes vena cava syndrome, in which BP would be decreased. However, BP will remain decreased until a position change occurs, therefore, taking the BP is not the priority. (B) The nurse should never leave a patient in distress unattended. (C) The weight of the pregnancy is compressing the inferior vena cava, causing the characteristic signs of decreased venous flow and BP drop. By taking the weight of the pregnancy off the vena cava, blood flow is restored and symptoms subside. (D) The client is complaining of dizziness. If you brought her to a sitting position, she could get off balance and sustain injury.

269. (D) Nursing process phase: analysis; client need: physiological integrity; content area: maternity nursing

Rationale
(A–C) The red blood cells increase in pregnancy but at a lower concentration than the plasma volume. (D) Both the plasma volume and red blood cells increase in pregnancy. Plasma increases by 1200 to 1500 ml while red cells increase 300 to 450 ml. Because of this imbalance, the ratio of RBCs to plasma (the hematocrit) will decrease. This is called psuedoanemia or hemodilution of pregnancy. The increased RBCs are usually adequate to accommodate the increased oxygen needs of the pregnant woman.

270. (B) Nursing process phase: analysis; client need: physiological integrity; content area: maternity nursing

Rationale
(A, C, & D) The UA and WBC are both within normal limits for the last trimester of pregnancy. A more appropriate follow-up may be a vaginal examination to determine if the fetus has descended into the pelvis. (B) A trace of protein is a normal finding in pregnancy due to the increased glomerular filtration rate. WBCs may increase to 18,000 in late pregnancy and be considered a normal finding.

271. (B) Nursing process phase: implementation; client need: physiological integrity; content area: maternity nursing

Rationale
(A) A normal increase for pregnancy is 15 to 20 beats per minute from the baseline heart rate. This client has an increase of 32 beats per minute over baseline, too high to be within normal limits. (B) When a pregnant client has a significant heart rate increase, this demonstrates an excess workload on the heart. The concern would be an undiagnosed heart condition, which typically causes symptoms on exertion. (C) This question would cause undue concern, and heart disease in the family does not address the most common heart conditions that occur in pregnancy. A better question might be to ask if the client has ever been diagnosed with a heart condition. (D) The client requires immediate follow-up. Waiting 2 weeks could place the client in acute distress.

272. (B) Nursing process phase: assessment; client need: physiological integrity; content area: maternity nursing

Rationale
(A) This is not a normal finding for the second trimester of pregnancy. Urinary frequency in the first and near the end of the third trimester (after lightening) are considered normal findings if no other symptoms accompany the frequency. (B) Because urinary frequency is not a normal finding in the second trimester, the nurse needs to follow up with questions that would assist the health-care provider in diagnosis. (C) The nurse cannot order these tests—the primary health-care provider provides the order; the nurse assists the client in obtaining the specimen. (D) The pregnant client should continue to drink appropriate amounts of fluid. Limiting fluids in general can lead to severe complications of dehydration and preterm labor due to the increased glomercular filtration rate. Limiting fluid after the evening meal may be appropriate if other findings are within normal limits.

273. (A) Nursing process phase: assessment; client need: physiological integrity; content area: maternity nursing

Rationale
(A) An increase of about 8 beats per minute occurs in the first trimester to accommodate the increased blood volume and work on the heart. By the third trimester, a client may increase heart rate up to 20 beats per minute over the baseline heart rate. (B) The blood pressure may actually drop 5 to 10 mm/Hg as a result of the relaxation of smooth vessels to accommodate increased blood volume that occurs in pregnancy. A rise in blood pressure is indicative of a hypertensive disorder. (C) There is a 20 percent increase in oxygen consumption during pregnancy to accommodate the demands of the products of consumption. Most clients increase their respiratory rate to help meet this increased oxygen demand, but a 20 percent increase would be indicative of respiratory distress. (D) The basal body temperature actually increases as a result of the energy demands of the products of conception.

274. (C) Nursing process phase: implementation; client need: health promotion and maintenance; content area: maternity nursing

Rationale
(A) The increased vaginal discharge is normal, but wearing tampons may increase the client's risk of developing a bacterial infection because of the normal change in vaginal flora that occurs in pregnancy. (B) The discharge the client describes is normal for pregnancy and is not indicative of a yeast infection. Also, the pregnant woman should not use any over-the-counter products without approval by the physician, nurse midwife, or practitioner. (C) By keeping her perineal area clean, she will feel fresh and decrease chance of skin irritation. (D) The pregnant client should never be advised to douche. Forceful instillation of fluid into the vaginal could cause miscarriage or other complications with the pregnancy.

275. (C) Nursing process phase: implementation; client need: health promotion and maintenance; content area: maternity nursing

Rationale
(A) The client should be instructed that she will experience an increase in vaginal discharge, white in color, and that this is normal for this stage of pregnancy. (B) The client should be instructed that occasional malaise and lethargy are common for the first trimester of pregnancy and these symptoms should improve by the second trimester. (C) Bleeding and cramping in the first trimester are indicative of miscarriage and the client should be instructed to report this immediately. (D) A weight gain of 2 to 3 pounds in a 6-week period is within normal limits for the first trimester of pregnancy. A gain of 1½ to 2 pounds per month is expected in the first trimester.

276. (A) Nursing process phase: planning; client need: health promotion and maintenance; content area: maternity nursing

Rationale
(A) The National Academy of Sciences Institute of Medicine recommends weight gain based on prepregnancy weight. For an underweight client, it may be recommended that the client gain 35 to 45 pounds; the average weight client, 25 to 35 pounds; and the overweight client, 15 to 25 pounds. (B) A client's expectations for weight gain may be unrealistic and not based on research. Some clients may feel they need to gain very little so they won't have to lose a great deal of weight after the pregnancy, while others may feel they are "eating for two" and gain an excessive amount of weight. Either situation can have dire effects on the pregnancy. (C) The client's age may be important in dietary patterns, but, in general, clients should follow the recommended weight-gain guidelines. (D) Cultural influences may affect the dietary pattern and overall nutritional state, but do not effect the desired weight gain.

277. (D) Nursing process phase: planning; client need: physiological integrity; content area: maternity nursing

Rationale
(A) In pregnancy, digestion slows down and moves more slowly through the system as a result of smooth muscle relaxation. (B) There is actually a decreased secretion of hydrochloric acid and pepsin in the first and second trimesters of pregnancy. It increases late in the third trimester. (C) Because of decreased motility, the client should be instructed to eat small, frequent meals to allow time for adequate digestion and minimize reflux. (D) There is relaxation of the smooth muscle, which decreases GI motility and cardiac sphincter control. Food remains in the stomach longer and the relaxed sphincter allows partially digested food and stomach acids to be refluxed, resulting in heartburn.

278. (A) Nursing process phase: assessment; client need: physiological integrity; content area: maternity nursing

Rationale
(A) At 20 weeks' gestation, the fundus of the uterus should be at umbilicus, about 20 cm fundal height. (B & C) After the 12th week, the fundus rises about 1 cm per week. These measurements would be between 16 and 18 weeks' gestation, but measurement is not accurate until about 20 weeks' gestation. (D) The fundus reaches the xiphoid process at about 36 weeks' gestation.

279. (D) Nursing process phase: assessment; client need: health promotion and maintenance; content area: maternity nursing

Rationale
(A–C) These changes can all be observed by the health-care provider and are considered objective findings. (D) This is a change that is reported by the client, a subjective symptom.

280. (C) Nursing process phase: implementation; client need: psychosocial integrity; content area: maternity nursing

Rationale
(A & D) Because ambivalence is normal at this stage of pregnancy, neither of these interventions would be appropriate. (B) Fetal movement is usually felt at 20 weeks' gestation. Ambivalence is typically resolved by that time. (C) Ambivalence occurs early in many pregnancies. Research has shown that there is no ill effect on the mother's ability to accept the pregnancy as it progresses or with bonding after the infant is born.

281. (C) Nursing process phase: implementation; client need: health promotion and maintenance; content area: maternity nursing

Rationale
(A) Weight gain is important. Even the overweight client should gain 15 to 25 pounds to accommodate the pregnancy. (B) This may frighten the client because she has already dieted in pregnancy. (C) Acknowledging her success while explaining the importance of weight gain during pregnancy will be most beneficial to the client. Explain that because she was overweight prior to pregnancy, she should gain 15 to 25 pounds. (D) Dieting in pregnancy should never be recommended. A healthy, balanced diet with adequate supplements of vitamins and minerals is needed for a healthy pregnancy.

282. (B) Nursing process phase: analysis; client need: safe, effective care environment; content area: maternity nursing

Rationale
(A) Glucose demands are increased because of the demands of the products of conception. (B) Changes in estrogen and progesterone cause beta-cell hyperplasia, enlarged insulin-secreting cells in the pancreas. (C) The client's diabetes will need to be followed closely due to the stresses that pregnancy will put on the body and the normal metabolic changes that occur in pregnancy. (D) Maternal insulin does not cross the placenta. The fetus has to produce its own insulin to accommodate increased glucose levels.

283. (D) Nursing process phase: implementation; client need: physiological integrity; content area: maternity nursing

Rationale
(A) Diet only may be successful with some client, but does not provide the full range of treatment options. (B & C) Oral hypoglycemics have been shown to have teratogenic effects on the fetus and are not recommended for treatment of diabetes in pregnancy. (D) A combination of diet and exercise is recommended for treatment of gestational diabetes. If medication is required, insulin is the drug of choice because it does not cross the placenta and has no direct effect on the fetus.

284. (B) Nursing process phase: evaluation; client need: safe, effective care environment; content area: maternity nursing

Rationale
(A) A lowered blood pressure may be a side effect of $MgSO_4$ because of the relaxation of smooth muscle, but is not the primary purpose of the medication. (B) A client with preeclampsia has increased neuromuscular irritability and is at risk for seizures, a potentially life-threatening condition for the client. Magnesium sulfate blocks the release of acetylcholine at the neuromuscular junction, thus decreasing neuromuscular irritability. (C) Because of magnesium sulfate's effect of peripheral vasodilatation, some decrease in peripheral edema may be seen. However, this is not a priority effect of the medication. More importantly, there may be a decrease in cerebral edema, which would increase cerebral perfusion. (D) Decreased urine output occurs as a result of smooth muscle relaxation effects of the medication. Decreased urine output will allow reabsorption of the medication, leading to toxic effects.

285. (C) Nursing process phase: implementation; client need: safe, effective care environment; content area: maternity nursing

Rationale
(A) It may be more comfortable for the client, but this is not the best answer. (B) Diastolic blood pressures changes very little during contractions, but may increase slightly. (C) Because of the increased workload on the heart during labor, the effect of pain, and the shift of blood from the uterus to the circulating blood volume during a contraction, systolic pressure will increase during contractions. (D) Blood pressure does change during contractions as a result of the stress response and the increased cardiac output during the contraction. The degree of change depends on the client's state and condition. After each contraction, BP should return to a normal range.

286. (B) Nursing process phase: evaluation; client need: safe, effective care environment; content area: maternity nursing

Rationale
(A) The pattern described in the scenario is a late deceleration and is caused by decreased placental perfusion. The pattern that occurs with fetal head compression is an early deceleration. (B) The pattern described occurs when there is decreased oxygen to the fetus and it cannot tolerate the deficit. (C) Variable decelerations are seen with cord compression. (D) Random accelerations are seen with fetal activity.

287. (C) Nursing process phase: assessment; client need: physiological integrity; content area: maternity nursing

Rationale
(A & B) Occipitoposterior positions typically prolong the first and second stages of labor. (C) OP positions present with a wider part of the fetal head, and the fetus typically descends through the pelvis more slowly. (D) The baby is delivered during the second stage of labor.

288. (C) Nursing process phase: implementation; client need: physiological integrity; content area: maternity nursing

Rationale
(A) It is normal for the hematocrit to decrease in pregnancy as a result of the imbalance in the ratio of the increased red blood cells to the plasma volume. (B) The laboratory values do not reflect a decrease that would be indicative of bleeding. (C) This drop in hematocrit occurs as a result of the imbalance between the red blood cells and the plasma volume. Both increase in pregnancy, but the plasma increases more rapidly and to a greater degree than the red blood cells, giving the picture of anemia. (D) Clotting factors will be increased somewhat in pregnancy as a natural protective mechanism; this should not be of concern in this case.

289. (A) Nursing process phase: assessment; client need: physiological integrity; content area: maternity nursing

Rationale
(A) Because of the positional change of the kidneys and the relaxation of the bladder caused by progesterone, the bladder frequently contains residual urine, which is a good medium for bacterial growth. (B) The ureters dilate in pregnancy, they do not engorge. (C) There is an increased excretion of protein in pregnancy, but that has not been shown to be a causative agent for UTIs. (D) There is actually no increase in urine output in pregnancy, only increased frequency with smaller amounts of urine each time.

290. (C) Nursing process phase: implementation; client need: safe, effective care environment; content area: maternity nursing

Rationale
(A) When the fetal head is not engaged and the membranes are ruptured, the client is at risk for a cord prolapse and should be on bedrest until the fetal part descends. (B) The client with ruptured membranes and minus 4 station should not be discharged. This client is also moving into the active phase of labor at 3 cm dilation. (C) When the fetal presenting part is not engaged into the pelvis, as with minus 4 station, and the membranes rupture, the cord can be "washed out" of the cervix, resulting in fetal distress. (D) A client with ruptured membranes should not get an enema because of the increased risk of infection from feces contamination. Also, the client is at risk for cord prolapse.

291. (B) Nursing process phase: evaluation; client need: safe, effective care environment; content area: maternity nursing

Rationale
(A) Although this may also be a good idea, the priority is to determine if the client is a gestational diabetic so that appropriate medical intervention can be initiated. (B) Any glucose screening results of greater than 140 mg/dl at 24 to 28 weeks' gestation should be followed with a glucose tolerance test to determine the presence of gestational diabetes. In clients undiagnosed and/or untreated with gestational diabetes, the potential for complications of pregnancy and infant morbidity increases significantly. (C) A hemoglobin A_{1c} is used to follow control of diabetics, and is not appropriate for an undiagnosed client. (D) This is out of range for normal findings for a pregnant client and needs to have follow-up laboratory work to establish the client's status as a diabetic.

292. (C) Nursing process phase: implementation; client need: safe, effective care environment; content area: maternity nursing

Rationale
(A) Pulmonary edema is the concern with this client. Prior to application of O_2, the client should be assessed and the physician notified. Also, 10 L/min is out of the normal protocol

range for nurse administration of O_2. (B) This is an adverse effect of this medication with this population. (C) The risk of using Brethine with a pregnant client is pulmonary edema. The client's breath sounds need to be evaluated for crackles and wheezes and the physician notified. Pulmonary edema is a potentially life-threatening condition for both the client and her fetus. (D) Medicating the client for pain could further depress the pulmonary function, increasing the distress. The scenario does not indicate the client is in pain at this time.

293. **(D)** Nursing process phase: assessment; client need: health promotion and maintenance; content area: maternity nursing

Rationale
(A–C) The numbers of syphilis, gonorrhea, and HIV cases reported in pregnant women are increasing, but these diseases will still remain below chlamydia in current statistics. (D) Currently, chlamydia is the most common STD in the general population as well as in pregnant women, according to the Center for Communicable Diseases.

294. **(C)** Nursing process phase: assessment; client need: safe, effective care environment; content area: maternity nursing

Rationale
(A) Fetal heart rate should be monitored continuously in clients with prolonged rupture of membranes. You may see an increase in fetal heart rate with maternal infection, but the FHR can increase for a number of reasons. This is not a good indicator of maternal infection. (B) Maternal blood pressure is not an early indicator of infection, which is the concern of a client with ruptured membranes for 20 hours. (C) After 20 hours, research has shown that the risk of infection to the client increases dramatically. Maternal temperature is one of the first indicators that an infection is present. (D) Uterine contractions are not an indicator of infection in the client.

295. **(B)** Nursing process phase: assessment; client need: physiological integrity; content area: maternity nursing

Rationale
(A & C) The nurse should be able to observe these complications during her assessment. (B) Because the hematoma is inside the vagina, there is initially no visible sign of edema. However, pressure on tissue and the accumulation of blood in the tissue can cause severe pain, outside what is expected with normal postpartum discomfort. As the hematoma progresses, there may be observable edema and discoloration, extending even to the client's inside thigh. (D) Anxiety can heighten the perception of pain, but the nurse must look at possible physical causes while supporting the client emotionally.

296. **(D)** Nursing process phase: evaluation; client need: safe, effective care environment; content area: maternity nursing

Rationale
(A) Weight is not an indicator of blood sugar control. (B) Monthly blood glucose levels are not good indicators of consistent glucose control. (C) This is another method of intermittent monitoring that does not look at the overall glucose levels. This would also rely on the client's compliance to perform accurate testing. This is still not the best indicator of glucose control. (D) This test is a measure of blood glucose levels over the past 4 to 6 weeks. There is an irreversible bond of glucose to hemoglobin protein. The life cycle for a red blood cell is about 120 days, so an elevated test indicates significant past hyperglycemia.

297. **(D)** Nursing process phase: implementation; client need: health promotion and maintenance; content area: maternity nursing

Rationale
(A) Oral hypoglycemics are contraindicated in pregnancy because of the teratogenic effects on the fetus. (B) Blood glucose home monitoring is the home-screening method that is considered to be most accurate and is recommended in pregnancy. (C) Based on the GST, a glucose test (GTT) is done. If that result is positive, the patient is diagnosed with gestational diabetes. (D) If medication is used to control diabetes, insulin is the drug of choice because it does not cross the placenta, therefore, it does not have teratogenic effects on the fetus.

298. **(C)** Nursing process phase: assessment; client need: physiological integrity; content area: maternity nursing

Rationale
(A) This may be an indication of some form of hypertension, but alone it does not indicate PIH. (B) Severe headaches and RUQ pain are significant if PIH is established, but are not the indicators for PIH. (C) These three symptoms are the classic triad that is diagnostic of the PIH process. (D) The first two symptoms, BP increase and edema, are of concern but there is not enough information to determine if it is PIH or related to some other disorder. Slight glycosuria is normal. If glycosuria is significant then it may indicate diabetes, not PIH.

299. **(B)** Nursing process phase: assessment; client need: health promotion and maintenance; content area: maternity nursing

Rationale
(A) Chromosomal disorders are evaluated best by maternal laboratory or fetal tests such as chorionic villa sampling. Ultrasound at this point would have no value. (B) An ultrasound is accurate in determining gestational age and is the most common purpose at this stage of pregnancy. (C) An ultrasound has a very slim chance of predicting the need for cesarean delivery. (D) The screening for gestational diabetes is a laboratory test ordered at about 25 weeks' gestation. An ultrasound has no merit in screening for this disorder.

300. **(D)** Nursing process phase: assessment; client need: physiological integrity; content area: maternity nursing

Rationale
(A–C) These are not landmarks for any presentation. (D) The mentum is the landmark for determining position in a face presentation.

301. **(A)** Nursing process phase: assessment; client need: physiological integrity; content area: maternity nursing

Rationale
(A) RSA stands for right sacroanterior. (B) Vertex is the presentation when the crown of the fetal head presents. (C) In an occipital presentation, the back of the fetal head presents first. (D) A face presentation has the mentum as the presenting part.

302. **(C)** Nursing process phase: assessment; client need: physiological integrity; content area: maternity nursing

Rationale

(A & B) Fetal heart tones are heard best at the fetus's upper back. LOA position refers to an occipital or head-down position, in which case fetal heart tones would be heard in the lower quadrant. Both of the upper locations would indicate a breech presentation, with the upper portion of the fetal head in the upper part of the maternal abdomen. (C) LOA indicates that the fetus's back is to the client's left side and "O" indicates an occipital, or head-down, presentation. Fetal heart tones would be found in the left lower quadrant. (D) Because the back of the fetus is to the left, fetal heart tones would be found on the left side, not the right.

303. **(B)** Nursing process phase: evaluation; client need: safe, effective care environment; content area: maternity nursing

Rationale

(A) Contractions become stronger and more regular as labor approaches. Clients will sometimes experience contractions for several hours that are 5 minutes apart but continue to be mild. Unless the cervix changes, labor cannot be verified. (B) Effacement and dilation of the cervix are the major indicators of true labor. (C) True labor contractions are usually described as starting in the low back and moving to the front low pelvic region. Upper abdominal pain may be an indicator of a complication of pregnancy. (D) In true labor, many times contractions will intensify with ambulation. However, this is not an accurate indicator of true labor.

304. **(D)** Nursing process phase: assessment; client need: health promotion and maintenance; content area: maternity nursing

Rationale

(A) This blood work is done at the first prenatal visit for a baseline and is usually repeated once or twice during pregnancy, not every visit. (B) A urinalysis is done to determine urinary tract infections and is only indicated when there are abnormal symptoms, such as burning or pain on urination. (C) A screening for blood glucose is typically done at 24 to 28 weeks' gestation to determine the possibility of gestational diabetes. This test is not routinely done. (D) A voided urine is obtained at each visit and dipsticks are used to determine the presence of protein or glucose, which could be indicative of underlying disease processes.

305. **(A)** Nursing process phase: implementation; client need: health promotion and maintenance; content area: maternity nursing

Rationale

(A) Depo-Provera prevents regular release of ova, inhibiting normal changes in the endometrial lining of the uterus. (B) Women more commonly report weight gain than weight loss. (B) May experience fatigue rather than increased metabolic activity. (D) Hypertension has not been reported in the literature as a side effect of Depo-Provera.

306. **(B)** Nursing process phase: implementation; client need: health promotion and maintenance; content area: maternity nursing

Rationale

(A) By 1 year of age, the incidence of undescended testes in all boys is less than 1 percent. (B) The testes descend into the scrotum in 90 percent of newborns by 36 to 40 weeks' gestation. (C) Although spermatogenesis does not occur until puberty, the higher temperature of the abdominal cavity causes deterioration of the sperm cells. (D) The ideal time frame for surgery for undescended testicles is 2 to 3 years of age.

307. **(C)** Nursing process phase: assessment; client need: health promotion and maintenance; content area: maternity

Rationale

(A) A trace of proteinuria and lower extremity edema are normal findings in pregnancy. A BP increase of this level would need to be followed closely but is not indicative of PIH. (B) Epigastric pain may be seen in PIH; however, dizziness is not a common symptom. (C) This is the classic triad of symptoms for PIH. (D) Mild glucose in the urine is a common finding in pregnancy. The hypertension is not specifically defined to meet the PIH criteria.

308. **(B)** Nursing process phase: implementation; client need: health promotion and maintenance; content area: maternity nursing

Rationale

(A) Formula supplementation is not recommended until the breast milk supply is well established. (B) Colostrum is uniquely suited to the needs of the newborn infant, providing vital antibodies and concentrated nutrition in the small volume typical of early feedings. (C) Colostrum gradually changes to breast milk between the third and fifth postpartum day. (D) Breast size is related to the amount of fatty tissue and gives no indication of the functional capacity of the breast.

309. **(D)** Nursing process phase: assessment; client need: health promotion and maintenance; content area: maternity nursing

Rationale

(A) Hyperreflexia is commonly seen with PIH. (B & C) Glucosuria is not a common finding in PIH. (D) Hypertension and proteinuria are two of the classic triad of symptoms found in PIH. The other symptom of this triad is greater than 1+ edema.

310. **(B)** Nursing process phase: assessment; client need: safe, effective care environment; content area: maternity nursing

Rationale

(A) Infection is not associated with eclampsia. (B) Eclampsia is characterized by seizure activity that often results in aspiration as a common complication. (C) Renal perfusion is decreased with hypertension resulting in decreased urine output. (D) Extremity injuries may occur with seizure activity but are not considered a major complication.

311. **(A)** Nursing process phase: assessment; client need: safe, effective care environment; content area: maternity nursing

Rationale

(A) Uterine atony, failure of the uterine muscle to contract firmly, is the most common cause of excessive bleeding following childbirth. It occurs in 75 to 85 percent of postpartum clients. (B) Retained placental fragments commonly cause late postpartum hemorrhage. (C) Cervical lacerations are seen less often and are characterized by slow, continuous bleeding with a contracted uterus. (D) Postpartum infection is not necessarily associated with postpartum hemorrhage. It occurs in only about 6 percent of postpartum women.

312. (A) Nursing process phase: implementation; client need: safe, effect care environment; content area: maternity nursing

Rationale

(A) MgSO$_4$ prevents seizures by blocking neuromuscular transmission. (B) With the administration of MgSO$_4$, a slight drop in BP may be seen as a result of the relaxation of smooth muscles. However, MgSO$_4$ is not an antihypertensive drug. (C) MgSO$_4$ treatment does not result in an increase urine output, but with toxicity may actually cause a decrease. (D) Decreasing edema as a result of diuresis caused by the increased perfusion of the kidneys is a positive sign. However, decreasing edema is not the primary purpose of MgSO$_4$ administration.

313. (C) Nursing process phase: analysis; client need: physiological integrity; content area: maternity nursing

Rationale

(A) Erythropoiesis normally increases after the first trimester but is unrelated to physiological anemia. (B) Dietary intake of iron is unrelated to the development of physiological anemia. (C) There is a 30 to 50 percent increase in maternal blood volume by the end of the first trimester. Although RBCs do increase at this time, plasma volume increases more rapidly, resulting in hemodilution. (D) The liver changes in size, structure, and form during pregnancy, but these changes have no impact on physiological anemia.

314. (C) Nursing process phase: analysis; client need: physiological integrity; content area: maternity nursing

Rationale

(A) At 12 hours' postpartum, the fundus should be midline and at the umbilicus. (B) At 12 hours' postpartum, a lazy uterus will generally be deviated to the left side but should be firm and at the umbilicus. (C) Bladder distention pushes the uterus up and generally to the right side. This may cause poor contraction of the uterine muscle, increasing the risk for postpartum hemorrhage. (D) Though postpartum hemorrhage may result from a boggy uterus caused by a distended bladder, this assessment does not necessarily indicate the presence of a hemorrhage.

315. (D) Nursing process phase: implementation; client need: safe, effective care environment; content area: maternity nursing

Rationale

(A) Sodium intake does not alter the disease process of pre-eclampsia and sodium restriction is typically not recommended. (B) Statistically, clients with mild pre-eclampsia who follow the home care recommendations deliver at term. (C) Bedrest is recommended for the mildly pre-eclamptic client, along with weekly urine and blood pressure checks. Ambulation typically causes an increase in the blood pressure and a decrease in the oxygen to the fetus. (D) Bedrest is recommended for the mildly pre-eclamptic client. This lowers the blood pressure and increases renal and fetal perfusion by taking the weight of the fetus off of the inferior vena cava.

316. (D) Nursing process phase: implementation; client need: safe, effective care environment; content area: maternity nursing

Rationale

(A) The client's BP is not within an acceptable range. She has experienced an increase of 36 mm Hg above her systolic and 16 mm Hg above her diastolic BP. This is one of the defining characteristics of pre-eclampsia and should be evaluated further. (B) The client's BP may increase slightly with contractions in the active phase of labor. In the latent phase contractions are usually mild and very well tolerated; a BP increase is not expected. (C) Client complaints should not be used as a basis for further assessment. The nurse must decide to further evaluate the client based on the objective findings. (D) The client has experienced an increase of 36 mm Hg above her systolic and 16 mm Hg above her diastolic BP. This is one of the defining characteristics of pre-eclampsia and should be evaluated further.

317. (C) Nursing process phase: evaluation; client need: safe, effective care environment; content area: maternity nursing

Rationale

(A) The client has had three abortions, and statistically this will not increase her risk of hemorrhage. (B) The nurse might assume that the client will be emotionally upset for this reason. There is not enough information to determine if the abortions were elective or to determine the client's state of mind. (C) In most females, the pelvis does not fully mature until the age of 15. The assessment of fundal height of 40 cm at 40 weeks' gestation and the −4 station indicates that the fetus has not dropped into the pelvis and engaged. The client is in labor, as indicated by the changes in the cervix. These findings indicate that the fetus is too large for the pelvis size. (D) None of the information given indicates that the fetus is small.

318. (C) Nursing process phase: assessment; client need: physiological integrity; content area: maternity nursing

Rationale

(A) This is too little fluid and would be considered oligohydraminos. There would be a concern over intrauterine growth retardation or placental insufficiency if this were found. (B) This is too little fluid and would be considered oligohydraminos. There would be a concern over intrauterine growth retardation or placental insufficiency if this were found. (C) At term, 800 to 1000 cc of amniotic fluid is a normal finding. (D) This is considered polyhydraminos, or too much amniotic fluid. There would be concerns of genetic disorders such as GI malformations if this were present.

319. (D) Nursing process phase: assessment; client need: physiological integrity; content area: maternity nursing

Rationale

(A & B) A pH of 7.00 and below carries a high risk for death from severe acidosis. (C) A pH of 7.19 and below indicates severe acidosis. (D) Normal pH for the fetus is more than 7.25.

320. (C) Nursing process phase: assessment; client need: physiological integrity; content area: maternity nursing

Rationale

(A) Perineal lacerations may occur for the laboring client, not the fetus. (B) Cephalohematomas are defined as bleeding between the periosteum and bone that does not cross the suture line. This may occur in about 6 percent of VE births but is not the most common trauma. (C) Scalp edema and bruising in a circular area as a result of the cup placement is the most common fetal trauma during a VE birth. Usually this resolves within 48 hours. (D) The vacuum cup does not apply pressure to the facial nerves and thus cannot cause damage. This trauma typically occurs with the use of forceps.

321. **(C)** Nursing process phase: assessment; client need: physiological integrity; content area: maternity nursing

Rationale

(A) Except for extension, the cardinal movements are completed by the second stage of labor. (B) The fetus does not begin the movements until it begins its passage through the true pelvis. (C) These movements allow the smallest part of the fetus to pass through first with the assistance of the forces of labor. (D) These movements do not determine position of the fetus, only the movements through the birth canal.

322. **(C)** Nursing process phase: analysis; client need: safe, effective care environment; content area: maternity nursing

Rationale

(A) Failure to descend is not indicative of a prolapsed cord, though failure of the fetus to engage could increase this risk. (B) The amount of amniotic fluid has nothing to do with progression through the pelvis. (C) The ischial spines are the narrowest part of the true pelvis. Failure to move below the spines is indicative of a fetal head that is too large in comparison to the pelvis. (D) Shoulder dystocia occurs after the fetus has passed through the true pelvis, and the head is delivered. The shoulders become locked on the symphysis.

323. **(B)** Nursing process phase: analysis; client need: physiological integrity; content area: maternity nursing

Rationale

(A) Hypotonic contractions are weak and infrequent, and usually are not effective in progressing labor. (B) The definition of precipitous labor is labor lasting less than 3 hours from the beginning of labor to delivery. This type of labor is characterized by frequent, intense contractions and rapid progression through the phases and stages of labor. (C) Prolonged labor is defined as labor that exceeds the normal. (D) Normal labor lasts about 8 to 12 hours, with less than 3 hours being the definition of precipitous labor.

324. **(C)** Nursing process phase: assessment; client need: content area: maternity nursing

Rationale

(A) This stands for artificial rupture of membranes. The amniotic bag is broken with an instrument by the health-care provider to allow the release of the fluid. (B) This is a procedure used to prevent loss of the products of conception. A suture is inserted at the cervix in a drawstring manner and the cervix is pulled closed. (C) An episiotomy is the incision made in the perineum to ease the second stage of labor and prevent tearing of the perineum. (D) This is the surgical cut made on the abdomen and through the uterus to deliver the infant surgically.

325. **(C)** Nursing process phase: analysis; client need: physiological integrity; content area: maternity nursing

Rationale

(A) Though the client may feel abdomen cramping similar to flatus discomfort, afterbirth pain is related to uterine cramping, not colon spasms. (B) Trauma will typically exhibit itself by tenderness in a specific area. Afterbirth pains are very common in all women, with or without traumatic deliveries. (C) Uterine contractions after delivery of the fetus and placenta prevent hemorrhage in the postpartum woman. They also help the uterus to return to close to its pre-pregnancy size. Af-

terbirth pains for a multipara, a woman who has experienced several births, are typically more uncomfortable than for a primipara, someone who has delivered just one baby. (D) A prolapsed uterus will be characterized by a feeling of pressure in the vaginal area and a feeling that "something is coming out." This is not related to afterbirth pains.

326. **(C)** Nursing process phase: assessment; client need: physiological integrity; content area: maternity nursing

Rationale

(A) Fertilization must occur before the ovum reaches the uterus, or the hormones needed to maintain the pregnancy will begin to degenerate and the fertilized egg cannot implant. (B) The ovum does not reach the vagina until it is expelled in a degenerated form. (C) The egg and the sperm meet in the fallopian tube and fertilization occurs. This can only occur within 1 to 2 days of ovulation, since the ovum and sperm cannot survive beyond that time. (D) This is the area between the uterine body and the cervix, and, again, the ovum does not reach this area until it is being expelled in a degenerated form.

327. **(B)** Nursing process phase: implementation; client need: health promotion and maintenance; content area: maternity nursing

Rationale

(A) Sex organs are not differentiated until 12 weeks' gestation. (B) By 12 weeks, sex organs are fully differentiated, and an ultrasound at 16 weeks should give a clear picture of the sex of the baby, especially if a vaginal probe is used. (C) Sex is determined at conception. (D) Ultrasounds are very reliable, depending on the skill of the person doing the ultrasound. Though not 100 percent accurate, most physicians are able to predict sex on a fairly regular basis.

328. **(C)** Nursing process phase: assessment; client need: health promotion and maintenance; content area: maternity nursing

Rationale

(A) "Morning sickness" is the term used to describe the normal nausea and vomiting that occurs in the first trimester of pregnancy, named such because it typically occurs in the morning. (B) This is not related to nausea and vomiting in pregnancy. (C) This is the term for nausea and vomiting after the first trimester. (D) This is a condition that is diagnosed based on a triad of symptoms; edema, elevated blood pressure, and proteinuria.

329. **(B)** Nursing process phase: assessment; client need: safe, effective care environment; content area: maternity nursing

Rationale

(A) A placenta previa is not implanted in the normal location. (B) This is the classic sign of a placenta previa. (C) This is the characteristic symptom of a placental abruption. (D) This is characteristic of a placental abruption.

330. **(D)** Nursing process phase: analysis; client need: safe, effective care environment; content area: maternity nursing

Rationale

(A) This cannot be made as a blanket statement. Depending on the deformity, such as heart or lung malformations, it may be contraindicated, but in most cases would be considered safe. (B) A macrosomic, or very large, fetus has a developed CNS and should be able to tolerate the effects of narcotic analgesics. (C) There have been no documented contraindications to the use of narcotics for persistent posterior positions, and many times the narcotic relaxant effect assists in the fetus turning. (D) Because the premature infant has an underdeveloped CNS, the narcotic knocks out any respiratory effort the premature neonate may have.

331. (B) Nursing process phase: planning; client need: health promotion and maintenance; content area: maternity nursing

Rationale

(A) One-on-one teaching is most appropriate for the very young adolescent. Developmentally, the teen under 15 may be too insecure to participate actively in a group session. (B) At this age, teens participate best in peer group activities. (C) According to research, teens of this age will not open up and participate as freely in a group with adults involved. (D) Written materials that are age-appropriate are acceptable, but a peer group has been proved to be more effective when educating this age group.

332. (C) Nursing process phase: analysis; client need: health promotion and maintenance; content area: maternity nursing

Rationale

(A) Women are more involved in the work force than ever before, especially in professional careers. (B) The teenage pregnancy rate has not decreased in recent years and has no influence on pregnancy in the woman over age 35. (C) Improvements in birth control measures allow the woman to delay pregnancy for education, work, or personal reasons. (D) The largest percentage of women who delay pregnancy until after the age of 35 are white, middle-class, and college-educated.

333. (C) Nursing process phase: implementation; client need: health promotion and maintenance; content area: maternity nursing

Rationale

(A) The mucus plug seals the cervix and is not attached to the amniotic bag. (B) The mucus plug seals the cervix but does not prevent premature opening of the cervix. (C) The mucus plug acts as a protective barrier for the fetus against both mechanical and bacterial invasion. It seals the entry of the cervix until labor occurs. As the cervix softens and opens up, the mucus plug separates and is expelled. (D) The mucus plug occurs as a result of the normal increase in cervical mucus and is not related to an infectious process.

334. (C) Nursing process phase: assessment; client need: physiological integrity; content area: maternity nursing

Rationale

(A) The uterus cannot be palpated externally below the symphysis because of the bony structure. The uterus is below the symphysis prior to the 12th week of gestation. (B) The uterus is palpated at the symphysis at about 12 weeks' gestation. (C) The uterus reaches the umbilicus at about 20 weeks' gestation. (D) The uterus reaches the xiphoid process near term gestation.

335. (A) Nursing process phase: assessment; client need: physiological integrity; content area: maternity nursing

Rationale

(A) During pregnancy, the vagina becomes increasingly vascular and congested with blood, causing the walls of the vagina to appear dark red or violet in color. (B) There is an increased blood flow to the vagina during pregnancy. (C) Estrogen production increases in pregnancy and contributes to an increased vascularization and congestion in the vagina. (D) These changes occur as early as 6 weeks' gestation and are related to increased blood flow, not pressure from the products of conception.

336. (C) Nursing process phase: implementation; client need: safe, effective care environment; content area: maternity nursing

Rationale

(A) A client at 38 weeks' gestation should not be advised to lie flat at any time. This causes vena cava syndrome and a subsequent drop in blood pressure. (B) The client at 38 weeks' gestation will naturally assume a feet-apart stance to balance. This widens her center of gravity and decreases her risk of falling. She should not be instructed to attempt to change this stance. (C) Because of the shift in the center of gravity that occurs, with the bulk in front, the client at 38 weeks risks getting off balance and falling is she leans forward to lift objects. (D) Back supporters designed for pregnancy use are very helpful in decreasing the fatigue that accompanies posture changes in pregnancy.

337. (C) Nursing process phase: analysis; client need: physiological integrity; content area: maternity nursing

Rationale

(A) The client would first be evaluated by her primary health-care provider if there is a concern. Ninety percent of women develop a physiological systolic murmur in pregnancy, and in most cases this is a normal finding. (B) This is the treatment for prolapsed valves. This type of recommendation should not be made without a further work-up. (C) Systolic murmurs occur in 90 percent of pregnancies and resolve after pregnancy. The heath-care provider should be informed so that he can determine if further work-up is needed. (D) Though systolic murmurs occur very commonly in pregnancy, all women do not develop murmurs.

338. (C) Nursing process phase: evaluation; client need: safe, effective care environment; content area: maternity nursing

Rationale

(A) Normally, there is a slight drop in BP that occurs from the relaxation effect of the hormones in pregnancy. Close to term, BP returns to normal pre-pregnant values. It is not normal to see an elevated BP, and this increase needs to be further evaluated. (B) An increase of 30 mm Hg above the systolic or an increase of 15 mm Hg above the diastolic is reason for concern and needs to be further evaluated. (C) Normally, there is a slight drop in BP that occurs from the relaxation effect of the hormones in pregnancy. Close to term, BP returns to normal pre-pregnant values. Anytime there is an increase, the client should be assessed for PIH or other BP-related conditions. (D) Hypertension is often called the "silent killer" and certainly can have detrimental effects without the client being aware of symptoms.

339. (C) Nursing process phase: analysis; client need: health promotion and maintenance; content area: maternity nursing

Rationale

(A) Indigestion at this stage of pregnancy is very common because of the increased intragastric pressure. Along with other symptoms, it may be indicative of other, more severe conditions, but certainly not always. (B) Hydrochloric acid and pepsin actually decrease in pregnancy. (C) There is decreased motility of the gastrointestinal tract as a result of the action of progesterone on smooth muscle. The tone of the esophagus is decreased, allowing stomach contents to reach the lower esophagus with the increase in intragastric pressure from the pregnancy. (D) Gastric motility is decreased in pregnancy. Reflux occurs because of the relaxation of the esophagus and increased intragastric pressure.

340. **(A)** Nursing process phase: implementation; client need: health promotion and maintenance; content area: maternity nursing

Rationale

(A) Epulides are nodules of vascular swelling that occur on the gums. The lesions bleed excessively if traumatized with a toothbrush or while eating. The cause is unknown but is probably related to high levels of estrogen. These lesions resolve spontaneously in the postpartum period. (B) Gingivitis is a gum disorder caused by a build-up of plaque, but is not exclusive to pregnancy and does not form nodules as in epulides. (C) Pica is a craving for, or ingestion of, nonfood items. (D) Ptyalism is an excessive production of saliva.

341. **(A)** Nursing process phase: implementation; client need: health promotion and maintenance; content area: maternity nursing

Rationale

(A) An increase in circulating estrogen occurs in pregnancy and causes palmar erythema. This is a common finding in pregnancy. (B) When the hematocrit is extremely high, the face and general skin tone may appear flushed. Hands may actually appear blanched. (C) Liver disease is one of several reasons that red palms may occur. It also occurs commonly in pregnancy. (D) Since this a normal pregnancy finding, the nurse should be aware that this is a normal finding.

342. **(B)** Nursing process phase: analysis; client needs: safe, effective care environment; content area: maturity nursing

Rationale

(A) There is a decrease in gastric motility in pregnancy. (B) The gallbladder becomes sluggish in pregnancy, causing an incomplete emptying and an increased risk of developing gallstones. (C) The blood volume in the liver does not increase in normal pregnancy. This condition occurs in pregnancy-induced hypertension and is an ominous finding. (D) There is a decrease in both hydrochloric acid and pepsid that occurs in pregnancy. There have been no studies to indicate that ulcers are more common in pregnancy.

343. **(C)** Nursing process phase: analysis; client need: health promotion and maintenance; content area: maternity nursing

Rationale

(A) Striae, commonly referred to as stretch marks, represent a tearing of connective tissue under the skin, usually occurring on the abdomen, buttocks, thighs, and breasts. (B) Increased blood flow causes a flushed appearance. (C) Because of the action of melanocyte-stimulating hormone, 50 to 70 percent of pregnant women experience a pigment change, especially noticeable on the face. The butterfly pattern appears very commonly among women who experience this disorder. After pregnancy, the discoloration typically fades, but may or may not disappear completely. (D) With lupus, there may also be a butterfly-shaped discoloration across the face, but it is typically reddish in color. This configuration does not mean the client has lupus.

344. **(D)** Nursing process phase: assessment; client need: health promotion and maintenance; content area: maternity nursing

Rationale

(A) Estrogen is a hormone normally present in women and is not indicative of a positive pregnancy test. (B) Progesterone is a hormone normally present in women and is not indicative of a positive pregnancy test. (C) FSH, or follicle stimulating hormone, is produced by the pituitary gland and stimulates follicles to grow, develop, and produce estrogen. Is not indicative of pregnancy. (D) hCG, or human chorionic gonadotropin, is the hormone produced by the trophoblastic cells of the developing placenta. It is excreted in the urine in increasing amounts as the placenta grows and gives a positive urine pregnancy test.

345. **(A)** Nursing process phase: assessment; client need: health promotion and maintenance; content area: maternity nursing

Rationale

(A) Cessation of menses; nausea and vomiting, especially in the morning; and breast tenderness are all subjective signs and symptoms that suggest, but do not prove, pregnancy. (B) Probably signs of pregnancy include objective signs such as Hegar's and Chadwick's signs and enlargement of the abdomen. These are highly indicative, but still do not prove pregnancy. (C & D) Positive or diagnostic signs of pregnancy include fetal heartbeat, fetus seen on ultrasound, and fetal movement felt by a trained examiner after 20 weeks' gestation.

346. **(B)** Nursing process phase: implementation; client need: health promotion and maintenance; content area: maternity nursing

Rationale

(A) The fetal heart should be heard at 10 to 12 weeks' gestation. (B) The fetal heart beat is usually picked up by Doppler at 10 to 12 weeks' gestation. (C) Ultrasound can pick up the heart motion much sooner than it can be heard by stethoscope, as early as 6 weeks' gestation. (D) Eight weeks is too early to hear a fetal heartbeat, trained ear or not. This is a condescending and incorrect statement.

347. **(C)** Nursing process phase: implementation; client need: health promotion and maintenance; content area: maternity nursing

Rationale

(A) Women are not immunized during pregnancy because of the risks of infection from the live virus. Rubella can have grave effects on the fetus, including blindness, deafness, and mental retardation. (B) This statement is inappropriate because it is frightening and demeaning for the client, and gives her no helpful information. (C) It is recommended that a client who is not immune to rubella be immunized during the immediate postpartal period. There is no risk if the client is breastfeeding. It is important to determine if the client has been in contact with anyone with rubella and to counsel her to avoid contact with anyone who is suspected of having rubella because of the possible detrimental effects on the unborn child if rubella is contracted during the first 12 weeks of pregnancy. (D) This has nothing to do with the mother's state of immunization. The newborn will receive immunization on a routine schedule.

348. (D) Nursing process phase: implementation; client need: safe, effective care environment; content area: maternity nursing

Rationale

(A) Because the client is Rh negative, she will receive a prophylactic injection of RhoGAM at about 24 weeks, which will prevent the formation of antibodies against the fetal blood cells. Depending on the newborn's blood type, the mother may receive another injection after delivery. (B) "Everyone" does not get an injection, only those who are Rh negative. This is inappropriate because it is incorrect information and flippant. (C) Because her husband, the father of the baby, is Rh positive, the infant may also be positive, which is what causes the incompatibility of blood types. (D) Because the client is Rh negative, the mother will receive a prophylactic injection of RhoGAM at about 24 weeks, which will prevent the formation of antibodies against the fetal blood cells. Depending on the newborn's blood type, the mother may receive another injection after delivery.

349. (C) Nursing process phase: implementation; client need: health promotion and maintenance; content area: maternity nursing

Rationale

(A) Routine glucose screening is done at 24 to 28 weeks' gestation, because this is the time during pregnancy when the body may have difficulty using glucose. (B) This should ideally be done prior to pregnancy so the woman can be immunized prior to pregnancy. Otherwise, it is drawn with the initial blood work, usually at 6 to 10 weeks' gestation. (C) This test is most accurate if drawn at 16 to 18 weeks' gestation. It is used to detect open neural defects or open abdominal wall defects. (D) This is not a blood test. The specimen is obtained by cervical and pharyngeal smears to determine the presence of group B strep, usually at the first prenatal visit along with the Pap test. If strep is present, the client is treated with antibiotics. The client may be tested again at term.

350. (A) Nursing process phase: implementation; client need: health promotion and maintenance; content area: maternity nursing

Rationale

(A) Urine is checked at each visit because the problems can occur in a short time frame. Presence of protein may indicate a problem with the renal system or PIH. Sugar may indicate a problem with undetected diabetes. Ketones are present when fat is being used for energy and may be present if the diet is insufficient to provide the calories needed for energy, as when there is excessive vomiting. (B) Urine is tested at each visit and is especially important toward the end of pregnancy. (C) A urinalysis is the test done for diagnosis of a urinary tract infection. This is done on the first visit and repeated only if the client has symptoms of infection. (D) This is a condescending statement. There is no reason why the nurse cannot give a factual answer to the client's question.

351. (B) Nursing process phase: evaluation; client need: safe, effective care environment; content area: maternity nursing

Rationale

(A) These symptoms would be indicative of a urinary tract infection, not metabolism of fat, which produces ketones as a byproduct. (B) Ketones are found when a client is not getting adequate amounts of food and fluid, and body fat is being used for energy. Typically this is related to nausea and vomiting in early pregnancy. (C) If the client were eating a lot of sugar, her ketones would be negative, since sugar is a source of energy. (D) Right upper quadrant pain may indicate gallbladder problems, which sometimes occur in pregnancy. Bile in the urine is the indicator for this disease process.

352. (D) Nursing process phase: implementation; client need: safe, effective care environment; content area: maternity nursing

Rationale

(A) This does not provide the client with an opportunity to get help. (B) This statement puts the blame on the client rather than the abuser. The client already has been made to feel that it is her fault—this statement supports that reasoning. (C) The client may feel threatened. With a questioning statement like this, she will most likely make up a story to cover for the bruises. (D) Confirming the injury followed by a generic statement related to abuse will typically get a response from the abused client.

353. (D) Nursing process phase: assessment; client need: safe, effective care environment; content area: maternity nursing

Rationale

(A) Most clients suffering abuse are afraid to report their abuser, either for fear of what he will do to her, or for fear that he will leave. (B) Most clients suffering chronic abuse will have injuries in areas not easily seen. During pregnancy, the chest and abdomen tend to be the targeted areas. (C) Most clients who suffer from chronic abuse are submissive and quiet. (D) Clients who are chronically abused tend to be evasive when answering questions. They will make up stories that do not make sense to cover for their abuser. They may appear very withdrawn and hopeless.

354. (C) Nursing process phase: implementation; client need: safe, effective care environment; content area: maternity nursing

Rationale

(A) Specimens are taken from the inside of the vagina. There would be little, if any, risk of contamination. (B) A full bladder may push the uterus up some, but not to the point that locating the cervix would be a problem. (C) A full bladder would cause increased discomfort, especially during the bimanual examination. (D) If the health-care provider is handling the instruments properly, there should be no possibility of bladder damage during a vaginal examination.

355. (C) Nursing process phase: assessment; client need: health promotion and maintenance; content area: maternity nursing

Rationale

(A) The uterus may be just beginning to rise out of the pelvis, and a measurement would be impossible. (B) The fetus is not large enough at this stage for age and fundal height to corre-late. (C) Research has shown that at 20 weeks' gestation, the gestational age and fundal height should correlate and should continue to correlate until about 38 weeks' gestation. This measurement is a noninvasive way of determining fetal growth. (D) Fundal height measurements need to begin at 20 weeks' gestation and continue throughout pregnancy.

356. (C) Nursing process phase: implementation; client need: health promotion and maintenance; content area: maternity nursing

Rationale
(A) First of all, 14 weeks is too soon to feel fetal movement; second, this statement would cause concern that something is wrong with her or her baby. (B) Some multigravidas may feel movement as early as at 16 weeks, but for most women, espe-cially primigravidas, it is closer to 18 to 20 weeks. (C) It is im-portant for the client to understand that the fetal movement will first feel more like a fluttery feeling than an actual kick, as she may expect. Most primigravidas feel this movement, called quickening, at 18 to 20 weeks. (D) The fetus has been moving practically since conception.

357. (A) Nursing process phase: analysis; client need: safe, effective care environment; content area: maternity nursing

Rationale
(A) Amniotic fluid is obtained and tested for lecithin-sphin-gomyelin ratio (LIS), which is an excellent indicator of fetal lung maturity. This client is at high risk for immature fetal lungs because of the preterm status of the pregnancy and the fact that she is a diabetic. (B) Amniocentesis to determine ge-netic deformities is typically done in the first half of preg-nancy. (C) An amniocentesis is not done for the purpose of determining meconium in the fluid, thought that would be noted on the report if found. (D) Volume of fluid is deter-mined by ultrasound, not amniocentesis.

358. (B) Nursing process phase: implementation; client need: safe, effective care environment; content area: maternity nursing

Rationale
(A) A positive test is recorded when the fetal heart rate base-line is not within normal limits and/or decelerations are noted with contractions. This would indicate the possibility of a poor fetal outcome. (B) A negative test is recorded when the fetal heart rate is within normal limits with no decelera-tions noted in the presence of contractions. This indicates a good fetal outcome. (C) *Reactive* is the term used for non-stress tests with a normal finding. (D) *Nonreactive* is the term used for nonstress tests with abnormal findings.

359. (C) Nursing process phase: implementation; client need: health promotion and maintenance; content area: maternity nursing

Rationale
(A) She should eat small, frequent meals to avoid overloading her GI system and assure adequate nutritional intake. (B) She should take small amounts of fluids with meals and be-tween meals. Too much fluid during a meal will increase the chance of nausea or vomiting. (C) Crackers have been found to decrease nausea by absorbing stomach acids and raising blood sugar, both problems that occur from not eating for 8 or more hours. (D) The client should be encouraged to eat a

high-protein diet before bedtime. This will prevent a rapid rise followed by drop in blood sugar, which occurs with car-bohydrates and is thought to contribute to morning sickness.

360. (C) Nursing process phase: implementation; client need: health promotion and maintenance; content area: maternity nursing

Rationale
(A) Because of the increased fluid needs of the body and in-creased risk for urinary tract infections during pregnancy, a pregnant client should never limit fluids, though she may de-crease her amount close to bedtime, as long as her total fluids are adequate. (B) Frequency is a normal occurrence in preg-nancy. As long as the client is not symptomatic, there is no rea-son to test for infection. (C) The client should be counseled that this is normal for the first trimester of pregnancy, but that she should report any signs of infection, such as burning, pres-sure, or pain with urination. (D) The client should be in-structed to void whenever the urge occurs. "Holding it in" will increase the risk of bacteria growth and an infection.

361. (D) Nursing process phase: implementation; client need: health promotion and maintenance; content area: maternity nursing

Rationale
(A) For normal vaginal discharge, this is accurate informa-tion; however, when the discharge smells bad and is itching and burning, it needs to be examined. (B) A pregnant woman should not wear tampons. (C) This is true, but she also needs to have the discharge evaluated, which is the best response. (D) An odorless discharge that does not cause itching or pain is normal in pregnancy. However, with these symptoms, the client needs to have an examination and have the discharge tested for STDs and other infectious processes.

362. (A) Nursing process phase: implementation; client need: health promotion and maintenance; content area: maternity nursing

Rationale
(A) By increasing the fiber and fluids, the stool will be softer and pass more readily. (B) Laxatives are habit-forming and should not be used on a regular basis. There is also a risk of electrolyte imbalance with chronic use of laxatives. (C) Min-eral oil interferes with the absorption of certain vitamins and nutrients and should not be used in pregnancy. (D) It is not advisable to use Fleet enemas on a regular basis. It is better to prevent the constipation than to treat it.

363. (C) Nursing process phase: implementation; client need: health promotion and maintenance; content area: maternity nursing

Rationale
(A) A client in the third trimester of pregnancy should not lay flat on her back. This causes vena cava syndrome, which is caused by the weight of the fetus applying pressure to her vena cava, and may cause a drop in blood pressure and decrease the blood supply to the fetus. (B) Pregnant women are en-couraged to have an average intake of salt. Sodium is needed in adequate amounts for the pregnancy. (C) Lying on the left lateral side will increase renal perfusion and help decrease edema. Also, lying down will decrease dependent edema in general. (D) Increasing the intake of fluids will actually help decrease edema.

364. (B) Nursing process phase: implementation; client need: safe, effective care environment; content area: maternity nursing

Rationale

(A) Hemoglobin represents the red blood cell volume, not total blood volume, which is what supports blood pressure. (B) During pregnancy, red blood cells normally increase in response to the increased oxygen demands of the products of conception. Hemoglobin, which is responsible for carrying oxygen to the body tissues, is attached to red blood cells. If red blood cells are too low, there will be inadequate oxygenation to the tissues. Research has shown that this contributes to preterm birth, low-birth-weight babies and fetal death. (C) Red blood cells' primary actions is to carry oxygen to the tissues. Besides, the question asks about hemoglobin, not red blood cells. (D) The hemoglobin is attached to the red blood cells, which carry oxygen to the maternal and fetal tissue.

365. (C) Nursing process phase: implementation; client need: health promotion and maintenance; content area: maternity nursing

Rationale

(A) Taking iron on an empty stomach can increase gastrointestinal upset in some people. (B) Some people do experience stomach upset with iron supplements and may have to take them with food. However, the maximum benefit is derived from taking the supplement between meals with orange juice. (C) Pairing iron supplements with orange juice between meals allows for maximum absorption of the iron. (D) Many times, the combination of iron supplements and milk will cause gastric upset, especially in pregnancy.

366. (A) Nursing process phase: implementation; client need: health promotion and maintenance; content area: maternity nursing

Rationale

(A) The redder the meat and darker green the vegetable, the higher the iron content. These are both excellent sources of iron, as well as of protein and B vitamins. (B) These are good sources of protein and vitamins. (C) Beans are an incomplete source of protein, not iron. (D) Milk is a good source of protein and calcium. However, most pregnant women do not need the fat in whole milk—2 percent, 1 percent, or skim all have the same calcium and protein, without the fat and calories. Whole wheat bread is a good source of fiber and may be iron-enriched, but is still not the best source of iron.

367. (C) Nursing process phase: implementation; client need: health promotion and maintenance; content area: maternity nursing

Rationale

(A) If she follows the ACOG recommendations for exercise, she should be safe in continuing her exercise routine. (B) Research has shown no link between problems in pregnancy and an intake of caffeine in moderate amounts. (C) There is a concern with toxoplasmosis, a virus found in cat feces, which can have teratogenic effects on the fetus. The client should be counseled to avoid exposure to cat feces, such as by changing the litter box, and to use good hand-washing techniques. (D) A nurse who uses universal precautions and good sense in practice should be able to carry a pregnancy safely.

368. (A) Nursing process phase: implementation; client need: safe, effective care environment; content area: maternity nursing

Rationale

(A) A woman working with children is at an increased risk for acquiring rubella, parvovirus, and cytomegalovirus. She should be tested prenatally and immunized for rubella. She also needs to be aware of how the infections are spread and make an informed decision based on this knowledge. (B) Actually, daycare workers tend to acquire viruses and other child-oriented infections just as easily as anyone else. (C) There have been no documented studies that show daycare workers to be at increased risk for injury over others in the service industry. (D) Cytomegalovirus is a herpes type virus often carried by children, but there is no immunization or treatment for it.

369. (C) Nursing process phase: implementation; client need: safe, effective care environment; content area: maternity nursing

Rationale

(A) There have been no documented connections between BP elevations and strep B infections. (B) It is not a nursing role to order laboratory work, but to monitor it. The physician may order laboratory values, but usually no more than twice daily. (C) Strep B can infect a woman, and she may have mild coldlike symptoms or no symptoms at all. Typically, there are no problems connected with this disease in pregnancy, until the rupture of membranes allows the infection to move into the uterine cavity, infecting the uterine lining and the fetus. The primary symptom of this infection after rupture of membranes is a rapidly rising maternal temperature. If this occurs, the physician should be notified immediately. Usually, the client who is known to be infected with strep B is given IV antibiotics as a preventative measure. (D) This should be done with all clients. If the fetus becomes infected or the mother has an elevated temperature, initially the FHR may exhibit tachycardia, and as reserves run out, you may see late decelerations.

370. (B) Nursing process phase: assessment; client need: safe, effective care environment; content area: maternity nursing

Rationale

(A) Homans' sign assesses for the presence of deep vein thrombosis, characterized by discomfort or cramping in the calf area of the leg, localized redness or edema. (B) This client is symptomatic of pyelonephritis, an infection in the kidneys. The costovertebral angle is in the flank area over the kidney. A gentle rap with the closed hand would elicit significant discomfort in this area in the presence of pyelonephritis. This is diagnostic along with urine cultures. (C) While this would be a nursing assessment you would perform, the client's symptoms should lead you to check for kidney pain first. (D) You would assess the client for contractions, but the symptoms do not point to preterm labor. This is not the priority nursing assessment.

371. (C) Nursing process phase: assessment; client need: physiological integrity; content area: maternity nursing

Rationale

(A) Normally there is no protein in the urine, and only a trace occurs in a normal pregnancy. Significant increases would indicate pregnancy-induced hypertension or other significant complications of pregnancy. (B) The bladder is actually compressed against the uterus in pregnancy, causing the capacity to be decreased. (C) The small amount of sugar that occurs normally in pregnancy supports the growth of bacteria, increasing the risk of urinary tract infection. Other changes that occur include a slight enlargement of the kidneys, dilation of the renal pelves and ureters, elongation of the ureters, and changes in bladder position. (D) The ureters actually lengthen slightly in pregnancy to accommodate the growing uterus.

372. (D) Nursing process phase: implementation; client need: health promotion and maintenance; content area: maternity nursing

Rationale
(A) Large amounts of carbohydrates will contribute to sugar in the urine and increase the risk of bacteria growth. (B) The pregnant client should void frequently, any time the urge occurs. "Holding urine" will increase the risk of bacteria growth. (C) The pregnant client should be encouraged to drink plenty of fluids, at least eight 8-oz glasses of water per day. (D) Voiding before and after intercourse will clear any of the glucose-rich semen from the area and help decrease the risk of bacteria growth.

373. (D) Nursing process phase: assessment; client need: safe, effective care environment; content area: maternity nursing

Rationale
(A) HIV is on the rise, but has not been rated first. (B) Chlamydia often coexists with gonorrhea, and tests are done for both when either is suspected. However, gonorrhea is not the most common type. (C) Syphilis is on the rise again in the United States, but still ranks behind chlamydia in reported cases. (D) This is the most common STD. More than half of women infected have no clinical signs. Symptoms that may occur include purulent vaginal discharge, postcoital bleeding, and diffuse low abdominal pain. Chlamydial infections are associated with premature rupture of membranes, preterm labor and birth, and low-birth-weight infants.

374. (C) Nursing process phase: implementation; client need: health promotion and maintenance; content area: maternity nursing

Rationale
(A) This would provide about 700 calories over the recommended number of calories, resulting in excessive weight gain and possible complications with the pregnancy. (B) This would provide 500 calories over the recommended caloric intake, most likely resulting in excessive weight gain above that required for a healthy pregnancy. (C) Based on an average weight, and activity level, 300 additional calories will meet the needs of most pregnancies without causing weight gain above the needs of the pregnancy. (D) This may be true of some women, but most women will need to increase the caloric intake some to provide adequate calories to maintain their health as well as the growth of the fetus and products of conception.

375. (B) Nursing process phase: implementation; client need: health promotion and maintenance; content area: maternity nursing

Rationale
(A) This approach would cause an adolescent to become more difficult to work with, and it takes away any control over the situation she may have. (B) This will allow the client to make choices and develop a meal plan she can stick with. This will allow for a happier client and a healthy pregnancy. It is also a much more positive way to deal with an adolescent. (C) An attempt to empathize will not help this situation. She already knows it is going to be hard; she needs help in gaining control and making appropriate decisions. (D) Supplements are not a substitute for a healthy diet.

376. (A) Nursing process phase: analysis; client need: safe, effective care environment; content area: maternity nursing

Rationale
(A) Pica is the consumption of nonfood items. This practice in pregnancy is of particular concern when it is something that interferes with nutrient absorption, as clay would. Other concerns are that these substances might be eaten in place of nutritious food, and parasites or bacteria may be ingested with dirt or clay. (B) People have theorized this to be true, but it has not been proved with research. (C) Baking the clay may kill the bacteria or parasites, but it can still interfere with absorption of nutrients. (D) This is a fairly common practice, but there are concerns surrounding this practice.

377. (B) Nursing process phase: analysis; client need: health promotion and maintenance; content area: maternity nursing

Rationale
(A) Age is a factor, but not the primary one. Diet preferences need to be looked at in terms of an overall healthy diet, as well as calorie intake. (B) Based on pre-pregnancy weight and height, the basal metabolic index (BMI) is calculated and the total expected weight gain is calculated. (C) Previous eating disorders need to be taken into account, since they can certainly influence weight gain in pregnancy. The weight gain for pregnancy will be calculated based on pre-pregnancy weight. (D) This is a factor that must be looked at in terms of the client being able to obtain adequate nutrition, but expected weight gain is calculated in the same way.

378. (C) Nursing process phase: implementation; client need: health promotion and maintenance; content area: maternity nursing

Rationale
(A) A client who is overweight at the beginning of pregnancy should be advised to gain less weight to avoid complications that can result from excess weight—15 to 25 lb is usually recommended. (B) If the pregnancy pulls from fat stores, this can result in ketonemia and ketonuria, which can be life-threatening to the fetus and can cause intellectual impairment. (C) Overweight women should be encouraged to gain 15 to 25 lb for a healthy pregnancy. (D) Excessive or minimal weight gain can both be detrimental to a healthy pregnancy and good perinatal outcomes.

379. (A) Nursing process phase: implementation; client need: health promotion and maintenance; content area: maternity nursing

Rationale
(A) Because of the extensive amount of energy expended from exercise, she will need to supplement her calories and carbohydrates to provide adequate nutrition for a healthy pregnancy. (B) If she continues this exercise without increasing her calories, she will not provide adequate nutrition for a

healthy pregnancy. (C) She should be able to continue her lifestyle if she provides adequate calories for the growth of the maternal and fetal tissue. (D) If she doubles the amount of calories, she will be taking in close to 5000 calories. She may actually have excessive weight gain despite her activity level. The client's diet needs to be reviewed and calories calculated based on her height, weight, and activity level.

380. **(C)** Nursing process phase: planning; client need: safe, effect care environment; content area: maternity nursing

Rationale

(A) Though this is the most important position in labor, it is not the best position to facilitate labor. (B) There is an increased risk of vena cava syndrome and reflex late decelerations when in this position. Studies have shown that contractions occur more frequently but are less effective in the supine position. (C) Standing and upright positions have been proved to be most efficient in dilating the cervix and progressing the fetal station. Unless there are complications, this position is very appropriate in the early stages of labor. (D) There have been no studies to prove whether this would facilitate labor or not, but lying on the abdomen would be very uncomfortable in labor.

381. **(B)** Nursing process phase: assessment; client need: physiological integrity; content area: maternity nursing

Rationale

(A) The diagonal conjugate is the distance from the lower margin of the symphysis pubis to the promontory of the sacrum. This is the diameter that can be measured on vaginal examination and is used to estimate the obstetric conjugate. (B) This is the shortest anteroposterior distance between the sacral promonitory and the symphysis pubis. It is the most significant diameter of the inlet, since the fetal presenting part must first pass successfully through this diameter before further descent can occur. (C) This is a combination of the anteroposterior (obstetrical conjugate), the transverse, and the two oblique diameters. (D) This consists of a line drawn between the two ischial tuberosities. This is the transverse diameter of the outlet.

382. **(D)** Nursing process phase: implementation; client need: health promotion and maintenance; content area: maternity nursing

Rationale

(A) This describes a baby in an attitude of flexion. (B) This leads the client to believe that the position is completely without concern. The fetus is coming head down but not "just as he should." (C) This describes an attitude of extension, where the face presents first. (D) This is correct and describes the attitude of flexion.

383. **(C)** Nursing process phase: implementation; client need: safe, effective care environment; content area: maternity nursing

Rationale

(A) Location of the fetus in an occipital posterior position is sometimes difficult, but adjustment of the fetal monitor would not be considered a comfort measure. (B) Most laboring clients benefit from ice chips but this is not a comfort measure specific to this fetal position. (C) Clients with a fetus in an occipital posterior position typically have terrible back pain, which can be relieved to some degree by counterpressure on the low back. (D) All clients in labor should change positions at least every 2 hours. This is not a comfort measure specific to this position.

384. **(C)** Nursing process phase: assessment; client need: safe, effective care environment; content area: maternity nursing

Rationale

(A) The latent phase is the early part of the first stage of labor and is characterized by excitement and the feeling that she can cope with labor. (B) The active phase of the first stage of labor is characterized by the woman's deep concentration and intense focus. She typically is in good control at this point. (C) This is the last phase of the first stage of labor and is characterized by the sudden loss of control, the feeling that she can no longer cope as the contractions get more intense. It is not unusual for the client to strike out, curse, or display other behaviors uncharacteristic and often surprising to the family. (D) This is the stage where the client may feel more relaxed and in control as she focuses to push the baby out.

385. **(C)** Nursing process phase: evaluation; client need: safe, effective care environment; content area: maternity nursing

Rationale

(A) These are not signs of labor. She may experience these signs for 2 to 3 days to a week before labor actually begins. (B) The nurse should identify these as premonitory signs of labor. (C) The nurse gave her feedback on what is happening now and what to expect. (D) While backache is common in late pregnancy, diarrhea is not a typical sign of late pregnancy or "overdoing" it. The nurse should recognize these as signs of approaching labor.

386. **(C)** Nursing process phase: implementation; client need: health promotion and maintenance; content area: maternity nursing

Rationale

(A) True labor contractions will increase in intensity with walking. (B) True labor contractions will be felt in the low back and come around to the low abdomen. (C) This describes a true labor contraction pattern. (D) Individuals do vary somewhat, but contraction patterns are very similar. Telling the client "she'll just know" can be very confusing to the client.

387. **(B)** Nursing process phase: analysis; client need: safe, effective care environment; content area: maternity nursing

Rationale

(A) While this would be considered, a temperature elevation is a better indicator of infection than an elevated heart rate alone. We are also looking for the normal response—infection would be considered a complication of labor. (B) A heart rate elevation on admission during the active phase of labor is most likely related to anxiety, pain, or excitement. After the client is admitted and calmed, the heart rate should decrease. (C) The heart rate does increase as much as 15 beats per minute from the prenatal heart rate, but this usually brings it up to 85 to 90 beats per minute. A rate of 120 would not be a normal elevation. (D) An elevated pulse is not one of the triad of symptoms that indicate pregnancy-induced hypertension (elevated BP, proteinuria, and edema), though heart rate may be increased secondary to increased cardiac output.

388. (A) Nursing process phase: analysis; client need: safe, effective care environment; content area: maternity nursing

Rationale

(A) An elevated pulse rate is the first indicator of maternal hemorrhage and precedes any drop in BP. This client needs to be evaluated closely for blood loss. (B) Heart rate increases during the perinatal period, then returns to the normal prelabor readings during the postpartum period. There should not be a heart rate elevation during postpartum, unless the client is in pain or there are other complications. (C) Since an elevated heart rate precedes a drop in BP with maternal hemorrhage, the heart rate is a concern. (D) While infection may be a concern, it is not the primary concern. A temperature elevation is a better initial indicator of infection, with an elevated heart rate secondary to the elevated temperature.

389. (A) Nursing process phase: assessment; client need: safe, effective care environment; content area: maternity nursing

Rationale

(A) In the low-risk, term client in the latent phase of labor, every hour is considered standard practice. (B) Unless complications are identified, the client does not have to be monitored every 30 minutes until the active phase of labor. (C) Unless problems are identified, the client does not have to have evaluation of fetal heart tones every 15 minutes until the second stage of labor. (D) Fetal heart tones only need to be evaluated every 5 minutes when complications are noted in the second stage of labor.

390. (C) Nursing process phase: evaluation; client need: safe, effective care environment; content area: maternity nursing

Rationale

(A) Baseline fetal heart rate is determined between contractions. (B) This is the method for evaluation of periodic changes in fetal heart rate. (C) Baseline fetal heart rate is determined between contractions, with fetal heart rate counted for 1 full minute between contractions. (D) Viewing a strip for 5 minutes both during and between contractions gives a brief picture of fetal status, but does not focus on baseline rate.

391. (C) Nursing process phase: analysis; client need: safe, effective care environment; content area: maternity nursing

Rationale

(A) In a normal labor pattern for a multipara, the latent phase should not exceed 14 hours. (B) In the latent phase of labor, the contractions are usually very mild and well tolerated by the client. (C) Even though the contractions are usually mild and well tolerated in the latent phase of labor, the client may become very frustrated, lose sleep, and become exhausted. Comfort measures need to be implemented, and the primary health-care provider should be made aware of the client's slow progress. (D) Because the contractions are typically mild, a healthy fetus should have no difficulty tolerating latent labor contractions for a long period of time.

392. (C) Nursing process phase: analysis; client need: safe, effective care environment; content area: maternity nursing

Rationale

(A) The fetus is not descending in the birth canal. At −2 station, the fetus is still well above the ischial spines. "Caput" indicates pressure on the fetal head by the bony pelvis. (B) Signs of caput should not normally appear until the fetus is at least at 0 station, going through the narrow portion of the pelvis. (C) If caput occurs before the fetal head is at 0 station, this is an indicator that there is pressure on the fetal scalp from the false pelvis, and the fetus may not be able to descend into the true pelvis. (D) This definition describes a cephalohematoma, rather than a caput. It is very unlikely that a fetus would experience a hematoma at −2 station.

393. (D) Nursing process phase: implementation; client need: safe, effective care environment; content area: maternity nursing

Rationale

(A) A prolonged contraction with inadequate rest time between contractions can contribute to fetal distress caused by decreased perfusion. Continuing to observe this pattern is negligent. (B) You will notify the midwife after other priority nursing measures are taken to protect the client and fetus. (C) These are not priority nursing actions for prolonged contractions; though after the main actions are taken, you may assess these to evaluate the client's tolerance of labor. (D) The first nursing measure is to turn off the oxytocin infusion when prolonged contractions and inadequate rest between contractions occur. Contractions should last no longer than 90 seconds and have a minimum of 30 seconds between contractions to allow adequate placental perfusion.

394. (B) Nursing process phase: implementation; client need: safe, effective care environment; area: maternity nursing

Rationale

(A) This position will assist in taking pressure off the back, but will not facilitate rotation of the fetus. (B) This position both relieves backache and assists in rotation of the fetus. By leaning forward, the heavier fetal back will turn to the maternal front. (C) This neither assists in rotation of the fetus nor in relief of back discomfort. (D) There may be some back relief with this position, but limited, if any, assistance in rotation of the fetus.

395. (C) Nursing process phase: analysis; client need: safe, effective care environment, content area: maternity nursing

Rationale

(A) This position aids in perfusion to the placenta and kidneys but does little to facilitate labor. (B) This position aids in perfusion to the placenta but does little to facilitate labor progression. (C) These positions take advantage of gravity during and between contractions and facilitate labor progression. (D) This position has many benefits but does not allow gravity to facilitate labor progression.

396. (A) Nursing process phase: implementation; client need: safe, effective care environment; content area: maternity nursing

Rationale

(A) The client is hyperventilating and will benefit from rebreathing her exhaled carbon dioxide. (B) While rebreathing with a paper bag works, it may be very frightening for the client in her current state. (C) The symptoms described do not constitute a vaginal examination. (D) This action would indicate that she is experiencing vena cava syndrome, but the symptoms are clearly related to hyperventilation and a side-lying position will not alleviate this.

397. **(D)** Nursing process phase: analysis; client need: safe, effective care environment; content area: maternity nursing

Rationale

(A) The client should make spontaneous vocalizations during pushing efforts. (B) The rectum should bulge during bearing down, rather than retract. (C) If the client feels very embarrassed with incontinence, she will "hold back" instead of pushing. (D) The client needs time to work through her feelings with her partner to prepare for pushing. This is a normal process that should be encouraged.

398. **(B)** Nursing process phase: implementation; client need: health promotion and maintenance; content area: maternity nursing

Rationale

(A) Most medications cross the placenta and affect the fetus in a potentially harmful way. The only drug considered safe for occasional use is acetiminophen. (B) It works as an antiprostaglandin but has less anti-inflammatory effect than aspirin or ibuprofen. It does cross the placenta and is metabolized by the fetal liver, so it should be used with caution. (C) Ibuprofen is not recommended with pregnancy because of its anti-inflammatory effect. Studies have shown that fetal prothrombin times and bilirubin concentrations are increased with the use of this drug. (D) Aspirin does cross the placenta and has an anticoagulant action, increasing the risk of fetal bleeding. The antiprostaglandin effect may cause closure of the ductus arteriosus before birth.

399. **(B)** Nursing process phase: implementation; client need: health promotion and maintenance; content area: maternity nursing

Rationale

(A) While pregnancy may increase a woman's introspection, it does not take away her ability to perform normally. This question was in regard to safety. (B) The concern with a job position that requires long hours of sitting in one position is the venous stasis and back strain that can occur. With proper instructions, she should be able to prevent these problems. (C) There have been some studies that indicate there may be some risk, but there are no definite studies that support this statement. (D) Again, we cannot decide what is "better" for the client. We need to give accurate information and allow the client to make informed decisions based on the facts.

400. **(C)** Nursing process phase: implementation; client need: health promotion and maintenance; maternity nursing

Rationale

(A) Never place the shoulder strap behind the back. This would cause a forward crushing injury to the abdomen and chest as well as the face. (B) The shoulder belt should fit snugly across the chest to prevent forward movement in the event of a crash. (C) Place the lap belt below the abdominal bulge snug across the pelvic bones. The shoulder strap should be snug across the chest and shoulder. (D) A pregnant woman should always wear her seatbelt in proper position while in a motor vehicle. Trauma to the abdomen can result

in fetal injury or death, separation of the placenta, rupture of the uterus as well as spinal cord, bladder, and other severe injuries.

401. **(D)** Nursing process phase: analysis; client need: safe, effective care environment; content area: maternity nursing

Rationale

(A) This is common practice for anyone receiving CPR. (B) The same ratio of chest compressions to breaths is used for pregnant women as for anyone else; 5:1 for two-man CPR, 15:2 for one-man CPR. (C) CPR should be initiated immediately and fetal heart tones assessed as soon as possible in an attempt to save both the mother and the fetus. (D) By placing the client wedged slightly to the side, the compressions will aid perfusion to the fetus as well. If the client is flat, the vena cava may be occluded and perfusion will be diminished, decreasing the chance of a good fetal outcome.

402. **(C)** Nursing process phase: implementation client needs: physiological integrity; content area: maternity nursing

Rationale

(A) The uterus, cervix, and perineum need at least 3 to 4 weeks to heal. Some couples may feel "physically ready" in less than a week, which would increase the risk of tissue trauma and infection. (B) While this has been the recommendation, it is not usually necessary to wait a full 6 weeks. If the client feels physically and psychologically ready as early as 3 to 4 weeks, and the lochia flow has stopped, it is considered safe to resume intercourse. (C) The most appropriate information is to wait for the lochia flow to stop, which takes 3 to 4 weeks, before resuming intercourse. This should allow adequate time for the uterus to heal, decreasing the risk of trauma or infection. (D) This is an opinionated and inappropriate response!

403. **(D)** Nursing process phase: implementation; client need: health promotion and maintenance; content area: maternity nursing

Rationale

(A) Pregnancy is "normal" in most cases, but some high-risk conditions can occur that will prevent the couple from safely having sexual intercourse during the pregnancy. (B) The enlarging maternal abdomen may require that the couple explore different positions for intercourse, but this is not a reason to suspend relations. (C) Many couples actually have an increased interest in sexual relations during pregnancy, and the issue should be addressed early in pregnancy. (D) Unless the client has a high-risk condition of pregnancy (preterm labor, previous preterm labor or threatened abortion, multiple gestation, placenta previa, pregnancy-induced hypertension, or diabetes), she and her husband should be able to continue sexual relations, though some alterations may be necessary, especially late in the pregnancy.

404. **(C)** Nursing process phase: implementation; client need: physiological integrity; content area: maternity nursing

Rationale

(A) Since a temperature up to 100.4°F is a normal finding in the first 24 hours after delivery, there is no need to contact the physician. (B) It is too early in the postpartum period for breast engorgement, which typically occurs on the second or third day postpartum. (C) A temperature elevation of up to 100.4°F in the first 24 hours' postpartum is considered a normal finding and is related to muscle exertion, dehydration, and hormonal changes. The best nursing action is to encourage fluids and rest and continue to observe. (D) Fundal and lochia checks are part of the routine postpartal assessment and are not related to the finding.

405. **(A)** Nursing process phase: implementation; client need: physiological integrity; content area: maternity nursing

Rationale
(A) A temperature elevation of greater than 100.4°F, especially after the first 24 hours' postpartum, is an indicator for infection, so the client's health-care provider should be notified prior to discharge. (B) Drinking large amounts of oral fluids is acceptable, but the client should not be discharged until the health-care provider is notified of the elevation, an abnormal finding. (C) Ordering laboratory work is not part of the nursing role in most institutions. (D) A temperature elevation of greater than 100.4°F, especially after the first 24 hours' postpartum, is an indicator for infection, so the client's health-care provider should be notified prior to discharge.

406. **(C)** Nursing process phase: implementation; client need: safe, effective care environment; content area: maternity nursing

Rationale
(A) This is important but not a priority in determining the cause of the increased heart rate. (B) This is an important assessment, but not the priority in determining the cause of the increased heart rate. (C) An increased heart rate (tachycardia) during the postpartal period is usually related to excessive vaginal bleeding (hemorrhage) or infection. (D) You need to assess the client's physical state first, then review the laboratory findings.

407. **(D)** Nursing process phase: implementation; client need: health promotion and maintenance; content area: maternity nursing

Rationale
(A) The lochia described is normal for this stage postpartum. Assessment of the heart rate and temperature are not indicated from these findings, though they may be part of a routine assessment. (B) The lochia described is normal for this stage postpartum. Evaluation of the client's abdomen for tenderness is not indicated from these findings. (C) The lochia described is normal for this stage postpartum. These findings are not indicative of an STD. (D) The lochia described is lochia serosa, which occurs on about day 4 to day 9 postpartum. This is a normal finding.

408. **(C)** Nursing process phase: assessment; client need: physiological integrity; content area: maternity nursing

Rationale
(A) The fundus should be evaluated every 15 minutes for the first hour after delivery, then if within normal limits, every 4 hours. (B) Since this client is past the initial recovery period, every 4 hours is the recommended time frame for routine assessments. (C) After the initial recovery period, the fundus should be assessed for location, consistency, and position every 4 hours. (D) While this is the practice in some facilities, this does not meet the current practice standard.

409. **(C)** Nursing process phase: assessment; client need: physiological integrity; content area: maternity nursing

Rationale
(A) This refers to a neurologic assessment and means: Pupils Equal Round Reactive to Light. (B) This refers to a total postpartum assessment and means: Breasts, Uterus, Bladder, Bowel, Lochia, Episiotomy, Homans', Emotions. (C) The mnemonic is used to remember the assessment for an episiotomy and means: Redness, Edema, Ecchymosis, Discharge, Approximation (of the edges). (D) This refers to Gravida, Term, Preterm, Abortions, Living children. This is used as part of the antenatal assessment.

410. **(B)** Nursing process phase: assessment; client need: physiological integrity; content area: maternity nursing

Rationale
(A) While this is an important assessment, it is not the priority based on the information. Also, blood pressure is one of the last parameters to show a change in most cases. (B) The patient's complaints of pressure and pain in the perineal area as well as the restlessness and anxiety are classic symptoms of a perineal hematoma. The nurse should visually inspect the perineum for signs of discoloration and edema. (C) It is highly unlikely that this is the client's cause of discomfort. (D) The signs of thrombus in the calf include pain, redness, and swelling in the calf area, as well as a positive Homans' sign. The symptoms listed do not relate.

411. **(C)** Nursing process phase: implementation; client need: safe, effective care environment; content area: maternity nursing

Rationale
(A) Aspirin is not typically used in the postpartum client, and if it were implemented, this is not part of the nursing role. (B) TED hose are sometimes used in the high-risk client, but they require a physician's order and are not the primary prevention. (C) Research has shown that early ambulation is the primary preventative treatment for thromboembolic disease. This is within the scope of nursing practice. (D) This could cause pressure in the popliteal area and restrict blood flow, contributing to clot formation.

412. **(C)** Nursing process phase: implementation client need: safe, effective care environment; content area: maternity nursing

Rationale
(A) Warfarin should not be used in pregnancy because it crosses the placenta and may cause hemorrhage in the products of conception, causing spontaneous abortion, abruption, and a number of other complications. (B) This is the antidote for heparin overdose. (C) Heparin does not cross the placenta and is considered safe for the mother and the pregnancy. (D) In rare cases, this drug may be used, but it is not the drug of choice. It is generally reserved for life-threatening cases of pulmonary embolism.

413. **(D)** Nursing process phase: implementation; client need: health promotion and maintenance; content area: maternity nursing

Rationale
(A & B) Research has shown that because of the molecular weight of heparin, it is unlikely to pass through breast milk, and even if it does, it cannot be absorbed through the baby's

gastrointestinal tract. It is considered safe to breastfeed while on heparin therapy. (C) This statement does not give enough information for the mother to make an informed decision. The client should be given factual information and allowed to make her own decision. (D) This is the best statement because it gives her the factual information and allows the client to make the final decision. The information is accurate and does not give the nurse's opinion of whether she should continue breastfeeding or not.

414. (D) Nursing process phase: implementation; client need: physiological integrity; content area: maternity nursing

Rationale
(A) Intermittent murmurs are common in the early neonatal period and may be heard at times, but not heard at other times. The nurse should notify the physician of her findings, realizing that this is a normal finding in most cases. (B) The newborn needs to be assessed by the physician, and information given by the physician on the condition of the newborn. The nurse is not in a position to state whether this is a normal or abnormal finding, or to order further tests if indicated. (C) While the nurse should document her findings, she should also notify the physician of the findings, because further evaluation may be indicated. (D) Intermittent murmurs usually occur secondary to the incomplete closure of the foramen ovale. However, because of the baby's other symptoms, the physician may decide other tests are indicated.

415. (B) Nursing process phase: analysis; client need: physiological integrity; content area: maternity nursing

Rationale
(A) Birth trauma and dehydration may place the low-risk infant at risk for an increased bilirubin level, but this typically shows up after the first 24 hours. The information given does not indicate this risk factor. (B) The newborn's weight and age place it at risk for thermoregulation problems. Because the newborn's temperature is decreased, she is attempting to compensate for increasing her heart rate and respiratory rate. This will use up energy stores and drop the baby's blood sugar, placing her at risk for hypoglycemia. (C) The newborn is 38 weeks' gestation, which is considered term. Below 37 weeks is preterm or premature. (D) This is the term used for a very large baby, usually associated with diabetic mothers. This is not applicable to this newborn.

416. (B) Nursing process phase: implementation; client need: psychosocial integrity; content area; maternity nursing

Rationale
(A) While this is true, the respiratory status is the primary concern. Thermoregulation is typically fairly easy to control. (B) It is important to verify the client's concerns and to give her answers in terms she can understand. At less than about 36 weeks' gestation, there is inadequate surfactant production to allow the baby's lungs to inflate during the inspiration phase and prevent collapse during the expiration phase. There are medications on the market that can be placed through an endotracheal tube directly into the baby's lungs that will lubricate the lungs and assist this process. (C) The organs are immature but functional in most cases. The baby will need close monitoring of systems to assure well-being, but typically the organs perform with minimal assistance. This comment is and would be frightening to the client. (D) With this comment

you are belittling her observation and concerns. You need to give factual information without overcompensating.

417. (C) Nursing process phase: evaluation; client need: health promotion and maintenance; content area: maternity nursing

Rationale
(A) Because the newborn's stomach only holds 20 to 40 cc initially, 30 cc is an adequate amount for a newborn on the first feeding. (B) This is demeaning for the client. The amount the baby took was adequate for the first feeding, and since the baby is sleeping, she is apparently satisfied with that amount. (C) On the first feeding, a newborn's stomach can generally hold 20 to 40 cc. The stomach distends easily, so within 3 to 4 days, capacity will increase to about 90 cc. (D) This should be done during the initiation of the first feed or if problems such as emesis or choking occurred. It is important to assure that the baby is being held upright and the bottle is not being propped. Since no problems were identified, this is not an appropriate intervention at this time.

418. (D) Nursing process phase: implementation; client need: health promotion and maintenance; content area: maternity nursing

Rationale
(A) The first period of reactivity is the time frame that lasts 15 to 30 minutes after birth. After 1 hour, the baby will be in an inactive period, and breastfeeding attempts are likely to be unsuccessful. (B) If there is a blood sugar drop after delivery, symptoms will occur before 2 hours of age. This answer does not respond to the period of reactivity. (C) The first period of reactivity is the time frame that last 15 to 30 minutes after birth. By 4 hours, the baby may be entering a second stage of reactivity. (D) The first period of reactivity is the time frame that last 15 to 30 minutes after birth. During this time the baby is alert and active with open eyes and a strong suck reflex. Research has shown that if the baby goes to breast during this time frame, the initial breastfeeding episode is usually successful. Also breastfeeding promotes uterine contraction and decreases vaginal bleeding.

419. (C) Nursing process phase: evaluation; client need: physiological integrity; content area: maternity nursing

Rationale
(A) Because of the irregular heart rate in a newborn, one should always listen for a full minute to get an accurate rate. (B) Because of the frequency of murmurs in the newborn and the need for accuracy in assessing, the apical pulse should be used. The brachial is used in CPR because it can be located without the need for a stethoscope. (C) Because of the irregular heart rate in a newborn, one should always listen for a full minute to get an accurate rate. By giving positive feedback to a new nurse, you will reinforce good practice. (D) She has not verbalized frustration with the skill. This statement would indicate that you found fault with her technique.

420. (A) Nursing process phase: assessment; client need: physiological integrity; content area: maternity nursing

Rationale
(A) Localized swelling of the scalp that does not cross the suture line is a characteristic finding. A cephalohematoma occurs as a result of blood accumulation in the soft tissue of the scalp, secondary to trauma, and may take several hours to appear. Depending on severity, it usually disappears in 2 to 3

days. (B) This is soft tissue swelling of the scalp as a result of pressure during the delivery. It is present at birth and crosses the suture line. (C) This term is used for thrush, a yeast infection of the mouth. (D) This is characterized by increasing head circumference caused by an abnormal accumulation of cerebrospinal fluid in the ventricles of the brain. Scalp edema is not characteristic of this disorder.

421. (C) Nursing process phase: analysis; client need: physiological integrity; content area: maternity nursing

Rationale
(A) The preterm newborn has thin, smooth skin. The sole creases, if present, only cover the anterior portion of the feet. (B) The term newborn's skin is thicker because of the increased fat deposits, but the skin should be smooth and soft. The sole creases are usually shallow and cover the entire sole. (C) The posterm newborn has dry, peeling skin that is leathery in consistency. The sole creases are deep and cover the entire sole. The baby's skin looks very much like an old person's skin. (D) This is a normal finding for a posterm newborn.

422. (D) Nursing process phase: assessment; client need: physiological integrity; content area: maternity nursing

Rationale
(A) This is done on a growth chart. (B) This is done on a conversion chart. (C) Determining head size in relation to the height, weight, and gestational age of the baby is charted on the growth chart. (D) The Ballard scale, a modified version of the Dubowitz scale, is used to assess gestational age. There are several assessments of both neuromuscular and physical maturity that are reviewed and a total score obtained.

423. (B) Nursing process phase: implementation; client need: physiological integrity; content area: maternity nursing

Rationale
(A) The NAACOG recommended temperature for a delivery room under normal conditions is 71°F. (B) A fan causes rapid heat loss from a wet newborn. NAACOG standards indicate that the room should be draft-free to effectively manage thermoregulation of the newborn. (C) The first action should be to turn off the fan. The mother may not tolerate being wrapped in a warm blanket at this point in delivery. (D) Significant heat loss can occur during the birth process if drafts are not minimized. Taking the baby to the warmer may be a measure to bring the temperature back up, but turning off the fan is the best initial action to prevent temperature problems.

424. (B) Nursing process phase: assessment; client need: physiological integrity; content area: maternity nursing

Rationale
(A) The deltoid muscle is not well developed in the newborn and should not be used. (B) This is the most highly developed muscle in the newborn and recommended for intramuscular injections. The rectus femoris, the anterior muscle in the leg, can also be used. (C) The gluteus maximum muscles in the buttocks are not well developed in the newborn and should not be used. (D) This is an area on the newborn foot. This is not a site for intramuscular injections.

425. (A) Nursing process phase: implementation; client need: physiological integrity; content area: maternity nursing

Rationale
(A) This baby is very dehydrated and needs to be admitted to the hospital for stabilization. (B) One PO feeding cannot reverse the baby's current poor status. The physician needs to be notified and the baby admitted for hydration. (C) This teaching will need to be done after the baby is stabilized in the hospital. (D) A nurse must have a physician's order for OG tube feedings. Sterile water would not be the fluid of choice for a baby in this condition.

426. (C) Nursing process phase: assessment; client need: physiological integrity; content area: maternity nursing

Rationale
(A, B, & D) The baby has a heart rate, but it is below 100, so he gets a score of 1 for heart rate. Reflex irritability receives a score of 1 for the grimace. The other assessments receive a 0, making the score a 2. (C) The Apgar is the assessment of 5 signs, each with a maximum score of 2 and a minimal score of 0, making the total score 0 to 10. This baby has a heart rate, but it is below 100, so he gets a score of 1 for heart rate. Reflex irritability receives a score of 1 for the grimace. The other assessments receive a 0, making the total score 2.

427. (D) Nursing process phase: implementation; client need: health promotion and maintenance; content area: maternity nursing

Rationale
(A) Isotretinoin is a teratogen. (B) It will not affect embryonic development because she stopped the medication 13 years ago. (C) This medication is a teratogen that can produce fetal malformation while taking the drug. (D) The medication does not have a long-term impact on embryonic development.

428. (A) Nursing process phase: implementation; client need: health promotion and maintenance; content area: maternity nursing

Rationale
(A) Between 7 and 10 days' postfertilization, the blastocyst implants itself in the endometrium, causing capillaries to be broken and subsequent bleeding. (B) Uterine bleeding, uterine contractions, and pain are signs of spontaneous abortion. (C) A hormonal decrease of estrogen after ovulation may cause midcycle bleeding. (D) Blastocyst formation is the embryonic structure developed from the morula.

429. (C) Nursing process phase: evaluation; client need: health promotion and maintenance; content area: maternity nursing

Rationale
(A) Pregnancy spans 40 weeks. (B) Pregnancy is divided into three trimesters. The first trimester is from week 1 to 13; the second trimester is from week 14 to 26; the third trimester is from week 27 to term (the 38th to 42nd week). (C) The average duration from time of conception is 9 1/2 lunar months, or from the first day of the last menstrual period the average is 10 lunar months. (D) Forty weeks multiplied by seven days is 280 days.

430. (B) Nursing process phase: analysis and planning; client need: health promotion and maintenance; content area: maternity nursing

Rationale
(A–D) To calculate Naegele's rule, count back 3 months from the first day of the last menstrual period and add 7 days. 8/1–3 months = 5/1, then add 7 days = 5/8.

431. (D) Nursing process phase: implementation; client need: physiological integrity; content area: maternity nursing

Rationale

(A) Increasing the rate of oxytocin infusion will increase the likelihood of the client's hyperstimulated contractions (duration of more than 60 seconds). Repositioning the client will not affect the duration of the contraction. (B) Decreasing the rate will not provide relief quickly enough. (C) Terminating the infusion rate alone will not compensate for the inadequate oxygen supply to the placenta related to the prolonged contraction. Membranes are ruptured and presenting part is −4 station. The client is at high risk for cord prolapse if she ambulates to the bathroom. (D) Hyperstimulated, tetanic contraction can lead to abruptio placentae or uterine rupture in addition to fetal hypoxia. Administering oxygen will facilitate perfusion of the placenta and fetus.

432. (B) Nursing process phase: assessment; client need: physiological integrity; content area: maternity nursing

Rationale

(A) In early fetal hypoxia, the fetus attempts to compensate for reduced blood flow with an increase in heart rate (above 160). (B) In late profound fetal hypoxia, myocardial activity becomes depressed and lowers the heart rate. (C) Maternal fever increases the metabolism of fetal myocardium. There can be an increase up to 2 hours before the mother is febrile. (D) An increased heart rate can be the first sign of an infection.

433. (A) Nursing process phase: implementation; client need: physiological integrity; content area: maternity nursing

Rationale

(A) Early decelerations are not pathological and do not require intervention. (B) The left lateral position provides the greatest potential for placental perfusion. (C) This is a normal fetal heart pattern. No current need exists for a cesarean birth. (D) Amnioinfusion is indicated to correct umbilical cord compression when membranes are ruptured.

434. (D) Nursing process phase: evaluation; client need: physiological integrity; content area: maternity nursing

Rationale

(A) Tonic neck reflex occurs when the newborn's head is turned to the side, the infant extends the arm on the side toward which the head is turned, and flexes the opposite arm. (B) Babinski's reflex occurs in response to the lateral aspect of the sole of the foot being stroked from the heel upward and across the ball of the foot. (C) When the newborn is supine and the head is slowly turned to the side, the infant's eyes remain stationary. (D) Moro reflex is in response to any intense stimulation.

435. (A) Nursing process phase: implementation; client need: psychosocial integrity; content area: maternity nursing

Rationale

(A) Sitting next to the client conveys support and concern, the beginning components of a trusting relationship. (B) This puts the potential abuser in a power position over the victim and in control of the client's responses to the nurse's questions. (C) Alerting security is not necessary at this time

because the spouse is in the waiting area. (D) Checking her records will not convey trust or support.

436. (D) Nursing process phase: analysis and planning; client need: physiological integrity; content area: maternity nursing

Rationale

(A) The left lateral position provides the best oxygen supply to the fetus. (B) The hands-and-knees position can alleviate cord compression. (C) Semisitting permits adequate oxygenation. (D) The dorsal recumbent position decreases venous return by producing pressure from the gravid uterus on the inferior vena cava and descending aorta.

437. (B) Nursing process phase: implementation; client need: physiological integrity; content area: maternity nursing

Rationale

(A) Skipping meals puts the mother at risk for malnutrition. (B) Foods high in carbohydrates will help reduce gastric acidity, thus minimizing the nausea and vomiting. (C) Brushing teeth before eating may bring on an episode of nausea and vomiting. (D) Carbohydrates will decrease the acidity but need to be consumed closer to the actual experience of the nausea.

438. (B) Nursing process phase: evaluation; client need: physiological integrity; content area: maternity nursing

Rationale

(A) Fresh fruits are high in vitamin C and iron. (B) Bran can inhibit the absorption of iron. (C) Caffeine inhibits the absorption of iron by the body. (D) The vitamin C in the tomato slice will enhance the body's ability to absorb the iron.

439. (C) Nursing process phase: implementation; client need; physiological integrity; content area: maternity nursing

Rationale

(A) Delivery is not imminent. The client is a primipara, in transition, and the fetus is at 0 station. (B) Administering a narcotic analgesic is risky because transition could be short, then the infant would have a peak drug level in his body. (C) Women can correct their breathing patterns with encouragement. The client has signs and symptoms of hyperventilation. Hyperventilation occurs because of an oxygen and carbon dioxide imbalance from irregular breathing. Transition is a prime time for this to occur because the client is tired and in pain. (D) Capillary refill assessment will provide information about impaired circulation. The client is hyperventilating.

440. (A) Nursing process phase: assessment; client need: psychosocial integrity; content area: maternity nursing

Rationale

(A) The client is not in immediate danger. This is the less threatening approach. (B) More information is needed from the client for a comprehensive assessment to be charted. (C) If the assessment identifies an abusive relationship, social services should be contacted. (D) Being this direct is less effective. The nurse will have a better chance to develop a therapeutic relationship using a less confrontational approach.

441. (B) Nursing process phase: assessment; client need: health promotion and maintenance; content area: maternity nursing

Rationale

(A) There is no evidence that intercourse in the last 3 months causes premature birth. (B) Ruptured membranes do not provide a protective barrier for the fetus and the risk of infection to the mother and to the fetus is greater. (C) Multiple gestation only as associated with premature labor would be a contraindication. (D) Vaginal discharge is a normal occurrence in pregnancy. Vaginal bleeding is an indication to abstain.

442. (A) Nursing process phase: analysis and planning; client need: physiological integrity; content area: maternity nursing

Rationale

(A) The nursing priority is to prevent infections. Most often the newborn of an HIV-positive mother will be asymptomatic in the hospital. (B) The nursing goal would be more specifically to gain weight at a steady rate. (C) There is nothing in the history that indicates a traumatic birth. (D) Promoting comfort is a goal suitable for an infant undergoing a surgical procedure, not at discharge.

443. (B) Nursing process phase: evaluation; client need: health promotion and maintenance; content area: maternity nursing

Rationale

(A) This action helps to prevent rectal bacteria from reaching the vagina. (B) Sitting in soapy bath water can irritate the uretha and increase exposure to infection. (C) Natural fabrics are more absorbent and less irritating. (D) Emptying the bladder after intercourse flushes out bacteria introduced via intercourse.

444. (B) Nursing process phase: evaluation; client need: psychosocial integrity; content area: maternity nursing

Rationale

(A) The fetus receives maternal antibodies between 38 and 40 weeks' gestation. (B) Fetal movements are felt by the mother at this time. (C) At 28 weeks, breathing motions are detected in the fetus. (D) Eyes open and close at 28 weeks.

445. (D) Nursing process phase: assessment; client need: physiological integrity; content area: maternity nursing

Rationale

(A) Increased flatulence is associated with second trimester increase in uterine size and decreased intestinal motility. (B) Backache is most common in the third trimester as the gravid uterus strains low back muscles. (C) Diastasis recti is associated with the third trimester. As the abdominal girth increases, the abdominal musculature separates. (D) Nasal stuffiness is a result of increased estrogen levels associated with the first trimester.

446. (A) Nursing process phase: evaluation; client need: health promotion and maintenance; content area: maternity nursing

Rationale

(A) The client has declared that cesarean birth is indicated due to small pelvis size. This comment needs clarification to ascertain understanding. (B) Risk for preterm labor does increase with age. (C) The afternoon is a warmer time of day with greater incidence of fluid loss during exercise. (D) Seeing the dentist during pregnancy is not contraindicated. Dental care is recommended without x-ray exposure.

447. (C) Nursing process phase: implementation; client need: psychosocial integrity; content area: maternity nursing

Rationale

(A) This is not a therapeutic response because it minimizes the client's feelings. (B) This response puts off the discussion of the client's immediate concern. (C) This is the best response because it opens the opportunity for exchange. (D) This response in not supportive and minimizes the client's concern.

448. (A) Nursing process phase: implementation; client need: physiological integrity; content area: maternity nursing

Rationale

(A) Uterine contractions are most efficient when the mother is upright and free to move. (B) The membranes are intact with the presenting part at zero station. There is no risk of cord prolapse. (C) Efficient uterine contractions facilitate the progress of labor. (D) Position changes have no effect on lack of bladder functioning.

449. (B) Nursing process phase: implementation; client need: psychosocial integrity; content area: maternity nursing

Rationale

(A) The client's feet are warm. This shows correct catheter placement. (B) The emotional needs are still present although discomfort may be absent. (C) Repositioning the client to a supine position will increase her risk of maternal hypotension. (D) Frequent vaginal exams are contraindicated due to increased infection rate after membranes have ruptured.

450. (D) Nursing process phase: implementation; client need: health promotion and maintenance; content area: maternity nursing

Rationale

(A) The infant should nurse at both breasts at each feeding to ensure continued levels of milk production. (B) Breastfed newborns nurse more often, about every 2 to 3 hours. This frequency is due to the more rapid digestion of breast milk. (C) It is difficult to compare milk ingestion because it is not available in a calibrated container for measure. (D) The intake and output will be comparable. Six to ten wet diapers per day is an indication of adequate hydration.

451. (B) Nursing process phase: evaluation; client need: health promotion and maintenance; content area: maternity nursing

Rationale

(A) Gradually increasing the number of supplemental bottles gradually slows milk production and lessens the intensity of breast engorgement. (B) Supplemental foods should be added to the baby's diet after 6 months of age. Supplements are started at this time to avoid food allergies, and the baby's ability to digest the foods is more mature. (C) During the weaning process, it is often less confusing to the infant to have someone else other than the mother give the bottle. The infant associates the mother with breastfeeding and may refuse to take the bottle. (D) It will be necessary for her to pump her breasts at work to prevent engorgement and to maintain milk production.

452. (B) Nursing process phase: implementation; client need: physiological integrity; content area: maternity nursing

Rationale

(A) The incidence of headache occurs after delivery. Treatment includes having the client lie flat, IV fluids, and, in severe cases, a blood patch over the epidural site. (B) Increased circulation fluid volume helps to prevent low blood pressure associated with regional anesthesia. (C) The IV infusion does maintain hydration; however, the bolus is intended to increase the volume of circulating fluid to prevent maternal hypotension as a result of the epidural. (D) The treatment for pruritus is IV administration of naloxone, which reverses the narcotic effect when an epidural narcotic is used.

453. (A) Nursing process phase: assessment; client need: physiological integrity; content area: maternal nursing

Rationale

(A) In a posterior presentation, the fetal head produces pressure against the lower maternal spine, causing low back discomfort. (B) Because the low back pain is persistent between contractions as well as during, it is indicative of posterior presentation as opposed to transitional labor discomfort. (C) Lower to mid-back pain is associated with urinary tact infections. Fever, pain on urination, and cloudy or blood-tinged urine also would be noted. (D) If the fetus is occiput posterior, lateral Sims' position encourages anterior rotation.

454. (D) Nursing process phase: implementation; client need: physiological integrity; content area; maternity nursing

Rationale

(A) This would be false reassurance. It is impossible to determine when an active mechanism will initiate and the subsequent birth will occur. (B) Additional assessment of the powers, passenger, passageway, and psyche need to be completed. (C) Discouraging maternal movement or mobility may in fact be contributing to ineffective contractions. (D) Walking has been shown to shorten the length of labor because it promotes the application of the presenting part against the cervix. It also encourages fetal descent into the birth canal.

455. (C) Nursing process phase: assessment; client need: physiological integrity; content area: maternity nursing

Rationale

(A) With prolonged rupture of membranes, there is an increased risk of infection. Pathogens from the vagina can be ascend into the amniotic sac. (B) After 42 weeks' gestation, the placenta will often start deteriorating in metabolic exchange, placing the fetus at risk. (C) With placenta previa there is increased risk of hemorrhage. If the mother were allowed to go into labor, the dilating cervix would decrease the amount of surface area of oxygen supply to the fetus. The placenta also blocks the cervical outlet. (D) With rapid deliveries, maternal and fetal complications such as uterine rupture and fetal hypoxia can occur.

456. (D) Nursing process phase: assessment; client need: physiological integrity; content area: maternity nursing

Rationale

(A) The fundus descends about 1 to 2 cm every 24 hours. One centimeter above the umbilicus is a finding consistent immediately after delivery. (B) One centimeter below is consistent with the first postpartal day. (C) Four centimeters below is equivalent to the fourth postpartal day. (D) Three centimeters below the umbilicus is consistent with the third day after delivery.

457. (B) Nursing process phase: implementation; client need: health promotion and maintenance; content area: maternity nursing

Rationale

(A) Because the mechanism described is related to the reversal of water metabolism, breastfeeding will not influence the physiological adjustment. (B) Diaphoresis is a method to reduce the acquired fluids maintained during pregnancy. (C) The large amount of urinary output and perspiration facilitates a large amount of initial weight loss in the puerperium. This compensatory mechanism is not related to an inflammation of the urinary tract. (D) A significant volume of urinary output may begin as soon as 12 hours after birth. In 2 to 3 days, night sweats develop to assist the body in eliminating the excess fluid. This is a normal process not associated with infection.

458. (C) Nursing process phase: assessment; client need: physiological integrity; content area: maternity nursing

Rationale

(A) The mucus plug is released in early labor. The plug is the same color and consistency as any other mucous membrane secretion. (B) The amniotic sac is a thin, transparent membrane. (C) The *Candida albicans* fungus produces a thick, white vaginal discharge. (D) The *Trichomonas vaginalis* protozoan yields a gray or yellow-green discharge.

459. (A) Nursing process phase: analysis and planning; client need: physiological integrity; content area: maternity nursing

Rationale

(A) The presence of a second-degree laceration extends through the perineal body and the transverse perineal muscle. The amount of tissue trauma produces significant discomfort. (B) Presence of a second-degree laceration does not increase the usual risk for infection. (C) Although urinary elimination may be affected by the tissue trauma associated with birth, the physiological need for comfort is greatest at this time. (D) Fear of further trauma to the episiotomy site may interfere with defecation. However, at this time bowel evacuation is not a priority.

460. (B) Nursing process phase: implementation; client need: physiological integrity; content area: maternity nursing

Rationale

(A) Temperature is below normal; there is no current indication of dehydration. (B) A relaxed uterus can fill with blood and clots. It must be palpated at regular intervals to verify that it is firm and not filling with blood. Because of the risk of hemorrhage, this is the priority. (C) The assessment data do not reflect a full bladder. (D) The data assessment does not reflect bleeding from any source other than the uterus.

461. (B) Nursing process phase: implementation; client need: physiological integrity; content area: maternity nursing

Rationale

(A) A vaginal delivery is not imminent. The client is 6 cm dilated. (B) The presenting part is pressing on the cord, which will decrease the amount of oxygen to the fetus. Pressing against the presenting part relieves the cord compression. (C) Placing the client in reverse Trendelenburg increases the pressure on the cord. (D) This will likely increase the severity of cord compression.

462. (B) Nursing process phase: analysis and planning; client need: physiological integrity; content area: maternity nursing

Rationale

(A) Energy levels are high after delivery because of increased adrenalin output related to the expulsive effort and anticipation of the baby. Encouraging the client to relax would be considered an unnecessary distraction. (B) The client should be encouraged to hold, touch, and examine her newborn. This is the highest priority because the client has verbalized a concern about the sex of her child. (C) The client is presently at low risk for discomfort. (D) Discharge teaching can be started once the patient is transferred to recovery.

463. (C) Nursing process phase: implementation; client need: physiological integrity; content area: maternity nursing

Rationale

(A) Massaging the lower leg is contraindicated because massaging could dislodge a blood clot. (B) Bedrest is indicated to prevent the clot from dislodging and causing pulmonary embolism. (C) A positive Homans' sign is pain in the calf when the foot is dorsiflexed. (D) Warmth is indicated because it increases blood flow to the area.

464. (C) Nursing process phase: analysis and planning; client need: physiological integrity; content area: maternity nursing

Rationale

(A) Bedrest is shown to minimize overstimulation that might precipitate a seizure. (B) Bladder fullness is not conclusive in the data assessment. (C) In severe pregnancy-induced hypertension, extensive kidney involvement impacts on renal functioning. Insertion of an indwelling catheter provides a mechanism to monitor renal functioning via output measurement. (D) Bladder catheterization actually promotes bladder atony.

465. (D) Nursing process phase: assessment; client need: physiological integrity; content area: maternity nursing

Rationale

(A) Complete placenta previa presents with painless, bright red vaginal bleeding. (B) Pregnancy-induced hypertension is a multisystem disorder often characterized by hypertension, proteinuria, and generalized edema. (C) HELLP syndrome exists when there is hemolysis of red blood cells, elevated liver enzymes, and a low platelet count. (D) Abruptio placentae exhibits with severe tenderness of the abdominal area, board-like abdomen, and vaginal bleeding.

466. (D) Nursing process phase: evaluation; client need: psychosocial integrity; content area: maternity nursing

Rationale

(A) Pregnancy-induced hypertension is not controlled by diet. This may be an indication of denial. (B) Being separated from family is most often perceived as stressful. The client is withdrawing. (C) This statement is not self-focused; the client is not discussing her feelings. (D) Women with illness in pregnancy are often hesitant to discuss their feelings. Often they feel powerless.

467. (C) Nursing process phase: analysis and planning; client need: psychosocial integrity; content area: maternity nursing

Rationale

(A) Leaving the client alone does not demonstrate caring and it discourages the discussion of her feelings, thus increasing her anxiety. (B) An announcement of need for an emergency cesarean section is a high-stress time. During high stress, it is extremely difficult to assimilate information. It is best to keep information simple and direct. (C) Describing cesarean birth as an alternative birth option helps to "normalize" the experience, thereby lowering anxiety levels. (D) No birth outcomes can be assured.

468. (B) Nursing process phase: analysis and planning; client need: physiological integrity; content area: maternity nursing.

Rationale

(A) Hydralazine is the drug of choice for patients close to delivery. Given in moderate to large does, it can interfere with placenta perfusion because maternal blood pressure drops. (B) Magnesium sulfate is an anticonvulsant that depresses the CNS. It prevents seizures by blocking the release of acetylcholine at the myoneural junction. Magnesium sulfate can also produce a transient drop in maternal blood pressure because it reduces muscle excitability. (C) IV labetalol, a beta blocker, lowers maternal blood pressure without maternal heart rate increases. (D) Diazoxide is vasodilator that causes a quick drop in blood pressure. Side effects include reduction of placental perfusion, sodium and water retention, and maternal-fetal hyperglycema.

469. (D) Nursing process phase: evaluation; client need: health promotion and maintenance; content area: maternity nursing

Rationale

(A) Breastfeeding is often initiated in the delivery room. (B) Colostrum is the first fluid secreted by the breasts until the milk comes in. (C) The more the baby nurses, the greater the milk produced. (D) Witch's milk is the fluid secreted by the breast in the newborn related to exposure to maternal hormones.

470. (C) Nursing process phase: implementation; client need: physiological integrity; content area: maternity nursing

Rationale

(A) Medical asepsis should be used with every peri-pad change after elimination and as saturated. (B) Ice packs are indicated in the first 24 hours. (C) Heat will increase circulation and subsequent healing and comfort. (D) Tampons are containdicated for after-delivery use because of the increased risk of toxic shock syndrome.

471. (C) Nursing process phase: assessment; client need: physiological integrity; content area: maternity nursing

Rationale

(A) Lochia rubra should be evidenced in lesser amounts and without clots after 1 week. (B) Endometritis is an infection of the uterine lining associated with fever and delayed involution of the uterus. (C) A return to bright red bleeding with clots is not within normal limits. Postpartum hemorrhage is indicated. (D) Delayed healing of the episiotomy would be evidenced with lack of wound approximation, redness, edema, and pain.

472. (A) Nursing process phase: evaluation; client need: health promotion and maintenance; content area: maternity nursing

Rationale

(A) In the healthy expectant mother, there is no risk of rupture of membranes due to intercourse. (B) Orgasmic contractions have not been found harmful to the fetus. (C) There is an increased risk of maternal-fetal infection once membranes rupture. (D) Often there is an increased interest in lovemaking as the expectant mother enters the second trimester. In the second trimester, the physical discomforts are somewhat lessened.

473. (B) Nursing process phase: assessment; client need: health promotion and maintenance; content area: maternity nursing

Rationale

(A) In true labor, contractions will continue even when there is a change of activity. (B) In false labor, particularly with a decrease of activity, the contractions will diminish. (C) In true labor, although a regular, textbook picture of labor may exist, the contractions will increase in strength. (D) The true labor contraction is wavelike. Braxton-Hicks contractions are felt in the back or upper abdomen.

474. (B) Nursing process phase: analysis and planning; client need: physiological integrity; content area: maternity nursing

Rationale

(A) Although traditional use of corticosteroids is to reduce inflammation, in this case it is to promote fetal lung maturity. (B) The glucocorticosteroids enhance the production of fetal pulmonary surfactant. (C) The glucocorticosteroids do not increase placental perfusion. (D) Hypertension is a side effect of glucocorticoid administration.

475. (C) Nursing process phase: assessment; client need: physiological integrity; content area: maternity nursing

Rationale

(A) The increased energy requirements of labor do not yield stabilized blood sugar levels. (B) The diabetic client's blood sugar levels do not increase during labor. (C) In labor, energy requirements increase. This need will deplete blood sugar levels. (D) Ketoacidosis occurs with elevated glucose and ketones.

476 (C) Nursing process phase: assessment; client need: physiological integrity; content area: maternity nursing

Rationale

(A) A toxic response to the anesthetic could range from palpitations to cardiac and respiratory arrest. (B) Cerebral edema is manifested by confusion and seizures. (C) After the birth of the infant, there is a sudden release of pressure on the pelvic nerves that may produce involuntary trembling. (D) Injection of anesthesia into a blood vessel is evidenced by convulsions and/or cardiac arrest.

477. (B) Nursing process phase: assessment; client need: physiological integrity; content area: maternity nursing

Rationale

(A) This is a low hemoglobin value (normal = 12–16 gm/dl). In HELLP syndrome, there is hemolysis of red blood cells, causing anemia. (B) This is a normal hematocrit value. In HELLP syndrome, the hematocrit is also a lower value due to hemolysis of red blood cells. (C) LDH (lactic dehydrogenase) is elevated in HELLP syndrome because of liver damage due to the deposition of fibrin within liver tissue. (D) A value less than $100,000/mm^3$ is indicative of HELLP syndrome. The low value is related to platelets adhering to collagen that is released from the vasospasm of blood vessels.

478. (C) Nursing process phase: analysis and planning; client need: psychosocial integrity; content area: maternity nursing

Rationale

(A) This goal is not specific or immediate. (B) This goal imposes an unrealistic expectation. (C) Verbalizing feelings is the most therapeutic and immediate goal. It must occur before any other goal can even be addressed. (D) Identifying contributing factors is not specific to the current situation.

479. (B) Nursing process phase: analysis and planning; client need: physiological integrity; content area: maternity nursing

Rationale

(A) It is apparent that the uncontrolled shaking does not foster a sense of well-being. (B) Chills or postdelivery shaking is a common occurrence. It is related to the sudden release of pressure on the pelvic nerves. Warm blankets promote comfort via relaxation of muscles. (C) Administering medication is a collaborative intervention. Assessment for pain should occur prior to administration of an analgesic. (D) Administering medication is a collaborative intervention. Diazepam may cause drowsiness that would interfere with the client processing the birth events.

480. (D) Nursing process phase: assessment; client need: physiological integrity; content area: maternity nursing

Rationale

(A) Spontaneous bruising is not related to magnesium sulfate administration. It is related to the destruction of red blood cells associated with pregnancy-induced hypertension. (B) The warm sensation is a result of the peripheral action of flushing and sweating. (C) Hourly urinary output is required to closely monitor renal functioning. Diminished urinary output (output of a minimum of 30 cc/hr is required) can result in an accumulation of magnesium sulfate in toxic levels. (D) Reduced deep tendon reflexes imply toxic levels of $MgSO_4$. This is often a first sign of toxicity. $MgSO_4$ is a central nervous system depressant.

481. (B) Nursing process phase: assessment; client need: physiological integrity; content area: maternity nursing

Rationale

(A) Walking during contractions is associated with first-stage labor, early to active. (B) Expressing a desire to hold and see the infant is evidenced with the second stage, the expulsive stage of labor. (C) Feeling unable to cope with contractions is associated with active labor, first stage. (D) Inability to concentrate and irritability is associated with transition, late first stage.

482. (B) Nursing process phase: analysis and planning; client need: safe, effective care environment; content area: maternity nursing

Rationale

(A–D) Gravidity—the number of times the uterus has been pregnant; T—the number of term births; P—the number of preterm births; A—the number of abortions; L—the number of living children. The client has been pregnant four times, so G = 4. The client has had 0 term births, so T = 0. The client has had one preterm birth, so P = 1. The client has had two spontaneous abortions, so A = 2. The client has one living child, so L = 1.

483. **(C)** Nursing process phase: analysis and planning; client need: health promotion and maintenance; content area: maternity nursing

Rationale

(A) The birth plan is generated from the expectant mother's or parents' perspective, not what the health-care team regiments. (B) The birth plan is a flexible tool to facilitate communication of desired outcomes between the expectant mother or parents and the health-care provider. (C) The birth plan facilitates the identification of labor and birth priorities for the couple or mother whereby she can begin dialoguing those ideas to the health-care provider. (D) A formalized birth plan does not have to be developed for parents to have input, but it is one way to clarify expectations.

484. **(B)** Nursing process phase: assessment; client need: physiological integrity; content area: maternity nursing

Rationale

(A) The uterine height at the level of the symphysis pubis is indicative of a pregnancy of about 10 weeks. (B) The uterine height at the level of the umbilicus is comparable to 20 weeks' gestation. (C) The uterine height that reaches the xiphoid process is indicative of 36 weeks' gestation. (D) The anatomical position of the uterus is above the level of the ischial spines.

485. **(A)** Nursing process phase: assessment; client need: physiological integrity; content area: maternity nursing

Rationale

(A) This is the bluish color of the cervix noted on visual inspection. (B) Goodell's sign is cervical softening that is palpated. (C) McDonald's sign is flexion of the fundus on the cervix, also palpated. (D) Piskacek's sign is palpated as a soft lateral bulge.

486. **(B)** Nursing process phase: assessment; client need: psychosocial integrity; content area: maternity nursing

Rationale

(A) An aversion to certain foods is related to changes in taste. (B) Requesting to baby-sit allows the expectant mother the opportunity to try out the maternal role. This is one component of the socialization process of role acquisition as specified by Rubin. (C) Wearing regular clothes is thought to delay maternal role acquisition. (D) Delay in reporting the news indicates a reluctance to acknowledge that the pregnancy exists, thereby delaying maternal role acquisition.

487. **(A)** Nursing process phase: implementation; client need: health promotion and maintenance; content area: maternity nursing

Rationale

(A) During the first trimester, the primary concerns of expectant parents relate to physical and emotional changes of pregnancy. These are the changes that they are presently experiencing. (B) Distinguishing true labor from false labor is a topic most relevant to a late pregnancy class. (C) The menstrual cycle would be best covered in a prepregnancy class. (D) Labor variations are more suitable for a late pregnancy class.

488. **(C)** Nursing process phase: assessment; client need: physiological integrity; content area: maternity nursing

Rationale

(A) The client's intake of water and sodium is not the most important assessment because she is already edematous. (B) Diuretics are not indicated because they further increase dehydration by decreasing intravascular volume and placenta perfusion. (C) Cerebral edema can lead to seizures and threaten the lives of both the mother and her fetus. (D) Urinary output is an indicator of circulating blood volume, but the priority is assessing the more life-threatening symptoms.

489. **(D)** Nursing process phase: implementation; client need: health promotion and maintenance; content area: maternity nursing

Rationale

(A) Vaginal delivery is only contraindicated within two consecutive positive HSV-II cultures close to time of delivery. (B) Herpes infections seems to be more severe in pregnant women. (C) Herpes transmission occurs by having close contact with another infected person. (D) The route of transmission is from mother to infant via an actively infected birth canal. If the cultures are not active, she should deliver vaginally.

490. **(D)** Nursing process phase: evaluation; client need: health promotion and maintenance; content area: maternity nursing

Rationale

(A) Contractions 60 seconds long, 3 to 5 minutes apart for 1 hour indicate that a good mechanism of labor is in place. (B) Giving her permission to call with any questions will lower her anxiety about being at home. (C) A warm shower is relaxing and appropriate for anyone in labor. (D) Loss of the mucous plug is associated with early effacement. That in itself does not necessitate a rush to the hospital.

491. **(C)** Nursing process phase: analysis and planning; client need: psychosocial integrity; content area: maternity nursing

Rationale

(A) Promoting maternal well-being is a nursing priority, not an intervention. (B) Describing the perioperative procedure is related to knowledge deficit. (C) The client may have distorted ideas about cesarean birth that will increase anxiety. (D) This promotes comfort, does not decrease anxiety.

492. **(B)** Nursing process phase: implementation; client need: health promotion and maintenance; content area: maternity nursing

Rationale

(A) Although the fetus may move down into the pelvis, there is still an expectation of regular fetal movement. (B) Placental insufficiency can be detected by a reduction in fetal movement. (C) This is nontherapeutic communication. It implies that the mother may be concealing information. (D) Answering a question with a question does not give the client factual information.

493. **(A)** Nursing process phase: evaluation; client need: health promotion and maintenance; content area: maternity nursing

Rationale
(A) Taking vitamins alone does not ensure a well-balanced diet. (B) Dark green leafy vegetables and red meats do have higher iron content. (C) Fresh fruits and vegetables are higher in vitamin content. (D) Bran inhibits the absorption of an iron supplement.

494. **(D)** Nursing process phase: implementation, client need: psychological integrity; content area: maternity nursing

Rationale
(A) Difficulty sleeping is associated with the third trimester. Because alcohol is a teratogenic substance, it is contraindicated in pregnancy. (B) This is confrontational and is a non-therapeutic response. (C) Ordinarily this is a good suggestion, but the expectant mother has expressed a concern that is not being addressed in this response. (D) This therapeutic response demonstrates a positive, supportive attitude toward the client without minimizing the problem.

495. **(B)** Nursing process phase: assessment; client need: physiological integrity; content area: maternity nursing

Rationale
(A) Membranes are often ruptured to facilitate labor progression. However, labor is progressing at a satisfactory rate of 1 cm/hr. (B) A prolapsed cord results when the presenting part is high in the pelvis (−3 station) and the membranes are ruptured. (C) The client is not completely dilated, and rupturing the membranes will not immediately bring her to 10 cm, necessary for a vaginal delivery. (D) Amniotic fluid emboli occurs most often after a rapid, difficult labor. A small tear is present in the amnion or the chorion that permits amniotic fluid into maternal circulation.

496. **(A)** Nursing process phase: implementation; client need: physiological integrity; content area: maternity nursing

Rationale
(A) No single position is best for all of labor. Walking utilizes gravity and provides an outlet for anxious energy. (B) The client's fetus is in vertex position, and the head is engaged at 0 station. She is not at risk for cord prolapse. She should be permitted to walk if she desires. (C) Bathing is contraindicated with ruptured membranes because of the risk of contamination since the barrier of protection is absent. (D) The client is coping and relaxing well between contractions. An epidural is not indicated at this time.

497. **(C)** Nursing process phase: evaluation; client need: physiological integrity; content area: maternity nursing

Rationale
(A) Transverse arrest is more common with an android pelvis. The narrow pelvic arch inhibits rotation. (B) Inlet delay is associated with the platypelloid pelvis. (C) The gynecoid pelvis yields a wide pubic arch, leading to spontaneous deliveries with productive uterine contractions. (D) The fetal head is more often posterior with the pelvis classification of android and anthropoid.

498. **(D)** Nursing process phase: evaluation; client need: physiological integrity; content area: maternity nursing

Rationale
(A) A vaginal examination would be indicated if dilation and/or effacement were suspected. (B) The current field intake has not been assessed. The urinary frequency and constipation are related to the increased pressure from the weight of the fetus. (C) The discomforts she is experiencing are related to the fetus moving further into the uterus. (D) Lightening is a subjective experience felt by the pregnant client toward the end of pregnancy. The cervix is taken up, and the isthmus becomes part of the lower uterine segment. The fetus assumes this space because there is more space in the lower uterus.

499. **(A)** Nursing process phase: assessment; client need: physiological integrity; content area: maternity nursing

Rationale
(A) Engagement occurs as the largest diameter of the presenting part passes through the inlet. In most clients it is determined when the presenting part is at, or nearly at, the level of the ischial spines. (B) Lightening is a subjective sensation felt by the expectant mother. It is not synonymous with engagement. (C) Floating describes the presenting part as being out of the pelvis and freely movable. (D) Dipping defines the presenting part as having passed through the plane of the inlet, but without engagement.

500. **(C)** Nursing process phase: evaluation; client need: physiological integrity; content area: maternity nursing

Rationale
(A) Dysfunctional labor is more often associated with a high station. The presenting part is not directly impacting the cervix for dilation and effacement. (B) Rapid descent of the fetal head is not usually associated with an abnormal or dangerous labor. (C) Lesser degrees of cervical dilations are associated with high stations, because there is less direct impact on the cervix to dilate and efface. (D) The incidence of pelvic disproportion is greater when the station is high at the onset of labor.

501. **(C)** Nursing process phase: evaluation; client need: health maintenance and promotion; content: maternity nursing

Rationale
(A) Petroleum-based products can weaken the rubber construction of the diaphragm. (B) A lower frequency of PID is found among women who use diaphragms and spermicide. (C) A decreased incidence of vaginitis, cervicitis, PID, and cervical intrapithelial neoplasia is found in women who use spermicide with the diaphragm. (D) The diaphragm must be left in place for at least 6 hours after the last intercourse. It takes 6 hours for the spermicide to kill the sperm.

502. **(D)** Nursing process phase: evaluation; client need: health promotion and maintenance; content area: maternity nursing

Rationale
(A) The ovaries are a major site of estrogen production. (B) The fallopian tubes provide a passageway for the ovum. The cilia and peristalsis propel the fertilized egg along the tube. (C) When a sperm penetrates the outer membranes of the egg, both become enclosed within the membrane. The ovum is then closed to other sperm. (D) The testes are homologous to the ovaries in the female. The clitoris is comparable to the male glans.

503. (C) Nursing process phase: implementation; client need: physiological integrity; content area: maternity nursing

Rationale

(A) The client will be well awake to begin the expulsive phase of labor. This intervention is suited for transition. (B) In the second stage, the client is completely effaced and dilated. (C) This is the stage of labor for the client to bear down. (D) The bladder status should have been previously determined.

504. (B) Nursing process phase: implementation; client need; physiological integrity; content area: maternity nursing

Rationale

(A) Jaundice and fever would be indicated for observation in the Rh-positive newborn of a Rh-negative mother. (B) 300 μg of Rh immunoglobulin IM is indicated for the client who has aborted after 8 weeks. (C) Rh immunoglobulin is *only* administered to the female client, not to the infant nor the father of the baby. (D) This treatment is a prophylactic approach to prevent antibody development. If one waits until the antibodies have developed, then subsequent pregnancies are at even greater risk.

505. (A) Nursing process phase: implementation; client need: health promotion and maintenance; content area: maternity nursing

Rationale

(A) Most inborn errors of metabolism are related to autosomal recessive inherited disorders. (B) An example of an autosomal dominant disorder is achondroplasia. (C) This order occurs in both males and females. An example is vitamin D–resistant rickets. (D) This disorder classification results from both genetic and environmental factors. They include neural tube defects.

506. (B) Nursing process phase: implementation; client need: health promotion and maintenance; content area: maternity nursing

Rationale

(A) A benefit of exercise is a heightened sense of well-being, but this is not the specific reason for exercising the pelvic floor postpartum. (B) The pelvic floor exercise is done to re-educate, to tone, and to strengthen the muscles that have been stretched during delivery. (C) Another benefit of exercise is increased peristalsis. This is not the specific rationale. Walking would be a better exercise choice for this purpose. (D) Lochia formation and flow are independent of the pelvis floor.

507. (C) Nursing process phase: implementation; client need: health promotion and maintenance; content area: maternity nursing

Rationale

(A) Suppressing urinary frequency is an unhealthy urination practice because it allows greater time for bacteria to increase in the bladder. (B) Because bacteria can be introduced during intercourse, fluid should be encouraged prior to intercourse to promote additional urination. (C) Emptying the bladder prior to a night's sleep lessons the amount of urine held in the bladder for a long time period. (D) Holding urine for longer time periods increases both discomfort and the client's risk for developing a urinary tract infection.

508. (D) Nursing process phase; evaluation; client need: physiological integrity; content area: maternity nursing

Rationale

(A) The suggested fluid intake of noncaffeinated fluids should be 2 to 3 quarts. (B) Wearing cotton panties increases moisture absorption in the genital area, but this alone is not a conclusive outcome. (C) Bathing every day will increase client comfort, but sitting in sudsy water can increased irritation of the urethra and allow bacteria to be vaginally introduced. (D) The absence of urinary tract infection in the client is the most definitive measure that the nurse's teaching was effective.

509. (B) Nursing process phase: analysis; client need: physiological integrity; content area: maternity nursing

Rationale

(A) Impaired gas exchange is related to alveolar-capillary changes or reduced capacity of the blood to carry oxygen. (B) High risk for injury is related to median nerve compression from changes in surrounding tissue. (C) Alterations in cardiac output are related to signs of PIH and pathological edema. (D) Activity intolerance is related to uterine irritability.

510. (D) Nursing process phase: assessment; client need: psycholosocial integrity; content area: maternity nursing

Rationale

(A) A positive interaction would be for the mother to refer to the infant by her name. This response indicates ambivalence. (B) The positive response would be for the mother to breastfeed her infant at this time. (C) The maternal process of becoming acquainted with the newborn is related to the mother holding, inspecting, and attaching to the infant herself. (D) This is an example of synchrony, a mutually rewarding activity.

511. (D) Nursing process phase: assessment; client need: psychosocial integrity; content: maternity nursing

Rationale

(A) A sleepy, closed-eye infant will not be able to establish eye-to-eye contact or track her parent's face. (B) The facilitating behavior of the infant would be that of clinging to the parent. (C) An infant with an unpredictable sleep-wake pattern is considered to exhibit an inhibiting behavior. (D) The infant who displays differentiated crying is better able to communicate his varying needs to his parents.

512. (A) Nursing process phase: assessment; client need: physiological integrity; content area: maternity nursing

Rationale

(A) Oxytocin is released as the infant nurses at the breast, causing uterine involution and subsequent noticeable abdominal cramping in the multigravida. (B) Transferring the baby to the nursery would probably cause the mother greater concern. (C) The process described by the client is one of normal limits. (D) The client has not requested pain management via medication.

513. (C) Nursing process phase: evaluation; client need: health promotion and maintenance; content area: maternity nursing

Rationale

(A) The colostrum produced by the mother will provide adequate nutritional and fluid intake until the milk comes in.

(B) The breasts should be cleansed with water only, because soap will dry the nipples. (C) Sore nipples can be prevented by positioning the infant such that there is less pulling on the nipple itself. (D) Breastfeeding mothers use the fat stored in their bodies during pregnancy.

514. (D) Nursing process phase: assessment; client need: physiological integrity; content area: maternity nursing

Rationale
(A) A blood loss of 300 to 400 cc is tolerated without consequence because of the hypervolemia acquired during pregnancy. (B) Aggressive attempts to deliver the placenta will be initiated if the placenta does not spontaneously deliver 30 minutes after the infant. Anything longer than 30 minutes increases the maternal risk for hemorrhage and infection. (C) Hypertension and headache may be related to PIH but are symptomatic of hypovolemia. (D) An increased heart rate and low blood pressure are classic indicators of hypovolemia secondary to hemophage.

515. (B) Nursing process phase: assessment; client need: physiological integrity; content area: maternity nursing

Rationale
(A) Rubra with clots is indicative of the first postpartum day. (B) Serosa is indicative of postpartum day 3. (C) Alba would be expected to occur after day 7. (D) The flow of lochia continues between 3 to 6 weeks.

516. (D) Nursing process phase: assessment; client need: physiological integrity; content area: maternity nursing

Rationale
(A) Ambulating her to the bathroom will facilitate emptying the bladder, but it does not guarantee the results of adequate elimination. (B) Ascertaining the fullness of the bladder does not ensure adequacy in emptying. (C) Catheterizing the bladder will give the nurse a measurable output, but it is a premature, perhaps unnecessary intervention at this point. (D) Measuring the first three voids for a volume of 150 cc at each void will ascertain an adequate emptying of the bladder.

517. (C) Nursing process phase: implementation; client need: health promotion and maintenance; content area: maternity nursing

Rationale
(A) The infant's most alert period is immediately after delivery. This is an opportune time to attempt to breastfeed. (B) The client's milk has not yet come in. There is no need to express colostrum for bottle feeding this time. (C) This is an excellent time to encourage the mother to breastfeed. She is motivated because she expressed a desire. The infant is alert. Breastfeeding will facilitate uterine involution and prevent bleeding. (D) The mother will not experience a let-down reflex until her milk comes in, 3 to 5 days after delivery.

518. (A) Nursing process phase: implementation; client need: health promotion and maintenance; content area: maternity nursing

Rationale
(A) Washing the perineum with water and mild soap will increase comfort and enhance healing. (B) It is a safe practice to use soap and water on the perineum. (C) Using tampons is not recommended, because of the increased risk of toxic shock syndrome and discomfort. (D) Perineal pads should be changed after each void or defecation or at least four times a day.

519. (C) Nursing process phase: implementation; client need: physiological integrity; content area: maternity nursing

Rationale
(A) Although cleaning will remove any contaminants present, it does not give the nurse additional data needed about the client's condition. (B) The amount of lochia is not conclusive information alone. (C) Delayed uterine involution is associated with infection. (D) Perineal care instruction may be redundant and unnecessary.

520. (B) Nursing process phase: analysis and planning; client need: physiological integrity; content area: maternity nursing

Rationale
(A) A puerperal infection such as endometritis would present with a fever of at least 100.4°F for 2 consecutive days, excluding the first 24 hours. (B) Persistent fever that does not respond to antibiotic treatment may indicate pelvic thrombophlebitis. (C) The three main clinical symptoms of toxic shock syndrome are fever of abrupt onset, hypotension, and diffuse rash. (D) Chorioamnionitis is related to prolonged rupture of membranes.

521. (A) Nursing process phase: implementation; client need: physiological integrity; content: maternity nursing

Rationale
(A) The upright, semi-Fowler's position will enhance the flow of lochia and uterine drainage. (B) A lateral position increases the client's comfort, but not drainage. (C) Vaginal irrigations increase the risk for infection after delivery. (D) The contractibility of the uterus will not enhance the drainage.

522. (B) Nursing process phase: evaluation; client need: physiological integrity; content area: maternity nursing

Rationale
(A) Antibiotic therapy should not be routinely administered without indication because of the elimination of the normal flora protecting the body from more harmful substances. (B) Good prenatal nutrition prevents anemia and subsequent hemorrhage. (C) Adequate prenatal fluid intake is not a priority for infection prevention in the postpartum period. (D) Ultrasounding the prenatal uterus is not an aid to detecting postnatal infections.

523. (A) Nursing process phase: implementation; client need: health promotion and maintenance; content area: maternity nursing

Rationale
(A) Whenever an oral contraceptive is missed, it should be taken as soon as it is remembered to sustain the hormonal level and prevent pregnancy. (B) A condom or an alternative form of contraception should be used if a pill is missed. However, the missed pill should be taken as soon as it is remembered. (C) It is not necessary to restart the cycle. (D) The best action is to take the missed dose and take the next single dose at the regularly scheduled time.

524. (B) Nursing process phase: evaluation; client need: health promotion and maintenance; content area: maternity nursing

Rationale
(A) There is an increased risk for cardiovascular problems after age 35 and in women who smoke. (B) Oral contraceptives are contraindicated in women with liver damage. There is sufficient concern about the relationship between liver cancer and oral contraceptives to advise against the use. (C) Shortness of breath and chest pain are early warning signs for the pill and should be reported immediately to the health-care professional. (D) One of the benefits of taking oral contraceptives is that they can lessen the cramping associated with the menstrual cycle.

525. (D) Nursing process: analysis; client need: physiological integrity; content area: maternity nursing

Rationale
(A) Intrauterine devices to prevent pregnancy are better suited by women who have had one child. There is an increased risk for PID—not thrombophlebitis. (B) Having irregular menses is not an indication for eliminating the IUD as a family planning option. The IUD will not impact the regulatory of the menstrual cycle. (C) Because the IUD does not have cardiovascular implications, smoking is not a contraindication for using a IUD. (D) Because there is an increased risk of pelvic infection, the best candidate is one who has one sex partner, has had one child, and has no evidence of any pelvic inflammatory disease.

526. (D) Nursing process phase: assessment; client need: physiological integrity; content area: maternity nursing

Rationale
(A) Citrus fruits are excellent sources of vitamin C. (B) Egg yolk, fish oil, and liver are sources of vitamins K and D. (C) Skim milk, dried beans, and cheese are sources of calcium. (D) Green leafy vegetables, whole wheat bread, and kidney beans are good sources of folic acid.

527. (A) Nursing process phase: assessment; client need: physiological integrity; content area: maternity nursing

Rationale
(A) Having three or more pregnancies within 3 years depletes the maternal nutritional reserves. (B) A maternal age of 30 is not considered a nutritional risk; however, an adolescent with less than 3 years postmenarche is considered to be at greater nutritional risk because her own body has not stopped growing. (C) This is considered to be the recommended exercise regimen and does not put a healthy expectant mother at risk. (D) The normal range for hemoglobin is 12 to 16 gms/dl for the child-bearing woman.

528. (A) Nursing process phase: assessment; client need: physiological integrity; content area: maternity nursing

Rationale
(A) Iron deficiency anemia makes up more than 75 percent of the anemia that occurs during pregnancy. (B) Folic acid deficiency is the most common cause of megaloblastic anemia during the prenatal period. (C) This is a genetic disease that occurs most often in persons of Mediterranean, Central African, or Asian descent. (D) This sickle-cell anemia is a disorder that presents in about 1 in 2000 pregnancies of African-American women.

529. (B) Nursing process phase: analysis and planning; client need: physiological integrity; content area: maternity nursing

Rationale
(A) The majority of fetal deaths for women with PIH are related to placenta problems: large placenta infarcts, small placenta size, and abruptio placenta. (B) PIH clients are extremely sensitive to blood loss at delivery. This may be related to the leakage of blood components into the extravascular space, which results in impaired coagulation. (C) The epigastric pain in severe pre-elampsia is possibly related to hepatic edema, subscapular edema, or hemorrhage. (D) Vascular changes and tissue hypoxia may impact many maternal organs throughout her body: retinas, liver, lungs, and brain.

530. (C) Nursing process phase: assessment; client need: physiological integrity; content area: maternity nursing

Rationale
(A) 1+ (B) 2+ (C) 3+ (D) 4+

531. (D) Nursing process phase: assessment; client need: physiological integrity; content area: maternity nursing

Rationale
(A) An increase in BUN is related to renal lesions, which impact the glomerular endothelial cells by swelling with fibrin deposits. The lumen is narrowed, and glomerular filtration is reduced. The renal tubules become ischemic and deposit protein substances, the end result being an increase in the BUN and creatinine levels. (B) An increase in the hematocrit is an ominous sign, because this indicates more fluid has moved from the blood vessels to the interstitial tissue as edema. (C) An increase in SGOT is consistent with hepatic congestion. (D) An increase in platelets would indicate an improvement, because in PIH, platelets are destroyed possibly because of blood vessel damage.

532. (A) Nursing process phase: assessment; client need: physiological integrity; content area: maternity nursing

Rationale
(A) Excess magnesium sulfate reduces the activity of CNS cells, thus causing depression of the respiratory rate. (B) Because magnesium sulfate is a CNS depressant, toxicity would produce diminished or absent reflexes. (C) An indicator of toxicity would be decreased urinary output of less than 25 to 30 cc/hr. (D) With toxicity, the nurse would expect to find signs of depressed CNS activity: lowered blood pressure, respiratory rate, and heart rate.

533. (B) Nursing process phase: assessment; client need: physiological integrity; content area: maternity nursing

Rationale
(A) This description best fits early or latent labor. (B) This description best fits active labor. (C) This description is most suitable for transitional labor. (D) This description is consistent with the expulsive stage of labor.

534. (C) Nursing process phase: implementation; client need: health promotion and maintenance; content area: maternity nursing

Rationale
(A) This response does not address the client's concerns. (B) The mechanism is known. See rationale C. (C) This is an accurate response communicated in a way that promotes the

client's understanding and ability to actively participate in decision making regarding her health care. (D) Although corticosteroids suppress the inflammatory response, this suppression does not activate the development of surfactant.

535. **(C)** Nursing process phase: implementation; client need: psychosocial integrity; content area: maternity nursing

Rationale

(A) Anxiety or fear about birth and the baby are often expressed in the form of dreams. Although dreams are common, they deserve to be addressed and not minimized. (B) This response both gives advice and changes the subject. Neither is therapeutic nor assesses maternal adaptation. (C) This response encourages the client to continue, allowing her to further express her concerns and move through the maternal tasks. (D) This response introduces another topic without addressing the client's concerns.

536. **(D)** Nursing process phase: implementation; client need: health promotion and maintenance; content area: maternity nursing

Rationale

(A) Physiological needs take priority over psychological needs. (B) This is important but is not of the highest priority. (C) An immunization schedule is good information, but it is not the most immediate choice. (D) Warning signs for physical problems such as hemorrhage, infection, and dehydration are important, because these conditions require early intervention to resolve.

537. **(B)** Nursing process phase: planning; client need: physiological integrity; content area: maternity nursing

Rationale

(A) The couple is undergoing the test now; they do not have enough information to make a decision. (B) A third-trimester ultrasound usually indicates a risk for a real or potential problem. The nurse should focus on the emotional needs of the client during the ultrasound. (C) There is insufficient information to make any decision at this point. (D) Third trimester is not considered a screening period.

538. **(B)** Nursing process phase: implementation; client need: physiological integrity; content area: maternity nursing

Rationale

(A) Vaginal examinations are avoided in clients with vaginal bleeding. (B) Bleeding may lead to hypovolemic shock, a life-threatening condition. (C) A vaginal examination would have to be performed to determine membrane status. (D) Labor progression is secondary to the bleeding.

539. **(B)** Nursing process phase: implementation; client need: health promotion and maintenance; content area: maternity nursing

Rationale

(A) Because the low-lying placenta may migrate upward there is no indication of a need for a cesarean birth related to the current status of the placenta. (B) Often the placenta migrates up and away from the cervical os as the placenta grows. (C) There is no established relationship between a low-lying placenta and abruptio placenta. (D) Spontaneous abortion is not specifically related to a low-lying placenta. It is estimated that almost half of all clients have a low-lying placenta in the first 30 weeks of pregnancy.

540. **(D)** Nursing process phase: analysis; client need: physiological integrity; content area: maternity nursing

Rationale

(A) Although it is necessary to assess the client's comfort level, this client is at risk for postpartum hemorrhage. (B) Shaking is a common phenomenon in recovery and is not unique to this client's history. (C) Assessing blood pressure and pulse every 15 minutes is routine postpartum care for the first hour after delivery. (D) The postpartum client with a low-lying placenta has an increased risk of postpartum hemorrhage, because uterine contraction is less effective at closing off the blood vessels of the placenta site.

541. **(A)** Nursing process phase: analysis; client need: physiological integrity; content area: maternity nursing

Rationale

(A) The replacement of fluids is started immediately to stabilize the client. (B) The client has a life-threatening situation that requires immediate intervention to stabilize. (C) Determining the fetal position is of little consequence, because the assessment data suggest uterine rupture. (D) This is an emergency situation that requires easy access to the client to institute life-saving measures. Lateral positioning would not provide that at this time.

542. **(B)** Nursing process phase: analysis; client need: physiological integrity; content area: maternity nursing

Rationale

(A) This is an emergency situation where the client's condition must be stabilized. Family members should be notified after intervention is initiated. (B) Uterine rupture requires a cesarean section. (C) The assessment data yield the clinical picture of uterine rupture, the source of bleeding. (D) Reassessment with fetal monitoring that would inhibit the intervention is contraindicated.

543. **(B)** Nursing process phase: analysis; client need: physiological integrity; content area: maternity nursing

Rationale

(A) Cesarean birth is performed when there is a failure to progress; presently this client is progressing. (B) Postpartum hemorrhage is a likely complication for the grand multipara because of her increased incidence of anemia, placenta previa, and abruptio. (C) The grand multipara is rarely induced because of the risks associated with rapid labor. (D) Retention of placenta is not a complication unique to the grand multipara.

544. **(D)** Nursing process phase: analysis; client need: physiological integrity; content area: maternity nursing

Rationale

(A) More than one fetus does not increase the rate of meconium-stained amniotic fluid. (B) An upright maternal position does not correspond to meconium-stained amniotic fluid. (C) Placenta anomalies do relate to meconium staining. (D) Fetal hypoxia results in the relaxation of the rectal sphincter, causing defecation.

545. **(C)** Nursing process phase: analysis; client need: physiological integrity; content: maternity nursing

Rationale

(A) Ineffective uterine contractions are weak and uncoordinated, failing to yield an effective labor pattern. (B) Small pelvic diameters can prolong labor. (C) Fetal bradycardia is not a dystocia category. (D) There is a relationship between the maternal psychosocial and physical variables and labor progress.

546. (B) Nursing processing phase: evaluation; client need: health promotion and maintenance; content area: maternity nursing

Rationale

(A–D) The paternal X or Y chromosome uniting with the X maternal chromosome determines the sex of the fetus.

547. (C) Nursing process phase: implementation; client need: psychosocial integrity; content area: maternity nursing

Rationale

(A) Giving the mother time along with her newborn will intensify her feelings without resolution. (B) Restricting family visitation is not appropriate when the new mother needs support. (C) A normal component of pregnancy is the development of a "fantasy baby." New parents give up their fantasy baby and take on their real baby—a normal attachment process. (D) The concern is immediate and requires a supportive nursing response now.

548. (B) Nursing process phase: implementation; client need: health promotion and maintenance; content area: maternity nursing

Rationale

(A) All alternatives need to be presented, otherwise they will not be making an informed choice. (B) Objective data, including benefits and limitations of each type of contraceptive, should be presented. (C) Ultimately, it affects both partners and should be a mutually agreed upon decision. (D) Effectiveness is an important factor to consider, however, all information should be presented.

549. (D) Nursing process phase: implementation; client need: health promotion and maintenance; content area: maternity nursing

Rationale

(A) The fat-soluble vitamins A and D in increased amounts have been associated with birth defects. (B) Additional sodium is not needed, because most expectant mothers easily meet or exceed the daily requirement. (C) Newborns whose mother took large doses of vitamin C exhibited scurvylike symptoms after their intrauterine supply was terminated. (D) Iron and folic acid are the most frequently advised supplements. They are difficult to acquire by diet alone.

550. (C) Nursing process phase: assessment; client need: physiological integrity; content area: maternity nursing

Rationale

(A) Amniocentesis is done after 14 weeks of pregnancy and yields information about genetic disorders, pulmonary maturity, and fetal hemolytic disease. (B) This test is performed between 10 to 12 weeks' gestation and yields the same information as the amniocentesis. (C) Between weeks 15 to 20, an alpha-fetoprotein test screens for neural tube defects. (D) A Coombs' test determines Rh incompatibility.

551. (A) Nursing process phase: evaluation; client need: health promotion and maintenance; content area: maternity nursing

Rationale

(A) As the uterus becomes gravid, the center of gravity moves away form the midline of the body, thus increasing the client's risk for falling while moving. (B) The pelvis can be unstable in the expectant mother so that double leg lifts are not recommended. (C) Expectant mothers should drink water before, during, and after a workout to replenish lost fluid. (D) Any pain that develops during exercise is reason to stop that activity and should be reported to the health-care provider.

552. (B) Nursing process phase: assessment; client need: health promotion and maintenance; content area: maternity nursing

Rationale

(A) Lamaze preparation for childbirth employs the use of several paced breathing techniques. (B) Dick-Read preparation focuses on the woman's ability to work with the forces of labor; the main breathing technique is abdominal. (C) Lowered lighting was considered less traumatic for the newborn during delivery. This method is attributed to Leboyer. (D) Deep mental relaxation and positive suggestion correspond to hypnosis.

553. (C) Nursing process phase: implementation; client need: psychosocial integrity; content area: maternity nursing

Rationale

(A) Support persons have been shown to reduce the need for medical interventions in the laboring woman. The nurse can role-model and provide the family with needed information. (B) A birth experience has the potential to enrich a family. Family-centered hospitals are more flexible with family support and not regimenting visitor quotas. (C) This response encourages the couple to concretize what they need from their family and how to get it. (D) This response dismisses the potential positive impact of the birthing experience on the family.

554. (A) Nursing process phase: implementation; client need: safe, effective care environment; content area: maternity nursing

Rationale

(A) Limiting visitors and quieting the environment reduce environmental factors that may stimulate convulsions. (B) Monitoring a fluid output of less than 50 cc/hr is an indicator of hypovolemia. (C) Determining the client's knowledge of the pathophysiology of PIH is more stimulation than the client's condition warrants. (D) Giving this information would be better suited for the client who is stable.

555. (A) Nursing process phase: evaluation; client need: health promotion and maintenance; content area: maternity nursing

Rationale

(A) The motion of travel and long sitting seem to stimulate uterine contractions. (B) Sexual activity also seems to augment uterine activity. (C) Plane travel with decreased oxygen and prolonged sitting correlate with increased uterine activity. (D) The lack of energy conservation and overexertion intensify uterine activity.

556. **(A)** Nursing process phase: planning; client need: psychosocial integrity; content area: maternity nursing

Rationale

(A) Because the words may have different meanings for the nurse and the client, it is important to ask the client for clarification. (B) This implies that the client's choice of words is unacceptable, which threatens the establishment of a therapeutic relationship. (C) The nurse risks losing credibility by using words with uncertain meanings. (D) If the nurse waits for clarification at a later time, the opportunity for an effective interaction is lost.

557. **(B)** Nursing process phase: planning; client need: physiological integrity; content area: maternity nursing

Rationale

(A) A prenatal client with class II functioning is not a high risk for PIH. (B) Because digitalis glycoside directly impacts the uterine muscle, early labor is a distinct possibility. (C) The effect of digitalis glycoside on the fetus is unclear; however, because glycosides slow the maternal heart rate, a slowing of the fetal heart rate is anticipated. (D) Hemodynamic changes are more likely to cause maternal cardiac stress.

558. **(D)** Nursing process phase: planning; client need: physiological integrity; content area: maternity nursing

Rationale

(A) Digitalis glycoside improves myocardial activity and slows the heart rate and atrioventricular conduction. (B) Aminophylline reduces bronchoconstriction and increases myocardial contractions. (C) Nitroglycerine reduces left ventricular afterload. (D) Oxytocin stimulates uterine contractions and also causes tachycardia and increased cardiac output, detrimental to the cardiac client.

559. **(A)** Nursing process phase: planning; client need: safe, effective care environment; content area: maternity nursing

Rationale

(A) Calcium gluconate rapidly reverses the side effects of magnesium sulfate. (B) Methylergonovine elevates central venous pressure and produces hypertension. It does not reverse the effect of magnesium sulfate. (C) Morphine sulfate is a CNS depressant and would compound the effects of magnesium sulfate. (D) Ergonovine elevates venous pressure and stimulates a rise in blood pressure.

560. **(D)** Nursing process phase: assessment; client need: physiological integrity; content: maternity nursing

Rationale

(A) Decreased urinary output is indicative of hypovolemia in the client with PIH. (B) In the client with PIH, increased urinary output is indicative of fluid shift into the vascular space. (C) Dyspena in the client with PIH is related to pulmonary edema. (D) Headache is the classic sign of cerebral edema and vasoconstriction.

561. **(A)** Nursing process phase: implementation; client need: health promotion and maintenance; content area: maternity nursing

Rationale

(A) Because of the elevated use of glucose and glycogen and low levels of insulin antagonist, human placental lactogen, hypoglycemia is often more pronounced in the first trimester.

(B) The risk of hyperglycemia is greatest during the second and third trimesters because insulin needs often double. (C) The development of ketoacidosis in the second and third trimesters is related to an increased resistance to insulin and elevated human placental lactogen. (D) Although metabolism and fetal and maternal needs vary greatly during pregnancy, the mother should not limit her normal physical activity to regulate her blood sugar.

562. **(B)** Nursing process phase: analysis; client need: physiological integrity; content area: maternity nursing

Rationale

(A) Fibrinogen levels are important to monitor in the client at high risk for hemorrhage. (B) Anemia is of special concern in clients with diabetes because increased glucose levels replace oxygen on the hemoglobin molecule, thus lowering the oxygen-carrying capacity. (C) Lowered estrogen levels correlate with spontaneous abortion. (D) LDH is important to monitor in the client at risk for PIH.

563. **(A)** Nursing process phase: planning; client need: physiological integrity; content area: maternity nursing

Rationale

(A) During the second trimester, the client's blood pressure is slightly lower than normal. The drop is associated with a decrease in peripheral resistance. (B) This is a low blood pressure reading not related to a normal prenatal finding. (C) This elevation is not associated with a normal finding of the second trimester. It could be related to anxiety. (D) This finding indicates no change, which is associated with the first trimester.

564. **(B)** Nursing process phase: analysis; client need: physiological integrity; content area: maternity nursing

Rationale

(A) Proteinuria is associated with PIH. (B) A significant number of women with asymptomatic bacteriuria develop kidney infections. (C) Decreased urinary output is associated with PIH. (D) Urine testing for glocuse would not be considered an adequate measure to diagnose gestational diabetes.

565. **(C)** Nursing process phase: planning; client need: physiological integrity; content area: maternity nursing

Rationale

(A) Protracted latent labor is related to cephalopelvic disproportion. (B) Candidates at high risk for cesarean birth are those cesarean section repeaters, those with failure to progress, and those with fetal distress. (C) There is an association between asymptomatic bacteriuria and preterm labor. (D) Relaxation of the pelvic floor occurs when the muscles are not toned because of delivery.

566. **(B)** Nursing process phase: planning; client need: physiological integrity; content area: maternity nursing

Rationale

(A) Altered health maintenance relates to ineffective coping skills and lack of support. (B) Risk for fluid volume deficit relates to the client's inability to ingest and retain fluids. Hyperemesis gravidarum results in dehydration, hypovolemia, and metabolic changes. All of these outcomes have a negative impact on fetal growth and development. (C) Risk for fatigue relates to increased carbohydrate metabolism. (D) Risk for infection relates to urinary stasis, poor hygiene, and so on.

567. (D) Nursing process phase: implementation; client need: psychosocial integrity; content area: maternity nursing

Rationale
(A) Reviewing the procedures will possibly lessen their anxiety, but the nurse should start where the couple's needs are. (B) Counseling referral is appropriate if their anxiety is not adequately lowered, however, the nurse should attempt to lower their anxiety if necessary. (C) This may relieve the anxiety that accompanies the unknown. (D) This will identify the couple's specific concerns and give direction for all other nursing interventions.

568. (B) Nursing process phase: implementation; client need: health promotion and maintenance; content area: maternity nursing

Rationale
(A) This is a premature referral since the couple have not yet made decisions about which testing is best for them. (B) This permits the couple to make informed choices based on an understanding of the long- and short-term problems associated with the genetic disorder in question. (C) This should be the couple's prerogative. (D) The couple should not feel rushed to make a major decision.

569. (B) Nursing process phase: implementation; client need: physiological integrity; content area: maternity nursing

Rationale
(A) This is the daily recommended amount of water necessary for adequate hydration. This fluid intake should not be decreased to minimize frequency. (B) Cola beverages contain caffeine, which has a diuretic effect that aggravates urinary frequency. (C) Acidic fruit juices do not impact urinary frequency during pregnancy. (D) Dairy products are an important source of calcium and vitamin D and should not be eliminated because they do not impact urinary frequency.

570. (C) Nursing process phase: implementation; client need: physiological integrity; content area: maternity nursing

Rationale
(A) Eating a diet high in fiber, thereby increasing gastric motility, will help prevent constipation and the straining that produces hemorrhoids. (B) Elevating the hips on a pillow reduces swelling. (C) Drinking caffeine drinks is not recommended during pregnancy. (D) Ice packs will increase comfort.

571. (C) Nursing process phase: implementation; client need: physiological integrity; content area: maternity nursing

Rationale
(A) The GTT screens for maternal gestational diabetes. (B) The GTT does not predict a client's ability to carry a pregnancy to term. (C) The GTT is used to screen pregnant women between the 24th and 28th weeks of pregnancy to manage the pregnancy without the complications that may develop. (D) The GTT is a determination of the client's blood sugar level and not a measure of calorie need.

572. (A) Nursing process phase: evaluation; client need: health promotion and maintenance; content area: maternity nursing

Rationale
(A) The elastic band of knee-high stockings would impede venous blood flow and increase the development of edema and additional varicosities. (B) Loose clothing promotes venous return. (C) Hip and leg elevation discourages dependent edema by promoting venous return. (D) Dorsiflexion improves circulation and promotes venous return.

573. (D) Nursing process phase: implementation; client need: psychosocial integrity; content area: maternity nursing

Rationale
(A) This response minimizes the client's statement and does not answer her question. (B) This statement is based on the assumption that the client is not pleased with her weight and implies that she has little control over what is happening. (C) This response implies that the client has not been practicing good self-care. (D) This response is the most supportive because it explains the rationale for the weigh-ins.

574. (C) Nursing process phase: implementation; client need: health promotion and maintenance; content area: maternity nursing

Rationale
(A) The pregnant client is least likely to experience Braxton Hicks contractions in the first trimester. (B) Multigravidas may note discomfort from Braxton Hicks contractions in the second and third trimesters. (C) Primigravidas are most likely to have Braxton Hicks contractions in the last trimester, when progesterone levels are lower and oxytocin levels are rising. (D) Primigravidas are most likely to have Braxton Hicks contractions in the third trimester.

575. (D) Nursing process phase: implementation; client need: physiological integrity; content: maternity nursing

Rationale
(A) A supine position encourages vena cava syndrome and decreases renal blood flow by as much as 50 percent. (B) A sitting upright position also diminishes renal blood flow and urinary output. (C) A standing position diminishes kidney perfusion and urinary output. (D) In the third trimester, the gravid uterus reduces bladder volume and impairs renal output. A left lateral position increases kidney perfusion and increases the glomerular filtration rate.

576. (A) Nursing process phrase: implementation; client need: health promotion and maintenance; content area: maternity nursing

Rationale
(A) Swimming is an acceptable form of exercise for the third-trimester client because it is non-weight-bearing and will be less likely to inhibit uterine blood flow. (B) Race-walking is a low-impact form of exercise. It may interfere with adequate oxygenation of the placenta. (C) Tennis is an aerobic form of exercise that may inhibit the oxygen supply to the fetus as well as increase the third-trimester client's own risk of injury related to falling. (D) Horseback riding is not recommended because of the risk of injury to the mother.

577. (B) Nursing process phase: analysis; client need: physiological integrity; content area: maternity nursing

Rationale
(A) BUN is elevated with dehydration because hypovolemia reduces renal perfusion and function. (B) The hematocrit el-

evates with maternal dehydration. This is related to hypovolemia and an increased concentration of red blood cells. (C) Hematocrit levels decrease in HELLP syndrome because of hemolysis of red blood cells. (D) An abnormally small amount of amniotic fluid is most often associated with postmaturity or a fetal anomaly such as a urinary tract obstruction.

578. (D) Nursing process phase: implementation; client need: physiological integrity; content area: maternity nursing

Rationale

(A) The safety of disulfiram (Antabuse) has not been established for pregnancy, so it is not a recommended treatment. (B) The client's immediate need for intervention would be best met via a 12-step program specific for expectant mothers. (C) At this point, the client is asking for professional help. Describing the effects of fetal alcohol syndrome would induce an unnecessary guilt response. (D) Disulfiram's safety has not been established for the fetus. Most Antabuse programs require female clients to have a negative pregnancy test and, if sexually active, to use a reliable form of contraception while taking the medication.

579. (D) Nursing process phase: implementation; client need: physiological integrity; content area: maternity nursing

Rationale

(A) Semi-Fowler's is beneficial for placenta previa because it allows the fetus to compress the placental vessels and reduce bleeding. (B) Supine with hips elevated ensures an adequate supply of oxygen to the brain. Hip elevation diminishes the effect of the vena cava syndrome. (C) Trendelenburg is the one position to be avoided in clients with vaginal bleeding because the position tends to jeopardize maternal respiratory effort. (D) Left lateral provides the best perfusion of the placenta.

580. (A) Nursing process phase: assessment; client need: physiological integrity; content area: maternity nursing

Rationale

(A) In the client with untreated gonorrhea, her infant is at high risk for contracting the disease during a vaginal delivery. (B) Most clients are asymptomatic and have a nonspecific vaginal discharge. (C) Gonorrhea can produce a puerperal infection in the postpartum client but causes relatively few problems for the prenatal client. (D) Reinfections occur at a rate of 11 to 30 percent in females with a history of gonorrhea.

581. (C) Nursing process phase: analysis and planning; client need: physiological integrity, content area: maternity nursing

Rationale

(A) Antibiotics used to treat GBS are nonteratogenic. (B) Antibiotics given to the mother after 38 weeks effectively treat the mother, but not the fetus. (C) After 38 weeks' gestation, treatment with antibiotics is effective because there is a reduced time for recolonization of the bacteria. (D) There are no data to suggest that there is an increased incidence of viral infections in the mother after a treatment regimen of antibiotics.

582. (B) Nursing process phase: evaluation; client need: health promotion and maintenance; content area: maternity nursing

Rationale

(A) The onset of contractions and subsequent dilation are ominous signs. (B) A contraction stress test is contraindicated because it may traumatize the cervix and disrupt the sutures. (C) Bedrest is advocated for 24 to 48 hours to reduce pressure on the cervix. (D) Ruptured membranes indicate that the sutures must be removed and the pregnancy terminated.

583. (C) Nursing process phase: analysis and planning; client need: physiological integrity; content area: maternity nursing

Rationale

(A) A missed abortion does not increase the risk for infertility. (B) HELLP syndrome develops from pre-elampsia and is characterized by hemolysis, elevated liver enzymes, and a low platelet count. (C) Fetal autolysis releases thromboplastin, which can precipitate DIC. (D) The treatment for pre-eclampsia is the birth of the fetus. Because the client has had a missed abortion, this eliminates her risk for pre-eclampsia.

584. (D) Nursing process phase: evaluation; client need: health promotion and maintenance; content area: maternity nursing

Rationale

(A) The use of tampons is not recommended because tampons are inserted into the vagina and left for a period of time such that bacteria may develop and increase the risk of an ascending infection. (B) No intercourse of any kind is permissible because of the possibility of bacteria being introduced into the vagina and uterus. (C) Baths are not recommended because the bath water retrogrades into the vagina. (D) A temperature over 100.4°F is a possible indication of an infection and should be reported to the healthcare provider.

585. (A) Nursing process phase: analysis and planning; client need: physiological integrity; content area: maternity nursing

Rationale

(A) Hydration is thought to suppress the distribution of oxytocin from the posterior pituitary gland. (B) An IV line is standard practice if the client is in a life-threatening situation; however, preterm labor is not necessarily a life-threatening situation. (C) Renal clearance is of particular importance with clients who have maternal hypovolemia. (D) The client's blood pressure is normotensive.

586. (B) Nursing process phase: implementation; client need: physiological integrity; content area: maternity nursing

Rationale

(A) Increasing the rate of infusion will complicate the situation. The client is exhibiting warning signs from the terbutaline sulfate. (B) This is the best action because the client is exhibiting pulmonary edema, an emergency situation. (C) Deep tendon reflexes should be monitored when magnesium sulfate is administered or the client has PIH. (D) Assessing uterine contractions is secondary to the existing emergency situation.

587. (B) Nursing process phase: analysis and planning; client need: physiological integrity; content area: maternity nursing

Rationale

(A) Multiple gestation is not a contradiction for steroid therapy. (B) PIH is a contradiction for steroid therapy, because the medication can suppress aldosterone and cause an elevation in blood pressure. (C) The side effects of steroid therapy do not negatively impact the client with placenta previa. (D) The side effects of steroid therapy do not negatively impact the client with hyperemesis gravidarum.

588. (B) Nursing process phase: implementation; client need: physiological integrity; content area: maternity nursing

Rationale

(A) The client's membranes have been ruptured for over 4 hours and assessment for infection should continue. (B) When amniotic fluid becomes infected, it has a strong odor and is yellow in color. After 4 hours of ruptured membranes, the incidence of infection increases. (C) The fluids will help to maintain hydration but do not confirm the development of an infection. (D) Monitoring intake and output does not give specific information about the development of chorioamnionitis.

589. (C) Nursing process phase: analysis and planning; client need: physiological integrity; content area: maternity nursing

Rationale

(A) The active phase of labor would not cause a sustained increase in FHR. The normal range is 120 to 160. (B) The assessment data are not consistent with maternal anxiety. (C) The maternal temperature is elevated. This fever can produce an elevated FHR. (D) An indication of cord prolapse would be a decrease in FHR.

590. (C) Nursing process phase: evaluation; client need: safe, effective care environment; content area: maternity nursing

Rationale

(A) A pH of less than 7.20 is an indication of frank acidosis, and surgical intervention is required to prevent CNS damage. (B) If the pH is over 7.25, labor continues and a repeat analysis is done if warranted. (C) This level indicates a mild preacidosis. A cesarean is not indicated, but sampling should be repeated in 30 minutes. (D) There should be routine fetal monitoring for a fetal blood pH over 7.25.

591. (A) Nursing process phase: evaluation; client need: physiological integrity; content area: maternity nursing

Rationale

(A) Vaginal show increases with fetal descent. Vaginal show is a blood-tinged, mucous discharge generated from the cervix. (B) Placenta previa would present with bright red vaginal bleeding. (C) Rupture of membranes should be confirmed with a gush or leakage of clear fluid. (D) Crowning is when a large portion of the fetal head is visible in the vaginal opening. It is representative of second stage.

592. (D) Nursing process phase: implementation; client need: psychosocial integrity; content area: maternity nursing

Rationale

(A) The decision should be based on the client's present needs, not those of others. This minimizes her experience. (B) This presents a nonobjective picture from which the client must decide. (C) This response gives approval and suggests the nurse's value system. (D) It is important to have the latest information on progression on which to base decision making. The client may have made more progress than she realizes.

593. (C) Nursing process phase: implementation; client need: physiological integrity; content area: maternity nursing

Rationale

(A) This position will increase the likelihood of vena cava syndrome and increase the client's discomfort. (B) Pushing at 8 cm increases the client' risk of cervical edema or lacerations. (C) Side-lying will help to minimize the urge to bear down and panting will distract her from bearing down. (D) Another examination is unnecessary at this time.

594. (A) Nursing process phase: implementation; client need: psychosocial integrity; content area: maternity nursing

Rationale

(A) Informing her of the beginning of each contraction will assist the client in dealing with the contraction and increase her sense of control. (B) Encouraging her to sleep will diminish her ability to successfully work with her labor. (C) The client is exhibiting behavior congruent with the transitional phase of labor. There is no need at present to give her oxygen. (D) If the fetus was having decelerations or the client was dehydrated, then increasing the IV would be effective intervention.

595. (B) Nursing process phase: implementation; client need: psychosocial integrity; content area: maternity nursing

Rationale

(A) Separating the client from her support is going to further impair her ability to manage. (B) Breaking the task of labor into manageable portions enhances the client's ability to cope. (C) This comment will add to her frustration and not assist her to cope with this difficult part of her labor. (D) During transition, discussing baby names would be too frustrating and overwhelming for this client.

596. (A) Nursing process phase: planning; client need: psychosocial integrity; content area: maternity nursing

Rationale

(A) The desire to push is often uncontrollable and signals the beginning of the bearing-down effort. This effort is accompanied by a sense of relief that birth is imminent. (B) Withdrawal and internal focus are characteristic of transition, when contractions are long with short intervals. (C) Anxiety is exhibited in the earlier phases of labor and has many causes, some of which are worrying about an inability to birth the baby or wondering whether the baby is healthy. (D) In late active labor, passivity is noted as contractions continue to increase in strength and labor persists.

597. (D) Nursing process phase: implementation; client need: physiological integrity; content area: maternity nursing

Rationale

(A) Identifying the idea of escalating pain is insufficient in helping the client to reduce her tension. (B) The client is most likely unaware of the tension she is harboring and will continue to exhibit the tension until it is confronted. (C) The observation of clenched fists and jaw is a beginning assessment that necessitates intervention. (D) Touching the tense areas and giving a verbal cue to release the tension are effective interventions.

598. (B) Nursing process phase: implementation; client need: physiological integrity; content area: maternity nursing

Rationale
(A) Uterine inversion is life-threatening. The fundus of the uterus should be replaced, so the Trendelenburg position would make this difficult. (B) Because blood loss may reach 1800 cc and maternal shock follows, volume replacement is necessary to offset this life-threatening situation. (C) Ergonovine is contraindicated because it will contract the cervix as well as the uterus, making it difficult to replace the uterus. (D) Oxytocin is administered intravenously to contract the uterus.

599. (D) Nursing process phase: implementation; client need: physiological integrity; content area: maternity nursing

Rationale
(A) Ambulating the client will stimulate uterine contractions, which are contraindicated for the client experiencing hypertonic uterine dysfunction. (B) Rest may correct a hypertonic contraction pattern. The lateral recumbent position is preferred to promote relaxation and increase uterine perfusion. (C) Oxytocin will stimulate the uterus to contract and often increase hypertonicity. (D) Management of hypertonic contractions is by therapeutic rest. This rest is achieved via administration of analgesics such as morphine or meperidine.

600. (B) Nursing process phase: implementation; client need: physiological integrity; content area: maternity nursing

Rationale
(A) Preparing the client for a cesarean delivery at this point is premature. Repositioning the client is suggested first. (B) Assuming a hands-and-knees position permits gravity to pull the fetus away from the maternal spine and facilitate turning to an anterior position. (C) Occult cord prolapse is more likely to occur in a breech presentation. (D) An occiput posterior presentation does not in and of itself elicit an abnormal fetal heart rate.

601. (D) Nursing process phase: analysis and planning; client need: physiological integrity; content area: maternity nursing

Rationale
(A) The client's labor was 12 hours. The average length of labor for a multigravida ranges between 1 and 15 hours. A prolonged labor results in myometrical fatigue, which may increase the incidence of uterine atony, thus increasing the risk for fluid deficit. (B) The client's gravity and parity are not extreme, which may put her at risk for uterine atony and subsequent hemorrhage. (C) Age alone is not a risk factor for fluid volume deficit. (D) Anesthesia may contribute to fluid volume deficit by altering blood pressure and impacting myometrial contractility.

602. (D) Nursing process phase: implementation; client need: physiological integrity; content area: maternity nursing

Rationale
(A) Gentle fundal massage stimulates uterine contractility and contains bleeding. (B) Using a firm, steady downward pressure helps to expel clots. Retained clots can impede uterine contractility. (C) A full bladder displaces the uterus and interferes with uterine contractions. (D) Lateral recumbent does not maximize the amount of blood flow to the brain and other vital organs. Dorsal recumbent is preferable.

603. (C) Nursing process phase: implementation; client need: physiological integrity; content area: maternity nursing

Rationale
(A) A warm, moist compress will increase vasocongestion and subsequent edema. (B) Because the vaginal outlet has been externally and internally traumatized, a topical spray will only be superficially effective. (C) Ice will promote vasoconstriction and lessen the development of edema. (D) Dry heat will increase vasocongestion and edema.

604. (B) Nursing process phase: assessment; client need: physiological integrity; content area: maternity nursing

Rationale
(A) Firm breasts suggest breast engorgement, which may occur 3 to 5 days postpartum if the client is breastfeeding. (B) Soft breasts without tenderness are an assessment that is within normal parameters for the first assessment. (C) The first postpartum assessment of the uterus should find it firm and at the level of the umbilicus. (D) Lochia should be rubra, moderate, and odorless.

605. (B) Nursing process phase: implementation; client need: physiological integrity; content area: maternity nursing

Rationale
(A) The nature and cause of the headache have not been completely determined. Giving an analgesic now may mask the symptoms further. (B) Determination of positional relief or intensification is associated with leakage of cerebrospinal fluid through the dura into the extradural space. This lowers the volume needed to support brain tissue and causes the brainstem to dip into the base of the skull when the client is upright. (C) Applying a cold compress to the forehead will cause vasoconstriction of the superficial vessels. Ultimately it will not alleviate the headache or improve the assessment data. (D) An elevated blood pressure accompanies the headache in the client with PIH.

606. (C) Nursing process phase: implementation; client need: health promotion and maintenance; content area: maternity nursing

Rationale
(A) Although breastfeeding with inverted nipples will take a bit more effort, the client should be supported by being instructed in ways to help the infant to latch on. (B) Analgesic administration is not usually necessary; the best interventions concern those that help the infant latch on. (C) Ice vasoconstricts and helps the nipple become erect. An erect nipple is easier for the infant to grasp. (D) Tea solutions are helpful to toughen nipples but do nothing to help the infant latch on.

607. (B) Nursing process phase: analysis and planning; client need: physiological integrity; content area: maternity nursing

Rationale

(A) The dangers associated with PIH exist for up to 72 hours or longer. (B) The client with PIH is at risk for fluid volume excess as related to fluid shifts. (C) The postpartum client is more likely to experience constipation than diarrhea. (D) Self-care deficit relates to the client's inability to care for herself, as in a client immediately following a cesarean birth.

608. (C) Nursing process phase: analysis and planning; client need: physiological integrity; content area: maternity nursing

Rationale

(A) The blood loss estimate is within normal limits for a vaginal delivery. The postpartum client tolerates this loss without consequence because of a pre-existing increase blood volume. (B) The action of oxytocin is to contract the uterus. There is no known rebound effect. (C) Magnesium sulfate is a CNS depressant, and it relaxes the uterine musculature. (D) The client experienced a blood pressure elevation because of vasoconstriction. The muscles of the uterus would be affected in the same way.

609. (B) Nursing process phase: analysis and planning; client need: physiological integrity; content area: maternity nursing

Rationale

(A) A diastasis recti is a separation of abdominal muscles that is a result of underlying uterine growth. It occurs gradually over the 9-month period of pregnancy without discomfort. (B) The separation of the two rectus muscles along the abdominal midline lessens the muscle tone needed for bowel evacuation. (C) The lack of abdominal tone is not sufficient to impair physical mobility. There is less support, however, to the internal abdominal organs. (D) There is no increased risk for injury related to diastasis recti.

610. (D) Nursing process phase: evaluation; client need: health promotion and maintenance; content area: maternity nursing

Rationale

(A) Discussion is a limited, passive form of learning and evaluation. The more senses and active involvement the increased chance of learning. (B) Although there is an objective form of evaluation involved, a test may be perceived as a threat to the learner. Focusing the discussion on the correct and missed answers reinforces total performance instead of the incorrect responses. (C) Repeating back an answer gives a limited view of the learner's knowledge base and limits the opportunity to build on the client's life experiences. (D) Return demonstration gives the nurse the opportunity to reinforce the desired behaviors and assist to modify the others. It has the best potential to lower the client's performance anxiety, because she has completed the task at least once with supervision.

611. (C) Nursing process phase; implementation; client need: physiological integrity; content area: maternity nursing

Rationale

(A) Ambulation enhances gastric motility, which will increase the movement of the gas out of the bowel. (B) The use of the left lateral recumbent position permits gas to move from the descending to the sigmoid colon. (C) Narcotic analgesics and hot or cold beverages compound the formation of gas by decreasing peristalsis. (D) Increasing physical activity by rocking enhances the expulsion of gas.

612. (D) Nursing process phase: implementation; client need; physiological integrity; content area: maternity nursing

Rationale

(A) Encouraging oral fluid intake prevents dehydration and increases the volume of circulation. However, the client is at risk for injury because of orthostatic hypotension. (B) Splinting the abdomen with pillows increases the client's comfort and effectiveness when performing deep breathing exercise. (C) Narcotic analgesics are not recommended for the client who is increasing her mobility because the risk of injury increases with altered sensorium. (D) Orthostatic hypotension may occur when moving from a supine to an upright position on beginning ambulation.

613. (C) Nursing process phase: evaluation; client need: physiological integrity; content area: maternity nursing

Rationale

(A) The normal value for fasting plasma glucose is <140 mg/dl. (B) During the first two postpartal days, proteolytic enzymes promote self-digestion of the protein substances from the endometrium. This process accounts for mild proteinuria. (C) Leukocytes are elevated during the early postpartum period. However, a significant increase suggests infection. (D) This is within the normal hemoglobin range (10 to 14 gms/dl) for a postpartum client.

614. (B) Nursing process phase: assessment; client need: physiological integrity; content area: maternity nursing

Rationale

(A) Foods ingested before the return of peristalsis encourage the development of a paralytic ileus. (B) Palpation for distention and discomfort is the next step in assessment of gas formation, collection, or potential paralytic ileus. Bowel sounds are usually actively present on the third postoperative day. (C) The administration of a soap-suds enema may be premature without further assessment. (D) Nasogastric tube insertion relieves distension from a paralytic ileus; however, this intervention is premature. Additional assessment of distension and discomfort should be determined.

615. (A) Nursing process phase; analysis and planning; client need: physiological integrity; content area: maternity nursing

Rationale

(A) Normal urinary output is greater than 30 cc/hr. The infusion rate should be increased. (B) Uterine fundal height after a cesarean is at the level of the umbilicus for up to 5 days. (C) Lochia flow should not be heavy; normal ranges from scant to moderate. (D) Reports of pain at the incision site are normal responses to the surgical procedure. Analgesics may be given the oral or intramuscular route.

616. (B) Nursing process phase: analysis and planning; client need: physiological integrity; content area: maternity nursing

Rationale

(A) Increasing the IV rate of infusion will not influence the wound drainage. (B) Outlining and indicating the date and time will objectively assist the nurse in monitoring the determination of increased drainage. (C) The physician should be notified if the oozing continues. (D) Changing the dressing is not indicated.

617. (C) Nursing process phase: evaluation; client need: health promotion and maintenance; content area: maternity nursing

Rationale
(A) Tightening the gluteals reduces stress and direct pressure on the perineum. (B) Reinsertion helps the hemorrhoid to regress. (C) Afterpains may continue as long as 2 to 3 days postdelivery in the multigravida. (D) Progressive ambulation improves the bladder and bowel functioning and promotes circulation.

618. (B) Nursing process phase: implementation; client need: psychosocial integrity; content area: maternity nursing

Rationale
(A) Making an appointment for the future does not help the client with coping meanwhile. (B) Inadequate rest negatively influences the client's ability to cope with her situation. This area needs addressing. (C) The maternal support group will not provide the client with the immediate feedback that she presently needs. (D) This reassurance is unfounded. There is no guarantee that they will subside quickly. Nor does the comment help the client cope better with her present situation.

619. (D) Nursing process phase: assessment; client need: physiological integrity; content area: maternity nursing

Rationale
(A) Normal uterine involution proceeds at a rate of approximately 1 cm/day. One week postpartum should find the uterus at the level of the symphysis pubis. (B) Lochia should be scant and odorless and pinkish brown in color. (C) The episiotomy edges should be touching with no note of drainage, swelling, or redness. (D) Breasts in the lactating mother should be of greater size. In the nonlactating mother, the breasts should be no larger than during pregnancy. Engorgement for the lactating mother may suggest feeding problems and requires additional assessment. Engorgement for the nonlactating mother may indicate that the breasts have been stimulated and that also needs further investigation.

620. (A) Nursing process phase: evaluation; client need: health promotion and maintenance; content area: maternity nursing

Rationale
(A) Oral intake for the lactating mother should be between 2500 and 3000 ml/day to produce quantity sufficient milk for the newborn. (B) An increased caloric support of 500 to 800 calories is necessary for milk production and supply. (C) Protein requirements are greater by 10 gms for pregnancy than for lactation. (D) Niacin-rich foods should be increased during lactation because niacin facilitates energy production.

621. (D) Nursing process phase: intervention; client need: health promotion and maintenance; content area: maternity nursing

Rationale
(A) Most couples can safely resume intercourse 3 to 4 weeks after a vaginal delivery. (B) If the couple has already attempted intercourse, asking them to delay 3 more weeks without the suggestion of alternatives does not promote the resumption of sexual expression. (C) Reassuring the client that everything is fine encourages self-doubt. (D) Vaginal dryness, especially in lactating mothers, may cause dyspareunia. The use of a water-soluble lubricant will increase the client's comfort.

622. (D) Nursing process phase: analysis and planning; client need: physiological integrity; content area: maternity nursing

Rationale
(A) Pressure from a full bladder is not felt in the vaginal area. Clients usually complain of low abdominal pain. (B) A prolapsed rectum causes feelings of fullness in the rectal area. (C) Lochia pools when the client is lying down but there is no feeling of fullness. When the client stands, the lochia exits through the vagina. (D) Prolonged pressure of the fetal head on vaginal mucosa can interfere with circulation, which in combination with a forceps delivery may result in vaginal lacerations and vaginal hematomas. Major symptoms include a feeling of fullness in the vagina or persistent perineal pain.

623. (B) Nursing process phase: implementation; client need: physiological integrity; content area: maternity nursing

Rationale
(A) Placing the infant in a well-heated isolette will contribute to apnea in the cold-stressed infant. (B) Wiping the newborn dry minimizes heat loss by evaporation. (C) Keeping the skin wet will place the infant at risk for cold stress, regardless of the water temperature. (D) Placing the infant on the examination table open to room air increases heat loss because some of the objects may be cooler then the infant's skin. The temperature of the delivery room is much cooler than intrauterine temperature.

624. (A) Nursing process phase: analysis and planning; client need: physiological integrity; content area: maternity nursing

Rationale
(A) The infant is exhibiting signs of hyperthermia related to the elevated temperature of the incubator. The desired temperature for a controlled heat source is above 36.5°C but not greater than 37°C. (B) A newborn's response to maternal narcotic analgesic administration will be a lowered heart rate, respiration, pulse, and blood pressure. (C) Hyperglycemia is exhibited by polyuria. (D) Symptoms of cold stress include irritability, pallor, respiratory distress, and cool skin.

625. (D) Nursing process phase: assessment; client need: physiological integrity; content area: maternity nursing

Rationale
(A) An Apgar score of 3 is indicative of a severely depressed infant who needs immediate resuscitation. (B) A score of 5 is also suggestive of a high infant mortality rate. (C) A score of 7 is on the lower end of the acceptable range for physiological status. (D) The only aspect of the five areas of assessment that was on the midrange of normal was the gray extremities. This is a common value because it takes a few minutes for the oxygenated blood to reach the extremities.

626. (D) Nursing process phase: implementation; client need: health promotion and maintenance; content area: maternity nursing

Rationale

(A) The newborn's hands are not indicative of body temperature. Wrapping the baby and covering the head will improve the increase or stabilization of body temperature. (B) The extremities of a newborn are not reliable indicators for newborn body temperature. (C) Cold hands do not conclusively indicate thermal heat loss. (D) Because there is more surface area exposed to room air, the hands will be cooler than the central body temperature.

627. (C) Nursing process phase: analysis and planning; client need: physiological integrity; content area: maternity nursing

Rationale

(A) During the first trimester, the expectant client is anemic when hemoglobin values are less than 11 gms/dl. (B) The client is considered to be anemic when her hematocrit is less than 33 percent. (C) A hemoglobin value of less than 10 gms/dl is considered to be anemia at any time during pregnancy. (D) A hematocrit of less than 35 percent is considered to be anemia at any point during pregnancy.

628. (A) Nursing process phase: assessment; client need: physiological integrity; content area: maternity nursing

Rationale

(A) Most expectant clients with mild to moderate anemia experience fatigue and are susceptible to infections. (B) Insomnia is symptomatic of third-trimester discomfort related to fetal movement, urinary frequency, or muscle cramping. (C) Shortness of breath is related to limited diaphragmatic expansion because of increased uterine size. (D) Headaches are associated with tension or sinus congestion.

629. (B) Nursing process phase: assessment; client need: physiological integrity; content area: maternity nursing

Rationale

(A) The client with hyperemesis gravidarum has a low level of activity tolerance because of an absence of energy from inadequate nutritional intake. Nursing interventions should include providing the client with a restful atmosphere and progressive activities as her condition permits. (B) Monitoring laboratory values is important because of the risk of metabolic acidosis and hypothrominemia. (C) Diet begins with limited amounts of oral fluids and bland foods and then is slowly advanced. (D) Hyperalimentation is initiated in severe cases after a slow dietary progression has failed.

630. (A) Nursing process phase: assessment; client need: physiological integrity; content area: maternity nursing

Rationale

(A) A copper-colored maculopapular rash covers the body of the infant with neonatal syphilis. (B) Pneumonitis is characteristic of HIV infection. (C) Microcephaly correlates with rubella and cytomegalovirus. (D) The incidence of cardiomyopathy is greater in infants of diabetic mothers.

631. (C) Nursing process phase: implementation; client need: health promotion and maintenance; content area: maternity nursing

Rationale

(A) Diaphragms are not contraindicated for the client with diabetes mellitus. (B) Condoms have no specific side effects or contraindications for a woman with diabetes mellitus. (C)

The side effects of oral contraceptives for the woman with diabetes mellitus include hypertension and hastening vascular disease. The estogren elevates cholesterol and triglyceride production while progesteron alters insulin activity. (D) Tubal ligation should be considered a viable alternative when considering the impact of diabetic complications.

632. (D) Nursing process phase: implementation; client need: physiological integrity; content area: maternity nursing

Rationale

(A) Bedrest should be encouraged because the client is at risk for thrombophlebitis. (B) Massaging the left leg is contraindicated because if a thrombus exists, it could dislodge it. (C) Any type of restrictive clothing impairs circulation, increasing trauma to the area. (D) Femoral vein thrombosis is associated with edema because the ileofemoral vein is associated with severe edema. Measurement will give objective data about the client's condition and guide the need for interventions.

633. (C) Nursing process phase: implementation; client need: psychosocial integrity; content area: maternity nursing

Rationale

(A) Finishing the teaching should not be the priority. Listening to the parents' concerns comes first. (B) This response does not allow the parents an opportunity to ventilate their feelings further. (C) Acknowledging their feelings and encouraging them to discuss their concerns is most therapeutic. (D) The parents are not ready to hear this; they are anxious about how to care for their baby.

634. (A) Nursing process phase: implementation; client need: psychosocial integrity; content area: maternity nursing

Rationale

(A) Acknowledging the client's feelings without being judgmental is critical. (B) This statement implies that strength only comes with difficult situations such as the death of a baby. (C) This information is irrelevant at this point. The client needs to have the grief process facilitated. (D) This is a punitive response indicating that because someone is capable, he or she will be given more challenges.

635. (B) Nursing process phase: analysis and planning; client need: physiological integrity; content area: maternity nursing

Rationale

(A) Alertness in the newborn is evidenced by brief attentiveness to a stimulus. (B) The occurrence of a wide-eyed stare is associated with long-term intrauterine hypoxia associated with postmature and premature infants. (C) Hypoglycemia is evidenced by poor muscle tone, eye movements, and tremors. (D) Hypothermia is evidenced by cold, mottled skin.

636. (D) Nursing process phase: analysis and planning; client need: physiological integrity; content area: maternity nursing

Rationale

(A) Cesarean birth is indicated only for obstetrical reasons. (B) Therapeutic abortions are rare. The spontaneous abortion rate is as high as 20 percent. (C) Congenital tuberculosis is uncommon. (D) Separation from the newborn is imperative to prevent the infant from contracting the disease. This is done until risk of infection is no longer a consideration.

637. (A) Nursing process phase: implementation; client need: physiological integrity; content area: maternity nursing

Rationale
(A) Starting early oral feedings institutes the normal intestinal flora needed for converting bilirubin to urobilinogen. (B) Delaying feedings causes hypoglycemia, which causes fat stores to be used for energy release. The energy-releasing fatty acids then compete with bilirubin for finding sites on albumin. (C) The infant should be brought to parents for feedings to promote bonding and offset the less-stimulating nursery environment. (D) The infant should be turned every 2 hours to prevent pressure areas.

638. (A) Nursing process phase: assessment; client need: physiological integrity; content area: maternity nursing

Rationale
(A) Nausea and vomiting are potential signs of hypotension. (B) Headache is characteristic of hypertension or of leakage of spinal fluid after a spinal puncture. (C) Fainting is related to vasomotor liability, however, the client is positioned on her left side and will not experience fainting in this position. (D) Nosebleed correlates with hypertension. In the pregnant client, vasocongestion of the upper respiratory tract precipitates nosebleeds.

639. (A) Nursing process phase: analysis and planning; client need: physiological integrity; content area: maternity nursing

Rationale
(A) The primary focus in transition to extrauterine life is to promote an effective cardiopulmonary effort. This determines the newborn's ability to oxygenate. (B) Maintaining body temperature is secondary to effective oxygenation. (C) Placing an infant in the parent's arms is secondary to verifying adequate cardiopulmonary functioning. (D) The vitamin K injection may be delayed until after the assessment in the nursery.

640. (A) Nursing process phase: implementation; client need: physiological integrity; content area: maternity nursing

Rationale
(A) Infants who undergo passive withdrawal are prone to convulsions from CNS stimulation. This increases the risk of injury, making this intervention the priority. (B) Oral nutrition will not be provided until the risk for seizure is absent. (C) The client's physiological needs have priority over psychosocial needs. (D) Turning the infant every 2 hours is secondary to the interventions to minimize risk of injury.

641. (C) Nursing process phase: implementation; client need: physiological integrity; content area: maternity nursing

Rationale
(A) Assessing dietary intake over 24 hours is helpful because it validates the foods that the client is actually consuming and any adjustments can be made from a reality base. (B) Determining protein requirement is necessary to maintain adolescent growth as well as that of the fetus. (C) Giving the client

a pamphlet to read without assessing her learning needs or desires is most likely to be ineffective. Generally, adolescents learn better peer to peer and they prefer watching videos to reading. (D) Selecting from foods the client already likes certainly will increase the likelihood that she will continue to take in those nutrients.

642. (A) Nursing process phase: evaluation; client need: physiological integrity; content area: maternity nursing

Rationale
(A) In Rh-negative mothers who have Rh-positive partners, Rh IgG lessens the risk of maternal isoimmunization in nonsensitized mothers. (B) There is no medical reason to terminate the pregnancy at this time. (C) Intrauterine fetal blood transfusions in Rh disease are often performed when the fetus has been determined to have a low hematocrit (cord blood sampling) or hydrops is present. Although this is a well-known form of treatment for Rh disease, this maternal-fetal unit is an unlikely candidate because the mother has not had a known opportunity to develop antibodies. Rh IgG would be the more effective, prophylactic, less-invasive treatment of choice. (D) Because isoimmunization occurs more often after the third trimester, Rh is administered during the 28th gestational week.

Focus on Obstetric-Gynecological Drug Dosages

643. (C) Nursing process phase: implementation; client need: safe, effective care environment; content area: maternity nursing

Rationale
400 mg divided by 200 mg $\times$ 1 tablet = 2 tablets
Math calculation explains incorrect answers.

644. (C) Nursing process phase: implementation; client need: safe, effective care environment; content area: maternity nursing

Rationale
10 units : 1000 ml = 10 mU/min : x : 60 min = 6 ml/hr
Math calculation explains incorrect answers.

645. (A) Nursing process phase: implementation; client need: safe, effective care environment; content area: maternity nursing

Rationale
1.25 mg : 1 tablet = 0.6 mg : x = 0.5 or ½ tablet
Math calculation explains incorrect answers.

646. (D) Nursing process phase: implementation; client need: safe, effective care environment; content area: maternity nursing

Rationale
25 mg : 1 ml = 10 mg : x = 0.4 cc
Math calculation explains incorrect answers.

647. (B) Nursing process phase: implementation; client need: safe, effective care environment; content area: maternity nursing

Rationale
2 mg : 1 ml = 0.4 mg : x = 0.2 ml
Math calculation explains incorrect answers.

648. (D) Nursing process phase: implementation; client need: safe, effective care environment; content area: maternity nursing

Rationale
2.5 mg : 1 tablet = 10 mg : x = 4 tablets
Math calculation explains incorrect answers.

649. (A) Nursing process phase: implementation; client need: safe, effective care environment; content area: maternity nursing

Rationale
2 mg : tablet = 1 mg : x = ½ tablet
Math calculation explains incorrect answers.

650. (C) Nursing process phase: implementation; client need: safe, effective care environment; content area; maternity nursing

Rationale
40 mg : 1 ml = 25 mg : x = 0.6 ml
Math calculation explains incorrect answers.

651. (C) Nursing process phase: implementation; client need: safe, effective care environment; content area: maternity nursing

Rationale
20 mg : 1 ml = 25 mg : x = 1.25 ml
Math calculation explains incorrect answers.

652. (B) Nursing process phase: implementation; client need: safe, effective care environment; content area: maternity nursing

Rationale
0.2 mg : 1 ml = 0.2 mg : x = 1 ml
Math calculation explains incorrect answers.

653. (C) Nursing process phase: implementation; client need: safe, effective care environment; content area: maternity nursing

Rationale
150 mg : 500 ml = x : 1 ml = 0.3 mg
Math calculation explains incorrect answers.

654. (C) Nursing process phase: implementation; client need: safe, effective care environment; content area: maternity nursing

Rationale
0.2 mg : 1 ml = 0.25 mg : x = 1.25 ml
Math calculation explains incorrect answers.

655. (D) Nursing process phase: implementation; client need: safe, effective care environment; content area: maternity nursing

Rationale
0.5 mg : 1 tablet = 1 mg : x = 2 tablets
Math calculation explains incorrect answers.

656. (D) Nursing process phase: implementation; client need: safe, effective care environment; content area: maternity nursing

Rationale
0.5 mg : 1 tablet = 1 mg : x = 2 tablets
Math calculation explains incorrect answers.

657. (D) Nursing process phase: implementation; client need: safe, effective care environment; content area: maternity nursing

Rationale
40 mg : 1 tablet = 320 mg : x = 8 tablets
Math calculation explains incorrect answers.

658. (D) Nursing process phase: implementation; client need: safe, effective care environment; content area: maternity nursing

Rationale
200 mg : 5 ml = 400 mg : x = 10 ml
Math calculation explains incorrect answers.

659. (A) Nursing process phase: implementation; client need: safe, effective care environment; content area: maternity nursing

Rationale
400 mg : 5 ml = 375 mg : x = 5 ml
Math calculation explains incorrect answers.

660. (B) Nursing process phase: implementation; client need: safe, effective care environment; content area: maternity nursing

Rationale
5 mg : 1 tablet = 20 mg : x = 4 tablets
Math calculation explains incorrect answers.

661. (B) Nursing process phase: implementation; client need: safe, effective care environment; content area: maternity nursing

Rationale
400 mg :1 ml = 400 mg : x = 1 ml
Math calculation explains incorrect answers.

662. (C) Nursing process phase: implementation; client need: safe, effective care environment; content area: maternity nursing

Rationale
400 mg : 1 ml = 500 : x = 1.25 ml
Math calculation explains incorrect answers.

663. (B) Nursing process phase: implementation; client need: safe, effective care environment; content area: maternity nursing

Rationale
50 mg : 1 tablet = 75 mg : x = 1.5 tablets
Math calculation explains incorrect answers.

664. (D) Nursing process phase: implementation; client need: safe, effective care environment; content area: maternity nursing

Rationale
17 IU : 1 ml = 75 IU : x = 5 ml
Math calculation explains incorrect answers.

665. (D) Nursing process phase: implementation; client need: safe effective care environment; content area: maternity nursing

Rationale
2.5 mg : 1 ml = 2 mg : x = 0.8 ml
Math calculation explains incorrect answers.

666. **(D)** Nursing process phase: implementation; client need: safe, effective care environment; content area: maternity nursing

Rationale
500 μg : 2 ml = 100 μg : x = 0.4 ml
Math calculation explains incorrect answers.

667. **(D)** Nursing process phase: implementation; client need: safe, effective care environment; content area: maternity nursing

Rationale
16 mg : 1 ml = 4 mg : x = 0.25 cc
Math calculation explains incorrect answers.

668. **(C)** Nursing process phase: implementation; client need: safe, effective care environment; content area: maternity nursing

Rationale
200 mg : 1 tablet = 300 mg : x = 1.5 tablets
Math calculation explains incorrect answers.

669. **(A)** Nursing process phase: implementation; client need: safe, effective care environment; content area: maternity nursing

Rationale
100 mg : 1 ml = 50 mg : x = 0.5 ml
Math calculation explains incorrect answers.

670. **(D)** Nursing process phase: implementation; client need: safe, effective care environment; content area: maternity nursing

Rationale
5 mg : 1 tablet = 25 mg : x = 5 tablets
Math calculation explains incorrect answers.

671. **(C)** Nursing process phase: implementation; client need: safe, effective care environment; content area: maternity nursing

Rationale
200 mg : 1 tablet × 4 tablets/day × 5 days = 20 tablets
Math calculation explains incorrect answers.

672. **(D)** Nursing process phase: implementation; client need: safe, effective care environment; content area: maternity nursing

Rationale
500 mg : 5 ml = 250 mg : x = 2.5 ml
Math calculation explains incorrect answers.

673. **(C)** Nursing process phase: implementation; client need: safe, effective care environment; content area: maternity nursing

Rationale
100,000 units : 1 ml = 400,000 units : x = 4 ml
Math calculation explains incorrect answers.

674. **(D)** Nursing process phase: implementation; client need: safe, effective care environment; content area: maternity nursing

Rationale
100 mg : 2.5 ml = 250 mg : x = 6.25 ml
Math calculation explains incorrect answers.

675. **(B)** Nursing process phase: implementation; client need: safe, effective care environment; content area: maternity nursing

Rationale
600,000 units : 1 ml = 2,400,000 units : x = 4 ml
Math calculation explains incorrect answers.

676. **(B)** Nursing process phase: implementation; client need: safe, effective care environment; content area: maternity nursing

Rationale
100 mg : 1 tablet = 200 mg : x = 2 tablets
Math calculation explains incorrect answers.

677. **(C)** Nursing process phase: implementation; client need: safe, effective care environment; content area: maternity nursing

Rationale
4 mg : 1 ml = 12 mg : x = 3 ml
Math calculation explains incorrect answers.

678. **(B)** Nursing process phase: implementation; client need: safe, effective care environment; content area: maternity nursing

Rationale
50 ml divided by 30 minutes × 10 gtts/min = 16 gtt/min
Math calculation explains incorrect answers.

679. **(C)** Nursing process phase: implementation; client need: safe, effective care environment; content area: maternity nursing

Rationale
300 mg : 1 ml = 450 mg : x = 1.5 ml
Math calculation explains incorrect answers.

680. **(C)** Nursing process phase: implementation; client need: safe, effective care environment; content area: maternity nursing

Rationale
0.25 mg : 1 ml = 0.5 mg : x = 2 ml
Math calculation explains incorrect answers.

681. **(D)** Nursing process phase: implementation; client need: safe, effective care environment; content area: maternity nursing

Rationale
4 gms divided by 50 gms × 100 ml = 8 ml
Math calculation explains incorrect answers.

682. **(B)** Nursing process phase: implementation; client need: safe, effective care environment; content area: maternity nursing

Rationale
2 mg : 1 ml = 0.5 mg : x = 0.25 ml
Math calculation explains incorrect answers.

683. **(C)** Nursing process phase: implementation; client need: safe, effective care environment; content area: maternity nursing

Rationale
10,000 units : 1 ml = 7,500 units : x = 0.75 ml
Math calculation explains incorrect answers.

684. (C) Nursing process phase: implementation; client
need: safe, effective care environment; content area:
maternity nursing

Rationale
10 mg : 1 tablet = 15 mg : x = 1.5 tablets
Math calculation explains incorrect answers.

685. (A) Nursing process phase: implementation; client
need: safe, effective care environment; content area:
maternity nursing

Rationale
100 units : 1 ml = 10 units : x = 0.1 ml
Math calculation explains incorrect answers.

686. (C) Nursing process phase: implementation; client
need: safe, effective care environment; content area:
maternity nursing

Rationale
10 mg : 0.5 ml = x : 1 ml = 20 mg
Math calculation explains incorrect answers.

687. (B) Nursing process phase: implementation; client
need: safe, effective care environment; content area:
maternity nursing

Rationale
300 mg : 1 tablet = 600 mg : x = 2 tablets
Math calculation explains incorrect answers.

688. (D) Nursing process phase: implementation; client
need: safe, effective care environment; content area: maternity nursing

Rationale
80 mg : 1 ml = 40 mg : x = 0.5 ml
Math calculation explains incorrect answers.

689. (B) Nursing process phase: implementation; client
need: safe, effective care environment; content area:
maternity nursing

Rationale
25 mg : 5 ml = 100 mg : x = 20 ml
Math calculation explains incorrect answers.

690. (D) Nursing process phase: implementation; client
need: safe, effective care environment; content area: maternity nursing

Rationale
1 mg : 1 ml = 2 mg : x = 2 ml
Math calculation explains incorrect answers.

691. (B) Nursing process phase: implementation; client
need: safe, effective care environment; content area:
maternity nursing

Rationale
1 mg : 1 ml = 0.4 mg : x = 0.4 ml
Math calculation explains incorrect answers.

692. (C) Nursing process phase: implementation; client
need: safe, effective care environment; content area:
maternity nursing

Rationale
10 mg : 1 ml = 15 mg : x = 1.5 ml
Math calculation explains incorrect answers.

693. (C) Nursing process phase: implementation; client
need: safe, effective care environment; content area:
maternity nursing

Rationale
1.5 mg : 1 ml = 0.5 mg : x = 0.3 ml
Math calculation explains incorrect answers.

694. (B) Nursing process phase: implementation; client
need: safe, effective care environment; content area:
maternity nursing

Rationale
250 mg : 1 ml = 100 mg : x = 0.4 ml
Math calculation explains incorrect answers.

695. (A) Nursing process phase: implementation; client
need: safe, effective care environment; content area:
maternity nursing

Rationale
1 mg : 1 tablet = 0.5 mg : x = ½ tablet
Math calculation explains incorrect answers.

chapter5

Pediatric Nursing Q & A

*by Rebecca Hall Cagle, Lola J. Case,
Donna J. Middaugh, Susan K. Pryor,
Susan I. Ray, Kathy A. Viator,
and Golden Tradewell*

1. A 1-day-old newborn of average gestational age is hospitalized in the well-baby nursery. Which of the following vital sign parameters is most important to report to the physician?
   A. Apical pulse 118 to 148 beats per minute
   B. Respirations 48 to 52 breaths per minute
   C. Axillary temperature 97.9°F to 98.1°F
   D. Blood pressure 65/41 (upper extremity) and 56/36 (lower extremity)

2. Which of the following explanations by the nurse is most accurate regarding the reason not to defrost frozen breast milk in the microwave?
   A. High-temperature microwaving significantly destroys the anti-infective factors.
   B. The baby can be burned by the hot breast milk.
   C. The glass container may explode from the heat.
   D. The warm milk may cause indigestion in the newborn.

3. The nurse is careful to fold the diaper down to lie below the level of the clamped umbilical cord. What is the correct reason for this action?
   A. To prevent infection at the cord site
   B. To prevent pain at the cord site
   C. To facilitate the dry gangrene process to <7 days
   D. To avoid irritation and prevent wetness on the cord site

4. Soft tissue trauma to the head of a newborn may be evident at birth or not evident until later. Which of the following signs would indicate caput succedaneum?
   A. An accumulation of serum and blood in the tissue, covering several bones and covered with petechiae
   B. Bilateral swelling over the parietal bones that was present minimally at birth and worsened by the second day
   C. Sunken fontanelles anteriorly and posteriorly with overlapping suture lines
   D. A sharply delineated swelling over the occipital bone, first evident at the third day

5. The nurse should monitor the results of which of the following laboratory tests in the client of average gestational age (AGA), who is breastfed and has multiple bruises from a forceps delivery?
   A. Blood glucose
   B. Bilirubin
   C. PKU
   D. WBC

6. The 2-day-old client has lesions that are 2 mm, white pustules on a reddened base. The physician documented erythema toxicum neonatorum on the chart. Which of the following is the best explanation to the mother by the nurse?
   A. It is a candidiasis infection commonly called "thrush."
   B. It is a benign, self-limiting rash commonly called "newborn rash."
   C. It is similar to acne in an adult and needs a mild antibiotic cream to avoid scarring.
   D. It may be indicative of a viral, bacterial, or fungal rash, and culture will be needed to confirm.

7. The client is an 8-hour-old newborn with O+ blood. Admission vital signs are stable. Which of the following laboratory reports indicates a worsening of a client's condition?
   A. Blood glucose of 80 mg/dl
   B. Serum calcium of 9 mg/dl
   C. Unconjugated bilirubin of 15 mg/dl
   D. Direct Coombs' test (negative)

170

8. What is the purpose of covering the genitals of an infant under phototherapy with a bikini diaper made from a face mask?
   A. To prevent burning of the genitals
   B. To prevent gonadal complications
   C. To protect the skin from diarrhea
   D. To measure urine output

9. Which of the following statements by the mother of an 8-month-old indicates a need for further teaching?
   A. "I should avoid regular, adult canned foods for the baby to prevent possible exposure to lead."
   B. "I should use fresh, home-prepared foods for the infant as much as possible."
   C. "I can use frozen, home-prepared foods for the infant."
   D. "I can add honey or corn syrup to food to increase the infant's acceptance of it."

10. Which of the following statements by the nurse is most accurate when teaching the 6-month-old client's mother about infant nutrition?
    A. Introduce combination rice-fruit cereals first along with formula.
    B. Begin whole milk with solid foods.
    C. Large quantities of fruit juices can be used between feedings.
    D. Breast milk and/or formula should continue as the primary source of nutrition.

11. Because of the client's history of being born prematurely, which of the following nursing measures is important in administration of childhood immunizations to the hospitalized infant of 2 months?
    A. Administer only half-doses until age 1.
    B. Immunization schedule should be adjusted based on the number of weeks the client was premature.
    C. Give oral polio vaccine (OPV) only while still in the nursery.
    D. Initiate at the appropriate, actual chronological age.

12. In determining the proper location to initiate chest compressions on an infant, which is the best technique for the nurse to use?
    A. Place the heel of one hand next to the index finger placed over the notch on the sternum.
    B. Place two hands next to the index finger placed over the notch in the sternum.
    C. Place two to three fingers on the sternum 1 finger's width below the imaginary line between the nipples.
    D. Place the middle finger only over the sternum 1 finger's width above the notch on the sternum.

13. Because of the possibility of mild local side effects from the DPT injection, the nurse should administer the medication using which technique?

A. Subcutaneously in the deltoid area
B. Deep intramuscular in the vastus lateralis or ventrogluteal
C. Using an air lock and a new sterile needle
D. After application of a topical anesthetic EMLA

14. Which of the following activities by the mother of an infant would indicate a need for additional teaching?
    A. Testing the warmed formula on the inner wrist
    B. Testing the warmed formula on her own tongue
    C. Testing the warmed formula on the top of her hand
    D. Providing formula cool to the touch

15. The nurse would expect to find which of the following cardinal symptoms in an infant with colic?
    A. A duration of crying >3 hours/day with drawing up of the legs
    B. A history of projectile vomiting and diarrhea
    C. Formula intolerance and weight loss
    D. Only late night, loud crying and fussiness

16. In determining the correct placement for the apnea monitor electrode, the nurse should conduct which measurements?
    A. Place the electrode 2 fingerwidths below the left nipple at the midaxillary line.
    B. Place the electrode midway between the nipples.
    C. Place the electrode 2 fingerwidths below the left nipple at the midclavicular line.
    D. Place the electrode 1 fingerwidth below the imaginary line between the nipples.

17. Which of the following explanations by the nurse would be most accurate regarding SIDS?
    A. A higher percentage of girls are affected.
    B. The peak time of year is fall (November).
    C. The time of death is typically during sleep in a supine position.
    D. The peak age is 2 to 4 months, with 95 percent occurring within the first 6 months.

18. Which of the following statements would indicate that the client had adequate teaching regarding use of baby powder?
    A. All forms of baby powder should be avoided in the diaper area.
    B. The powder should be placed in the hand to then apply to the diaper area.
    C. Talc powder is safer than corn starch products.
    D. Powder does not help to keep the skin dry.

19. The physician has ordered topical corticosteroids for a client's atopic dermatitis. The nurse correctly identifies the purpose of applying topical corticosteroids to atopic dermatitis is:
    A. To dry the area
    B. To moisten the area
    C. To decrease inflammation
    D. To decrease pruritus

20. Which of the following approaches by the nurse toward the physical examination of the toddler is best?
    A. Complete as much as possible while the toddler is in the parent's lap.
    B. Begin with the rectal temp to "get the worst over with first."
    C. Ask the parent to leave the room before initiating the examination.
    D. Never perform the complete physical, only the area of chief complaint.

21. The nurse explains to a mother the purpose of waiting until 18 to 24 months to initiate toilet training for her infant as:
    A. The toddler is not psychologically ready until that age.
    B. The toddler is not physiologically ready until that age.
    C. The toddler is not psychologically or physiologically ready until that age.
    D. The toddler is not able to hold urine for a full hour until that time.

22. Which of the following physical examination procedures would the nurse expect to save until toward the end of the examination of a toddler?
    A. Otoscopic examination of the ears
    B. Auscultation of the lungs
    C. Pulse, temperature, and respiration
    D. Percussion of the abdomen

23. Which of the following statements by the nurse is most accurate in teaching about the typical play behavior of a toddler?
    A. They prefer solitary play.
    B. They prefer parallel play.
    C. They prefer associative play.
    D. They prefer team sports.

24. The nurse is explaining basic car safety to a class of parents. What is the meaning of the "rule of fours" in regard to child safety seats?
    A. The child must be 4 years old to be restrained in the regular restraint system.
    B. The child must be 4 feet tall to be restrained in the regular restraint system.
    C. The child must be 40 inches or 40 pounds to be restrained in the regular restraint system.
    D. The child must be traveling less than 4 miles to be restrained in a regular restraint system.

25. To promote optimal health for the deciduous teeth, the nurse should instruct the parents in which dental care techniques for their preschooler?
    A. Don't worry about the baby teeth, begin brushing with permanent ones.
    B. Take the child for yearly dental examinations once school starts.
    C. Supervise brushing and assist with flossing throughout the preschool years.
    D. Allow the child to assume self-care for brushing and flossing.

26. Which one of the following families needs instruction in possibly using unfluorinated bottled water to reduce fluorine intake?
    A. An exclusively breastfed infant
    B. A child with no fluoride in the drinking water
    C. A child who drinks formula mixed with fluorinated well water
    D. A child who drinks formula made from tap water from a city water system

27. Which approach by the nurse is best in obtaining a health history of a 13-year-old girl?
    A. Direct all questions to the mother.
    B. Direct all questions to the child.
    C. Allow the parent to stay in the room to decrease the child's fear.
    D. Question the mother and child together and separately.

28. Which of the following explanations of the sociogram is the most accurate?
    A. It is a technique of drawing circles to signify the important people in one's life and is appropriate for ages 5 years and older.
    B. It is a form of family Apgar that measures adaptation, partnership, growth, affection, and resolve.
    C. It is a family-doing-something picture that describes the client's perspective of family.
    D. It is exactly the same as a genogram, which is used to diagrammatically record a family medical history.

29. The nurse explains to a mother that in which of the following moral development stages identified by Kohlberg does the child first begin to be concerned with conformity?
    A. Stage 1, the punishment obedience orientation
    B. Stage 2, the instrumental relativist orientation
    C. Stage 3, the interpersonal concordance orientation
    D. Stage 4, the law-and-order orientation

30. Which of the following notations is more accurate for the nurse to chart on a child who is lying quietly in bed watching television yet who states his pain is a 4 on a scale of 1 to 5?
    A. Client rates pain a 4 on the scale of 1 to 5.
    B. Client rates pain incorrectly on the scale for pain.
    C. Client resting quietly without pain.
    D. Client is faking pain.

31. Assessment of pain is subjective to the degree that it is what the client says it is; however, pain rating scales may be used in clients beginning at which age?
    A. 1 year old
    B. 2 years old
    C. 3 years old
    D. 4 years old

32. The nurse correctly identifies that the most common of the opiate-induced side effects in a child is:
    A. Constipation
    B. Respiratory depression
    C. Nausea and vomiting
    D. Anaphylaxis

33. Because of the possibility of air entering the pleural cavity after removal of a chest tube in a 3-year-old after surgery, the nurse would have which supply available?
    A. A Telfa dressing
    B. A petrolatum-covered gauze
    C. An elastic (Ace) bandage
    D. An adhesive bandage (Band-Aid)

34. Which of the following nursing interventions would best monitor fluid levels in an immediately postoperative child who had undergone cardiac surgery?
    A. Strictly measuring the intake of all oral fluids and urine output every shift
    B. Strictly measuring the intake of all oral and IV fluids and urine output hourly via Foley catheter
    C. Asking the parents to count all diapers used and bottles given
    D. Restrict all fluids and place the child on the bedpan hourly

35. Which of the following signs in a pediatric client would indicate to the nurse that the client's condition is worsening and renal failure may be present?
    A. Less than 1 ml/kg per hour of urine output
    B. Decreased blood urea nitrogen (BUN) levels
    C. Decreased serum creatinine levels
    D. Fewer (<6) wet diapers per day

36. To prevent accidental overdosage of digoxin in the child, the nurse should carefully calculate and question any one dosage greater than which amount?
    A. 1 teaspoon (tsp)
    B. 25 micrograms (μg)
    C. 0.025 milligrams (mg)
    D. 1 milliliter (ml)

37. Which of the following statements by the mother indicates the need for further teaching about the administration of digoxin to her infant?
    A. "If my child vomits, I should not give a second dose."
    B. "I can place the medication in a small amount of milk."
    C. "I should administer the medication slowly to the side and back of the mouth."
    D. "If I forget a dose and only 3 hours has passed since the scheduled time, I should give the medication."

38. To promote optimal respirations and maximum chest expansion, the nurse places the infant with cardiovascular disease in which position?
    A. Supine
    B. Side-lying
    C. Prone with the head down
    D. With head of the bed up 45 degrees

39. Which of the following explanations is best, regarding the implications of findings of a hyperoxia test in a cyanotic newborn?
    A. In a 100% oxygen environment, an arterial oxygen pressure (PaO_2) of less than 100 mm Hg suggests cardiac disease.
    B. In a 100% oxygen environment, a PaO_2 of less than 100 mm Hg suggests respiratory disease.
    C. In a 100% oxygen environment, a PaO_2 of less than 100 mm Hg suggests metabolic disease
    D. In a 100% oxygen environment, a PaO_2 of less than 100 mm Hg suggests hematologic disease

40. The nurse should teach the family and child at risk for hyperlipidemia and hypercholesterolemia that the diet should include which of the following substitutes?
    A. Red meat
    B. Hot dogs
    C. Turkey
    D. Regular milk

41. Which of the following explanations of the etiology secondary hypertension (HTN) in children is most accurate?
    A. It is caused by renal disease.
    B. It is caused by cardiovascular disease.
    C. It is caused by endocrine disorders.
    D. It is caused by neurological disorders.

42. The nurse would expect to find the greatest evidence of cyanosis in a child with which cardiovascular condition?
    A. A defect of decreased pulmonary flow like tricuspid atresia
    B. An obstructive defect like coarctation of the aorta
    C. A defect of increased pulmonary blood flow like atrioventricular canal defect
    D. A mixed defect like transposition of the great vessels (TGV) with a large patent ductus arteriosus (PDA)

43. The nurse would expect to find which of the following clients on the hospital unit for clients with increased pulmonary blood flow defects?
    A. A 3-month-old with coarctation of the aorta
    B. A 4-year-old with aortic stenosis
    C. A newborn with pulmonic stenosis
    D. A 3-week-old with an atrial septal defect

44. The nurse would expect to first find which of the following in a child experiencing the acute phase of Kawasaki disease (KD)?
    A. Reddened, bulbar conjuctiva with dry eyes
    B. Cracked lips and a strawberry tongue
    C. A vesicular rash accentuated in the perineum

D. An abrupt onset of high fever unresponsive to antipyretics or antibiotics

45. The nurse correctly identifies that the purpose of giving the client with KD aspirin for 6 to 8 weeks is:
    A. To prevent the fever from returning
    B. To control the associated pain
    C. To serve as an antiplatelet agent
    D. To decrease inflammation

46. Which of the following statements would indicate that the parent of a child with a newly applied cast needs further instructions?
    A. "I should allow the cast to air-dry."
    B. "I should use my fingertips to handle the cast."
    C. "I should check distal extremities for temperature and color."
    D. "I should keep the affected extremity elevated."

47. Which of the following traction procedures might a nurse expect to use to prepare a client with a fractured humerus?
    A. Dunlop traction
    B. Bryant's traction
    C. Buck's extension traction
    D. Russell traction

48. To prevent trauma and complications, the nurse may not release which type of traction?
    A. Skeletal
    B. Skin
    C. Cervical (non-Crutchfield)
    D. Buck's

49. Because of the possibility of pulmonary emboli in an adolescent with multiple long-bone fractures, the nurse would have which of the following supplies readily accessible for initial treatment?
    A. Oxygen
    B. Heparin
    C. Corticosteroids
    D. IV fluids

50. Which of the following approaches by the nurse is best for the immediate treatment of a common grade II muscle strain?
    A. Rest, heat, cast, and elevation
    B. Range of motion (ROM) check, iodine, warm compress, and elastic bandage
    C. Restriction, heat, crutches, and exercise
    D. Rest, ice, compression, and elevation

51. To prevent sports injuries, the nurse should recommend which one of the following sports as less likely to produce an injury?
    A. Football
    B. Gymnastics
    C. Running
    D. Golf

52. With which of the following physical activities in which girls participate would the nurse be the least concerned about delayed menarche?
    A. Swimming
    B. Figure skating
    C. Running
    D. Ballet dancing

53. Which of the following explanations about scoliosis by the nurse would be most accurate?
    A. It is an abnormal increase in the convex curvature of the thoracic spine.
    B. It is an accentuated curvature of the lumbar spine.
    C. It is a spinal deformation involving lateral curvature.
    D. It is the forward slipping of a vertebra onto another.

54. Which of the following approaches by the nurse is best in assessing for the presence of hip dislocation in the newborn?
    A. An Allis test
    B. An Ortolani's maneuver
    C. The bulge sign
    D. The Phalen's maneuver

55. Because of the tendency for this condition to occur and be insignificant, the nurse is *most* likely to notify the physician of which of the following musculoskeletal findings?
    A. The appearance of pes planus in a 2-year-old
    B. The appearance of pronation in a 15-month-old
    C. The appearance of genu varum (less than 2.0 cm) between the knees in a 13-month-old
    D. The appearance of genu valgum (greater than 3.0 cm) between the medial malleoli in a 3-year-old

56. Which of the following diagnostic tests provides definitive diagnosis for juvenile rheumatoid arthritis (JRA)?
    A. Sedimentation (sed rate) rate elevation
    B. The positive latex fixation test
    C. Antinuclear antibodies (ANA) positive
    D. Clinical exclusion of other similar conditions

57. Because of the usual presenting signs and symptoms in a client with osteogenesis imperfecta (OI), the nurse should provide nonjudgmental support and realize that OI is often confused with what occurrence?
    A. Hemophilia
    B. Child abuse
    C. JRA
    D. Sprains

58. When assessing a child, which of the following information is more reliable in determining if a child has a fracture?
    A. The child will not be able to move a broken extremity.
    B. The child who refuses to walk should be strongly suspected of having a fracture.
    C. Radiological examination with a comparison film of the unaffected extremity is diagnostic.

D. If bruising and swelling are present, it is soft-tissue trauma only.

59. Which of the following information is most important in promoting hydration in a client with a fever and upper respiratory infection?
  A. Oral rehydration solutions such as Pedialyte should be considered for infants.
  B. Sports drinks such as Gatorade should be considered for children.
  C. Parents should be encouraged to measure all intake and output.
  D. Liquids should not be forced or the child awakened for fluids.

60. Which of the following procedures would the nurse expect to prepare for a client with acute otitis media?
  A. Otoscopic examination with possible tympanometry
  B. A complete blood count (CBC) with differential
  C. A culture of the external auditory canal
  D. X-rays of the face and skull

61. Which of the following rationales is the correct reason for the nursing action of not observing the posterior pharynx of a client with excessive agitation, drooling, and absence of a cough reflex?
  A. It would only upset a frightened child.
  B. The signs and symptoms are diagnostic.
  C. Only a throat culture is needed.
  D. It may totally occlude the airway.

62. The nurse would expect to find which of the following in a client experiencing acute group A β-hemolytic streptococci infection of the throat and tonsils?
  A. A gradual onset of headache, fever, and abdominal pain
  B. Red throat with posterior pharynx drainage
  C. Inflamed tonsils with exudate
  D. Post auricular lymphadenopathy

63. Which of the following is the first early response for the child with an impending airway obstruction?
  A. Decreasing pulse and respirations
  B. Substernal, suprasternal, and intercostal retractions
  C. Decreasing responsiveness
  D. Nasal congestion and drainage

64. Which of the following statements by the nurse is most accurate when teaching the client about asthma?
  A. It is an irreversible airway obstruction.
  B. It is a reversible airway obstruction.
  C. It is more prevalent in boys than girls.
  D. It has usually an onset at 4 to 5 years of age.

65. The nurse correctly identifies the purpose of giving an asthmatic client a β-2 agonist as:
  A. To decrease inflammation
  B. To assist in smooth-muscle relaxation

C. To block reflex bronchial constriction
D. To provide nonsteroidal anti-inflammatory benefits

66. The nurse correctly identifies the purpose of giving the client with asthma a corticosteroid as:
  A. The anti-inflammatory effects
  B. To decrease bronchospasms
  C. To prevent infection
  D. To provide nonsteroidal properties

67. Which of the following diagnostic tests is commonly used to measure the asthmatic client's greatest flow velocity during an acute asthmatic attack?
  A. Peak expiratory flow rate (PEFR)
  B. Arterial blood gases (ABGs)
  C. Peripheral oxygen saturation (SaO_2)
  D. Auscultation of anterior and posterior lung fields

68. Which of the following statements is more accurate regarding respirations throughout the lifetime?
  A. Respirations slow and become more abdominal.
  B. Respirations increase and become more abdominal.
  C. Respirations slow and become more thoracic.
  D. Respirations increase and become more thoracic.

69. In preparing to teach the client about using a metered-dose inhaler, the nurse would include which of the following in the plan of care?
  A. The canister should not be shaken before use.
  B. Two quick inspirations should occur as the top of the canister is mashed.
  C. The breath should be held for 5 to 10 seconds after medication is instilled.
  D. A full canister will float sideways on the surface.

70. The nurse should teach the client with any type of upper respiratory infection (URIs) which of the following?
  A. Allergies cause many URIs, and shots are always indicated.
  B. Prevention of attacks is not possible.
  C. Children will outgrow URIs.
  D. Avoid active and passive smoking.

71. Which of the following statements would indicate that the teenage client needs further instructions?
  A. "I should not share my nose spray with anyone else."
  B. "I should use my spray only as directed."
  C. "I can save the nose spray for my own personal use with subsequent infections."
  D. "I should not use the spray for more than three consecutive days."

72. Which of the following *observations* would indicate that the client in the immediate postoperative

5-10

period after tonsillectomy and adenoidectomy (T&A) was *worsening*?
A. Frequent swallowing
B. Complaints of moderate pain
C. Pulse of 100 to 110
D. Dark brown blood in the emesis

73. The nurse correctly identifies which of the following as usually the earliest detectable sign of dehydration?
A. Tachycardia
B. Dry skin and mucous membranes
C. Sunken fontanelles
D. Delayed capillary refill

74. Which of the following isotonic IV fluids would the nurse expect to prepare for a dehydrated client?
A. 5% dextrose in water or 0.9% normal saline
B. Lactated Ringer's or dextrose solution ½ NS
C. D5W or saline solution ½ NS
D. 0.9% NS or LR

75. Which of the following statements by the nurse is most accurate when teaching the parents of a dehydrated child about replacement fluids?
A. Any cola or juice is considered a clear liquid.
B. Diluted formula is considered clear liquid.
C. Water is the only true clear liquid.
D. Clear fluid is one through which newsprint can be read.

76. In selecting a site to place the IV in a child, which of the following considerations is most important?
A. Development, cognitive, and mobility needs of the client
B. Nurse's preference and experience with the site
C. The ability not to have to disrupt other structures (hair)
D. The ability to secure the IV with a transparent dressing

77. Which of the following commonly used nursing actions best determines the amount of urine and stool excreted by a hospitalized infant in diapers?
A. An external collection bag to measure exact milliliters
B. Counting the number of soiled diapers per day
C. Weighing the diapers and subtracting a dry diaper weight (1 gm = 1 cc lost)
D. An internal Foley catheter measured hourly

78. Which of the following interventions is the first therapeutic management approach in the treatment of mild acute diarrhea in the pediatric client?
A. Parenteral fluids
B. Oral rehydration therapy (ORT)
C. A BRAT diet (bananas, rice, applesauce, toast, and tea)
D. Antidiarrheal agents

79. Which of the following nursing interventions would best provide the daily maintenance fluid requirements for a child weighing 25 kg?
A. 100 ml/kg per day
B. 1000 ml/kg plus 50 ml/kg for each kilogram over 10 kg
C. 500 ml/kg plus 20 ml/kg for each kilogram over 15 kg
D. 1500 ml/kg plus 20 ml/kg for each kilogram over 20 kg

80. Which of the following laboratory reports indicates that the client may have partially compensated respiratory acidosis?
A. Plasma pH decreased, plasma PO_2 increased, and plasma HCO_3 increased
B. Plasma pH increased, plasma PO_2 decreased, and plasma HCO_3 decreased
C. Plasma pH decreased, plasma PO_2 decreased and plasma HCO_3 decreased
D. Plasma pH increased, plasma PO_2 increased and plasma HCO_3 increased

81. Because of the 8-year-old's history of an abrupt onset of symptoms (within 4 to 6 hours) after eating at a community picnic, the nurse anticipates which of the following organisms as causing the onset of the acute diarrhea?
A. Salmonella
B. Norwalklike organisms
C. *Clostridium botulinum*
D. Staphylococcus

82. The nurse would expect to find which of the following in a client experiencing a first-degree burn?
A. Blisters
B. Pain
C. Waxy white or brown skin
D. Dull and dry wounds

83. Which of the following statements would indicate the need for further teaching in the emergency treatment of minor burns?"
A. "I should *not* apply butter."
B. "I should *not* rupture the blisters."
C. "I should immediately apply a loose gauze dressing."
D. "I should run cool water over the area."

84. In preparing to apply a topical preparation over a burn, the nurse would question the application of which agent to a child allergic to sulfa?
A. Silver nitrate
B. Silver sulfadiazine (Silvadene)
C. Povidone-iodine (Betadine)
D. Bacitracin

85. To increase the infant's resistance to infection, the nurse should provide which of the following information to the mother on feeding?
A. Promote breastfeeding for the first year of life through objective information.

B. Remain entirely neutral—offer no information to the mother on breast or bottle.
C. Provide written informational packets only and ask for the mother's decision.
D. Take the infant a bottle, and if the mother wants to use it, she can.

86. In general to promote adequate nutrition throughout puberty, it is best to encourage the increase of which of the following foods?
A. Calcium, zinc, protein, and iron
B. Calcium, fat, vitamin C, and folic acid
C. Calcium, zinc, B complex vitamins, and folate
D. Calcium, carbohydrate, protein, and vitamin C

87. The nurse would expect to find which of the following nail manifestations in a teenager with iron deficiency anemia?
A. Smooth, pink nails
B. Brittle or spoon-shaped nails
C. Splinter hemorrhages
D. Beau's lines

88. Which of the following information is most accurate to teach parents in regard to nutrition for toddlers?
A. A rigid schedule of meals and snacks should be provided.
B. The toddler should sit and eat every entire meal with the family.
C. Skim milk or low-fat milk may be used.
D. In general, 1 tablespoon of solid food per year of age per serving.

89. Which of the following questions is most important to ask the mother of a 4-year-old with uncomplicated erythema infectiosum (fifth disease)?
A. Has she ever had it before?
B. Does she take her child to daycare?
C. Is she pregnant now?
D. Will she be able to isolate the child at home?

90. In a 6-year-old client with iron deficiency anemia, the nurse should observe the laboratory values for which of the following abnormal findings?
A. Mean corpuscular volume (MCV), 79 μm^3
B. Mean corpuscular hemoglobin concentration (MCHC), 35 percent hemoglobin(Hb)/cell
C. Hematocrit (HCT), 30 percent
D. Hemoglobin (Hgb), 11.5 gms/dl

91. The nurse identifies which of the following organisms as the agent leading to scarlet fever in a child?
A. *Bordetella pertussis*
B. Enteroviruses
C. Rubella virus
D. Group B hemolytic streptococci

92. Which of the following parent statements indicates a proper understanding of when the child with chickenpox may return to school?
A. When vesicles have dried
B. When crusts have fallen off
C. When new lesions have stopped appearing
D. When 7 days have passed since the first vesicle appeared

93. The nurse would expect to find which of the following on the first day of a child experiencing scarlet fever?
A. A red strawberry tongue
B. Flushed cheeks
C. Positive Schultz-Charlton test
D. Increased rash density in axilla

94. What is the purpose of applying lotions such as calamine (Caladryl) sparingly over open lesions?
A. Excessive absorption may lead to toxicity.
B. It prevents the oatmeal baths from being soothing.
C. It keeps the area moist and prevents crusting.
D. It prolongs the period of outbreak.

95. Which of the following medications should be avoided in a healthy child with varicella?
A. Aspirin
B. Acyclovir
C. Acetaminophen (Tylenol)
D. Diphenhydramine (Benadryl)

96. Which of the following parental statements indicates accurate knowledge of bacterial conjunctivitis's clinical manifestations?
A. Eyes are itchy with inflamed conjuctiva and watery discharge bilaterally
B. Unilateral pain, tearing, and inflamed conjuctiva
C. Severe photophobia and subconjunctival bleeding bilaterally
D. Purulent drainage with early-morning crusting bilaterally

97. Which of the following tests is the most common in diagnosing pinworms in the child?
A. A rectal swab and culture
B. The tape test
C. A skin scraping
D. A stool specimen

98. The nurse would monitor the results of which of the following since the client has plumbism (lead poisoning) and is receiving edetate calcium disodium chelation therapy?
A. CBCs
B. Serum lead levels
C. Urine output
D. HCT and Hgb

99. Which of the following information would be most important to remember in assessing a child with poisoning?
A. Determine any allergies to medications
B. Determine what was taken and any treatments initiated by parents
C. Give ipecac before activated charcoal

D. Place sweetener in the activated charcoal to improve palatability

100. Which of the following nursing actions would be best when documenting a child's allegations of sexual abuse?
A. Use exact quotes verbatim.
B. Use summary statements for clarification.
C. Do not document anything but objective data.
D. Use only closed-ended questions to ease the use of a flow sheet.

101. Which of the following statements would indicate that the parent of a school-aged child needs further instructions on bike safety?
A. A safety helmet should always be worn.
B. The child should be able to place both feet flat when straddling the bar.
C. The child should be able to touch the tiptoes to the ground when on the seat.
D. The child should be carefully supervised while riding between 4 and 8 P.M. as most accidents occur at that time.

102. Because of the child's need for conformity during the school-age years, play is often influenced by which dominant concept.
A. Rigid rules
B. Physical skill
C. Intellectual expansion
D. Fantasy

103. Which of the following information would be important in developing play therapy for a 7-year-old?
A. Girls prefer to play with boys
B. Boys prefer to play with girls
C. Each prefers mixed-group play
D. Boys prefer to play with boys and girls with girls

104. The nurse should observe the hospitalized school-age child for common sleep problems, which include:
A. Night terrors
B. Nightmares
C. Sleep walking and talking
D. Enuresis

105. The nurse should be careful to assess a child brought to the ER with an in-line skate injury for which condition?
A. Ankle sprains
B. Femur fractions
C. Wrist or forearm injuries
D. Skull concussions

106. Which of the following explanations by the nurse is most accurate regarding dental care of the school-aged child?
A. The child should begin regular visits to the dentist.
B. The child can expect to begin losing the deciduous teeth.

C. Teeth will appear smaller than normal because of the rapid growth of facial bones.
D. Fluoride is no longer needed because permanent teeth are already formed.

107. Which of the following words is best to describe an elevated, solid, irregular-shaped area of cutaneous edema caused by an insect bite on the leg of a 10-year-old?
A. Macule —flat
B. Wheal
C. Papule —firm like a wart
D. Vesicle—blister c fluid

108. Which of the following explanations is most accurate for describing the way in which the surgical incision from the appendectomy of a 9-year-old will heal?
A. Primary intention is the way in which wounds that are well approximated will heal with minimal scarring.
B. Secondary intention is the way in which wounds that heal from inside out close. Scarring is increased.
C. Tertiary intention is the way in which wounds that had delayed suturing heal. There is more granulation scarring.
D. Surgical wounds are fully sutured and are considered immediately healed.

109. Because of a child's diagnosis with scabies, the nurse anticipates the need to provide instruction to the family on which topic first?
A. The application of the lindane or permethrin (Elimite) cream with precautions
B. The fact that itching will continue for weeks
C. The fact that all close contacts may need to be treated
D. The proper laundering of linens and cloths for the family

110. Which of the following statements by the parent of a child indicates the need for further teaching in regard to poison ivy exposure?
A. "The oil in the plant is the offending substance."
B. "The area should be scrubbed with warm water and strong soap immediately."
C. "The rash is not spread by the fluid in the blisters leaking out."
D. "Even burning piles of poison ivy can cause a rash in some people."

111. Because sun exposure is a common problem for children, which of the following explanations is best to a parent of a child who asks what SPF 15 means on the sun block?
A. The 15 means that the child will not receive any sun damage for 15 minutes.
B. The 15 means that it must be applied 15 minutes before exposure, but it is good for all day.

C. The 15 means that it lowers skin cancer risk 15 percent.

D. The 15 means that the person can remain in the sun 15 times longer than usual before burning.

112. What is the purpose of giving the adolescent client information about injury prevention?
    A. Adolescents are accident prone and need to be safe.
    B. The primary cause of death in adolescence is unintentional injury.
    C. Homicide is the leading cause of death in all adolescents.
    D. As the adolescent expands her world and is around strangers, she is more likely to get a gunshot wound.

113. Which of the following approaches by the nurse toward a health interview with an adolescent is best?
    A. Explain that all information will be kept confidential.
    B. Ask close-ended questions to facilitate communication.
    C. Explain that most information will be kept confidential.
    D. Allow the parent to remain throughout.

114. When the nurse is assessing an adolescent boy, which of the following would indicate Tanner stage 1?
    A. No pubic hair, much like that of childhood
    B. Initial scrotal testes enlargement, straight sparse hair
    C. Initial enlargement of penis, dark curly hair over pubic area
    D. Development of the glans with increased penis diameter

115. Which of the following explanations by the nurse to the parents of adolescents aged 13 and 17 would be most accurate regarding psychological health?
    A. Expect wide mood swings and intense daydreaming in both teens.
    B. Expect the 13-year-old to be more introspective and withdrawn when feelings get hurt.
    C. Expect the 13-year-old to have feelings of inadequacy but does not ask for help.
    D. Expect the 17-year-old to maintain more consistent emotions and control anger while the 13-year-old may have outbursts of anger.

116. When assessing an adolescent girl, which of the following signs would indicate Tanner stage 3 in an adolescent girl?
    A. Breast bud stage with enlarged areolar diameter
    B. No separation of breast and areola contours
    C. Projection of areola and papilla to form a secondary mound
    D. Mature configuration

117. Because of the client's age and risk for substance abuse, which of the following items should nursing measures target to provide health teaching because of its being the most frequently abused substance by adolescents?
    A. Alcohol
    B. Cigarettes
    C. Marijuana
    D. Other drugs

118. Because of the extensiveness of severe cystic acne, the nurse should anticipate the dermatologist to order:
    A. Isotretinoin (Accutane)
    B. Tretinoin (Retin-A)
    C. Benzoyl peroxide
    D. A topical antibiotic

119. Which of the following procedures would the nurse anticipate preparing an adolescent girl with a request for a prescription contraceptive?
    A. Pelvic examination
    B. Abdominal sonogram
    C. Gonorrhea and chlamydia cultures
    D. Endometrial biopsy

120. Which of the following explanations by the nurse would be more accurate in describing how oral contraceptives work?
    A. They inhibit ovulation.
    B. They kill sperm.
    C. They prevent implantation.
    D. They trap and block sperm.

121. Which of the following adolescent client statements indicates the need for further instruction?
    A. "I may gain weight on Depo-Provera shots."
    B. "I may have irregular or no periods while on Depo-Provera."
    C. "I must return every 3 months for an injection."
    D. "I will have sexually transmitted disease (STD) protection with the Depo-Provera."

122. Which of the following statements about rape is most accurate?
    A. Male rape victims are more likely to report the incident than female victims.
    B. The typical victim is tall with seductive clothing.
    C. Rape is defined as actual penile penetration of the vagina.
    D. Half of the rape cases occur to 15- to 19-year-old females.

123. Which of the following signs and symptoms would indicate an untreated chlamydia infection in the adolescent girl?
    A. A thin, milky white, malodorous vaginal discharge
    B. Lower abdominal pain with fever and dysuria
    C. A raised, firm, flesh-colored rash on the perineum
    D. A thick, cheesy-like discharge with pruritus

124. A 6-year-old is admitted to the hospital with a fractured femur. Which one of the following techniques for assessing pain would be most effective for the nurse to use when caring for an early school-age child?
    A. Question him about his pain.
    B. Observe him for restlessness.
    C. Listen for pain clues in his cries.
    D. Consider the cause of his pain.

125. A mother brings her 18-month-old daughter to the clinic. Which of the following tasks is most typical of a normally developed 18-month-old?
    A. Copying a circle
    B. Building a tower of eight or more blocks
    C. Pulling toys behind her
    D. Playing tag with other children

126. The mother of a 21-month-old is recently divorced and is seeking employment. She brings her child to the clinic because she eats "ashes, crayons, paper—almost anything she can get into her mouth." As a possible cause, the nurse should first direct her attention to determining whether the child may possibly be:
    A. Having an inappropriate diet of too much soft, low-roughage food
    B. Suffering from a hormonal deficiency due to a genetic defect
    C. Relieving discomfort due to cutting large teeth
    D. Showing signs of anxiety due to a change in the home environment

127. The father of a normally developed 3-year-old male brings him to the clinic for a check-up in preparation for enrolling him in preschool. Which one of the following tasks can the nurse expect a child of this age to be most skilled with?
    A. Tying his shoelaces
    B. Copying a circle
    C. Identifying five body parts
    D. Hopping on one foot

128. The grandmother of a 24-month-old brings her grandson to the clinic. She tells the nurse she is having problems with toilet training. Which of the following explanations by the nurse would be most accurate?
    A. "He is not ready to be trained."
    B. "The rewards for him are too limited."
    C. "The training equipment that you are using for him is inappropriate."
    D. "He is demonstrating his own individuality."

129. A 2½-year-old is brought to the clinic for his yearly physical. The child becomes uncooperative when procedures must be performed on him. If the following courses of action are possible, which one would be best for the nurse to try first?
    A. Obtain another nurse to assist.
    B. Allow a parent to assist.
    C. Wait until the child calms down.
    D. Use restraints during the procedure.

130. The mother of a 4-year-old is being taught by the nurse how to instill eardrops. Which of the following statements by the mother would indicate understanding of the procedure?
    A. "I will pull the earlobe up and forward."
    B. "I will pull the earlobe up and backward."
    C. "I will pull the earlobe down and forward."
    D. "I will pull the earlobe down and backward."

131. The mother of a 6-week infant brings him to the clinic for his 6-week examination. She is concerned about the "soft spot near the front of his head" and wants to know when it will close. Which of the following explanations by the nurse is accurate?
    A. The anterior fontanelle closes when the infant's age is between 2 and 4 months.
    B. The anterior fontanelle closes when the infant's age is between 4 and 8 months.
    C. The anterior fontanelle closes when the infant's age is between 8 and 12 months.
    D. The anterior fontanelle closes when the infant's age is between 12 and 18 months.

132. The grandmother of a 3-year-old brings her granddaughter to the clinic because she is concerned about her nutritional status. She described that for the last week she has refused to eat anything except animal crackers and peanut butter and jelly sandwiches. Which of the following would be most appropriate for the nurse to suggest?
    A. "You need not be overly concerned because this food fad will probably only last for a short period."
    B. "You should insist that your granddaughter eat small portions of the family's meal sufficient to maintain adequate nutrition."
    C. "You need to consult a physician, because this kind of food intake will cause nutritional deficiencies."
    D. "You need to offer your granddaughter extra time to play outside if she eats what the family eats at mealtime."

133. A 2½-year-old was brought to the clinic by her father. In obtaining a history the father stated, "She is afraid of the dark and says 'No' to everything she is asked to do." The nurse, in planning care, is aware that the negativism demonstrated by this age child is frequently an expression of:
    A. Hyperactivity
    B. Sibling rivalry
    C. Separation anxiety
    D. Autonomy establishment

134. The mother of a 2-year-old asks the nurse for some suggestions on how to discipline her child. Which of the following approaches would be best for the nurse to suggest?
    A. Corporal punishment in the form of spanking to eliminate unacceptable behavior.

B. Structured interactions to prevent or minimize unacceptable behavior.
C. Reasoning and scolding to eliminate unacceptable behavior.
D. No form of discipline because the negativism demonstrated will soon pass.

135. The mother of a 2-month-old asks the nurse what is the best way to protect her infant son while riding in the car. Which one of the following statements would indicate the mother's understanding of the nurse's instruction regarding infant safety while riding in a car?
A. Infant should be lying on car seat with seat belt around infant. Best to have infant facing driver.
B. Infant seat sitting flat on car seat with infant facing driver. Seat belt around infant seat.
C. Infant seat facing forward with seat belt around infant and seat.
D. Infant seat facing rear of the car with infant facing back of car with seat belt in place.

136. The father of a 3-year-old expresses concern of his son's fear of the dark. Which of the following concepts of Piaget's theory would assist the nurse in explaining the child's fear?
A. Reversibility
B. Conservation of matter
C. Object permanence
D. Animism

137. In obtaining a history upon hospital admission, the mother describes that her 4-year-old often falls while running. In preparing to teach the mother about vision for this age child, the nurse would include which of the following in her plan of care?
A. Vision for this age child is normally myopic.
B. Vision for this age child is normally hyperopic.
C. Vision for this age child is normally presbyopic.
D. Vision for this age child is normally amblyopic.

138. The nurse is preparing to teach a community class on care of the newborn and infant. In preparing to teach the class regarding normal growth and development for this age, the nurse would include which of the following in her plan of care for the normally developed 6-month-old?
A. He should be able to drink from a cup.
B. He should have thumb-finger grasp.
C. He should be able to roll over.
D. He should be able to say "mama" or "dada" specific.

139. A 13-month-old is admitted to the pediatric day surgery unit for a bilateral tympanotomy tube insertion. In the past 7 months the child has had multiple middle ear infections that have not responded to antibiotic therapy. In obtaining a history, the nurse's initial assessment would most likely find which of the following signs and symptoms that are most characteristic of otitis media?

A. Vomiting, diarrhea, and yellow tympanic membrane
B. Pulling at the ears, earache, and gray tympanic membrane
C. Cough, irritability, and inverted tympanic membrane
D. Rhinorrhea, fever, and bulging tympanic membrane

140. The nurse practitioner prescribed amoxicillin for an 8-month-old diagnosed with acute otitis media. The primary purpose of this medication is to:
A. Shrink swollen tissues in the eustachian tube
B. Reduce the severe pain
C. Treat the probable organism, *Haemophilus influenzae*
D. Reduce the fever

141. The parents of a child being treated for acute otitis media with antibiotic therapy were instructed by the nurse to bring the child back to the clinic for a recheck after completing the medication. The purpose of the recheck is to:
A. Document that the infection was completely cleared
B. Obtain a prescription for another course of antibiotics
C. Make certain that the child had been given all of the antibiotic
D. Determine whether the ear infection had affected hearing

142. A 12-month-old was admitted to the day surgery unit for placement of tympanotomy tubes for chronic otitis media. A postoperative intervention planned by the nurse was to teach the parents to apply external heat or cool compresses and not to allow chewing by offering liquids and soft foods. Which of the following nursing diagnoses do these interventions address?
A. Potential for impairment in skin integrity related to ear drainage
B. Alteration in comfort: Pain related to the inflammatory process
C. Knowledge deficit (parents) related to unfamiliarity with the situation
D. Hyperthermia related to infectious process

143. A normal 4-year-old has been admitted to the pediatric unit for a tonsillectomy and adenoidectomy. The child asks the nurse if it will hurt to have his tonsils out. Which of the following responses would be best for the nurse to make?
A. "It will hurt, but we can give you medicine to help you feel better."
B. "It will hurt, but not that bad."
C. "It will not hurt because you're a big boy."
D. "It will hurt because of the incisions in the throat."

144. The nurse discusses the postoperative care of a 4-year-old scheduled for a tonsillectomy and adenoidectomy (T&A) with the child's mother.

Which of the following statements by the mother indicates the need for further instruction?

A. "My son can have sips of clear liquids when awake."

B. "My son should be asked to cough frequently to prevent breathing problems."

C. "My son can have something for pain if needed."

D. "My son should be kept on his abdomen or side immediately upon return from surgery."

145. The mother of a 2-month-old brings the infant to the clinic for his first series of immunizations. The nurse in preparing the diphtheria, pertussis, and tetanus (DPT) vaccine will plan to administer the vaccine using the:

A. Oral route

B. Intradermal route

C. Intramuscular route

D. Subcutaneous route

146. An 8-year-old male is being evaluated at the clinic with a medical diagnosis of Legg-Calvé-Perthes disease. In preparing to teach the boy's parents, the nurse would include which of the following in the plan of care?

A. Teaching gentle stretching exercises for both legs

B. Teaching diet planning for weight reduction

C. Teaching relaxation techniques to help control the pain

D. Teaching care and management of the corrective appliance

147. In addition to a detailed history and physical examination, which one of the following diagnostic methods would be most helpful in confirming a diagnosis of Wilms' tumor?

A. An elevated antibody level

B. Computerized tomography

C. A low hemoglobin count

D. A high leukocyte count

148. Surgery is performed on a 3-year-old male with a diagnosis of Wilms' tumor. The tumor was classified as a stage II malignancy. In planning postoperative care, the nurse is aware that the tumor:

A. Has bilateral renal involvement

B. Has extended beyond the kidney but is completely resected

C. Is limited to the kidney and is completely resected

D. Has metastasized to the lung, liver, bone, and brain

149. The nurse caring for a child postoperatively with a diagnosis of Wilms' tumor stage II is aware that the optimum treatment protocol at stage II would include:

A. Surgery, radiation, and chemotherapy

B. Surgery and radiation

C. Surgery and chemotherapy

D. Radiation and chemotherapy

150. The parents of a 3-year-old child bring him to the hospital for corrective surgery for hypospadias. Which of the following nursing interventions would not be appropriate in caring for the child preoperatively?

A. Administering muscle relaxants to the child as ordered

B. Preparing the parents and the child for possible bladder spasms

C. Explaining to the child that the condition is something he was born with and not punishment

D. Discussing with the parents the expected cosmetic results

151. A 2-month-old male is admitted for surgery because of an inguinal hernia with a communicating hydrocele. Which one of the following statements is not true concerning these congenital anomalies?

A. Hydrocele is opaque by transillumination; a hernia is translucent by transillumination.

B. Hydrocele usually cannot be reduced; a hernia is generally easily reduced.

C. Hydrocele cannot be produced by a sudden increase in intra-abdominal pressure; a hernia can be produced by a sudden increase in intra-abdominal pressure.

D. An irreducible or strangulated hernia should be evaluated by a surgeon. Surgical repair may be indicated for a communicating hydrocele if not resolved by 1 year of age.

152. The nurse has been teaching the parent of a newborn male with bladder exstrophy proper care. Which of the following statements by the parent indicates a need for further health teaching?

A. "After surgery and the baby grows he will be able to urinate normally."

B. "It will be important for me not to put him in the bath water."

C. "I should inspect the skin around the defect for any skin irritation or breakdown."

D. "It would be helpful to talk with other parents who have a child like mine."

153. A 3-year-old male is hospitalized with idiopathic nephrosis for supportive care. In addition to proteinuria, the three clinical features that he is most likely to exhibit include:

A. Hyperproteinemia, hyperlipidemia, and foamy urine

B. Hyperproteinemia, hypolipidemia, and edema

C. Hypoproteinemia, hypolipidemia, and foamy urine

D. Hypoproteinemia, hyperlipidemia, and edema

154. The nurse is preparing the parents of a child with idiopathic nephrosis for discharge. In teaching the parents how to care for him at home, the nurse should include information about how to prevent

relapses of nephrotic syndrome. Such relapses can be precipitated by:
A. Mechanical trauma
B. Emotional stress
C. Acute infections
D. Dietary restrictions

155. A 16-year-old with chronic glomerulonephritis (CGN) is being evaluated at the pediatric outpatient clinic. Which of the following laboratory findings would be indicative of deteriorating renal function?
A. Fixed specific gravity of the urine, increased BUN and creatinine
B. Fixed specific gravity of the urine, increased BUN and decreased creatinine
C. Impaired nerve conduction, increased sodium (Na), and decreased potassium (K)
D. Impaired nerve conduction, decreased Na, and increased calcium

156. A nurse caring for a hospitalized child with a diagnosis of CGN assesses that the child's blood pressure is elevated and that she has not voided in over 14 hours. Which of the following would be the most appropriate initial nursing action?
A. Encouraging her to eat a low-sodium diet
B. Encouraging her to drink more water so a urine specimen can be obtained for routine analysis
C. Assessing her neurological status
D. Assisting her to ambulate to increase her glomerular infiltration rate

157. The nurse is teaching the parents of a child with nephrotic syndrome the potential complications of steroid therapy. The nurse could evaluate the effect of teaching if the parents could repeat which of the following complications of steroid therapy?
A. Growth retardation, hypertension, and infections
B. Growth retardation, hypotension, and infections
C. Diabetes mellitus, hypotension, and gastrointestinal bleeding
D. Diabetes mellitus, hypertension and growth acceleration

158. A common symptom that the nurse would assess for in the care of a child with nephrotic syndrome would include which of the following?
A. Increase in appetite
B. Increase in constipation
C. Decrease in weight
D. Decrease in urination

159. In administering oxygen therapy to a child in respiratory difficulty, a preventive measure to be taken by the nurse in regard to the untoward effects of oxygen therapy is:
A. Padding elastic bands of the face mask
B. Taking the apical pulse before starting therapy
C. Humidifying the gas before delivery
D. Placing the client in the orthopneic position

160. The nurse is to administer the Denver Developmental Screening Test (DDST) to a 2-year-old male child. She would explain to the child's mother that the four areas to be tested with the DDST include:
A. Personal-social, fine motor, receptive-expressive, and gross motor
B. Personal-social, language, psychological, and gross motor
C. Personal-social, language, fine motor, and gross motor
D. Personal-social, gross motor, receptive-expressive, and fine motor

161. The nurse is administering the DDST to a 3-year-old child who is being evaluated for the Early Periodic Screening and Development Testing (EPSDT). When administering the test, the nurse will:
A. Praise him at the end of the test, after all items have been completed.
B. Praise him only for correct performances.
C. Praise him whether or not he correctly performs the item.
D. Ask the parent not to interfere by praising him.

162. A 2-year-old client is recovering from shunt insertion surgery to relieve hydrocephalus. One appropriate nursing diagnosis is a high risk for injury related to the rapid reduction of intracranial pressure. Which of the following would be an appropriate nursing intervention?
A. Position the child flat on the operated side.
B. Position the child on the unoperated side.
C. Position the head of the bed in semi-Fowler's (45 degrees).
D. Position the bed in the low Trendelenburg position.

163. The nurse is caring for a newborn on the pediatric unit with an unrepaired myelomeningocele. Which one of the following nursing interventions is appropriate?
A. Placing her in a supine position
B. Aspirating accumulated fluid from the defect daily
C. Providing visual stimulation at her eye level
D. Range-of-motion (ROM) exercises to lower extremities

164. A 16-year-old male is admitted to the hospital with a diagnosis of encephalitis. The nurse anticipates that his treatment will include:
A. Strict protective isolation
B. Partial exchange transfusions
C. Peritoneal or hemodialysis
D. Parenteral antibotics

165. A 3-year-old child is admitted to the pediatric unit

with a diagnosis of bacterial meningitis. Nursing interventions immediately on admission would include which of the following?
A. Provision of a private room
B. Application of restraints
C. Insertion of a Levin's tube
D. Administration of antacids

166. The nurse is preparing to teach the parents of a child with a seizure disorder about the side effects of phenytoin (Dilantin). The nurse will emphasize the importance of:
A. Restricted activity
B. Adequate rest
C. Adequate diet
D. Dental hygiene

167. An 18-year-old high school student has suffered an injury to the cervical spine. When the client is brought into the emergency room, a primary goal of nursing care would be:
A. Prevention of spinal shock
B. Provision of pain relief
C. Maintenance of orientation
D. Maintenance of respiration

168. The nurse is planning a tracking program for a 16-year-old adolescent female with type I diabetes mellitus. Which of the following factors will have the greatest influence on the success of the teaching?
A. Teaching periods limited to 1-hour blocks
B. One nurse implementing the teaching plan
C. Her parents acceptance of her diagnosis
D. The adolescent's acceptance of her diagnosis

169. An adolescent with insulin-dependent diabetes mellitus asks the nurse if she can still go with her friends to get pizza and ice cream. The most appropriate response by the nurse would be:
A. "You can have pizza if you omit a similar amount of food from your next meal. You should avoid ice cream because sweets aren't good for you."
B. "Being with your friends is important. I will teach you how to select your foods so that you can have pizza and ice cream."
C. "Both pizza and ice cream have valuable nutrients. Don't eat all of the crust."
D. "You can go with them; however, you should not eat pizza and ice cream. Your friends will learn that you can't have these things."

170. A 13-year-old female has been diagnosed with hyperthyroidism. She has been placed on propylthiouracil (PTU). The nurse explains that the therapeutic effect of the drug for her is to:
A. Reduce iodine stored in the thyroid gland
B. Depress activity of stored thyroid hormone
C. Inhibit formation of thyroxine
D. Lower metabolic rate

171. The nurse is working on an endocrine nursing unit. She has to do many finger-stick glucose checks. The most appropriate time to do the glucose checks is:
A. Bedtime
B. Midmorning and midafternoon
C. Before meals (AC)
D. After meals (PC)

172. A 15-year-old male on the pediatric unit has Cushing's disease. Which one of the following defining characteristics best describes a client with this disease?
A. External tan, moon face, buffalo hump, soft bones
B. Abdominal striae, moon face, buffalo hump, obesity
C. Anorexia, cold intolerance, moon face, buffalo hump
D. Obesity, cold intolerance, moon face, buffalo hump

173. An adolescent client is scheduled for an adrenalectomy. Which one of the following drugs is most important for this client?
A. Cortisol
B. Desoxycorticosterone (Cortate)
C. Insulin
D. Vasopression

174. An 18-year-old diabetic male has been admitted to pediatric intensive care in severe chronic renal failure (CRF). At times he is very confused and lethargic. The nurse assesses that these mental changes are primarily due to:
A. Elevated blood pH
B. Azotemia
C. Hypertension
D. Bradycardia

175. An adolescent client with severe CRF is on a restricted diet. Based on the severity of CRF, what nutrients will be restricted in the diet?
A. Fats
B. Proteins
C. Calcium
D. Carbohydrates

176. Addison's disease, however rare in children, was diagnosed in an adolescent female client. Which one of the following signs would be evident with this disease?
A. Weight gain
B. Hypertension
C. Hyperglycemia
D. Hyperpigmentation

177. A 14-year-old client with hyperthyroidism had a subtotal thyroidectomy. In the immediate postoperative period, the nurse assesses for laryngeal nerve damage. Which one of the following assessment findings indicates laryngeal nerve damage?
A. Hoarseness
B. Hemorrhage

C. Wheezing
D. Facial twitching

178. A 4-year-old female is hospitalized to receive chemotherapy for neuroblastoma. Which of the following effects would the nurse expect to find after chemotherapy begins?
A. Increase in the leukocyte count
B. Painful lesions in the mouth
C. Swelling in weight-bearing joints
D. Brittle, ridged nails

179. A 1-year-old is hospitalized with eczema. The doctor orders Burow's soaks continuously for 2 days. The nurse explains to the mother the purpose of the soaks is to:
A. Reduce inflammation and edema
B. Promote bacteriostasis and reduce itching
C. Aid in removing crusted area
D. Promote healing and prevent scratching

180. The nurse is evaluating the teaching of a parent of a 3-year-old male child in regard to instilling eye medication. Which of the following statements by the parent would indicate a need for further teaching?
A. "I will have his head extended."
B. "I will ask him to look up."
C. "I will pull the lower lid upward."
D. "I will rest my hand holding the dropper on his forehead."

181. A 15-year-old adolescent with acute lymphocytic leukemia (ALL) is receiving chemotherapy for cancer. The nurse is encouraging her to eat. Which one of the following foods will this client most likely select?
A. Hamburger
B. Orange juice
C. French fries
D. Plain yogurt

182. The school nurse is teaching a class of high school females about prevention of breast cancer. She informs the students that the most effective diagnostic tool with breast cancer is:
A. Mammogram
B. Breast self-examination
C. Thermogram
D. Biopsy

183. A 17-year-old male client was recently diagnosed with bone cancer. Which one of the following symptoms is experienced by clients with bone cancer?
A. Pain and swelling in tumor area of affected extremity
B. Pain in extremity, which is relieved by extended position
C. Increased motion of affected extremity
D. Shortening of affected extremity

184. A 17-year-old male client with bone cancer (osteogenic sarcoma) had an amputation of the affected extremity. He experienced a great deal of blood loss and a blood transfusion is ordered. In preparing the transfusion, the nurse knows that the only appropriate IV solution to run with blood is
A. Dextrose 5% in water
B. Ringer's lactate
C. Normal saline
D. Plasmalyte

185. After surgery for amputation of the affected extremity, a 17-year-old male with bone cancer has become withdrawn. Which intervention by the nurse is most likely to be successful in assisting this client to feel less isolated?
A. Telling him to sit in the visitors' lounge.
B. Encouraging him to look at himself in the mirror.
C. Arranging for a visit from another adolescent with the same surgery.
D. Allowing his family to remain with him constantly.

186. A 15-year-old female with cancer is being treated with radiation therapy. The nurse teaches her to protect her skin between treatments. Which of the following statements indicates a need for further teaching?
A. "I need to handle the skin in the area gently."
B. "I need to wear loose-fitting clothes."
C. "I need to avoid irritation of the skin with soap."
D. "I need to use a heat lamp on the skin area daily."

187. A 6-year-old female is recently diagnosed with acute lymphocytic leukemia. After her chemotherapy is initiated, the nurse carefully monitors her for frequency of bowel elimination in order to:
A. Recognize the possible side effects of chemotherapy.
B. Estimate the degree of fluid balance.
C. Note the adequacy of her nutritional intake.
D. Determine if she has developed a gastroenteritis.

188. A 5-year-old hospitalized for chemotherapy has had difficulty in maintaining adequate nutrition. In planning an intervention for this problem, which one of the following interventions would be most appropriate?
A. Selecting the child's menu to ensure proper nutritional balance
B. Allowing her to eat her meals with a group of preschoolers
C. Providing high-calorie, low-protein between-meal snacks
D. Maintaining a rigid schedule for mealtimes and snacks

189. The nurse is preparing to teach a class of high school male seniors about testicular examination. Which of the following instructions would she plan to include?

A. Examine both testicles simultaneously.

B. Testicular examination should be done daily.

C. Gently stroke the testicles with your fingers to detect abnormalities.

D. The best time for examination is after a shower.

190. The mother of a 3-year-old male who had surgery for Wilms' tumor expresses concern about potential behavioral problems during the recovery period at home. She asks for some suggestions on how to discipline her child. Which of the following interventions would be best for the nurse to suggest?

A. Corporal punishment in the form of spanking to eliminate unacceptable behavior

B. Structured interactions that focus on the consequence to prevent or minimize unacceptable behavior

C. Reasoning and scolding to eliminate unacceptable behavior

D. No form of discipline is needed because the negativism will soon pass

191. A 16-year-old male recovering from drug addiction has been diagnosed with hepatitis B. In planning care for him, the nurse will need to include teaching him:

A. To increase his daily exercise activities

B. To eat a diet high in fats

C. The associated dangers of the parenteral mode of transmission of hepatitis

D. To limit his fluid intake

192. An 11-year-old client is diagnosed with hepatitis A. In planning care, the nurse knows that the period of communicability is:

A. During the preicteric phase

B. During the icteric phase

C. During the posticteric phase

D. Not known

193. A 16-year-old male is admitted to the hospital with a suspected diagnosis of ulcerative colitis (UC). In addition to diarrhea and abdominal cramps, this client might be expected to exhibit which of the following signs and symptoms?

A. Weight gain, nausea, abdominal mass, low-grade fever

B. Weight gain, vomiting, abdominal mass, normal temperature

C. Anorexia, vomiting, extreme thirst, normal temperature

D. Anorexia, nausea, extreme thirst, low-grade fever

194. A 16-year-old male after admission to the hospital with a diagnosis of UC continues to have bloody diarrhea. His oral intake of fluids and solid foods is poor. The doctor orders total parenteral nutrition (TPN). When administering TPN, the nurse would keep in mind that it is:

A. A hypertonic solution used mainly to increase osmotic pressure of blood plasma

B. A hyperosmolar solution used mainly to reverse negative nitrogen balance

C. A hypotonic solution used mainly for hydration

D. An alkalyzing solution used to treat metabolic acidosis and cellular edema

195. A client receiving TPN has a potential for several systemic imbalances. In planning care, the nurse is aware that a common metabolic alteration that must be assessed regularly is:

A. Septicemia

B. Hyperglycemia

C. Acidosis

D. Alkalosis

196. A 5-year-old child is seen at the clinic with a chief complaint of diarrhea for 2 days. Care of the child with diarrhea would include which of the following interventions?

A. Encouraging frequent feedings

B. Encouraging a high-fiber, high protein diet

C. Reintroduction of regular foods slowly

D. Encouraging a diet high in calories

197. A 15-year-old female was seen at the children's clinic with chest congestion and a persistent and unproductive cough. She has drunk large amounts of citrus juice, attempted to get more rest, and has taken a cough medicine with codeine. She is now experiencing abdominal discomfort and states that she is constipated. Which of the following is most likely the biggest contributor to the constipation?

A. Codeine in the antitussive medication

B. Persistent, unproductive cough

C. Excessive amounts of fruit juice

D. Intermittent bedrest

198. The mother of a 2-year-old child rushed him to the pediatric emergency room with a chief complaint of, "He ate a large leaf off of one of my potted plants." What is the first step by the nurse in the treatment of poisoning in a child?

A. Terminating the exposure to the toxic substance

B. Preventing the absorption of poison

C. Locating the poison

D. Assessing the child

199. A 3-year-old has been admitted to the pediatric emergency room with ingestion of a corrosive substance. Which of the following is part of the emergency care of the child who has ingested a corrosive substance?

A. Administer syrup of ipecac with warm water.

B. Dilute the corrosive with milk unless vomiting occurs.

C. Dilute the corrosive with water.

D. Allow oral intake.

200. A 1-year-old male child is admitted to the hospital with a diagnosis of celiac disease. The signs and symptoms associated with celiac disease are related to:
    A. Malformation of the ileum
    B. Inoculation of the sprue virus
    C. Congenital absence of trypsin
    D. Sensitivity to gluten products

201. In planning nutritional needs with the mother of a child diagnosed with celiac disease, the nurse would teach which one of the following diets?
    A. A salt-free diet
    B. A diet low in gluten
    C. A diet free of phenylalanine
    D. A diet high in calories, high in protein, and low in fat

202. A 10-year-old male with sickle-cell anemia is admitted to the hospital with a vasoocclusive crisis. Which one of the following assessment findings does the nurse identify as distinguishing this type of crisis?
    A. Jaundice
    B. Heart murmur
    C. Pain
    D. Lethargy

203. The nurse is discussing home care with the parents of a 9-year-old child with sickle-cell disease. The nurse teaches the parents that prompt medical attention should be sought for any:
    A. Difficulty with schoolwork
    B. Eruption of 12-year molars
    C. Vomiting and/or diarrhea
    D. Increase in appetite

204. The parents of a 9-year-old diagnosed with sickle-cell disease have expressed concern that their 8-month-old child may also have sickle-cell disease. Which of the following laboratory studies would yield the most definitive information about this situation?
    A. Hemoglobin electrophoresis
    B. Fibrinogen activity
    C. Lactate dehydrogenase (LDH)
    D. Sickle-cell screening examination

205. An 18-month-old child has been hospitalized with a diagnosis of gastroenteritis. In teaching the parents diet discharge instructions, the nurse would teach that which one of the following foods would be reintroduced last?
    A. Bananas
    B. Rice
    C. Applesauce
    D. Ice cream

206. A 9-year-old male with the diagnosis of a ruptured appendix is returning from surgery after an appendectomy was performed. Postoperative nursing care of the client following surgery for a ruptured appendix is likely to include:
    A. Applying wet-to-dry dressings to the incision site for several days
    B. Administering antibiotics for 24 to 72 hours
    C. Encouraging the client to resume normal physical activities as soon as possible
    D. Positioning the client on his right side

207. The nurse is planning preoperative care for a 2-month-old diagnosed with pyloric stenosis. What measures should the nurse teach the parents to use in feeding an infant with pyloric stenosis preoperatively?
    A. Feed the infant with a Breck feeder.
    B. Burp the infant between feedings.
    C. Handle the infant as little as possible after feedings.
    D. Increase the frequency and amount of the feeding.

208. The nurse is planning a discharge teaching session for the parents of a 2-year-old child who has undergone colostomy for Hirschsprung's disease. Which of the following is an appropriate teaching intervention for this family?
    A. Toddler-sized colostomy bags can be obtained from most medical supply companies.
    B. The child should have a liberal fluid intake.
    C. It is normal for the colostomy site to ooze blood for 5 to 7 days postoperatively.
    D. Always position the child so that there is no pressure on the colostomy site.

209. A 9-year-old male comes to the clinic with his father "to get his immunizations." His father reports that he has had two diphtheria, pertussis, tetanus (DPT) immunizations and one oral polio vaccine (OPV). Which one of the following would the nurse prepare to administer?
    A. DPT, OPV, MMR (measles, mumps, rubella)
    B. Td (tetanus with less diphtheria), MMR, OPV, TB (tuberculin) skin test
    C. MMR, TB skin test
    D. TB skin test, Td

210. The nurse is assessing the development of a 3-year-old male child. The mother reports that the child can climb stairs, can speak in three- to four-word sentences, shares toys, but cannot button his shirt. Which one of the following responses by the nurse would be most appropriate?
    A. "All children do not develop at the same pace. Although he is ahead in some areas, he is a little behind in a few as well."
    B. "It would be helpful to practice some of the fine motor skills with your child such as buttoning his shirt."
    C. "It would be beneficial for you to make an appointment with the pediatrician because he is behind in all areas of development."
    D. "Your child is at the appropriate level of development for his age."

211. The nurse is preparing anticipatory guidance classes for the parents of infants and toddlers. Which one of the following topics would be most appropriate for the nurse to include?
    A. Discussion of injury prevention
    B. Discussion of sibling rivalry
    C. Discussion of limiting TV viewing time
    D. Discussion of day-care and kindergarten programs

212. The nurse is caring for a 12-year-old female hospitalized for a fractured arm. During the assessment and morning bath, the girl expressed concern to the nurse that she had not started her menstrual periods. The nurse noted that she had breast buds and some axillary and pubic hair growth. Which of the following responses by the nurse would be most appropriate?
    A. "You need to make an appointment with your doctor for a laboratory work-up for delayed puberty."
    B. "You need to have radiographs done for bone age."
    C. "Your development is normal for your age."
    D. "You need to discuss this with your mother."

213. The mother of a 4-year-old male expressed concern to the nurse regarding the child's stuttering. Which one of the following comments by the mother would indicate a need for language evaluation?
    A. "He has been stuttering for the past 4 months."
    B. "He stutters more when he is excited."
    C. "He avoids speaking."
    D. "He does not like to play with other children."

214. Which one of the following describes an attempt to reduce the negative effects of hospitalization for children?
    A. Parents are encouraged to leave and take care of other family members at home.
    B. Children are encouraged to leave their schoolwork at home and enjoy a vacation from studying.
    C. Children are placed in 2- to 4-bed wards so they will have someone to play with.
    D. Hospitals sponsor prehospitalization parties for preschoolers when surgery has been scheduled.

215. Concerning children's legal rights and ethical considerations for their care, which of the following statements is true?
    A. Children are regarded as possessions of their parents and therefore under total parental control.
    B. Children do not have the right of confidentiality or access to their medical records.
    C. Children over 13 years of age are considered "mature minors."
    D. Most states allow minors to obtain birth control and treatment for sexually transmitted disease (STD) without parental consent.

216. Which of the following should be included in a child's health history as part of the family profile section?
    A. Maternal grandfather with type I diabetes mellitus
    B. Three-day history of nasal congestion and temperature elevation to 102°F rectally
    C. Attentive adolescent with mother providing interview information
    D. Fifteen-month-old with history of multiple otitis media infections "just like his brother"

217. Which nursing action will reduce anxiety in the child and family when assessing the genitalia as part of the physical exam?
    A. Performing this part of the examination after explaining the procedure
    B. Encouraging the family to leave the room during this part of the examination
    C. Approaching this part of the examination in a matter-of-fact manner while exposing only the area to be examined
    D. De-emphasizing the importance of this part of the examination because most children have normal genitalia

218. If a nurse made all of the following observations on a full-term infant, which one should suggest to the nurse that an abnormality may be present?
    A. Regurgitates food after breastfeeding
    B. Lacks a sucking reflex
    C. Unable to follow a light
    D. Engorged breasts

219. The nurse is ready to begin a physical examination on an 8-month-old. The child is sitting contentedly on his mother's lap, chewing on a toy. Which of the following should the nurse do first?
    A. Auscultate heart and lungs.
    B. Elicit reflexes.
    C. Move the child to the examination table.
    D. Examine head, systematically moving toward the feet.

220. Sarah has just been admitted to your unit with a tentative diagnosis of immune suppression. One nursing action you will initiate is to:
    A. Establish strict isolation to limit the spread of infections.
    B. Screen visitors to prevent exposure to known cases of influenza and varicella.
    C. Offer a diet high in raw fruits and vegetables to promote good nutrition.
    D. Ask her parents to bring her stuffed animals in from home to establish a sense of normalcy.

221. Jason had a history of fever (102°F) after the second DPT vaccine. What nursing action would be appropriate when he returns for his third DPT injection?

A. Continue with the DPT immunization but give aspirin before administering the vaccine.

B. Give pediatric diphtheria and tetanus (DT) alone.

C. Discontinue all further DPT immunizations.

D. Continue routine immunizations according to schedule.

222. When teaching a group of parents of preschoolers about sleep disturbances in children, the nurse should recommend which of the following actions for management of sleep terrors?

A. Awaken the child and encourage discussion of the terror to alleviate fear.

B. Help the child who wakens from a sleep terror to feel secure by allowing co-sleeping with parents.

C. Awaken the child gently and make a fuss over the events of the terror to encourage expression of anxiety.

D. Check to be certain the child is OK and provide reassurance if the child awakens.

223. Immediately following their child's hospitalization, the parents who would be most likely to have difficulty coping with their feelings about the child's diagnosis would be the parents of:

A. Jill, who has been hospitalized with a recent diagnosis of diabetes mellitus

B. Stephen, who has been hospitalized for surgical correction of undescended testicles

C. Lauren, who has been hospitalized due to sepsis resulting from an untreated injury

D. Mary, who has been hospitalized with juvenile rheumatoid arthritis

224. Robert, aged 24 months, has a special blanket, hugs and kisses, and a drink of juice at bedtime. Based on your understanding of growth and development, you know that:

A. Robert is prolonging the bedtime routine.

B. He should not be allowed to become too attached to a special possession.

C. The game is harmless when there is time but he should be put to bed quickly.

D. This developing ritualism is important to the toddler's sense of security and autonomy.

225. The child who is at the greatest risk for sensory overload is one who:

A. Is critically ill in an intensive care unit (ICU)

B. Has frequent visits by his family

C. Has been on bedrest for 2 weeks

D. Is on isolation precautions

226. Which one of the following is correct regarding verbal communication with children?

A. A word such as "dye" may be frightening to children whose cognitive functioning is still very concrete.

B. The quickest way to stop undesirable behavior is to forcefully say, "Stop that!"

C. Urinary tract infections in preschoolers provide an appropriate time to correct childish words such as "pee-pee."

D. Children relate to verbal communication because nonverbal communication is too sophisticated conceptually.

227. In assessing pain in children, the nurse should remember that:

A. Kids tolerate pain better than adults.

B. If kids are active, they don't hurt very much.

C. Kids don't always tell the truth about pain.

D. If narcotics are not effective they can be replaced by paralyzing agents and reduce the risk of addiction.

228. Which of the following policies on the hospital unit might the nurse question?

A. All intravenous infusions given to infants must be placed on an intravenous infusion pump.

B. Side rails are to be fully raised on cribs with small newborns.

C. Age is the only criterion utilized when assigning a child to cribs or beds.

D. All restraints, if used, must be tied to the main bed frame.

229. Tina is an active 8-month-old who already pulls up to stand and is beginning to walk holding on. From this assessment data, the nurse may diagnose:

A. Altered growth and development related to developmental precocity

B. Potential for infection

C. Impaired physical mobility related to confinement in a crib

D. Potential for injury

230. Seven-month-old Robert's temperature goes up to 102°F and he needs antipyretic medication. The nurse administers the appropriate dose of medication by:

A. Mixing it in a bowl of applesauce and allowing his mother to feed him

B. Holding Robert semiupright and placing the medication syringe in the side of his mouth

C. Handing the medication cup to Robert and asking him to drink

D. Making the decision to give the medication IM

231. Mimi has just been admitted with pertussis. Therapeutic actions include:

A. Deep suctioning to remove mucus plugs

B. Administering pertussis vaccine

C. Encouraging participation in active play

D. Maintaining an atmosphere of high humidity

232. Care of a child with chickenpox is directed primarily toward the prevention of:

A. Anemia and dehydration

B. Anorexia and malnutrition

C. Infection at the site of lesions

D. Infection in the respiratory system

233. Jenny Heartfull is 2 years old and has been admitted for repair of a tetralogy of Fallot defect. A compensatory mechanism that decreases venous return and is common in patients with Jenny's diagnosis is:
    A. Squatting
    B. Clubbing
    C. Dyspnea
    D. Polycythemia

234. Which of the following data would likely be present on a 10-year-old patient who has a congenital heart defect that produces systemic cyanosis?
    A. A small heart size on x-ray
    B. White blood cell count of 1000
    C. Height and weight below 10th percentile
    D. Apical heart rate of 60 beats/minute

235. Which of the following explanations regarding cardiac catheterization is appropriate for a 4-year-old?
    A. Postural drainage will be performed every 4 hours for 24 hours after the test.
    B. It is necessary to be completely put to sleep during the test.
    C. The test is very short, usually taking less than 1 hour.
    D. When the special medicine is put into the tubing, it will feel warm.

236. Early diagnosis of coarctation of the aorta may be facilitated by:
    A. Close observation for cyanosis
    B. Blood pressure in all extremities
    C. Chest x-ray
    D. Cardiac catheterization

237. The primary rationale for encouraging the mother of a toddler with croup to stay at the bedside as much as possible is that:
    A. Mothers of hospitalized toddlers often experience guilt.
    B. The mother's presence will reduce anxiety and ease the child's respiratory efforts.
    C. Separation from the mother is a major development threat at this age.
    D. The mother can provide constant observations of the child's respiratory efforts.

238. Five-year-old Mark is seen in his home by the home health nurse. She finds him sitting upright on the bed supporting his trunk with his arms. He has a runny nose, fever, and circumoral pallor. He complains of a sore throat in a muffled voice and his mother says he refuses to eat or drink. The most appropriate action by the nurse would be to:
    A. Carefully examine his oropharynx with a tongue depressor.
    B. Arrange for transportation to the nearest pediatric emergency care facility.
    C. Advise the mother to give Mark acetaminophen and call tomorrow if he isn't better.

D. Call the local health clinic to arrange for an appointment later in the day.

239. An appropriate nursing intervention when caring for an infant with an upper respiratory infection and an elevated temperature would be:
    A. Give small amounts of clear fluids frequently to prevent dehydration.
    B. Push solid food intake to maintain caloric needs.
    C. Dress the child in heavy clothing to prevent chilling.
    D. Give the child cold-water baths to reduce fever.

240. Angela, age 3, has just been admitted with a history of progressive respiratory distress with an abrupt onset. She is making a "froglike" croaking sound on inspiration, is restless, and is drooling. The most important action by the nurse would be to:
    A. Examine her oropharynx and report findings to the physician.
    B. Insist that Angela lie down and rest quietly to increase respiratory efficiency.
    C. Auscultate her lungs and place her in a croup tent with humidified oxygen.
    D. Notify the physician immediately and be prepared for a tracheostomy or intubation.

241. Congenital hip dislocation in the infant may be recognized during physical assessment as:
    A. Shortening of the leg on the unaffected side
    B. Hyperextension of the tibial ligaments
    C. Restricted abduction of the affected hip
    D. Equalized skin folds of the thighs on adduction of the hips

242. A spica cast is applied for the correction of a fractured femur. In the immediate postcasting hours, a primary nursing goal would be to prevent:
    A. Respiratory impairment
    B. Neurovascular impairment
    C. Altered skin integrity
    D. Urinary stasis

243. During assessment of a child with suspected hyperthyroidism, the nurse could expect to obtain a history of:
    A. Arrested skeletal development
    B. Weight loss in spite of a hearty appetite
    C. Chronic constipation and distention
    D. Cold intolerance and febrile episodes

244. Iron-deficiency anemia is a common nutritional problem of young children. The major reason for this is:
    A. Most mothers introduce solid foods too early, causing inadequate absorption of nutrients.
    B. Young children are subject to bleeding disorders, leading to a decrease in red blood cells.
    C. Children are allowed to consume too much milk, leading to inadequate intake of foods rich in iron.

D. Many infants have an inability to utilize fetal stores of iron due to malabsorption syndrome.

245. Oral iron supplements are often prescribed for children with iron-deficiency anemia. Which of the following would indicate correct understanding of a mother administering oral iron supplements to her child?
A. "I will give the iron supplement with orange juice."
B. "I will give the iron in ice cream to disguise the taste."
C. "I will mix the iron in her formula and give it at nap time."
D. "I will give the iron preparation with meals."

246. Wilma, age 6 weeks, has just returned to the pediatric unit following surgical repair of her cleft lip. Which nursing action will best protect Wilma's operative site?
A. Applying bilateral elbow restraints
B. Cleansing the wound with warm normal saline
C. Providing a pacifier to reduce restlessness and crying
D. Positioning on either side with blanket rolls

247. The formation of crusts on the suture line of a repaired cleft lip must be inhibited in order to:
A. Minimize pain
B. Prevent pharyngitis
C. Facilitate suture removal
D. Prevent scarring and uneven healing

248. The nursery nurse observed that a newborn responded to initial feeding attempts with signs characteristic of tracheoesophageal fistula (TEF). Attempts to feed were discontinued because:
A. His sucking attempts were poorly coordinated and ineffective.
B. He gagged after several swallows, choked, and became apneic and cyanotic.
C. His sucking and rooting reflexes were immature and he ignored the nipple.
D. He fell asleep after taking a few cc's of formula and refused to take more

249. While an infant is awaiting corrective surgery for tracheoesophageal fistula (TEF), he is placed in an Isolette with his head and shoulders elevated. The rationale for this position is to:
A. Reduce the cardiac workload that has been increased by the anomaly
B. Relieve the pressure on the diaphragm precipitated by the abdominal distention
C. Reduce the reflux of gastric secretions into the trachea through the fistula
D. Allow air to escape from the fistula into the trachea to reduce gastric distention

250. The parents of 2-year-old Melissa ask the nurse why their daughter needs a lumbar puncture (LP) to diagnose possible *Haemophilus influenzae* menin-

gitis. The nurse tells the parents the purpose of an LP is to:
A. Obtain a sample of cerebrospinal fluid for laboratory analysis and to measure spinal fluid pressure
B. Visualize cerebrospinal fluid pathways and identify tumors or abscesses
C. Inject contrast media into the cerebrospinal fluid to visualize the cerebral circulation
D. Inject contrast media to visualize the structures surrounding the spinal canal and subarachnoid space

251. In preparing for a lumbar puncture (LP) on 2-year-old Melissa, the nurse should:
A. Expect general anesthesia to be used for sedation during the test.
B. Expect to set up a tray with equipment the same size as for adults.
C. Expect to support the child in a side-lying position with the head flexed and knees drawn up.
D. Reassure the parents that the test is simple, painless, and risk-free.

252. Johnny had a febrile seizure when he was 18 months old. What conclusions might you draw from this?
A. He is more likely to develop a seizure disorder when he gets older.
B. There is no relationship to developing a future seizure disorder.
C. His newborn sister will have febrile seizures.
D. He is likely to be learning disabled as a result of the seizure.

253. Which nursing intervention should be included in the plan of care for a male infant following surgical repair of hypospadias?
A. Sterile dressing changes every 4 hours
B. Removal of the suprapubic catheter on the first postoperative day
C. Frequent inspection of the tip of the penis
D. Urethral catheterization if voiding does not occur over an 8-hour period

254. The child with vesicoureteral reflux is at risk for which of the following:
A. Hemolytic-uremic syndrome
B. Glomerulonephritis
C. Chronic renal infections and scarring
D. Nephrotic syndrome

255. Masturbation, urinary stasis, bubble baths, and constipation all may be contributing factors to which of the following genitourinary problems in children?
A. Urinary tract infection
B. Wilms' tumor
C. Bladder spasms
D. Hypospadias

256. Which of the following reflects recommended

procedure for cardiopulmonary resuscitation of the pediatric patient?

A. To check for a pulse in an infant under 1 year of age, the brachial artery is palpated.

B. The compression-to-ventilation ratio for children under the age of 8 years is 15:2.

C. If an infant is not breathing, give four quick breaths followed by a pause to allow for exhalation.

D. The cardiac compression rate for children between the ages of 1 and 8 years should be 120 per minute.

257. Which of the following is the best way for the nurse to assess tissue perfusion in the child with multiple injuries?

A. Measure blood pressure and count pulse.

B. Inspect skin color and measure capillary refill.

C. Observe respiratory pattern and monitor temperature.

D. Determine level of consciousness and evaluate neurological status.

258. The father of a toddler who is eating a hot dog suddenly yells, "Help! He's choking to death!" Which of the following signs would indicate that lifesaving measures are necessary?

A. Gagging

B. Coughing

C. Pulse over 100

D. Inability to speak

259. Six-year-old Tommy is admitted to the hospital in respiratory distress. The best rationale for not giving sedatives is that sedatives in this child could:

A. Lead to shock

B. Cause tachycardia through vagal stimulation

C. Alter blood gas concentrations

D. Depress the respiratory center

260. Ten-year-old Mark is being discharged in a plaster cast. When teaching to support home management for Mark, the nurse should include which instruction?

A. Wash the cast daily with soap and warm water.

B. Gently knock on the cast at the injury site to assess for pain.

C. Check the skin at the cast edges for redness or swelling each morning and night.

D. Use a yardstick padded with gauze to scratch under the cast.

261. Clark, age 16, has an open fracture of his left femur. The femur has been stabilized by pinning the bone and setting up balanced suspension traction. The primary purpose of the traction is to:

A. Protect his injury from contamination.

B. Maintain the reduction of the femoral fracture.

C. Mobilize his fractured leg.

D. Improve joint function in the unaffected leg.

262. Countertraction to support a child's position and alignment in bed is primarily supplied by:

A. Weights, pulleys, and ropes

B. Elevation of the foot of the bed

C. Gravity and body weight

D. Elevation of the knee gatch

263. The most reliable guide to the adequacy of fluid replacement for an 80-pound child with burns is:

A. A falling hematocrit

B. Urine output of 30 to 40 cc per hour

C. Absence of thirst

D. Increased seepage from burn wound

264. Which home care procedure, if stated by parents of a child with a minor burn, indicates correct understanding?

A. Give analgesic medication immediately after changing the burn wound dressing.

B. Observe the unburned skin surrounding the wound for redness and swelling.

C. Wash the burn wound three times a day with dilute Betadine solution and leave it uncovered to promote drying.

D. Scrub the wound vigorously with soap and water and apply a dry gauze dressing.

265. An appropriate nursing intervention for care of the unconscious child would be:

A. Changing the child's position infrequently to minimize the chance of increased intracranial pressure

B. Continuous administration of narcotics or sedatives to provide comfort and pain relief

C. Monitoring fluid intake and output carefully to avoid fluid overload and cerebral edema

D. Administration of solid foods when chewing motions have returned

266. Which of the following is a clinical manifestation of increased intracranial pressure in children?

A. A low-pitched cry

B. A sunken fontanelle

C. Diplopia and/or blurred vision

D. Increased blood pressure

267. When assessing the level of consciousness in an acutely ill child, the nurse should collect data concerning:

A. The child's ability to recall and state events from the past

B. Any recent changes in the child's bowel and bladder patterns

C. The loss of any previously acquired developmental skills

D. The child's response to environmental stimuli and degree of arousal

268. When assisting a family to reduce risk and vulnerability in their child who has a chronic illness, the nurse should consider which goal to be most important?

A. Maintaining control of the symptoms of the illness

B. Organizing a support group for families with children who have similar conditions

C. Restricting the child's physical environment to eliminate exposure to pollution, bacteria, and viruses

D. Providing instruction in reducing constitutional factors that impact on the child's response to stressors

269. Regardless of age, children with congestive heart failure should be placed in which position to maximize cardiac function?

A. Semi-Fowler's
B. Prone
C. Supine
D. Trendelenburg's

270. Nursing interventions for the infant with congestive heart failure would include:

A. Forcing fluids to at least 1500 cc per day
B. Monitoring respirations during active periods
C. Giving four large feedings to conserve energy
D. Organizing activities to allow for uninterrupted rest

271. The most common organism causing bacterial endocarditis is:

A. *Staphylococcus albus*
B. *Pseudomonas*
C. *Streptococcus viridans*
D. *Staphylococcus aureus*

272. The parents of a 6-year-old child with congenital heart disease are afraid to let her play with other children because she might overexert herself. The nurse should reply that the:

A. Child needs the stimulation of playing with peers for normal growth and development.
B. Parents, with guidance, can meet the child's needs for normal growth and development.
C. Child needs constant parental supervision to avoid overexertion.
D. Child needs to understand that her peer's activities are too strenuous.

273. Which of the following statements is descriptive of bronchial asthma in children?

A. It is also called hyperactive airway disease.
B. It occurs more than twice as often in girls as in boys.
C. The single cause of asthma is an allergic hypersensitivity.
D. Severe respiratory alkalosis can result from respiratory failure in asthma.

274. Which of the following medications is the most important in the treatment of an acute, severe attack of asthma in a young child?

A. Ephedrine
B. Corticosteroids
C. Epinephrine
D. Cough syrup with codeine

275. Which of the following factors is the most essential to the nursing care of a child with cystic fibrosis?

A. Diuretics, prevention of diarrhea, and adequate nutrition
B. Protection against pulmonary infection, adequate nutrition, and rest
C. Prevention of dehydration, cleanliness, and medications
D. Prevention of dehydration, protection against pulmonary infection, and diet regulation

276. The nurse's plan of care to meet self-concept needs in the adolescent with cystic fibrosis should include strategies for:

A. Clothing selection that compensates for protuberant abdomen and emaciated extremities
B. Attractive hairstyling, hats, or wigs that mask areas of alopecia
C. Discrete use of facial makeup that covers red blotches
D. Activity or exercise routine that incorporates aerobics and long-distance running

277. Nursing interventions for the child with muscular dystrophy should include strategies for:

A. Increasing caloric intake
B. Promoting strenuous exercise
C. Preventing respiratory infections
D. Limiting physical activity

278. A nurse is participating in a screening program for musculoskeletal disorders among schoolchildren. Which position taken by the children will help most to detect scoliosis?

A. Lying flat on the floor while extending the legs straight from the trunk
B. Sitting in a chair while lifting the feet and legs to a right angle with the trunk
C. Standing against a wall while pressing the length of the back against the wall
D. Bending forward at the waist while allowing the head and arms to fall freely

279. Which of the following skills is it most reasonable to expect a 5-year-old with type I diabetes to be able to perform?

A. Selecting foods based on exchange lists
B. Selecting the injection site and assisting with the insulin injection
C. Performing blood glucose testing independently
D. Preparing and administering insulin independently

280. Helen, age 5 years, was diagnosed with type I diabetes mellitus at age 3 years. During a check-up for an ear infection, her mother asked the nurse, "Why has Helen's insulin dosage been increased since last year? Is she getting worse?" Which response is most appropriate for the nurse to make?

A. "It may not be that she is deteriorating. Diabetes that begins in childhood is always more severe and harder to regulate."

B. "Since insulin dosage in childhood is based on body weight, insulin needs will increase as she grows."

C. "Her insulin requirement has increased only because of her infection."

D. "Her underlying problem is no more severe than before, but you have not controlled her nutrition rigidly enough."

281. Ima is 5 years old and has come to the hospital complaining of severe pain in her left knee. She has been diagnosed with sickle-cell anemia and is in pain crisis. Priorities for management at this time would include which of the following:
A. Physical therapy and ambulation
B. Place in reverse isolation
C. Platelet transfusion
D. Increase fluids and give analgesics

282. During a sickle-cell crisis, there is often tissue damage resulting from vaso-occlusion. Vaso-occlusion is best explained physiologically as:
A. Blockage of small blood vessels by sickled red blood cells so that ischemia and infarction to distal tissues and cells occur
B. Pooling of blood in the spleen, resulting in increased abdominal pressure, shock, and death
C. Reduction of red blood cell formation, resulting in hypoxia and destruction of tissue
D. Rupture of small blood vessels as a result of increased production of red blood cells

283. Children receiving radiation therapy and chemotherapy have an increased susceptibility to infection, which is attributable to:
A. Mucosal changes
B. Polycythemia
C. Edema
D. Bone marrow depression

284. Prednisone is administered for children with nephrotic syndrome nephrosis until:
A. The urine is free from protein.
B. The urinary tract infection is gone.
C. The generalized edema subsides.
D. The hypertension is resolved.

285. Children with nephrotic syndrome are placed on bedrest during the edematous phase. A priority nursing intervention while the child is on bedrest is to:
A. Keep the child quiet in bed.
B. Change positions every few hours.
C. Limit the parent from holding the child.
D. Do active range of motion every few hours.

286. Which of the following assessments is most significant in diagnosing fluid retention in a child with either nephrotic syndrome or glomerulonephritis?
A. Increasing daily weight
B. Increasing specific gravity
C. Decreasing urine output
D. Decreasing fluid intake

287. Which of the following statements is most accurate for acute glomerulonephritis?
A. It is a syndrome in which there is impaired reabsorption of bicarbonate and/or excretion of hydrogen ions.
B. It often occurs following an antecedent streptococcal infection.
C. It is a clinical disorder that results in massive urinary protein loss.
D. It is a disorder associated with a defect in the ability to concentrate urine.

288. During the acute phase of glomerulonephritis in a child, which of the following nursing interventions would be appropriate?
A. Encourage oral intake of pretzels and bananas.
B. Place the child in strict isolation.
C. Arrange for the child to be taken to the playroom to play pool.
D. Assess the child's appearance for signs of cerebral complications.

289. One-month-old Sally has just had a shunt insertion for hydrocephalus. The nurse would know that the discharge teaching was effective if the parents said which of the following?
A. "I know to expect uncontrolled eye movements."
B. "I will only lay her on her stomach to protect the shunt."
C. "If she starts vomiting, I will call the neurology clinic immediately."
D. "I will never touch the shunt area so I won't dislodge it."

290. Ricky, a 2-year-old, starts to have a tonic-clonic (generalized) seizure while in his crib in the hospital. His jaws are clamped. What is the *most* important nursing activity at this time?
A. Place a padded tongue blade between Ricky's jaw.
B. Prepare suction equipment.
C. Restrain Ricky to prevent injury.
D. Observe the seizure and protect Ricky from harming himself.

291. Jenny, age 8, has been diagnosed with epilepsy since age 5. She has been seizure-free for the past 2 years on antiepileptic therapy. The most common cause of a recurrence of her seizures would be:
A. Withdrawal of antiepileptic drugs
B. A degenerative disease
C. Cerebrovascular accident
D. A head injury

292. Deby, age 6 weeks, is admitted to the hospital for treatment of congenital hip dysplasia. Initial treatment for this condition will most likely involve a(n):

A. Open reduction

B. Abduction splint or harness

C. Tenotomy of the contracted muscles

D. Osteotomy to reconstruct the acetabular roof

293. Tad, age 5 months, is fitted for a Pavlik harness, which he will wear for 5 to 6 months in an attempt to correct his congenital hip dysplasia. The best way to validate that the mother understands how to use the harness is to:

A. Ask her to tell you the purpose of the harness and how she will put it on.

B. Ask her to show you how she removes and replaces the harness.

C. Ask the mother to tell you what the doctor has told her about the harness.

D. Demonstrate the removal and application of the harness while the mother watches.

294. Jeffery Brown has just been admitted to the term nursery. Routine assessment indicates that he probably has bilateral club feet. Initial treatment for Jeffery will probably consist of:

A. Passive exercises four times a day to overcorrect the defect

B. Adhesive strapping to hold the feet in an overcorrected position

C. Application of casts to the feet as soon as the diagnosis is made

D. The use of a Denis Browne splint after discharge

295. Ten-year-old Leo had osteomyelitis that did not respond to the antibiotic therapy and the periosteum ruptured, resulting in sepsis of the knee joint. He is started on another round of antibiotic therapy. The major goal of therapy for Leo at this time is:

A. Preservation of joint function

B. Improving his nutritional status

C. Promoting rest to facilitate healing

D. Prevention of infection

296. Mike, age 2½, has been placed in 90-90 traction for the reduction of a fractured femur. Which of the following will be most helpful during the period of immobilization?

A. Letting him wear clothing from home

B. Placing few behavioral limitations on him

C. Taking him to the playroom in his bed

D. Placing him in a quiet room with reduced stimuli

297. The primary purpose of putting a child's fractured femur in traction is to:

A. Keep the child from moving the leg until it has a chance to heal.

B. Stabilize the fracture site until a cast can be applied.

C. Prevent muscle spasms in the thigh.

D. Allow the child more freedom of movement than casting would.

298. Fractures that involve the epiphyseal plate of a long bone present a special problem in children because they:

A. Are difficult to reduce and immobilize

B. Heal more slowly than fractures in other areas of the bone

C. Are difficult to detect and may be mistaken for dislocation

D. Have an increased incidence of longitudinal growth problems

299. The factor that is most likely to put children at risk for traumatic injury is:

A. Their curiosity and immature judgment, which lures them into places of danger

B. Their parents are unaware of developmental factors that make them susceptible to injury.

C. They generally have a low center of gravity, which causes them to fall awkwardly.

D. Their play is often unsupervised and playgrounds are often unsafe.

300. Nine-year-old Marty has been placed in a hip spica cast for the treatment of a fractured femur. When elevating Marty's head, it is important to remember to:

A. Limit her length of stay in this position to 1 hour.

B. Raise the entire mattress and frame at the head of the bed.

C. Use at least two pillows under the shoulders to elevate her head.

D. Put her in a nighttime (extra-absorbent) diaper to absorb urine.

301. An important principle to keep in mind when examining the musculoskeletal system in a child is that:

A. Individual variations can be detected by comparing one side of the body with the other.

B. Percussion and palpation are the basis of the physical examination.

C. Clothing does not need to be removed during the examination.

D. The examination of other body systems rarely contributes to the musculoskeletal examination.

302. A complication of immobility in children that is easily prevented by astute nursing care is:

A. Swelling of extremities

B. Bone pain

C. Constipation

D. Disease atrophy in a casted extremity

303. Ortolani's maneuver is performed in a newborn to assess:

A. Range of motion

B. Hip stability

C. Degree of joint flexion

D. Foot stability

304. Johnny is a newborn with bilateral cleft lip and

palate. Johnny will require which of the following adjustments of his feeding procedure?
A. Thickened bottle feedings to facilitate sucking
B. Larger quantities of formula than a baby without the defect
C. More frequent burping than a baby without the defect
D. More frequent feedings than a baby without the defect

305. Which of the following interventions is appropriate for an 18-month-old child immediately after cleft palate repair?
A. Elbow restraints on at all times except for brief, supervised exercise periods
B. Permit the child to meet autonomy needs by feeding himself finger foods
C. Suction the child at frequent intervals to prevent wound infection
D. Cleanse the child's mouth with oral antiseptic using cotton swabs after meals

306. Which of the following methods of taking fluids would be most appropriate for an 18-month-old on the second day after cleft palate repair?
A. A drinking straw
B. A large-holed nipple
C. An asepto syringe
D. A cup

307. The herniation of abdominal viscera and intestines into the base of the umbilical cord in a newborn is called:
A. Congenital diaphragmatic hernia
B. Gastroschisis
C. Omphalocele
D. Umbilical hernia

308. The nursery nurse observes that a newborn responds to initial feeding attempts with signs characteristic of tracheoesophageal fistula (TEF). Feeding attempts should be discontinued because:
A. His sucking attempts are poorly coordinated and ineffective with excessive swallowing.
B. He gags after several swallows, chokes, and becomes apneic and cyanotic.
C. His sucking and rooting reflexes are immature and he ignores the nipple.
D. His abdomen becomes very distended and he falls asleep, refusing more formula.

309. While an infant is awaiting the initial surgery for TEF, he is placed in an infant warmer with his head and shoulders elevated. The rationale for this position is to:
A. Reduce the cardiac workload that has been increased by the anomaly.
B. Relieve the pressure on the diaphragm precipitated by abdominal distention.
C. Reduce the reflux of gastric secretions from the esophagus into the trachea.

D. Allow air to escape from the fistula into the trachea to reduce abdominal distention.

310. Billy, age 6 months, is admitted to the hospital for a rectal biopsy to confirm a suspected diagnosis of Hirschsprung's disease. The nurse would expect to note which of the following symptoms when assessing his health status?
A. History of constipation, abdominal distention, palpable fecal mass
B. Rectal bleeding, diarrhea, prolonged jaundice at birth
C. Irritability, vomiting, dehydration
D. History of colic, bloody diarrhea, nausea

311. An infant with Hirschsprung's disease is scheduled for surgery to create a temporary colostomy. Priorities in his postoperative care should include strategies for:
A. Limiting physical activity
B. Dilating the stomach
C. Preventing prolapse of the rectum
D. Assessing bowel function

312. Three-month-old Kent has been admitted to the hospital with diarrhea and dehydration from frequent watery stools for the past 2 days. The most common cause of death in infants with diarrhea is:
A. Infection in the gastrointestinal tract
B. Loss of body fluids and salts
C. Destruction of red blood cells during the early phase
D. Secondary infection

313. Mat is a 6-week-old infant admitted to the hospital with pyloric stenosis. Pyloric stenosis can best be described as:
A. Dilation of the pylorus
B. Hypertrophy of the pyloric muscle
C. Hypertonicity of the pyloric muscle
D. Reduction of tone in the pyloric muscle

314. Which of the following observations made of the exposed abdomen is most indicative of pyloric stenosis?
A. Abdominal rigidity
B. Substernal retraction
C. Visible peristalsis
D. Marked distention of lower abdomen

315. A nursing responsibility when caring for an infant with suspected pyloric stenosis would be which of the following?
A. Observe for projectile vomiting
B. Monitor for signs of respiratory alkalosis
C. Administer large, infrequent feedings to allow for rest
D. Place the infant in the supine position after feedings

316. An infant that is unrestrained in a motor vehicle accident is at greater risk for which type of injury?
A. Fractured femur

B. Aspiration pneumonia
C. Head injury
D. Kidney trauma

317. On a cool, rainy day you come upon a motor vehicle accident and find a mother and her 4-month-old infant lying beside the road. Which of the following is more likely to be a problem for the infant than the mother?
A. Infection
B. Compound skeletal fractures
C. Hyperthermia
D. Hypothermia

318. Primary assessment of the injured child includes which of the following?
A. Weight estimation, blood pressure measurement, body inspection
B. Allergic history, symptom analysis, head-to-toe survey
C. Airway patency, respiratory effectiveness, circulatory status
D. Temperature measurement, medication history, mode of injury

319. Mike was hit on the head with a baseball, losing consciousness for several minutes. He now appears fine. As the school nurse, your plan of action is to:
A. Perform a brief neurological examination, and then refer him to his primary care provider.
B. Give him acetaminophen and suggest that he take a short nap.
C. Place ice on his head and then allow him to go about this normal activities.
D. Suggest that his parents keep him NPO and wake him every 4 hours for the next 24 hours.

320. The parents of a child who suffered a recent concussion are concerned that their son cannot recall what happened immediately before and after the accident. Which of the following answers is most accurate?
A. "That is a little unusual; I'll mention it to the neurosurgeon."
B. "It is not unusual for children to have amnesia for that period of time."
C. "Usually the amnesia is just for the time period after the accident."
D. "Children vary in their response to a head injury."

321. The nurse is assessing a child for postconcussion syndrome. Which of the following is not typical of this disturbance?
A. Blackouts
B. Sleep disturbances
C. Emotional disturbances
D. Poor school performance

322. Joey is brought to the emergency room with a head injury and transient loss of consciousness. At the hospital, he is awake and responsive and his vi-

tal signs are stable. Which of the following criteria would necessitate Joey's hospitalization?
A. Loss of consciousness
B. An area of swelling greater than 2 cm
C. Bleeding from a wound
D. Vomiting of undigested food

323. A 7-month-old is hospitalized with severe diarrhea and dehydration. Which of the following orders on the chart should the nurse question?
A. Enteric precautions
B. NPO
C. Vital signs q 4 hours
D. IV of D5W

324. Two-year-old Jan has a generalized seizure that is tentatively diagnosed as a febrile seizure. She is hospitalized for diagnostic work-up and treatment. Her mother asks the nurse if Jan should be on continuous anticonvulsant medication at home. The nurse should base a response on the fact that children who have febrile seizures:
A. Do not usually need long-term anticonvulsant therapy
B. Need long-term anticonvulsant therapy
C. Need anticonvulsants only when they have upper respiratory infections
D. Need anticonvulsants if the seizures lasted 15 seconds or less

325. Children who have a history of febrile seizures:
A. Are often found to have the Arnold-Chiari defect
B. Require treatment for underlying infection
C. Require long-term maintenance on anticonvulsant medications
D. Frequently benefit from a ketogenic diet

326. Robby had a febrile seizure when he was 18 months old. What conclusions might the nurse draw from this?
A. He is more likely to develop a seizure disorder when he gets older.
B. His newborn sister will have febrile seizures.
C. There is no significant relationship to developing a future seizure disorder.
D. He is likely to be learning disabled as a result of these seizures.

327. Three-year-old Mindy is admitted to the hospital with a tentative diagnosis of bacterial meningitis. Nursing care for Mindy should include:
A. Providing a well-lighted environment
B. Maintaining isolation for a minimum of 72 hours
C. Assessing for changes in level of consciousness
D. Forcing fluids

328. A significant aspect of the history of a toddler with bacterial meningitis would be the finding that a couple of weeks before onset of the illness the toddler had:
A. Shown no signs of illness

B. Contacted otitis media
C. Received booster shots
D. Developed a fine red macular rash

329. The cremasteric reflex is responsible for which physiological response in infants?
A. Penile erection
B. Tightening of perineal muscles when scrotum is touched
C. Urination
D. Withdrawal of testes into the inguinal canal

330. Tim, a newborn, is noted to have hypospadias and chordee. His parents are advised not to have him circumcised. The nurse knows that the rationale for this advice is:
A. The poorly developed penile vasculature makes the surgical procedure too risky.
B. The associated chordee is very difficult to remove during circumcision.
C. The foreskin is used to repair the deformity surgically.
D. The meatus can become stenosed, leading to symptoms of urinary obstruction.

331. Glen, aged 12 months, is returned to his hospital room following surgical repair of his hypospadias. He has an IV infusion and both a urethral and a suprapubic catheter in place. The nurse tells Glen's parents that the primary purpose of the suprapubic catheter is to provide:
A. An entry port for bladder irrigation
B. An alternate urinary elimination route
C. Accurate measurement of urinary output
D. An opportunity to observe the color of the urine

332. Billy, 18 months old, has been diagnosed with cryptorchism. The nurse explains that the major complication of untreated cryptorchism is:
A. Sterility
B. Infection
C. Torsion of the testes
D. Inguinal hernia

333. Congenital defects of the genitourinary tract such as hypospadias are usually repaired as early as possible to:
A. Prevent mental illness
B. Prevent separation anxiety
C. Promote acceptance of hospitalization
D. Promote development of normal body image

334. Children being treated for nephrotic syndrome are at particular risk for infection because of:
A. The immunosuppressive effect of steroids
B. Generalized edema
C. Electrolyte imbalance
D. The idiopathic nature of the illness

335. Eight-year-old Lisa has been hospitalized for treatment of nephrotic syndrome. Her weight is 30 kg, and she has generalized edema. What data support the nursing diagnosis of fluid volume excess related to compromised regulatory function for Lisa's care plan?
A. Extreme restlessness
B. Hematocrit level of 37 percent
C. Intake of 1500 ml in 24 hours
D. Urine output of 100 ml in 8 hours

336. Mark has been diagnosed with nephrotic syndrome for 3 months and was doing well until a relapse 2 days ago forced his rehospitalization. In talking with his parents, the nurse would want to emphasize that:
A. The prognosis is now much worse.
B. This will probably be Mark's last hospitalization.
C. Exacerbations and remissions are characteristic of this disease.
D. If his medication had been taken properly, the relapse would not have occurred.

337. Mimi, age 3, has been diagnosed with a urinary tract infection. Her parents will be caring for her at home during the treatment period. They should be told to:
A. Decrease her oral fluid intake.
B. Encourage her to void frequently.
C. Give her warm bubble baths.
D. Wash her perineum with soap after every void and defecation.

338. Two weeks after being diagnosed, 2-year-old Tara is seen in the clinic to determine if her urinary tract infection has been cured. The most significant data for making this determination is:
A. She no longer complains of abdominal pain.
B. Her urine is negative for bacteria.
C. She has completed 10 full days of antibiotics.
D. She has become much less irritable.

339. Six-year-old Ted is admitted to the hospital with suspected glomerulonephritis. This diagnosis is most strongly supported by which of the following data?
A. Three pound weight gain in the past 2 weeks
B. Irritability
C. Documented strep throat 1 week ago
D. Increased urine output with decreased specific gravity

340. Eleven-year-old John is resisting the restriction of sodium and fluids placed on him with his diagnosed glomerulonephritis. Which would be the best plan for John?
A. Select his diet and fluids for him since he would not know what to choose.
B. Have him eat by himself so he will not be reminded of what he cannot have to eat.
C. Tell him that if he will eat what is provided, you will see if the doctor will let him have a little bite of a favorite, but restricted food.
D. Involve him in the plan, allow him to select

from permitted foods, and make a game of recording his fluids.

341. Asthma is more likely to become persistent if its onset occurs in which age group?
   A. School age
   B. Infants
   C. Adolescent
   D. Preschooler

342. Which of the following would the nurse expect to be used immediately for the wheezing child on presentation in the emergency room?
   A. Oxygen
   B. Epinephrine
   C. Theophylline
   D. Corticosteroids

343. Which of the following is an indication of a *potential complication* in the asthmatic child?
   A. Increase in PaO_2
   B. Decrease in wheezing
   C. Decrease in $PaCO_2$
   D. Increase in O_2 saturation

344. Which of the following test results aids in the diagnosis of cystic fibrosis in children?
   A. Elevated plasma protein
   B. Decreased plasma protein
   C. Elevated plasma cholesterol
   D. Elevated sweat chloride

345. When teaching the parents of a child diagnosed with acute rheumatic fever (ARF), it is important to stress that prophylactic antibiotic therapy is continued for ——— or until the child is 20 years of age.
   A. Six months
   B. Two years
   C. Five years
   D. Ten days

346. Which procedure will place a child at the highest risk for subacute bacterial endocarditis (SBE)?
   A. Root canal
   B. Chest x-ray
   C. Immunizations
   D. Barium swallow

347. Braces are often ordered for the treatment of scoliosis in children when the curvature is less than 40 degrees. Satisfactory results of this treatment depend primary on:
   A. Fit and appearance of the brace
   B. Teaching and counseling by the nursing personnel
   C. Reinforcement by the parents
   D. Compliance and cooperation of the child

348. Discharge planning for parents of an 8-year-old with rheumatic fever should include which of the following as toxic symptoms of sodium salicylate?
   A. Tinnitus and nausea
   B. Chills and an elevation of temperature
   C. Dermatitis and blurred vision
   D. Unconsciousness and acetone breath odor

349. Gowers' sign, distinctive movements observed when a child goes from a sitting to a standing position, is seen when children are diagnosed with:
   A. Structural scoliosis
   B. Legg-Calvé-Perthes disease
   C. Congenital hip dysplasia
   D. Duchenne's muscular dystrophy

350. Conner, who is 4 years old, is newly diagnosed as having Legg-Calvé-Perthes disease. The nurse would expect initial symptoms of this disease to include:
   A. A limp
   B. Leg-length discrepancy
   C. Waddling gait
   D. Pain after climbing stairs

351. Tad, age 6, has been diagnosed as having Legg-Calvé-Perthes disease. The left femur is involved. While he is undergoing therapy, the major emphasis is to:
   A. Prevent flexion of the left hip
   B. Control pain, which is especially acute during the night
   C. Prevent weight bearing on the head of the left femur
   D. Encourage Tad to walk despite discomfort at the left hip

352. Nursing care of the child with muscular dystrophy should include strategies for:
   A. Increasing caloric intake
   B. Preventing respiratory infections
   C. Promoting strenuous exercise
   D. Limiting physical activity

353. A teaching plan for a child or family concerning hemophilia would include that:
   A. Hemophilia is primarily an X-linked recessive disorder.
   B. Hemophilia involves a decrease in platelets.
   C. The primary therapy is replacement of coagulation factors III or IV.
   D. Replacement therapy will always require hospitalization.

354. Rick, a hemophiliac, fell on his left arm while playing at home. There is no overt bleeding, but the arm is swelling. In addition to specific replacement treatment, appropriate home measures would be to:
   A. Apply warm, moist compresses
   B. Apply pressure for at least 5 minutes
   C. Begin passive range of motion unless pain is severe
   D. Elevate area above the level of the heart

355. Which of the following findings would most likely be observed when initially assessing a hemophiliac child who has just sustained an injury to his right knee?

A. Petechiae
B. Dehydration
C. Hemarthrosis
D. Neutropenia

356. Which of the following interventions is contraindicated during the initial care of a child with hemophilia, following acute traumatic injury to the knee?
A. Bedrest
B. Active range-of-motion exercises
C. Elevation of the affected knee
D. Ice bags to the knee

357. If ordered for a child with hemophilia, which of the following analgesics should the nurse question?
A. Codeine
B. Meperidine (Demerol)
C. Acetylsalicylic acid (aspirin)
D. Acetaminophen (Tylenol)

358. A 6-year-old is hospitalized with 2nd degree burns on her face. Which of the following activities by the nurse would provide the child the greatest degree of support concerning her self-concept?
A. Reassuring her repeatedly that the burns will heal quickly, leaving no scars.
B. Encourage her to look at her wounds during cleaning and debridement.
C. Showing her photographs illustrating progressive healing of other children's burns.
D. Pointing out to her each evidence of healing in various burn wounds.

359. The clinical manifestations of sickle-cell disease in children are the result of:
A. Vaso-occlusion
B. Hypertension
C. Hypotension
D. Edema

360. The parents of a child in sickle-cell pain crisis tell the nurse that they are worried about the narcotic analgesics causing addiction. The nurse should explain which of the following concerning the use of narcotics with their child?
A. Narcotics are often ordered but not usually needed.
B. When medically indicated, children rarely become addicted.
C. Narcotics are given as a last resort because of the threat of addiction.
D. Narcotics are used only if other measures, such as ice packs, are ineffective.

361. Robin, age 4 years, is experiencing alopecia, nausea, and stomatitis from her chemotherapy for acute lymphocytic leukemia (ALL). These side effects of chemotherapy are related to:
A. Toxins resulting from the dying cells build up in the body.

B. Slow-growing cells respond best to the chemotherapy.
C. Chemotherapy kills both normal and abnormal cells.
D. Chemotherapy is mostly absorbed in the GI tract.

362. After a complete course of therapy, Robin is determined to be in remission from her ALL. Remission for a leukemic patient is best defined by which of the following?
A. Recovery from alopecia occurs.
B. There is a decrease in nausea and vomiting.
C. Blast cells are reduced by 40 percent in the bone marrow.
D. Tumor cells are not evident microscopically.

363. Your terminally ill child's mother asks, "How should I talk with my son about his illness?" Which of the following should the nurse consider most important when responding to the mother?
A. The child's age and cognitive development
B. The child's physical condition
C. The child's relationship with the assigned nurse
D. The child's past illness history

364. The nurse notices that a terminally ill child's parents are not visiting very frequently or providing needed support. Which of the following measures should be implemented?
A. Call the parents in and have them explain to the child why they are not visiting as they should.
B. Spend as much time with the child as possible, recognizing that the parents may need to withdraw temporarily to cope.
C. Tell the child that it is good to have time alone to think and prepare for things to come.
D. Warn the parents that if they do not visit the child frequently now, they may experience intense guilt later.

365. Jane is an 8-year-old girl with type I diabetes. She experiences polyuria, polydipsia, and polyphagia during ketoacidotic periods. Her family could correctly be taught that:
A. Polydipsia is a symptom resulting from the body's attempt to recover from polyuria.
B. Polyphagia is secondary to an increase in the cellular uptake of glucose.
C. Polyuria results when the kidneys retain fluid because of low levels of glucose filtered from the blood.
D. All three symptoms occur as a result of Jane's hypoglycemic state during ketosis.

366. Teaching the parents of a child with type I diabetes about the relationship between the results of urine tests for ketones and blood glucose levels is based on the knowledge that ketones will begin to

appear in the urine when the blood glucose level reaches approximately:
A. 120 mg/dl
B. 150 mg/dl
C. 180 mg/dl
D. 250 mg/dl

367. If a type I diabetic child takes her regular insulin at 7 A.M., what time during the day should her parents be taught that the peak action from the regular insulin should be expected?
A. 7:30 A.M.
B. 10 A.M.
C. 1 P.M.
D. 3 P.M.

368. Your client is a 12-year-old diagnosed with new-onset type I diabetes. Your teaching plan for insulin injections should be based on which of the following?
A. The parents do not need to learn the procedure.
B. Self-injections will be possible when the client is closer to adolescence.
C. The client can learn to give self-injections as soon as he can reach all injection sites.
D. The client is old enough to give most of his own injections.

369. Stan, age 11, has had type I diabetes for 3 years. Recently he developed an infection, fever of 102°F, and blood glucose levels ranging from 200 to 300 mg/dl. Stan may require insulin every 4 hours. Which form of insulin is appropriate for this schedule?
A. Neutral protamine Hagedorn (NPH)
B. Humulin N
C. Regular
D. Ultralente

370. Terry, age 8, is brought to the emergency room after experiencing his first seizure. His mother tells the nurse that she cannot believe her child has epilepsy. The nurse's best response would be:
A. "Epilepsy is easily treated."
B. "Very few children have actual epilepsy."
C. "The seizure may or may not mean that your child has epilepsy."
D. "Your child has had only one convulsion; it probably won't happen again."

371. A 11-year-old boy, without a history of seizures, experiences a tonic-clonic seizure at school. Breathing is not impaired, but there is some postictal confusion. Following the seizure, the most appropriate initial action by the school nurse is which of the following?
A. Call the emergency medical service (EMS).
B. Notify the parent and regular practitioner.
C. Notify the parent that the child should go home.
D. Stay with the child, offering calm reassurance.

372. An infant with hydrocephalus is hospitalized for surgical placement of a ventriculoperiteoneal shunt. Postoperative nursing care should include which of the following?
A. Monitor closely for signs of infection.
B. Pump the shunt reservoir to maintain patency.
C. Administer sedation to decrease irritability.
D. Maintain Trendelenburg's position to decrease pressure on the shunt.

373. An important nursing intervention when caring for an infant with myelomeningocele in the preoperative stage is which of the following?
A. Place the infant on side to decrease pressure on the spinal cord.
B. Apply a heat lamp to facilitate drying and toughening of the sac.
C. Keep the skin clean and dry to prevent irritation from diarrheal stools.
D. Watch for signs of increased intracranial pressure that might indicate developing hydrocephalus.

374. The most common problem of infants born with a myelomeningocele is which of the following?
A. Mental retardation
B. Neurogenic bladder
C. Respiratory compromise
D. Limited use of extremities

375. The major determinant of neonatal (under 28 days of life) mortality in the United States is:
A. Infectious diseases
B. Accidental injuries
C. Poor nutrition
D. Low birth weight

376. Knowledge of infant and child mortality and morbidity statistics assist nurses in:
A. Developing a commitment to families
B. Identifying age groups at risk for certain diseases or injuries
C. Recognizing changes in adaptation
D. Alleviating parental anxiety related to childhood illness

377. In the United States, the leading cause of death in children aged 1 to 19 years is:
A. AIDS
B. Homocide
C. Cancer
D. Accidents and injury

378. The advancement of pediatric nursing practice through contributions to nursing research is the responsibility of:
A. Nurse educators
B. Sigma Theta Tau International Nursing Honor Society
C. Nurse researchers
D. All nurses

379. One role of the pediatric nurse is defined as prac-

ticing within the framework of preventative health principles. The best approach to prevention is education and anticipatory guidance. This describes the pediatric nursing role of:
A. Family advocacy
B. Support and counseling
C. Illness prevention and health promotion
D. Health-care planning

380. The most common childhood illness is:
A. Rotavirus
B. Tonsillitis
C. The common cold
D. Respiratory syncytial virus

381. Which of the following would be an accurate statement about parents of hospitalized children?
A. Because adolescents need to increase their independence, it is appropriate to ask their parents to go home.
B. Parents' participation in care facilitates their coping with their child's illness.
C. Parents should bring children new toys to distract them from their anxiety about separation.
D. Parents who cannot stay with their hospitalized child should be reassured that the child's nurse will be with him or her all the time.

382. What is the most important therapeutic value of play for hospitalized children?
A. Release of surplus energy
B. Helps child distinguish between fantasy and reality
C. Encourages creativity
D. Facilitates communication of needs and fears

383. To elicit information about previous pain experiences, the nurse should ask the child which of the following questions?
A. "Do you know what pain is?"
B. "Whose fault do you think it is when you get hurt?"
C. "How bad has your pain been?"
D. "Tell me about hurts you have had before."

384. Which of the following pain assessment strategies may be used by the nurse to gather objective information about a child's pain experience?
A. Behavioral observation
B. Pain intensity rating scales
C. Drawings
D. Parent interviews

385. Lee, age 10, has an order for morphine sulfate for the relief of pain on the first postoperative day. In assessing her for pain, it is important to remember that:
A. Children do not feel pain or feel pain less than adults.
B. Children always tell the truth about whether or not they are experiencing pain.
C. Whatever is painful to an adult should be con-

sidered painful to a child unless proven otherwise.
D. It is better to undertreat pain in a child than to risk respiratory depression or addiction to opioids.

386. Six-year-old Toni is to undergo a cardiac catheterization next week. An effective method of preparing her for the experience would be to:
A. Provide her parents with the necessary information so they can tell her what to expect.
B. Give her a book to take home and read the night before the procedure.
C. Not tell her anything because she would not understand and would become too anxious.
D. Take Toni and her parents on a tour of the procedure room and explain equipment.

387. A major concern of nurses working with well children is the prevention of communicable disease. Primary prevention is best achieved by:
A. Ensuring current and complete immunizations for all children
B. Isolating children who have been diagnosed as having a communicable disease
C. Boiling drinking water during outbreaks of communicable disease
D. Avoiding exposure of susceptible children during the prodromal stage of the illness

388. Lamar, age 2, has varicella. You advise his mother to cut his nails short, give him colloidal oatmeal baths, dress him in loose clothing, and apply calamine (Caladryl) to the lesions. The *best* rationale for your recommendations is:
A. By reducing the itching and scratching, less scarring from the lesions will occur.
B. By reducing itching and scratching, the likelihood of bacterial invasion of the lesions is decreased.
C. By reducing the itching and scratching, faster healing will occur.
D. By reducing the itching and scratching, he will be made comfortable and will be more pleasant to live with.

389. Measles vaccine is not given before 15 months of age because:
A. The infant would become too ill from the vaccine.
B. The infant is not susceptible to measles until this age because of innate immunity.
C. The infant may have too high a passive antibody titer to generate a response.
D. If given earlier, it will create a false-positive response to the tuberculin test.

390. Ms. Williams tells you that she is going to breast-feed her infant son Shane to "keep him from getting sick easily." You know that the type of immunity that occurs through breastfeeding is:
A. Naturally acquired passive

B. Naturally acquired active
C. Artificially acquired passive
D. Innate

391. When immunity in a child is obtained from exposure to the invading agent, this is called:
A. Innate immunity
B. Natural immunity
C. Passive immunity
D. Acquired immunity

392. When Ms. Brown brings Missy for her 2-month examination, she tells you that she has read that the DPT may not be safe and she is not sure whether Missy should receive it. Your *best* response is:
A. "It's your decision. You must do what you feel comfortable with."
B. "There is some risk involved, but it is still less than the risk to Missy if she should contract pertussis."
C. "The pertussis portion of the vaccine is the risky part. If you like, we can give her just the DT."
D. "Please don't worry about such sensationalism. We will take good care of Missy."

393. Infants are prone to developing middle ear infections (otitis media) because:
A. They cannot blow their nose.
B. Frequent milk feedings are a culture medium for bacteria.
C. Teething causes an increase in oral bacteria.
D. Infants have short, straight eustachian tubes.

394. Six-year-old Karen has tetralogy of Fallot. She is admitted to your unit. Her mother asks you why Karen has clubbed fingers. You should base your response on the knowledge that the clubbing of her fingers is caused by:
A. Elevated WBC count
B. Peripheral hypoxia
C. Elevated hematocrit
D. Destruction of bone marrow

395. Infants and children with an uncomplicated ventricular septal defect are not usually cyanotic because with this type of anomaly:
A. Pressure in the right side of the heart is greater than it is in the left side.
B. The left ventricle enlarges to accommodate an increased volume of blood.
C. Pressure is decreased in an abnormally dilated pulmonary artery.
D. Blood is shunted from the left to the right ventricle.

396. The pathological changes of sickle cell anemia could be described as which of the following?
A. Sickle-shaped cells carry excessive oxygen.
B. Red blood cell destruction is decreased.
C. Sickle-shaped RBCs cause obstruction, causing local hypoxia.
D. The life span of sickled red blood cells increases.

397. A 7-year-old child is admitted with vaso-occlusive sickle cell crisis. The child's care should include which of the following?
A. Correction of alkalosis
B. Administration of heparin
C. Administration of meperidine (Demerol)
D. Promotion of hydration

398. A school-age child has a diagnosis of β-thalassemia or Cooley's anemia. As a result, the child is undergoing chelation therapy. Which of the following laboratory results would evaluate the effect of the chelating therapy?
A. Arterial blood gases
B. Serum iron
C. Hemoglobin
D. Red blood cells

399. While at school, a 12-year-old with hemophilia fell on his arm in the classroom. The school nurse would initiate which of the following supportive measures until factor replacement therapy can be instituted?
A. Apply a warm compress
B. Begin active range of motion
C. Elevate the injured area above the level of the heart
D. Apply pressure for at least 3 minutes

400. An 8-year-old child arrives at the school nurse's office with epistaxis. Which of the following is the most appropriate nursing action to stop an occasional episode of epistaxis?
A. Have the child sit up and lean forward.
B. Apply ice to the bridge of the nose.
C. Apply pressure to the bridge of the nose for at least 3 minutes.
D. Have the child lie down quietly.

401. A child is being evaluated for renal disease. The nurse correctly identifies that the glomerular filtration is estimated by which one of the following tests?
A. Serum protein
B. Creatine
C. pH
D. Osmolality

402. A 4-year-old girl is admitted with acute glomerulonephritis. Which of the following results of the urinalysis would indicate the child is still in the acute phase?
A. Hematuria and decreased specific gravity
B. Bacteriuria and increased specific gravity
C. Proteinuria and hematuria
D. Bacteriuria and proteinuria

403. A mother asks the nurse what would be the first indication that her 4-year-old daughter's acute glomerulonephritis is improving. The nurse's best response would be which of the following?
A. Blood pressure increases.
B. The urine specific gravity will be increased.

C. Urine will be free of protein.

D. Urine output will increase.

404. A 9-year-old girl with the diagnosis of acute glomerulonephritis is to have daily weights. The nurse notes after 3 days that the child has lost 6 pounds. This is most likely the result of which of the following?
   A. Lack of exercise
   B. Poor appetite
   C. Reduction of edema
   D. Increased salt intake

405. A child is experiencing severe edema associated with acute glomerulonephritis. The nurse, when teaching about his diet, should include which of the following?
   A. Moderate sodium restriction
   B. Increased calories
   C. Increased potassium
   D. Forcing fluids

406. A 2-year-old, who is not potty trained, has been diagnosed with nephrotic syndrome. The nurse would choose which of the following as the best way to detect fluid retention in this child?
   A. Daily weights
   B. The number of wet diapers every 24 hours
   C. Abdominal girth measurements every 3 days
   D. Urine testing for hematuria

407. A hospitalized child diagnosed with nephrosis is receiving high doses of prednisone. Nursing interventions should facilitate obtaining which of the following as related to prevention of a complication from prednisone use?
   A. Stimulation of appetite
   B. Detection of edema
   C. Increase in osmotic pressure
   D. Prevention of infections

408. The nurse is teaching a mother that her infant needs a vaporizer for treating an upper respiratory infection. Why does the nurse recommend a cool-mist vaporizer rather than a steam vaporizer?
   A. They are safer.
   B. They are less expensive.
   C. They do not heat the environment.
   D. Respiratory secretions are dried with its use.

409. In the recovery room, the nurse caring for a 3-year-old following a tonsillectomy should implement which of the following?
   A. Watch for continuous swallowing.
   B. Encourage gargling with cool water to reduce discomfort.
   C. Position the child on his back for sleeping.
   D. Apply warm compresses to the throat.

410. A 24-month-old child has been diagnosed with acute otitis media. Trimethoprim/sulfamethoxazole (Bactrim) is prescribed. Parent teaching should include which of the following?

A. Continue medication until all of the symptoms subside.
B. Stop giving medication if hearing loss develops.
C. Administer all of the prescribed medication.
D. Stop giving medication and return to the clinic if the fever still exists in 24 hours.

411. A 6-year-old is seen in the clinic complaining of pain in the outer ear. The nurse suspects otitis externa. Which of the following would the nurse assess, knowing it is the most common cause of otitis externa?
   A. Trauma
   B. Swimming
   C. Foreign object obstruction
   D. Acute otitis media

412. When planning care for a child with croup, the nurse correctly identifies that a medical emergency always exists with which of the following types of croup?
   A. Spasmodic croup
   B. Laryngitis
   C. Laryngotracheobronchitis
   D. Epiglottis

413. The nurse identified a goal for a 6-year-old asthmatic to be prevention of respiratory infection. The rationale for this goal is that respiratory infections will result in which of the following?
   A. Increases sensitivity to allergens.
   B. Liquefies bronchial secretions.
   C. Can trigger or aggravate asthmatic state.
   D. Potentiates the effectiveness of medications.

414. Which of the following interventions should the nurse teach the mother for providing care to a newborn with oral candidiasis ("thrush")?
   A. Apply medication to oral mucosa, being careful none is ingested.
   B. Continue medication for prescribed number of days.
   C. Remove white patches with a soft cloth.
   D. Avoid use of a pacifier.

415. The nurse is explaining to a mother some basic principles of growth and development. Growth and development is best described by which of the following statements?
   A. Development occurs at predictable rates.
   B. The sequence of development milestones is predictable.
   C. The rate of growth among children is predictable.
   D. The rate of growth and achievement of developmental milestones are correlated.

416. A nurse is performing a physical assessment on a toddler. An appropriate approach is which of the following?
   A. Always proceed in a head-to-toe direction.
   B. Perform traumatic procedures first.

C. Demonstrate use of equipment.

D. Use minimal physical contact initially.

417. In order for the nurse to correctly take a child's blood pressure, the blood pressure cuff should cover what percentage of the child's upper arm when taking the child's blood pressure?
A. 25 percent
B. 33 percent
C. 50 percent
D. 75 percent

418. When testing preschool children for visual acuity, the nurse would plan to use the most appropriate test for this age group. The nurse would select which of the following?
A. Cover test
B. Snellen's E chart
C. "Lazy E" test
D. Picture acuity chart

419. In order to assess a child's capillary filling time, the nurse would do which of the following?
A. Palpate the carotid artery.
B. Inspect the buccal membranes.
C. Ascultate the heart.
D. Palpate the skin to produce a slight blanching.

420. A 2-year-old child is to have a Denver II administered. Prior to administration, the nurse explains to the mother that the purpose of this test is which of the following?
A. It tells what a child can do at a particular age.
B. It is an intelligence test for young children.
C. It measures a child's development.
D. It is a way to determine if a child's development is normal.

421. The community health nurse correctly identifies the leading cause of death in an infant under 1 year of age as:
A. Pneumonia and influenza
B. Respiratory distress syndrome
C. Sudden infant death syndrome
D. Congenital anomalies

422. The community health nurse correctly identifies the leading cause of death in children over the age of 1 year as which of the following?
A. Injuries
B. Congenital anomalies
C. HIV infection
D. Cancer

423. The community health nurse correctly identifies the leading cause of death in children from injuries as:
A. Fires
B. Drowning
C. Motor vehicle
D. Bicycling

424. When planning health promotion teaching for a group of high school students, the nurse identifies that following motor vehicle injuries, which of the following are leading causes of death during late adolescence?
A. HIV infections
B. Cancer
C. Suicide
D. Homicide

425. A 6-month-old infant is being seen for well-child care. The mother asks what immunizations the baby will receive. After reviewing the chart and finding that the infant is current with the recommended childhood immunization schedule, the nurse would respond to the mother by identifying which of the following immunizations?
A. Hepatitis B and oral poliovirus (OPV) vaccines
B. Mumps-measles-rubella (MMR) and *Haemophilus influenzae* type B (HIB) vaccines
C. Hepatitis B, DTP, HIB, and OPV vaccines
D. Diphtheria-pertussis-tetanus (DTP), OPV, and varicella-zoster virus (VZV) vaccines

426. A newly admitted 4-month-old has an order for a blood sugar. The nurse knows a proper location for the puncture site is which of the following locations?
A. Femoral artery
B. Center of the dorsal heel
C. The center of the finger pad of the index finger
D. The outer aspects of the heel

427. A 1-month-old infant with a ventricular septal defect is being monitored with pulse oximetry. The infant's consistent SaO_2 is 90%. Which of the following would the nurse evaluate this finding as?
A. This is within normal range.
B. SaO_2 of 90% equals a PO_2 of 45 mm Hg.
C. SaO_2 of 90% signifies developing hypoxia.
D. The infant ate 30 minutes ago so the SaO_2 is not accurate.

428. An infant with spina bifida is scheduled for surgery in 24 hours. Care of the infant with a myelomeningocele sac would include which of the following?
A. Apply a sterile, moist, nonadherent dressing over the defect.
B. Place the infant in a supine position.
C. Frequent diapering is necessary to prevent contamination.
D. All clothing and covers need to be kept clean and dry.

429. The nurse caring for an infant with spina bifida is concerned when which of the following signs of increased intracranial pressure occurs?
A. The infant quiets when picked up or handled.
B. There is maintenance of the occipitofrontal circumference.
C. The sagittal fontanelle is present.
D. The cranial sutures are separated.

430. Children who have spina bifida are prone to develop an allergy to latex. The most important nursing intervention related to this is which of the following?
A. Administer antihistamines and steroids daily.
B. Educate caregivers about the child's exposure to medical products that contain latex.
C. Educate parents that latex allergies are rare and not a serious health hazard.
D. Provide a nonlatex environment to avoid contact with latex products.

431. A 2-week-old infant is returning to the nurse's care following the placement of a ventriculoperitoneal (VP) shunt. Postoperative care would include which of the following nursing interventions?
A. Position the infant carefully on the operative side.
B. Observe for abdominal distention.
C. Elevate the head of the crib at least 6 inches.
D. Routinely pump the shunt to assess its function.

432. A 4-year-old boy with spina bifida is to begin a clean, intermittent catheterization program. When teaching the parents how to catheterize their son, the mother asks what is to be done to clean the catheter after the procedure. The appropriate response is which of the following?
A. "Throw the catheter away, and use a new one with each catheterization."
B. "Wash the catheter, then place it in boiling water for 2 minutes to kill germs."
C. "Wash the catheter with soap and water, rinsing the inside of the tube well with clear water."
D. "Dry the catheter with a paper towel and store it in a clean dry container."

433. A 5-year-old is found unresponsive, not breathing, and without a pulse. The nurse begins CPR. The proper depth for chest compressions is which of the following?
A. ½ to 1 inch
B. 1 to 1½ inches
C. 1½ to 2 inches
D. 2 to 2½ inches

434. A 3-month-old infant is found in the crib and appears to be cyanotic and unresponsive. The nurse begins CPR. The nurse will check for circulation by assessing which of the following?
A. Carotid pulse
B. Brachial pulse
C. Femoral pulse
D. Radial pulse

435. A 6-year-old girl is in respiratory arrest. Following the steps for CPR, the nurse gives two slow breaths and sees the chest rise. Although the girl does have a pulse, she is still not breathing. The nurse would continue rescue breathing at which of the following rates?

A. 1 breath every 3 seconds
B. 1 breath every 5 seconds
C. 30 times per minute
D. 45 times per minute.

436. When performing the proper technique for chest compressions on a 5-month-old infant, the nurse would use:
A. The heel of one hand with the other hand on top
B. The heel of one hand
C. The index, middle, and ring fingers
D. The index and middle fingers

437. A 2-year-old is eating a hot dog. He begins to choke. He is conscious, coughing, and making a high-pitched sound. The appropriate nursing action would be which of the following?
A. Open the child's mouth and look for a foreign object.
B. Perform the Heimlich maneuver.
C. Stay with the child, but do not perform any intervention.
D. Perform a combination of back blows and chest thrusts.

438. Physicians have diagnosed a mother's 2-day-old infant boy with an atrial septal defect, caused by a functioning foramen ovale. When explaining the diagnosis to the mother, the nurse includes in the discussion the function of the foramen ovale. In fetal circulation, the foramen ovale allows part of the blood to bypass the:
A. Left ventricle
B. Pulmonary system
C. Liver
D. Superior vena cava

439. When assessing the infant with possible coarctation of the aorta, the nurse would most likely find:
A. A fourth heart sound
B. A diastolic murmur
C. Pulse pressure difference between the upper and lower extremities
D. Bounding femoral pulses

440. The nurse correctly identifies the most common cyanotic heart defect caused by the classic combination of four anomalies, which results in decreased pulmonary blood flow, right-to-left shunting, and deoxygenated blood reaching the systemic circulation, as:
A. Tetralogy of Fallot
B. A ventricular septal defect
C. Patent ductus arteriosus
D. Transposition of the great arteries

441. A 4-month-old infant with tetralogy of Fallot has returned to the unit following a heart catheterization. The nurse assesses the infant, who has become acutely cyanotic and hyperapneic. Appropriate nursing actions in this situation would include which of the following?

A. Decrease the IV infusion to keep an open rate.
B. Administer meperidine (Demerol) as needed.
C. Apply a nasal cannula and begin oxygen administration at 0.05 L/min.
D. Place the infant in a knee-chest position.

442. With right-to-left shunting in tetralogy of Fallot, the nurse evaluates IV infusions carefully. Which of the following complications may occur readily because of the right-to-left shunt?
A. Septicemia
B. Occlusion of the catheter
C. Air embolism to the brain
D. Fluid overload

443. A 2-year-old will be having a cardiac catheterization tomorrow to evaluate his atrial septal defect. Based on his developmental stage, the nurse:
A. Uses pictures to explain the procedure to the child and his parents that evening.
B. Explains the procedure, using simple words and sentences, just before the preoperative sedation.
C. Asks the parents to explain the procedure to the child after the nurse explains it to them.
D. Asks the parents to leave the room while the preoperative medication and instructions are given.

444. Home care instructions for the 5-year-old child following a cardiac catheterization should include:
A. If a small bruise develops around the insertion site, notify the physician.
B. Use tub bathing for 7 to 10 days.
C. Give aspirin if the child complains of pain at the insertion site.
D. Remove the pressure dressing in 24 hours and keep a clean, dry bandage on the insertion site for several days.

445. Parent care for the family of a child with a congenital heart defect would include:
A. Encouraging the parents not to tell the child about the seriousness of the congenital heart defect, so the child will function as normally as possible.
B. Acknowledging the fear and concern surrounding their child's health and assisting the parents through the grieving process as they mourn the loss of their fantasized healthy child.
C. Identifying anger and resentment as destructive emotions that serve no purpose.
D. Expressing to the parents after the corrective surgery is completed and successful, all these feelings will be resolve.

446. An infant with a congenital heart defect is being discharged on digoxin elixir every 12 hours. The nurse teaches the parents when administering digoxin to the infant:

A. If the infant vomits within 30 minutes of the digoxin administration, repeat the dose.
B. Mix it with formula so the infant swallows it easily.
C. If the infant vomits two or more consecutive doses, or becomes listless or anorexic, notify the physician.
D. If a dose of digoxin is skipped for more than 6 hours, a new timetable for administration must be developed.

447. A 4-year-old child with a history of sickle-cell anemia is admitted to the nursing unit where assessment findings reveal tenderness and swelling in the hands and feet. The nurse correctly identifies the child as most likely experiencing a/an:
A. Aplastic crisis
B. Vaso-occlusive crisis
C. Dactylitis crisis
D. Sequestration crisis

448. The focus of nursing interventions for the child experiencing sickle-cell crisis is aimed toward:
A. Maintaining an adequate level of hydration
B. Providing pain relief
C. Preventing infection
D. Oxygen therapy

449. A week-old infant has been diagnosed with coarctation of the aorta. The nurse is aware that congestive heart failure (CHF) is a possible clinical consequence. The early signs of CHF in an infant would include which of the following?
A. Bradycardia
B. Weight loss
C. Apnea
D. Profuse scalp sweating

450. A 4-week-old infant is admitted in CHF related to an atrial septal defect. On admission, the heart rate (HR) is 164, the respiratory rate (RR) is 82, BP is 74/40, and oxygen saturation is 96 percent. He is tired, irritable, and having mild retractions, but no edema is observed. He has been feeding poorly for several days. Medications that have been ordered include digoxin and furosemide (Lasix). In planning fluid and nutrition for the next 12 hours, the nurse would expect which of the following interventions to be ordered?
A. Push bottle feedings every 3 hours.
B. Begin infant on high calorie formula and bottle feed every 4 to 5 hours.
C. Place a nasogastric feeding tube and institute gavage feedings to meet maintenance fluid requirements.
D. Make the infant NPO and run IV fluids at one-half maintenance.

451. A 4-week-old infant in CHF from a ventricular septal defect is being digitalized. The order reads that the infant is to receive a total 30 μg/kg of body weight of digoxin in four divided doses over 24

hours. The infant weighs 11 lb. Digoxin is available as an elixir with a concentration of 50 μg/ml. The correct quantity to be administered is which of the following?
A. 0.5 ml
B. 0.75 ml
C. 1.0 ml
D. 3.0 ml

452. A 4-week-old infant in CHF from an atrial septal defect is receiving furosemide and digoxin. When reviewing the infant's laboratory findings, the serum potassium level is 3.6 mmol/L. Which of the following would be the appropriate intervention?
A. The potassium level is normal.
B. The potassium level is too low and the practitioner needs to be notified.
C. The potassium level is too high and the practitioner needs to be notified immediately.
D. The potassium level is not significant in this client.

453. When planning care for an infant in CHF, one of the identified goals is to decrease the cardiac demand. To lessen the workload on the heart, the plan includes which of the following to minimize metabolic needs?
A. Provide a neutral thermal environment.
B. Place the infant in a supine position while sleeping.
C. Avoid sedation through medication.
D. Increase environmental stimuli.

454. A 4-week-old infant with CHF from an atrial septal defect is placed on accurate intake and output. The output for the last 4 hours was recorded as one wet diaper weighing 18 cc. The infant weighs 8 lb. The nurse evaluates this information as which of the following?
A. The amount of urine is adequate and continued accurate input and output will continue.
B. The amount of urine is above the normal range.
C. The amount of urine is below the normal range.
D. Four hours is too short a time frame to determine output by using wet diapers.

455. A 2-year-old girl undergoing chemotherapy for leukemia has recently been hospitalized for pneumonia. Her platelet count is 50,000 mm³. Which of the following requires further assessment because of its potential risk of bleeding?
A. She has an intermittent infusion device in her hand.
B. A tympanic thermometer is present in the room.
C. A sign stating no IM injections are to be administered is hanging in the room.
D. She is receiving 6 L of oxygen via nasal cannula.

456. A 3-year-old boy has leukemia and is undergoing chemotherapy. He has developed stomatitis from the chemotherapy. Which of the following interventions would be helpful related to the stomatitis?
A. Provide a bland, moist, soft diet.
B. Use lemon glycerin swabs.
C. Administer viscous lidocaine.
D. Limit oral care to once a day.

457. A 13-year-old with leukemia is receiving chemotherapy. A frequent complication is infection secondary to neutropenia. This child is susceptible to infection during immunosuppressive therapy, which causes an absolute neutrophil count (ANC) of less than 100/mm³. When the nurse is assessing the following laboratory data, which of the following indicates that the ANC is below 100/mm³?
A. WBC = 1000, neutrophils = 7 percent, bands = 7 percent
B. WBC = 1300, neutrophils = 5 percent, non-segmented neutrophils = 8 percent
C. WBC = 1200, neutrophils = 4 percent, non-segmented neutrophils = 6 percent
D. WBC = 1100, neutrophils = 5 percent, bands = 4 percent

458. A nurse observes an adolescent being hit by a car while rollerblading. She stops to assist and is told the emergency medical system has been activated. Until the paramedics arrive, which of the following should be considered in providing care for the adolescent who has experienced severe trauma?
A. Move the adolescent off the side of the road and into a less congested area.
B. Apply a blanket because temperature maintenance is more difficult in this age group.
C. Assess the injured area first; assessment of other areas can wait.
D. Rapid assessment begins with the level of consciousness.

459. A school-aged girl was a passenger in a car involved in a motor vehicle accident. She responds to verbal stimuli, has a pulse of 140, and has a breathing rate of 32 per minute. The emergency medical system has been activated. A large laceration is found on the girl's left lower leg. A tourniquet was applied by the first person providing assistance. Which of the following should the nurse implement related to the tourniquet?
A. Leave the tourniquet in place.
B. Remove the tourniquet and apply direct pressure if bleeding occurs.
C. Elevate the affected extremity prior to removing the tourniquet.
D. Apply pressure to the appropriate pressure point prior to loosening the tourniquet.

460. A 9-year-old girl was a passenger in an automobile accident. She sustained a spinal cord injury result-

ing in paralysis. Which of the following is a physiological effect of immobilization in children?

A. Bone calcium increases, depleting serum calcium, resulting in hypocalcemia.

B. Increased joint mobility leads to the formation of contractures.

C. Dependent edema develops, which results in tissue that is prone to infection and trauma.

D. The workload on the heart decreases as a result of the redistribution of the blood volume from the reduction of gravity pressure.

461. A child who is a quadriplegic has been admitted to the pediatric unit. The child is hypercalcemic. The nurse correctly identifies which clinical manifestation as suggestive of hypercalcemia?

A. Anuria

B. Polydipsia

C. Increased neuronal permeability

D. Hyperreflexia

462. A quadriplegic child is to be placed in an upright position on a tilt table twice a day. The mother asks the nurse what the reason is for putting the child on the tilt table. The nurse replies that it reduces which of the following effects of immobility?

A. Impaired healing

B. Bone demineralization

C. Negative nitrogen balance

D. Thrombus formation

463. An 11-year-old sustained a fracture in the epiphyseal plate of his left radius from a fall during physical education. The nurse is teaching his parents about the fracture. Which of the following should be included in this discussion?

A. Epiphyseal injuries are unusual because it is the strongest point of the long bone.

B. Healing is usually delayed in this type of fracture.

C. Bone growth can be affected with this type of fracture.

D. Medical management with this type of fracture is the same as for other fractures.

464. A 5-year-old boy was seen in the emergency room for a complete fracture of the left femur. The child was casted, and the nurse is providing cast care instructions for the parents. Which of the following should be included in the parent's education?

A. A blow-dryer on the heat setting may be used to facilitate drying the cast.

B. The movement and sensation in the child's left toes should be checked frequently for the first day.

C. Expect to observe swelling and discoloration of the left toes for the first 3 to 5 days.

D. The left leg should be kept in a dependent position for the first 24 hours.

465. A 3-year-old has just returned from surgery in a spica cast. Which of the following assessment findings would cause a nurse to suspect that an infection has developed under the cast?

A. Numbness in the toes of the left foot

B. Toes of the right foot that are cold to touch

C. Normal movement of the toes

D. Hot spots felt on the cast surface

466. A 3-year-old in a spica cast is a client on the pediatric unit. Considering both safety and development, the most appropriate play activity for this child would be which of the following?

A. A toy telephone

B. Bean bag toss

C. Game of checkers

D. Marbles

467. The role of the school nurse in relation to sports injuries is directed toward prevention, treatment, and rehabilitation. Which of the following statements is correct regarding sports injuries during adolescence?

A. The increased strength during adolescence helps to prevent injuries related to fatigue.

B. Rapidly growing bones, muscles, and tendons offer protection from unusual strain.

C. Adolescents do not possess the insight and judgment to recognize when a sport activity is beyond their capability.

D. More injuries take place in organized athletic competition than during recreational sport activities.

468. In soft-tissue injuries such as sprains or strains, the therapeutic treatment is to ice the injury immediately. When ice is applied, which of the following results?

A. The pain threshold is increased.

B. The tissues have increased metabolism.

C. More histaminelike substances are released.

D. Deep-tissue vasodilatation is produced.

469. A 14-year-old male is sent to the school nurse after experiencing shin splints during a track practice. Which of the following is the appropriate nursing intervention?

A. Tell the boy shin splints are not a serious injury.

B. Walking is the best method for reducing the pain.

C. Ice, rest, and a nonsteroidal anti-inflammatory over-the-counter medication usually relieve the pain.

D. Explain to the adolescent that shin splints are a form of stress fracture.

470. A 10-year-old male with hypopituitarism will receive growth hormone therapy. In preparing for home care, the nurse should teach the family which of the following?

A. Treatment is most successful if growth hormone therapy is started in adolescence.

B. Replacement therapy will be needed throughout the rest of the boy's life.

C. Daily subcutaneous injections will be required for replacement therapy.

D. If replacement therapy is successful, the boy will attain his adult height at the same rate as his peers.

471. A school nurse is reviewing information parents have provided on children's health records. The nurse would identify sexual development in girls and boys as precocious and needing investigation before which of the following ages?
A. Nine years of age in both girls and boys
B. Girls—9 years of age; boys—11 years of age
C. Ten years of age in both girls and boys
D. Girls—8 years of age; boys—9 years of age

472. A teacher seeks the school nurse to discuss her concerns about a 12-year-old girl. The girl has gradually changed her behaviors over the school year. The girl has become hyperactive, irritable, developed a decreased attention span, and the shape of her eyes appears to be changing. The nurse tells the teacher which of the following?
A. The symptoms are characteristic of a prepubescent female. She will outgrow it.
B. The symptoms may be indicative of hyperthyroidism and need further evaluation. Most cases of Graves' disease occur in children between 12 to 14 years of age.
C. The symptoms may be indicative of hypothyroidism and need further evaluation. Hypothyroidism is the most common endocrine problem in childhood.
D. The symptoms may be indicative of diabetes insipidus. A family history is necessary, as well as further evaluation.

473. A camp nurse recognizes the signs of heatstroke in a 13-year-old boy. His temperature is 104°F. He is confused, but is able to drink water safely. While waiting to transport the boy to the hospital, nursing interventions would include which of the following?
A. Continue to ambulate slowly and with assistance.
B. Administer antipyretics.
C. Administer salt tablets.
D. Apply towels wet with cool water.

474. The nurse is providing preoperative education to an adolescent girl who will be experiencing Harrington instrumentation to treat scoliosis. Interventions the girl can expect following surgery would include which of the following?
A. The surgery eliminates the need for casting and bracing.
B. Nasogastric intubation and urinary catheterization may be required.
C. Little discomfort will follow the surgery, and pain will be controlled nonpharmacologically.

D. Ambulation will not be allowed for approximately 4 months.

475. A 6-year-old boy has been admitted to the pediatric unit with a diagnosis of acute osteomyelitis. An appropriate nursing intervention when caring for this child would be which of the following?
A. Move and turn the child gently and carefully to minimize discomfort.
B. Apply warm compresses to the affected extremity.
C. Encourage frequent ambulation.
D. The child will be NPO until the acute symptoms subside.

476. A nursing diagnosis relevant for a child with juvenile rheumatoid arthritis is pain related to joint inflammation. A planned nursing intervention useful to reduce the pain caused by the inflammation would include which of the following?
A. Apply ice packs to relieve acute swelling and pain.
B. Administer acetaminophen to reduce the inflammation.
C. Encourage range-of-motion exercises during periods of inflammation.
D. Provide a well-balanced diet.

477. A 3-year-old girl is admitted to the unit with a diagnosis of short-bowel syndrome. The parents sought medical assistance because stools were increasing in frequency and their consistency was becoming watery over the last 24 hours. The child's temperature is 102.6°F, and she has vomited several times. During the initial nursing assessment, the nurse would monitor which of the following?
A. Stool pH, BUN, and vital signs
B. Urine specific gravity, stool for blood, electrolytes
C. Vital signs, stool-reducing substance, stool culture
D. Vital signs, weight, urine specific gravity, and input-output

478. A 6-year-old child had heart surgery today and a mediastinal tube was inserted. The last set of vital signs were BP 80/50, P 94, R 22, and T 98.4°F. The nurse evaluates the vital signs and correctly identifies which of the following as indicating a cardiac tamponade?
A. Blood pressure of 78/50
B. Decreased breath sounds
C. Jugular vein distention
D. Pulse of 100

479. A 12-year-old child developed a pneumothorax from trauma experienced during a motor vehicle accident. A left pleural tube was inserted in the emergency room. After chest tube insertion, the nurse is assessing the child's vital signs, which are BP 100/60, P 96, and R 24. Which of the following

would be most indicative of developing a tension pneumothorax?
A. Blood pressure decrease to 98/56
B. Complaints of pain on the left side
C. Decreased air movement on the left side of the chest
D. Pulse rate increasing to 100

480. A child was admitted to the pediatric unit, diagnosed with Kawasaki disease. The pediatrician ordered intravenous gamma globulin. Which of the following symptoms would the nurse identify as being the most important in determining a problem with the gamma globulin infusion?
A. Chest tightness
B. Dysuria
C. Increased blood pressure
D. Tenderness at the IV site

481. A child has been receiving high doses of aspirin therapy for Kawasaki disease. Which of the following would the nurse recognize as indicating an adverse effect of aspirin therapy?
A. Increase in platelet aggregation
B. Peripheral edema
C. Tinnitus
D. Urticaria

482. An 11-month-old is being discharged from the hospital after receiving IV gamma globulin and aspirin therapy for Kawasaki disease. Which of the following should the nurse include in the discharge teaching to the mother?
A. Daily temperatures should be recorded for 1 month; elevations should be reported to the physician.
B. Delay the administration of the MMR immunization for 5 months.
C. Low-dose aspirin therapy can be stopped in 1 month.
D. Notify the physician if your child persists with irritability.

483. A 10-year-old male took a dose of regular insulin at 9 P.M. At which times would the nurse expect a hypoglycemic reaction?
A. 9:30 P.M. to 10:30 P.M.
B. 11 P.M. to 1 A.M.
C. 3 A.M. to 5 A.M.
D. 6 A.M. to 8 A.M.

484. At 4 P.M., a child's capillary glucose level was 66. How many grams of carbohydrates are initially recommended for this level of hypoglycemia?
A. 15
B. 30
C. 45
D. None are required.

485. A 9-year-old female diagnosed with insulin-dependent diabetes mellitus (IDDM) is in the clinic for a regular check-up. Among the blood work drawn today was the glycosylated hemoglo-bin. Her mother tells the nurse she doesn't understand what this test measures. Which of the following explanations by the nurse would be most accurate?
A. This test is done to determine the accuracy of the child's daily glucose monitoring.
B. This test is done when the physician thinks the client is nonadherent with the treatment regimen.
C. Glucose molecules attach to hemoglobin and measuring this indicates to the physician how well the body utilizes insulin.
D. Glucose molecules attach to hemoglobin. By measuring this, the average glucose level is determined, which indicates how well the diabetes was controlled over the past 3 months.

486. A 7-year-old female diabetic client takes a combination of NPH and regular insulin every morning at 7:30. The nurse is teaching the mother the usual times that children who are on mixed insulin dosages experience hypoglycemia. Which of the following times do the usual hypoglycemic episodes occur in children?
A. 8 A.M. and 11 P.M.
B. 9:30 A.M. and 2 P.M.
C. 10 A.M. and 1 P.M.
D. 11:30 A.M. and 2:30 P.M.

487. A 12-year-old diabetic male is experiencing a mild hypoglycemic episode. Which of the following food sources equals 15 gms of carbohydrates?
A. One-half cup of apple juice
B. One-half cup of whole milk
C. One-half cup of orange juice with 2 teaspoons of sugar
D. One cup of orange juice

488. The mother of a child with leukemia brings her in for a check-up. The mother says her little girl does not seem to have any energy. The WBC count indicates neutropenia. Which of the following is indicative of neutropenia?
A. Absolute neutrophil count between 500 and 1000
B. Absolute neutrophil count between 2500 and 3000
C. Absolute neutrophil count between 5000 and 7000
D. Absolute neutrophil count >10,000

489. A 7-year-old child has been diagnosed with thrombocytopenia. The nurse can expect spontaneous bleeding in the child if the platelet count is at which level?
A. 18,000
B. 46,000
C. 100,000
D. 150,000

490. A 15-year-old female has a platelet count of 88,000. Which of the following nursing actions would be

the most appropriate to include in this client's care plan?
A. Assessing temperature elevations by rectal thermometers
B. Promoting good oral hygiene by brushing teeth after each meal and bedtime
C. Restricting aspirin intake to once a day
D. Teaching the client how to use creams to remove hair on legs

491. A 6-year-old female with sickle cell disease came to the emergency room for pain management. The ER physician diagnosed her with a vaso-occlusive episode. The physician ordered IV hydration and morphine sulfate for pain management. The mother asks the nurse why oxygen was not ordered. Which of the following explanations by the nurse would be the most accurate?
A. "Oxygen is only helpful if hypoxemia is apparent."
B. "Hydration is necessary to prevent dehydration that causes sickling."
C. "Hydration with IV fluids and pain medication are more beneficial for the type of crisis your child is having."
D. "Oxygen will not decrease sickling or pain that is occurring now; however, hydration will decrease the sickling and the pain."

492. A 2-year-old male was admitted to the pediatric unit 5 days ago due to a sickle cell crisis. The child will be discharged in a few days. Which of the following would take first priority in discharge planning?
A. Assess the parents's knowledge of pain management for their child.
B. Consult social services so that they can follow up postdischarge for any complications.
C. Refer parents to a support group for families of chronically ill children.
D. Teach the child and parents measures that can prevent sickle cell crisis.

493. A 10-year-old female returned from surgery this morning. The surgeon ordered meperidine (Demerol) for severe pain every 4 hours with acetaminophen with codeine (Tylenol #3) for mild to moderate pain. Which of the following information is the most important to know about Demerol?
A. Demerol orally is as effective as intramuscular injections.
B. It should not be administered longer than 48 hours.
C. Demerol has fewer adverse effects than morphine.
D. Narcan should be used to reverse adverse effects of Demerol.

494. A father brings his 3-year-old daughter to the clinic because he says she doesn't play as much as she used to and appears fatigued. After a history

and assessment, the physician tells the father he thinks she may have juvenile dermatomyositis (JDMS). The nurse correctly identifies which of the following behaviors as being the most characteristic of a child with JDMS?
A. Difficulty walking up steps
B. Distal, symmetrical muscle weakness
C. Rigidity in the neck
D. Weight gain from limited activity

495. A 16-year-old male brings a letter to the school nurse stating that he has been diagnosed with ankylosing spondylitis and has been started on indomethacin (Indocin) 25 mg twice a day. Long term, which of the following actions by the nurse would assist him with the adaptation to this disease?
A. Referral to a career counselor
B. Restricting physical activities during school hours
C. Teaching measures to prevent GI bleeding
D. Supplying a second set of books at home, so he will not have to carry them back and forth to school

496. A 9-year-old child has been immobilized in skeletal traction for 6 weeks because of a fracture in the right femur from trauma sustained in a motor vehicle accident. The last laboratory results revealed hypercalcemia. What is the essential nursing action in this case?
A. Administer at least 2500 ml of fluids orally to this child daily.
B. Consult the physical therapist for exercise suggestions.
C. Monitor the calcium level of the child daily.
D. Notify the physicians to see if any action should be taken.

497. A 12-year-old returned to the pediatric unit after an open reduction to the left ulna. Which of the following circumstances would indicate that the child may be developing compartment syndrome?
A. Pain that is radiating toward the left fingers
B. Increasing pain in the left arm responsive to medications
C. Pain that is nonresponsive to a narcotic analgesic
D. Pain specific to the wrist that requires a narcotic for relief

498. The nurse is assessing a 16-year-old male who weighs 60 kg and is 15 hours' postoperative from a reduction of a compound fracture to the right femur. The nurse would give immediate attention to which of the following?
A. Blood pressure of 100/60
B. Petechiae noted on the chest
C. Minimal relief of pain after administration of a narcotic
D. Total urine output of 600 ml since surgery

499. A 6-year-old female is being admitted to the pediatric surgery unit for the application of an Ilizarow external fixation device. Which statement is the most accurate regarding this device?
A. The Ilizarow external fixation device allows for lengthening of the bone because it properly aligns the bone so fusion can occur.
B. The Ilizarow external fixation device is used to correct improperly healed fractures by providing immobilization to the bone after it has been reset.
C. The Ilizarow external fixation device is used for traumatic fractures that usually require a longer time to heal.
D. The Ilizarow external device allows manual distraction of the bone so that new bone can develop in the space created.

500. A 4-year-old has been placed in Buck's extension traction to reduce a simple fracture to the left tibia. Which of the following nursing actions would be the most important in maintaining the traction?
A. Assessing the weights frequently to make sure they are hanging freely
B. Doing neurovascular checks every 4 hours to ensure adequate circulation to the extremity
C. Monitoring the effectiveness of the muscle relaxant that was administered
D. Readjusting the fit of the Ace bandage daily to promote countertraction

501. An immobilized child has developed hypercalcemia. Which of the following selections of foods would be most appropriate for the child's evening meals?
A. Chicken, peas, cornbread, and plums
B. Tuna salad sandwich, carrots, and low-fat milk
C. Boiled shrimp, rice, watermelon, and ice tea
D. Grilled cheese sandwich, strawberries, and ice cream

502. An 8-year-old child recently was diagnosed with polyarticular juvenile rheumatoid arthritis. Which of the following goals would be the most important in the collaborative management of the disease process?
A. Limiting physical deformities
B. Maintaining growth within parameters for age group
C. Preserving joint function
D. Preventing side effects from corticosteroid therapy

503. A 6-year-old with pauciarticular juvenile rhematoid arthritis has been fitted with a splint for her right knee. As the nurse planning care, when would be the most appropriate time for the splint to be worn?
A. During rest periods and at night
B. During play activities with other children
C. During school hours
D. During any painful episodes

504. A 10-year-old male with juvenile rheumatoid arthritis has been admitted to the pediatric unit. What is the best rationale for positioning the child in prone position?
A. Allows for posterior assessment of the skin
B. Places the hips and knees in proper alignment
C. Prevents skin breakdown
D. Reduces pain through natural positioning

505. A 10-year-old female with juvenile rheumatoid arthritis complains of morning stiffness. The mother says she is frequently late for school because of this. What would be the best strategy for the nurse to teach the mother-client how to deal with the morning stiffness?
A. Have the child do limbering-up exercises 30 minutes before time to dress for school.
B. Have the child sleep on a warm waterbed to prevent morning stiffness.
C. Wake the child 1 hour early in the morning, administer medications, and then allow the child to sleep another hour before rising.
D. Wake the child 1 hour early, then place her in a warm bath to limber the joints.

506. The nurse is teaching the mother of a 9-year-old male newly diagnosed with systemic lupus erythematosus (SLE) measures to regulate his activity. Which is the most important factor to consider in regulating activity to reduce the risk of an exacerbation of the disease process?
A. Continuing the same physical education activities at school as before the diagnosis of lupus, but with closer supervision
B. Promoting 8 to 10 hours of sleep at night, with one or two rest periods during the day
C. Rescheduling school hours, so half the number of school hours are home-bound, directed by a tutor
D. Supervising after-school and weekend activities to ensure that excessive fatigue does not occur

507. A nurse is teaching a 16-year-old female diagnosed with SLE self-care measures. Which of the following would be the best measure to teach regarding sun protection?
A. Avoid the sun between 10 A.M. and 2 P.M.
B. Dress with long-sleeve shirts and pants when exposed to the sun between 10 A.M. and 2 P.M.
C. Reapply sunscreen every 8 hours and after becoming wet.
D. Between the hours of 10 A.M. and 2 P.M., wear a hat to avoid excessive sun rays.

508. A 17-year-old client has been diagnosed with SLE. What is the primary goal of the nurse teaching the client about SLE?
A. Adjustment to the treatment plan
B. Managing limitations to social activities
C. Recognizing limitations caused by disease
D. Understanding potential side effects of medications

509. A 12-year-old female diagnosed with SLE is experiencing an exacerbation of the disease. Her rheumatologist has prescribed prednisone. Which of the following diets would be the most important to teach to this client?
A. Acid ash diet
B. High protein diet
C. Reduced fat diet
D. Low sodium diet

510. A 12-year-old male with SLE is being seen in the rheumatology clinic. Which of the following symptoms could indicate the presence of disease activity?
A. Complaints of sun sensitivity
B. Excessive fatigue
C. Puffy eyes and edematous ankles
D. Presence of a malar rash

511. An 11-year-old male has been treated over the last year for episodes of allergic rhinitis. Assessment during this clinic visit indicates no symptoms of rhinitis. The doctor instructs the child and mother to continue with the cromolyn sodium nasal spray once a day. The mother says to the nurse, "I don't understand why he has to take medicines when he's not having any problems." Which response best indicates the nurse understands the rationale for this treatment?
A. "Cromolyn sodium must be taken for a long time before it is effective."
B. "Cromolyn sodium stabilizes the eosinophil count."
C. "Cromolyn sodium reduces inflammation when taken over a period of time."
D. "Cromolyn sodium is used as a prophylactic to prevent allergic symptoms once exposed to an allergen."

512. A 12-year-old female has been receiving immunotherapy for 1 year. The parents report their child continues to have allergic symptoms, without any improvement. Which of the following statements by the nurse would be the most accurate?
A. "Allergy testing must be redone to determine if new allergies have developed."
B. "It can take as long as 48 months before symptoms improve."
C. "No improvement in 1 year indicates the immunotherapy is ineffective."
D. "The strength of the immunotherapy must be increased for more benefit."

513. Skin testing on a 7-year-old client indicated an allergy to dust mites. What measures would the nurse teach the mother to reduce exposure to the dust mite?
A. Clean bath and shower areas daily with a disinfectant.
B. Do not allow tobacco smoke in the home.
C. Limit the child's exposure to animals.
D. Restrict child from playing on carpeted floors.

514. A 4-year-old child has allergies to milk and wheat. Which of the following foods could trigger an allergic response in this child?
A. Cocoa
B. Popcorn
C. Tuna
D. Wieners

515. A 10-year-old child experienced an anaphylactic reaction to eggs. It is important to teach the child and family foods that contain eggs. What food below should the nurse teach to avoid?
A. Cola beverages
B. Gravy
C. Instant breakfast drinks
D. Mayonnaise

516. A 12-year-old client received her monthly allergy shot today. Fifteen minutes after the shot was given, a raised edematous area, 8 by 10 cm, was present at the injection site. Which response by the nurse demonstrates the best nursing judgment?
A. "Allergy shots must be discontinued when local reactions occur."
B. "I'll ask the physical for an order for a medication to reduce itching."
C. "Next time she is due for an allergy shot, I will not increase the dosage, but remain at the same strength."
D. "The edematous area is what is expected, so we can continue with increasing the dosage."

517. A mother asks the nurse about feeding cereal to her 5-month-old. Which cereal should a nurse teach the mother to introduce first in the infant's diet?
A. Barley
B. Oats
C. Rice
D. Wheat

518. A mother brings her 8-month-old infant to the clinic for a check-up. The physician tells the mother to begin mixing the infant's cereal with fruit juice instead of milk. The mother says to the nurse, "I don't understand why I should mix the cereal with juice." Which of the following explanations by the nurse would be the most accurate?
A. "At this age, formula does not provide enough iron."
B. "Fruit juice contains vitamin C, which increases the absorption of iron in the cereal."
C. "Since solid foods are being introduced, milk should be decreased."
D. "The juice improves the flavor of the cereal."

519. A mother is in the clinic with her 10-month-old infant. So far, the mother only feeds her infant formula and baby cereal. In preparing to teach the mother methods for introducing solid foods, the

nurse would include which of the following statements in her plan of care:
A. "Baby cereals should be discontinued at 1 year of age when the infant is eating other sources of foods."
B. "Eggs are the best source of protein to introduce initially."
C. "Introduce one new food at a time, trying this food at least 4 days before adding any new foods."
D. "Once cereals are added to your child's diet, iron supplements can be stopped."

520. The mother brought her 12-month-old into the clinic for a well-baby check-up. During the assessment, the nurse discovers the mother is giving the infant fruit juice through a bottle. Which of the following explanations by the nurse would be the most accurate?
A. "Fruit juice given through a bottle should be diluted with water."
B. "Giving your child fruit juice by a cup reduces dental caries."
C. "It is best to give fruit juice mixed with cereal."
D. "Using a cup will promote the development of your child."

521. The nurse is preparing to suction a 6-year-old client with a tracheostomy. Which of the following vacuum-pressure ranges is recommended for suctioning the child?
A. 50 to 70
B. 70 to 90
C. 80 to 100
D. 100 to 120

522. A 6-year-old child is going to be discharged home with a tracheostomy. The nurse is teaching the parents principles of tracheostomy suctioning. To prevent trauma to the respiratory tract, the nurse should teach the parents which of the following?
A. One suction catheter may be used for a 24-hour period without introducing bacteria, as long as it is rinsed with sterile solution after use and kept in a sterile container.
B. Premeasure the depth the catheter should be inserted, not exceeding the length of the tracheostomy tube.
C. Hyperventilate the child with 100 percent oxygen before and after suctioning.
D. Use a suction catheter that is one-half the diameter of the tracheostomy tube.

523. A 6-year-old client with cerebral palsy requires frequent suctioning because of copious amounts of secretions. During the suctioning procedure, which of the following would indicate a need for oxygenation:
A. An episode of coughing
B. An oxygen saturation decreasing to 95 percent from 97 percent

C. An inability to obtain secretions because of the thickness of the mucus
D. The client develops bradycardia.

524. The parents of a 9-month-old infant with a tracheostomy tube are going to take their child home. The nurse should teach the parents to limit suctioning to:
A. 5 seconds
B. 15 seconds
C. 20 seconds
D. 30 seconds

525. A 3-year-old had a tracheostomy performed on her 5 days ago. Which of the following signs would indicate that the child needs suctioning?
A. Blood pressure of 80/50
B. Heart rate of 120
C. Oxygen saturation of 95 percent
D. Respiratory rate of 22

526. A child with pneumonia has been admitted to the pediatric unit. The physician ordered continuous pulse oximetry. Which of the following circumstances could give an inaccurate pulse oximetry reading?
A. A client whose capillary refill is less than 3 seconds in the extremity the probe is on
B. A client who has been diagnosed with iron deficient anemia
C. A sedated client
D. Covering the client's extremity that has the pulse oximetry probe.

527. Parents bring their 2-year-old to the emergency room because of noisy respirations. Assessment by the nurse reveals wheezing with a respiratory rate of 32, heart rate of 120, and weight of 14 kg. The physician orders ephinephrine hydrochloride (1:1000), 0.01 mg/kg subcutaneously now. The medicine is supplied in 1 mg/1 ml ampules. Which of the following is the correct dose to administer according to weight?
A. 0.014 ml
B. 0.14 ml
C. 1.4 ml
D. 14.0 ml

528. A child was just given a subcutaneous injection of epinephrine. The nurse is responsible for assessing the child's status. When would the nurse expect the epinephrine to begin working?
A. Less than 5 minutes
B. Five to 10 minutes
C. Twenty minutes
D. Twenty to 30 minutes

529. A 1-year-old was admitted to the pediatric unit diagnosed with respiratory infection. The nurse observes intermittent nasal flaring while the child is sleeping. The mother asks the nurse what the nasal flaring means. Which of the following state-

ments by the nurse is the most accurate explanation?

A. Nasal flaring assists small children by enabling them to breath more easily.

B. Nasal flaring indicates an increased effort in breathing brought about by the respiratory infection.

C. Nasal flaring occurs when there are increased secretions in the tracheobronchial tree.

D. Nasal flaring is a mechanism that reduces the resistance of air flow in the respiratory tract.

530. A 3-year-old has been admitted to the pediatric unit for mild dehydration. The physician has ordered IV fluids. Which of the following locations would be the most appropriate to assess for placement for the initial IV site:

A. Nondominant hand

B. Top of the foot

C. Antecubital fossa

D. Scalp

531. A 6-year-old is receiving a blood transfusion after orthopedic surgery. He begins to complain of nausea and vomiting, and chills with leg pains. These symptoms indicate what kind of transfusion reaction?

A. Allergic

B. Circulatory overload

C. Hemolytic

D. Septic

532. The physician wrote an order to give one unit of packed red blood cells to a 10-year-old diagnosed with anemia. Which of the following actions would be appropriate by the nurse when administering blood products?

A. Blood should be warmed to 37°C when being infused.

B. Discontinue the blood after 4 hours, whether it is completed or not.

C. Hang the blood within 1 hour of receiving it from the blood bank.

D. Infuse 5% dextrose in water (D5W) before and after the blood transfusion.

533. A 3-month-old infant is in intensive care because of pneumonia. The child has been very irritable and hard to console. At this stage in his treatment, low concentrations of oxygen have been sufficient to maintain oxygen saturation above 95 percent. Which of the following oxygen delivery systems would be best for this infant at this stage of his illness?

A. Blow-by method

B. Mask

C. Nasal cannula

D. Tent

534. A physician has ordered gentamycin 2 drops OD four times a day for a 2-year-old child. Which of the following actions is appropriate by the nurse?

A. Pull the left lower eyelid down, instill drops, then repeat with the other eye.

B. Pull the left pinna back and upward to instill drops.

C. Pull the right lower eyelid down to form a reservoir, then instill the drops.

D. Pull the right pinna straight back and down to instill drops.

535. An order was written to give a 10-year-old female prednisone, one drop every 8 hours both ears. Which of the following is the appropriate procedure for instilling ear drops?

A. Keep the child's head in the same position for 10 minutes after the drop is instilled.

B. Pull the pinna back and upward to instill drops.

C. Raise the head of the bed to a 45-degree angle after the drops are instilled.

D. Tape a piece of cotton in the ear canals.

536. Ampicillin has been ordered IV push for an 8-year-old child. In comparing the IV push method to the IV piggyback method, which of the following differences would be the most evident?

A. IV push medication administration takes less than 10 minutes.

B. IV piggyback medication must be diluted with a certain amount of IV solution.

C. The IV piggyback method reduces allergic responses.

D. The IV push method is recommended because it is less confining to the child.

537. A nurse is administering an immunization by intramuscular method to a 6-year-old. Which of the following is an appropriate action by the nurse?

A. Administer the vaccine into the vastus lateralis muscle.

B. Insert the needle at a 90-degree angle.

C. Omit aspiration when administering immunizations.

D. Use a ⅝-inch needle.

538. A nurse is administering a subcutaneous medication to a 15-month-old female. Which of the following approaches by the nurse is best?

A. Choosing the vastus lateralis muscle for the injection site.

B. Inserting the needle at a 90-degree angle.

C. Pulling the skin taut before inserting the needle.

D. Using a ⅝-inch 25-gauge needle to administer the medicine.

539. The nurse is preparing to administer an intramuscular injection to a 4-year-old child. Which of the following muscles would be the most appropriate site to use?

A. Deltoid

B. Vastus lateralis

C. Dorsogluteal

D. Ventrogluteal

540. Meperidine (Demerol) has been ordered for a 43-kg adolescent who is 24 hours' postoperative from an appendectomy. The recommended dosage for pediatric pain management is 1 to 1.8 mg/kg. Which of the following doses will be allowed for maximum pain control?
A. 43 mg
B. 60 mg
C. 77 mg
D. 100 mg

541. A 7-year-old has been receiving packed red blood cells for 2 hours. The vital signs are: BP = 92/56, RR = 24, P = 100, and T = 98.8°F. Which of the following would alert the nurse that the child might be having a transfusion reaction?
A. Chest and back pain
B. Tarry stools
C. Dysuria
D. Increase in urine output

542. A 2-year-old weighting 12 kg was admitted to the pediatric unit with septicemia. The pediatrician orders ampicillin (50 mg/kg) to be administered IV every 8 hours. Ampicillin, which is available in 250 mg vials, needs to be reconstituted with 5 ml saline. What is the ordered dose in milliliters?
A. 2.4 ml
B. 5 ml
C. 10 ml
D. 12 ml

543. The physician has ordered gentamycin, 18 mg, to be infused in 50 ml of D5W over 45 minutes. The nurse is going to use a pump setup that delivers milliliters per hour. What would the nurse set the pump on to infuse 50 ml in 45 minutes?
A. 8
B. 45
C. 50
D. 67

544. A 1-year-old male is being treated with gentamycin IV. Which of the following information is most important to know when administering gentamycin?
A. The effects are enhanced if it is administered along with a penicillin.
B. Irreversible deafness can occur if the client receives toxic doses.
C. Low dosages of gentamycin can produce photosensitivity.
D. Nausea and vomiting are the usual side effects.

545. A 4-year-old female has been receiving gentamycin for 3 days. Which of the following signs and symptoms should alert the nurse that the child might be toxic?
A. BP = 78/45
B. Decreased urine output
C. Heart rate = 110
D. Tarry stool

546. A 10-year-old male has been on theophylline for 5 days. Which of the following would indicate the need for immediate action?
A. Hyperactivity
B. Resting heart rate of 120
C. Respiratory rate of 24
D. Theophylline level of 18

547. A 14-year-old was started on total parenteral nutrition (TPN) 24 hours ago. Which nursing action would receive the highest priority?
A. Assessing glucose levels
B. Checking central line site for infection every 8 hours
C. Monitoring intake and output
D. Weighing the client daily

548. A surgeon has ordered an enema for a 10-year-old who is scheduled for surgery. According to his age, the volume of fluid should not exceed how many milliliters?
A. 100
B. 300
C. 500
D. 700

549. The nurse is conducting visual screenings at the local health department. From the nurse's knowledge of growth and development, what is the earliest age a child could have a visual acuity of 20/20?
A. 4 years old
B. 6 years old
C. 8 years old
D. 10 years old

550. A 10-year-old child was admitted to the pediatric unit with a fever ranging from 102 to 103.5°F, nonresponsive to acetaminophen (Tylenol) for 2 days. During rounds, the nurse observes that the child is listless with substernal retractions. The pediatrician who is on the unit immediately assesses the child and requests an endotracheal tube and supplies for an emergency intubation. Which of the following information is the quickest for obtaining an appropriate sized endotracheal tube?
A. Measuring the length of the child with the Broselow resuscitation tape
B. Memorizing the standard endotracheal tube sizes for age
C. Knowing that any uncuffed tube would be the appropriate size during an emergency
D. Using the child's little finger to determine endotracheal tube size

551. An 11-year-old child has been receiving TPN for 3 days. The central line infiltrated approximately 2 hours ago. Which of the following symptoms could be expected in this situation?
A. Bradycardia
B. Flushed skin
C. Irritability
D. Labored breathing

552. A gastrostomy tube was placed in a 5-year-old 5 days ago. He has been receiving full-strength gavage feedings every 4 hours for 24 hours. The nurse is responsible for administering the next feeding. When checking the residual, she finds more than half the amount of the last feeding. Which of the following is the most appropriate action by the nurse?
A. Reinsert the residual, then notify the physician.
B. Hold this feeding and make another attempt in 4 hours.
C. Reinsert the residual and make another attempt at feeding in 30 minutes.
D. Reinsert the residual, subtract this amount from the amount due this feeding, and instill the remaining amount.

553. A toddler has been admitted to the pediatric unit for a nutritional assessment and calorie count. Which of the following toys would be best to promote the toddler's development?
A. Board games
B. Coloring books and crayons
C. Push-pull toys
D. Puzzles

554. A preschooler is in the playroom. What behavior by the preschooler would the nurse expect to observe during play?
A. Playing a board game with another child
B. Playing on the floor with a music box
C. The child talking to an imaginary friend
D. The child sitting close to another child, but playing with toys alone

555. The nurse has been asked to conduct a workshop for parents on "The Appropriateness of Play in the Developing Child." Which of the following would be the most important guideline to discuss with parents?
A. Buying toys that are structured for a specific developmental task
B. Making play an educational experience
C. That play teaches skills which stimulate a child's intelligence
D. Using older persons as baby-sitters

556. A group of children are in the playroom located on the hospital unit. What age children does the nurse expect to be playing with toys?
A. Late-stage infancy
B. Preschoolers
C. School age
D. Adolescents

557. A 24-month-old was admitted to the pediatric unit with suspected meningitis. Which of the following laboratory results on the spinal fluid specimen distinguish bacterial meningitis from viral meningitis?
A. Cloudy, purulent appearance

B. Normal glucose
C. Normal protein count
D. Slightly elevated white blood cell count (WBC)

558. Parents bring their 22-month-old child to the emergency room because their child will not eat and seems to have no energy. The physician suspects meningitis. On initial assessment, what signs and symptoms would the nurse expect to find that indicate meningitis?
A. Fontanelle even with scalp
B. Nuchal rigidity
C. Pupils that react to light
D. Temperature of 99°F

559. A 2-month-old infant was admitted to the pediatric unit to rule out gastroesophageal reflux. Diagnostic testing supported the diagnosis of gastroesophageal reflux. During discharge teaching, the parents ask the nurse if they should continue to put their child in an infant seat after feedings? What is the most appropriate response by the nurse?
A. The infant seat increases intra-abdominal pressure and is discouraged.
B. The infant seat is a good measure to prevent your infant from aspirating vomitus.
C. The infant seat should be used for 1 hour after feeding, then place your infant on his stomach in the crib.
D. The infant seat is outdated, and it is recommended to put infants on their backs in cribs with the head elevated 30 degrees after feedings.

560. A 4-year-old was placed on a pulse oximeter to monitor her oxygen saturation (SaO$_2$). The nurse's initial response to an alarm and an SaO$_2$ of <80 would be:
A. Check the placement of the pulse oximetry probe.
B. Note the child's skin color.
C. Initiate oxygen via face mask.
D. Observe for restlessness.

561. Proper suctioning of a tracheostomy tube is important to prevent atelectasis and decrease hypoxia from the suctioning procedure. Which vacuum pressure range should the nurse choose?
A. 20 to 40 mm Hg
B. 40 to 60 mm Hg
C. 60 to 80 mm Hg
D. 80 to 100 mm Hg

562. Children and parents should be taught measures to prevent otitis externa. Which nursing measure would be appropriate to prevent this occurrence?
A. Using a solution of white vinegar and rubbing alcohol (50/50) in both ear canals after each swim and at bedtime
B. Ordering bacitracin ointment for the child or parent to place in the external canal tid

C. After showering, having children dry their ear canals thoroughly using a cotton swab

D. Insisting that the parents keep their child's hair cut short and cropped above the ears

563. Upon assessment of a 4-year-old child, the nurse notes the absence of a spontaneous cough, persistent drooling, and extreme agitation. The clinical observations suggest the presence of:
A. Croup
B. Epiglottitis
C. Pneumonia
D. Asthma

564. Vigilant observation and assessment of respiratory status is necessary when monitoring children with acute laryngotracheobronchitis. The nurse would observe for early signs of impending airway obstruction including:
A. Increased pulse and respiratory rate; substernal, suprasternal, and intercostal retractions; nasal flaring; and increased restlessness
B. Decreased pulse; increased respiratory rate; substernal, suprasternal, and intercostal retractions; nasal flaring; and increased restlessness
C. Increased pulse and respiratory rate; substernal, suprasternal, and intercostal retractions; cyanosis; and increased restlessness
D. Increased pulse; decreased respiratory rate; substernal, suprasternal, and intercostal retractions; cyanosis; and increased restlessness

565. The nurse providing care to the infant with respiratory syncytial virus (RSV) must utilize consistent hand-washing and avoid touching her own nasal mucosa or conjunctiva. Which rationale would justify such action?
A. The transmission of RSV is predominantly through direct contact with respiratory secretions.
B. RSV may be spread through small particle aerosols (airborne transmission).
C. RSV transmission is known to occur either through direct contact with mucosal secretions or airborne transmission.
D. Although RSV transmission is through direct contact with respiratory secretions, the organism survives only 2 minutes on the skin.

566. Which nursing action would be appropriate for the nurse providing care to a child receiving ribavirin through a mist tent if the tent must be opened?
A. The nurse may open the mist tent by using the zipper.
B. Gloves and gowns are recommended for the nurse.
C. Masks, gowns, and gloves are recommended for the nurse.
D. Temporarily stop the aerosol administration.

567. Immediate nursing action for children with peak expiratory flow rate in the red zone should be:
A. Continue the routine treatment plan.
B. Notify the physician because maintenance therapy may need to be decreased.
C. If symptoms arise, then routine therapy may need to be increased.
D. The physician should be notified immediately because severe airway narrowing may be occurring.

568. The nurse checks the child's metered-dose inhaler to note how much medication is left in the canister. When the canister is placed in a cup of water and sinks to the bottom, then the canister is:
A. Empty
B. Half-full
C. Full
D. Cannot determine

569. Which signs would alert the nurse of theophylline toxicity?
A. Nausea, tachycardia, irritability, seizures, and dysrhythmia
B. Nausea, headache, irritability, insomnia, and hyperactivity
C. Headache, diaphoresis, fever, nausea, and irritability
D. Diaphoresis, fever, muscle cramping, and vertigo

570. Close monitoring of serum theophylline concentrations is an important nursing action. A serum concentration between 10 and 20 μg/ml would indicate what information to the nurse?
A. The child's serum level is below the therapeutic level.
B. The child's serum level is above the therapeutic level.
C. The child's serum level is within the therapeutic range.
D. Currently there is no true established therapeutic level.

571. Bronchial drainage is generally performed:
A. Three to four times a day immediately after meals
B. Three to four times a day before meals
C. Twice a day before meals
D. Twice a day after meals

572. Upon assessment of the child with an acute asthma exacerbation, the nurse notes cyanosis, inaudible breath sounds, diminished LOC, increased respiratory rate, nasal flaring, moderate retractions, and PCO_2>40. What would the nurse assess as the severity of this episode?
A. Mild
B. Moderate
C. Moderate to severe
D. Severe

573. A 2-year-old was admitted to the hospital with possible bacterial pneumonia. Her quantitative sweat chloride test (pilocarpine iontophoresis) returned with a level of 70 mEq/L. What is the most appropriate initial nursing response for this test result?

A. Counsel the parents regarding the genetic inheritance of cystic fibrosis.

B. Order another sweat chloride test because false positives are often seen in children with pneumonia.

C. Feel relieved because the child's test results do not indicate she has cystic fibrosis.

D. Notify the physician of the child's positive test results for cystic fibrosis.

574. A 4-year-old child has cystic fibrosis. The physician has ordered chest physiotherapy (CPT) and bronchodilator medication to be administered via aerosol. Based on the nurse's knowledge of the disease and its management, which should come first: the CPT or bronchodilator medication?

A. Chest physiotherapy

B. Bronchodilator medication

C. Really does not matter which comes first

D. CPT is usually not recommended for children with cystic fibrosis

575. Genetic counseling provided by the nurse for parents with cystic fibrosis children should include:

A. Cystic fibrosis is a known inherited disease as an autosomal recessive trait. Both parents contribute the defective gene to the affected child; their children have a 1:4 chance of inheriting this disease.

B. Cystic fibrosis is a known inherited disease as an autosomal recessive trait. Both parents contribute the defective gene to the affected child; their children have a 1:2 chance of inheriting this disease.

C. Cystic fibrosis is a known inherited disease as an autosomal dominant inheritance. One parent contributes the defective gene to the affected child; his or her children have a 1:2 chance of inheriting this disease.

D. Cystic fibrosis is a known inherited disease as an X-linked dominant inheritance. Affected children have one affected parent. From an affected male parent, all daughters will be affected. From an affected female parent, half of the sons and daughters will be affected.

576. The nurse would expect that the hospitalized child with cystic fibrosis would be placed on what type of diet?

A. Low calorie, low fat, high salt, supplement with a fat-soluble vitamins A, D, E, and K

B. High calorie, low fat, low salt, supplement with water-miscible forms of vitamins A, D, E, and K, and pancreatic enzymes

C. High calorie, high protein, supplement with water-miscible forms of vitamins A, D, E, and K, and pancreatic enzymes

D. Low calorie, high protein, low fat, supplement with fat-soluble vitamins of A, D, E, and K, and pancreatic enzymes

577. A child has cystic fibrosis. He takes three pancreatic enzymes with regular meals and one enzyme with snacks. He remains at the 50th percentile for height and weight according to the standardized growth charts, and also continues to have one to two stools per day. What action should the nurse take in relation to this child's enzyme intake?

A. Increase his enzymes to five with regular meals and three with snacks.

B. Increase his enzymes to five with regular meals and remain at one for snacks.

C. Decrease his enzymes to two with regular meals and continue one for snacks.

D. Continue his current enzyme therapy with no changes because he is growing normally and having only two stools per day.

578. A child has been hospitalized to evaluate her bowel elimination status. Her physician suspects the child may have Hirschsprung's disease. Which of the following signs and symptoms are present in Hirschsprung's disease?

A. Chronic constipation, fecal impaction, poor appetite, abdominal distention, and poor growth

B. Passage of ribbonlike stool, abdominal distention, hearty appetite, weight gain, and irritability

C. Bloody diarrhea, fever, and severe lethargy

D. Increased thirst, increased appetite, and weight loss

579. The most appropriate nursing action to decrease the stress of frequent abdominal circumference measurements in children is:

A. Play soft music during the procedure.

B. Use a brightly colored tape measure.

C. Leave the tape measure in place beneath the child.

D. Administer acetaminophen (Tylenol) as needed to diminish the stress.

580. Dietary modifications are essential in the treatment of children with Hirschsprung's disease. Which one of the following food groups should the nurse suggest to parents as high-fiber foods.

A. Corn, beans, bananas, avocado, and all meats

B. Whole-grain cereal, peaches, cooked broccoli and cabbage, and popcorn

C. Prunes, raisins, rolls, lettuce, spinach, and candy bars

D. Apples, bananas, raisins, potatoes, and dairy products

581. When planning care for an infant with gastroesophageal reflux, the nurse should position the infant:

A. Flat prone or head-elevated prone following feeding and at night
B. Side-lying following feeding and during sleep
C. Back only during sleep
D. Upright in an infant seat

582. Infants with gastroesophageal reflux may also be treated with prokinetic medications such as metoclopramide (Reglan). Which of the following are known side effects associated with prolonged or high doses of Reglan?
A. Diarrhea, nausea, and foul-smelling stool
B. Wheezing, bowel inflammation, and irritability
C. Restlessness, drowsiness, and extrapyramidal reaction
D. Gas-bloating, increased nasal secretions, and increased gastric emptying

583. When assessing the child for acute appendicitis, the nurse should know the most common initial symptoms are:
A. Poor feeding, diarrhea, and lethargy
B. Colicky abdominal pain and tenderness
C. A temperature greater than 39°C (102.2°F) and absent bowel sounds
D. Absence of abdominal pain and presence of abdominal distention

584. A sudden relief from pain in the child with appendicitis would be recognized by the nurse as:
A. An indication that the child's condition is improving
B. An indication that pain-relieving drugs are no longer needed by the child
C. An indication that the child is not being completely honest regarding his pain
D. An indication of perforation and a worsening of the child's condition

585. Which signs and symptoms of peritonitis caused by a ruptured appendix should the nurse monitor for?
A. Temperature greater than 39°C (102.2°F), absent bowel sounds, increased diffuse abdominal pain, and tachycardia
B. Tachycardia, tachypnea, low-grade fever, and hyperactive bowel sounds
C. Abdominal distention, absent bowel sounds, vomiting, and diarrhea
D. Tachycardia, rapid and deep breathing, pallor, and chills

586. The nurse must design an appropriate plan of care for the child with acute appendicitis. Based on nursing knowledge, which nursing diagnosis would be highest in priority?
A. Fluid volume deficit
B. Pain
C. Risk for infection
D. Altered family processes

587. The nurse is planning care for a 3-year-old with appendicitis. Which pain rating scale would be most appropriate?
A. Word graphic scale
B. Color tool
C. Numeric scale
D. FACES pain rating scale

588. Inflammatory bowel disease (IBD) in children includes two chronic intestinal disorders: ulcerative colitis and Crohn's disease. In coordinating the therapeutic plan in children, the nurse would anticipate the use of which drugs as being considered the most effective for treating moderate to severe IBD?
A. Corticosteroids
B. Gentamicin
C. Diphenhydramine (Benadryl)
D. Acetaminophen

589. When assessing the client with inflammatory bowel disease (IBD), the nurse would identify a unique problem associated with the pediatric population with IBD as:
A. Weight gain
B. Growth failure
C. Early sexual maturation
D. Tall stature

590. Which nursing action would be appropriate in providing nasogastric tube feedings to a child with Crohn's disease?
A. Place the child supine with the chin directed toward the chest when inserting the nasogastric tube.
B. To stabilize the tube, tape it to the child's forehead.
C. Use only preheated formula for all feedings.
D. The child should be positioned on the right side or abdomen for 1 hour after feedings.

591. A 4-week-old infant was admitted to the hospital with projectile vomiting, lethargy, dehydration, and weight loss. The admitting nurse suspects hypertrophic pyloric stenosis (HPS). What other signs would alert the nurse to this possible diagnosis?
A. Bile-stained emesis
B. Visible gastric peristalsis
C. Respiratory distress
D. Diarrhea

592. Infants with HPS suffer from fluid and electrolyte imbalances from a loss of hydrogen ions and depletion of potassium, sodium, and chloride. The nurse correctly identifies this as what type of acid-base imbalance?
A. Metabolic alkalosis
B. Respiratory alkalosis
C. Metabolic acidosis
D. Respiratory acidosis

593. The main goal of nursing care for the child with celiac disease should be which of the following?

A. Assisting the child to adhere to dietary restrictions
B. Enhancing the child's ability to cope with the disease
C. Enabling the child to eat the foods he or she desires
D. Promoting weight loss to achieve a normal weight

594. A child is diagnosed as having sickle-cell disease. When explaining the disease to his parents, the nurse notes that:
A. The presence of fetal hemoglobin (HbF) delays the disease symptoms.
B. The presence of adult hemoglobin (HbA) in infants prevents the occurrence of disease-related symptoms.
C. HbF is composed of two α and two β chains, which lack the defect.
D. The combination of HbF and Hbs prevent the sickling episodes from occurring.

595. After teaching parents regarding sickle-cell anemia, the nurse allows the parents to make comments. Which of the following indicates a need for further teaching?
A. "My child should drink plenty of fluids daily."
B. "I should make sure my child does not become overheated."
C. "My child should not be around other people who are sick."
D. "I know my child will grow out of this disease."

596. A 2-year-old child was brought to the emergency room experiencing a vaso-occlusive sickle-cell crisis without hypoxemia. The child was treated with IV fluids and analgesics. The child's father questioned why his son was receiving no oxygen. How should the nurse respond initially?
A. Advise the father to talk with the child's physician.
B. Tell the father you will set up oxygen therapy for the child.
C. Question the father about how he believes the oxygen will help his son.
D. Teach the father about vaso-occlusive crises.

597. A 14-year-old Quaker girl comes to the emergency room with an asthma exacerbation. What beliefs about medical care may impact on her treatment in the hospital?
A. No special rites or restrictions exist in the Quaker religion regarding medical care.
B. Illness or injury is thought to be a result of sins committed in a previous life.
C. Quakers are opposed to the use of blood and blood products in illness treatment.
D. Quakers believe in divine healing through church leaders.

598. A child of the Muslim faith is gravely ill and expected to die. What action would the nurse expect from the family after the child's death?
A. The family may wish to wash and prepare the body by turning the face toward Mecca.
B. The body will be ritually washed by the Ritual Burial Society.
C. No special rites are given, but the presence of church elders is a comfort.
D. Water is poured by a priest into the dead child's mouth. A blessing is then given by tying a thread around the child's neck or wrist.

599. When designing play activities for the preschooler, the nurse would select:
A. Pat-a-cake or peek-a-boo
B. Ring-around-a-rosy, London Bridge, or simple board games
C. Cards, checkers, or chess
D. Baseball, football, or soccer

600. The mother of a 6-month-old infant returned to the pediatrician's office with her baby. The baby is becoming more physically mobile. The nurse should provide the parent with anticipatory guidance regarding toy safety. Which one of the following answers is appropriate?
A. Toys making loud noises are more stimulating for young children.
B. Toys should be constructed well enough to resist rough play.
C. Toys should be heavy for playing.
D. To be challenging, the toys chosen should be above the child's age group.

601. Like other age groups, school-age children have typical childhood fears. Identify which group of fears is particular to the school-age child:
A. Separation from the parent, loud or sudden noises, strangers, and animals
B. Separation from the parent, "monsters or ghosts," animals, "bad" people, death
C. Separation from the parent, staying alone, the dark, tests and school failure, death
D. Poor social ability, social isolation, public speaking, gossip, sexuality, death

602. Nurses must help parents learn how to assist their children in overcoming their fears. What advice should the nurse give a parent with a child who is fearful of swimming in deep water?
A. The parent should openly display disapproval for the child's fear of the water.
B. Parents should encourage the child's unreasonable fear.
C. Parents should aggressively attack the child's fear by throwing the child into deep water.
D. The parent should gradually desensitize the child by bringing the child out into shallow and then deeper water.

603. Parents often question nurses regarding the effects of TV viewing on their children. What infor-

mation is appropriate for parents? Select the answer that is appropriate for parental guidance:
A. Limit the child's viewing to 2 hours or less daily.
B. Allow the child to watch TV programs alone.
C. Encourage the child to choose an alternate activity (i.e., bike riding, reading, drawing) after watching TV.
D. Have the child develop a list of TV programs to watch each week.

604. The nurse must elicit information from the parents regarding their child's feeding behavior. Which questions would provide the nurse with more information?
A. "Does your child have a good appetite?"
B. "Did your child have any vomiting in the last 24 hours?"
C. "Is your child still taking formula with iron?"
D. "What do you think about your child's eating habits?"

605. A 4-year-old has returned to the public health clinic for her preschool physical examination. The child reacts to the nurse's presence by displaying shy behaviors. Which response initially by the nurse would enhance communication with the child?
A. Be honest with the child.
B. Talk with the child while the parent is not present.
C. First talk with the parent in the presence of the child.
D. Speak in a calm, unhurried voice.

606. The office nurse must prepare to examine a 2-year-old. Which nursing action is least appropriate when performing a physical examination on a toddler?
A. Praise the child for cooperative behaviors.
B. Have the parent leave the room.
C. If restraint is needed, then use it. The parent may also assist in restraining the child.
D. Perform procedures quickly.

607. A 15-year-old athlete reported to the public health clinic for her annual sports physical examination. What age-specific approaches should the nurse use during the physical examination process?
A. Allow the child to undress in the presence of the nurse.
B. Perform the examination quickly by exposing the child's entire body.
C. Emphasize abnormal findings during the examination to enhance the child's understanding.
D. Use a matter-of-fact approach when discussing the child's sexual growth and development.

608. Visualization of the tympanic membrane is difficult in children less than 3 years of age. To enhance visualization during an otoscopic examination, the nurse initially should:
A. Pull the pinna up and back.
B. Pull the pinna down and back.
C. Use an ear irrigation method to remove occluding wax.
D. Play an ear game with the child to elicit his or her cooperation.

609. A 6-year-old male was admitted to the pediatric unit with right middle lobe pneumonia. Which area of the lungs should his nurse auscultate to hear adventitious breath sounds?
A. Right posterior, between the second and fifth intercostal space
B. Right posterior, between the third and sixth intercostal space
C. Right anterior, between the second and fourth intercostal space
D. Right anterior, between the fourth and fifth intercostal space

610. While auscultating a 6-year-old's breath sounds, the nurse should use other measures to enhance effective auscultation. Which action would be least effective?
A. Auscultate while the child is relaxed.
B. The stethoscope should be warm when placed on the skin.
C. Place the stethoscope firmly on the chest.
D. Auscultate through clothing, rather than possibly awakening a sleeping child.

611. A 15-year-old adolescent mother has recently returned to the public health clinic with her infant. Her baby is now 3 months old. The mother is alarmed because her baby's "soft spot" (anterior fontanelle) appears to bulge when she cries, coughs, and lies down. In this situation, what should the nurse's initial response be?
A. "From what you have described, it sounds as though your baby's soft spot is perfectly normal. Let me examine the baby to make sure everything is all right."
B. "Well, what do you think your baby's anterior fontanelle is supposed to do?"
C. "You need to talk to the baby's pediatrician regarding what you observed."
D. "I really cannot discuss this with you now. Can you come back this afternoon and I will check the baby then?"

612. As part of the newborn neurological assessment, a Babinski reflex should be elicited. What type of normal response would the nurse expect to see when testing for the presence of a Babinski reflex?
A. Finger tapping on the glabella produces eyes tightly shut.
B. The arm and leg extend on the side toward which the infant's head is turned. The opposite arm and leg are flexed.

C. When palms of the hands and soles of feet are touched, flexion of the fingers and toes occurs.

D. When the sole of the foot is stroked upward, the toes fan and dorsiflexion of the great toe.

613. Currently, vitamin K administration is part of routine newborn treatment. What rationale best describes why the nurse should administer this vitamin?

A. Vitamin K is absolutely necessary to the synthesis of prothrombin for normal blood clotting and coagulation. In newborns, the supply of vitamin K is poor during the first week of life.

B. Vitamin K is needed for the bone marrow to produce thrombin and prothrombin for clotting. Although the supply of vitamin K is adequate, the newborn may not effectively use available vitamin K.

C. Vitamin K is normally synthesized by the liver. However, the newborn's liver is immature and benefits from vitamin K supplements.

D. Vitamin K not only prevents hemorrhagic disease, but it also assists in the development of immunity against gastrointestinal parasites and bacteria.

614. A mother and father have chosen not to have their infant son circumcised. In planning for discharge, what information should the nurse provide the parents regarding hygiene?

A. The foreskin should be retracted fully to the glans penis three times a day for cleansing.

B. Retraction of the foreskin is not a necessary practice to ensure good hygiene.

C. The foreskin should be gently retracted only as far as it will go during cleansing and then returned to a normal position.

D. The foreskin should be retracted gently and left in a retracted position at least three times a day.

615. A 1-month-old infant's formula must be supplemented with a carbohydrate source to enhance her caloric intake. Which dietary supplement should the nurse add to her formula?

A. Polycose

B. Casec

C. MCT oil

D. Soyalac

616. A 3-day-old newborn was brought to her pediatrician's office for swelling on her scalp. The nurse's assessment revealed left parietal edema within the boundaries of the parietal bone and normal neurological signs. The mother stated that this was her first baby and the physician used forceps to assist with the delivery. How should the nurse interpret this information?

A. The infant probably has some caput succedaneum, which requires no treatment.

B. The infant has a cephalohematoma resulting from a forceps delivery.

C. A subgaleal hemorrhage is possible since the baby has normal neurological signs and parietal edema.

D. The use of forceps has caused a parietal skull fracture and edema.

617. What nursing actions can prevent breastfeeding jaundice?

A. Encourage early introduction of feedings, breastfeeding every 2 hours, and avoidance of supplementation.

B. Encourage early introduction of feedings, breastfeeding alternating with the use of supplementation.

C. Allow mothers to bottle-feed.

D. Have mothers breastfeed on demand by the infant.

618. A 16-week-old infant requires the insertion of a ventriculoperitoneal (VP) shunt for the treatment of hydrocephalus. The nurse is keenly aware of the problems associated with hydrocephalus. What is the most serious complication of VP shunts?

A. Mechanical malfunction

B. Obstruction of the shunt

C. Shunt infection

D. Subdural hematoma

619. The nurse knows that signs of increased intracranial pressure (ICP) in older children are more subtle. Which is the most valuable indicator of increasing ICP for his age group?

A. Changes in the child's level of consciousness (LOC) and interaction with the environment

B. Increasing complaints of headache

C. Nausea and vomiting

D. Diplopia and blurred vision

620. A baby was discharged from the hospital 4 weeks ago. He is now 6 weeks' postoperative for VP shunt placement. Up until this morning, the child has nippled 4 ounces of formula every 4 hours without difficulty. The mother reports that the baby has vomited each feeding since this morning. Additionally, the mother notes that the baby has been unusually fussy and irritable today. Given the above information, what nursing action is most appropriate when admitting the infant to the hospital pediatric unit?

A. Notify the child's pediatrician of the infant's fussiness and irritability so that sedation can be ordered.

B. Place the child on NPO status until an antiemetic can be given.

C. Assess the infant's neurological status; measure the child's head circumference; note the appearance of the surgical site; take the infant's vital signs; and then notify the infant's neurosurgeon.

D. Note the infant's hydration status by measuring urine specific gravity, noting skin turgor and mucous membranes, assessing intake and output status, and then notify the infant's pediatrician.

621. While assessing a 4-hour-old baby, the nursery nurse notes an excessive amount of frothy saliva in the mouth, coughing, gagging, and a short episode of cyanosis. After the nurse suctions the oropharynx, the infant has no further signs of respiratory distress and requires no oxygen. The nurse's next response should be:
    A. Monitor the infant closely to note any further signs of respiratory distress.
    B. Notify the physician immediately for further medical evaluation of the infant for possible tracheoesophageal fistula.
    C. Since the infant is not at risk, report the occurrence to the physician during her routine rounds.
    D. Feed the infant plain water and then notify the physician of any feeding difficulty.

622. Fetal alcohol syndrome (FAS) is the number one cause of mental retardation. Which statement is the rationale for nurses to educate women of child-bearing age regarding this preventable syndrome?
    A. During pregnancy, there is no known safe amount of alcohol consumption.
    B. Some individuals are known to be at risk for the genetic development of FAS.
    C. Only heavy alcohol consumption by the mother will place an unborn child at risk for FAS.
    D. Only drinking alcohol during the first trimester of pregnancy will cause FAS

623. A mother has brought her infant son into the clinic to receive his immunizations. The nurse notes that during the physical assessment, the infant has considerable head lag. What nursing action should the nurse initiate?
    A. Instruct the mother to return to the clinic in 4 weeks to recheck the infant's head lag.
    B. Complete the child's developmental and neurological assessment and send the child with your findings to the physician for further evaluation.
    C. Teach the mother infant-stimulation exercises to enhance the child's ability to maintain head control.
    D. During history taking, question the mother regarding the existence of any familial neurological disease.

624. An infant's primary nurse is teaching the parents some activities to stimulate the child's development. Identify play activities appropriate for an 11-month-old infant:
    A. Play music, hang mobiles with black-on-white contrasting designs, cuddle the infant, or use a stroller to walk with the infant.
    B. Offer brightly colored toys for grasping, put a rattle or noise maker in the infant's hand, use soft toys made of multiple texture, or use a stroller to walk with the infant.
    C. Encourage imitation of sounds, repeat the words "dada" and "mama," state body parts, use simple commands, or place toys far enough out of reach to encourage seeking.
    D. Use pictures in books to discuss people, places, animals, and objects; show how to build a two-block tower; imitate animal sounds; encourage eating finger foods; or provide large push-pull toys.

625. Early introduction of solid foods to infants can lead to allergy development, weight gain, and gastrointestinal difficulties. Nurses should encourage parents to:
    A. Delay the introduction of citrus fruits, meats, and eggs until after 6 months of age. These foods may impact allergy development in the infant.
    B. Offer finger foods such as grapes, cheese, and raw vegetables to children by 6 months of age.
    C. Introduce whole milk to infants as young as 6 months of age.
    D. Encourage large quantities of fruit juices such as apple, pear, peach, and grape.

626. An 18-month-old toddler was admitted to the pediatric unit from the emergency room (ER). Her mother brought her to the ER because the baby was fussy, irritable, and had a subjective (felt as though she was febrile) temperature. While in the ER, the nurse noted the child to be well below the fifth percentile for height and weight, and unable to turn over, crawl or walk, and unresponsive to the nurse's interventions. The child was diagnosed as nonorganic failure to thrive. Identify the priority nursing goal for this child?
    A. The child's intake will be sufficient to enhance growth and development.
    B. The mother will understand normal growth and development expectations for an 18-month-old child.
    C. The mother will gain the skills needed to effectively parent this child.
    D. The child will achieve appropriate developmental milestones.

627. The most significant nursing intervention in preventing and controlling diaper dermatitis is:
    A. Removing the diaper to facilitate air drying.
    B. Changing soiled diapers as soon as possible.
    C. Applying a skin barrier such as zinc oxide or petrolatum.
    D. Using superabsorbent disposable diapers, which can decrease skin wetness.

628. When an infant becomes apneic, the nurse must initiate actions to stimulate breathing. Below are a list of nursing actions. Identify the appropriate

nursing action that should be used to stimulate an infant:
A. Use vigorous stimulation by patting or rubbing the trunk or flicking the feet.
B. Use gentle stimulation to initiate spontaneous respirations.
C. Maintain the infant in a prone position.
D. Spend only 45 seconds of time on stimulation, before initiating CPR.

629. On a routine visit to the pediatrics clinic, a client discusses her frustration with toilet training. She complains that her 12-month-old son frequently soils his diaper and refuses to use the commode. She further explains that she recently required her son to sit on the commode for 20 minutes. The child still refused to toilet on the commode. How should the nurse respond to this client's comments regarding toilet training?
A. "Did you try offering your son a reward for successful toileting?"
B. "Perhaps your son will respond better to a potty chair rather than a free-standing toilet."
C. "Your son is not physically or emotionally ready to toilet train at this time."
D. "I can't understand why your son will not train, he's plenty old enough."

630. Sibling rivalry is a natural feeling of jealousy when a new child is added to a family. As the nurse, identify which child is more likely to experience sibling rivalry:
A. A toddler without siblings
B. A school-age child without siblings
C. A school-age child with two preschool siblings
D. A set of preschool twins

631. Identify the appropriate schedule for routine active vaccination of infants at birth:
A. Hepatitis B only
B. Hepatitis B and *Haemophilus influenzae* type B (HIB)
C. DPT and OPV
D. DPT, OPV, and HIB

632. A mother visited the community health clinic with her 1-year-old son. Her son is scheduled to receive his first measles, mumps, and rubella (MMR) vaccination. After receiving the vaccine, the client questions the nurse regarding further immunizations. The mother asks, "When should my son receive his next MMR?" What nursing response would be appropriate?
A. "Since your son was 12 months old when he received the MMR vaccine, no further immunization is necessary."
B. "The only time your son may need further immunization is in the presence of a measles outbreak."
C. "Your son will receive a second MMR when he returns for his DPT at 15 months of age."

D. "Your son will need to receive his second MMR at age 11 to 12 years."

633. As the nurse, identify which statement is true regarding child sexual abuse:
A. Sexual abuse in children is easily identified because of the high number of obvious physical indications.
B. Incidents of sexual abuse are reported more frequently since adults are more willing to believe children.
C. The medical diagnosis is easily made since there is a typical profile of the child victim.
D. Sexually abused children may not possess more knowledge of sexual activity than children who have not been victimized.

634. The nurse has instructed a mother on methods to dust-proof and allergen-proof her home. The mother states she wants to prevent her child from having future asthma attacks. However, the mother insists she has little extra money for purchasing the plastic mattress pad and pillow covers. What immediate response would be appropriate for the nurse to make?
A. "If you really care about the health of your child, you will find the extra money needed."
B. "You can make your own mattress pad and pillow cover by using heavy-weight plastic garbage bags and duct tape."
C. "Let me refer you to our social worker, so she can assist you with your financial needs."
D. "Can you explain your financial situation further?"

635. A fourth grader at the local elementary school is being monitored by the school health nurse since he has asthma. Which nursing intervention is most appropriate for this child considering he has asthma?
A. In cooperation with the teachers and school administration, have the child store his medication in an accessible site.
B. Place all the child's medications in a locked closet.
C. Instruct the child and parent that no medications can be given by school personnel. Only a parent can give the child medication.
D. Medications should be placed in the school nurse's office for safety purposes.

636. Maintaining IV therapy in children continues to be a challenge for pediatric nurses. Infiltration of IV sites occurs with relative frequency. What signs of infiltration should the nurse be aware of?
A. Erythema, pain, edema, blanching, and streaking at the vein site.
B. Fever, chills, poor feeding, and lethargy
C. Limited ability to move the affected extremity and pain on movement.
D. Backflow of blood at the IV site and IV tubing

637. A baby was born 24 hours ago with a myelomeningo-cele. The nursery nurse notes the baby is irritable and lethargic, and has an elevated temperature and possible nuchal rigidity. These signs should alert the nurse to:
     A. Early signs of infection, possibly involving the CNS
     B. Developing hydrocephalus
     C. Respiratory infection
     D. Genitourinary infection

638. When a child is diagnosed with diabetes, the nurse must provide the family with education. School-age children have the ability to administer their own insulin. The sites chosen for injections will impact the onset and duration of insulin action. Which statement is true regarding the leg as an injection site?
     A. The rate of onset is fast, but the duration is long.
     B. The rate of onset is fast, but the duration is short.
     C. Both the rate of onset and the duration are very fast.
     D. The rate of onset is very slow, and the duration is very long.

639. A 4-year-old was admitted to the pediatric unit to rule out intussusception. A complete nursing history would assist the physician in making the diagnosis. Which signs and symptoms point to intussusception?
     A. Severe colicky abdominal pain, vomiting, and currant jelly–like stools
     B. Frequent diarrhea stools, mild dehydration, and elevated temperature
     C. Vomiting, diarrhea, and generalized red rash
     D. Diarrhea, abdominal cramping, and moderate dehydration

640. A 6-year-old was recently admitted to the hospital with new-onset seizures. His primary nurse designs a plan of care suitable for him. While hospitalized, he has a generalized cerebral seizure. What is the priority nursing action during this seizure episode.
     A. Observe and record the characteristics of his seizure activity.
     B. Protect the child's privacy by pulling the curtains shut and closing the door.
     C. Place the child on his side to prevent aspiration and maintain a patent airway.
     D. Press the call light for further nursing assistance.

641. A 6-year-old continues to have prolonged seizure activity. His physician states that the child is in status epilepticus and orders diazepam IV push. What specific knowledge regarding diazepam should guide the nurse's administration of the drug?
     A. Because of the drug's multiple incompatibilities, diazepam should be administered intra-

venously directly into the vein or the closest insertion site on the IV tubing.
     B. When given too slowly, the drug causes anorexia, nausea, and vomiting in some children.
     C. Some children develop leukopenic aplastic anemia with too high doses of the drug.
     D. If given too fast, the drug will further initiate seizure activity.

642. The nurse notes that an order for diazepam IV push is above the recommended safe range for a child's weight. What nursing response should be initiated?
     A. Give the safe dosage, but avoid telling the physician.
     B. Look for another reference to recalculate the dosage.
     C. Give the physician-ordered dosage.
     D. Alert the physician that the dosage ordered is above the recommended safe range.

643. The school nurse has been invited by a fourth-grade teacher to educate students regarding healthy food choices. According to the food pyramid, which daily food choices would the nurse recommend to school-age children?
     A. 2 to 3 servings of the milk group, 2 to 3 servings of the meat group, 2 to 4 servings of the fruit group, 3 to 5 servings of the vegetable group, 6 to 11 servings of the bread group
     B. 2 to 3 servings of the milk group, 4 to 5 servings of the meat group, 2 to 3 servings of the fruit group, 3 to 5 servings of the vegetable group, 6 to 8 servings of the bread group
     C. 4 to 5 servings of the bread group, 4 to 5 servings of the meat group, 4 to 5 servings of the fruit group, 4 to 5 servings of the vegetable group, 6 to 11 servings of the bread group
     D. 1 to 2 servings of the milk group, 1 to 2 servings of the meat group, 1 to 2 servings of the fruit group, 1 to 2 servings of the vegetable group, 4 to 5 servings of the bread group

644. Urinary tract infections in the neonatal period are difficult to identify. Which signs and symptoms would alert the nurse to a possible urinary tract infection in the neonate?
     A. Poor feeding, vomiting, poor weight gain, frequent urination, crying on urination
     B. Foul-smelling urine, crying on urination, frequent urination, fever, persistent diaper rash
     C. Enuresis, pain on urination, frequent urination, fever, pallor
     D. Incontinence, painful urination, back pain, excessive thirst, growth failure

645. New parents must be taught appropriate techniques for bottle-feeding and formula preparation. Which of the following parent responses indicates a need for further teaching?

A. "I should not dilute the formula to further extend the amount."
B. "I can't use the microwave to warm formula bottles."
C. "I will use a clean technique for preparing bottles and formula."
D. "In some situations, I can prop the bottle when feeding by baby."

646. Nurses should initiate parent education aimed at preventing sudden infant death syndrome (SIDS). Which of the following statements indicates a need for further teaching?
A. "Healthy infants should be placed in the prone position for sleep."
B. "Infants should be placed on a firm mattress to sleep."
C. "Infants should never sleep on sheepskins, quilts, comforters, and pillows."
D. "Infants should be placed on their side or back to sleep."

647. Toilet training is a major developmental task for the toddler to achieve. Nurses must provide parents with the appropriate knowledge to train their children. Which answer reflects a need for further teaching?
A. "Children accomplish bowel control before urinary control."
B. "Even after training, children may have daytime accidents."
C. "Nighttime bladder training is usually achieved by age 2."
D. "Children should be limited to 10 minutes on the potty when toilet training is first initiated."

648. An 18-month-old is diagnosed with lead poisoning. Her blood lead level is 25 mg/dl. The nurse understands that infants and young children are at highest risk for developing mental retardation and neurological deficits as a result of lead toxicity. A complete nursing history must be done in order to identify potential environmental sources of lead. Which question would identify the leading source of lead?
A. "Does your residence contain any chipping or flaking paint?"
B. "Do you own any pets?"
C. "From what grocery store do you purchase your vegetables?"
D. "Can you describe your child's eating habits?"

649. Parents and children with asthma must be educated to recognize the early warning signs of an exacerbation. Which of the following signs indicates a need for further teaching of the parents to recognize an early warning sign of an exacerbation?
A. Headache, cough, itchy chin, behavioral changes, runny nose, allergic shiners under the eyes
B. Audible inspiratory and expiratory wheezing within the child's chest

C. The child's peak flow meter numbers will change from green to yellow zone
D. Exposure to a known trigger

650. To auscultate a child's breath sounds, the nurse should use measures to enhance effective auscultation. Which nursing action would effectively enhance auscultation?
A. Auscultate while the child is relaxed.
B. The stethoscope should be cold when placed on the skin.
C. Place the stethoscope loosely on the skin.
D. To avoid awakening a sleeping child, auscultate through the child's clothing.

651. If nurses are unfamiliar with the features of fetal alcohol syndrome (FAS), then many infants and children will go unidentified. Which answer reflects major features of FAS?
A. Hypoplastic philtrum, short upturned nose, thinned upper lip, macrocephaly, mental retardation
B. Microcephaly, enhanced coordination and motor ability, hypotonia, mental retardation
C. Irritability, hypoactivity, rapid growth, mental retardation
D. Hearing disorders, seizures, mental retardation, hypotonia, microcephaly

652. In identifying realistic goals in working with the parents of a 3-year-old abused child, the nurse should understand abusive parents have not mastered the task of:
A. Developing a trusting relationship
B. Role gratification
C. Functioning outside the home
D. Developing a value system

653. A 5-year-old was diagnosed with asthma at age 2. This hospital stay marks the child's sixth hospital admission this year. Which nursing response would best assist the nurse in gathering information from the child's parents regarding possible triggers?
A. "Identify family members who smoke in your home."
B. "Are cockroaches a pest control problem in your home?"
C. "Does your child prefer to play indoors or outdoors."
D. "Describe your child's room to me."

654. Heparin locks are popular venous access devices for use in pediatrics. Choose the answer that best describes appropriate nursing action for flushing this device in children.
A. If a heparin flush is used, the recommended flush ratio is 1:1000 units per milliliter.
B. A positive-pressure technique for flushing should be used to prevent the backflow of blood into the lock.
C. Heparin locks should always be flushed with a heparin solution.

D. Saline is used to flush the lock only after medication is administered.

655. The nurse has provided nursing care to a premature infant in the neonatal intensive care unit. The infant's parents visit infrequently and rarely touch the baby. As the nurse, what rationale would offer an explanation for the parents' reaction to their premature infant?
A. Parents of premature infants often do not want their child prior to its birth.
B. Mothers of premature infants usually do not seek out prenatal care.
C. The physical separation of premature infants and parents may lead to parental emotional separation.
D. Premature infants usually have birth defects, which frighten parents.

656. Infants exposed to narcotic substances while in utero can display signs of neonatal narcotic withdrawal. Which acute signs would alert the nurse to possible neonatal narcotic withdrawal?
A. Tremors, restlessness, hyperactive reflexes, increased muscle tone, sneezing, tachypnea, high-pitched shrill cry
B. Sleepiness, good feeders, frantic sucking of hands, vomiting, diarrhea, sneezing, tachypnea
C. Sleepiness, lethargy, hypotonicity of muscles, frequent yawning, vomiting, diarrhea, tremors
D. Poor feeding, constipation, irritability, tremors, shrill cry, hyperactivity, sweating

657. The drug-addicted infant requires specialized nursing care. Identify the most appropriate nursing action for the infant with narcotic abstinence syndrome:
A. Use only bright lighting to monitor and record infant responses.
B. Cover infants loosely with a light-weight blanket.
C. Space individual nursing activities throughout the day.
D. Maintain a calm and quiet care environment.

658. Special care must be taken to protect an exposed myelomeningocele sac in a newborn. Identify the nursing strategy designed to protect the infant's fragile myelomeningocele sac.
A. The infant is maintained in the side-lying position.
B. The infant is placed in a warmer or incubator.
C. Moist, sterile, adherent dressings are placed over the sac.
D. When the sac becomes soiled, vigorous cleansing of the sac is needed.

659. As a method for preventing seizures, children are often maintained on phenytoin at home. Prior to discharge, the nurse must educate the family regarding this medication. Which statement indi-

cates a need for further teaching concerning phenytoin?
A. "I must take my child to the dentist frequently."
B. "I shouldn't worry if my child starts to snore."
C. "My child's school performance should improve."
D. "My child will develop more motor (ataxia) and rash symptoms."

660. A 3-year-old child was admitted to the hospital for acute gastroenteritis. The mother states the child has had vomiting and diarrhea for the last 2 days. The nurse's assessment for dehydration should include:
A. Head circumference, assessment of anterior fontanelle, baseline weight
B. Urine specific gravity, head circumference, anterior fontanelle assessment
C. Baseline weight, skin turgor, head circumference
D. Urine specific gravity, baseline weight, skin turgor

661. At the local community health clinic, the nurses teach a parenting class on toddler accident prevention. Which information would be appropriate for parents in this class?
A. Inform the parents of traffic rules for cycling that they can teach to their toddler.
B. Rules for interacting with strangers should be targeted. Parents can then teach these rules to their children.
C. Household cleaners can be stored in low cabinets. Toddlers can then be taught that these cabinets are off limits.
D. The handles of pots and pans on stove tops should be placed out of reach for the toddler.

662. An infant has returned to the public health clinic to receive immunizations. Which answer is a true contraindication and would delay the child receiving immunizations?
A. A mild acute illness with a low-grade fever
B. Presently receiving antimicrobial therapy
C. Prematurity
D. Anaphylactic reaction to a vaccine

663. A mother complains that her 6-week-old infant cries with colic several hours a day. What nursing measures can the nurse offer this mother to relieve her infant's colic?
A. Increase the volume of infant formula and provide less frequent feedings.
B. Burp the infant before and after feedings.
C. If crying persists, take the infant for a car ride.
D. Place the infant prone to burp.

664. Hospitalized infants with nonorganic failure to thrive present the nurse with multiple feeding challenges. Feeding guidelines must be established by the nursing staff. Which feeding guide-

line would be most appropriate for the infant with nonorganic failure to thrive?

    A. All nurses should be allowed to feed the infant, to identify which nurses seem to enhance the child's intake of nutrients.

    B. Provide a feeding environment with multiple forms of stimulation.

    C. Offer the child a variety of foods to identify the child's likes and dislikes.

    D. During the feeding, state only simple verbal instructions.

665. A physician has ordered home phototherapy for a newborn with an elevated bilirubin. Once the home health nurse sets up the equipment, she instructs the parents on infant care. Identify the home instructions the nurse should verbalize to the parents.

    A. Eye shields should only be placed on the infant during daylight hours.

    B. A small diaper may be worn when the infant is receiving phototherapy.

    C. Phototherapy provides warmth, thus parents need not be concerned regarding the infant's temperature.

    D. The infant should be removed from phototherapy treatment for 1 hour at least every 2 hours.

666. A preschool Head Start program will obtain vision screening through the local public health clinic. Which equipment must the public health nurses obtain to perform vision screenings at this preschool?

    A. Snellen's letter acuity charts

    B. Occluders

    C. Flashlights

    D. One-foot ruler

667. A client is undecided whether to breastfeed or bottle-feed her infant. The nurse should provide this client with the information she needs to make an informed choice. What information correctly compares the differences between breast milk and formula?

    A. Breastfed infants have normal stools, while formula-fed infants tend to have very loose stools.

    B. Breast milk prevents infection, while formula has no immunological benefits.

    C. Breast milk contains very few vitamins, while formula is fortified with vitamins.

    D. Formula has added calcium and phosphorus for bone growth, while breast milk does not contain these minerals.

668. A 7-year-old boy is receiving a blood transfusion. The nurse assesses that he has developed precordial pain, dyspnea, distended neck veins, and a cough. These findings are indicative of which of the following complications?

    A. Allergic reaction

    B. Air embolism

    C. Hemolytic reaction

    D. Circulatory overload

Focus on Pediatric Drug Dosage Calculation

669. A 3-year-old was admitted with aseptic meningitis. The physician ordered 40 mg chewable tablets of acetaminophen. On hand were 80 mg tablets. How many tablets will the nurse administer?

    A. ½ tablet

    B. 1 tablet

    C. 1½ tablets

    D. 2 tablets

670. A 2-year-old was admitted with otitis media. The child weighed 10 kg. The physician ordered amoxicillin 250 mg every 12 hours PO times 10 days. On hand was 125 mg/5 ml liquid suspension. How many milliliters will the nurse administer?

    A. 1 ml

    B. 5 ml

    C. 10 ml

    D. 15 ml

671. The physician ordered dactinomycin (actinomycin-D) 15 mg/kg IV for a child who weighs 5 kg with osteogenic sarcoma. Using a 0.5 mg/ml vial, how many milliliters did the nurse administer IVPB?

    A. 50 ml

    B. 100 ml

    C. 150 ml

    D. 200 ml

672. A 1-year-old child was admitted with herpes simplex encephalitis. The child had a BSA of 1.0 m^2. The physician ordered acyclovir 500 mg/m^2. Using a 500 mg/5 ml vial, the nurse administered how many milliliters IV?

    A. 1 ml

    B. 2.5 ml

    C. 4.0 ml

    D. 5.0 ml

673. A 15-month-old recovering from an automobile accident was crying with pain. The physician ordered meperidine (Demerol) 5 mg every 4 hours PRN for pain. The baby's BSA is 0.57 m^2. On hand was Demerol 25 mg/0.5 ml ampule. How many milliliters did the nurse administer?

    A. 0.1 ml

    B. 0.2 ml

    C. 0.3 ml

    D. 0.4 ml

674. A 10-year-old was admitted with the diagnosis of Wilms' tumor. The BSA of this child was 1.3 m^2. The adult dose of doxorubicin (Adriamycin) is 60 mg. How many milligrams will the child receive?

    A. 30 mg

    B. 36 mg

    C. 40 mg

    D. 46 mg

675. A newborn weighing 4 kg was admitted with a severe infection. The physician ordered vancomycin 10 mg/kg every 12 hours. The newborn could receive 40 mg every 12 hours. Using a 500 mg/10 ml vial, how many milliliters did the nurse administer IM?
A. 0.2 ml
B. 0.4 ml
C. 0.6 ml
D. 0.8 ml

676. The physician ordered gentamicin 2 mg/kg of body weight IVPB every 8 hours on a 26-pound child. Converting to kilograms, the nurse found that the child weighed 12 kg and required 24 mg of medication. On hand was 20 mg/2 ml. How many milliliters will be needed to administer the required amount?
A. 1.0 ml
B. 1.4 ml
C. 2.0 ml
D. 2.4 ml

677. The physician ordered cefotaxime (Claforan) 200 mg every 12 hours to a 10-day-old infant weighing 4 kg. The vial reconstitutes to make 95 mg/ml. How many milliliters will the nurse add to the IV solution every 12 hours?
A. 1.0 ml
B. 2.0 ml
C. 3.0 ml
D. 4.0 ml

678. The physician ordered amikacin (Amikin) 40 mg every 8 hours for a 2-year-old child. On hand is a 100 mg/2 ml vial. How many milliliters will the nurse administer?
A. 0.4 ml
B. 0.6 ml
C. 0.8 ml
D. 1.0 ml

679. The physician ordered diphenhydramine 15 mg every 6 hours today for a 3-year-old weighing 40 pounds. Using a 50 mg/ml vial, how many milliliters did the nurse administer?
A. 0.1 ml
B. 0.2 ml
C. 0.3 ml
D. 0.4 ml

680. A 10-year-old was admitted with severe edema secondary to nephrotic syndrome. The physician ordered 3.3 mg/kg/day of spironolactone (Aldactone). This child weighed 45.45 kg. How many milligrams will the child receive daily?
A. 50 mg
B. 100 mg
C. 150 mg
D. 200 mg

681. A 7-year-old was seen in the ER with hyperuricemia. The physician ordered allopurinol (Zyloprim) 300 mg every day. The nurse instructed the mother to give the child how many 100 mg tablets?
A. ½ tablet
B. 1 tablet
C. 2 tablets
D. 3 tablets

682. A 15-year-old was seen by her local family physician with chills, fever, and general malaise. The physician diagnosed her with influenza Type A. The physician ordered amantadine (Symmetrel) 200 mg PO for the symptoms. The nurse instructed the client to take how many 100 mg tablets?
A. ½ tablet
B. 1 tablet
C. 2 tablets
D. 3 tablets

683. A 10-year-old was diagnosed with leukemia. The physician ordered 3.3 mg/m² of methotrexate IV. The client had a BSA of 1.7 m². How many milliliters will the nurse administer from a 25 mg/ml vial?
A. 0.12 ml
B. 0.22 ml
C. 1.12 ml
D. 1.22 ml

684. The physician ordered imipramine 25 mg for a 6-year-old who was having enuresis. The pharmacist dispensed 50 mg tablets. The nurse instructed the mother to administer how many tablets?
A. ½ tablet
B. 1 tablet
C. 1½ tablets
D. 2 tablets

685. A child seen at the local pediatric clinic was diagnosed with otitis media. The child weighed 10 kg. The physician ordered amoxicillin 200 mg. Using a 250 mg/5 ml suspension, how many milliliters would the nurse administer?
A. 2 ml
B. 4 ml
C. 6 ml
D. 8 ml

686. A child weighing 34 kg was admitted with severe meningitis. The physician ordered 8.5 mg phenytoin (Dilantin) to be given IV. Using a 50 mg/ml vial, how many milliliters would the nurse administer?
A. 0.1 ml
B. 0.2 ml
C. 0.3 ml
D. 0.4 ml

687. A child weighing 10 kg was admitted with meningitis secondary to *H. influenzae* virus. The physician ordered ampicillin 200 mg/kg/day to be divided into four doses. How many milligrams would be in each dose?

A. 200 mg
B. 300 mg
C. 400 mg
D. 500 mg

688. A 10-year-old with bronchial asthma was seen in the ER. The child weighed 39 kg. The physician ordered aminophylline 7.5 mg/kg IV (290 mg). How many milliliters would the nurse administer using a 250 mg/ml vial?
   A. 1.0 ml
   B. 1.2 ml
   C. 1.5 ml
   D. 2.0 ml

689. A 7-year-old had developed a nonproductive cough. The child weighed 23 kg. The physician ordered benzonatate 8 mg/kg (184 mg) in three to six divided doses. How many 100 mg tablets would the nurse instruct the mother to give?
   A. ½ tablet
   B. 1 tablet
   C. 1½ tablets
   D. 2 tablets

690. A 14-year-old was having severe diarrhea. The physician ordered bismuth subsalicylate 300 mg. Using a 262 mg/15 ml suspension, the nurse administered how many milliliters?
   A. 10 ml
   B. 15 ml
   C. 17 ml
   D. 20 ml

691. A 9-year-old was admitted for severe constipation. The physician ordered bisacodyl 10 mg tablets. The nurse instructed the mother to give how many 5-mg-tablets?
   A. ½ tablet
   B. 1 tablet
   C. 1½ tablets
   D. 2 tablets

692. A 6-year old was admitted to the local ER with severe rhinitis. The physician ordered brompheniramine (Dimetane) 2 mg tid. How many tablets would the nurse administer from 4 mg stock?
   A. ½ tablet
   B. 1 tablet
   C. 1½ tablets
   D. 2 tablets

693. A 12-year-old with chronic myelocytic leukemia was given busulfan 6 mg PO. The pharmacist dispensed 2 mg tablets. The nurse instructed the mother to give how many tablets?
   A. 1 tablet
   B. 2 tablets
   C. 3 tablets
   D. 4 tablets

694. A 10-year-old was admitted for generalized seizures. The child weighted 46 kg. The physician ordered

15 mg/kg (690 mg) IV. Using a 50 mg/ml vial, how many milliliters did the nurse administer?
   A. 10.8 ml
   B. 11.8 ml
   C. 12.8 ml
   D. 13.8 ml

695. An 8-year-old was admitted with severe diarrhea secondary to irritable bowel syndrome. The physician ordered Mitrolan 500 mg PO bid PRN. The nurse instructed the mother to administer how many 500 mg tablets?
   A. ½ tablet
   B. 1 tablet
   C. 1½ tablets
   D. 2 tablets

696. A 1-year-old was admitted with tonsillitis. The child weighed 10 kg. The physician ordered cefprozil (Cefzil) 15 mg/kg (150 mg) tid. Using a 250 mg/5 ml liquid suspension, how many milliliters did the nurse administer?
   A. 1 ml
   B. 2 ml
   C. 3 ml
   D. 4 ml

697. A 13-year-old was experiencing trigeminal neuralgia. The physician ordered carbamazepine 400 mg bid PO. The nurse instructed the teen to take how many 100 mg tablets?
   A. 1 tablet
   B. 2 tablets
   C. 3 tablets
   D. 4 tablets

698. A 2-year-old was being prepped for an abdominal exploratory surgery. The physician ordered 5.0 ml of castor oil. Each capful contained 0.62 ml. How many capfuls would the nurse administer?
   A. 2 capfuls
   B. 4 capfuls
   C. 6 capfuls
   D. 8 capfuls

699. A 5-year-old was admitted with pneumonia. The child weighed 18 kg. The physician ordered ceftazidine (Fortaz) 30 mg/kg per day (540 mg) IV. Using a 1 gm/1 ml vial, how many milliliters would the nurse administer daily?
   A. 0.44 ml
   B. 0.54 ml
   C. 0.64 ml
   D. 0.74 ml

700. A 12-year-old was admitted with petit mal seizures. The physician ordered methsuximide (Celontin) 300 mg PO daily. Using 150 mg tablets, how many tablets would the nurse administer?
   A. ½ tablet
   B. 1 tablet
   C. 1½ tablets
   D. 2 tablets

701. A 3-year-old was being evaluated for constipation. The physician ordered Citrucel 5 ml bid with water. How many milligrams would the child receive from a 450 mg/5 ml liquid suspension?
    A. 150 mg
    B. 250 mg
    C. 350 mg
    D. 450 mg

702. A 5-year-old was admitted for acute iron intoxication. The physician ordered deferoxamine 1 gm IV. Using a 500 mg/1 ml vial, how many milliliters did the nurse administer?
    A. 0.5 ml
    B. 1 ml
    C. 1½ ml
    D. 2 ml

703. A 14-year-old was being evaluated for insomnia. The teenager weighted 50 kg. The physician ordered chloral hydrate 50 mg/kg (2500 mg) at the hour of sleep. Using a 500 mg/5 ml liquid, how many milliliters would the nurse instruct the teenager to take?
    A. 10 ml
    B. 15 ml
    C. 20 ml
    D. 25 ml

704. A 5-year-old was diagnosed with a mycoplasma infection. The child weighed 21 kg. The physician ordered chlorambucil 50 mg/kg per day to be divided every 6 hours. Each dose was 265 mg. Using a 150 mg/5 ml vial, how many milliliters would the nurse administer?
    A. 8.0 ml
    B. 8.8 ml
    C. 2.0 ml
    D. 2.8 ml

705. A 15-year-old was being given chlordiazepoxide (Librium) 5 mg as a preprocedure sedation. With 10 mg tablets on hand, how many tablets did the nurse administer?
    A. ½ tablet
    B. 1 tablet
    C. 1½ tablets
    D. 2 tablets

706. A 2-year-old was seen in the local ER with nausea and vomiting. The child weighed 44 kg. The physician ordered chlorpromazine (Thorazine) 0.55 mg/kg (24 mg) IV. Using a 25 mg/ml vial, how many milliliters did the nurse give the child IV?
    A. 0.66 ml
    B. 0.76 ml
    C. 0.86 ml
    D. 0.96 ml

707. A 3-year-old was traveling with her family to Mexico. The physician was immunizing the family members against malaria. The child weighed 23 kg. The physician ordered chloroquine 5 mg/kg per week (115 mg). Using a 50 mg/ml vial, how many milliliters would the child receive?
    A. 0.3 ml
    B. 1.3 ml
    C. 2.3 ml
    D. 3.3 ml

708. A 10-year-old was admitted with severe edema secondary to prednisone. The physician wanted to diurese the child. The child weighed 46 kg. The physician ordered chlorothiazide 20 mg/kg per day to be divided into two doses (460 mg each). Using a 500 mg/ml vial, how many milliliters would the nurse administer?
    A. 0.72 ml
    B. 0.82 ml
    C. 0.92 ml
    D. 1.0 ml

709. A 15-year-old was seen in the local ER with intractable hiccups. The physician ordered chlorpromazine (Thorazine) 50 mg in 500 ml of normal saline IV. Using a 25 mg/ml vial, how many milliliters must be added to the IV solution?
    A. 0.5 ml
    B. 1.0 ml
    C. 1.5 ml
    D. 2.0 ml

710. A 15-year-old was diagnosed with a vitamin E deficiency secondary to sickle-cell anemia. The physician ordered 75 IU every day. The nurse instructed the teenager to take how many 50 IU tablets?
    A. 0.5 tablet
    B. 1.0 tablet
    C. 1.5 tablets
    D. 2.0 tablets

711. A 12-year-old was admitted with heat exhaustion and became very hypotensive. The child weighed 57 kg. The physician ordered ephedrine sulfate 3 mg/kg (171 mg) IV. Using a 50 mg/ml vial, how many milliliters would the nurse administer IV?
    A. 1.4 ml
    B. 2.4 ml
    C. 3.4 ml
    D. 4.4 ml

712. A 13-year-old was treated for juvenile rheumatoid arthritis. The physician ordered choline salicylate 1000 mg PO. Using an 870 mg/5 ml vial, how many milliliters will the nurse administer?
    A. 2 ml
    B. 4 ml
    C. 6 ml
    D. 8 ml

713. A 4-year-old, weighing 22 kg, was being treated with oxitriphylline (Choledyl) 4 mg/kg (88 mg) every 6 hours for acute bronchial asthma. Using a 100 mg/5 ml suspension, how many milliliters did the nurse administer?

A. 4.4 ml
B. 5.4 ml
C. 6.4 ml
D. 7.4 ml

714. A 17-year-old was being treated prophylactically with cimetidine to prevent the formation of a duodenal ulcer. The physician ordered 400 mg HS. How many 200 mg tablets must the teenager take?
A. 1 tablet
B. 2 tablets
C. 3 tablets
D. 4 tablets

715. A 2-year-old was admitted with pneumonia. The physician ordered clindamycin 10 mg/kg per day (57 mg) to be divided every 8 hours. The child weighed 17 kg. Using a 150 mg/ml vial, how many milliliters would the nurse administer for one dose?
A. 0.2 ml
B. 0.4 ml
C. 0.6 ml
D. 0.8 ml

716. A 13-year-old received methotrimeprazine (Levoprome) 10 mg IM as a preoperative sedation. Using a 20 mg/ml vial, how many milliliters did the nurse administer?
A. 0.5 ml
B. 0.6 ml
C. 0.7 ml
D. 0.8 ml

717. A 3-year-old was admitted for a diazepam overdose. The child weighed 23 kg. The physician in the ER ordered physostigmine salicylate 0.02 mg/kg (0.46 mg) IV to reduce CNS depressant effects. Using a 1 mg/ml vial, how many milliliters did the nurse administer?
A. 0.26 ml
B. 0.36 ml
C. 0.46 ml
D. 0.56 ml

718. A 6-year-old was being treated with thiabendazole 25 mg/kg for pinworms. The child weighed 34 kg. How many milligrams would the child receive?
A. 660 mg
B. 750 mg
C. 850 mg
D. 950 mg

719. A 7-year-old was being treated for a vitamin B_1 deficiency. The physician ordered thiamine hydrochloride 50 mg IM. Using a 100 mg/ml vial, how many milliliters did the nurse administer?
A. 0.5 ml
B. 1.0 ml
C. 1.5 ml
D. 2.0 ml

720. A 12-year-old was being treated with imipramine 25 mg PO for depression. The pharmacist dispensed 50 mg tablets. The nurse instructed the client to take how many tablets?
A. ½ tablet
B. 1 tablet
C. 1½ tablets
D. 2 tablets

721. An 8-year-old with cerebral palsy was being treated with dantrolene (Dantrium) 1 mg/kg per day IM for spasticity. The client weighed 34 kg. Each dose will contain 17 mg. Using a 20 mg/ml vial, how many milliliters would the nurse administer?
A. 0.75 ml
B. 0.85 ml
C. 0.95 ml
D. 1.0 ml

722. A 14-year-old was being treated with mefenamic acid (Ponstel) 500 mg PO for severe dysmenorrhea. The nurse instructed the teenager to take how many 250 mg capsules?
A. 1 capsule
B. 2 capsules
C. 3 capsules
D. 4 capsules

Answers

1. **(D)** Nursing process phase: assessment; client need: health promotion and maintenance; content area: pediatric nursing

Rationale
(A) A normal heart rate for a newborn is 120 to 140 bpm. Crying may increase it and sleeping may decrease it. (B) The normal respiratory rate for a newborn is 30 to 60/min. Crying may increase it and sleeping may decrease it. (C) Axillary temperature is 97.9°F to 98°F in the newborn and may be altered by environmental factors. (D) Coarctation of the aorta may be present if the systolic blood pressure in the upper extremity is 6 to 9 mm Hg > the lower extremity. This discrepancy, as well as weaker femoral pulses, needs to be reported.

2. **(A)** Nursing process phase: implementation; client need: safe, effective care environment; content area; pediatric nursing

Rationale
(A) High temps from microwaves destroy the anti-infective properties. Lower temps are also questionable. (B) The risk of burns to the newborn is true for breast milk or formula heated in a microwave. (C) There is risk of exploding glass containers for any food or milk product if microwaved at too high a temperature. (D) Breast milk is warm by nature and does not increase indigestion.

3. **(D)** Nursing process phase: implementation; client need: physiologycal integrity; content area: pediatric nursing

Rationale
(A) It is true that infection should be prevented, but many other factors contribute to infection besides diaper placement. (B) There are no nerves in the umbilicus to cause pain. (C) The dry gangrene process takes 7 to 14 days, depending on the preparations applied to the cord, other perinatal events, and type of delivery. (D) The wetness from diaper soiling and subsequent irritation can be prevented by securing the diaper below the cord.

4. **(A)** Nursing process phase: assessment; client need: health promotion and maintenance; content area: pediatric nursing

Rationale
(A) Caput succedaneum, the most common scalp lesion of the newborn delivered vaginally, is characterized by swelling extending beyond the borders of a single bone and may include overlying bruising. (B) The cephalhematoma is the condition of bleeding into the area between bone and periosteum. It may be bilateral and is often minimal at birth, increases in size on the second day, and is sharply delineated by the third day. (C) Sunken fontanelles indicate dehydration. Suture lines may be overlapping. (D) This describes a cephalhematoma.

5. **(B)** Nursing process phase: assessment; client need: safe, effective care environment; content area: pediatric nursing

Rationale
(A) Blood glucose is monitored in infants of diabetic mothers. Those who are large or small for gestational age or have additional signal systems of jitteriness, twitching, and decreased activity levels need glucose levels checked. (B) The bilirubin should be monitored closely because the client is at risk for hyperbilirubinemia due to breastfeeding-associated jaundice and due to excessive production of bilirubin from the breakdown of blood held in bruises. (C) Phenylketonuria (PKU) is monitored to detect the autosomal recessive trait to prevent mental retardation. It is unrelated to breastfeeding or bruising. (D) The WBC denotes infection that abrasions and other factors, but not necessarily bruises, may precipitate.

6. **(B)** Nursing process phase: implementation; client need: psychosocial integrity; content area: pediatric nursing

Rationale
(A) Oral thrush is characterized by white patches on the tongue and mouth that resemble milk, but cannot be easily wiped off and may bleed if removed. (B) "Newborn rash" is characterized by these firm, pale yellow or white pustules 1 to 3 mm in size. The condition resembles flea bites, but is benign and self-limiting. (C) Although the pustules may resemble acne, acne treatment is not indicated. No treatment is indicated. (D) If the diagnosis is questionable, cultures may be done; however, the diagnosis can be made on clinical presentation.

7. **(C)** Nursing process phase: evaluation; client need: physiological integrity; content area: pediatric nursing

Rationale
(A) Blood glucose should be between 40 and 125 mg/dl. Less than 40 is hypoglycemia; more than 125 is hyperglycemia. (B) Serum calcium is normally 8 to 10 mg/dl. (C) Unconjugated bilirubin increases rapidly with blood incompatibilities. Normal values for unconjugated bilirubin are 0.2 to 1.4 mg/dl.

Pathological jaundice occurs usually at <24 hours of age. The physician should be notified. (D) The direct Coomb's test is a method of testing blood incompatibilities. A positive test indicates that antibodies are attached to the circulating erthrocytes of the newborn.

8. **(B)** Nursing process phase: analysis and planning; client need: physiological integrity; content area: pediatric nursing

Rationale
(A) The Plexiglas shield protects from undesirable UV rays from the phototherapy lights. (B) Because no long-term research has studied the gonadal function of men treated with phototherapy, many health-care providers seek to protect the gonads. (C) A small diaper is used for absorbency if diarrhea is a real problem. (D) Although hydration status may be monitored by weighing diapers in some clients, the mask would not effectively absorb all of the urine for an accurate measurement.

9. **(D)** Nursing process phase: evaluation; client need: safe, effective care environment; content area: pediatric nursing

Rationale
(A) Unless the canned food was especially prepared for infants, excessive sodium, salt, and additives may be transferred to the infant. (B) & (C) Home-prepared foods, fresh or frozen, are the preferred foods to decrease the risk of unwanted additives. (D) Refined sugar may be used but honey and corn syrup should be avoided because of the risk of botulism.

10. **(D)** Nursing process phase: implementation; client need: safe, effective care environment; content area: pediatric nursing

Rationale
(A) New foods should be introduced one at a time. Usually, plain rice cereal is the suggested first solid food. (B) Whole milk should not be introduced within the first year. (C) Large quantities of juice may cause abdominal pain, bloating, or diarrhea. It may be substituted for a milk feeding one time per day. (D) Breast milk and/or formula are primary sources of nutrition for infants up to 12 months.

11. **(D)** Nursing process phase: analysis and planning; client need: safe, effective care environment; content area: pediatric nursing

Rationale
(A) Full-strength doses are recommended for premature as well as full-term infants. (B) Dosages should be given based on the actual, not corrected, chronological age. These may be initiated in the hospital. (C) The OPV is the one vaccine *not* given in the hospital due to the risk of transmission to other infants in the nursery. (D) The actual chronological age is used to administer vaccines to preterm infants.

12. **(C)** Nursing process phase: evaluation; client need: physiological integrity; content area: pediatric nursing

Rationale
(A) The one-hand method is appropriate for a child 1 to 8 years old. (B) The two-hand method is appropriate for anyone over 8 years old. (C) The drawing of an imaginary line between the nipples and placing two to three fingers below

the line is appropriate for infants. (D) In infants, the sternal notch is not palpated as the point of origin to determine finger placement.

13. (B) Nursing process phase: analysis and planning; client need: safe, effective care environment; content area: pediatric nursing

Rationale

(A) Subcutaneous injection is not recommended for DPT. Deep intramuscular injection is recommended. The deltoid is used only after 18 months of age. (B) Deep intramuscular injection with an appropriate-length needle into the ventrogluteal or vastus lateralis is the recommended method. (C) An air lock is theoretically helpful but not proven to be beneficial. The needle change after drawing up the medicine does not decrease local reactions. (D) The application of a local anesthetic may decrease pain, but not local reactions.

14. (A) Nursing process phase: evaluation; client need: safe effective care environment; content area: pediatric nursing

Rationale

(A) Testing of the formula temperature is always indicated. The inner wrist is not an appropriate site for accurate measurement. The mother's own tongue or back of hand should be used. (B & C) The mother's own tongue or back of hand should be used to test formula temperature. (D) Formula should be cool to the touch. Warm formula to touch is often too hot to be served.

15. (A) Nursing process phase: assessment; client need: physiological integrity; content area: pediatric nursing

Rationale

(A) The typical colicky infant does cry more than usual and does have abdominal cramping. (B) Although abdominal pain and gastric distention may be present, projectile vomiting and diarrhea are not typical. (C) Typically, the formula is tolerated well and infant thrives with adequate weight gain. (D) Some studies will indicate late evening fussiness in infants. For some infants, the time is altered.

16. (A) Nursing process phase: evaluation; client need: safe, effective care environment; content area: pediatric nursing

Rationale

(A) The proper placement of the apnea monitor electrode is 1 to 2 fingerwidths below the left nipple in the midaxillary line. (B) The measurement of the midway between the 2 nipples is taken in determination of placement for chest compressions. (C) The measurement of 2 fingerwidths below the left nipple is taken, but the electrode is not to be placed at that point. (D) One fingerwidth below the level of the imaginary line between the nipples is the proper placement for chest compressions.

17. (D) Nursing process phase: implementation; client need: health promotion and maintenance; content area: pediatric nursing

Rationale

(A) Boys and girls are both affected. Males are affected at higher percentages. (B) The peak time of year is winter (January). (C) The time of death is usually during sleep but most often in a prone, not supine, position. (D) The peak age is 2 to 4 months, with 95 percent occurring in the first 6 months.

18. (B) Nursing process phase: evaluation; client need: safe, effective care environment; content area: pediatric nursing

Rationale

(A) Powder, especially talc, may be dangerous, but corn starch products may be useful in keeping skin dry. (B) Proper technique is to avoid "puffs of powder" in the air, risking aspiration. It is appropriate to put small amounts of powder in the hand first. (C) Talc is very dangerous if inhaled, but corn starch-based products are safer. (D) Powder, especially talc, may be dangerous, but corn starch products, especially, may keep skin dry.

19. (C) Nursing process phase: analysis and planning; client need: physiological integrity; content area: pediatric nursing

Rationale

(A) Nonlipid hydrophillic agents such as Cetaphil and baths may be used in the dry method of treatment. (B) Frequent oil or oil-based oatmeal baths may be used to moisten. (C) Corticosteroids decrease inflammation, which may then decrease itching. Cream products may add moisture. (D) Hydroxyzine (Atarax) and diphenhydramine (Benadryl) are often used to decrease pruritus.

20. (A) Nursing process phase: implementation; client need: safe, effective care environment; content area: pediatric nursing

Rationale

(A) Less invasive procedures and approaches should be used. The parent is a source of comfort to the toddler. (B) Invasive procedures such as rectal temps cause fear of losing blood or body parts to the toddler and are very upsetting to the toddler. (C) The parents are needed to provide information needed by the health-care provider (HCP) and support needed by the toddler. (D) A full history and physical is needed for health maintenance and assessment of proper growth and development at periodic intervals during the life.

21. (C) Nursing process phase: analysis and planning; client need: health promotion and maintenance; content area: pediatric nursing

Rationale

(A & B) Because more than psychological or physiological readiness alone is required for toilet training (motivation, ability to communicate need, and physical readiness as to the ability to identify the need to void or defecate), the answers are not complete. (C) Both physiological and psychological readiness are needed, therefore the choice is more complete. Toddlers should be assessed individually for readiness and not hurried. (D) The toddler may be able to hold urine for 2 hours as evidenced by staying dry for that long and/or waking up dry from naps before that age.

22. (A) Nursing process phase: assessment; client need: safe, effective care environment; content area: pediatric nursing

Rationale

(A) Due to fear of losing blood and "insides" leaking out, invasive procedures such as otoscopic examination are threatening and are best left to later in the physical examination. (B) Auscultation is less invasive and can be performed while the parent holds the toddler in the lap. (C) Vital signs can be taken using less invasive procedures such as axillary instead of rectal temperatures. (D) Percussion of the abdomen can be made into a game and is not as threatening.

23. **(B)** Nursing process phase: assessment; client need: health promotion and maintenance; content area: pediatric nursing

Rationale
(A) Infancy is the period of solitary play. (B) Toddlers prefer parallel play. This play is alongside another child but not with that child. (C) Early childhood is the time for associative play in groups, but limited formal structural rules are needed. (D) Team sports with more rigid rules occur later in childhood.

24. **(C)** Nursing process phase: analysis and planning; client need: safe, effective care environment; content area: pediatric nursing

Rationale
(A & B) The child must be 40 pounds *or* 40 inches to use regular restraints; age is not considered in the factor. The midpoint of the head should be higher than the vehicle backseat while sitting in the booster chair, before the booster chair is omitted. (C) The rule is 40 pounds or 40 inches before the regular restraint system is used. (D) Mileage is never considered because many serious accidents occur near the home.

25. **(C)** Nursing process phase: implementation; client need: health promotion and maintenance; content area: pediatric nursing

Rationale
(A) Cleaning and brushing should begin with the first tooth. (B) Dental examinations are recommended twice per year. (C & D) Parents should supervise brushing and assist with flossing because fine motor skills are not refined.

26. **(C)** Nursing process phase: evaluation; client need: safe, effective care environment; content area: pediatric nursing

Rationale
(A) A breastfeeding infant *always* needs fluorine. (B) A child with *no* fluoride in the drinking water does not need a reduction. (C) A child who drinks from a known fluorinated water supply needs the amount of fluoride determined and may need unfluorinated water if the level is too high. (D) A child who drinks from city water system may receive a range of fluoride levels from none to excessive. Supplements of fluoride or a reduction in fluoride may be needed.

27. **(D)** Nursing process phase: implementation; client need: psychological integrity; content area: pediatric nursing

Rationale
(A) The mother can provide or place most of the information needed but not all. (B) The child can provide a lot of the needed information, but possibly not all of the historical or other background needed. (C) The parent may remain if the child wants but should be asked to leave at some point to further interview the child. (D) Do interview the parent and child together and separately to allow each to share any "confidential" information that the other is not wanted to hear.

28. **(A)** Nursing process phase: implementation; client need: psychological integrity; content area: pediatric nursing

Rationale
(A) A sociogram is the drawing of circles to signify important people in one's life. (B) The family Apgar measures adaptation, partnership, growth, affection, and resolve. (C) The kinetic family drawing is the technique of drawing the family doing something. (D) A genogram is a diagram of family medical history and is not interchangeable with a sociogram.

29. **(C)** Nursing process phase: assessment; client need: psychological integrity; content area: pediatric nursing

Rationale
(A) At stage 1, the child seeks to avoid punishment but has no understanding of the underlying moral orders. (B) At stage 2, the elements of fairness are evident but practically applied. (C) Stage 3, the beginning of the conventional level, is when one is concerned with conformity, loyalty, and actively maintaining social order. (D) At stage 4, the person does his or her duty, respects laws, and values order.

30. **(A)** Nursing process phase: implementation, client need: psychological integrity, content area: pediatric nursing

Rationale
(A) This option is to the point and accurate. (B) The fact that your opinion of the client's pain and the client's opinion of the pain differ should not be considered. If physical appearance differs from the stated value, chart the stated value. (C) The client may be lying in bed, but he states that he is in pain, which is what should be documented. (D) The statement that the client is faking pain is a judgment and should not be documented.

31. **(C)** Nursing process phase: assessment; client need: health promotion and maintenance; content area: pediatric nursing

Rationale
(A) During infancy the client presents generalized responses to pain by crying loudly and assuming a look of pain, but she cannot "objectify" it. (B) A young child can anticipate painful procedures and try to resist, but cannot objectively describe it. (C) By age 3 the Faces pain scale can be used to point to the face best depicting the child's own pain. (D) By age 4 the child can associate meaning with numbers and can use tools like the poker-chip tool or numerical-value tool.

32. **(A)** Nursing process phase: analysis and planning; client need: physiological integrity; content area: pediatric nursing

Rationale
(A) Constipation is such a common side effect that ordering prophylactic laxatives for someone in need of long-term therapy is understood. (B) Respirations may decrease but not usually to a state of respiratory depression. (C) Nausea and vomiting are side effects that are less common than constipation. (D) Anaphylaxis is rare.

33. **(B)** Nursing process phase: implementation; client need: safe, effective care environment; content area: pediatric nursing

Rationale
(A) A Telfa dressing would not provide the airtight seal. (B) A petrolatum-covered gauze secured on all four sides is used to form an airtight seal. (B) An Ace bandage would not provide the airtight seal. (D) A Band-Aid would not provide the airtight seal.

34. **(B)** Nursing process phase: analysis and planning; client need: physiological integrity; content area: pediatric nursing

Rationale
(A) Because the child is often NPO for the first 24 hours, this option does not include measuring the primary fluid intake of parenteral fluids. (B) Strictly measuring the intake of all oral and IV fluids, including medication diluents and flushes for lines in addition to hourly Foley catheter measurements, gives the best input and output picture. (C) Parents should not be requested to keep accurate counts in the immediate postoperative period and numbers of bottles or diapers is not exact. (D) Fluids are restricted, but offering the bedpan hourly would be inaccurate, inappropriate, unnecessary, and tiring for the immediate postoperative period.

35. **(A)** Nursing process phase: evaluation; client need: physiological integrity; content area: pediatric nursing

Rationale
(A) The sign of renal failure is a urine output of 1 ml/kg per hour with an increased BUN and serum creatinine. (B) BUN is increased with renal failure. (C) Serum creatinine is increased with renal failure. (D) Fewer than six wet diapers per day may indicate mild dehydration.

36. **(D)** Nursing process phase: implementation; client need: safe and effective care environment; content area: pediatric nursing

Rationale
(A) A teaspoon is five times higher than the dose the nurse should first question. (B) A nurse should question any microgram dose greater than 50 μg. (C) A nurse should question any milligram dose greater than 0.05 mg. (D) A nurse should question any one dose greater than 1 ml.

37. **(B)** Nursing process phase: evaluation; client need: safe, effective care environment; content area: pediatric nursing

Rationale
(A) If vomiting occurs, the doses should not be repeated. (B) Because of binding, the medication should not be given with milk products. It should be given 1 hour before meals or 2 hours after meals. (C) Oral medication is properly administered to the side and back. (D) If a dose is forgotten and less than 4 hours has passed, the dose can be given.

38. **(D)** Nursing process phase: evaluation; client need: physiological integrity; content area: pediatric nursing

Rationale
(A) Supine is a position recommended by the American Association of Pediatrics (AAP) for well infants. Infants with cardiovascular problems breathe more easily if the head of bed is elevated. (B) Side lying is a position recommended by the AAP for well infants. Infants with cardiovascular problems breath more easily if the head of bed is elevated. (C) Prone is recommended for infants, with a tendency to spit up or with respiratory problems, but not with the head down. (D) The head of bed up 45 degrees or an infant seat is recommended along with loose clothing for optimal chest expansion.

39. **(A)** Nursing process phase: implementation; client need: physiological integrity; content area: pediatric nursing

Rationale
(A) Because cyanosis can be caused by many reasons (cardiac, respiratory, metabolic, or hematological), tests are done to differentiate. In a 100% oxygen environment, a PaO_2 less than 100 mm Hg suggests cardiac disease. (B) A PaO_2 greater than 150 mm Hg suggests respiratory disease. (C) Other tests are used to differentiate metabolic disease. (D) Other tests are used to differentiate hematologic disease.

40. **(C)** Nursing process phase: implementation; client need: health promotion and maintenance; content area: pediatric nursing

Rationale
(A) Red meat is high in cholesterol and saturated fats. (B) Low-fat hot dogs are a good substitute, but not regular hot dogs. (C) Turkey, skinless chicken, or tofu are good substitutes for red meat. (D) Skim milk is a better choice than regular milk, which is 4 percent fat.

41. **(A)** Nursing process phase: evaluation; client need: health promotion and maintenance; content area: pediatric nursing

Rationale
(A) Renal disease causes more than 90 percent of the cases of secondary HTN in the child. (B–D) Less frequent causes of secondary HTN are cardiovascular disease and endocrine and neurological disorders.

42. **(A)** Nursing process phase: assessment; client need: physiological integrity; content area: pediatric nursing

Rationale
(A) A newborn with tricupsid atresia is usually cyanotic. (B) Infants with obstructive defects often have the sign and symptoms of congestive heart failure (CHF). Mild cases may be asystematic. (C) With conditions like atrioventricular canal defect, cyanosis may be mild but worsened with crying. A characteristic murmur is present and CHF may be severe. (D) Infants with TGV who have minimal mixing of the blood become severely cyanotic, however, if a large PDA is present, the signs and symptoms of CHF are more characteristic than those of cyanosis.

43. **(D)** Nursing process phase: assessment; client need: physiological integrity; content area: pediatric nursing

Rationale
(A) Coarctation of the aorta is an obstructive defect. (B) Aortic stenosis is an obstructive defect. (C) Pulmonic stenosis is an obstructive defect. (D) Arterial septal defects are associated with an increase in pulmonary blood flow.

44. **(D)** Nursing process phase: assessment; client need: physiological integrity; content area: pediatric nursing

Rationale
(A) The reddened conjunctiva and dry eyes occur later in the acute phase. (B) The cracked lips and strawberry tongue occur later in the acute phase. (C) Rashes related to KD vary but

are never vesicular. (D) A high fever for 5 days or more is characteristic of KD. Initial antipyretics and antibiotics do not seem to affect it.

45. **(C)** Nursing process phase: analysis and planning; client need: health promotion and maintenance; content area: pediatric nursing

Rationale
(A) Initially, aspirin helps control fever. (B) Analgesic therapy is not usually in the therapeutic management plan. (C) Later on, the aspirin serves as an antiplatelet agent and is continued until platelet counts are normal or indefinitely if coronary abnormalities develop. (D) The anti-inflammatory effects are for the initial treatments, maintenance doses are for platelet and cardiovascular benefits.

46. **(B)** Nursing process phase: evaluation; client need: safe, effective care environment; content area: pediatric nursing

Rationale
(A) Heated fans or dryers are not used to dry the cast because then the cast will be dry on the outside and wet underneath, which will cause mold to form. (B) The palms should be used to prevent indentations. (C) Distal area should be checked for signs of impaired blood flow and neurological integrity. (D) To prevent swelling, the extremity should not be in a dependent position for greater than 30 minutes at a time.

47. **(A)** Nursing process phase: assessment; client need: safe, effective care environment; content area: pediatric nursing

Rationale
(A) The Dunlap traction with either skin or skeletal traction suspends the arm horizontally. (B) Bryant's traction is an older form of traction once used on fractured femurs, but which is no longer recommended because of the possible tourniquet effects. (C) Buck's traction is a skin traction used to extend the legs. (D) The Russell traction is a skin traction of the lower leg and sling of the knee.

48. **(A)** Nursing process phase: implementation; client need: safe, effective care environment; content area: pediatric nursing

Rationale
(A) Skeletal traction involves a pin or wire placement into the bone. The weight should not be released or lifted for moving the child in bed. (B) Skin traction may be released and weights lifted as instructed by the physician's orders. (C) Plain cervical traction is a form of skin traction. (D) Buck's is a form of skin traction.

49. **(A)** Nursing process phase: analysis and planning; client need: safe, effective care environment; content area: pediatric nursing

Rationale
(A) Oxygen via mask or cannula needs to be administered *immediately* to treat the severe dyspnea. (B) Heparin may be given as part of the management plan. (C) Corticosteriods may be given as part of the management plan. (D) An IV will be established to treat shock and administer medication.

50. **(D)** Nursing process phase: implementation; client

need: safe, effective care environment; content area: pediatric nursing

Rationale
(A) Heat is usually not used initially because it would increase the blood supply and swelling. A cast is not indicated. (B) Iodine may be applied on an abrasion but has no benefits for a sprain. The ability to move, or range of motion, is part of assessment, and not treatment. Heat is not used initially. (C) The activity is restricted through the use of crutches at times. Gradual weight-bearing exercises begin after a period of rest, ice, compressions, and elevation. (D) Rest and ice (especially through a wet bandage), compression with an elastic bandage, and elevation higher than the level of the heart are beneficial.

51. **(D)** Nursing process phase: implementation; client need: safe, effective care environment; content area: pediatric nursing

Rationale
According to the AAP, sports have been divided into categories based on how strenuous the sport is and the probability of collision. Collision sports have the greatest risk of injury, followed by contact sports. (A) Football is a collision contact sport. (B) Gymnastics is a limited contact and collision sport. (C) Running is a strenuous noncontact sport. (D) Golf is a nonstrenuous noncontact sport and would hence have the least likely chance of threat for injury.

52. **(A)** Nursing process phase: implementation; client need: safe, effective care environment; content area: pediatric nursing

Rationale
(A) Because swimmers have a heavier body weight than the other three, they are less likely to have delayed menarche. (B & D) Figure skaters, gymnasts, and ballet dancers have the highest mean age of menarche. (C) Track runners' menarche is delayed but not as much as that of the others.

53. **(C)** Nursing process phase: implementation; client need: safe, effective care environment; content area: pediatric nursing

Rationale
(A) Kyphosis is an abnormality with an increased convex curvature of the thoracic spine. (B) Lordosis is the accentuated curvature of the lumbar spine. (C) Scoliosis is a defect in the lateral curvature. (D) Spondylolisthesis is the condition of one vertebra slipping forward onto another.

54. **(B)** Nursing process phase: assessment; client need: health promotion and maintenance; content area: pediatric nursing

Rationale
(A) The Allis test is a less reliable method to assess hip dislocation by placing the infant's feet flat on the table and flexing the knees to compare height. (B) Ortolani's maneuver involves flexing the knees of the infant and then abducting the hips of the infant outward. A pop or click may indicate a dislocated hip. (C) The bulge sign is used to test for swelling of the suprapatellar pouch. (D) Phalen's maneuver is used to test for carpal tunnel syndrome of the wrists.

55. **(D)** Nursing process phase: implementation; client need: health promotion and maintenance; content area: pediatric nursing

Rationale

(A) Fat pads are present to conceal the arch for up to 3 years. The appearance is normal. (B) Pronation is caused by the broad-based stance of a 12- to 30-month-old and is normal. (C) Genu varum (less than 2.5 cm between the knees) is common for 1 year after walking is initiated. (D) A physician would need to be aware if the medial malleoli measurement were greater than 2.5 cm; up to 2.5 cm, that is, "knock knees," is normal and common in the 2- to 3.5-year-old.

56. (D) Nursing process phase: evaluation; client need: physiological integrity; content area: pediatric nursing

Rationale

(A) The sed rate may be elevated or not. (B) The latex fixation test is negative in 90 percent of JRA cases. (C) The ANA are not found consistently in the subtypes of JRA. (D) JRA is a disease of exclusion by ruling out other possibilities.

57. (B) Nursing process phase: analysis and planning; client need: psychological integrity; content area: pediatric nursing

Rationale

(A) Multiple bruises may occur over fractures, but no acute bleeding. (B) Often abuse is a common misconception because even holding the ankles to change the diaper can result in a fractured bone. (C) JRA presents differently than OI. (D) Sprains are ligament damage, not bone fractures.

58. (C) Nursing process phase: assessment; client need: physiological integrity; content area: pediatric nursing

Rationale

(A) A child may be able to use the affected extremity. (B) A child who does not want to walk may have a fracture, it should not be ruled out, but it is not diagnostic. (C) An x-ray with comparison films is still the best way to compare extremities for fractures. (D) Bruising and swelling may be present over fractures.

59. (D) Nursing process phase: assessment; client need: physiological integrity; content area: pediatric nursing

Rationale

(A) Drinks such as Pedialyte or Infantile can be used in infants. (B) Sports drinks such as Gatorade or Exceed can be used in children. (C) Parents should observe the frequency of voiding and notify the practitioner if input appears to be insufficient. (D) It is important to remember that forcing fluids creates the difficulties of trying to force food. Gentle persuasion with preferred or favorite liquids is sufficient. The child should not be awakened for fluids.

60. (A) Nursing process phase: assessment, client need: safe, effective care environment; content area: pediatric nursing

Rationale

(A) Otitis media is usually based on clinical manifestations of a bright red bulging tympanic membrane with no light reflex or landmarks. (B) A CBC can be done, but many times it is not, because diagnosis is based on clinical physical examination. (C) Cultures to identify the organism are done if there is any drainage in the ear. (D) X-rays are not beneficial.

61. (D) Nursing process phase: assessment; client need: safe, effective care environment; content area: pediatric nursing

Rationale

(A) It may upset a frightened child, but physiological safety is greater than psychological safety. (B) They are diagnostic, but the answer is not complete. (C) A throat culture would be contraindicated because of the risk of airway obstruction. (D) The person who examines the posterior pharynx should be prepared to intubate immediately because of the risk of occluding the airway.

62. (C) Nursing process phase: assessment; client need: safe, effective care environment; content area: pediatric nursing

Rationale

(A) The onset is most often abrupt. (B) The throat is red, but sinusitis usually causes a postnasal drip. (C) In 50 to 80 percent of cases, the tonsils and pharynx will be inflamed with exudate. (D) Very tender anterior cervical lymphadenopathy may be present.

63. (B) Nursing process phase: assessment; client need: physiological integrity; content area: pediatric nursing

Rationale

(A) Pulse and respirations typically increase with early airway obstructions. (B) Retractions are a common finding in early airway obstruction. (C) Restlessness usually increases early. (D) Nasal flaring is evident but not necessarily congestion and drainage.

64. (B) Nursing process phase: implementation; client need: health promotion and maintenance; content area: pediatric nursing

Rationale

(A & B) Asthma is reversible with treatment or spontaneously. Chronic obstructive pulmonary disease (COPD) or emphysema is nonreversible. (C) Asthma is not influenced by sex. (D) Asthma usually beings *before* 4 to 5 years old.

65. (B) Nursing process phase: analysis and planning; client need: health promotion and maintenance; content area: pediatric nursing

Rationale

(A) Corticosteroids decrease inflammation. (B) B-2 Agonists are bronchodilators and are used frequently. (C) Helium blocks reflex bronchial constriction. (D) Cromolyn is the best nonsteroidal anti-inflammatory agent.

66. (A) Nursing process phase: analysis and planning; client need: safe, effective care environment; content area: pediatric nursing

Rationale

(A) Corticosteroids have anti-inflammatory properties. (B) B-2 agonists decrease spasms and bronchodilate. (C) Antibiotics prevent and reduce infection. (D) Cromolyn provides nonsteroidal anti-inflammatory effects.

67. (A) Nursing process phase: analysis and planning; client need: safe, effective care environment; content area: pediatric nursing

Rationale

(A) PEFR measures peak flow velocity and is compared to the client's personal best. (B) ABGs measure artery blood gases of PaO_2, $PaCO_2$, pH, and base excess. (C) SaO_2 measures peripheral oxygen saturation and is presented in a percentage.

(D) Auscultation will help determine wheezing and any decrease in breath sounds.

68. **(C)** Nursing process phase: assessment; client need: physiological integrity; content area: pediatric nursing

Rationale
(A–D) Respirations are 30 to 60 at birth and slow to about 16 to 20 in adulthood. Respirations are more abdominal in the neonate and become *more* thoracic in adulthood.

69. **(C)** Nursing process phase: analysis and planning, client need: health promotion and maintenance, content area: pediatric nursing

Rationale
(A) The canister should be shaken. (B) One breath lasting 3 to 5 seconds is indicated. (C) The breaths should be held 5 to 10 seconds after inspiration of the medication. (D) An empty canister floats on the surface, a full container sinks to the bottom.

70. **(D)** Nursing process phase: implementation, client need: health promotion and maintenance, content area: pediatric nursing

Rationale
(A) Allergies are a factor in many URIs, but shots are not always indicated. Testing helps determine allergies. (B) Prevention of attacks may be possible if triggers are identified and avoided or prophylactic medications are given. (C) Children do have decreased URIs by age 5 years. Infant infections soar at 3 to 6 months. But people of all ages may get URIs. (D) Smoking of any type should be avoided because it is not beneficial.

71. **(C)** Nursing process phase: evaluation; client need: safe, effective care environment; content area: pediatric nursing

Rationale
(A) The spray bottle should be retained for one person. (B) Overuse may lead to rebound congestion. (C) The spray should be used for the one infection only, not to prevent recurrent infections. (D) The spray should be discarded after 3 days.

72. **(A)** Nursing process phase: evaluation; client need: physiological integrity; content area: pediatric nursing

Rationale
(A) An early sign of bleeding and potential hemorrhage in a T & A client is frequent swallowing. (B) Moderate pain is common, especially in the first 24 hours. (C) A pulse of greater than 120 beats per minute may indicate hemorrhage. (D) Dark brown blood is expected in emesis secretions and in the nose and teeth. Bright red blood is indicative of hemorrhage.

73. **(A)** Nursing process phase: assessment; client need: physiological integrity; content area: pediatric nursing

Rationale
(A–D) The order of clinical signs of dehydration is usually tachycardia (the earliest detectable sign), dry skin and mucous membranes, sunken fontanelles, circulatory failure, loss of elasticity, and delayed capillary refill.

74. **(D)** Nursing process phase: assessment; client need: safe, effective care environment; content area: pediatric nursing

Rationale
(A–C) Any dextrose product is not isotonic. They are contradicted in the treatment stages of diabetic ketocidosis. (D) The IV fluids 0.9% NS and LR are close to the body's osmolality and are isotonic in nature.

75. **(D)** Nursing process phase: assessment; client need: safe, effective care environment; content area: pediatric nursing

Rationale
(A) Many colas are dark, and a newspaper cannot be read through them. (B) Formula and milk products are not considered a liquid because they curd on contact with resin in the stomach. (C) Other fluids such as commercial sports drinks or fluid replacers are considered clear. (D) Any liquid that is clear enough for a newspaper to be read through it is considered to be clear.

76. **(A)** Nursing process phase: assessment; client need: safe, effective care environment; content area: pediatric nursing

Rationale
(A) Accessibility and convenience are considered, but the child's developmental, cognitive, and mobility needs must receive the most attention. (B) The ability of the nurse to locate and secure a site is important, but the child's needs are priority. (C) Shaving the hair for scalp veins may be upsetting to parents and should always be preceded by a full explanation. (D) A transparent dressing is preferred, but if opaque is used, hourly checks are indicated.

77. **(C)** Nursing process phase: analysis and planning; client need: safe, effective care environment; content area: pediatric nursing

Rationale
(A) An infant often has an external urine collection bag to retrieve urine specimens. (B) The number of wet diapers gives a broad estimate as to whether output is adequate. (C) A diaper can be weighed to better determine the milliliters of fluid lost (1 gm = 1 cc). Because evaporation is possible, frequent checks are needed, especially if the client is under a radiant warmer or if the diaper leaks. (D) Catheters are not routinely inserted without adequate rationale.

78. **(B)** Nursing process phase: analysis and planning; client need: health promotion and maintenance; content area: pediatric nursing

Rationale
(A) Parenteral fluids are used for severe dehydration. (B) ORT is first-line treatment as long as the child can take fluids orally. (C) The BRAT diet is low in electrolytes and has little nutritional value since it is low in protein and energy. (D) Antidiarrheal agents are usually not given in infancy or toddlerhood because of the potential adverse effects.

79. **(D)** Nursing process phase: implementation; client need: safe, effective care environment; content area: pediatric nursing

Rationale
(A) A child of 1 to 10 kg needs 100 ml/kg. (B) A child of 11 to 20 kg needs 1000 ml/kg plus 50 ml/kg for each kilogram

over 10 kg. (C) The 500 ml/kg plus 20 ml/kg for each kilogram over 15 kg is not a formula applied to various weight groups. (D) A child over 20 kg needs 1500 ml/kg plus 20 ml/kg for each kilogram over 20 kg.

80. (A) Nursing process phase: evaluation; client need: physiological integrity; content area: pediatric nursing

Rationale

(A) Respiratory acidosis results in decreased pH, increased PO_2, and increased HCO_3. (B) Respiratory alkalosis results in increased pH, decreased PO_2, and decreased HCO_3. (C) Metabolic acidosis results in decreased pH, decreased PO_2 and decreased HCO_3. (D) Metabolic alkalosis results in increased pH, increased PO_2, and increased HCO_3.

81. (D) Nursing process phase: evaluation; client need: physiological integrity; content area: pediatric nursing

Rationale

(A) Salmonella's incubation period is 6 to 72 hours, and usually less than 24 hours. (B) Norwalklike organisms have an incubation period of 1 to 3 days. (C) *Clostridum botulinum* has an incubation period of 12 to 26 hours, with a range of 6 hours to 8 days. (D) Staphylococcus has an incubation period of 4 to 6 hours and is often caused by contaminated food such as mayonnaise or custards.

82. (B) Nursing process phase: assessment; client need: physiological integrity; content area: pediatric nursing

Rationale

(A) Blisters occur in second-degree burns. (B) Pain is the predominant symptom in first-degree burns. (C) Waxy white skin may be present in second- or third-degree burns. Brown skin is present in third-degree burns. (D) Burns of full thickness, fourth-degree burns, appear dull and dry with bones or ligaments noted.

83. (C) Nursing process phase: evaluation; client need: health promotion and maintenance; content area: pediatric nursing

Rationale

(A) Butter and oils should not be applied. (B) Blisters should be left intact. (C) Loose gauze is not necessarily applied. (D) Cool water should be run over the burn.

84. (B) Nursing process phase: evaluation; client need: health promotion and maintenance; content area: pediatric nursing

Rationale

(A) Silvadene contains sulfa and should not be used in those who are allergic. Silver nitrate would be used. (B) Silvadene contains sulfa and should not be used in those who are allergic. (C) Silvadene contains sulfa and should not be used in those who are allergic. Betadine would be contraindicated in those allergic to iodine. (D) Silvadene contains sulfa and should not be used in those who are allergic. Bacitracin may be used in those allergic to silvadene.

85. (A) Nursing process phase: implementation; client need: health promotion and maintenance; content area: pediatric nursing

Rationale

(A) Benefits to mother and infant should be provided, and the parents of the infant should be allowed to make an in-

formed decision. (B) *No* information will not lead to an informed decision. (C) Written packets would not allow for questions and answers. (D) The mother should have some input into the type of formula used if she opts to bottle. The nurse should not assume bottle feeding.

86. (A) Nursing process phase: implementation; client need: health promotion and maintenance; content area: pediatric nursing

Rationale

(A) Because of the rate of physical growth in puberty, the nutritional intake of iron, calcium, zinc, and protein should almost be doubled. (B & C) Overall nutrition and a well-balanced diet are important, but fat content should not exceed 30 percent. Folate (folic acid) is important, especially for girls and women before and during pregnancy. (D) Overall nutrition and a well-balanced diet are important. Vitamin C needs do not necessarily increase.

87. (B) Nursing process phase: assessment; client need: physiological integrity; content area: pediatric nursing

Rationale

(A) Smooth, pink nails are normal. (B) Brittle or spoon-shaped nails may be indicative of iron deficiency. (C) Splinter hemorrhages are evident of vitamin C deficiency. (D) Beau's lines may be caused by trauma.

88. (D) Nursing process phase: implementation; client need: health promotion and maintenance; content area: pediatric nursing

Rationale

(A) A rigid schedule should not be enforced. The toddler may eat more or less each day. (B) A toddler is not developmentally ready to sit through long meals. Family meals are important but should not be prolonged. (C) Skim milk and low fat milk may be used for children after 2 years old, but the toddler period is 12 to 36 months. Whole milk is needed at 12 to 24 months. (D) In general, 1 tablespoon for each year is adequate for a solid food serving. This is in accordance with the number of servings per food group.

89. (C) Nursing process phase: assessment; client need: health promotion and maintenance; content area: pediatric nursing

Rationale

(A) This may be of interest but is not as critical as if she is currently pregnant. (B) This is important to know for other mothers to be aware of, but isolation is not necessary. (C) If the mother is pregnant and contracts the disease, it may be harmful or fatal to the fetus. (D) Isolation of the unhospitalized child is not necessary.

90. (C) Nursing process phase: assessment; client need: physiological integrity; content area: pediatric nursing

Rationale

(A) Mean corpuscular volume is usually less than 77 to 95 μm^3. (B) MCHC is normally 31 to 37 percent. (C) HCT is normally 35 to 45 percent. A 30 percent reading is low. (D) Hgb is normally 11.5 to 15.5.

91. (D) Nursing process phase: assessment; client need: physiological integrity; content area: pediatric nursing

Rationale
(A) *Bordetella pertussis* causes whooping cough. (B) Enterovirus causes polio. (C) Rubella virus causes German measles. (D) Streptococci cause scarlet fever.

92. **(A)** Nursing process phase: evaluation; client need: physiological integrity; content area: pediatric nursing

Rationale
(A) When the vesicles have dried, the child can be released from home isolation. (B) Crusts may still be present when the child returns to school. Support and conferences with the teacher may be needed for the child's psychological security. (C) New lesions may appear for a few days. When they are dry, the child may be removed from isolation. (D) It does take an average of 1 week for lesions to dry. Look at the lesions.

93. **(B)** Nursing process phase: assessment; client need: physiological integrity; content area: pediatric nursing

Rationale
(A) A white strawberry tongue is present on day 1 and a red strawberry tongue on day 3. (B) On day 1 the cheeks are flushed, and it progresses to a circumoral pallor by day 3. (C) The Schultz-Charlton blanching test is positive on day 3. (D) The density of the rash is increased in the neck and groin on day 1 and in the axilla on day 3.

94. **(A)** Nursing process phase: analysis and planning; client need: safe, effective care environment; content area: pediatric nursing

Rationale
(A) If oral diphenydramine is given simultaneously, toxicity can result from the increased topical absorption. (B) Cool baths with oatmeal or soap are still comforting according to some. (C) Calamine does not prevent crusting. (D) Calamine may be very comforting or helpful and does not prolong the outbreak, according to the literature.

95. **(A)** Nursing process phase: implementation; client need: safe, effective care environment; content area: pediatric nursing

Rationale
(A) Aspirin should be avoided because of the risk for Reye's syndrome. (B) Acyclovir is controversial because it causes a milder case and may lead to less immunity. (C) Acetaminophen is controversial because it does not really decrease the mild fever or fussiness the child has and may delay drying and scabbing of the vesicles. (D) Diphenhydramine is recommended for the itching.

96. **(D)** Nursing process phase: evaluation; client need: physiological integrity; content area: pediatric nursing

Rationale
(A) Allergic conjunctivitis usually presents with watery discharge, itching, and inflamed conjunctiva. (B) Foreign-body conjunctivitis usually presents unilaterally with pain, swelling, tearing, and inflammation. (C) Viral-hemorrhage conjunctivitis presents with photophobia and subconjunctivial bleeding. (D) Bacterial conjunctivitis (pink eye) presents bilaterally with purulent drainage that often mats the eyes shut on awakening.

97. **(B)** Nursing process phase: assessment; client need: safe, effective care environment; content area: pediatric nursing

Rationale
(A) Rectal swabs are used to determine the causative organisms of diarrhea. (B) The tape test, which involves placing transparent (not magic or frosted) tape, sticky side out, around a tongue depressor, which is then secured to the anus of the sleeping child. Specimens are collected in the early morning, before stooling or awakening. (C) A skin scraping is used for many rashes and infestations like scabies. (D) A stool specimen is often used for diarrhea complaints.

98. **(C)** Nursing process phase: assessment; client need: safe, effective care environment; content area: pediatric nursing

Rationale
(A) CBCs are monitored, but urine output is most critical. (B) Serum lead levels are monitored to determined when to begin therapy and to follow the effectiveness of the therapy. (C) Urine output *must* be adequate to administer $CaNa_2$ EDTA injections. (D) Hematocrit and hemoglobin are a part of the CBC.

99. **(B)** Nursing process phase: assessment; client need: safe, effective care environment; content area: pediatric nursing

Rationale
(A) Allergies are important to know; however, first what was taken and when it was taken needs to be determined to plan treatment. (B) Because there is no universal antidote for "poison," what was taken, amount, when, and anything that caregivers may have done to improve or worsen the situation all need to be determined. (C) Ipecac is given before activated charcoal, if both are to be given. However, ipecac is contraindicated if the client takes calcium channel blockers, benzodiazepines, and other drugs. (D) Activated charcoal is black, tasteless, and odorless medicine that may hold sweetener, but it is lower priority.

100. **(A)** Nursing process phase: analysis and planning; client need: safe; effective care environment; content area: pediatric nursing

Rationale
(A) Exact quotes are best for presenting the child's picture. (B) Summary statements would reflect your *analysis* of all the information, but would not allow others to later see the subjective and objective data independently for evaluation. (C) Both subjective and objective data need to be used. Both need to be presented in a professional, nonjudgmental, objective way. (D) Some open-ended questions provide better and more complete explanations. Certain closed-ended questions are also appropriate.

101. **(C)** Nursing process phase: evaluation; client need: health promotion and maintenance; content area: pediatric nursing

Rationale
(A) A helmet should be worn by anyone riding a bicycle. (B) When straddling the bar, both feet should touch the ground. (C) The child should be able to touch the entire ball of the foot (not just the toes) to the ground while sitting on the seat. (D) Most motor vehicle accidents involving bicycles occur between 4 and 6 P.M., accidents involving just bicycles occur between 4 and 8 P.M. Supervision is helpful to reduce risk.

102. **(A)** Nursing process phase: analysis and planning;

client need: physiological integrity; content area: pediatric nursing

Rationale
(A) Rules that are often extremely rigid are developed by the children for their games. The rules are also present in language and behavior. (B–D) Physical skill, intellectual ability, and fantasy are all components but are subject to the children's rigid rules and rituals.

103. (D) Nursing process phase: assessment; client need: health promotion and maintenance; content area: pediatric nursing

Rationale
(A–D) Girls prefer to play with girls and boys prefer to play with boys.

104. (C) Nursing process phase: assessment; client need: physiological integrity; content area: pediatric nursing

Rationale
(A) Night terrors are more common in the preschooler. (B) Nightmares are less common in this age group than in the preschooler. A traumatic event may cause one. (C) Sleep walking and sleep talking happen as stage 4 to stage 1 of non-REM sleep occurs. This is usually 90 to 120 minutes after going to sleep. They are both common in the school-aged child. (D) Bed wetting is a common problem for this age group. In the hospital, bed wetting is less likely to cause physical danger than wandering about the hospital sleep walking. Patience and support should be provided to reduce psychological upset.

105. (C) Nursing process phase: assessment; client need: physiological integrity; content area: pediatric nursing

Rationale
(A, B, & D) Although a child should be assessed for any chief-complaint injuries, upper extremity injuries are most common. Ankle sprains, femur fractures, and concussions would be examined based on client presentation. (C) Upper extremity injuries are most common with in-line skate accidents as the child tries to break the fall.

106. (B) Nursing process phase: implementation; client need: health promotion and maintenance; content area: pediatric nursing

Rationale
(A) The child should have already begun dental visits and should continue these. (B) The deciduous teeth (crowns only, roots have dissolved) will become loose and begin to be lost at 6 years old. (C) Permanent teeth appear too large for the small facial features. (D) Fluoride is still important, and fluoride treatments may decrease the enamel breakdown.

107. (B) Nursing process phase: analysis and planning; client need: physiological integrity; content area: pediatric nursing

Rationale
(A) A macule is flat and nonpalpable (freckle). (B) A wheal is the elevated, solid, irregularly shaped, cutaneous edema area (insect bite). (C) A papule is an elevated, circumscribed firm area (wart). (D) A fluid-filled, superficial elevation is a vesicle (blister).

108. (A) Nursing process phase: implementation; client need: physiological integrity; content area: pediatric nursing

Rationale
(A) Surgical wounds not contaminated by infection heal by primary intention. All edges are well approximated. (B) A third-degree burn may heal from the inside out as infected areas are debrided away. A more severe scar is left. (C) Deep lacerations that had delayed suturing or no suturing heal from excessive granulation and have deeper scars. (D) The surgical wound may be repaired but is not healed. Proper care should be given to avoid infection so the site can heal by primary intention.

109. (A) Nursing process phase: analysis and planning; client need: safe, effective care environment; content area: pediatric nursing

Rationale
(A) All of the topics will be taught. It is critical to teach proper application, especially of lindane, because prolonged exposure can cause neurological symptoms (seizures). (B) Itching will continue and should be treated. (C) Close contacts will need to be treated because the length of time from exposure to the appearance of symptoms is delayed. (D) Hot water will need to be used to launder all clothes and linens.

110. (B) Nursing process phase: evaluation; client need: health promotion and maintenance; content area: pediatric nursing

Rationale
(A) It is the oil in the plant that causes the irritation. (B) Cool water and either no soap or mild soap should be used. The cool water neutralizes the oil not bonded to the skin. Harsh soaps remove protective skin oils and scrubbing irritates skin. (C) The rash is not spread by the blisters but by the oil, which may still be present on clothes or animal fur. (D) The smoke from the burning of poison ivy can lead to reactions and rashes.

111. (D) Nursing process phase: implementation; client need: safe, effective care environment; content area: pediatric nursing

Rationale
(A & D) If properly applied, the 15 means that the child can remain in the sun 15 times normal before burning occurs (if burning usually occurred in 20 minutes, he could stay out 300 minutes before burning occurred). (B) The lotion must be applied 15 to 20 minutes before, but it should be applied frequently and liberally. (C) Any decrease in sunburns, especially in early life, will decrease the risk of skin cancer later. The 15 does not mean by 15 percent. There may be a greater reduction if all sunburns were avoided.

112. (B) Nursing process phase: analysis and planning; client need: health promotion and maintenance; content area: pediatric nursing

Rationale
(A) Adolescents are not particularly more accident prone. They do tend to believe "nothing bad can happen to me." (B) The primary cause of death in adolescents is unintentional injury, primarily motor vehicle accidents (MVAs). (C) Homicide is the leading cause of death in African-American adolescences, but second in overall adolescents. (D) Actually more homicides occur with friends and family members.

113. **(C)** Nursing process phase: implementation; client need: psychological integrity; content area: pediatric nursing

Rationale

(A) *All* information cannot be kept confidential. Many things are mandated by law to be reported to state health departments or the Department of Health and Human Services. (B) Asking open-ended questions allows the adolescent to share more and decrease stereotyping. (C) Most information can be kept confidential. Life-threatening issues that must be reported to parents will be done with the client's knowledge. (D) The parent should be excused for most of the interview.

114. **(A)** Nursing process phase: assessment; client need: physiological integrity, content area: pediatric nursing

Rationale

(A) At Tanner stage 1 there is no pubic hair. (B) Tanner stage 2 involves initial scrotal testes enlargement. (C) Tanner stage 3 involves initial enlargement of the penis. (D) Tanner stage 4 involves development of the glans and an increase in diameter.

115. **(D)** Nursing process phase: implementation; client need: psychological integrity; content area: pediatric nursing

Rationale

(A) Mood swings and daydreaming are common in 11- to 14-year-olds. (B) The 14- to 17-year-old will be more introspective and withdrawn. (C) The 14- to 17-year-old will also exhibit more feelings of inadequacy but will find it hard to ask for assistance. (D) The 18-year-old should be calmer, controlling anger and other emotions, while the 13-year-old has outbursts of anger with verbal insults and name calling.

116. **(B)** Nursing process phase: assessment; client need: psychological integrity; content area: pediatric nursing

Rationale

(A) Stage 2 is breast bud development. (B) Stage 3 is the separation of contours. (C) Stage 4 is a secondary mound formation. (D) Stage 5 is mature configuration.

117. **(A)** Nursing process phase: analysis; client need: health promotion and maintenance; content area: pediatric nursing

Rationale

(A) By 12th grade, 89.5 percent of students have tried alcohol. (B) By 12th grade, 64.4 percent of students have tried cigarettes. (C) By 12th grade, 40.7 percent of students have tried marijuana. (D) Although of a serious nature, fewer students used other drugs. Alcohol is considered the "gate keeper" to the use of other drugs.

118. **(A)** Nursing process phase: analysis and planning; client need: safe, effective case environment; content area: pediatric nursing

Rationale

(A) Accutane is reserved for severe cystic acne and should be managed by a dermatologist. (B) Retin-A is commonly used to treat any acne. (C) Benzoyl peroxide is often used in combination with Retin-A: one every morning and one every evening. (D) Topical antibiotics may be prescribed for any acne that is inflammatory.

119. **(A)** Nursing process phase: implementation; client need: safe, effective care environment; content area: pediatric nursing

Rationale

(A) A pelvic examination is indicated for the first-time request of oral contraceptives. (B) An abdominal sonogram is indicated for diagnosis of menstrual disorders in some instances. (C) Gonorrhea and chlamydia cultures, as well as other STD evaluation, is mandated by client exposure and risk factors. The girl may not be sexually active yet. (D) Endometrial biopsy is reserved for unusual or problematic bleeding or amenorrhea.

120. **(A)** Nursing process phase: implementation; client need: health promotion and maintenance; content area: pediatric nursing

Rationale

(A) Oral combination contraceptives inhibit ovulation, if used properly. (B) Spermacides kill sperm. (C) Postcoital contraceptive pills, which are known as "morning after" pills, prevent implantation, but this is not the way that oral contraceptives taken daily work. (D) Condoms trap the sperm.

121. **(D)** Nursing process phase: evaluation; client need: health promotion and maintenance, content area: pediatric nursing

Rationale

(A) Weight gain is common on Depo-Provera therapy. (B) Periods may be irregular or amenorrhea present. (C) Injections are repeated every 12 weeks on average. (D) There is *no* STD protection on Depo-Provera. Condoms would be needed for STD protection.

122. **(D)** Nursing process phase: implementation; client need: health promotion and maintenance; content area: pediatric nursing

Rationale

(A) Male victims are *less* likely to report the rape. (B) There is no typical victim. Victims include members of all ethnic groups and all ages. The seductive clothing, or the "woman asked for it by what she was wearing," explanation is a myth. (C) Rape involves any sexual activity—penile penetration of the vagina or anus, sodomy, and so on. (D) Fifty percent of rape victims are estimated to be between 15 and 19 years old.

123. **(B)** Nursing process phase: assessment; client need: physiological integrity; content area: pediatric nursing

Rationale

(A) Bacterial vaginosis presents with a milky white, thin, fishy odor. (B) With pelvic inflammatory disease, which is often the result of chlamydia, there is lower abdominal pain, fever, and dysuria. (C) Human papillomavirus (HPV), or genital warts, presents with a raised, flesh-colored rash. (D) Candida (yeast) is often thick and cheesy with itching.

124. **(A)** Nursing process phase: assessment; client need: physiological integrity; content area: pediatric nursing

Rationale

(A) Children's verbal statements and descriptions of pain are the most important factors is assessing their pain. (B) Restlessness is a physiological response to pain; however, it may also be produced by emotions such as fear, anger, or anxiety. (C) Listening for pain clues in cries would not be as appropriate for this age child because a child of this age can verbally describe his pain. (D) Pathology may give clues to the expected intensity and type of pain; however, it is a mistake to believe that certain conditions or procedures always produce a standard amount of pain.

125. (C) Nursing process phase: assessment; client need; health promotion and maintenance; content area: pediatric nursing

Rationale
(A) Copying a circle is a typical behavior of a 3-year-old. (B) Building a tower of eight or more blocks is a typical behavior of a 3-year-old. (C) Pulling toys behind is a typical task expected of a normally developed 18-month-old. (D) Playing tag requires cooperative play and the ability to follow rules, which develops at about 5 years of age.

126. (D) Nursing process phase: analysis; client need: psychosocial integrity; content area: pediatric nursing

Rationale
(A) Eating nonfood substances is called pica. Having a diet of soft, low-roughage foods is an unlikely cause of pica. However, pica has been found to be associated with both iron and zinc deficiencies. Controversy exists regarding whether pica is the cause or a result of the deficiency. (B) Suffering from a hormonal deficiency due to a genetic defect is not a likely cause of pica. Pica has been reputed to be the presenting symptom with celiac disease thought to be caused by iron deficiency. (C) Relieving discomfort due to cutting large teeth is not a likely cause of pica. (D) The child may be relieving anxiety through oral gratification. In this situation, the change in the home environment may be the cause of anxiety.

127. (C) Nursing process phase: assessment; client need: health promotion and maintenance; content area: pediatric nursing

Rationale
(A) The normally developed 3-year-old is not expected to be able to tie his shoelaces. He will probably not do this well until he is 5 or 6 years old. (B) Only 25 percent of normally developed 3-year-olds can copy a circle. (C) A normally developed 3-year-old should be able to identify five body parts. Ninety percent of children age 30 months can identify five body parts. (D) Twenty-five percent of normally developed 3-year, 3-month-old children can hop on one foot.

128. (A) Nursing process phase: implementation; client need: psychosocial integrity; content area: pediatric nursing

Rationale
(A) The most common reason for failing when toilet training toddlers is that they are not ready for training. (B) Even with rewards, if the child is not ready to be trained he will not learn voluntary control. (C) Even with proper equipment, if the child is not ready to be trained he will not learn voluntary control. (D) It is possible, but unlikely, that a child is demonstrating individuality when there are reports of having difficulty with toilet training.

129. (B) Nursing process phase: analysis; client need: psychosocial integrity; content area: pediatric nursing

Rationale
(A) Obtaining another nurse to assist may be necessary but

would not be the best first course of action. (B) Most authorities recommend that a parent be allowed to assist when a child is unable to cooperate during a procedure. Poor cooperation is due to fright and the child will feel more secure with the parent present. (C) Waiting until the child calms down may be an alternative but is not recommended as a first course of action. (D) Using restraints during the procedure may be necessary but is not recommended as a first course of action.

130. (B) Nursing process phase: evaluation; client need: health promotion and maintenance; content area: pediatric nursing

Rationale
(A) Pulling the earlobe up and forward is not the correct method for instilling eardrops in either the adult or the child. (B) Pulling the earlobe up and backward is the correct way to instill eardrops for a child older than 3 years of age, because the auditory canals are directed inward, forward, and down. (C) Pulling the earlobe down and forward is not the correct method for instilling eardrops in either the adult or the child. (D) Pulling the earlobe down and backward is not correct for instilling eardrops in either the adult or the child.

131. (D) Nursing process phase: implementation; client need: health promotion and maintenance; content area: pediatric nursing

Rationale
(A) The anterior fontanel does not close between 2 and 4 months. The small posterior fontanel usually closes by the end of the second month. (B) The anterior fontanel does not close between 4 and 8 months. (C) The anterior fontanel does not close between 8 and 12 months. (D) The most common time for the anterior fontanel to close is between 12 and 18 months of age.

132. (A) Nursing process phase: implementation; client need: health promotion and maintenance; content area: pediatric nursing

Rationale
(A) Appetite and food preferences are sporadic during the toddler years. A child may enjoy one food for several days in a row and suddenly refuse to eat it again for days. It is best to accept such extremes and offer other foods in small portions. (B) Insisting that she eat small portions of the family's meals or any other attempt to alter such food fads is met with resentment and obstinacy. (C) It would not be necessary to consult a physician because this food fad will pass. (D) Offering the child extra time to play outside is not an appropriate nutritional strategy.

133. (D) Nursing process phase: planning; client need: psychosocial integrity; content area: pediatric nursing

Rationale
(A) Hyperactivity is a behavior that may be demonstrated by the toddler, but does not necessarily explain the negativism demonstrated by a toddler. (B) Sibling rivalry is a behavior that may be demonstrated by the toddler, but does not necessarily explain the negativism demonstrated by a toddler. (C) Separation anxiety is a behavior that may be demonstrated by the toddler, but does not necessarily explain the negativism demonstrated by a toddler. (D) According to Erikson, the developmental task of toddlerhood is acquiring a sense of autonomy while overcoming a sense of doubt and shame. Characteristics of negativism and rituals are typical of behaviors in the toddler's quest for autonomy.

134. (B) Nursing process phase: implementation; client need: psychosocial integrity; content area: pediatric nursing

Rationale
(A) Corporal punishment (spanking) does cause a dramatic decrease in behavior but has serious flaws. It teaches children that violence is acceptable, may physically harm the child as a result of parental rage, and children often become accustomed to spanking, requiring more severe corporal punishment each time. (B) The best approach toward discipline is to minimize misbehavior by using structured interactions so that unacceptable behavior is prevented or minimized. (C) Reasoning is more appropriate for older children, especially when moral issues are involved. Reasoning combined with scolding many times takes the form of shame or criticism. Unfortunately, children take such remarks seriously believing that they are "bad." (D) Limit-setting and discipline are positive, necessary components of child rearing.

135. (D) Nursing process phase: evaluation; client need: health promotion and maintenance; content area: pediatric nursing

Rationale
(A) It would be very unsafe to have infant lying on car seat even with seat belt in place. (B) Using infant seat is safer but not flat and not with infant facing driver. (C) If the infant seat were facing forward the head would whip forward, creating enormous stress on the neck. (D) A rear-facing infant seat provides the very best protection for the heavy head and weak neck of a young child.

136. (D) Nursing process phase: implementation; client need: health promotion and maintenance; content area: pediatric nursing

Rationale
(A) Children in the concrete operational state of Piaget's theory (school-age) comprehend the concept of reversibility—that an act can be undone by performing an opposite act or a change in relations can be compensated for by performing another manipulation on something. (B) School-age children also understand the concept of conservation—that things are the same even when their form and shape change. (C) Object permanence is a milestone of the sensorimotor period of Piaget's theory. It is demonstrated at 6 to 9 months of age when the infant reaches for a hidden object. (D) According to Piaget's theory, at approximately 2 years of age the child enters the preconceptual phase of cognitive development, which lasts until 4 years of age. Animism is a concept of preconceptual thought in which the child attributes to inanimate objects lifelike qualities.

137. (B) Nursing process phase: analysis; client need: health promotion and maintenance; content area: pediatric nursing

Rationale
(A) Myopia, or nearsightedness, is the ability to see objects at close range but not at a distance. (B) Hyperopia, or farsightedness, is the ability to see objects at a distance. Most children are normally hyperopic until about 7 years of age. (C) presbyopia is a defect of vision in advancing age, usually between 40 and 45 years of age. The defect involves loss of accommodation or recession of near point. (D) Amblyopia, also called "lazy eye," is reduced visual acuity in one eye despite appropriate optical correction.

138. (C) Nursing process phase: planning; client need: health promotion and maintenance; content area: pediatric nursing

Rationale
(A) Drinking from a cup usually begins around 8 months of age and most normally developed children do this well by 17 months of age. (B) The thumb-finger group usually begins around 7 months of age and most normally developed infants can do this by 10 months of age. (C) Rolling over usually begins as early as 3 months of age and most normally developed infants can do this before 6 months of age. (D) Being able to say "mama" or "dada" specific usually beings at a little over 6 months of age and most normally developed infants can do this well by 13 months.

139. (D) Nursing process phase: assessment; client need: physiological integrity; content area: pediatric nursing

Rationale
(A) Vomiting and diarrhea may be signs of otitis media but the tympanic membrane would not be yellow in color. (B) Pulling at the ears and earache are common signs and symptoms of otitis media but the tympanic membrane would not be gray in color. (C) Cough is not a sign of otitis media; irritability may be present but the tympanic membrane is not inverted. (D) Rhinorrhea, fever (a temperature as high as 40°C [104°F]), and a bulging tympanic membrane are common signs and symptoms of otitis media.

140. (C) Nursing process phase: analysis; client need: physiological integrity; content area: pediatric nursing

Rationale
(A) Reducing inflammation of the eustachian tube will occur but this is not the primary purpose for treatment with amoxicillin. (B) Treating the ear infection will reduce the pain but is not the primary purpose for treatment with amoxicillin. (C) Acute otitis media is frequently caused by the *H. influenzae* and *Streptococcus pneumonia* bacteria. The primary purpose of amoxicillin is to treat the infection caused by these two organisms. (D) As the infection is treated the fever will be reduced, but this is not the primary reason for treatment with amoxicillin.

141. (A) Nursing process phase: implementation; client need: physiological integrity; content area: pediatric nursing

Rationale
(A) Evaluating the effectiveness of the treatment is the primary reason for the follow-up appointment. (B) Obtaining a prescription for another antibiotic would not be necessary unless the treatment was determined to be ineffective. (C) Ascertaining whether the child had received all of the antibiotic would be important in determining the effectiveness of the treatment but is not the primary reason for the recheck appointment. (D) Identifying potential complications such as effusion or hearing impairment are also important but determining effectiveness of the treatment is the primary reason for the initial return appointment.

142. (B) Nursing process phase: implementation; client need: physiological integrity; content area: pediatric nursing

Rationale
(A) Potential for impairment in skin integrity related to ear

drainage should be considered as a potential nursing diagnosis but is not addressed in the intervention of teaching the parents not to allow chewing. (B) The application of heat may reduce pain in some children but may cause discomfort for others. An ice compress placed over the affected ear may also provide comfort because it reduces edema. These interventions are appropriate for the nursing diagnosis. Alteration in comfort: Pain related to infectious process. (C) Knowledge deficit of parents related to unfamiliarity of the situation may be an appropriate nursing diagnosis but is not specifically related to these interventions. (D) Hyperthermia related to infectious process may be an appropriate nursing diagnosis but is not specifically related to these interventions.

143. (A) Nursing process phase: analysis; client need: psychosocial integrity; content area: pediatric nursing

Rationale
(A) This response is best because it is an honest response and you want the child to know he can get medicine to make the pain better. (B) This would not be an honest response and could cause the child to mistrust the nurse. (C) This would not be an appropriate response because it is not a truthful statement. (D) This response would not be appropriate for the cognitive development of a normal 4-year-old.

144. (B) Nursing process phase: implementation; client need: safe, effective care environment; content area: pediatric nursing

Rationale
(A) This comment by the mother would indicate an understanding of food and fluids restrictions immediately after T&A surgery. (B) This comment by the mother would indicate a need for further instruction because coughing frequently, clearing throat, and blowing nose may aggravate the operative site. (C) This comment by the mother would indicate understanding of the need for pain medication post-T&A. (D) This comment by the mother would indicate an understanding of immediate postoperative position until child is fully awake to facilitate drainage of secretions.

145. (C) Nursing process phase: planning; client need: safe, effective care environment; content area: pediatric nursing

Rationale
(A) Poliomyelitis vaccine is the only immunization given by the oral route. (B) None of the immunizations is given by the intradermal route. The tuberculin skin test, however, is given by this route. (C) Diphtheria, pertussis, and tetanus (DPT) immunization is given deep into the largest muscle available. The best muscle to use in a 2-month-old infant is the vastus lateralis. (D) Measles, mumps, and rubella (MMR) immunization is given by the subcutaneous route.

146. (D) Nursing process phase: analysis; client need: health promotion and maintenance; content area: pediatric nursing

Rationale
(A) Gentle stretching exercises would be inappropriate because the child is usually treated conservatively by containment accomplished by non-weight-bearing devices on the affected limb. (B) Weight is not a causative factor of this disease, and even if weight reduction is needed it would not be the major emphasis of nursing care. (C) Pain is usually not a factor after treatment is initiated and would not be the ma-

jor emphasis in planning care. (D) The aim of treatment for Legg-Calvé-Perthes disease is to keep the head of femur contained in the acetabulum. Containment can be accomplished by non-weight-bearing devices on the affected limb such as abduction brace, leg casts, or a leather harness sling. Conservative therapy is usually continued for 2 to 4 years. Because most of the child's care is on an outpatient basis, the major emphasis for nursing care is to teach the family the care and management of the corrective appliance.

147. (B) Nursing process phase: analysis; client need: safe, effective care environment; content area: pediatric nursing

Rationale
(A) An elevated antibody level would help document a recent infection but is not diagnostic of a Wilms' tumor. (B) Computerized tomography is one diagnostic study that may assist in the diagnosis of Wilms' tumor. (C) The client may have a low hemoglobin count due to anemia that would have to be combined with more definitive studies to confirm a diagnosis of Wilms' tumor. (D) A high leukocyte count may be present due to the metastasis of the disease. The leukocyte count would also have to be combined with more definitive studies to confirm a diagnosis of Wilm's tumor.

148. (B) Nursing process phase: planning; client need: physiological integrity; content area: pediatric nursing

Rationale
(A) Bilateral renal involvement is classified as stage V. (B) Tumor that extends beyond the kidney and is completely resected is stage II. (C) A tumor that is limited to the kidney and completely resected is stage I. (D) A tumor that has metastasized to lung, liver, bone, and brain is classified as stage IV.

149. (A) Nursing process phase: implementation; client need: physiological integrity; content area: pediatric nursing

Rationale
(A) Surgery is scheduled as soon as possible after confirmation of a renal mass. Postoperative radiation is indicated for all children with Wilms' tumor except those with stage I disease and favorable histology. Chemotherapy is indicated for all stages. (B) Radiation would be included if child was staged beyond stage I. Surgery and chemotherapy are included for all stages; therefore, excluding chemotherapy is not correct. (C) Surgery, radiation, and chemotherapy would be included for stage II. (D) Radiation and chemotherapy is not correct because it excludes surgery.

150. (A) Nursing process phase: analysis; client need: safe, effective care environment; content area: pediatric nursing

Rationale
(A) Administering muscle relaxants is not an appropriate nursing intervention preoperatively for a child having hypospadias. (B) Bladder spasms are a potential complication for a child having a hypospadias repair. The nurse would want to explain this to the parents and child preoperatively. (C) The preschool-age child may think getting sick is punishment for some wrongdoing. It is important to explain to the school-age child that the illness is not punishment. (D) It would be an appropriate nursing intervention to discuss the expected cosmetic results with the parents.

151. (A) Nursing process phase: analysis; client need: physiological integrity; content area: pediatric nursing

Rationale
(A) A hydrocele is translucent by transillumination and a hernia is opaque by transillumination. (B) The hydrocele is usually not reducible, but a hernia can usually be reduced. Parents should be taught simple measures (warm bath, avoidance of upright positioning) to reduce the hernia. (C) Unlike a hernia, the hydrocele may not be reducible and may not be produced by a sudden increase in intra-abdominal pressure (such as straining). (D) These are true statements.

152. (A) Nursing process phase: evaluation; client need: safe, effective care environment; content area: pediatric nursing

Rationale
(A) Parents should be instructed regarding a realistic outcome of surgery. Surgical closure of the defect does not ensure normal urination and urinary diversion may be necessary. (B) Until the defect is repaired the caregiver will need to sponge bathe because there should be no immersion in water. (C) It would be important to check the skin periodically around the defect because constantly draining urine may contribute to skin necrosis. (D) Support groups to parents and children are usually very useful in promoting psychological adjustment and coping.

153. (D) Nursing process phase: analysis; client need: physiological integrity; content area: pediatric nursing

Rationale
(A) Hyperproteinemia is not a clinical feature of idiopathic nephrosis. The hyaline casts form high protein and sluggish flow, and oval fat bodies as well as red blood cells may give the urine a foamy appearance. Hyperlipidemia is a feature of idiopathic nephrosis. (B) Hyperproteinemia and hypolipidemia are not clinical features of idiopathic nephrosis. Edema is associated with idiopathic nephrosis. (C) Hypolipidemia is not a clinical feature of idiopathic nephrosis. Hypoproteinemia and foamy urine are present with idiopathic nephrosis. (D) Hypoproteinemia, hyperlipidemia, and edema are all clinical features associated with idiopathic nephrosis.

154. (C) Nursing process phase: implementation; client need: health promotion and maintenance; content area: pediatric nursing

Rationale
(A) Mechanical trauma is not associated with relapses of idiopathic nephrosis. (B) The child with idiopathic nephrosis often does experience emotional stress because of the nature of frequent relapses; however, frequent relapses are not usually precipitated by emotional stress. (C) Acute infections in children with idiopathic nephrosis can precipitate relapses. Prompt treatment is essential. (D) Salt is restricted to no additional salt during relapses and steroid therapy. Regular diet is permissible during remission. Salt restriction does not precipitate a relapse.

155. (A) Nursing process phase: analysis; client need: physiological integrity; content area: pediatric nursing

Rationale
(A) As CGN progresses, urine specific gravity stabilizes or becomes fixed at an isotonic state (about 1.012) as a result of the inability of the kidney to reabsorb solutes or respond to an-

tidiuretic hormone. Failing renal function is evidenced by elevated BUN, creatinine, and uric acid levels. (B) Fixed specific gravity of the urine, and increased BUN and creatinine (not decreased creatinine) are indicative of deteriorating renal function. (C) Impaired nerve conduction, decreased NA (not increased NA), and elevated K (not decreased K) are some of the alterations associated with CGN. (D) Impaired nerve conduction, decreased NA, and decreased calcium (not increased calcium) levels are alterations associated with CGN.

156. (C) Nursing process phase: analysis; client need: safe, effective care environment; content area: pediatric nursing

Rationale
(A) The nurse would encourage this client to eat a low-sodium diet, but this would not be the most important initially. (B) The nurse would not encourage this client to drink more water because she is experiencing oliguria, and fluids are often restricted during the acute phase of the disease. (C) A complication during the acute phase of glomerulonephritis is hypertensive encephalopathy. If this occurs, it would result in transient loss of vision and/or hemiparesis, disorientation, and generalized grand mal convulsions. In this situation the nurse should expect the possibility of this complication and initiate a neurological assessment and seizure precautions. (D) The nurse would not want to encourage ambulation during the acute phase because bedrest is usually recommended to decrease glomerular infiltration rate.

157. (A) Nursing process phase: evaluation; client need: health promotion and maintenance; content area: pediatric nursing

Rationale
(A) Corticosteroids are therapeutic agents used in the management of nephrotic syndrome. Children who require frequent courses of steroid therapy are highly susceptible to the complications of steroid administration. Some of these complications are growth retardation, hypertension, gastrointestinal bleeding, Cushing's syndrome, bone demineralization, infection, and diabetes mellitus. (B) Growth retardation, hypertension (not hypotension), and infections are some of the complications of steroid therapy. (C) Diabetes mellitus, hypertension (not hypotension), and gastrointestinal bleeding are some of the complications of steroid therapy. (D) Diabetes mellitus, hypertension, and growth retardation (not acceleration) are some of the complications of steroid therapy.

158. (D) Nursing process phase: assessment; client need: physiological integrity; content area: pediatric nursing

Rationale
(A) Edema of the intestinal mucosa associated with nephrotic syndrome may result in diarrhea, loss of appetite, and poor intestinal absorption. Increase in appetite, therefore, is not a symptom of nephrotic syndrome. (B) Constipation is usually not a symptom of nephrotic syndrome. (C) The child with nephrotic syndrome has weight gain, which usually progresses insidiously over a period of days or weeks. Decrease in weight, therefore, is not a symptom seen with nephrotic syndrome. (D) The volume of urine is decreased and appears frothy—symptoms of nephrotic syndrome.

159. (C) Nursing process phase: implementation; client need: safe, effective care environment; content area: pediatric nursing

Rationale

(A) Padding the elastic bands is not usually done because the bands need to fit snuggly and can be adjusted to prevent skin irritation. (B) The nurse may take the pulse before starting therapy but this is not a preventive measure in reference to the untoward effects of oxygen therapy. (C) Humidifying the oxygen gas before administration is a protective measure of oxygen administration because it helps to prevent drying of the nose and mouth mucosa. (D) If client is experiencing severe difficulty with breathing, placing him or her in the orthopneic position may facilitate easier breathing, but this is not a protective measure of oxygen therapy.

160. **(C)** Nursing process phase: implementation; client need: health promotion and maintenance; content area: pediatric nursing

Rationale

(A) The four areas tested with the DDST are personal-social, language, fine motor, and gross motor. It does not include testing the receptive-expressive ability of the child. (B) The four areas tested with the DDST are personal-social, language, fine motor, and gross motor. It does not directly assess psychological development. (C) These are the four areas tested with the DDST. (D) The four areas tested with the DDST are personal-social, language, fine motor, and gross motor. It does not include testing for the receptive-expressive ability of the child.

161. **(C)** Nursing process phase: implementation; client need: health promotion and maintenance; content area: pediatric nursing

Rationale

(A) It would be acceptable to praise him at the end of the test, but during administration, you would want to praise him after each item, whether or not he correctly performs the item. (B) It would not be best to praise him only for correct performances. (C) It would be best to praise him whether or not he correctly performs the item because this would contribute to the child's confidence. (D) The nurse would not want to ask the parent not to interfere by praising. The nurse would explain that she would praise the child at the completion of each item.

162. **(B)** Nursing process phase: analysis; client need: safe, effective care environment; content area: pediatric nursing

Rationale

(A) Postoperatively after shunt placement, the child is carefully positioned on the unoperated side to prevent pressure on the shunt valve. You would not position the child flat on the operated side. (B) Postoperatively after shunt placement, the child is carefully positioned on the unoperated side to prevent pressure on the shunt valve. (C) Postoperatively after shunt placement, the child is kept flat to help avert complications resulting from too rapid reduction of intracranial fluid. If there is increased ICP, the surgeon will prescribe the head of the bed to be elevated. (D) Postoperatively after shunt placement, the child is kept flat to help avert complications resulting from too rapid reduction of intracranial fluid. The low Trendelenburg position would not be an appropriate intervention because it would enhance rapid reduction of intracranial fluid.

163. **(D)** Nursing process phase: implementation, client need: safe, effective care environment; content area: pediatric nursing

Rationale

(A) The newborn with an unrepaired myelomeningocele would be positioned on the stomach, not the supine position. You would want to position the newborn so as not to cause pressure on the defect. (B) Aspirating fluid from the defect would be an inappropriate and unsafe nursing intervention. (C) It would be an appropriate nursing intervention to provide visual stimulation to a newborn with an unrepaired myelomeningocele. Black-and-white drawings or geometric shapes can be placed within the infant's view. (D) Gentle ROM exercises are sometimes performed but restricted to the foot, ankle, and knee joint.

164. **(D)** Nursing process phase: planning; client need: physiological integrity; content area: pediatric nursing

Rationale

(A) Isolation of the child with encephalitis is not necessary. However, good handwashing technique must be followed. (B) Partial exchange transfusions are not appropriate interventions for a child with encephalitis. (C) Peritoneal or hemodialysis are necessary when there is renal injury. Encephalitis involves cerebral injury. (D) Parenteral antibiotics are used to treat the infection. Encephalitis can be caused by a variety of organisms including bacteria, spirochetes, fungi, protozoa, helminths, and viruses.

165. **(A)** Nursing process phase: implementation; client need: safe, effective care environment; content area: pediatric nursing

Rationale

(A) The initial therapeutic management of bacterial meningitis would include isolation precautions. A private room would be necessary. (B) The child being treated for bacterial meningitis is usually not restrained. Restraints would only be necessary if it was determined that the child would interrupt therapeutic measures such as pulling out the intravenous line. (C) The initial therapeutic management of bacterial meningitis does not include insertion of a Levin tube. (D) The therapeutic management of bacterial meningitis does not include administration of antacids.

166. **(D)** Nursing process phase: planning; client need: physiological integrity; content area: pediatric nursing

Rationale

(A) Restricted activity is not a measure that has to be implemented when a child is receiving phenytoin. (B) Adequate rest is a measure that is important for all children and is not directly related to receiving phenytoin. (C) Adequate diet is a measure that is important for all children and is not directly related to receiving phenytoin. (D) A side effect of phenytoin is hyperplasia of the gums, so dental hygiene is very important.

167. **(D)** Nursing process phase: planning; client need: physiological integrity; content area: pediatric nursing

Rationale

(A) Prevention of spinal shock is important, but maintenance of respiration is the primary goal. (B) With cervical spine injury, pain is not a problem. (C) Maintenance of orientation is not a primary goal after spinal injury. (D) Maintenance of respiration is of primary importance with a cervical spine injury. The child with a high-level injury will require continuous ventilating assistance.

168. **(D)** Nursing process phase: planning; client need:

health promotion and maintenance; content area: pediatric nursing

Rationale

(A) An appropriate and effective teaching-learning strategy is to limit the teaching sessions. However, this strategy would not have the greatest influence on the success of teaching. (B) An appropriate and effective teaching-learning strategy is to have one person implement the plan. However, this strategy would not have the greatest influence on the success of teaching. (C) The parent's acceptance of the client's diagnosis is also important. However, it would not have the greatest influence on the success of teaching. (D) The adolescent's acceptance of her diagnosis would ultimately have the greatest influence of the success of the teaching.

169. (B) Nursing process phase: implementation; client needs: psychosocial integrity; content area: pediatric nursing

Rationale

(A, C, & D) This is not a therapeutic response. The ADA diet allows for flexibility and the incorporation of preferred foods in most instances. (B) This would be a therapeutic response. As the nurse works with the adolescent and family to use the exchange system with the ADA diet, the incorporation of preferred foods can occur in most instances.

170. (C) Nursing process phase: implementation; client need: physiological integrity; content area: pediatric nursing

Rationale

(A) The therapeutic effects of PTU are not to reduce iodine stored in thyroid gland. (B) The therapeutic effects of PTU are not to depress the activity of stored thyroid hormone. (C) The therapeutic effects of PTU are to inhibit formation of thyroxine. (D) The therapeutic effects of PTU are not to lower metabolic rate.

171. (C) Nursing process phase: implementation; client need: safe, effective care environment; content area: pediatric nursing

Rationale

(A) Bedtime is not the most appropriate time to check for finger-stick glucose. (B) Midmorning and midafternoon are not the most appropriate times to check for finger-stick glucose. (C) Before meals (AC) is the most appropriate time. Glucose would rise in the blood after food intake. Sliding scale insulin is often adjusted according to AC blood glucose checks. (D) After meals (PC) is not the appropriate time to check for finger-stick glucose.

172. (B) Nursing process phase: analysis; client need: physiological integrity; content area: pediatric nursing

Rationale

(A) External tan is evident with Addison's disease; however, moon face, buffalo hump, and obesity are evident with Cushing's disease. (B) These are all defining characteristics of Cushing's disease because of the increased appetite and deposition of fat. (C) Anorexia, weight loss, and low blood pressure are opposite of the characteristics usually seen with Cushing's disease, since the characteristics are increased appetite, weight gain, and hypertension. There are abdominal striae because of weight gain. (D) Cold intolerance is not a characteristic of Cushing's disease; however, obesity, moon face, and buffalo hump are evident with Cushing's disease.

173. (A) Nursing process phase: analysis; client need: physiological integrity; content area: pediatric nursing

Rationale

(A) Treatment of Cushing's disease after adrenalectomy involves replacement of glucocorticoids (cortisol) and mineralocorticoids (aldosterone). (B) Desoxycorticosterone (Cortate) is a topical hydrocortisone used to treat inflammatory skin disorders. (C) Insulin is used in the management of diabetes mellitus. (D) Vasopressin is an angiotensin-converting enzyme (ACE) inhibitor used to treat hypertension.

174. (B) Nursing process phase: assessment; client need: physiological integrity; content area: pediatric nursing

Rationale

(A) In CRF, although there is continual hydrogen ion retention and bicarbonate loss, the plasma pH is maintained at a level compatible with life by other buffering mechanisms. (B) A decrease in renal function is associated with a rise in fasting BUN and creatinine concentration and products of protein metabolism. This is an azotemic state. The retention of these waste products can alter mental status. (C) The sodium excess with CRF may cause hypertension, but this does not usually alter mental status unless it is severe. (D) Bradycardia is not a symptom of CRF.

175. (B) Nursing process phase: analysis; client need: safe, effective care environment; content area: pediatric nursing

Rationale

(A) Fats in the diet are not usually restricted in CRF. Because fat-soluble vitamins can accumulate in clients with CRF, vitamins A, E, and K are not supplemented beyond normal dietary intake. (B) Dietary intake of protein in CRF is limited to the recommended daily allowance (RDA) for the child's age. The goal of the diet in CRF is to provide sufficient calories and protein for growth while minimizing the excretory demands on the kidney. (C) Calcium is not restricted in CRF. Calcium carbonate preparations are used as phosphorus binders and to correct calcium-phosphorus imbalance. (D) Carbohydrates are not restricted in CRF.

176. (D) Nursing process phase: analysis; client need: physiological integrity; content area: pediatric nursing

Rationale

(A) Weight loss, not weight gain, is seen with Addison's disease because of dehydration and anorexia from impaired gastrointestinal functioning. (B) Hypotension, not hypertension, is seen with Addison's disease. (C) Hypoglycemia, not hyperglycemia, is evident with Addison's disease. (D) Hyperpigmentation over pressure points, such as the elbows, knees, or waist, is common with Addison's disease. Pigmentary changes of previous scars, palmar creases, mucous membranes, and hair are also evident.

177. (A) Nursing process phase: assessment; client need: safe, effective care environment; content area: pediatric nursing

Rationale

(A) Severe stridor and hoarseness usually indicate damage to the laryngeal nerve, although some hoarseness is to be expected. (B) Hemorrhage is a potential complication with any surgery but does not indicate laryngeal nerve damage. (C) Wheezing is not indicative of laryngeal nerve damage after thyroidectomy. (D) Facial twitching is not indicative of laryngeal nerve damage after thyroidectomy.

178. **(B)** Nursing process phase: assessment; client need: physiological integrity; content area: pediatric nursing

Rationale
(A) An increase in the leukocyte count is not a side effect of chemotherapy. (B) Many chemotherapeutic agents cause stomatitis (painful lesions in the mouth). (C) Arthralgia and myalgia may occur with the use of procarbazine, but this effect is not as common as stomatitis when considering chemotherapeutic agents in general. (D) Ridging of the nails may occur with the use of cyclophosphamide (Cytoxan), but in general this effect is not as common as stomatitis.

179. **(B)** Nursing process phase: implementation; client need: safe, effective care environment; content area: pediatric nursing

Rationale
(A) Burow's solution does not have an anti-inflammatory effect. (B) Burow's solution is bacteriostatic and has a drying, antipruritic effect on weeping lesions. (C) Burow's solution does not remove crusted areas. (D) Burow's solution, through its bacteriostasis action, can aid healing; however, it does not prevent scratching.

180. **(C)** Nursing process phase: evaluation; client need: safe, effective care environment; content area: pediatric nursing

Rationale
(A) To instill eye medication, the child is placed supine or sitting with the head extended. (B) To instill eye medication, the child while supine or sitting with the head extended is asked to look up. (C) To instill eye medication, one hand is used to pull the lower lids downward, not upward. This response would indicate a need for further teaching. (D) The hand that holds the dropper rests on the head so that it may move synchronously with the child's head.

181. **(D)** Nursing process phase: analysis; client need: physiological integrity; content area: pediatric nursing

Rationale
(A) Hamburgers are a favorite food of adolescents. However, a complication of chemotherapy is stomatitis, so a hamburger would be hard to eat. (B) Orange juice would not be chosen because the acidic nature would burn the painful lesions in the mouth usually caused by chemotherapy. (C) French fries are a favorite food of adolescents. However, with the complication of stomatitis with chemotherapy, french fries would most likely be too difficult to eat. (D) Plain yogurt would most likely be the choice because it is soft, not spicy, and would be the most easily eaten with stomatitis.

182. **(B)** Nursing process phase: implementation; client need: health promotion and maintenance; content area: pediatric nursing

Rationale
(A) The mammogram is a useful diagnostic tool for breast cancer; however, in the early detection of breast cancer, it is not as useful as the monthly breast self-examination. (B) The breast self-examination is the most effective diagnostic tool with breast cancer. The monthly breast self-examination is most useful in the early detection of lesions that may be malignant. (C) A thermogram is not indicated as a diagnostic tool for breast cancer. (D) A biopsy is useful once a lesion is found. However, it is not as effective as a breast self-examination in the early detection of breast cancer.

183. **(A)** Nursing process phase: assessment; client need: physiological integrity; content area: pediatric nursing

Rationale
(A) Most malignant bone tumors produce localized pain and swelling in the tumor area of the affected extremity. The pain may be severe or dull and may be attributed to trauma or the vague complaint of "gravity pains." (B) Pain in the extremity affected by bone cancer is often relieved by assuming the flexed position, rather than the extended position, which relaxes the muscle overlying the stretched periosteum. (C) In the extremity affected by bone cancer there is a limitation of motion rather than increased motion. (D) There is no shortening of the extremity affected by bone cancer.

184. **(C)** Nursing process phase: implementation; client need: safe, effective care environment; content area: pediatric nursing

Rationale
(A) Dextrose 5% in water is not a safe solution for blood administration because it would facilitate the hemolysis of RBCs. (B) Ringer's lactate is not a safe solution for blood administration because it would facilitate the hemolysis of RBCs. (C) Normal saline is the only safe solution for blood administration because it does not cause hemolysis of RBCs. (D) Plasmalyte is not a safe solution to be used for blood administration because it would cause hemolysis of RBCs.

185. **(C)** Nursing process phase: implementation; client need: psychosocial integrity; content area: pediatric nursing

Rationale
(A) Telling him to sit in the visitors' lounge may not necessarily help the client with the feeling of isolation. (B) Encouraging him to look at himself in the mirror would not help the client with feelings of isolation. (C) Arranging for a visit from another adolescent with a similar surgery would assist the client in dealing with his feelings of isolation because he could share his fears and concerns with someone with similar problems. (D) In assisting the client to deal with feelings of isolation, allowing the family to stay with the client would not be as effective as choice C.

186. **(D)** Nursing process phase: evaluation; client need: safe, effective care environment; content area: pediatric nursing

Rationale
(A) A client receiving radiation therapy would be taught to handle the skin in the area gently. (B) A client receiving radiation therapy would be taught to wear loose-fitting clothes. (C) A client receiving radiation therapy would be taught to avoid irritation of the skin with soap. (D) A client would not be taught to use a heat lamp because this would promote further drying and excoriation of the skin.

187. **(A)** Nursing process phase: implementation; client

need: safe, effective care environment; content area: pediatric nursing

Rationale
(A) An ileus is often a common complication of chemotherapy; therefore, it is important for the nurse to carefully monitor bowel elimination. (B) It may also be important to assess fluid balance with chemotherapy, but this is not the reason for monitoring bowel elimination. (C) It is also important to note nutritional intake with chemotherapy, but it is not the reason for monitoring bowel elimination. (D) It is common for clients receiving chemotherapy to have nausea and vomiting as well as diarrhea, which are symptoms of gastroenteritis, but gastroenteritis is either viral- or bacterial-induced nausea, vomiting, and diarrhea.

188. (B) Nursing process phase: planning; client need: physiological integrity; content area: pediatric nursing

Rationale
(A) Planning the child's menu does not ensure proper nutritional balance because it may include foods that she does not like. (B) Allowing her to eat meals with children of her own age may encourage her to eat as she observes the other children eating. (C) While the client is receiving chemotherapy, the nurse would want to encourage light, low protein snacks. A light, low protein meal followed by candy of a distinctive flavor may be helpful. (D) It would not be conducive to good nutrition to maintain a rigid schedule for mealtimes and snacks.

189. (D) Nursing process phase: planning; client need: health promotion and maintenance; content area: pediatric nursing

Rationale
(A) When examining the testicles, the nurse teaches the client to palpate one testicle and then the other—not both simultaneously. (B) Testicular examination is taught by the nurse to be done monthly by the client. (C) The client is taught to firmly palpate the testicles with his fingers to detect any abnormalities. (D) The client is taught that the best time to perform the testicular examination is monthly after a shower.

190. (B) Nursing process phase: implementation; client need: psychosocial integrity; content area: pediatric nursing

Rationale
(A) Corporal punishment as a form of discipline is not recommended because it has the serious flaw of teaching the child that violence is acceptable. If the spanking is a result of rage, the child may be physically harmed. Furthermore, children become accustomed to spanking, requiring more severe corporal punishment each time. (B) Structured interactions that focus on the consequences is an effective form of discipline to minimize or eliminate unacceptable behavior. (C) Reasoning, which involves explaining why an act is wrong, is usually appropriate for older children. It should not be combined with scolding, which sometimes takes the form of shame or criticism. (D) It would not be best to not discipline because children need the security of knowing that they will be given guidance.

191. (C) Nursing process phase: implementation; client need: physiological integrity; content area: pediatric nursing

Rationale
(A) During periods of active hepatitis, the client is taught to get plenty of rest and not to increase his daily exercise activities. (B) Eating a diet high in fats would be contraindicated in the treatment of hepatitis. Special high protein, high carbohydrate, low fat diets are generally not of value. (C) In young people with a history of drug abuse, the nurse has the additional responsibility of stressing the parenteral mode of transmission of hepatitis. (D) Limiting fluid intake would be contraindicated in the treatment of hepatitis.

192. (D) Nursing process phase: planning; client need: safe, effective care environment; content area: pediatric nursing

Rationale
(A) The period of communicability for a client with hepatitis A is not known. The preicteric phase is the period when there are prodromal symptoms and the absence of jaundice (which usually lasts 5 to 7 days). (B) The period of communicability for a client with hepatitis A is not known. The icteric phase is when the prodomal symptoms disappear and the jaundice begins. (C) The period of communicability for a client with hepatitis A is not known. The posticteric phase is after the prodromal symptoms and jaundice disappear. (D) The period of communicability for a client with hepatitis A is not known.

193. (C) Nursing process phase: analysis; client need: physiological integrity; content area: pediatric nursing

Rationale
(A) Weight gain and abdominal mass are not evident with ulcerative colitis (UC). Nausea is usually present. Some children and adolescents do present with fever. (B) Weight gain and abdominal mass are not present with UC. Vomiting is usually present. It is common for a client with UC to have normal temperature. (C) Common presenting symptoms of UC are anorexia, vomiting, extreme thirst, and normal temperature. UC often presents with the insidious onset of diarrhea and usually without fever or weight loss. (D) Some children with UC present with gross bloody diarrhea, cramps, urgency with defecation, mild anemia, fever, anorexia, weight loss, and moderate signs of systemic illness.

194. (B) Nursing process phase: implementation; client need: physiological integrity; content area: pediatric nursing

Rationale
(A) TPN is not a hypertonic solution, which is used to increase the osmotic pressure of the blood plasma. (B) TPN is a hyperosmolar solution that is used mainly to reverse negative nitrogen balance. TPN includes a concentrated solution of protein, glucose, lipids, and other nutrients. (C) TPN is not a hypotonic solution used mainly for hydration. (D) TPN is not an alkalyzing solution used to treat metabolic acidosis and cellular edema.

195. (B) Nursing process phase: planning; client need: safe, effective care environment; content area: pediatric nursing

Rationale
(A) Septicemia is a catheter-related complication of TPN but is not a metabolic alteration. (B) Hyperglycemia is a common metabolic disorder caused by the excessive glucose intake from the TPN solution. It may occur during the first few days as the child adapts to the high glucose load. Nursing respon-

sibilities include blood glucose testing. (C) Acid-base disorders may occur but are not as common with a metabolic disorder as hyperglycemia. (D) Alkalotic disorders may occur but are not as common with a metabolic disorder as hyperglycemia.

196. **(C)** Nursing process phase: implementation; client need: safe, effective care environment; content area: pediatric nursing

Rationale
(A) It is an appropriate intervention to encourage frequent feedings, but these feedings should be very small. (B) It would not be an appropriate nursing intervention to encourage a high-fiber, high protein diet during an acute episode of diarrhea. (C) It is an appropriate intervention to reintroduce a regular diet slowly. (D) It is not an appropriate intervention to encourage a diet high in calories during an acute episode of diarrhea.

197. **(A)** Nursing process phase: analysis; client need: physiological integrity; content area: pediatric nursing

Rationale
(A) A side effect of codeine use is constipation. (B) Persistent nonproductive cough has no relationship with constipation. (C) Excessive amounts of fruit juice would not cause constipation. (D) Prolonged bedrest or inactivity may contribute to constipation but not intermittent bedrest.

198. **(D)** Nursing process phase: analysis; client need: safe, effective care environment; content area: pediatric nursing

Rationale
(A) While terminating the exposure to the toxic substance is important, it is not the first step in treatment of poisoning in a child. (B) While preventing the absorption of poison is important, it is not the first step in the treatment of poisoning in a child. (C) If not known, locating the poison would be very important but is not the first step in the treatment of poisoning in a child. (D) Assessing the child is the most important initial step in treatment of a child with poisoning.

199. **(C)** Nursing process phase: analysis; client need: safe, effective care environment; content area: pediatric nursing

Rationale
(A) Inducing emesis is contraindicated because vomiting redamages the mucosa. (B) The corrosive is not diluted with milk, which coats membranes, making assessment difficult. (C) The corrosive is diluted with water, unless vomiting occurs. (D) Oral intake is not allowed.

200. **(D)** Nursing process phase: analysis; client need: physiological integrity; content area: pediatric nursing

Rationale
(A) The signs and symptoms of celiac disease are not associated with malfunction of the ileum. (B) The signs and symptoms of celiac disease are not associated with inoculation against the sprue virus. (C) The signs and symptoms of celiac disease are not related to the congenital absence of trypsin. (D) The signs and symptoms of celiac disease are associated with an intolerance of the protein gluten, found in the grain of wheat, barley, rye, and oats.

201. **(B)** Nursing process phase: implementation; client need: physiological integrity; content area: pediatric nursing

Rationale
(A) A salt-free diet is not indicated for a child with celiac disease. A salt-free diet is often necessary in the treatment of hypertension and renal disease. (B) A diet low in gluten products is required in the management of celiac disease. Gluten is found in the grain of wheat, barley, rye, and oats. (C) A diet free of phenylalanine is not indicated in the treatment of celiac disease. A diet free of phenylalanine is indicated in the treatment of phenylketonuria. (D) A diet high in calories, high in protein, and low in fat is not indicated for a child with celiac disease. This kind of diet is indicated in the treatment of children with cystic fibrosis.

202. **(C)** Nursing process phase: assessment; client need: physiological integrity, content area: pediatric nursing

Rationale
(A) Jaundice is not a clinical manifestation of vaso-occlusive crisis with sickle-cell disease. (B) Heart murmur is not a clinical manifestation of vaso-occlusive crisis with sickle-cell disease. (C) Pain occurs with the vaso-occlusive crisis of sickle-cell disease as a result of the sickled cells obstructing the blood vessels causing occlusion, ischemia, and potentially necrosis. (D) Lethargy may occur as a result of the pain experienced with vaso-occlusive crisis with sickle-cell disease.

203. **(C)** Nursing process phase: implementation; client need: safe, effective care environment; content area: pediatric nursing

Rationale
(A) Difficulty with schoolwork would be a concern of parents of a child with sickle-cell disease but does not necessitate prompt medical attention. (B) Eruption of 12-year molars would also be of interest but would not require prompt medical attention. (C) Vomiting and/or diarrhea would require prompt medical attention by the parents of a child with sickle-cell disease because dehydrating state would most likely precipitate a vaso-occlusive crisis. (D) An increase in appetite would probably be welcomed by the parents of a child with sickle-cell disease and certainly is not a condition that requires prompt medical attention.

204. **(A)** Nursing process phase: analysis; client need: physiological integrity; content area: pediatric nursing

Rationale
(A) Hemoglobin (Hgb) electrophoresis is a test that enables abnormal forms of Hgb to be detected. Hgb S is an abnormal form of Hgb associated with sickle-cell disease. (B) Fibrinogen activity is primarily used in the diagnosis of suspected bleeding disorders. (C) The enzyme LDH is found in many blood tissues, especially the heart, liver, kidneys, skeletal muscle, brain, red blood cells, and lungs. The serum LDH rises within 24 to 72 hours after a myocardial infarction. (D) Both sickle-cell disease, homozygous for Hgb S, and sickle-cell trait, heterozygous for Hgb S, can be detected by this study.

205. **(D)** Nursing process phase: implementation; client need: physiological integrity; content area: pediatric nursing

Rationale
(A–C) Following an acute episode of gastroenteritis, solid foods are introduced slowly. Reintroduction is usually done with a BRAT diet (bananas, rice, applesauce, and toast) for a short time only since this diet is low in energy and protein. (D) Initially the gut cannot tolerate the high amount of glucose in the ice cream.

206. (A) Nursing process phase: implementation; client need: physiological integrity; content area: pediatric nursing

Rationale
(A) In some instances of ruptured appendix, the wound is closed following irrigation of the peritoneal cavity. Many surgeons, however, leave the wound open to prevent wound infection and abscess formation. A wet-to-dry dressing over the open wound is often ordered. (B) Systemic antibiotic is ordered for a much longer period of time. Twenty-four to 72 hours would not be appropriate systemic antibiotic treatment. (C) Encouraging the client to resume normal physical activities is generally important but would not be appropriate in the immediate postoperative period. (D) It is not necessary to position the client on the right side during the postoperative care of ruptured appendix.

207. (C) Nursing process phase: implementation; client need: safe, effective care environment; content area: pediatric nursing

Rationale
(A) It is not necessary to feed the infant with a Breck feeder. Breck feeders are used in the feeding of children with cleft lip or palate. (B) In most instances, burping after feedings is important. This must be done very gently, if at all, because the infant should be handled as little as possible after feedings. (C) It is most important to teach the parents to handle the infant as little as possible after feedings to help prevent emesis. (D) Usually the infant is allowed nothing by mouth and given IV fluids to correct electrolyte imbalance. If feedings are continued, the infant is handled as little as possible after feedings to help prevent emesis.

208. (D) Nursing process phase: implementation; client need: safe, effective care environment; content area: pediatric nursing

Rationale
(A) It would be important to inform the parents where additional supplies can be obtained. Initially the supplies for discharge can be provided by the hospital. (B) Fluid intake should be normal for child's physiological needs. Restriction or forcing fluids is not appropriate treatment. (C) It is not normal for the colostomy site to ooze blood for 5 to 7 days postoperatively. (D) The child should always be positioned so that there is no pressure on the colostomy site. This facilities drainage of the colostomy.

209. (B) Nursing process phase: implementation; client need: safe, effective care environment; content area: pediatric nursing

Rationale
(A) It is not appropriate to administer the DPT immunization to a child over 6 years of age. The older child does not receive pertussis and needs a smaller amount of diphtheria (Td). (B) It is appropriate to administer the Td, MMR, OPV, and TB skin test. He had not received all of the DPT immunizations and would need Td. He would also need the first MMR, the second OPV, and the TB skin test. (C) It would not be appropriate just to administer the MMR and the TB skin test because he would also need the Td and the OPV. (D) It would not be appropriate just to administer the TB skin test and the Td because he would also need the MMR and the OPV.

210. (D) Nursing process phase: implementation; client

need: health promotion and maintenance; content area: pediatric nursing

Rationale
(A) It is true that all children do not develop at the same pace; however, it would be best not to emphasize the strengths and weaknesses of the child. (B) It would not be best to emphasize the practice of any skill that the child cannot perform. (C) It would not be necessary for the mother to make an appointment with the pediatrician because the child is not behind in his development. (D) The child is performing tasks that are appropriate for his age.

211. (A) Nursing process phase: planning; client need: health promotion and maintenance; content area: pediatric nursing

Rationale
(A) It would be most important for the nurse to include the topic of prevention of injury, such as teaching the importance of car seats. (B) It would be important to include the topic of sibling rivalry, but not as important as injury prevention. (C) It would be important for parents of toddlers to include a discussion of limiting TV viewing time, but not as important as injury prevention. (D) It would be important to discuss factors that would assist in identifying appropriate day-care and kindergarten programs, but not as important as injury prevention.

212. (C) Nursing process phase: analysis; client need: health promotion and maintenance; content area: pediatric nursing

Rationale
(A) It would not be an appropriate response to tell her to make an appointment with her doctor because her development is normal. (B) It would not be an appropriate response to tell her to get radiographs for bone age because her development is normal. (C) It would be the most appropriate response to tell her that her development is normal for her age. This adolescent is at Tanner's stage II of sexual development. (D) It would not be an appropriate response to tell her to discuss this with her mother. This statement would discourage communication between the client and the nurse. However, it would good for her to discuss concerns with her mother.

213. (C) Nursing process phase: analysis; client need: health promotion and maintenance; content area: pediatric nursing

Rationale
(A) Stuttering for the past 4 months does not indicate a need for language evaluation because stuttering for this age child is normal. (B) It is normal for a child of his age to stutter more when he is excited and does not indicate a need for language evaluation. (C) Avoiding speaking would indicate a need for language evaluation because it is not normal for a child of this age to avoid speaking. (D) Not liking to play with other children is not normal for a child of this age, but would not indicate a need for language evaluation.

214. (D) Nursing process phase: implementation; client need: psychosocial integrity; content area: pediatric nursing

Rationale
(A) Parents are encouraged to stay with their child throughout all phases of the hospitalization. (B) Children are en-

couraged to maintain their current schoolwork in the hospital if physically able. Most hospitals for children have in-house schoolteachers. (C) While placing a child in a 2- to 4-bed ward will provide diversion, this is not the best answer for this question. (D) A prehospitalization party for preschoolers is an excellent method of orienting children to the hospital prior to admission.

215. **(D)** Nursing process phase: implementation; client need: health promotion and maintenance; content area: pediatric nursing

Rationale
(A) Children are not regarded as possessions of their parents and legally may be given emancipation rights or placed under the guardianship of another adult. (B) All clients have the right of confidentiality and access to their medical records, preferably under the supervision of a health-care professional who can clarify and answer questions appropriate for the client. (C) Children over the age of 15, if deemed able to understand medical interventions and risks, may be considered mature minors. (D) Most states allow minors to obtain birth control and treatment for STDs without parental consent.

216. **(A)** Nursing process phase: assessment; client need: safe, effective care environment; content area: pediatric nursing

Rationale
(A) This is pertinent information to be included in the family profile, because it may alert caregivers to a potential predisposition to type I diabetes mellitus. (B) Although this is important physical assessment data, this information is not pertinent to be included in the family profile section of the admission history. (C) Although this is important assessment data, this information is not pertinent to the family profile section. (D) It is important to know this family has had experience with otitis media; however, this information is not essential to the family profile.

217. **(C)** Nursing process phase: assessment; client need: physiological integrity; content area: pediatric nursing

Rationale
(A) Although it is important to explain the process for the physical exam to the child and family, it is not necessary to draw undue attention to examination of the genitalia with additional explanation. (B) The examination of the genitalia should be done swiftly while preserving modesty, thus eliminating the need to ask family to leave. (C) This method preserves dignity and reduces undue anxiety. (D) The genitalia should be included in the complete physical examination of all clients.

218. **(B)** Nursing process phase: assessment; client need: physiological integrity; content area: pediatric nursing

Rationale
(A) Occasional regurgitation after breastfeeding is a normal finding in newborn infants. (B) This finding is abnormal in a full-term and could signal an underlying neurological dysfunction. (C & D) These findings are normal in full-term infants.

219. **(A)** Nursing process phase: assessment; client need: physiological integrity; content area: pediatric nursing

Rationale
(A) Auscultating the heart and lungs while the infant is quiet and relaxed will yield accurate rates and allow for clear auscultation of sounds. (B) Eliciting reflexes will most likely get the infant excited or upset, not allowing for accurate auscultation. (C) Moving the infant of this age away from his mother's lap may cause undue stress and not allow for accurate data. (D) It is best to get accurate heart and lung sounds before approaching the head and manipulating the infant.

220. **(B)** Nursing process phase: planning; client need: safe, effective care environment; content area: pediatric nursing

Rationale
(A) Strict isolation is not indicated at this time for Sarah. (B) All visitors should be screened for symptoms of influenza and varicella, because these are highly contagious and could present significant risk to Sarah. Visitors should also observe careful handwashing. (C) Raw fruits and vegetables may transmit disease organisms to Sarah. All fruits and vegetables should be canned or cooked. (D) Stuffed animals can harbor infectious organisms. Toys that can be easily disinfected should be encouraged.

221. **(D)** Nursing process phase: implementation; client need: health promotion and maintenance; content area: pediatric nursing

Rationale
(A) No infant should be given aspirin, due to the potential for Reye's syndrome. Prophylactic administration of acetaminophen at the time of the immunization and every 4 to 6 hours may minimize urticaria and soreness. (B) A mild fever is not a contraindication to giving the DPT immunization. Benefits of the vaccines outweigh the risks of fever and other common complications of vaccines. (C) Fever is not sufficient reason to discontinue all DPT immunizations. (D) Provide immunizations as scheduled, being alert for possible side effects.

222. **(D)** Nursing process phase: implementation; client need: psychosocial integrity; content area: pediatric nursing

Rationale
(A) Intervene only if necessary to protect the child from injury. Unlike with nightmares, children experience only a partial arousal from very deep nondreaming sleep and are calm and return to sleep quickly. (B) The child will generally have no memory of a dream, yelling, or thrashing about during the terror, and can be easily put back to sleep after the terror. (C) It is difficult to keep children awake following a sleep terror. The child will have no memory of the events. (D) Stress to parents that sleep terrors are a normal, common phenomenon in preschoolers that requires relatively no intervention.

223. **(C)** Nursing process phase: analysis; client need: psychosocial integrity; content area: pediatric nursing

Rationale
(A) Although a diagnosis of diabetes mellitus would cause great concern in parents, there is little or no cause for guilt for having potentially contributed to the diagnosis, as with answer C. (B) Undescended testicles are fairly common and are not present as a result of care by parents. (C) Lauren's diagnosis is a direct result of an injury that has not been treated, thus potentially causing guilt in the parents for not seeking prior care and contributing to difficulty coping. (D) See rationale A.

224. **(D)** Nursing process phase: assessment; client need: psychosocial integrity; content area: pediatric nursing

Rationale
(A) Although Robert may not want to go to bed, it is important to him to have the same series of events occur each night. (B) Robert should be allowed to keep his special possession as a source of comfort and familiarity. (C) It is important to maintain home rituals and routines as much as possible to promote security and autonomy. (D) Toddlers will progress to more advanced stages of development when allowed to develop a strong sense of security and autonomy.

225. **(A)** Nursing process phase: analysis; client need: psychosocial integrity; content area: pediatric nursing

Rationale
(A) The intensive care unit is a source of almost constant stimuli: sounds, sights, smells, touch, etc. The unit can be very frightening for a child and can easily produce sensory overload. (B) Frequent visits by family will help to lessen sensory overload and provide familiarity and comfort. (C) Bedrest for 2 weeks can produce sensory deprivation. (D) Isolation can produce sensory deprivation.

226. **(A)** Nursing process phase: implementation; client need: psychosocial integrity; content area: pediatric nursing

Rationale
(A) Young children may hear the word "dye" and only know the meaning "die." Careful use of words and phrases in concrete-thinking children will help eliminate misunderstandings. (B) A better approach to stop undesirable behavior is to show children what to do or not to do and tell them why. (C) Urinary tract infections in preschoolers can be frightening and elicit regressive behavior. This is not a time to stress children into giving up familiar words. (D) Nonverbal communication, showing young children, is much easier for them to understand.

227. **(C)** Nursing process phase: assessment; client need: physiological integrity; content area: pediatric nursing

Rationale
(A) Children do not tolerate pain better than adults. They may demonstrate different ways of coping with pain. (B) Many times, increased activity is a child's method of dealing with pain. (C) Kids don't always tell the truth about pain. They may be too young to express their pain verbally or may be frightened of getting a "shot" or other painful intervention. (D) Paralyzing agents would require the child to be placed on a ventilator. These agents do not stop pain, only movement.

228. **(C)** Nursing process phase: analysis; client need: safe, effective care environment; content area: pediatric nursing

Rationale
(A) Placing infant intravenous infusions on a pump serves as a safeguard to prevent fluid overload. (B) As a standard precaution, side rails must be kept fully raised on all cribs. (C) Age should not be the only criterion for assigning a child to a crib. Size, home experience, and developmental level should be considered as well. (D) Restraints should be tied to the main bed frame, not the side rails, where injury could occur when the rails are lowered.

229. **(D)** Nursing process phase: assessment; client need: safe, effective care environment; content area: pediatric nursing

Rationale
(A) There is no altered growth and development. (B) No data suggest potential for infection. (C) Tina displays no impaired physical mobility. (D) Falls and the ability to reach more objects will increase Tina's chances of injury with her newfound mobility.

230. **(B)** Nursing process phase: implementation; client need: physiological integrity; content area: pediatric nursing

Rationale
(A) Although Robert may be able to eat applesauce, you would not want to mix medications in a large amount of food or fluid, because the infant may not ingest all of the medication. (B) This is a safe, effective method of delivering oral medications to infants. (C) Robert will most likely not be able to drink the medication from the cup himself. (D) Oral medications are less traumatic than IM.

231. **(D)** Nursing process phase: implementation; client need: physiological integrity; content area: pediatric nursing

Rationale
(A) Deep suctioning should be avoided, because it will stimulate the "whooping" cough and further irritate the airway. (B) The pertussis vaccine is not therapeutic in the presence of the disease. (C) Bedrest, not activity, should be encouraged to minimize coughing and stress. (D) High humidity will liquefy airway secretions and reduce airway irritation.

232. **(C)** Nursing process phase: planning; client need: health promotion and maintenance; content area: pediatric nursing

Rationale
(A) Anemia and dehydration are not primary concerns with chickenpox. (B) Anorexia and malnutrition are not primary concerns with chickenpox. (C) Infection at the site of lesions, from scratching, is a primary concern. Nursing interventions to minimize itching and scratching should be implemented. (D) Infection in the respiratory system is not a primary concern with chickenpox.

233. **(A)** Nursing process phase: analysis; client need: physiological integrity; content area: pediatric nursing

Rationale
(A) Squatting is a compensatory mechanism that decreases venous return from the legs and is common to this congenital heart defect. (B) Clubbing is commonly found in children with chronic hypoxia; however, it does not decrease venous return. (C) Dyspnea may be present but it does not decrease venous return. (D) Polycythemia is commonly found in children with chronic hypoxia; however, it does not decrease venous return.

234. **(C)** Nursing process phase: assessment; client need: physiological integrity; content area: pediatric nursing

Rationale
(A) Congenital heart defects that involve a right-to-left shunt generally produce an enlarged heart. (B) White blood cell counts should be normal unless an infection is present. (C)

Congenital heart defects that involve hypoxemia generally result in growth rates below the 10th percentile. (D) Apical heart rates would most likely be elevated.

235. **(D)** Nursing process phase: implementation; client need: psychosocial integrity; content area: pediatric nursing

Rationale
(A) Postural drainage is not indicated after this test and this terminology and talk of time will have no meaning for a 4-year-old. (B) Using the words "put to sleep" may have frightening connotations to a 4-year-old and should be avoided. (C) The 4-year-old will most likely not understand the concepts of 1 hour's time. (D) This is an accurate statement, given in terms the 4-year-old can understand.

236. **(B)** Nursing process phase: assessment; client need: health promotion and maintenance; content area: pediatric nursing

Rationale
(A) Cyanosis is not a primary feature of this disorder (B) Coarctation of the aorta frequently produces diminished blood supply to the lower extremities and may be diagnosed early by careful comparison of blood pressure and pulses in all four extremities. (C) Chest x-ray is not used to facilitate early diagnosis. (D) Cardiac catheterization may be used to confirm the diagnosis of coarctation of the aorta, but it is not for early diagnosis.

237. **(B)** Nursing process phase: planning; client need: physiological integrity; content area: pediatric nursing

Rationale
(A) This is not a rationale for having the mother of a child with croup at the bedside. (B) A primary plan is to reduce anxiety and ease respirations of children with croup to minimize airway irritation and inflammation. (C) Although this may be true, it is not the primary rationale for a child with croup. (D) The mother is not given the responsibility for constant observation of the child's respirations, and this is not the primary rationale for this situation.

238. **(B)** Nursing process phase: assessment; client need: physiological integrity; content area: pediatric nursing

Rationale
(A) Mark is experiencing epiglottitis. Examination of the oropharynx, especially with a tongue depressor, is contraindicated until in an equipped emergency room. (B) This is a potential emergency situation because Mark is exhibiting signs of restricted airway. (C) Mark needs emergency medical attention and antibiotics. (D) Mark will need emergency attention immediately.

239. **(A)** Nursing process phase: implementation; client need: physiological integrity; content area: pediatric nursing

Rationale
(A) Infants can experience dehydration easily when losing body fluids through respirations and with fever, and should be given small, frequent feedings of clear fluids. (B) Solid foods will be difficult to swallow with potentially elevated respiratory rate and will not replenish the lost fluid. (C) Heavy clothing will hold in body heat, thus further elevating the temperature. (D) Cold-water baths will cause vasoconstriction

and serve to further hold in body heat and elevate core temperature. Tepid sponging is recommended.

240. **(D)** Nursing process phase: implementation; client need: physiological integrity; content area: pediatric nursing

Rationale
(A) Angela is experiencing severe airway compromise with croup and requires an immediate airway. (B) Angela can breathe much better in a sitting position and should not be forced to lie down. (C) Although these are important interventions, getting immediate medical intervention to secure an airway is of priority. (D) Angela has demonstrated a narrowing airway and is restless, a key signal that she may be hypoxic.

241. **(C)** Nursing process phase: assessment; client need: health promotion and maintenance; content area: pediatric nursing

Rationale
(A) Congenital hip dislocation produces a shortening of the leg on the affected side. (B) There is no hyperextension of the tibial ligaments. (C) The affected hip has restricted abduction. (D) There are unequal skin folds of the thighs on adduction.

242. **(B)** Nursing process phase: assessment; client need: physiological integrity; content area: pediatric nursing

Rationale
(A) Respiratory impairment is not of primary concern. (B) Neurovascular checks should be made frequently in the postcasting hours to identify any signs of compromised circulation. (C) Although the client does have altered skin integrity; this is not a primary nursing goal in the immediate postcasting period. (D) Urinary stasis is not of primary concern in this time frame.

243. **(B)** Nursing process phase: assessment; client need: physiological integrity; content area: pediatric nursing

Rationale
(A) Bone development should not be affected by hyperthyroidism. (B) Hyperthyroidism increases metabolism and children frequently experience weight loss while maintaining a hearty appetite. (C) This would be a symptom associated with hypothyroidism. (D) Cold intolerance is a symptom associated with hypothroidism.

244. **(C)** Nursing process phase: evaluation; client need: health promotion and maintenance; content area: pediatric nursing

Rationale
(A) This is not an explanation of iron-deficiency anemia in young children. (B) Young children are not subject to bleeding disorders. (C) Ingestion of large volumes of milk may result in decreased food intake, thus leading to iron deficiency. (D) Malabsorption syndromes are not common in young children.

245. **(A)** Nursing process phase: evaluation; client need: health promotion and maintenance; content area: pediatric nursing

Rationale
(A) Orange juice enhances iron absorption. (B) Calcium can

inhibit iron absorption, so ice cream should be avoided. (C) Iron preparations should not be mixed with dairy products, and the iron would change the taste of the formula and possibly cause an infant to reject the formula. (D) Iron is best given on an empty stomach.

246. (A) Nursing process phase: implementation; client need: physiological integrity; content are: pediatric nursing

Rationale
(A) A key objective in protecting the operative site is to keep Wilma's hands away from her mouth. Elbow restraints are an effective method. (B) This action is not best directed to protect the operative site. (C) Although it is true that Wilma should be kept from crying, a pacifier is contraindicated because sucking and friction could disrupt the operative site. (D) Placing Wilma on her side or prone could cause her to rub the operative site and disrupt integrity.

247. (D) Nursing process phase: assessment, client need: physiological integrity; content area: pediatric nursing

Rationale
(A) This is not a rationale for inhibiting crust formation. (B) Pharyngitis is not a concern with cleft lip repair. (C) This is not a key rationale for inhibiting crust formation. (D) Prevention of scarring and uneven healing are of prime importance and will be facilitated if crusts are not allowed to form.

248. (B) Nursing process phase: evaluation; client need: physiological integrity; content area: pediatric nursing

Rationale
(A) These are not signs found in newborns with TEF. (B) Infants with TEF will choke, gag, and exhibit signs of aspiration with feeding. (C & D) These are not signs characteristic of TEF.

249. (C) Nursing process phase: evaluation; client need: physiological integrity; content area: pediatric nursing

Rationale
(A) Cardiac workload is not significantly increased by this anomaly. (B) Although there may be abdominal distention, the primary rationale for the head elevation is to minimize gastric acid reflux into the airway. (C) This position helps minimize gastric-secretion reflux into the trachea and lungs. (D) This is not a rationale for this positioning.

250. (A) Nursing process phase: implementation; client need: physiological integrity; content area: pediatric nursing

Rationale
(A) This is the primary purpose of performing a LP. (B) Spinal fluid pathways are not visualized with a LP to diagnose meningitis. (C & D) Contrast media are not introduced and pathways are not visualized with an LP to diagnose meningitis.

251. (C) Nursing process phase: implementation; client need: physiological integrity; content area: pediatric nursing

Rationale
(A) General anesthesia is not used for sedation; however, local anesthesia may be injected prior to insertion of the lumbar needle. (B) Pediatric-size lumbar needles will be used. (C) This is the most common position to facilitate widening of the vertebral spaces. (D) Lumbar punctures are not painless and do carry some degree of risk, especially in the presence of increased intracranial pressure.

252. (B) Nursing process phase: analysis; client need: health promotion and maintenance; content area: pediatric nursing

Rationale
(A) Less that 5 percent of children with febrile seizures go on to develop future seizure disorders. (B) There is little chance that a future seizure disorder will develop as a result of having a febrile seizure. (C) It cannot be said that his newborn sister will develop febrile seizures also. (D) Febrile seizures do not cause learning disabilities.

253. (C) Nursing process phase: planning; client need: physiological integrity; content area: pediatric nursing

Rationale
(A) Dressings are usually not placed on the penis, to allow for continuous inspection. (B) Although a suprapubic catheter may be present, it will most likely remain in place for several days. (C) The tip of the penis must be frequently inspected to ensure continued perfusion. (D) Urethral catheterization is contraindicated postoperatively to prohibit damage of the reconstructed urethra. The infant will return from surgery with a urine catheter in place.

254. (C) Nursing process phase: analysis; client need: health promotion and maintenance; content area: pediatric nursing

Rationale
(A) This is not a manifestation of urine refluxing into the ureters. Hemolytic-uremic syndrome usually follows an acute gastrointestinal or upper respiratory tract infection. (B) Glomerulonephritis is not known to occur with vesicoureteral reflux. (C) Urine is constantly refluxing from the bladder back up the ureters to the kidney, thus introducing potential bacteria directly into the kidneys, producing kidney damage and scarring. (D) Nephrotic syndrome is not known to occur with vesicoureteral reflux.

255. (A) Nursing process phase: analysis; client need: health promotion and maintenance; content area: pediatric nursing

Rationale
(A) Masturbation may introduce organisms into the urethra, causing an infection. Urinary stasis is the single most important host factor influencing the occurrence of urinary tract infections, because urine that remains in the bladder allows bacteria from the urethra to grow. Constipation may cause displacement of the bladder and posterior urethra, causing obstruction, incomplete micturition, and urinary stasis. The essential oils in bubble baths and shampoos can irritate the urethra, causing itching, pain, and frequent urination. (B) Wilms' tumor is a cancerous tumor surrounding the kidney and has no relation to these conditions. (C) Bladder spasms are not caused by these conditions. (D) Hypospadias is a condition present at birth in which the urethral opening is located below the glans penis.

256. (A) Nursing process phase: implementation; client need: physiological integrity; content area: pediatric nursing

Rationale

(A) The brachial pulse is felt for infants under 1 year of age. The carotid pulse is difficult to palpate in infants. (B) The compression-to-ventilation ratio for children under the age of 8 is one breath to every five compressions. (C) If an infant is not breathing, give two slow breaths (1–1 ½ seconds each). Observe chest rise and allow lung deflation between breaths. (D) The cardiac compression rate for children between the ages of 1 and 8 years should be 100 per minute.

257. **(B)** Nursing process phase: assessment; client need: physiological integrity; content area: pediatric nursing

Rationale

(A) Blood pressure and pulse rate are important cardiovascular assessment parameters, but will not give an accurate picture of tissue perfusion. (B) Inspecting skin color, capillary refill, and temperature will given an accurate picture of tissue perfusion. (C) Respiratory pattern and temperature will not give data specific to tissue perfusion. (D) Level of consciousness and neurological status will not give data about tissue perfusion.

258. **(D)** Nursing process phase: assessment; client need: physiological integrity; content area: pediatric nursing

Rationale

(A) Gagging indicates that the toddler still has a patent airway. The toddler should be watched carefully to see that he can still speak. No lifesaving measures are necessary at this time. (B) Coughing indicates that the toddler can exchange air. The toddler should be watched to make sure that he can clear the food from his throat by coughing. Should he suddenly not be able to speak, lifesaving measures are indicated. (C) A pulse over 100 is appropriate for a toddler and does not indicate the need for lifesaving measures. The key parameter to observe with choking is the ability to speak. (D) Inability to speak indicates an obstructed airway. Lifesaving measures are indicated at this time to clear the obstruction from the airway.

259. **(D)** Nursing process phase: analysis; client need: safe, effective care environment; content area: pediatric nursing

Rationale

(A) Sedatives will probably not lead to shock, but could significantly depress the child's already labored respirations, leading to possible respiratory arrest. (B) Sedatives most likely will cause a reduced heart rate. No vagal stimulation is involved. (C) Blood gas concentrations may be affected after the child has suffered depressed respirations. Therefore, depression of the respiratory center is the primary reason for withholding sedatives. (D) Sedatives frequently have a depressive effect on the respiratory center. Tommy is already suffering respiratory distress, and nothing should be given that might further compromise his oxygen exchange.

260. **(C)** Nursing process phase: implementation; client need: safe effective care environment; content area: pediatric nursing

Rationale

(A) Plaster casts should be kept dry. A plastic bag or wrap can be used to protect the cast from water during bathing. (B) It is not necessary to knock on the cast to assess for pain. Mark should be asked to describe his discomfort intensity and location. (C) Mark and his family members should be taught to check skin at the top and bottom edges for redness, swelling,

decreased sensation, and temperature. (D) Nothing should be inserted into a cast. Severe trauma to tissue under the cast surface may result and go undetected until the cast is removed weeks later. Itching may be controlled with diphenhydramine hydrochloride (Benadryl).

261. **(B)** Nursing process phase: evaluation; client need: health promotion and maintenance; content area: pediatric nursing

Rationale

(A) Clark's injury should be protected from contamination; however, this is not the primary purpose of traction. (B) The primary purpose of traction is to maintain alignment of the bone. (C) Clark's fractured leg is immobilized, but that is not the primary purpose of the traction. (D) Traction serves no purpose for the unaffected leg.

262. **(A)** Nursing process phase: implementation; client need: physiological integrity; content area: pediatric nursing

Rationale

(A) Weights, pulleys, and ropes help maintain countertraction to support position and alignment of a fracture. (B) Elevation of the foot of the bed will not maintain position or alignment. (C) Gravity and body weight alone do not support position and alignment of a fracture. (D) Elevation of the knee gatch will not support position and alignment of a fracture.

263. **(B)** Nursing process phase: evaluation; client need: physiological integrity; content area: pediatric nursing

Rationale

(A) A falling hematocrit will not be a reliable guide to the adequacy of fluid replacement. (B) A urine output of 30 to 40 cc per hour is the minimal acceptable output of the approximately 1 cc per kg per hour guideline. A urine output less than this would indicate inadequate fluid replacement. (C) The absence of thirst is not a reliable indicator of adequate fluid replacement, especially in a burn victim who may be in shock and significantly fluid depleted. (D) Increased seepage from burn wounds may indicate the need for additional fluid replacement.

264. **(B)** Nursing process phase: implementation; client need: health promotion and maintenance; content area: pediatric nursing

Rationale

(A) Minor burns do not require a dressing nor analgesic medication for wound care. (B) The skin should be observed for redness, swelling, and signs of infection and left open to the air. (C) The burn does not need to be washed with Betadine iodine solution. (D) The burn does not need vigorous scrubbing, which may destroy the wound integrity or a dressing.

265. **(C)** Nursing process phase: implementation; client need: safe, effective care environment; content area: pediatric nursing

Rationale

(A) Although interventions that directly increase intracranial pressure should be avoided or minimized (suctioning, coughing, gagging, head or neck bent, lying flat, etc.), it is important to change the child's position frequently to avoid skin breakdown. (B) The unconscious child should be assessed for signs of discomfort; however, continuous narcotics or sedatives will not allow for accurate neurological assessment and may delay signs of deteriorating neurological status. (C) Intake and output should be monitored carefully to avoid fluid overload and cerebral edema. These children are kept on one-half to two-thirds maintenance fluids. (D) Chewing motions do not indicate ability to take solids.

266. **(C)** Nursing process phase: assessment; client need: health promotion and maintenance; content area: pediatric nursing

Rationale
(A) A high-pitched cry is characteristic of increased intracranial pressure in infants. (B) A bulging fontanel is indicative of increased intracranial pressure. (C) Diplopia (double vision) and/or blurred vision may be signs of increased intracranial pressure. (D) A widening pulse pressure (the difference between systolic and diastolic) is indicative of possible increased intracranial pressure.

267. **(D)** Nursing process phase: assessment; client need: health promotion and maintenance; content area: pediatric nursing

Rationale
(A) The ability to recall events from the past is not a reliable indicator of level of consciousness. Orientation to person, place, and time should all be assessed, if possible, as well as behavioral changes. (B) Recent changes in the child's bowel and bladder patterns are not reliable assessments of level of consciousness. (C) The loss of developmental skills does not accurately assess current level of consciousness. Regression of skills can occur with a variety of causes, not affecting level of consciousness. (D) The child's response to environmental stimuli and degree of arousal are accurate assessments, along with vital signs and neurological system assessment, of level of consciousness.

268. **(A)** Nursing process phase: planning; client need: health promotion and maintenance; content area: pediatric nursing

Rationale
(A) This is the most important goal to be met with children experiencing chronic illnesses. (B) Although support groups are very helpful, the most important goals involve maintenance of physical well-being. (C) Restrictions in the physical environment should be confined only to those things that directly worsen physical symptoms. As normal a physical environment as possible should be maintained. (D) Although this may be helpful, it is not the most important goal listed.

269. **(A)** Nursing process phase: implementation; client need: physiological integrity; content area: pediatric nursing

Rationale
(A) This position will facilitate respirations and decrease cardiac workload. (B) A prone position will not facilitate respiratory effort and may increase cardiac workload. (C) A supine position will not facilitate respirations and may increase cardiac workload. (D) Trendelenburg's position, although useful in cases of shock, will not assist the child in congestive heart failure and may worsen respirations and cardiac function.

270. **(D)** Nursing process phase: implementation; client need: physiological integrity; content area: pediatric nursing

Rationale
(A) Fluids are usually restricted to lessen cardiac workload and reduce circulating volume. (B) Respirations should be continuously monitored, not just during active periods. (C) Large feedings should be avoided because they may create undue cardiac stress. Frequent, small feedings are ordered if the patient is not NPO. (D) It is important to organize all nursing activities to get them done and then allow for prolonged periods of uninterrupted rest.

271. **(C)** Nursing process phase: analysis; client need: physiological integrity; content area: pediatric nursing

Rationale
(A) This organism is not usually responsible for bacterial endocarditis. (B) *Pseudomonas* is not usually associated with bacterial endocarditis. (C) Strep infections are the primary cause of bacterial endocarditis, as well as acute glomerulonephritis, in children. (D) This organism is not usually associated with bacterial endocarditis.

272. **(A)** Nursing process phase: implementation; client need: health promotion and maintenance; content area: pediatric nursing

Rationale
(A) As near a normal environment as possible should be maintained. Children with these conditions will usually pace their own activities. (B) Contact with other children will be one of the best ways to meet some growth and development needs. (C) Constant parental supervision should be avoided, to avoid overprotectiveness. (D) The child needs to understand that she should stop and rest from her activities when she feels tired or out of breath.

273. **(A)** Nursing process phase: analysis; client need: health promotion and maintenance; content area: pediatric nursing

Rationale
(A) True (B) The occurrence is greater in boys than girls. (C) Allergic hypersensitivity is only one cause of asthma. (D) Severe respiratory acidosis can result from respiratory failure in asthma.

274. **(C)** Nursing process phase: implementation; client need: physiological integrity; content area: pediatric nursing

Rationale
(A) Ephedrine, not to be confused with epinephrine, is a sympathiomimetric but is not as effective for immediate relief of asthma as epinephrine. (B) Corticosteroids are used to decrease inflammation; however, they are not the most important drugs listed for use in acute asthma attacks. (C) Epinephrine (Adrenalin) is given by injection or inhalation in acute asthma attacks. (D) Cough suppressants, especially containing codeine, are not used for acute asthma attacks. Priority must be given to relieving the bronchial spasms.

275. **(B)** Nursing process phase: planning; client need: physiological integrity; content area: pediatric nursing

Rationale
(A) Diuretics are not a routine part of the care in cystic fibrosis. The child with cystic fibrosis will have bulky, foul-smelling

stools, but prevention of diarrhea is not essential care. Adequate nutrition is essential care. (B) Each of these is essential to the care of all children with cystic fibrosis. (C) Although each of these is important, they are not the most essential part of care. (D) Although these are important, they are not the most essential part of care.

276. **(A)** Nursing process phase: planning; client need: psychosocial integrity; content area: pediatric nursing

Rationale
(A) Clothing that does not accentuate these physical traits will increase the adolescent's self-image. (B) Alopecia is not a common problem with cystic fibrosis. (C) Red blotches are not a common problem with cystic fibrosis. (D) The adolescent with cystic fibrosis will not have the energy to take part in strenuous, long exercises.

277. **(C)** Nursing process phase: implementation; client need: health promotion and maintenance; content area: pediatric nursing

Rationale
(A) Children with muscular dystrophy frequently have a problem with weight gain and have to limit caloric intake. (B) Strenuous exercise is not appropriate or feasible for children with muscular dystrophy. (C) Prevention of respiratory infections is a primary goal. Due to the limited thoracic muscle movement, these children will not be able to take deep breaths and cough effectively and are susceptible to respiratory infections. (D) Physical activity is self-limited by the disease process.

278. **(D)** Nursing process phase: assessment; client need: health promotion and maintenance; content area: pediatric nursing

Rationale
(A & B) These positions will not facilitate observation of a curvature of the spine. (C) This position will not allow direct visualization of the spine. (D) This position will provide the best visualization of a curvature of the spine and unequal height of the scapulae.

279. **(B)** Nursing process phase: planning; client need: health promotion and maintenance; content area: pediatric nursing

Rationale
(A) A 5-year-old will not be able to read or understand the concept of food exchange lists. (B) True. A 5-year-old should be encouraged to select the appropriate injection site and assist with preparing the site and pushing in the plunger of the syringe. Children should be encouraged to participate in all aspects of their care and to assume greater responsibilities of their self-care as they grow and mature. (C) The average 5-year-old will have difficulty sticking himself or herself and operating the glucometer. They should be encouraged to watch and help so they can assume this task in the future. (D) Reading the insulin labels, manipulating the syringe to maintain aseptic technique, and withdrawing the appropriate amounts of insulin will be difficult for a 5-year-old.

280. **(B)** Nursing process phase: evaluation; client need: health promotion and maintenance; content area: pediatric nursing

Rationale
(A) This is not a therapeutic response and is does not answer

why Helen's insulin dosage was increased. (B) Correct. Insulin must be regulated as the child grows. (C) Insulin may be decreased during times of infection if the child is not eating well. (D) We have no data that Helen's nutrition was not regulated.

281. **(D)** Nursing process phase: planning; client need: physiological integrity; content area: pediatric nursing

Rationale
(A) Physical therapy and ambulation will not address the need to reduce the sickling and clumping of cells. (B) Isolation is not needed because there is no contagion. (C) Platelet transfusions are not effective in reducing the effects of sickle-cell crisis. (D) True. Hydration and analgesia are the key therapies to reduce the clumping of sickled cells and reduce pain.

282. **(A)** Nursing process phase: analysis; client need: health promotion and maintenance; content area: pediatric nursing

Rationale
(A) True. Sickled red cells will often block small vessels, causing the death of surrounding distal tissue. (B) This is not a cause of tissue damage with sickle-cell disease. (C) There is increased production of sickled red cells, which cause vaso-occlusion. (D) Vaso-occlusion is caused by the sickled cells, not by increased numbers of red cells.

283. **(D)** Nursing process phrase: analysis; client need: health promotion and maintenance; content area: pediatric nursing

Rationale
(A) Mucosal changes will involve the potential for breakdown and development of opportunistic infections, such as thrush, but these changes do not themselves increase susceptibility to infection. (B) Polycythemia is an increase in red blood cells. This would not increase susceptibility to infection. (C) Edema may be present, but does not increase susceptibility to infection. (D) Correct. Bone marrow suppression will increase susceptibility to infection.

284. **(A)** Nursing process phrase: analysis; client need: physiological integrity; content area: pediatric nursing

Rationale
(A) Correct. The absence of protein in the urine signals the return of normal kidney function. It is essential that the child remain on steroids until the urine is free of protein and remains normal for 10 days to 2 weeks. (B) A urinary tract infection is not a component of nephrotic syndrome. (C) Generalized edema may subside before the urine is free from protein; therefore, this is not used as an indicator for stopping the steroid therapy. (D) The hypertension is usually minimal with nephrotic syndrome; therefore, this would not be an indicator for stopping steroid therapy. Note: Severe hypertension can be found in children with acute glomerulonephritis.

285. **(B)** Nursing process phase: implementation; client need: health promotion and maintenance; content area: pediatric nursing

Rationale
(A) While it is important that the child get rest, this is not a priority intervention. (B) Correct. Edema can be severe and generalized with nephrotic syndrome, causing severe skin breakdown on pressure points, genitalia, and areas of friction. (C)

Parents can hold and comfort their child, but must be careful not to irritate the skin, causing breakdown. (D) Active range-of-motion exercises are not indicated. This is a time of rest.

286. **(A)** Nursing process phase: analysis; client need: physiological integrity; content area: pediatric nursing

Rationale
(A) Correct. Accurate daily weights are indicators of fluid retention in infants and children. (B) Increasing specific gravity indicates the kidneys are concentrating the urine. This is not a significant factor for diagnosing fluid retention in nephrotic syndrome or gluomerulonephritis. (C) Decreasing urine output may indicate fluid retention, but this is not the most significant indicator. (D) Decreasing fluid intake does not indicate fluid retention.

287. **(B)** Nursing process phase: analysis; client need: physiological integrity; content area: pediatric nursing

Rationale
(A) These symptoms are not present in acute glomerulonephritis. (B) True. Titers for antistreptolysin-O (ASO) are drawn as part of the diagnostic work-up for acute glomerulonephritis. A strep infection commonly has occurred 10 to 14 days before the onset of the glomerulonephritis. (C) Small to moderate proteinuria may occur with acute glomerulonephritis. Massive proteinuria is a classic finding with nephrotic syndrome. (D) Diabetes insipidus is characterized by the inability to concentrate urine.

288. **(D)** Nursing process phase: assessment; client need: physiological integrity; content area: pediatric nursing

Rationale
(A) Because of the hypertension, these children are frequently placed on low sodium and potassium diets during the oliguric phase. (B) There is no indication for strict isolation. (C) Bedrest is important during the acute phase. (D) Correct. Seizure activity and cerebral complications are possible with the severe hypertension associated with acute glomerulonephritis.

289. **(C)** Nursing process phase: evaluation; client need: health promotion and maintenance; content area: pediatric nursing

Rationale
(A) Uncontrolled eye movements should not be present and should be reported to the physician, because they may signal seizure activity. (B) Sally can be placed on her back or side. A donut-shaped ring is used in the immediate postoperative period to protect the suture site. Stomach positioning is not recommended for any infant because of the possible correlation with sudden infant death syndrome (SIDS). (C) Correct. Vomiting could be a sign of increased intracranial pressure, signaling a shunt malfunction. (D) The shunt site may be touched and cleaned without fear of dislodgment.

290. **(D)** Nursing process phase: implementation; client need: safe, effective care environment; content area: pediatric nursing

Rationale
(A) Forcing a padded tongue blade into the mouth of anyone having a generalized seizure can be very dangerous. Bite blocks are used only in anticipation of a seizure. (B) Suction equipment may be needed, but the priority action is to protect Ricky from injury during the seizure. (C) Restraining Ricky could cause extensive injury during forceful tonic-clonic movement. Do not restrain, only cushion the areas that Ricky's head and extremities may hit. (D) Correct. Protect Ricky from hitting his head and extremities on the crib rail and from falling. Observe Ricky for a patent airway, color, and pattern of seizure activity.

291. **(A)** Nursing process phase: evaluation; client need: health promotion and maintenance; content area: pediatric nursing

Rationale
(A) Correct. The antiepileptic drugs are keeping Jenny's seizures under control. Withdrawal of these will lower the seizure threshold and initiate seizure activity. It is important to teach clients and families not to stop the child's medications unless directed to do so. (B) A degenerative disease is not a likely cause of recurrent seizures in children. (C) A cerebrovascular accident (stroke) is not a likely cause of recurrent seizures in children. (D) A head injury may cause seizure activity, but it is not the most likely cause of recurrent seizure activity.

292. **(B)** Nursing process phase: planning; client need: health promotion and maintenance; content area: pediatric nursing

Rationale
(A) An open reduction is usually not the initial treatment for congenital hip dysplasia. (B) Correct. A splint or harness that keeps the hips in abduction is usually the initial treatment of choice. (C) A tenotomy of contracted muscles is not indicated with congenital hip dysplasia. (D) An osteotomy is not an initial treatment choice for congenital hip dysplasia.

293. **(B)** Nursing process phase: evaluation; client need: health promotion and maintenance; content area pediatric nursing

Rationale
(A) The best way to validate learning is to see the mother perform the necessary tasks. She may be able to tell you the purpose, yet not be able to use the harness. (B) Correct. This method allows you to visualize the mother taking off and putting on the harness. You can see technique, thus validating what the mother has learned. (C) This will not allow you to know if the mother knows how to use the harness. (D) You need to see the mother perform the tasks to validate learning.

294. **(C)** Nursing process phase: planning; client need: physiological integrity; content area: pediatric nursing

Rationale
(A) Passive exercises may be used in later stages. The initial treatment of choice is usually the application of casts. (B) Adhesive strapping is not a successful method of treatment. Casting is much more effective. (C) Correct. Bilateral casts will be applied to keep the feet in an overcorrected position. Casts will have to be changed at least every week initially, as the baby grows. (D) A Denis Browne splint may be used after removal of the casts.

295. **(A)** Nursing process phase: analysis; client need: physiological integrity; content area: pediatric nursing

Rationale
(A) Correct. The major goal is to preserve his joint function.

This is the reason for the aggressive antibiotic therapy. (B) We have no knowledge of Leo's nutritional status, and the major goal of this therapy is to preserve his knee joint. (C) While promoting rest will facilitate healing, the major goal of therapy is to preserve his knee joint. (D) Leo already has an infection, and the major goal of therapy must be to preserve life and limb.

296. (C) Nursing process phase: planning; client need: psychosocial integrity; content area: pediatric nursing

Rationale
(A) This may or may not be possible with the traction in place; and of the choices available, this is not the most helpful to Mike during immobilization. (B) It is important to maintain structure to help the child cooperate with physical limitations. (C) Correct. Taking Mike to the playroom will help reduce his isolation and allow him to feel a part of play activities while keeping his traction in place. Mike can participate in activities that involve his upper body from his bed. (D) This will only serve to further increase his isolation.

297. (B) Nursing process phase: evaluation; client need: physiological integrity; content area: pediatric integrity

Rationale
(A) The primary purpose of traction is to stabilize the fracture until a cast can be applied. (B) Correct. This is the primary purpose of traction for fractured femurs. (C) The primary purpose of traction is not to prevent muscle spasms. (D) This is not the primary purpose of traction. Casting may have to be delayed until swelling and surgical sites have healed and the bone is shown to be in proper alignment.

298. (D) Nursing process phase: analysis; client need: physiological integrity; content area: pediatric nursing

Rationale
(A) These fractures are not difficult to reduce and immobilize. (B) They do not heal more slowly than other fracture sites. (C) They are not more difficult to detect. (D) Correct. Because these fractures occur at the "growth plate," they may affect growth of the long bone.

299. (A) Nursing process phase: analysis; client need: safe, effective care environment; content area: pediatric nursing

Rationale
(A) Correct. The innate curiosity and lack of judgment as to what may be unsafe leads young children into situations that may produce traumatic injuries. (B) This is not the factor that is most likely to put children at risk for injury. (C) Children have a high center of gravity because of their heads being proportionately large for their bodies. This puts them at risk for head injury with falls and motor vehicle accidents. (D) While this may be true in some cases, this is not the factor that is most likely to put them at risk for injury.

300. (B) Nursing process phase: implementation; client need: physiological integrity; content area: pediatric nursing.

Rationale
(A) It is not necessary to limit the time in this position, so long as the correct position is achieved with the entire mattress and frame raised. (B) Correct. To maintain comfortable positioning with a hip spica cast (which extends from the foot to the chest), Marty must have the entire mattress and frame elevated. She is unable to bend at the waist. (C) Two pillows under her head would force her head to be bent severely forward and would be very uncomfortable since she cannot bend from the waist. (D) This answer does not answer the question regarding elevating Marty's head.

301. (A) Nursing process phase: assessment; client need: health promotion and maintenance; content area: pediatric nursing

Rationale
(A) Correct. A good musculoskeletal system examination will compare the right side of the body and extremities with the left. Muscle tone, color, size, reflexes, circulation, and so on, should be compared between extremities. (B) Inspection and palpation are the basis of the musculoskeletal examination. (C) Clothing will need to be removed to accurately visualize all musculoskeletal areas. (D) The examination of all body systems will contribute to the musculoskeletal system. No system assessment should be considered in isolation from other systems.

302. (C) Nursing process phase: evaluation; client need: health promotion and maintenance; content area: pediatric nursing

Rationale
(A) Often swelling cannot be prevented during times of immobilization. (B) Bone pain can be minimized with pain medications but may not be able to be prevented. (C) Correct. Astute nursing assessment of bowel function, fluid and nutrition status, and the use of stool softeners can prevent the complication of constipation during immobilization. (D) Disuse atrophy of a casted extremity cannot be prevented, because the muscles cannot be used.

303. (B) Nursing process phase: assessment; client need: health promotion and maintenance; content area: pediatric nursing

Rationale
(A) Ortolani's maneuver assesses stability of the hip joint to help diagnoses developmental dysplasia of the hip. (B) Correct. If the femoral head can be felt to slip forward into the acetabulum on pressure from behind, it has been dislocated. This is Ortolani's test. Often an audible click can be heard on exit or entry of the femur out of or into the acetabulum. (C) Ortolini's maneuver does not test for degree of joint flexion. (D) Ortolani's maneuver does not test for foot stability.

304. (C) Nursing process phase: implementation; client need: physiological integrity; content area: pediatric nursing

Rationale
(A) Thickened bottle feedings are usually used in infants to help prevent gastroesophageal reflux. This is not a routine with infants with cleft lip and palate. (B) There is no physiological reason this baby would need a higher intake of formula than other infants. (C) Correct. The bilateral cleft lip and cleft palate will cause the infant to take in a great deal of air with each swallow, thus causing possible gastric distention. Frequent burping is necessary to remove the air and hopefully reduce the chance of vomiting and aspiration. (D) This baby will not require more frequent feedings, but will require different methods of feeding, using special appliances or feeding devices.

305. (A) Nursing process phase: implementation; client need: safe, effective care environment; content area: pediatric nursing

Rationale
(A) Correct. It is essential that nothing be allowed to enter the child's mouth, including his hands, that might disrupt the newly repaired palate. (B) In the immediate postoperative period, the child is not allowed to put his fingers or irritating foods into his mouth, which might disrupt the palate sutures. (C) Suction catheters or wands are not allowed in the child's mouth because they might disrupt the palate sutures. (D) Cotton swabs are contraindicated inside the mouth to eliminate potential damage to the sutures.

306. (D) Nursing process phase: implementation; client need: physiological integrity, content area: pediatric nursing

Rationale
(A) Nothing is allowed to enter the child's mouth in the immediate postoperative period. A straw could damage the integrity of the palate sutures. (B) A nipple entering the child's mouth and the child sucking could damage the palate sutures. (C) An asepto syringe could damage the palate sutures. Anything entering the child's mouth is contraindicated in the immediate postoperative period. (D) Correct. A cup is a successful method of delivering fluids orally in the immediate postoperative period. Nothing enters the mouth and the child does not suck, which could damage the palate repair.

307. (C) Nursing process phase: analysis; client need: health promotion and maintenance; content area: pediatric nursing

Rationale
(A) Congenital diaphragmatic hernia is failure of the diaphragm to form completely, causing the intestines and other abdominal structures to enter the thoracic cavity. (B) Gastroschisis occurs when the bowel herniates through a defect in the abdominal wall to the right of the umbilical cord and through the rectus muscle. (C) Correct. Omphalocele occurs when there is herniation of the abdominal contents through the hernia of the umbilical cord, usually with an intact peritoneal sac. (D) Umbilical hernia is present when fusion of the umbilical ring is incomplete at the point where the umbilical vessels exit the abdominal wall, causing a portion of bowel to protrude.

308. (B) Nursing process phase: analysis; client need: physiological integrity; content area: pediatric nursing

Rationale
(A & D) This is not characteristic of an infant with TEF. (B) Correct. The infant will most likely have an esophagus that ends in a blind pouch with a fistula connecting the lower esophagus and trachea. Each attempt to swallow a liquid results in gagging and choking with possible aspiration. These infants are immediately placed NPO until a thorough evaluation is made. (C) This is characteristic of a premature infant, not an infant with TEF.

309. (C) Nursing process phase: analysis; client need: physiological integrity; content area: pediatric nursing

Rationale
(A) Cardiac workload has not been directly increased by this anomaly. The positioning is to reduce gastric reflux. (B)

There may or may not be abdominal distention. This position is designed to reduce gastric reflux into the trachea. (C) Correct. Elevating the head and shoulders will reduce the reflux of gastric content into the lungs through the fistula. This is essential to try and minimize lung damage from this reflux aspiration. (D) The fistula connects the trachea and esophagus. This position will not help air to escape from the fistula.

310. (A) Nursing process phase: assessment: client need: physiological integrity; content area: pediatric nursing

Rationale
(A) Correct. Hirschsprung's disease is a congenital anomaly that results in mechanical obstruction from inadequate motility of part of the intestine. There is an absence of autonomic parasympathetic ganglion cells in one or more areas of the colon. These are symptoms seen with this disorder. (B–D) These are not symptoms seen with Hirschsprung's disease.

311. (D) Nursing process phase: planning; client need: health promotion and maintenance; content area: pediatric nursing

Rationale
(A) Physical activity does not have to be limited in this infant. (B) There is no need to dilate the stomach after surgery for Hirschsprung's disease. (C) Preventing prolapse of the rectum is not a concern with this surgery. (D) Correct. It is essential to assess bowel function with the newly created colostomy. This should include evaluation of the return of bowel sounds; the consistency, color, and amount of stool; and assessment of the stoma.

312. (B) Nursing process phase: analysis; client need: physiological integrity; content area: pediatric nursing

Rationale
(A) Infection in the gastrointestinal tract may have caused the diarrhea, but death occurs from the rapid loss of body fluids and salts. (B) Correct. The dehydration, electrolyte imbalance, and metabolic acidosis that acute diarrhea cause is fatal for approximately 400 children a year in the United States. It is essential to promptly correct fluid and electrolyte imbalances in infants and young children. (C) This is not characteristic with diarrhea and dehydration and is not the usual cause of death. (D) A secondary infection is not the usual cause of death with severe diarrhea and dehydration.

313. (B) Nursing process phase: analysis; client need: physiological integrity; content area: pediatric nursing

Rationale
(A & C) The pyloric muscle is hypertrophied, not dilated. (B) Correct. Hypertrophic pyloric stenosis occurs when the circular muscle of the pylorus becomes thickened, causing constriction of the pylorus and obstruction of the gastric outlet. (D) There is hypertrophy of the pyloric muscle, not a reduction in tone.

314. (C) Nursing process phrase: assessment; client need: physiological integrity; content area: pediatric nursing

Rationale
(A) Abdominal rigidity is characteristic of bowel perforation and peritonitis, not pyloric stenosis. (B) Pyloric stenosis should not cause respiratory distress, which would be indicated by substernal retractions. (C) Correct. Because the food or formula is trying to get past the hypertrophied pyloric

muscle, often strong peristalsis waves may be visible on the abdomen. (D) Because little food or formula can pass beyond the hypertrophied pyloric muscle, you would not expect to see marked distention of the lower abdomen.

315. (A) Nursing process phase: implementation; client need: physiological integrity; content area: pediatric nursing

Rationale
(A) Correct. Projectile vomiting is characteristic of hypertrophic pyloric stenosis, caused by the inability of food or fluids to pass the hypertrophied pyloric muscle. (B) Respiratory alkalosis is not an expected result of pyloric stenosis. (C) These infants should be fed small, frequent feedings in an upright position to allow for more formula to pass the pyloric muscle. (D) These infants should be placed in a head-elevated, right-side-lying position after feedings to facilitate gastric emptying and protect their airway from aspiration with vomiting.

316. (C) Nursing process phase: analysis; client need: safe, effective care environment; content area: pediatric nursing

Rationale
(A) Infants are at most risk for head injuries in motor vehicle accidents. (B) Aspiration pneumonia is not a usual risk of accidents. (C) Correct. Infant's large heads take the brunt of impact when propelled forward in an accident. (D) Kidney trauma is not the greatest risk during an accident involving infants.

317. (D) Nursing process phase: assessment; client need: physiological integrity; content area: pediatric nursing

Rationale
(A) Infection would not be a problem at the accident site. (B) The infant would not be more prone to compound skeletal fractures, because his bones are more flexible than an adult's. (C) Hyperthermia will not be a problem for the infant, but hypothermia will. (D) Correct. The infant will not be able to keep his body temperature up in cool, damp conditions as well as an adult. Hypothermia can be a significant factor with infants and must be addressed quickly.

318. (C) Nursing process phase: assessment; client need: physiological integrity; content area: pediatric nursing

Rationale
(A, B, & D) These are not primary assessment parameters for an injured child. (C) Correct. The ABC's (airway, breathing, and circulation) are the primary assessments to make of anyone who has been injured. These take priority over all other parameters.

319. (A) Nursing process phase: implementation; client need: physiological integrity; content area: pediatric nursing

Rationale
(A) Correct. Your responsibility as a school health nurse is to assess Mike's neurological status and then to make sure that he is seen by a physician. Since Mike lost consciousness, he needs to have a thorough assessment for a concussion and to rule out further neurological injury, such as subdural hematoma. (B) You would not want Mike taking a nap prior to being assessed by a physician for concussion. (C) You would not want Mike to continue with his activities until he

has been assessed for concussion. (D) These instructions may be given to the parents after he is thoroughly evaluated for the concussion.

320. (B) Nursing process phase: analysis; client need: health promotion and maintenance; content area: pediatric nursing

Rationale
(A) The symptom of amnesia before and after concussion is not unusual for children and is benign if it is the only neurological symptom. (B) Correct. It is normal for children to have amnesia for events prior to and just after their concussion. It does not represent neurological impairment. (C) The amnesia that occurs is usually before and after concussion. (D) While this may be true statement, it does not answer the parent's question regarding the amnesia.

321. (A) Nursing process phase: assessment; client need: physiological integrity; content area: pediatric nursing

Rationale
(A) Correct. Blackouts are not a normal finding with postconcussion syndrome, and could signal neurological dysfunction that must be assessed. Sleep disturbances, emotional disturbances, and poor school performance are all typical findings of postconcussion syndrome. (B–D) This is a finding of postconcussion syndrome.

322. (A) Nursing process phase: analysis; client need: physiological integrity; content area: pediatric nursing

Rationale
(A) Correct. Further loss of consciousness would indicate serious head injury with possible intracranial bleeding or swelling. Joey should be admitted to the hospital and given further testing and observation to determine the cause of the loss of consciousness. (B) An area of swelling from the head injury would not in itself be an indication for hospitalization. (C) Scalp wounds can bleed profusely and must be controlled, but bleeding from the head wound would not in itself necessitate hospitalization. (D) Vomiting of undigested food in the emergency room is common after a head injury in response to pain. If the vomiting continues long after the time of injury, this could indicate increasing intracranial pressure and would necessitate immediate follow-up.

323. (D) Nursing process phrase: analysis; client need: physiological integrity, content area: pediatric nursing

Rationale
(A & B) This is appropriate for an infant with diarrhea. (C) This is appropriate for a hospitalized infant. (D) Correct. Infusion of hypotonic solutions can lead to hyponatremia and be life-threatening.

324. (A) Nursing process phase: planning; client need: health promotion and maintenance; content area: pediatric nursing

Rationale
(A) Correct. Children with febrile seizures do not usually need long-term anticonvulsant medications because these seizures are directly related to febrile illnesses and are short in duration. (B) These children do not usually require anticonvulsant therapy. (C) Anticonvulsants are usually not required for febrile seizures. (D) Febrile seizures that last less than 15 seconds do not require anticonvulsant therapy.

325. (B) Nursing process phase: planning; client need: health promotion and maintenance; content area: pediatric nursing

Rationale
(A) Febrile seizures are associated with febrile illnesses. The Arnold-Chiari defect is associated with hydrocephalus in infants. (B) Correct. Febrile seizures are associated with the presence of a febrile illness. Treating the illness with antibiotics will reduce the incidence of febrile seizures. (C) Long-term anticonvulsant therapy is not indicated for febrile seizures. (D) A ketogenic diet may be beneficial for various forms of epileptic seizures, but is not effective for febrile seizures.

326. (C) Nursing process phase: analysis; client need: health promotion and maintenance; content area: pediatric nursing

Rationale
(A) When he gets older, it is not likely that Robby will develop a seizure disorder from having had a febrile seizure as a small child. (B) Febril seizures are not familial, and it cannot be predicted whether his newborn sister will have febrile seizures or not. (C) Correct. The incidence of developing a future seizure disorder is less than 3 percent. (D) There is no cause for development of a learning disorder from a febrile seizure.

327. (C) Nursing process phase: implementation; client need: physiological integrity; content area: pediatric nursing

Rationale
(A) Bright lights are often irritating to the child with meningitis and should be used only when necessary. In general, stimulation should be minimized during the acute phase. (B) Isolation is usually maintained 24 hours after the initiation of antibiotic therapy. (C) Correct. Changes in the level of consciousness would indicate a worsening neurological status with increasing intracranial pressure, and would require prompt intervention. (D) Fluids are frequently kept at maintenance or below maintenance levels to minimize increased intracranial pressure. They should not be forced during acute neurological conditions.

328. (B) Nursing process phase: analysis; client need: health promotion and maintenance; content area: pediatric nursing

Rationale
(A) Bacterial meningitis in a toddler is usually preceded by otitis media or other upper respiratory infection. (B) Correct. Otitis media frequently precedes bacterial meningitis in young children. (C) There is no relationship between bacterial meningitis and booster immunization shots. (D) A fine red macular rash would most likely indicate a contact dermatitis or other contagious disorder that would not be linked to the development of bacterial meningitis.

329. (D) Nursing process phase: analysis; client need: health promotion and maintenance; content area: pediatric nursing

Rationale
(A) The cremasteric reflex does not cause penile erection. (B) Tightening of the perineal muscles is not associated with the cremasteric reflex. (C) Urination is not affected by the cremasteric reflex. (D) Correct. The cremasteric reflex is the withdrawal of the testes into the inguinal canal with stroking of the inner thigh area. A hyperactive cremasteric reflex in infants may cause the testes to remain in the inguinal canal.

330. (C) Nursing process phase: analysis; client need: physiological integrity; content area: pediatric nursing

Rationale
(A) Poor penile vasculature is not usually associated with hypospadias and chordee. (B) While this is a true statement, the hypospadias defect must be repaired using the foreskin, so circumcision is not performed. (C) Correct. Hypospadias is the presence of the urethral opening along the ventral shaft of the penis. Chordee are fibrous bands of skin that often result. Circumcision removes the foreskin. The foreskin is necessary for reconstruction during the repair of the hypospadias defect. (D) This is not a rationale for not circumcising the infant with hypospadias and chordee.

331. (B) Nursing process phase: implementation; client need: physiological integrity; content area: pediatric nursing

Rationale
(A) Bladder irrigation will not be performed after hypospadias repair. (B) Correct. The suprapubic catheter is placed as an alternate urinary elimination route following the reconstruction of the meatus. This ensures that the bladder will not become distended if the primary urinary catheter should become blocked. (C) While a suprapubic catheter would allow for accurate urine measurement, this is not the reason it is placed following hypospadias repair. (D) While this is true, this is not the reason a suprapubic catheter is placed following hypospadias repair.

332. (A) Nursing process phase: evaluation; client need: health promotion and maintenance; content area: pediatric nursing

Rationale
(A) Correct. Cryptorchism is the retention of the testes in the inguinal canal. If left untreated, sterility can result from intense body heat. (B) Infection is not associated with untreated cryptorchism. (C) Torsion of the testes is not the major complication of untreated cryptorchism. (D) Inguinal hernia is not associated with untreated cryptorchism.

333. (D) Nursing process phase: analysis; client need: psychosocial integrity; content area: pediatric nursing

Rationale
(A) This is not a rationale for early repair of genitourinary defects. (B) Separation anxiety will be avoided in part for small infants; however, they are repaired early to promote normal body image. (C) These defects are repaired early to promote normal body image, not to promote acceptance of hospitalization. (D) Correct. The goal is to produce as near normal looking and functioning genitourinary organ as early as possible to promote development of normal body image.

334. (A) Nursing process phase: analysis; client need: physiological integrity; content area: pediatric nursing

Rationale
(A) Correct. Nephrotic syndrome is treated with steroids, which may cause immunosuppression and put the child at risk for infection. (B) Generalized edema does not put the child at risk for infection. (C) Electrolyte imbalance does not put

the child at particular risk for infection with nephrotic syndrome. (D) The idiopathic nature of the illness does not put the child at risk for infection.

335. **(D)** Nursing process phase: planning; client need: health promotion and maintenance; content area: pediatric nursing

Rationale

(A) Extreme restlessness may indicate any number of things and does not give the best indication of the diagnosis of fluid volume excess of the choices given. (B) This value falls within the normal parameters. You would expect a low hematocrit level as the blood cells become more dilute with excess fluid volume. (C) An intake of 1500 ml in 24 hours for a 30-kg child is not excessive and would not support the diagnosis of fluid volume excess. (D) Correct. You would expect a 30-kg child to have a minimal urine output of at least 1 to 2 ml/kg per hour, giving Lisa an average output of at least 240 to 480 ml in 8 hours. An output this low (100 ml/8 hr) supports the diagnosis of fluid volume excess.

336. **(C)** Nursing process phase: evaluation; client need: health promotion and maintenance; content area: pediatric nursing

Rationale

(A) Relapses with nephrotic syndrome are common and do not indicate a worsening prognosis. (B) Exacerbations and remissions are common, and the nurse cannot predict future hospitalizations. (C) Correct. Exacerbations and remissions may occur for many months following the diagnosis of nephrotic syndrome. (D) Excerbations and remissions occur even while on correct medications. This is also not a therapeutic statement to emphasize to the family.

337. **(B)** Nursing process phase: implementation; client need: health promotion and maintenance; content area: pediatric nursing

Rationale

(A) The family should be encouraged to increase, not decrease, Mimi's oral fluid intake to keep urine passing through the urinary tract. (B) Correct. Mimi should avoid stasis of urine in her bladder. An increased fluid intake and encouraging her to void frequently will help keep the system "flushed." (C) Bubble baths should be avoided. The bubble bath solution causes irritation of the urinary meatus and frequently is linked to urinary tract infections in young children. (D) While proper cleanliness is important, especially for little girls, it is more important at this time to keep Mimi's urinary tract flushed with fluids and frequent voiding.

338. **(B)** Nursing process phrase: assessment; client need: health promotion and maintenance; content area: pediatric nursing

Rationale

(A) Abdominal pain is not a reliable indicator of the presence of a urinary tract infection. (B) Correct. The absence of bacteria in the urine is a true indication of the effectiveness of the therapy. (C) Completion of a full course of antibiotic therapy will not in itself tell if an infection is no longer present. (D) Irritability and other symptoms are not reliable indicators of the presence of an infection.

339. **(C)** Nursing process phase: assessment; client need:

health promotion and maintenance, content area: pediatric nursing

Rationale

(A) A weight gain does not strongly support the diagnosis of glomerulonephritis. (B) Irritability can be present with many different factors and does not strongly suggest glomerulonephritis specifically. (C) Correct. The majority of children have been diagnosed with a strep infection prior to the onset of glomerulonephritis. (D) An increase in urine output and decreased specific gravity are not signs of glomerulonephritis. Urine output is less with a rise in specific gravity.

340. **(D)** Nursing process phase: planning; client need: physiological integrity; content area: pediatric nursing

Rationale

(A) This action will likely cause further stress and rebellion. John should be made an active part of his care planning. (B) Isolation from others will not be therapeutic for John. He may be more willing to eat a proper diet if he is allowed to be around friends or family. (C) This is not an acceptable mode of treatment. It is important that John adhere to his dietary restrictions during the acute phase of glomerulonephritis. (D) Correct. These actions will garner support and cooperation from John.

341. **(B)** Nursing process phase: analysis; client need: health promotion and maintenance; pediatric nursing

Rationale

(A) This is the time of common onset of asthma in children; however, the younger the onset, the more likely it is to become persistent. (B) Correct. Infants who demonstrate hyperactive airway disease are more likely to have persistent airway problems. (C) An onset of asthma at this age does not have as great a chance of becoming persistent as with an onset in infancy. (D) While the onset of asthma during the preschool years can become persistent, of the answer choices, infancy would have the greatest potential.

342. **(A)** Nursing process phase: implementation; client need: physiological integrity; content area: pediatric nursing

Rationale

(A) Correct. While these other medications may be used at some point, oxygen is given immediately to children demonstrating compromised air exchange. (B) While epinephrine may be used in the treatment of a disorder causing wheezing, oxygen will be used immediately. (C) Theophylline will not be used immediately for the child presenting with wheezing. (D) Steroids will not be used immediately for the treatment of the wheezing child.

343. **(B)** Nursing process phase: analysis; client need: physiological integrity; content area: pediatric nursing

Rationale

(A) An increase in PaO_2 would not be a sign of a complication, but a sign of increased oxygen delivery to tissues. (B) Correct. While we often assume a decrease in wheezing is a good sign, it could, in fact, signal a worsening airway, such that the child is no longer able to move enough air to even wheeze. This would be an emergency situation requiring immediate mechanical ventilation. (C) A decrease in $PaCO_2$ would indicate that the child is now able to blow off more carbon dioxide, thus an improvement. (D) An increase in oxygen saturation would be an improvement, not a complication.

344. (D) Nursing process phrase: analysis; client need: health promotion and maintenance; content area: pediatric nursing

Rationale
(A) Elevated plasma protein is not associated with cystic fibrosis. (B) Plasma protein is not used in the diagnosis of cystic fibrosis. (C) Plasma cholesterol is not used in the diagnosis of cystic fibrosis. (D) Correct. An elevated sweat chloride level is key to the diagnosis of cystic fibrosis.

345. (C) Nursing process phase: implementation; client need: health promotion and maintenance; content area: pediatric nursing

Rationale
(A) This is not of long enough duration for prophylactic antibiotic therapy following ARF. (B) Five years is the recommended duration. (C) Correct. Five years is the recommended duration for prophylactic antibiotic therapy following acute rheumatic fever. (D) This is the normal recommended duration for acute antibiotic therapy for common infections. ACF requires a much longer duration of therapy to prevent recurrence.

346. (A) Nursing process phrase: analysis; client need: health promotion and maintenance; content area: pediatric nursing

Rationale
(A) Correct. The most common portal of entry of the causative organisms is from dental work. (B) The chest x-ray will not place the child at risk for SBE. (C) Immunizations do not place the child at risk for SBE. (D) A barium swallow does not place the child at risk for SBE.

347. (D) Nursing process phase: evaluation; client need: physiological integrity; content area: pediatric nursing

Rationale
(A) While fit and appearance of the brace are important, they are not the most important factor to achieve satisfactory results. (B) Teaching and counseling are important, but if the child is not compliant, the therapy will not be successful. (C) Reinforcement by the parents is important, but if the child is not compliant and cooperative in using the brace as prescribed, therapy will not be successful. (D) Correct. Compliance and cooperation with the prescribed therapy is key to success. The child must often wear the brace for several years, up to 23 hours a day to achieve a reduction in the spinal curve.

348. (A) Nursing process phase: implementation; client need: health promotion and maintenance; content area: pediatric nursing

Rationale
(A) Tinnitus and nausea are common toxic symptoms. (B–D) These are not toxic symptoms of sodium salicylate.

349. (D) Nursing process phase: assessment; client need: health promotion and maintenance; content area: pediatric nursing

Rationale
(A) Gowers' sign is not seen with structural scoliosis. (B) Gowers' sign is not seen with Legg-Calvé-Perthes disease.

(C) Gowers' sign is not seen with congenital hip dysplasia. (D) Correct. Children with Duchenne's muscular dystrophy attain standing positions by assuming a kneeling position, then gradually pushing their torso upright by "walking" their hands up their legs. This is known as Gowers's sign.

350. (A) Nursing process phrase: assessment; health promotion and maintenance; content area: pediatric nursing

Rationale
(A) Correct. Legg-Calvé-Perthes disease is a self-limiting disorder in which there is aseptic necrosis of the femoral head. Initial symptoms are a limp and pain in the affected hip. (B) Leg-length discrepancy is not seen with this disease. (C) Waddling gait is not characteristic of this disease. (D) Pain is most evident on arising and at the end of a long day of activities. It is not specific to climbing stairs.

351. (C) Nursing process phase: planning; client need: physiological integrity; content area: pediatric nursing

Rationale
(A) It is a major emphasis to prevent weight bearing on the head of the femur involved, not to prevent flexion. (B) While pain may become a concern, it is most important to prevent further damage to the femur by preventing weight bearing. (C) Correct. With the necrosis, it is essential to prevent weight bearing on the head of the femur to prevent further damage. (D) Tad should be prevented from bearing weight on the affected femur.

352. (B) Nursing process phase: implementation; client need: physiological integrity; content area: pediatric nursing

Rationale
(A) Children with muscular dystrophy often have a problem with increased weight gain as their activity level diminishes. It is important to balance caloric intake. (B) Correct. As the muscles used for respiration become weak, children with muscular dystrophy will have increasing difficulty coughing and clearing secretions. Respiratory infections are a major contributor to morbidity and mortality in these children. (C) While muscles should remain active as long as possible, strenuous exercise should not be promoted in children with muscular dystrophy. (D) Physical activity should be maintained as long as possible.

353. (A) Nursing process phase: analysis; client need: health promotion and maintenance; content area: pediatric nursing

Rationale
(A) Correct. Approximately 80 percent of all cases of hemophilia are demonstrated as X-linked recessive. (B) Hemophilia involves a deficiency in clotting factor VIII or factor IX, not a decrease in platelets. (C) The primary therapy is replacement of coagulation factor VIII or IX. (D) Replacement therapy does not always require hospitalization and is most frequently accomplished at home.

354. (D) Nursing process phase: implementation; client need: physiological integrity; content area: pediatric nursing

Rationale
(A) It is most important to try to stop the bleeding. Warm,

moist compresses will not assist in stopping the bleeding. (B) Pressure may cause additional damage and will not be as beneficial for the hemophiliac. (C) Movement of the involved extremity should be avoided until the danger of bleeding has passed. (D) Correct. Elevation of the extremity above the level of the heart, combined with giving replacement factor will help to stop the bleeding.

355. (C) Nursing process phase: analysis; client need: physiological integrity; content area: pediatric nursing

Rationale

(A) Petechiae are characteristic of low platelets. The child with hemophilia has a coagulation factor deficiency, not platelet deficiency. (B) There is not enough loss of fluid in this child to cause dehydration. (C) Correct. This child will bleed into the knee joint, producing hemarthrosis. (D) There is no cause for neutropenia in this child.

356. (B) Nursing process phrase: implementation; client need: physiological integrity; content area: pediatric nursing

Rationale

(A) Bedrest is indicated during the acute phase to minimize further bleeding and trauma to the tissues. (B) Correct. Active range-of-motion exercises may damage tissue and cause further bleeding. (C) Elevation of the affected knee is an appropriate intervention to minimize bleeding. (D) Ice bags to the knee are appropriate to help slow bleeding.

357. (C) Nursing process phase: analysis; client need: safe, effective care environment; content area: pediatric nursing

Rationale

(A) Codeine would be an appropriate analgesic for a child with hemophilia. (B) Demerol would not be contraindicated for a child with hemophilia. (C) Correct. Aspirin would be contraindicated for a child with hemophilia because it may further increase bleeding. (D) Tylenol would be an appropriate analgesic for a child with hemophilia.

358. (D) Nursing process phase: implementation; client need: psychological integrity; content area: pediatric nursing

Rationale

(A) Burns do not heal quickly and can leave scars. (B) Cleaning and debridement are painful. She will not be interested in looking in a mirror. (C) At her age this is not the most helpful action. (D) Correct. Tangible evidence that she is healing is the most supportive action.

359. (A) Nursing process phase: analysis; client need: physiological integrity; content area: pediatric integrity

Rationale

(A) Correct. The entanglement of sickle-shaped cells with one another blocks the microcirculation, causing vaso-occlusion. This causes hypoxia, ischemia, and infarction of the tissue. (B) Hypertension is not a factor in sickle-cell disease. (C) The clinical manifestation of sickle-cell disease is not the result of hypotension. (D) The clinical manifestation of sickle-cell disease is not the result of edema.

360. (B) Nursing process phase: analysis; client need: physiological integrity; content area: pediatric nursing

Rationale

(A) This is not a factual statement. Narcotics are an important intervention in relieving the pain crisis with sickle-cell disease. (B) Correct. When narcotics are indicated for pain, children rarely become addicted. Less than 1 percent of children who receive opioids for severe pain become behaviorally addicted. The goal is prevention of pain, and often this requires high doses of opioids, round the clock. (C) Narcotics are an essential first-line intervention for children in pain crisis. (D) Narcotics are used as a primary intervention, along with non-pharmacologic methods of pain relief.

361. (C) Nursing process phase: evaluation; client need: physiological integrity; content area: pediatric nursing

Rationale

(A) Toxins are not responsible for her alopecia, nausea, and stomatitis. (B) This answer does not relate to the cause of alopecia, nausea, and stomatitis. (C) Correct. Chemotherapy kills both cancer cells and normal cells, resulting in the loss of hair, irritation of the stomach lining, and ulcers in the mouth. (D) Chemotherapy is mostly delivered intravenously. Gastric absorption is not responsible for these side effects.

362. (D) Nursing process phase: evaluation; client need: health promotion and maintenance; content area: pediatric nursing

Rationale

(A) Regrowth of hair is not a measure of remission. (B) A decrease in nausea and vomiting does not define remission. (C) Blast-cell reduction does not define remission. (D) Correct. The absence of tumor cells microscopically will be a true measure of remission.

363. (A) Nursing process phase: analysis; client need: psychosocial; content area: pediatric nursing

Rationale

(A) Correct. The child's age and cognitive development will guide the nurse and mother for how to explain his illness and treatments. Explanations should be appropriate for his developmental level. (B) His physical condition is not the primary determinant for how to talk with him about his illness. (C) The child's relationship with the nurse is not the most important factor to consider when responding to the mother. (D) While the child's past illnesses may influence how much explanation is necessary, it is more important to gear explanations to his developmental level.

364. (B) Nursing process phase: implementation; client need: psychosocial integrity; content area: pediatric nursing

Rationale

(A) This would not be therapeutic for the child or family. (B) Correct. The parents may need some time alone to gather strength for the impending death of the child. The nurse's role is to support both the child and family. (C) This is not therapeutic for the child and does not recognize the needs of the parents. (D) This is judgmental and not therapeutic for child or family.

365. (A) Nursing process phase: analysis; client need: physiological integrity; content area: pediatric nursing

Rationale

(A) Correct. High levels of glucose in the blood will cause increased urination (polyuria), which will cause increased thirst (polydipsia). (B) Polyphagia is secondary to decreased (not increased) uptake of glucose. (C) Polyuria is an increased excretion of urine, not retention. (D) These symptoms occur as a result of Jane's hyperglycemic (not hypoglycemic) state during ketosis.

366. (D) Nursing process phase: analysis; client need: health promotion and maintenance; content area: pediatric nursing

Rationale
(A) This is a normal glucose level and would not cause the release of ketones in the urine. (B) No ketones would be spilled in the urine with this blood glucose level. (C) Although this is an elevated blood glucose level, ketones would not yet be present in the urine. (D) Correct. Ketones will be present in the urine with blood glucose levels of approximately 250 mg/dl or greater.

367. (B) Nursing process phase: analysis; client need: physiological integrity; content area: pediatric nursing

Rationale
(A) Regular insulin peaks in 2 to 4 hours. Onset of the insulin begins in approximately 30 minutes. (B) Correct. The peak blood concentrations of regular insulin occur 2 to 4 hours after injection. This is the time that the child would be at most risk for experiencing hypoglycemia and should be prepared to have a snack. (C) The peak time has already occurred for regular insulin. (D) The regular insulin is almost gone from the child's system by 8 hours.

368. (D) Nursing process phase: implementation; client need: health promotion and maintenance; content area: pediatric nursing

Rationale
(A) It is important for all close family members to know and understand all procedures needed to care for the child with type I diabetes. (B) Many young children can learn and understand the concepts of self-injection prior to adolescence. (C) The client should be able to reach all necessary injection sites by this age. (D) Correct. Most children can learn the techniques of self-injection by the age of 10. By this age, they have the necessary fine motor coordination and can understand the principles involved in drawing up and injecting insulin.

369. (C) Nursing process phase: analysis; client need: physiological integrity; content area: pediatric nursing

Rationale
(A) NPH insulin is an intermediate-acting insulin and will not act quickly enough to treat acute hyperglycemia. It does not peak until 6 to 8 hours after injection. (B) Humulin N is an intermediate-acting insulin also and would not act quickly enough to treat acute hyperglycemia. (C) Correct. Regular insulin is a short-acting insulin and will act within 30 minutes and peak within 2 to 4 hours of administration, making it the insulin of choice to treat acute hyperglycemia. (D) Ultralente is a super long-acting insulin and would never be used to treat acute hyperglycemia.

370. (C) Nursing process phase: analysis; client need: health promotion and maintenance; content area: pediatric nursing

Rationale
(A) This answer assumes that the child does indeed have epilepsy and does not address the parent's concern. (B) This answer does not address the mother's concern for this child and is not therapeutic. (C) Correct. This answer is factual and tells the mother that not all seizures signal the diagnosis of epilepsy. (D) The nurse has no knowledge whether the seizures will reoccur or not. This is not a therapeutic answer.

371. (A) Nursing process: implementation; client need: physiological integrity; content area: pediatric nursing

Rationale
(A) Correct. EMS should be called to transport the child to the hospital for further evaluation. Since this child has no history of seizures, a thorough physical examination and neurological evaluation must be done immediately. EMS personnel will be prepared to treat the child, should a seizure begin during transport. (B) While these people should be notified, the child should be transported ASAP to the hospital by EMS personnel. (C) The child must be evaluated immediately for this first seizure, and it is the nurse's responsibility to see that the child is transported to the hospital by EMS. (D) EMS should be notified ASAP to transport the child. The school nurse can remain with the child after EMS has been notified.

372. (A) Nursing process phase: implementation; client need: physiological integrity; content area: pediatric nursing

Rationale
(A) Correct. The child is at risk for an infection from the surgery, which could lead to meningitis. (B) The shunt reservoir does not need to be pumped to maintain patency. (C) Sedation is not administered, because it may impede neurological assessment. (D) Trendelenburg's position would be contraindicated, because it would place the infant in a head-down position and increase intracranial pressure.

373. (D) Nursing process phase: implementation; client need: physiological integrity; content area: pediatric nursing

Rationale
(A) The infant should be placed in the prone position to minimize tension on the sac and the risk of trauma. (B) The sac should be kept warm and moist, wrapped in sterile, moist, nonadherent dressings, until the infant goes to surgery. The sac should not be allowed to dry. (C) The infant will be NPO and will not have diarrheal stools. The sac should be kept sterile and moist prior to surgery. (D) Correct. Hydrocephalus is common in infants with myelomeningocele, so the infant should be assessed frequently for signs of increased intracranial pressure.

374. (B) Nursing process phase: analysis; client need: health promotion and maintenance; content area: pediatric nursing

Rationale
(A) Mental retardation may occur, but is not the most common problem. (B) Correct. Neurogenic bladder is the most common problem associated with myelomeningocele, and myelomeningocele is one of the most common causes of neurogenic bladder. (C) Respiratory compromise is not a common problem with myelomeningocele. (D) The degree of musculoskeletal impairment in extremities varies widely with the extent and location of the defect.

375. (D) Nursing process phase: evaluation; client need: health promotion and maintenance; content area: pediatric nursing

Rationale

(A) Infectious diseases are not the major determinant of neonatal death in the United States. (B) Accidental injuries are the leading cause of death in children 1 to 19 years of age, but not the major determinant of neonatal mortality. (C) Poor nutrition is not the major determinant of neonatal mortality in the United States. (D) Correct. Low birth weight is the number one determinant of neonatal death in the United States.

376. (B) Nursing process: evaluation; client need: health promotion and maintenance; content area: pediatric nursing

Rationale

(A) Mortality and morbidity statistics will not affect commitment to families. (B) Correct. Knowledge of the leading causes of death and morbidity will identify age groups at risk for diseases and injuries and lead to prevention techniques. (C) Knowledge of mortality and morbidity statistics will not assist in recognizing changes in adaptation. (D) Knowledge of mortality and morbidity statistics will lead to prevention of illness and injury, not the alleviation of parental anxiety.

377. (D) Nursing process phase: analysis; client need: health promotion and maintenance; content area: pediatric nursing

Rationale

(A) While the number of deaths from AIDS is increasing, accidental injury still accounts for the majority of deaths of children. (B) Homicide is one cause of accidental death, but it alone is not the leading cause of death. (C) Cancer is not the leading cause of death in this age group. (D) Correct. Because of their physical and developmental characteristics, children aged 1 to 19 years are most vulnerable to accidents and injury that can cause death.

378. (D) Nursing process phase: analysis; client need: health promotion and maintenance; content area: pediatric nursing

Rationale

(A) Contributions to nursing research are not the sole responsibility of nurse educators. (B) While Sigma Theta Tau International plays a leading role in nursing research and scholarship, it is the responsibility of all nurses. (C) Nurse researchers play a vital part in the advancement of nursing research, but it is the responsibility of all nurses. (D) Correct. All nurses must participate in the advancement of nursing practice through contributions to nursing research, whether by initiating, facilitating, or evaluating nursing research.

379. (C) Nursing process phase: evaluation; client need: health promotion and maintenance; content area: pediatric nursing

Rationale

(A) This describes the nursing role of prevention and health promotion, not family advocacy. (B) Prevention and health promotion are described, not support and counseling. (C) Correct. The question describes the role of illness prevention and health promotion. (D) The question describes the role of prevention and promotion, not health-care planning.

380. (C) Nursing process phase: analysis; client need: health promotion and maintenance; content area: pediatric nursing

Rationale

(A) Rotavirus is not the most common childhood illness. (B) While prevalent, tonsillitis is not the most common childhood illness. (C) Correct. The common cold, or upper respiratory infection, is the most common childhood illness. (D) While very prevalent during winter months, respiratory syncitial virus (RSV) is not the most common childhood illness.

381. (B) Nursing process phase: implementation; client need: psychosocial integrity; content area: pediatric nursing

Rationale

(A) This is not a therapeutic intervention. (B) Correct. Parents who are allowed to participate in their child's care cope better with their illness. (C) New toys as distraction are not therapeutic in dealing with the anxiety of separation. (D) It is not reasonable to reassure parents that the nurse will be with their child at all times.

382. (D) Nursing process phase: analysis; client need: psychosocial; content area: pediatric nursing

Rationale

(A) While play may release surplus energy, this is not the most important therapeutic value of play in the hospital. (B) This may take place with play; however, the facilitation of communication of needs and fears is the most therapeutic value of play in the hospital. (C) Creativity may be encouraged, but this is not the most therapeutic value of play. (D) Correct. Therapeutic play will allow the child to communicate his or her needs, fears, and thoughts through the actions of dolls, puppets, drawings, and so on.

383. (D) Nursing process phase: assessment; client need: physiological integrity; content area: pediatric nursing

Rationale

(A) This statement will not give the nurse information about the child's previous pain experience. (B) This statement links pain with guilt and will not give the nurse therapeutic information about previous pain. (C) Children cannot often quantify pain and will be unable to say how bad pain has been. (D) Correct. Asking children to tell about "hurts" they have had before will allow them to describe past pain and let the nurse assess their methods of coping.

384. (A) Nursing process phase: assessment; client need: physiological integrity; content area: pediatric nursing

Rationale

(A) Correct. This is the only objective choice listed. (B) Pain-intensity rating scales are subjective, not objective. (C) Drawings are subjective, not objective. (D) Parent interviews are subjective, not objective.

385. (C) Nursing process phase: assessment; client need: physiological integrity; content area: pediatric nursing

Rationale

(A) This statement is false. Infants and children do feel pain and should be treated appropriately. (B) Children may not tell the truth about experiencing pain because they may fear getting a "shot" or other procedure, which they imagine to be more painful than what they are experiencing. (C) Correct.

Whatever is painful to an adult should be considered painful to an infant or child. Pain should be anticipated and treated early and aggressively. (D) Undertreating pain leads to playing catch-up and never eliminating the pain. The fear of respiratory depression or addiction to opioids is unfounded if proper dosages and methods of administration are used.

386. **(D)** Nursing process phase: implementation; client need: psychosocial integrity; content area: pediatric nursing

Rationale
(A) Toni needs to be shown and told what to expect on a tour of the facility prior to the procedure date. Toni's parents can then reinforce what she saw and what will happen. (B) A book is not as effective in preparing her as letting her see and touch the actual environment herself. (C) A 6-year-old is quite capable of understanding simple explanations. A lack of information will lead to anxiety. (D) Correct. Toni and her parents should be taken on a tour to see the area and equipment and should be allowed a chance to meet and talk with personnel involved in the procedure.

387. **(A)** Nursing process phase: implementation; client need: health promotion and maintenance; content area pediatric nursing

Rationale
(A) Correct. Immunizations are the best way to achieve primary prevention (before the diseases occur). (B) Isolating children with communicable diseases is not a method of primary prevention. (C) Boiling drinking water during outbreaks is not a method of primary prevention. (D) This is not a method of primary prevention.

388. **(B)** Nursing process phase: analysis; client need: physiological integrity; content area: pediatric nursing

Rationale
(A) These measures will reduce itching and scratching, but the primary rationale is to decrease infection, not reduce scarring. (B) Correct. Bacterial infections can occur with continued scratching of the lesions; therefore, measures are taken to reduce itching and scratching. (C) Faster healing may occur, but the best rationale is to avoid infection. (D) This may be true; however, it is not the best rationale for the actions listed.

389. **(C)** Nursing process phase: analysis; client need: health promotion and maintenance; content area: pediatric nursing

Rationale
(A) This is not true. (B) This is not the rationale for giving the vaccine after age 15 months. (C) Correct. After age 15 months, or so, infants no longer have passive antibodies from their mother to generate a response to the vaccine and build their own antibodies. (D) This is incorrect.

390. **(A)** Nursing process phase: analysis; client need: health promotion and maintenance; content area: pediatric nursing

Rationale
(A) Correct. Natural passive immunity is temporary immunity by transfusing immunoglobulins or antitoxins naturally from the mother to the baby. The infant receives natural antibodies from the mother's breast milk passively while breastfeeding. (B) Naturally acquired active immunity would come from actively forming immune bodies either from having had the disease or by introducing the antigen into the individual. (C) This is temporary immunity by transfusing immune globulins or antitoxins artificially. (D) Innate immunity does not describe how the infant received the immunity.

391. **(D)** Nursing process phase: analysis; client need: health promotion and maintenance; content area: pediatric nursing

Rationale
(A) Innate immunity, or resistance to infection, is not obtained from exposure to the invading agent. (B) Natural immunity is innate immunity or resistance to infection or toxicity. (C) Passive immunity is temporary immunity by transfusing immunoglobulins or antitoxins either artificially or naturally. (D) Correct. Acquired immunity is from exposure to the invading agent, either bacteria, virus, or toxin.

392. **(B)** Nursing process phase: analysis; client need: health promotion and maintenance; content area: pediatric nursing

Rationale
(A) This answer does not address Ms. Brown's concerns nor provide her with any information concerning the vaccine. (B) Correct. This addresses Ms. Brown's concerns and informs her of the risks of contracting pertussis. (C) Pertussis is very dangerous in young infants, so this would not be a wise option, or within the nurse's role. (D) This answer is patronizing and does not address Ms. Brown's concerns.

393. **(D)** Nursing process phase: analysis; client need: health promotion and maintenance; content area: pediatric nursing

Rationale
(A) The inability to blow their noses does not influence the prevalence of otitis media infections in infants. (B) The culture medium for bacteria from milk does not influence otitis media infections. (C) Teething and increased oral bacteria do not influence the prevalence of otitis media infections. (D) Correct. The short, straight eustachian tubes in infants make the presence of bacteria to the middle ear more prevalent, thus increasing the incidence of otitis media infections.

394. **(B)** Nursing process phase: analysis; client need: health promotion and maintenance; content area: pediatric nursing

Rationale
(A) Elevated white blood counts do not cause clubbing of fingers. (B) Correct. Clubbing, or increased tissue surface area on fingers and toes, is a compensatory response to lack of oxygen and perfusion (peripheral hypoxia) to the tissues. (C) An extremely elevated hematocrit may cause some clogging of small arteries and arterioles, but clubbing is a physiological response to chronic hypoxia. (D) Destruction of bone marrow does not produce clubbing.

395. **(D)** Nursing process phase: analysis; client need: health promotion and maintenance; content area: pediatric nursing

Rationale
(A) Pressure in the left side of the heart is greater than it is in the right side, thus no unoxygenated blood from the right

ventricle passes to the left ventricle. (B) The right ventricle enlarges to accommodate an increased volume of blood. (C) Pressure is increased in the pulmonary artery. (D) Correct. Since pressures are higher on the left side of the heart than the right side, blood is shunted from the left to the right. Thus, a small amount of oxygenated blood returns to the right ventricle to be recirculated. No unoxygenated blood goes to the left ventricle and out to the general circulation.

396. (C) Nursing process phase: assessment, client need: physiological integrity; content area: pediatric nursing

Rationale
(A) Red blood cells that are sickled have decreased capacity to carry oxygen. (B) As the red blood cells sickle, there is increased hemolysis and destruction. (C) Obstruction is caused by the sickled RBCs. The resultant absence of blood flow to adjacent tissues causes local hypoxia, leading to tissue ischemia and infarction. (D) With the formation of sickled RBCs, mechanical fragility is increased, thereby decreasing the life span of the RBC.

397. (D) Nursing process phase: analysis and planning; client need: physiological integrity; content area: pediatric nursing

Rationale
(A) The client will not be in a state of alkalosis. Instead, he will be in a state of metabolic acidosis from the hypoxia. (B) The occlusive process is a result of sickled RBCs. Heparin has no effect on minimizing the sickling process. However, heparin could lead to internal hemorrhage. (C) Demerol is not recommended because normeperidine, a metabolite of meperidine, is a stimulant to the central nervous system that produces seizures when it accumulates with repetitive dosing. Clients with sickle cell disease are at risk for normeperidine-induced seizures. (D) Hydration is promoted for hemodilution through oral and intravenous therapy. The hemodilution decreases the entanglement and enmeshing of sickle-shaped cells that lead to vaso-occlusion.

398. (B) Nursing process phase: evaluation; client need: physiological integrity; content area: pediatric nursing

Rationale
(A) ABGs measure the PO$_2$ level in arterial blood. (B) Chelating therapy involves giving an iron-chelating agent to remove excess iron. Excess iron may develop from frequent blood transfusion. Therefore, serum iron levels evaluate the effect of chelating therapy. (C) Hemoglobin does not evaluate iron levels. (D) RBC level does not correlate to increased iron levels.

399. (C) Nursing process phase: implementation; client need: physiological integrity; content area: pediatric nursing

Rationale
(A) A cold compress would be applied to promote vasoconstriction. (B) Immobilizing the arm would be appropriate to decrease blood flow. (C) Elevating the arm above the level of the heart is appropriate to decrease blood flow to the area. (D) Pressure should be applied for 10 to 15 minutes to allow clot formation.

400. (A) Nursing process phase: implementation; client need: physiological integrity; content area: pediatric nursing

Rationale
(A) Having the child sit up and lean forward is the appropriate position to decrease bleeding and prevent aspiration. (B) Ice is applied to the bridge of the nose only if the bleeding persists. (C) Continuous pressure to the nose with the thumb and forefinger should occur for 10 minutes. (D) A lying down position increases blood flow to the area and increases the possibility of aspiration.

401. (B) Nursing process phase: analysis and planning; client need: physiological integrity; content area: pediatric nursing

Rationale
(A) Blood protein forms the largest portion of plasma solutes. It includes albumin, fibrogen, and globulins, but does not estimate the glomerular filtration rate. (B) Glomerular filtration is a measure of the amount of plasma from which a given substance is totally cleared in 1 minute. Creatine, an end product of protein metabolism in muscle, is freely filtered by the glomerulus and is the most useful clinical estimation of glomerular filtration. (C) The pH is an indicator of acid-base balance. The kidney can regulate the acid-base balance by regulating serum bicarbonate. The pH level does not estimate glomerular filtration. (D) Osmolality measures the osmotic pressure and is the accepted term used to describe the osmotic force of solute per unit of weight in a solvent. It does not estimate glomerular filtration.

402. (C) Nursing process phase: assessment; client need: physiological integrity; content area: pediatric nursing

Rationale
(A) In AGN, hematuria is present but the specific gravity is moderately elevated, not decreased. (B) Bacteria are not seen in the urine of children with AGN. (C) During the acute phase, the urinalysis characteristically shows proteinuria, hematuria, and increased specific gravity. (D) Bacteria are not seen in the urine and urine cultures are negative.

403. (D) Nursing process phase: evaluation; client need: physiological integrity; content area: pediatric nursing

Rationale
(A) Usually a moderate elevation in blood pressure exists with the onset of acute glomerulonephritis. (B) Specific gravity is increased in AGN, indicating concentrated urine. (C) Slight to moderate proteinuria may persist for several weeks. (D) The first sign of improvement is a small increase in urinary output with a corresponding decrease in body weight.

404. (C) Nursing process phase: analysis; client need: physiological integrity; content area: pediatric nursing

Rationale
(A) Ambulation does not have an adverse affect on the course of the disease. Children will naturally restrict their activity due to malaise. Yet this restriction would not result in a 6-pound weight loss in 3 days. (B) A regular diet is permitted, but the intake of Na+ is restricted. (C) After urine output increase, a copious diuresis begins 1 to 2 days later. One liter of fluid weighs approximately a pound. As the diuresis begins and the edema resolves, the child will lose weight. (D) This child would be placed on sodium restriction, which would decrease salt intake.

405. (A) Nursing process phase: implementation; client need: physiological integrity; content area: pediatric nursing

Rationale
(A) A moderate sodium restriction is placed on the diet of a child with severe edema to prevent further retention of fluids. (B) Calorie count will not be altered from a regular diet. (C) Foods with large amounts of potassium are restricted during the period of oliguria. (D) Forcing fluids would be contraindicated. Fluid restriction is necessary when the output is significantly reduced.

406. **(A)** Nursing process phase: implementation; client need: physiological integrity; content area: pediatric nursing

Rationale
(A) Daily weight is the best method to detect fluid retention in infants and small children. (B) The number of diapers is not as significant as the weight of the diapers to measure output. (C) Abdominal girth will measure ascites; however, it should be completed daily. (D) Hematuria is not present with nephrotic syndrome.

407. **(D)** Nursing process phase: analysis and planning; client need: safe, effective care environment; content area: pediatric nursing

Rationale
(A) Stimulation of appetite is not a necessary intervention. Prednisone causes an increase in appetite as a side effect and obesity may result with prolonged use. (B) The purpose for administering the prednisone is to decrease urinary excretion of protein. As this occurs the client's diuresis begins and the edema resolves. (C) Because the prednisone decreases the urinary excretion of protein, the osmotic pressure will increase due to the retention of protein. (D) Nursing interventions should be taken to prevent infections. A complication of prednisone is an increased susceptibility to infections.

408. **(A)** Nursing process phase: implementation; client need: health promotion and maintenance; content area: pediatric nursing

Rationale
(A) Steam vaporizers are discouraged because of the hazards related to burns and little evidence exists to support their efficacy. (B) Both vaporizers cost about the same amount of money. (C) Heating the environment occurs regularly during the winter months and is not the problem for recommending a cool-mist vaporizer. (D) The moisture from vaporizers soothes inflamed membranes. It does not dry respiratory secretions.

409. **(A)** Nursing process phase: implementation; client need: physiological integrity; content area: pediatric nursing

Rationale
(A) The nurse assesses for frequent swallowing or clearing of the throat, which would be a sign of hemorrhage in young children. (B) Gargling of any kind may initiate bleeding. (C) The child is placed on his abdomen or side to facilitate drainage of secretions until the child is fully awake. (D) An ice collar may be applied to provide pain relief and vasoconstriction.

410. **(C)** Nursing process phase: implementation; client need: health promotion and maintenance; content area: pediatric nursing

Rationale
(A) Antibiotics must be given until all the prescribed medication is taken even though the child is asymptomatic in 24 to 48 hours. (B) Parents require anticipatory guidance regarding the temporary hearing loss. Medication should be continued. If persistent difficulty in hearing continues beyond the acute stage, the child should be reevaluated. (C) All of the prescribed Bactrim should be given to eradicate the infection completely. (D) Symptoms and fever take 24 to 48 hours to subside. The medication should be continued.

411. **(B)** Nursing process phase: assessment; client need: physiological integrity; content area: pediatric nursing

Rationale
(A) The environment of the outer ear is altered with otitis externa, not traumatically injured. (B) Otitis externa results from normal ear flora that assume pathogenic characteristics under conditions of excessive wetness or dryness. Swimming is the most common cause of otitis externa. (C) Foreign object obstruction does not cause the normal flora to become pathogenic. (D) Acute otitis media is an infection of the middle ear and does not cause otitis externa.

412. **(D)** Nursing process phase: analysis; client need: physiological integrity; content area: pediatric nursing

Rationale
(A) Spasmodic croup usually occurs in young children ages 3 months to 3 years and is a benign condition causing upper airway obstruction. (B) Laryngitis is a common illness in older children and adolescents which is almost always self-limiting, requiring symptomatic treatment. (C) Laryngotracheobronchitis is the most common type of croup experienced by children less than 5 years of age. Usually, children respond to therapy and recovery is prompt. (D) Epiglottis is a serious obstructive inflammatory process requiring immediate attention. The obstruction is supraglottic and the onset is abrupt. The diagnosis of epiglottitis constitutes an emergency.

413. **(C)** Nursing process phase: analysis and planning; client need: safe, effective care environment; content area: pediatric nursing

Rationale
(A) There is no correlation between respiratory infections and an increase in sensitivity to allergens. (B) Respiratory infections can lead to inflammation and narrowing of airways. Also, bronchial secretions may increase and thicken, not liquefy. (C) Respiratory infections can trigger or aggravate the asthmatic state, especially in young children, whose airways are mechanically smaller and more reactive. (D) Respiratory infections do not potentiate the effectiveness of medications.

414. **(B)** Nursing process phase: implementation; client need: health promotion and maintenance; content area: pediatric nursing

Rationale
(A) The medication is applied over the surface of the tongue and oral mucosa and the remainder is swallowed by the infant. (B) Medication therapy is continued for about 1 week even if lesions have disappeared. (C) The white patches cannot be removed and attempts at removal usually will result in bleeding from the scraped surface areas. (D) Pacifiers may be used; however, they should be boiled once a day for at least 20 minutes because candidal spores are heat resistant.

415. (B) Nursing process phase: analysis; client need: health promotion and maintenance; content area: pediatric nursing

Rationale

(A) Development does not progress at the same rate or pace in children. The focus of development shifts at successive stages. One type of development seems to take precedence over another during various periods of growth. (B) There is a fixed, precise order to development. (C) The rate of growth among children is unpredictable. There are periods of accelerated growth and periods of decelerated growth. (D) There is no correlation between developmental milestones and the rate of growth.

416. (D) Nursing process phase: analysis and planning; client need: health promotion and maintenance; content area: pediatric nursing

Rationale

(A) Ordinarily, a head-to-toe assessment provides a guideline for assessment and minimizes omitting segments of the exam. However, when examining children, alter the sequence to accommodate the child's developmental needs. (B) Perform all traumatic procedures last. (C) Allow the toddler to inspect equipment; however, demonstrating the use of equipment is usually ineffective. (D) Minimal physical contact should be used initially, then inspect body area through play, for example, counting fingers and tickling toes.

417. (D) Nursing process phase: analysis and planning; client need: health promotion and maintenance; content area: pediatric nursing

Rationale

(A–C) The most important factor in accurately measuring the BP is the use of an appropriate size cuff. Two measure methods may be used, the limb length and limb circumference. If using the limb length, a width sufficient to cover 75 percent of the upper arm is necessary. Coverages of 25, 33, and 50 percent are all too small and would result in a falsely high BP measurement. (D) The BP cuff should cover 75 percent of the child's upper arm to obtain an accurate measurement.

418. (D) Nursing process phase: analysis and planning; client need: health promotion and maintenance; content area: pediatric nursing

Rationale

(A) The cover test is used to assess binocularity and to determine if strabismus exists. (B) Snellen's E chart uses the capital letter E pointing in four directions. It may be used with preschoolers; however, preschool children often have difficulty with direction despite adequate vision. (C) The "Lazy E" acuity chart is not ideal because preschoolers may not have the perceptual abilities needed to determine in which direction the "legs" of the E are pointing. (D) A picture acuity chart or the Blackbird system should be used with this population.

419. (D) Nursing process phase: assessment; client need: physiological integrity; content area: pediatric nursing

Rationale

(A) Palpating the carotid artery provides information concerning the pulse. (B) Inspecting the buccal membranes provides assessment data related to cyanosis. (C) Auscultating the heart provides assessment data concerning heart sound.

(D) Press the skin lightly on a central site, such as the forehead, or the top of the hand to produce a slight blanching. The time it takes for the blanched area to return to its original color is the capillary refill time.

420. (A) Nursing process phase: implementation; client need: health promotion and maintenance; content area: pediatric nursing

Rationale

(A) The Denver II tells what a child can do at a particular age if the child's behavior is typical of his or her behavior at other times. (B) The Denver II does not measure intelligence. (C & D) The Denver II is a screening test. It does not measure development. Development is a dynamic process. The Denver II should be used as one part of a developmental surveillance. The child's "whole picture" needs to be assessed and one should not rely solely on the information from a screening procedure.

421. (D) Nursing process phase: analysis and planning; client need: health promotion and maintenance; content area: pediatric nursing

Rationale

(A) Pneumonia and influenza account for 1.6 percent of the deaths of infants and rank as the ninth leading cause of death. (B) Respiratory distress syndrome is the fourth leading cause of death and is responsible for 7 percent of the deaths of infants. (C) Sudden infant death syndrome is the second leading cause of death with 14.5 percent of all deaths being attributed to this cause. (D) Congenital anomalies are the leading cause of infant mortality, accounting for over 20 percent of those deaths.

422. (A) Nursing process phase: analysis and planning; client need: health promotion and maintenance; content area: pediatric nursing

Rationale

(A) Injuries are the leading cause of death until people reach their forties. Injuries account for 45 percent of all childhood death from ages 1 to 14. (B) Congenital anomalies are second among children ages 1 to 14, accounting for 12 percent of deaths. (C) Deaths as a result of HIV infections account for 1.8 percent among children ages 1 to 14; however, this rate is increasing. (D) In children between 1 and 14, 9.2 percent of deaths are caused by cancer.

423. (C) Nursing process phase: analysis and planning; client need: health promotion and maintenance; content area: pediatric nursing

Rationale

(A) Fires and burns are the third leading cause of mortality in children aged 1 to 14. (B) The second leading cause of death in childhood is drowning. (C) The overwhelming cause of death in children over the age of 1 is motor vehicle accidents. The majority of the fatalities involve occupants who are unrestrained. (D) Bicycle injuries are another important cause of childhood deaths, especially from head injuries. Children infrequently wear helmets and parents are often unaware of their importance.

424. (D) Nursing process phase: analysis and planning; client need: health promotion and maintenance; content area: pediatric nursing

Rationale
(A) Although growing, HIV infections are the sixth leading cause of death in late adolescence. (B) In late adolescence, 11.9 percent of deaths are caused by cancer. (C) Suicide rates have increased sharply—75 percent for ages 10 to 14 and 34.5 percent for ages 15 to 19. Suicide is the third leading cause of death in this age group. (D) Homicide is the second leading cause of death in late adolescence. Firearm homicide is the leading cause of death among black males aged 15 to 19 years.

425. (C) Nursing process phase: implementation; client need: health promotion and maintenance; content area: pediatric nursing

Rationale
(A) Both are administered at 6 months, but there are other vaccines also to be given. This is an incomplete answer. (B) MMR is not given until 12 months of age. (C) These four immunizations are recommended at 6 months of age if the child is current with the recommended schedule. (D) VZV is not recommended for administration until 12 months of age.

426. (D) Nursing process phase: implementation; client need: physiological integrity; content area: pediatric nursing

Rationale
(A) Arterial blood sampling is painful and unnecessary for accurate blood sugars. (B) The center of the heel is not appropriate because more nerve endings are located there. (C) In infants, the heel is recommended. Also, a finger stick site is to the side of the finger pad because there are more blood vessels and fewer nerves lateral to the finger pad. (D) The boundaries for a heel puncture can be marked by an imaginary line extending posteriorly from a point between the fourth and fifth toes running parallel to the lateral aspect of the heel and another line extending posteriorly from the middle of the great toe and running parallel to the medial aspect of the heel. The puncture sites are the outer aspects of the heel defined by the identified lines.

427. (C) Nursing process phase: evaluation; client need: physiological integrity; content area: pediatric nursing

Rationale
(A) The normal SaO_2 range is 95–99%. (B) An SaO_2 of 80% equals PO_2 of 45 mm Hg. (C) A consistent SaO_2 of 90% signifies developing hypoxia and equals a PO_2 of 60 mm Hg. (D) Eating does not affect the accuracy of the SaO_2 measurement.

428. (A) Nursing process phase: implementation; client need: physiological integrity; content area: pediatric nursing

Rationale
(A) The myelomeningocele is prevented from drying by the application of a sterile, moist, nonadherent dressing over the sac. (B) Before surgery, the infant is kept in the prone position to minimize tension on the sac and the risk of trauma. (C) Diapering the infant is contraindicated until the defect has been repaired and healing is well advanced. (D) The infant is placed in an incubator or warmer so that temperature can be maintained without clothing or covers, which may irritate the delicate lesion.

429. (D) Nursing process phase: evaluation; client need: physiological integrity; content area: pediatric nursing

Rationale
(A) An increased intracranial pressure would be indicated if the infant cries when picked up or handled, and quiets when lying still. (B) An increased occipitofrontal circumference indicates increased intracranial pressure. (C) A sagittal fontanelle may be present in infants with Down syndrome. It does not represent an increase in intracranial pressure. (D) Separated cranial sutures are a sign of increased intracranial pressure.

430. (D) Nursing process phase: implementation; client need: physiological integrity; content area: pediatric nursing

Rationale
(A) Antihistamines and steroids may be given to children who are allergic to latex before and after surgery to reduce the possibility of a serious reaction. (B) Caregivers need to be educated about medical items and nonmedical items that will expose the child to latex. (C) Latex allergies in children with spina bifida range from an estimated 18 to 60 percent. Latex allergy is identified as being a serious health hazard. (D) Avoiding latex products is the most important nursing intervention. The establishment of a nonlatex environment is necessary.

431. (B) Nursing process phase: implementation; client need: physiological integrity; content area: pediatric nursing

Rationale
(A) The infant is positioned on the unoperated side to prevent pressure on the shunt valve. (B) Abdominal distention needs to be assessed because the CSF may cause peritonitis or a postoperative ileus as a complication of distal catheter placement. (C) The infant is kept flat to help avert complications resulting from a too rapid reduction of intracranial fluid. If the ventricular size is reduced too rapidly, the cerebral cortex may pull away from the dura and tear small veins, resulting in a subdural hematoma. (D) The shunt should not be pumped to assess function because this may pull choroid plexuses into the ventricular slits of the shunt tubing, possibly causing obstruction. The physician is the only person who should pump the shunt.

432. (C) Nursing process phase: implementation; client need: health promotion and maintenance; content area: pediatric nursing

Rationale
(A) This is a clean catheterization. A sterile catheter is not necessary with each catheterization. (B) Boiling the catheter is not advocated. (C) The catheter is to be washed thoroughly with soap and water, and rinsed completely with clear water. (D) Drying the catheter and storing it take place after the catheter has been washed.

433. (B) Nursing process phase: implementation; client need: physiological integrity; content area: pediatric nursing

Rationale
(A) This is the proper depth to use with infants under the age of 1 year. (B) This is the proper depth for a child from 1 year through 8 years of age. (C) This is the proper depth from 8 years of age through adulthood. (D) This is too deep and not advocated for any age person.

434. (B) Nursing process phase: implementation; client need: physiological integrity; content area: pediatric nursing

Rationale

(A) The carotid pulse is assessed in children over the age of 1 year. (B) The brachial pulse is used to assess circulation in infants from birth to 1 year of age. (C) The femoral pulse is not used in CPR. (D) The radial pulse is not used in CPR.

435. (A) Nursing process phase: implementation; client need: physiological integrity; content area: pediatric nursing

Rationale

(A) For infants through age 8, the breathing pattern is 1 breath every 3 seconds or 20 times per minute. (B) Children over 8 years of age through adulthood would use the rate of 1 breath every 5 seconds or 12 breaths a minute. (C & D) Thirty and 45 breaths per minute are too fast for any age person.

436. (D) Nursing process phase: analysis; client need: physiological integrity; content area: pediatric nursing

Rationale

(A) The use of both hands is done from 8 years of age through adulthood. (B) The heel of one hand is used in children from 1 to 8 years of age. (C) Three fingers are never used. (D) The index and middle fingers are used on newborns to the age of 1 year.

437. (C) Nursing process phase: analysis; client need: physiological integrity; content area: pediatric nursing

Rationale

(A) This would be appropriate if the child becomes unconscious. (B) This would be appropriate if the child is conscious, but unable to cough, talk, or make sounds. (C) This is appropriate because the child is conscious and can still cough and make sounds. The airway is not completely obstructed. (D) These actions would be appropriate for an infant whose airway is obstructed.

438. (B) Nursing process phase: implementation; client need: health promotion and maintenance; content area: pediatric nursing

Rationale

(A) The foramen ovale permits most of the blood to shunt from the right atrium to the left atrium. The blood then goes to the left ventricle, permitting systemic fetal circulation with blood containing a higher oxygen saturation. (B) As the blood shunts from the right atrium to the left atrium, the pulmonary system is bypassed. The fetus receives oxygen from the maternal circulation, therefore permitting the partial bypass of the pulmonary system. (C) The foramen ovale is found in the atrial septum of the heart and does not affect the liver. (D) The superior vena cava returns blood to the heart, bringing the blood to the location of the foramen ovale.

439. (D) Nursing process phase: assessment; client need: safe, effective care environment; content area: pediatric nursing

Rationale

(A) The first and second heart sounds in an infant with coarctation of the aorta are usually normal. Third and fourth sounds do not exist with this diagnosis. (B) Either no murmur will be heard or a systolic murmur from an associated cardiac defect will be heard along the left upper sternal border. A diastolic murmur is not associated with coarctation of the aorta. (C) Pulse pressure differences of 20 mm Hg or greater exist between the upper extremities and the lower extremities. Evaluating the upper and lower extremities with the appropriate-sized cuffs is important. (D) Femoral and pedal pulses will be diminished or absent in infants with coarctation of the aorta.

440. (A) Nursing process phase: analysis; client need: physiological integrity; content area: pediatric nursing

Rationale

(A) Tetralogy of Fallot is the most common cyanotic heart defect, which in its classic form consists of four anomalies—a ventricular septal defect, pulmonary stenosis, an overriding aorta, and ventricular hypertrophy. The blood flow is obstructed from the pulmonary stenosis, decreasing the pulmonary blood flow and shunting blood through the ventricular septal defect, creating a right-to-left shunt, allowing deoxygenated blood to reach the systemic circulation. (B) A ventricular septal defect alone creates a left-to-right shunt. The pressure in the left ventricle is greater than that of the right; therefore, the blood will shunt from the left ventricle to the right ventricle, increasing the blood flow to the lungs. No deoxygenated blood will reach the systemic circulation. (C) In patent ductus arteriosus, the pressure in the aorta is greater than in the pulmonary artery, creating a left-to-right shunt. Oxygenated blood from the aorta flows into the unoxygenated blood of the pulmonary artery. (D) Transposition of the great arteries results in two separate and parallel circulatory systems. The only mixing or shunting of blood is based on the presence of associated lesions.

441. (D) Nursing process phase: implementation; client need: physiological integrity; content area: pediatric nursing

Rationale

(A) The cyanotic infant is well hydrated to keep the hematocrit and blood viscosity within acceptable limits to reduce the risk of CVA. Intravenous fluid replacement and volume expansion would be initiated if needed. Fluids would not be restricted. (B) Meperidine would not be administered because it may cause respiratory depression. Morphine is administered and is helpful in reducing the infundibular spasm that is causing decreased pulmonary blood flow. (C) The infant should be placed in a 100 percent oxygen environment. Usually the oxygen is delivered by face mask. (D) The knee-chest position is helpful in relieving hypoxia. The squatting position is helpful because flexing the legs (1) reduces the return of venous blood from the lower extremities, which is very desaturated, and (2) increases systemic vascular resistance, which diverts more blood flow into the pulmonary artery.

442. (C) Nursing process phase: evaluation; client need: physiological integrity; content area: pediatric nursing

Rationale

(A, B, & D) Although possible complications from the mismanagement of IV infusions, these complications are not related to a right-to-left shunt. (C) Intracardiac shunting of blood from the right side to the left side of the heart allows air in the venous system to go directly to the brain, resulting in an air embolism. Therefore, all IV lines should have filters in place to prevent air from entering the system, and the entire tubing and any syringes used for flushing or administering medications are checked for air. Any air is removed, and all connections are taped securely.

443. (B) Nursing process phase: implementation; client need: health promotion and maintenance; content area: pediatric nursing

Rationale
(A) A toddler is not capable of conceptualizing about the inside of his or her body and is concerned about body intactness; therefore, diagrams would not be useful. Also, the previous evening is too far from the procedure for the toddler to remember the instructions. (B) Simple explanations the morning of the procedure with the parents present are the best developmental strategy to use. Explanations focus on the toddler's need for parental support, body intactness, and short attention span. (C) A relationship between the nurse and the child needs to develop. Also, misinformation may be given to the child. (D) The parents are the child's support system and need to be there to strengthen the child.

444. (D) Nursing process phase: implementation; client need: health promotion and maintenance; content area: pediatric nursing

Rationale
(A) A small bruise may develop around the insertion site and is not a reason for alarm. (B) The site should be kept clean and dry. Tub baths should be avoided for several days; however, the child may shower. (C) Acetaminophen or ibuprofen is the drug of choice if there is pain at the insertion site—not aspirin. (D) The pressure dressing should be removed the day after the catheterization. The site should then be covered with an adhesive bandage for several days.

445. (B) Nursing process phase: implementation; client need: psychosocial integrity; content area: pediatric nursing

Rationale
(A) It is important to discuss with parents the need to treat the child normally, as you do any other children. Be truthful and honest with the child about the heart defect. (B) Parents of children with congenital heart defects go through a grieving process over the loss of their "healthy" child. The nurse needs to recognize these feelings and give the parents a role in the child's care when they are ready. (C) Anger and resentment are normal feelings that must be dealt with appropriately. (D) Parents may go through a second grieving process after the repair of the cardiac defect. During this grieving period, they mourn the loss of the defective child who now may be essentially normal.

446. (C) Nursing process phase: implementation; client need: health promotion and maintenance; content area: pediatric nursing

Rationale
(A) Occasionally the child may vomit. Do not repeat the dose because the amount of digoxin that was absorbed is unknown and serum levels of digoxin that are too high are more dangerous than those that are temporarily to low. (B) To ensure that the entire dose of digoxin is received, never mix it with food or formula. (C) Vomiting, anorexia, and listlessness are all signs of digoxin toxicity and should be reported to the practitioner immediately. (D) If a dose is forgotten for more than 4 hours, advise the parents to skip that dose and continue the next dose as scheduled.

447. (C) Nursing process phase: assessment; client need: safe, effective care environment; content area: pediatric nursing

Rationale
(A) Aplastic crisis is characterized by a lack of reticulocytes in the blood. Platelet and white blood cell counts are usually not depressed. It is usually self-limiting, lasting 5 to 10 days. (B) Vaso-occlusive crisis is the most common type of crisis. Sickled cells become clogged, leading to distal tissue hypoxia and infarction. Joints and extremities are the most commonly affected areas. (C) Dactylitis crisis, or "hand-foot syndrome," causes symmetrical infarction of the bones in the hands and feet, resulting in painful swelling in the soft tissues of the hands and feet. (D) Sequestration crisis occurs as enormous volumes of blood pool within the spleen. The spleen enlarges, causing tenderness. Signs of shock including pallor, tachypnea, and faintness result related to the deficient intravascular volume. This type of crisis is potentially fatal.

448. (A) Nursing process phase: analysis; client need: physiological integrity; content area: pediatric nursing

Rationale
(A) Maintaining the hydration level is the focus for nursing intervention because dehydration enhances the sickling process. Both oral and parenteral fluids are used. (B) The pain is a result of the sickling process. Analgesics or narcotics will be used for symptom relief, but the underlying etiology of the pain will be resolved with hydration. (C) Serious bacterial infections may result because of splenic dysfunction. This is true at all times, not just during the acute period of a crisis. (D) Oxygen therapy is used as a symptomatic relief for the hypoxia resulting from the sickling process. Hydration is the primary intervention to alleviate the dehydration that enhances the sickling process.

449. (D) Nursing process phase: assessment; client need: physiological integrity; content area: pediatric nursing

Rationale
(A) Tachycardia, especially during rest and slight exertion, is an early sign of CHF. (B) A sudden weight gain would be indicative of fluid retention accompanying CHF. (C) Tachypnea is the early assessment finding in CHF. (D) Profuse scalp sweating is an early indicator of CHF, especially in infants.

450. (C) Nursing process phase: analysis; client need: physiological integrity; content area: pediatric nursing

Rationale
(A & B) The infant is in mild respiratory distress with tachypnea. Bottle feeding would be too tiring, and he would not receive adequate fluids and nutrition. (C) Gavage feedings will allow the infant to rest and will supply the needed nutrition. Enteral feedings are preferred over IV hydration because more calories can be given. (D) Fluid restriction is not needed, because the infant is behind in fluid intake and furosemide therapy has begun. Further fluid restriction would risk dehydration.

451. (B) Nursing process phase: implementation; client need: physiological integrity; content area: pediatric nursing

Rationale
(A, C, & D) 0.5 ml is too little, and 1.0 ml and 3.0 ml are too much. (B) To begin with, the body weight is converted to

kilograms: $11/2.2 = 5$ kg. The infant is to receive 30 μg for each kilogram of body weight: $30 \times 5 = 150$ μg of digoxin in 24 hours. The 150 μg of digoxin is to be given in four equally divided doses: $150/4 = 37.5$ μg in each dose. The elixir available is 50 μg of digoxin in each milliliter: $37.5/50 = 0.75$ ml. Therefore, the correct quantity to be administered is 0.75 ml.

452. (A) Nursing process phase: evaluation; client need: physiological integrity; content area: pediatric nursing

Rationale
(A) The serum potassium level falls within the normal range of 3.5 to 5.5 mmol/L. Careful monitoring should be continued because the level of serum potassium will enhance or diminish the effect of digoxin. (B) If the potassium level was low, it would enhance the effects of digoxin and increase the risk for digoxin toxicity. (C) If the potassium level was too high, an increased serum potassium level diminishes digoxin's effect. (D) The potassium level is significant because of its effect on digoxin. Also, furosemide causes the excretion of potassium; therefore, the infant is at risk for developing a potassium imbalance.

453. (A) Nursing process phase: analysis; client need: safe, effective care environment; content area: pediatric nursing

Rationale
(A) A neutral thermal environment is necessary to prevent cold stress in infants, which would increase the metabolic demand. (B) The proper position in which to place the infant to decrease metabolic needs would be a semi-Fowler's position. This is accomplished by elevating the head of the infant's crib or by placing the infant in an infant seat. This position would reduce the effort to breath. (C) If an infant is irritable and cannot be soothed, medication may be required to sedate the infant to decrease the metabolic demand. (D) Environmental stimuli should be decreased to promote rest for the infant.

454. (C) Nursing process phase: evaluation; client need: physiological integrity; content area: pediatric nursing

Rationale
(A) An infant should produce 2 to 3 ml/kg per hour of urine. When calculated, the amount of urine the infant should have excreted would be 7 to 11 cc/hr or 28 to 44 cc over the 4-hour period. Therefore, the amount of urine is not adequate. (B) As calculated in part A, the amount of urine does not exceed the normal range. (C) The amount of urine produced falls below the expected range. The practitioner should be notified of the oliguria. (D) Infants younger than 1 year of age normally void every 1 to 2 hours. Four hours is an adequate time frame to use to assess output.

455. (D) Nursing process phase: assessment; client need: safe, effective care environment; content area: pediatric nursing

Rationale
(A) The intermittent infusion device maintains access to a vein if needed without multiple venipunctures being necessary. (B) The tympanic thermometer prevents using the rectal route and possible rectal damage. (C) Special care is given to avoid performing skin punctures, so finger sticks, IM injections, venipunctures, and bone marrow tests are avoided whenever possible. (D) The nurse needs to assess whether the oxy-

gen is being humidified. The nose is vascular and can bleed easily if the mucosa is dried by the oxygen. Also, the placement of the nasal prongs needs to be inspected to determine if signs of irritation exist.

456. (A) Nursing process phase: implementation; client need: physiological integrity; content area: pediatric nursing

Rationale
(A) Bland, moist, soft diets should be provided to prevent irritation and further trauma to the mucosa. (B) Lemon glycerin swabs should not be used because of the drying effect on the mucosa and the irritation of the lemon on the eroded tissue. (C) Viscous lidocaine is not recommended for young children because it may depress the gag reflex, increasing the risk for aspiration. (D) Mouth care is done routinely before and after every meal and as often as every 2 to 4 hours to rid the mucosal surface of debris, which is an excellent medium for bacterial and fungal infections.

457. (D) Nursing process phase: assessment; client need: physiological integrity; content area: pediatric nursing

Rationale
(A) The formula is to determine the total percentage of neutrophils and multiply it by the WBC count: $(0.07 + 0.07) \times 1000 = 140$ ANC. (B) $(0.05 + 0.08) \times 1300 = 169$ ANC. (C) $(0.04 + 0.06) \times 1200 = 120$ ANC. (D) $(0.05 + 0.04) \times 1100 = 99$ ANC

458. (D) Nursing process phase: implementation; client need: physiological integrity; content area: pediatric nursing

Rationale
(A) Do not move the child until emergency personnel arrive and appropriate steps to maintain spinal stability may be followed to prevent further injury. (B) Temperature maintenance is difficult in young children, who have a larger surface area related to body mass. This is not true in adolescents. (C) The area of injury would be assessed following level of consciousness, ABC's (airway, breathing, circulation), and hemorrhage. (D) The first assessment should be of the level of consciousness using the AVPU method (alert, responds to verbal stimuli, responds to painful stimuli, and unresponsive to stimuli).

459. (A) Nursing process phase: analysis; client need: physiological integrity; content area: pediatric nursing

Rationale
(A) Once applied, a tourniquet is not removed or loosened. Below the tourniquet site, the skin and tissue have begun to necrose. If the tourniquet is removed or loosened, this allows the release of high concentrations of toxins into the circulation, which may induce a systemic, deadly, tourniquet shock. (B) If a tourniquet had *not* been applied, the first step in controlling bleeding would be to apply direct pressure to the wound site. (C) If a tourniquet had *not* been applied, the second step in controlling bleeding is to elevate the wound site. (D) If a tourniquet had *not* been applied, the third step in controlling bleeding is to apply pressure to the appropriate arterial pressure point.

460. (C) Nursing process phase: analysis; client need: physiological integrity; content area: pediatric nursing

Rationale
(A) The daily stresses on bones created by motion and weight bearing maintain the balance between bone formation and bone reabsorption. With immobility, the stresses are diminished, and bone formation ceases. Bone calcium becomes severely depleted, making the skeletal structures prone to pathological fractures and increasing serum calcium ion concentrations, or hypercalcemia. (B) Joint mobility is decreased and leads to the formation of contracture. (C) Without muscle contraction, the venous stasis and increased intravascular pressure in the extremities lead to dependent edema. Edematous tissue is prone to infection and trauma. (D) An increased workload on the heart is the result of the horizontal position and immobility, which alter the distribution of blood within the body. There is an increase in venous return and the volume of blood to be handled by the heart, resulting in an increase in blood pressure and heart rate.

461. **(B)** Nursing process phase: analysis; client need: physiological integrity; content area: pediatric nursing

Rationale
(A) Symptoms of hypercalcemia associated with bone catabolism include nausea and vomiting, polydipsia, polyuria, and lethargy. (B) Polydipsia is a symptom of hypercalcemia. (C) High levels of serum calcium decrease neuronal permeability, which can lead to the depression of the central and peripheral nervous system. (D) Symptoms of nervous system involvement include smooth and skeletal muscle fatigue, diminished reflexes, and atony of the gastrointestinal tract.

462. **(B)** Nursing process phase: implementation; client need: safe, effective care environment; content area: pediatric nursing

Rationale
(A) Frequent position changes and TED stockings help to prevent dependent edema, which impairs healing. (B) Placing the child in an upright position on a tilt table increases the stress on bones, which promotes bone formation and prevents bone demineralization. (C) A negative nitrogen balance develops as a result of catabolism, which may occur if the child does not consume adequate quantities of protein to meet the metabolic needs of the body. (D) Thrombus develops as a result of circulatory stasis combined with hypercoagulability. Muscle contraction promotes venous return and prevents venous stasis—not an upright position.

463. **(C)** Nursing process phase: implementation; client need: physical integrity; content area: pediatric nursing

Rationale
(A) The epiphyseal plate is the weakest point in long bones and, consequently, is a frequent site of damage during trauma. (B) Healing is usually prompt with epiphyseal injuries. (C) The epiphyseal plate plays a major role in the longitudinal growth of the developing child. Therefore, early and correct assessment is essential to minimize the incidence of longitudinal growth problems and angular deformities. (D) The medical management is different from that for other fractures because an open reduction and internal fixation are often employed to prevent complications.

464. **(B)** Nursing process phase: implementation; client need: health promotion and maintenance; content area: pediatric nursing

Rationale
(A) Heated driers are not to be used, since they cause the cast to dry on the outside and remain wet underneath, thus becoming moldy. They also cause burns from heat conduction by way of the cast to underlying tissue. (B) The movement and sensation of the visible extremities are to be checked frequently to determine if neurovascular complications are developing. (C) Observations of pain, swelling, discoloration of the exposed extremity, lack of pulsation and warmth, or the inability to move the exposed parts are to be reported immediately. The cast can become like a tourniquet, shutting off circulation and producing neurovascular complications. (D) The casted extremity should be kept elevated on pillows or similar support for the first 24 hours to decrease edema and to facilitate venous return.

465. **(D)** Nursing process phase: assessment; client need: physiological integrity; content area: pediatric nursing

Rationale
(A & B) An assessment finding indicating possible circulatory compromise leading to neurovascular complications should be reported immediately. (C) This assessment finding is normal and requires no action. (D) If hot spots develop, they may indicate infection and should be reported. A window may be made in the cast to observe the site.

466. **(A)** Nursing process phase: analysis; client need: psychosocial integrity; content area: pediatric nursing

Rationale
(A) A toy phone is safe, and children from 1 to 7 years of age enjoy imitating adult behavior with replicas of adult tools. (B) The child does not have the mobility to retrieve the bean bags and could become frustrated. (C) The game of checkers is too advanced developmentally. Rules exist to be followed, and waiting is necessary for alternating turns. Children 8 to 12 become more interested in playing games. (D) Marbles are a safety issue. They are small and, if placed in the child's mouth, could result in choking.

467. **(C)** Nursing process phase: assessment; client need: physiological integrity; content area: pediatric nursing

Rationale
(A) The increased strength and vigor during adolescence may tempt adolescents to overextend themselves. (B) Rapidly growing bones, joints, muscles, and tendons are especially vulnerable to unusual strain. (C) Adolescents may not possess the insight or judgment to recognize when an activity is beyond their capability. (D) More injuries occur during recreational sports participation than in organized athletic competition.

468. **(D)** Nursing process phase: analysis; client need: physiological integrity; content area: pediatric nursing

Rationale
(A) Icing the injury reduced the pain threshold. (B) The decreased temperature slows the tissue metabolism. (C) Edema formation is reduced as fewer histaminelike substances are released. (D) Nine to 15 minutes of ice exposure produce a deep-tissue vasodilation without increasing metabolism.

469. **(C)** Nursing process phase: implementation; client need: health promotion and maintenance; content area: pediatric nursing

Rationale

(A) Shin splints are a serious injury experienced by athletes who run extensively. (B) Walking will not reduce the pain—rest is necessary. (C) Ice, rest, and a nonsteroidal anti-inflammatory medication are the treatment for pain. (D) Shin splints are not a form of stress fractures. Shin splints result from the ligaments tearing away from the tibial shaft.

470. (C) Nursing process phase: implementation; client need: health promotion and maintenance; content area: pediatric nursing

Rationale

(A) Administration of growth hormone should begin in pre-pubertal children. (B) Replacement therapy is based on radiological evidence of epiphyseal closure, which is a criterion for ending therapy. (C) Therapy for growth hormone replacement requires daily subcutaneous injections administered at bedtime. (D) Even when hormone replacement is successful, these children attain their eventual adult height at a slower rate than their peers.

471. (D) Nursing process phase: assessment; client need: physiological integrity; content area: pediatric nursing

Rationale

(A–C) The listed ages are too old to be classified as precocious puberty. (D) Manifestations of sexual development before age 9 in boys and age 8 in girls are considered precocious and should be investigated.

472. (B) Nursing process phase: analysis; client need: physiological integrity; content area: pediatric nursing

Rationale

(A) The gradual development of hyperactivity, irritability, short attention span, and exophthalmos are not related to, or characteristic of, prepubescence. (B) The stated symptoms match the clinical features of hyperthyroidism. The most common cause of hyperthyroidism in children is Graves' disease, with a peak incidence at 12 to 14 years of age. (C) Impaired growth and development are the presenting symptoms of hypothyroidism. (D) Polyuria and polydipsia are the primary clinical manifestations of diabetes insipidus.

473. (D) Nursing process phase: implementation; client need: physiological integrity; content area: pediatric nursing

Rationale

(A) Immediate care would include relocating to a cooler environment and resting. (B) Antipyretics are of no value. (C) Sweating may or may not be present. Until the sodium level can be accurately evaluated, replacement of sodium is not recommended. (D) To cool the boy, after moving to a cooler environment, extra clothing is removed, cool towels are applied, and fans may be used if available.

474. (B) Nursing process phase: implementation; client need: psychosocial integrity; content area: pediatric nursing

Rationale

(A) A plastic molded jacket will be worn following surgery to provide external stabilization of the spine while the girl resumes activities. (B) There is usually some degree of paralytic ileus following the surgery, creating the need for nasogastric intubation. Urinary retention is common, so an indwelling catheter is frequently used for the first 48 hours. (C) Considerable pain is often experienced for the first few days following the surgery and requires the administration of pain medication, preferably the use of opioids administered on a regular schedule, as opposed to "as needed." (D) Activity is begun by instructing the girl to roll from a side-lying position to a sitting position. Next, walking slowly with the aid of a walker and safety belt is allowed. Finally, unassisted ambulation is allowed and is usually achieved by the sixth postoperative day.

475. (A) Nursing process phase: implementation; client need: physiological integrity; content area: pediatric nursing

Rationale

(A) During the acute phase, any movement of the affected limb will cause discomfort. Therefore, moving and turning are carried out carefully and gently to minimize discomfort. (B) Warm compresses are not recommended. Pain medication or sedation may be necessary for pain control. (C) The affected limb should be supported and casts may be required to immobilize the affected limb. (D) The child may have a poor appetite. High-calorie liquids should be encouraged. During convalescence, adequate nutrition must be maintained to aid healing and reconstitution of new bone.

476. (D) Nursing process phase: planning; client need: physiological integrity; content area: pediatric nursing

Rationale

(A) Providing moist heat to the joints has been found to be the best for relieving pain and stiffness. (B) Administering anti-inflammatory drugs, not acetaminophen, helps suppress the inflammatory process leading to pain. (C) Exercising painful swollen joints will aggravate the pain. (D) Provision of a well-balanced diet will avoid excess weight gain, which will cause additional strain and further inflammation of the joints.

477. (D) Nursing process phase: assessment; client need: safe, effective care environment; content area: pediatric nursing

Rationale

(A) Stool pH would detect carbohydrate malabsorption, and BUN will provide information concerning fluid and electrolyte balance. However, obtaining these tests is not an independent nursing function. (B) Again, drawing blood for electrolytes and testing stool for blood are not independent nursing interventions. (C) Stool-reducing substance and stool cultures must be ordered from their physician. (D) Since dehydration and electrolyte imbalances are common with diarrhea, important initial nursing interventions include assessment of the child's hydration status, including vital signs, weight, urine specific gravity, and input-output. All of these assessment finding are independent nursing actions.

478. (C) Nursing process phase: analysis; client need: physiological integrity; content area: pediatric nursing

Rationale

(A) A blood pressure of 78/50 is an acceptable low reading for a 6-year-old. (B) Decreased breath sounds are more consistent with a pneumothorax than heart surgery, mediastinal tubes and tamponade. (C) Jugular vein distention means that there are increased pressures associated with the cardiovascular system. This is an emergency and needs immediate attention. (D) A pulse rate of 100 is an acceptable high limit for a resting 6-year-old.

479. (C) Nursing process phase: analysis; client need: physiological integrity; content area: pediatric nursing

Rationale
(A) This is an acceptable blood pressure for the child's age and is only slightly decreased from post chest tube insertion vital signs. (B) Pain on the left side is expected due to the trauma received on that side. (C) Decreased movement on the left side of the chest is indicative of a tension pneumothorax and is a medical emergency. There is an increase in intrathoracic pressure, resulting in a decrease of air movement in the left lung. (D) This is an increase above normal and should be watched. An elevated pulse is indicative of respiratory problems as well as pain.

480. (A) Nursing process phase: analysis; client need: physiological integrity; content area: pediatric nursing

Rationale
(A) Chest tightness is a symptom of an allergic reaction that can occur with the infusion of gamma globulin. Gamma globulin is considered a blood product. (B) Dysuria is not a symptom of an immediate reaction to gamma globulin. (C) An adverse reaction to gamma globulin is a decrease in blood pressure, not an increase. (D) Tenderness at the IV site does occur with the infusion of gamma globulin and should be closely watched.

481. (C) Nursing process phase: assessment; client need: physiological integrity; content area: pediatric nursing

Rationale
(A) With high doses of aspirin therapy, there will be a decrease in platelet aggregation. (B) Peripheral edema is not associated with high doses of aspirin. (C) Tinnitus is a classic adverse reaction in aspirin therapy and should be reported to the physician. (D) Urticaria is a symptom of an allergic reaction, but this is not an occurrence seen in aspirin therapy.

482. (B) Nursing process phase: implementation; client need: health promotion and maintenance; content area: pediatric nursing

Rationale
(A) It is important to record the child's temperature because symptoms can recur; however, it is only recommended to take temperature for several days after the last elevation. (B) The MMR should be delayed for approximately 5 months because the antibodies acquired during gamma globulin infusion can decrease the effectiveness of the live virus. (C) Low-dose aspirin therapy can be indefinite, depending on the severity of the coronary involvement. (D) Parents should be notified that irritability in their child can occur for up to 2 months from the onset of symptoms.

483. (B) Nursing process phase: assessment; client need: safe, effective care environment; content area: pediatric nursing

Rationale
(A) The onset of regular insulin is one-half to 1 hour; hypoglycemia expected with peak. (B) The peak of regular insulin occurs in 2 to 4 hours and this is the time the nurse can expect the reaction if it occurs. (C) The duration of the regular insulin is 6 to 8 hours. (D) NPH insulin peaks in 6 to 8 hours.

484. (A) Nursing process phase: analysis, client need: safe, effective care environment; content area: pediatric nursing

Rationale
(A) Fifteen grams of carbohydrates are recommended for a glucose level between 60 and 80. (B) Thirty grams of carbohydrates are recommended for a glucose level between 40 and 60. (C) Forty-five grams total may need to be given eventually, but the initial amount for this glucose level is 15 grams. In 30 minutes, recheck the glucose level and if it is still between 60 and 80 give another 15 grams of carbohydrates. This process may be repeated until an appropriate glucose reading is obtained. (D) This glucose will continue to drop if no action is taken and could eventually produce coma.

485. (D) Nursing process phase: implementation; client need: physiological integrity; content area: pediatric nursing

Rationale
(A) This is part of what the test indicates, but the test is to measure the average glucose for the last 3 months, which determines control of diabetes. (B) This test is accepted as indicating indirectly the adherence of the client, but the rationale for the test is to measure control. (C) This test does measure the control of diabetes, but is not a direct measure of insulin utilization. (D) This is the best answer because it includes specifics as to why the test is done.

486. (D) Nursing process phase: implementation; client need: safe, effective care environment; content area: pediatric nursing

Rationale
(A) The onset of the regular insulin is just beginning at this time and the NPH insulin is just beginning to peak. Therefore, hypoglycemia will not occur until later. (B) Both the regular and NPH insulins are just beginning to peak. Therefore, hypoglycemia would not occur until later. (C) The regular insulin is peaking, but the NPH insulin has not reached the peak stage. (D) Both insulins are peaking. The regular insulin is reaching the end of the peak stage and the NPH insulin is just beginning to peak.

487. (A) Nursing process phase: implementation; client need: physiological integrity; content area: pediatric nursing

Rationale
(A) A half-cup of apple juice is 15 gms of carbohydrates. (B) One cup of milk is equal to 15 gms of carbohydrates; therefore, a half-cup is 8 gms. (C) This combination is approximately 45 gms of carbohydrates. The orange juice (½ cup) is 15 gms and the sugar is 30 gms. (D) One cup of orange juice is equal to 30 gms of carbohydrates.

488. (A) Nursing process phase: analysis; client need: physiological integrity; content area: pediatric nursing

Rationale
(A) The client is considered to be neutropenic when the absolute neutrophil count is 1000 or less. (B) The result 2500 is the low side of normal and should be watched closely. (C) Normal neutrophil count falls between 2500 and 7000. (D) The level 10,000 is above the normal range.

489. (A) Nursing process phase: assessment; client need: physiological integrity; content area: pediatric nursing

Rationale

(A) A platelet count of <20,000 can result in spontaneous bleeding. (B) A platelet count of <50,000 indicates thrombocytopenia and precautions must be taken to decrease the chance of bleeding. (C) A platelet count of 100,000 is below normal and the client is considered to be thrombocytopenic, but signs and symptoms are usually not apparent if the count is above 50,000. (D) A normal platelet count is considered to be between 150,000 and 450,000.

490. (D) Nursing process phase: implementation; client need: safe, effective care environment; content area: pediatric nursing

Rationale

(A) Rectal thermometers should not be used on clients with thrombocytopenia. (B) Caution should be taken when brushing teeth. The brushing can cause gum bleeding. Usually, symptoms do not occur until platelet count is <50,000. (C) Aspirin or aspirin-containing products should be prohibited. Aspirin can decrease platelet agglutination. (D) Caution should be taken when using a razor because if a cut occurs, excessive bleeding can result.

491. (D) Nursing process phase: implementation; client need: physiological integrity; content area: pediatric nursing

Rationale

(A) This is a true statement but it doesn't give the mother an explanation and she may not understand what hypoxemia is. (B) Hydration is necessary in dehydration as well as with sickle cell crisis, but we do not know that this client is dehydrated. (C) This statement is true, but it doesn't explain why hydration is more beneficial. (D) This statement is more specific and tells the mother why oxygen is not used and hydration is.

492. (D) Nursing process phase: implementation; client need: physiological integrity; content area: pediatric nursing

Rationale

(A) It is important to assess the parents' knowledge of pain management; however, prevention of crisis and pain should be taught first. (B) This is an appropriate part of the plan, but parents must be taught prevention first. (C) Support groups are beneficial for families, but physiological needs should take priority. (D) Measures to prevent disease activity are the priority because they promote physiological needs and safety for the client.

493. (B) Nursing process phase: analysis; client need: safe, effective care environment; content area: pediatric nursing

Rationale

(A) To get the same effect from oral medicine as intramuscular, it takes approximately four times the dose. (B) Demerol should not be administered longer than 48 hours due to a toxic metabolite, normeperidine. (C) Demerol becomes toxic in 48 hours, but morphine sulfate can be given for a longer duration. (D) Although naloxone (Narcan) is the antidote for Demerol, this is not the most important response relating to Demerol's use in controlling pain.

494. (A) Nursing process phase: assessment; client need: safe, effective care environment; content area: pediatric nursing

Rationale

(A) Muscles are weak and inflamed and these children exhibit difficulty climbing stairs. (B) Muscle weakness occurs symmetrically in the proximal muscles. (C) There is weakness in the neck muscles and the child may have trouble holding head up. (D) These children are often thin and under their normal growth scale with poorly developed muscles.

495. (A) Nursing process phase: implementation; client need: physiological integrity; content area: pediatric nursing

Rationale

(A) Long-term career counseling would be very important. Pain and stiffness that he will experience in the hips and lower back from the disease will limit him to certain career choices. (B) All activities should not be restricted. Heavy sports and activities that would stress the hips and lower back should be restricted. (C) Preventing GI disturbances would be important, but these should be under control early in the disease process. (D) Children and adolescents with rheumatoid arthritis are allowed to have a second set of books, by law.

496. (A) Nursing process phase: implementation; client need: physiological integrity; content area: pediatric nursing

Rationale

(A) A primary action for correcting hypercalcemia is vigorous hydration to promote removal of calcium from the body. (B) Stress to the bone through exercise is important for reabsorption of calcium in the bone. Consulting the physical therapist is appropriate, but exercises must be performed for this to occur. (C) Monitoring the calcium level allows information for assessment, but there is no action for correcting the problem. (D) Notifying the physician is appropriate, but action should be taken to correct the hypercalcemia. The primary action is hydration.

497. (C) Nursing process phase: assessment; client need: safe, effective care environment; content area: pediatric nursing

Rationale

(A) Pain is expected with a fracture due to edema and pressure to the tissue. Pressure on a nerve can cause pain radiation. (B) Pain in the entire extremity can be the result of edema and trauma. Relief from medication is the desired effect. (C) Pain in the area nonresponsive to medication is indicative of a deteriorating neuromuscular status. This would require immediate attention to relieve pressure in the area. (D) Fractures can produce severe pain. Therapeutic management of moderate to severe pain is the administration of narcotics.

498. (B) Nursing process phase: assessment; client need: physiological integrity; content area: pediatric nursing

Rationale

(A) Acceptable range for blood pressure readings for a 16-year-old male is 98/49 to 136/85. The blood pressure, 100/60, falls between the 5th and 50th percentile range for age. (B) Petechiae on the chest is a classic symptom of shock related to pulmonary fat embolism. Immediate attention should be given to this sign. Adolescents are the most likely pediatric population to develop pulmonary emboli. They usually occur within 12 to 24 hours of injury. (C) Control of pain is very important. The nurse should plan a different strategy for pain management. (D) The range for urinary output for a 60 kg client is 30 to 120 ml/hr depending on hydration status. An assessment formula for calculating urinary output is 0.5 to 2 ml/kg/hr. Because this client is 15 hours' postoperative, an appropriate range for this time period is 450 to 1800 ml.

499. (D) Nursing process phase: assessment; client need: physiological integrity; content area: pediatric nursing

Rationale
(A) One reason for using this device is to assist with lengthening the bone. However, lengthening is achieved through distraction, not fusion. The device will keep the bone properly aligned. (B) The Ilizarow external fixation device is designed for manual manipulation to distance the separated bone and allow the new bone tissue to fill in the space. (C) The Ilizarow external fixation device is not used to reduce fractures. It can be used to correct deformities in the bone from the fracture healing at inappropriate angles. (D) The Ilizarow external fixation device is an appliance that allows bone distraction. Separation of bone encourages regeneration of new bone in the space created.

500. (A) Nursing process phase: implementation; client need: physiological integrity; content area: pediatric nursing

Rationale
(A) In order to get the desired traction from the weights applied, they must be hanging freely. If they are not, then the force of pull is less than desired. (B) Neurovascular checks are conducted to assess circulation to the extremity, but they have no effect on the traction's functioning. (C) There are no effects to maintain traction. Checking the effectiveness of the muscle relaxant is important so that a level of comfort can be obtained. However, a purpose of traction is to stress the muscle to fatigue so that the muscle can relax, promoting alignment of the bone. (D) Countertraction is achieved by the body weight, not tightness of the Ace bandage.

501. (A) Nursing process phase: implementation; client need: physiological integrity; content area: pediatric nursing

Rationale
(A) Each of these foods is low in calcium and acceptable on an acid-ash diet. (B) Tuna, carrots, and low-fat milk are considered to be sources of calcium. (C) Shrimp and watermelon are sources of calcium. (D) Cheese, strawberries, and ice cream are sources of calcium.

502. (C) Nursing process phase: planning; client need: health promotion and maintenance; content area: pediatric nursing

Rationale
(A) A goal of collaborative management of juvenile rheumatoid arthritis is to prevent deformities. Once deformities have occurred, then the goal would be to limit further deformities. (B) Maintaining normal growth is important. In order to maintain growth, the joint must maintain functioning so that deformities do not occur. (C) This disease directly affects joint capsules; therefore, the goal would be directed to preserving the joint functioning. If this is maintained, then physical deformities are less likely to occur. (D) Side effects of corticosteroids can't be prevented, but can be minimized. For example, one side effect of corticosteroids is fluid retention. Low-sodium diet is encouraged to reduce fluid retention.

503. (A) Nursing process phase: implementation; client need: safe, effective care environment; content area: pediatric nursing

Rationale
(A) Splints are used to immobilize joints for pain reduction and to prevent flexion contractures during rest and acute inflammatory episodes. (B) The joints should be exercised. Using the joints during normal activities is encouraged. Splints would prevent movement and decrease participation in activities. (C) The child will be active and moving the joints during school. Only during rest or inflammatory periods would the splints be used to decrease pain and contractures. (D) The joints are going to be painful for some children every day. For others it may be episodic. For example, in the morning the joints will be stiff and painful on rising, but the joint should be used rather than put on a splint.

504. (B) Nursing process phase: implementation; client need: safe, effective care environment; content area: pediatric nursing

Rationale
(A) Placing a client in the prone position does expose the posterior side. A posterior assessment of skin can be done side lying as well. This position is not necessary to assess skin posteriorly. (B) Positioning on the abdomen naturally straightens the hips and knees in alignment. (C) The prone position will prevent skin breakdown posteriorly, but pressure points can develop anteriorly; therefore, the position must be changed every few hours. (D) Changing positions can relieve pain when joints have been in one place too long and become stiff.

505. (C) Nursing process phase: implementation; client need: safe, effective care environment; content area: pediatric nursing

Rationale
(A) Exercises before school are good, but taking medication first before attempting exercises would be easier for the child. (B) The warmth is a good strategy, but the joints will be stiff from no movement. (C) Giving the medicine will be the best strategy for combating morning stiffness. (D) A warm bath will help the client move the joints more easily. This, in combination with the onset of medicine, will make it easier.

506. (B) Nursing process phase: planning; client need: health promotion and maintenance; content area: pediatric nursing

Rationale
(A) When establishing an activity level, begin with a small amount and work up to the prior activity level, if possible. Pay close attention so the child does not become fatigued. Excessive fatigue can cause an exacerbation. (B) Rest is of vital importance. The routine for rest is to get 8 to 10 hours at night with one or two rest periods during the day, preferably one in the morning and the next during the afternoon. (C) Rescheduling school for home-bound status and tutoring may be necessary. If possible, it is best for the child to go to school and plan rest periods at school with the assistance from his teachers and school nurse. (D) It is wise to supervise activi-

ties, but if gradual activity is added back to a tolerance level along with scheduled rest periods, then fatigue will be avoided.

507. (A) Nursing process phase: implementation; client need: health promotion and maintenance; content area: pediatric nursing

Rationale
(A) Sun exposure should be avoided between 10 A.M. and 2 P.M. (B) Clothes should be worn to cover as much of the body as possible, but the sun should be avoided between 10 A.M. and 2 P.M. (C) Sunscreen should be reapplied every 4 hours or when the body becomes wet. (D) Hats are a measure to prevent direct exposure to the sun, but avoiding any sun exposure between 10 A.M. and 2 P.M. is better.

508. (A) Nursing process phase: planning; client need: safe, effective care environment; content area: pediatric nursing

Rationale
(A) Adjustment to the treatment plan promotes adherence, which controls the symptoms and complications of the disease. (B) Managing limitations to social activities is important for psychological needs and role identity. However, the physiological goal is priority goal. (C) Recognizing limitations is part of the importance of adjusting to the treatment plan. (D) It is important to understand adversity to medications, so that if side effects occur, one can take action. If an individual adjusts to the treatment plan, then this is part of that.

509. (D) Nursing process phase: implementation; client need: health promotion and maintenance; content area: pediatric nursing

Rationale
(A) An acid ash diet assists with increasing urine acidity and reducing calcium intake. (B) Often people who have chronic illness need a high protein diet to aid in the repair of tissues and to increase protein levels. However, this question gives no information that the client is protein deficit. (C) A reduced fat diet is good for SLE clients, because if they become overweight, this increases the stress on their joints. However, this question gives the nurse no indication that there is a problem with weight. (D) A low sodium diet is the best diet to choose, because clients on prednisone have a tendency to retain fluid.

510. (B) Nursing process phase: assessment; client need: physiological integrity; content area: pediatric nursing

Rationale
(A) Lupus clients are prone to sun sensitivity. Excessive exposure to sun can trigger an exacerbation. (B) Fatigue is a major indicator of disease activity and should be avoided. Adequate rest enables the body to fight disease and assist with preventing exacerbations. (C) Puffy eyes and edematous ankles are often seen in the client on prednisone therapy. They are not signs of lupus. (D) Malar rash is the classical sign of lupus and the only clinical sign that can confirm the diagnosis. The rash can still be apparent when there is less than a full flare-up.

511. (D) Nursing process phase: implementation; client need: health promotion and maintenance; content area: pediatric nursing

Rationale
(A) It can take up to 4 weeks before there is a therapeutic effect, but the purpose of continuing this drug is to prevent further symptoms. (B) Eosinophils can be increased during allergic reactions. Cromolyn sodium does not work to stabilize eosinophil count; however, it may prevent a rise in the eosinophil count if an allergic reaction is prevented. (C) Cromolyn sodium stabilizes the membranes of sensitized mast cells, thus preventing the release of chemical mediators after an antigen–immunoglobulin E (IgE) interaction. (D) Cromolyn sodium prevents an allergic reaction by stabilizing the membranes of sensitized mast cells, thus prohibiting the release of chemical mediators after exposure to an antigen.

512. (B) Nursing process phase: implementation; client need: safe, effective care environment; content area: pediatric nursing

Rationale
(A) New allergies can develop during immunotherapy. If this were the case, then vaccines for the new allergies must be added to the immunotherapy. One year is not a long enough time period in which to test the effectiveness. (B) The usual time period before symptoms improve is 24 to 48 months. (C) Improvement may take as long as 2 years. (D) The immunotherapy is on a schedule where vaccines are gradually increased as meant until maintenance is obtained.

513. (D) Nursing process phase: implementation; client need: health promotion and maintenance; content area: pediatric nursing

Rationale
(A) Disinfecting the bath and shower reduces the growth of molds. (B) Avoid smoking around children to reduce respiratory infection and improve pulmonary function test. Cigarette smoke is an irritant to the respiratory tract. (C) Exposure to animals will not trigger allergies if someone is not allergic to the animals. (D) One place where dust mites live is carpets. A child playing on carpet has an increased chance of exposure, especially the closer the face and nose are to the carpet.

514. (D) Nursing process phase: implementation; client need: health promotion and maintenance; content area: pediatric nursing

Rationale
(A) Cocoa products will have no effect on those with milk or wheat allergies, unless the cocoa is put in the milk. (B) Popcorn should be avoided by those with corn hypersensitivities. (C) Fish is a common allergen, but tuna has no effect on those with wheat or milk allergies. (D) Wieners should be avoided because they contain milk and wheat products.

515. (D) Nursing process phase: implementation; client need: health promotion and maintenance; content area: pediatric nursing

Rationale
(A) Cola beverages should be avoided by those with chocolate allergy. (B) Gravy should be avoided by those with wheat allergy. (C) Instant breakfast beverages should be avoided by those with milk allergy. (D) Mayonnaise is made with eggs and therefore should be avoided.

516. (C) Nursing process phase: implementation; client need: safe, effective care environment; content area: pediatric nursing

Rationale
(A) Local restrictions do occur, indicating there is an immune response, which is expected. (B) To treat the symptoms it is appropriate to have a medicine ordered that will relieve the discomfort from itching; however, this will not do anything for reactivity. (C) When a client has a local reaction from an allergy shot, it is appropriate to stay at the same dosage the next time. (D) It is not advised to increase the dosage since the client is reacting to extract and could have an anaphylactic reaction.

517. (C) Nursing process phase: implementation; client need: safe, effective care environment; content area: pediatric nursing

Rationale
(A) Barley cereal is fed to infants, but not initially. (B) Oat cereal is another type of cereal that is prepared for infants, but not initially. (C) Rice cereal is the first choice for cereal to be fed to infants because it is easily digested and has low allergenic properties. (D) Wheat has a strong tendency to produce an allergic reaction; therefore, it is not started until later and, even then, alone to see whether the infant will tolerate it.

518. (B) Nursing process phase: implementation; client need: health promotion and maintenance; content area: pediatric nursing

Rationale
(A) Most formulas are iron fortified, and cereals have a high iron content. (B) Cereals are a good source of iron for infants, and vitamin C enhances the absorption of iron. (C) When increasing the amount of solid foods in an infant's diet, the milk is decreased. However, the cereal is dry and must be prepared with a liquid. (D) Mixing two foods together to improve the taste of food is done on a limited basis to promote eating a variety of foods.

519. (C) Nursing process phase: implementation; client need: health promotion and maintenance; content area: pediatric nursing

Rationale
(A) Because of their high iron content, baby cereals should be continued until the child is 18 months old. (B) Eggs are a good source of protein. In order to detect any allergic reaction, the yolk should be introduced first; then egg whites should be introduced in small quantities when the child is close to a year old. (C) This is the appropriate method by which to introduce foods so that allergies can be detected. (D) This is true; however, it does not teach the mother how to introduce solid foods.

520. (B) Nursing process phase: implementation; client need: health promotion and maintenance; content area: pediatric nursing

Rationale
(A) Initially, to prevent abdominal cramping and diarrhea, fruit juice should be diluted until the child adapts. (B) This practice is promoted to avoid prolonging the bottle feeding habit. Prolonged bottle feeding promotes dental caries. (C) The vitamin C in fruit juice enhances iron absorption from cereal; however, fruit juice can be given in another way, especially when the child is eating a variety of foods. (D) Allowing the child to hold and drink from a cup does promote growth and development, but juice from a bottle promotes dental caries.

521. (C) Nursing process phase: implementation; client need: safe, effective care environment; content area: pediatric nursing

Rationale
(A) The pressure range of 50 to 70 would not create enough vacuum. If this range was used initially, it would require insertion of another suction catheter at a higher range, creating unnecessary trauma. (B) The upper range might be adequate if secretions were thin. (C) The recommended range of pressure is 80 to 100 for children. The lower range would be appropriate for thin secretions and the upper range for thick secretions. (D) This pressure range is too high, which could create an hypoxic state and/or atelectasis.

522. (B) Nursing process phase: implementation; client need: safe, effective care environment; content area: pediatric nursing

Rationale
(A) It is an acceptable practice to reuse suction catheters for a 24-hour period if cleaning and sterilizing the catheter are maintained. The absence of sterile technique could result in bacterial infection, but not trauma. (B) To prevent trauma to the respiratory tract, the catheter tip should not exceed the end of the tract tube by more than 0.5 cm. Premeasuring is the best way to decrease trauma. (C) This is one measure to use to prevent hypoxia. Hypoxia can result in tissue damage, but does not cause direct trauma. (D) This is another measure that can cause hypoxia, but not direct trauma.

523. (D) Nursing process phase: implementation; client need: safe, effective care environment; content area: pediatric nursing

Rationale
(A) Coughing suggest the catheter was inserted too far. (B) A decrease in oxygen saturation indicates the need for oxygen. However, this decrease is not a major decrease. (C) Secretions can decrease oxygen saturation; however, to loosen secretions, saline and a ventilating (Ambu) bag are recommended. (D) Bradycardia is a direct indication that the client should be ventilated with high oxygen concentration.

524. (A) Nursing process phase: implementation; client need: safe, effective care environment; content area: pediatric nursing

Rationale
(A) The American Heart Association recommends that suctioning take no more than 5 seconds. (B) This is considered too long a period of time on children. (C) Twenty seconds can result in hypoxia. (D) Thirty seconds can result in hypoxia.

525. (B) Nursing process phase: assessment; client need: physiological integrity; content area: pediatric nursing

Rationale
(A) An acceptable BP range for a 3-year-old is 72/40 to 110/73. (B) An acceptable heart rate for an awake 3-year-old is 70 to 110. A heart rate above this range would indicate tachycardia. Tachycardia is an indication that a tracheostomy client needs suctioning. (C) An oxygen saturation of 95 percent is acceptable. (D) A respiratory rate of 22 for a 3-year-old is acceptable.

526. (D) Nursing process phase: implementation; client

need: safe, effective care environment; content area: pediatric nursing

Rationale

(A) A capillary refill of less than 3 seconds is acceptable. Adequate blood flow is necessary for pulse oximetry to give an accurate reading. (B) Pulse oximetry measures hemoglobin saturation. A person who has low hemoglobin can be easily saturated, which would not reflect a true oxygenation status. (C) Excessive movement can interfere with pulse oximetry readings because the oximeter reads pulsations through blood flow. (D) Bright lights on the sensor can alter the readings because the oximeter is designed to measure light.

527. **(B)** Nursing process phase: implementation; client need: safe, effective care environment; content area: pediatric nursing

Rationale

(A) This dose is less than ordered. (B) The appropriate calculation for this is:

(1) Recommended dose × weight = dose for client
0.01 mg/kg × 14 kg = 0.14 mg

(2) $\dfrac{\text{Dose desired}}{\text{Dose on hand}}$ × quantity in volume = volume to be administered

$$\frac{0.14 \text{ mg}}{1 \text{ mg}} \times 1 \text{ ml} = 0.14 \text{ ml}$$

(C) This dose is too large.
(D) This dose is too large.

528. **(B)** Nursing process phase: evaluation; client need: safe, effective care environment; content area: pediatric nursing

Rationale

(A) Epinephrine administered subcutaneously has a time of onset of at least 5 minutes. (B) The time of onset for subcutaneous epinephrine is between 5 and 10 minutes. (C) The peak time for subcutaneous epinephrine is 20 minutes. (D) The duration of subcutaneous epinephrine is 20 to 30 minutes.

529. **(D)** Nursing process phase: assessment; client need: safe, effective care environment; content area: pediatric nursing

Rationale

(A) Nasal flaring is an effort that assists with a more efficient gas exchange, but it also indicates an increased effort in breathing. (B) Nasal flaring indicates an increased effort in breathing caused by the infection, but more specifically because there is an increase in resistance to air flow. (C) Nasal flaring can occur when there are increased secretions. Nasal flaring can occur without increased secretions when resistance to air flow is present. (D) This statement is the most accurate because it specifically explains the purpose of nasal flaring—to reduce resistance to air flow. Nasal flaring occurs because there is resistance to air flow, and it is compensatory to reduce resistance.

530. **(A)** Nursing process phase: implementation; client need: safe, effective care environment; content area: pediatric nursing

Rationale

(A) Since it is the most distal site, this site is best for an initial

attempt. (B) The feet should be avoided in the child who is walking. (C) The antecubital fossa should be avoided because it restricts movement. (D) Scalp veins are usually reserved as sites in infants.

531. **(D)** Nursing process phase: assessment; client need: safe, effective care environment; content area: pediatric nursing

Rationale

(A) Allergic reactions produce symptoms such as rash, itching, urticaria, wheezing, and signs of respiratory edema and possibly anaphylaxis. (B) Circulatory overload reactions include signs and symptoms such as labored breathing, coughing, lung congestion, increased edema; venous pressure; and chest or back pain. (C) Hemolytic reactions consists of symptoms such as restlessness, fever, chills, increased respiratory rate and heart rate, decreased BP, hematuria, and shock. (D) Septic shock includes signs and symptoms such as chills, fever, headache, decreased BP, nausea and vomiting, and leg and back pain.

532. **(B)** Nursing process phase: implementation; client need: safe, effective care environment; content area: pediatric nursing

Rationale

(A) Nurses should warm blood for trauma clients with large replacement needs. (B) Blood should not be hung longer than 4 hours because there is an increased chance of reaction and infection. (C) Blood should be hung within 30 minutes of receiving it from the blood bank. (D) It is appropriate to hang normal saline, not D5W, along with the blood to prevent clotting.

533. **(A)** Nursing process phase: analysis; client need: safe, effective care environment; content area: pediatric nursing

Rationale

(A) Blow-by is a good method of delivering low concentrations of oxygen and is less confining than other delivery systems. (B) Masks are difficult to fit properly on infants. (C) Infants can tolerate nasal cannulas, but they are more restrictive than other mechanisms. (D) With infants, oxygen hoods are used more frequently than tents. With a tent, assessment of the child is difficult. Furthermore, infants and children are confined and are away from their parents more.

534. **(C)** Nursing process phase: implementation; client need: safe, effective care environment; content area: pediatric nursing

Rationale

(A) The abbreviation OD means right eye, not both eyes. (B) The order is to instill drops into the right eye, not the left ear. (C) The abbreviation OD refers to the right eye, and pulling the lower lid down and forming a reservoir in the conjunctival sac is proper. (D) The order is to instill drops into the right eye, not the right ear. However, this is an appropriate procedure for instilling drops into the ear of a child younger than 3 years old.

535. **(B)** Nursing process phase: implementation; client need: safe, effective care environment; content area: pediatric nursing

Rationale

(A) It is appropriate to keep the child in the same position for a few minutes, but 10 minutes is not required. (B) This is the proper way to expose the ear canal in an older child. (C) Raising the head of the bed is not required. (D) Placing a piece of cotton in the ear is acceptable, but not required.

536. (A) Nursing process phase: implementation; client need: safe, effective care environment; content area: pediatric nursing

Rationale
(A) IV push medicine administration should take less than 10 minutes. (B) The IV piggyback method confines the child more, but the route chosen is in accordance with pharmaceutical recommendations. (C) If medicines are given too fast, an allergic response can occur. (D) When there is a choice, this is good consideration for children with certain problems.

537. (B) Nursing process phase: implementation; client need: safe, effective care environment; content area: pediatric nursing

Rationale
(A) Once a child has been walking for a year or is past 5 years old, the dorsogluteal muscle is developed and is the preferred site. (B) A 90-degree angle is appropriate for an intramuscular injection. (C) Aspiration should be done with vaccines as with other medications. (D) For intramuscular injections, 0.5 to 1-inch needles are recommended.

538. (A) Nursing process phase: implementation; client need: safe, effective care environment; content area: pediatric nursing

Rationale
(A) The vastus lateralis is appropriate for an intramuscular injection in a child of this age. (B) A 90-degree angle is recommended for an intramuscular injection in order to pass through subcutaneous tissue and reach the muscle. (C) Pulling the skin taut is recommended for intramuscular instead of subcutaneous injections. (D) A ⅜- to ⅝-inch, 25- or 26-gauge needle is recommended subcutaneously.

539. (A) Nursing process phase: analysis; client need: safe, effective care environment; content area: pediatric nursing

Rationale
(A) The deltoid muscle has developed and is an acceptable site. (B) The vastus lateralis muscle is appropriate, but can make the leg sore and thus interrupt walking. (C) The dorsogluteal muscle is not recommended until after the child is 5 years old. (D) The gluteal muscles are not ideal sites even though the muscles may be developed by 4 years old.

540. (C) Nursing process phase: analysis; client need: safe, effective care environment; content area: pediatric nursing

Rationale
(A) This is the minimum recommended dose for pain relief. (B) This is the middle range recommended dose for pain control. (C) This is the maximum recommended dose allowed. (D) This exceeds the maximum dose recommended.

541. (A) Nursing process phase: analysis; client need: physiological integrity; content area: pediatric nursing

Rationale
(A) Chest and lower back are indicative of a reaction caused by circulatory overload. Chest pain can also indicate a hemolytic reaction. (B) Gastrointestinal symptoms such as bleeding are usually not associated with blood transfusion reactions. (C) Hematuria followed by anuria can be associated with a hemolytic reaction, especially if the condition progresses to shock. (D) An increased intake of fluids can create an increased urine output. However, the symptoms of a reaction are a reduction in output or hematuria.

542. (D) Nursing process phase: analysis; client need: safe, effective care environment; content area: pediatric nursing

Rationale
(A) This incorrect dose was derived by omitting the last step in the calculation of the problem, which is dividing dose in milligrams by quantity. (B) This incorrect data was derived by dividing 50 mg into 250 (how the medication supplied). Furthermore, the recommended dose by weight was not obtained first, nor was the quantity per kilogram. (C) This incorrect answer was obtained only by dividing the quantity by the dose per kilogram. (D) To obtain the correct answer, use the following formulas:
Step 1. Recommended dose × wt = dose for client
$$50 \text{ mg/kg} \times 12 \text{ kg} = 600 \text{ mg}$$
Step 2. $\frac{\text{Dose desired}}{\text{Dose on hand}} \times$ quantity in ml = volume to be administered
$$\frac{600 \text{ mg}}{250 \text{ mg}} \times 5 \text{ ml} = 12 \text{ ml}$$

543. (D) Nursing process phase: analysis; client need: safe, effective care environment; content area: pediatric nursing

Rationale
(A) The answer, 8 ml, is derived by the following equations:
$$\frac{50 \text{ ml}}{60} = 8.33 \text{ ml}$$
(B) This answer, 45 ml, would deliver 50 ml in 30 minutes. (C) Setting the pump on 50 would deliver 50 ml/hr. (D) The formula for the pump set-up is:
$$\frac{\text{ml}}{\text{min}} \times \frac{60 \text{ min}}{1 \text{ hr}} = \text{ml/hr}$$
$$\frac{50 \text{ ml}}{45 \text{ min}} \times \frac{60 \text{ min}}{1 \text{ hr}} = \frac{3000}{45} = 66.66 \text{ ml/hr} = 67 \text{ ml/hr}$$

544. (B) Nursing process phase: analysis; client need: safe, effective care environment; content area: pediatric nursing

Rationale
(A) This is a true statement, but the nurse is not responsible for prescribing the medicine. (B) This is the most important factor to know, so signs and symptoms of ototoxicity can be assessed early to prevent permanent damage. (C) Photosensitivity is an adverse reaction when gentamycin is administered topically. (D) Nausea and vomiting are adverse reactions and can be relieved with antiemetics.

545. (B) Nursing process phase: analysis; client need: safe, effective care environment; content area: pediatric nursing

Rationale
(A) This is an acceptably low BP in a 4-year-old. (B) The

nurse should be alert to a decreasing urine output, which can cause renal problems. (C) This is an acceptably high heart rate for an awake 4-year-old. (D) Tarry stools indicate bleeding in the gastrointestinal (GI) tract, which is not noted as an adverse reaction with gentamycin.

546. (B) Nursing process phase: analysis; client need: safe, effective care environment; content area: pediatric nursing

Rationale

(A) Hyperactivity is a common occurrence with children on theophylline. (B) Tachycardia is indicative of a toxic level of theophylline. (C) A respiratory rate of 24 is slightly elevated and should be watched closely. Tachypnea is an adverse effect. (D) A theophylline level of below 20 usually produces no side effects.

547. (A) Nursing process phase: assessment; client need: safe, effective care environment; content area: pediatric nursing

Rationale

(A) During the first few days of TPN administration, the child might not tolerate the high dose of dextrose. Therefore, glucose levels should be monitored to detect hyperglycemia. (B) Infection can be introduced at the catheter insertion site, but signs and symptoms usually are not apparent for 48 to 72 hours after contamination. (C) It is important to monitor input and output—changes can be indicative of an electrolyte imbalance. (D) Excessive weight gain can indicate fluid and electrolyte imbalance.

548. (C) Nursing process phase: implementation; client need: safe, effective care environment; content area: pediatric nursing

Rationale

(A) This is the maximum amount suggested for an infant. (B) This is the maximum amount suggested for a preschooler. (C) This is the maximum amount recommended for a school-age child. (D) This is the maximum amount recommended for an adolescent.

549. (B) Nursing process phase: assessment; client need: health promotion and maintenance; content area: pediatric nursing

Rationale

(A) The normal visual acuity at age 4 years is 20/40. (B) The normal visual acuity at age 6 years is 20/20. Therefore, this would be earliest age at which a child could have this visual acuity. (C) Visual acuity can be 20/20 at age 8 years. (D) Visual acuity can be 20/20 at age 10 years.

550. (D) Nursing process phase: assessment; client need: safe, effective care environment; content area: pediatric nursing

Rationale

(A) This is a measure to determine the appropriate sized endotracheal tube, but would take too long during an emergency. (B) Children above 3 years old are less likely to have a standard size. (C) Uncuffed endotracheal tubes are usually not used in children over 9 years old. (D) The "pinky rule" is a quick measure to determine the appropriate sized endotracheal tube.

551. (C) Nursing process phase: assessment; client need: physiological integrity; content area: pediatric nursing

Rationale

(A) In hypoglycemia, the client would have tachycardia. (B) Skin that has pallor is a sign of hypoglycemia. Flushed skin is a sign of hyperglycemia. (C) In hypoglycemia, clients exhibit irritability and nervousness. (D) Labored breathing is seen in hyperglycemia, and shallow respirations occur in hypoglycemia.

552. (A) Nursing process phase: implementation; client need: safe, effective care environment; content area: pediatric nursing

Rationale

(A) When the residual is greater than half, the residual should be replaced, the physician notified, and another attempt made in 30 minutes. (B) Skipping feedings means a reduction in nutrients and calories in a child who has a compromised GI system. (C) This is appropriate if the residual is between one-quarter and one-half the last feeding. (D) This is appropriate if the residual is less than one-quarter of the amount of the last feeding.

553. (C) Nursing process phase: implementation; client need: health promotion and maintenance; content area: pediatric nursing

Rationale

(A) Board games are good for school-age children. Rules and regulations and playing with others are important at this age. (B) Coloring books and crayons are good for preschoolers to enhance creative expression. (C) Push-pull toys are good for toddlers to enhance walking skills. (D) Puzzles aid preschoolers to develop fine motor skills and stimulate the imagination.

554. (C) Nursing process phase: assessment; client need: psyhcological integrity; content area: pediatric nursing

Rationale

(A) School-age children are at a competitive play stage, so board games played with another child are appropriate play. (B) Infants are learning to manipulate toys, so a music box promotes this and stimulates auditory system. (C) Preschool children are creative; imaginary friends are usual for this age. (D) This is an example of parallel play, which toddlers engage in.

555. (C) Nursing process phase: implementation; client need: psychological integrity; content area: pediatric nursing

Rationale

(A) Do not be too structured with toys. Play should be fun and include the child's favorite toys. (B) Play should be fun and enjoyable, and the emphasis should not always be put on educational aspects. (C) Play is how children learn new skills and abilities that foster intelligence. (D) The choice of baby-sitters should include a person who can act as a playmate.

556. (B) Nursing process phase: assessment; client need: psychological integrity; content area: pediatric nursing

Rationale

(A) Infants are just beginning to learn to manipulate objects and hold things. Some toys can be manipulated such as an activity box in the crib. (B) Preschool children are the age group that the nurse will see playing with the toys the most. Toys aid in social development and promote creativity. (C) School-age children will engage in games and activities that are competitive and promote playing with other children. (D) Adolescents focus on their peer groups and identifying with others.

557. (A) Nursing process phase: assessment; client need: physiological integrity; content area: pediatric nursing

Rationale
(A) The normal appearance for bacterially infected spinal fluid is cloudy and purulent. Virally infected spinal fluid is usually clear. (B) The glucose is elevated in bacterial meningitis and is normal in viral meningitis. (C) In bacterial meningitis, the protein is usually elevated. In viral meningitis, it is normal or only slightly elevated. (D) In bacterial meningitis, the WBC is elevated much higher than in viral cases, where there is only a slight elevation.

558. (B) Nursing process phase: assessment; client need: physiological integrity; content area: pediatric nursing

Rationale
(A) The fontanelle in children with severe inflammation will be bulging; however, the anterior fontanelle in this infant should have closed. There is usually complete closure of the anterior fontanelle by 18 months. (B) Nuchal rigidity caused by meningeal irritation is a classic sign in children with meningitis. (C) Pupils that are equal and react briskly are a normal and desired finding. With increased intracranial pressure, the pupils will become sluggish to react and possible unequal. (D) A temperature of 100°F or above is elevated, which is a symptom of meningitis. However, for this elevation, an antipyretic is usually not prescribed. A temperature is often not treated until it reaches 101.5°F.

559. (A) Nursing process phase: implementation; client need: safe, effective care environment; content area: pediatric nursing

Rationale
(A) The infant seat is no longer used because it increases intra-abdominal pressure, causing an increase in the symptoms associated with gastroesophageal reflux. (B) The position encouraged is prone with the head of bed elevated 30 degrees. (C) The infant seat is no longer used, but the prone position with the head of bed elevated is encouraged. (D) The prone position is advocated over supine position.

560. (B) Nursing process phase: implementation; client need: physiological integrity; content area: pediatric nursing

Rationale
(A) The probe may have become displaced or have poor contact. However, the nurse should initially visually assess the child. (B) Skin color will give a more direct indication of oxygenation. (C) Oxygen should only be administered after noting cyanosis and finding probe placement intact. As with any medication, a physician should order the oxygen first. (D) Restlessness is a subtle indicator of poor oxygenation.

561. (D) Nursing process phase: implementation; client need: safe, effective care environment; content area: pediatric nursing

Rationale
(A–C) These ranges are too low. (D) This is an accurate range.

562. (A) Nursing process phase: implementation; client need: health promotion and maintenance; content area: pediatric nursing

Rationale
(A) The solution will maintain a dry environment and is effective in preventing any recurrence. (B) The application of a medication would require a physician's order and thus would not be considered a nursing measure. The intervention does not focus on prevention. (C) Children should avoid using cotton swabs in the ear canal in order to prevent injury. (D) This drastic measure is not encouraged. Parents should be instructed to pull long hair back and dry the hair and ears thoroughly.

563. (B) Nursing process phase: assessment; client need: physiological integrity; content area: pediatric nursing

Rationale
(A) A brassy cough and some degree of agitation may be present in croup syndrome. (B) These three clinical signs are predictive of epiglottitis. (C) Persistent drooling is not expected with pneumonia. Some degree of agitation in the presence of hypoxia may be noted. Coughing is expected. (D) Asthmatic children may experience coughing. Some degree of agitation may be noted with hypoxia. Drooling is not expected.

564. (A) Nursing process phase: assessment; client need: physiological integrity; content area: pediatric nursing

Rationale
(A) All are early signs of impending airway obstruction. (B) Increased pulse is an early sign. (C) Cyanosis is a late sign. (D) Decreased respiratory rate and cyanosis are late signs.

565. (A) Nursing process phase: implementation; client need: physiological integrity; content area: pediatric nursing

Rationale
(A) The nurse may inoculate herself by direct contact from hand to eye, nose, or other mucous membrane. (B & C) Airborne transmission has never been documented. (D) RSV in secretions may survive for 30 minutes on the skin.

566. (D) Nursing process phase: implementation; client need: physiological integrity; content area: pediatric nursing

Rationale
(A) The small particle aerosol generator must be turned off before opening the tent. (B & C) Gloves and gowns are not essential due to negligible dermal absorption. (D) Stopping the aerosol temporarily limits the nurse's environmental exposure to ribavirin.

567. (D) Nursing process phase: implementation; client need: physiological integrity; content area: pediatric nursing

Rationale
(A) The child will need more aggressive treatment because the red zone indicates severe airway narrowing. (B & C) Notify the physician immediately because the red zone indicates a need for more aggressive therapy. (D) Notify the physician because severe airway narrowing may be occurring.

568. (C) Nursing process phase: assessment; client need:

health promotion and maintenance; content area: pediatric nursing

Rationale

(A) If empty, the canister would float to the top of the cup in a side-lying position. (B) The canister would tend to float to the top of the cup if partially empty. (C & D) When placed in a cup of water the canister would sink to the bottom if full.

569. (A) Nursing process phase: assessment; client need: physiological integrity; content area: pediatric nursing

Rationale

(A) All of these signs are indicative of theophylline toxicity. (B) These are known side effects of the medication, not toxic effects. (C) Only nausea is considered a sign of theophylline toxicity. (D) None of these symptoms indicates theophylline toxicity.

570. (C) Nursing process phase: evaluation, client need: safe, effective care environment; content area: pediatric nursing

Rationale

(A–D) Theophylline has a therapeutic level of 10 to 20 μg/ml.

571. (B) Nursing process phase: implementation; client need: physiological integrity; content area: pediatric nursing

Rationale

(A) To diminish the risk of vomiting, bronchial drainage is performed before meals or 1 to 1½ hours after meals. (B) Bronchial drainage is preferred before meals to prevent nausea and vomiting. (C) Bronchial drainage is performed three to four times a day. (D) Bronchial drainage is performed three to four times a day, usually before meals.

572. (D) Nursing process phase: assessment; client need: physiological integrity; content area: pediatric nursing

Rationale

(A–D) All the signs and symptoms suggest a severe acute exacerbation of asthma.

573. (D) Nursing process phase: implementation; client need: physiological integrity; content area: pediatric nursing

Rationale

(A) This action is an appropriate later nursing action, once the parents are aware of the diagnosis. (B) A diagnosis of pneumonia does not cause a false-positive sweat chloride result. (C) A chloride concentration of above 60 mEq/L is diagnostic for cystic fibrosis. (D) The nurse's initial response should be to notify the physician of the test results.

574. (B) Nursing process phase: implementation; client need: physiological integrity; content area: pediatric nursing

Rationale

(A & B) The bronchodilator medication will open the bronchi to enhance expectoration and should be given before CPT. (CPT will loosen and move secretions toward the glottis in order to facilitate expectoration.) (C) Bronchodilator medication should be initiated prior to CPT. (CPT will loosen and move secretions toward the glottis in order to facilitate expectoration.) (D) CPT remains an extremely important part

of the management of children with cystic fibrosis. (CPT will loosen and move secretions toward the glottis in order to facilitate expectoration.)

575. (A) Nursing process phase: implementation; client need: physiological integrity; content area: pediatric nursing

Rationale

(A–D) Cystic fibrosis is a known inherited disease as an autosomal recessive trait. Both parents contribute the defective gene to the affected child; their children have a 1:4 chance of inheriting this disease.

576. (C) Nursing process phase: implementation; client need: physiological integrity; content area: pediatric nursing

Rationale

(A) These children need high-calorie diets with water-miscible forms of vitamin A, D, E, and K. Restriction of fat is not necessary. Extra salt may be added to foods, especially during warm weather months. (B) Restriction of fat and salt is not necessary. (C) High-calorie and high-protein diets are needed for these children to receive all the recommended daily allowances, due to their impaired intestinal absorption. Water-miscible forms of vitamins A, D, E, and K are given, because the absorption of fat-soluble vitamins is decreased. These children receive supplements of pancreatic enzymes because obstruction of the pancreatic ducts limits release of digestive enzymes into the duodenum. (D) High-calorie diets are needed for these children to receive all the recommended daily allowances. Dietary fat does not need to be restricted. Water-miscible forms of vitamins A, D, E, and K are recommended because they have limited absorption of fat-soluble vitamins.

577. (D) Nursing process phase: implementation; client need: health promotion and maintenance; content area: pediatric nursing

Rationale

(A & B) He is continuing to grow normally and having no more than two stools per day. He needs no increase in enzyme therapy. (C) Do not decrease the number of enzymes because the child continues to grow well and has no more than two stools per day. The decrease in enzymes will cause the child to experience poor absorption of nutrients from the GI tract. (D) The number of enzymes given is determined by the child's ability to obtain normal growth and regular stools one to two times a day.

578. (A) Nursing process phase: assessment; client need: physiological integrity; content area: pediatric nursing

Rationale

(A) All these signs and symptoms occur in Hirschsprung's disease. (B) These children typically have poor appetites and poor weight gain. (C) These symptoms indicate enterocolitis, which may cause death in children with Hirschsprung's disease. (D) Only weight loss suggests Hirschsprung's disease.

579. (C) Nursing process phase: implementation; client need: physiological integrity; content area: pediatric nursing

Rationale

(A) Playing soft music only during the procedure will not necessarily decrease the child's stress. (B) Attractive, bright colors may not decrease stress and in some situations may increase stress. (C) By leaving the tape measure in place, the child can remain undisturbed during the circumference measurement. Otherwise, the child must be lifted or turned for each check, which may awaken or disturb a resting child. (D) Tylenol should not be administered simply to eliminate stress. A more suitable method to provide comfort should be identified.

580. (B) Nursing process phase: implementation; client need: health promotion and maintenance; content area: pediatric nursing

Rationale
(A) Only beans are considered a high-fiber food. (B) All the foods listed are high-fiber foods. (C) Regular candy bars are not high in fiber. (D) Milk products do not contain high-fiber content.

581. (A) Nursing process phase: planning; client need: safe, effective care environment; content area: pediatric nursing

Rationale
(A) The American Academy of Pediatrics (AAP) Task Force on Infant Positioning and SIDS (1992) recommends healthy infants being positioned on their back or side during sleep. However, the prone position may be more suitable for infants with GER. (B & C) The AAP recommends these positions for healthy infants during sleep. (D) This is no longer recommended for infants with GER because this position has not been proven to be more effective than the prone position.

582. (C) Nursing process phase: assessment; client need: safe, effective care environment; content area: pediatric nursing

Rationale
(A) These are not common side effects. (B & D) These are not side effects. (C) These are known side effects of prokinetic medication.

583. (B) Nursing process phase: assessment; client need: physiological integrity; content area: pediatric nursing

Rationale
(A) These symptoms are not common symptoms of appendicitis and may suggest other childhood illnesses. (B) These symptoms are the most common initial symptoms of acute appendicitis. (C) These symptoms occur later with appendicitis and indicate perforation. (D) These symptoms reflect signs of peritonitis from a perforated appendix.

584. (D) Nursing process phase: assessment; client need: physiological integrity; content area: pediatric nursing

Rationale
(A) Sudden pain relief is usually associated with perforation and worsening of the child's condition. (B) Pain relief with medication is usually more gradual in onset. This pain relief is occurring without medication. (C) Children in pain will verbalize as complete information as possible regarding their pain. (D) Sudden pain relief is associated with perforation and worsening of the child's condition.

585. (A) Nursing process phase: assessment; client need: physiological integrity; content area: pediatric nursing

Rationale
(A) These signs and symptoms are indicative of peritonitis. (B) In peritonitis, bowel sounds are absent and temperature greater than 39°C (102.2°F) is expected. (C) Vomiting and diarrhea are symptoms associated with appendicitis. (D) Shallow breathing is expected because the child will refrain from the use of abdominal muscles.

586. (B) Nursing process phase: planning; client need: safe, effective care environment; content area: pediatric nursing

Rationale
(A) These children typically have decreased oral intake and fluid loss from vomiting. However, pain is the number one problem. (B) Pain is the most common symptom of acute appendicitis and the highest priority problem. (C) Children are at risk for infection due to the potential for rupture. Pain is an actual, persistent problem. (D) The family is in need of support for their hospitalized child. The child's pain is a higher priority need.

587. (D) Nursing process phase: implementation; client need: physiological integrity; content area: pediatric nursing

Rationale
(A) This scale uses descriptive words to associate the varying degrees of pain intensity. The scale is not suitable for children less than 5 years of age. (B) This tool allows children to construct their own pain scale on a body outline. The tool requires cooperation of the child and knowledge of colors. The scale is not recommended for children younger than 4 years of age. (C) Children are asked to rate their pain on a scale of 0 (no pain) to 10 (worst pain). To participate, the child must understand the concept of numbers and counting. The tool is not appropriate for children younger than 5 years. (D) This scale is appropriate for 3-year-old children. Children rate their pain according to happy and sad faces.

588. (A) Nursing process phase: implementation; client need: safe, effective care environment; content area: pediatric nursing

Rationale
(A) Intravenous steroids are the most effective drugs for treating moderate to severe IBD because of their ability to reduce the inflammatory process. (B) Antibiotics have not been found useful in treating IBD. (C & D) These have not been found to be useful in treating IBD.

589. (B) Nursing process phase: assessment; client need: physiological integrity; content area: pediatric nursing

Rationale
(A) Weight loss an malnutrition are typical complications of these diseases. (B) Growth failure is a serious pediatric complication of IBD. (C) Delayed sexual maturation is related to malnutrition in these children. (D) Retarded height associated with growth failure is notable in this population.

590. (D) Nursing process phase: implementation; client need: physiological integrity; content area: pediatric nursing

Rationale
(A) The head should be slightly hyperflexed or the nose pointed toward the ceiling. (B) Taping the tube to the child's

forehead may cause damage to the nostril. The tube should be taped to the child's cheek. (C) Only room temperature formula should be utilized for feedings. (D) This position diminishes the possibility of regurgitation and aspiration.

591. (B) Nursing process phase: assessment; client need: physiological integrity; content area: pediatric nursing

Rationale

(A) The emesis of HPS infants contains milk or formula without bile. (B) During a physical examination of the abdomen, gastric peristalsis may be visible. (C) Symptoms of respiratory distress are not associated with this condition. (D) Diarrhea is not associated with this condition.

592. (A) Nursing process phase: assessment; client need: physiological integrity; content area: pediatric nursing

Rationale

(A) Metabolic alkalosis: increased plasma pH; normal plasma PCO_2; increased HCO_3 (B) Respiratory alkalosis: increased plasma pH; decreased plasma PCO_2; normal HCO_3 (C) Metabolic acidosis: decreased plasma pH; normal plasma PCO_2; decreased HCO_3 (D) Respiratory acidosis: decreased plasma pH; increased plasma PCO_2; normal HCO_3

593. (A) Nursing process phase: implementation; client need: health promotion and maintenance; content area: pediatric nursing

Rationale

(A) The family must be educated regarding the disease process and the effect of gluten. Food sources of gluten and dietary restrictions are emphasized to ensure the child's health status. (B) This goal will be achieved when the first goal is met. (C) The child must adhere to dietary restriction to maintain symptom-free health status. (D) These children may have anorexia, vomiting, and diarrhea that already result in weight loss.

594. (A) Nursing process phase: implementation; client need: health promotion and maintenance; content area: pediatric nursing

Rationale

(A) Fetal hemoglobin (HbF) prevents sickling, since it contains no β chains. These β chains found in Hbs carry the defect causing sickling. HbF is rapidly replaced by HbA and Hbs during infancy. (B) The newborn has about 80 percent fetal hemoglobin, which decreases in the first year. While HbF is present, no sickling will occur. (C) HbF is composed of two α and two γ polypeptide chains that do not contain the defect. (D) Hbs contains β chains that carry the defect and thus cause disease symptoms.

595. (D) Nursing process phase: implementation; client need: health promotion and maintenance; content area: pediatric nursing

Rationale

(A) Adequate hydration is necessary to prevent sickling episodes. (B) Overheating will cause fluid loss and hemoconcentration. A goal of therapy is hemodilution to prevent sickling. (C) Illness can also trigger sickling episodes. Any source of infection should be avoided. If the child becomes even mildly ill, parents should obtain medical help. (D) Sickle-cell anemia is an inherited disease for which there is no cure.

596. (C) Nursing process phase: implementation; client need: physiological integrity; content area: pediatric nursing

Rationale

(A) The nurse should address directly the father's concerns. (B) Oxygen therapy cannot be initiated by the nurse unless requested by the physician. (C) The nurse should explain to the father that oxygen has not been proved useful in vaso-occlusive crisis without hypoxemia. (D) The nurse must first assess what the father's knowledge base is and then clarify misconceptions.

597. (A) Nursing process phase: implementation; client need: psychosocial integrity; content area: pediatric nursing

Rationale

(A) This child's religious beliefs will not impact her medical treatment. (B) The Hindu religion embraces this belief. (C) The Jehovah's Witness faith strongly opposes the use of transfusions. (D) Devout Mormons believe that divine healing is possible.

598. (A) Nursing process phase: implementation; client need: psychosocial integrity; content area: pediatric nursing

Rationale

(A) This action is true of the Muslim faith. (B) Only members of the Jewish faith use the Ritual Burial Society. (C) The Muslim faith contains several death rituals. (D) This death ritual belongs to the Hindu religion.

599. (B) Nursing process phase: planning; client need: psychosocial integrity; content area: pediatric nursing

Rationale

(A) These simplistic games are inappropriate for infants and toddlers since they have limited cognitive and physical ability. (B) Preschool children are able to participate in simple, repetitive games with few flexible rules. (C) These games are more suitable for the school-age child or adolescent since they require rules of play to be followed. (D) Preschoolers do not handle competition well. They lose poorly and will try to change the rules to meet their own needs.

600. (B) Nursing process phase: implementation; client need: health promotion and maintenance; content area: pediatric nursing

Rationale

(A) Loud-noise toys are not recommended since these toys may be damaging to the child's hearing. (B) Small pieces, parts, and seams should be securely fastened or sewn. (C) A heavy toy can injure a child if the toy falls on the child. (D) All toys should be labeled and designed for specific age groups.

601. (C) Nursing process phase: assessment; client need: psychosocial integrity; content area: pediatric nursing

Rationale

(A) These fears are typical of the toddler. (B) These fears are particular to the preschooler. (C) These fears are particular to the school-age child. (D) These fears are present in the adolescent.

602. (D) Nursing process phase: implementation; client need: psychosocial integrity; content area: pediatric nursing

Rationale
(A) Creating feelings of shame in the child will serve to decrease the child's self-esteem, but not his or her fear. (B) When parents encourage the child's fear or overprotect the child from the fear itself, then parents reinforce the child's unrealistic fear. (C) This action will only increase the child's fear of the water. (D) The parent should gradually desensitize the child by bringing the child out into shallow water and then into deeper water.

603. **(A)** Nursing process phase: implementation; client need: psychosocial integrity; content area: pediatric nursing

Rationale
(A) Children should have less than 2 hours per day of TV viewing. (B) When parents watch TV programs, they have a better understanding of the type of content and appropriateness for their child. Also, this viewing provides the parent and child the opportunity to discuss the program. (C) This strategy allows TV viewing to always be a primary activity. TV viewing should be a secondary activity. (D) The parent should design a list of approved TV programs from which the child can choose. This list allows the child to choose only parent-approved programs for viewing.

604. **(D)** Nursing process phase: assessment; client need: physiological integrity; content area: pediatric nursing

Rationale
(A–C) A closed-ended question offers only a yes or no response. (D) An open-ended question will always provide the nurse with more information. This question allows the parents to respond with more detail.

605. **(C)** Nursing process phase: assessment; client need: health promotion and maintenance; content area: pediatric nursing

Rationale
(A) This strategy is always appropriate with children. However, this response would not be appropriate initially. (B) Removing the parent may only serve to increase the child's shyness and fear. (C) By talking initially with the parent, the child is allowed time to become at ease with the caregiver. (D) A calm, unhurried voice is always effective in communicating with children. This response, however, is not used initially.

606. **(B)** Nursing process phase: implementation; client need: physiological integrity; content area: pediatric nursing

Rationale
(A) Good positive response by the nurse. (B) Young children are more cooperative when their parents are allowed to remain with them. (C) Restraint is acceptable when the child's actions place her at risk for injury to herself. (D) When children are uncooperative, performing procedures quickly is imperative.

607. **(D)** Nursing process phase: implementation; client need: psychosocial integrity; content area: pediatric nursing

Rationale
(A) The nurse must respect the adolescent's right of privacy by allowing her to undress in private. (B) The nurse must respect the adolescent's right of privacy and expose only the area to be examined. (C) Emphasis should be placed on normal findings; however, abnormal findings must be discussed. (D) Using a matter-of-fact approach will serve to place the adolescent at ease when sexual development is discussed.

608. **(B)** Nursing process phase: assessment; client need: physiological integrity; content area: pediatric nursing

Rationale
(A) This mechanism is appropriate for children older than 3 years of age. (B) In children younger than 3 years of age, the auditory canal is curved. This curvature prevents visualization of the tympanic membrane. The canal must be straightened by pulling the pinna down and back to improve visualization. (C) This action would not be an initial response by the nurse. (D) This action may prove to enhance cooperation, but it will not improve visualization.

609. **(D)** Nursing process phase: assessment; client need: physiological integrity; content area: pediatric nursing

Rationale
(A & B) The right middle lobe cannot be auscultated posteriorly. (C & D) The right middle lobe can only be auscultated effectively between the fourth and fifth intercostal space.

610. **(D)** Nursing process phase: implementation; client need: physiological integrity; content area: pediatric nursing

Rationale
(A) If the child is crying, talking, laughing, or moving, your ability to auscultate effectively is impaired. (B) The child will react negatively to a cold stethoscope. (C) Vibrations and sound transmissions can be prevented when the stethoscope sits firmly on the chest. (D) The movement of clothing and sliding of fingers with the stethoscope can falsely mimic pathological breath sounds.

611. **(A)** Nursing process phase: assessment; client need: physiological integrity; content area: pediatric nursing

Rationale
(A) The fontanelle may bulge or feel taut when coughing, crying, or lying down. (B) This response does not reassure the mother and may force the mother to respond defensively. Also, the nurse should use the mother's terminology to enhance communication. (C) This response does not calm the mother's fears regarding a perfectly normal finding. (D) This response delays action and sets the stage for the mother not to return with her infant.

612. **(D)** Nursing process phase: assessment; client need: physiological integrity; content area: pediatric nursing

Rationale
(A) Glabellar reflex (B) Tonic neck reflex (C) Grasp reflex (D) Babinski reflex

613. **(A)** Nursing process phase: implementation; client need: physiological integrity; content area: pediatric nursing

Rationale
(A) Vitamin K prevents hemorrhagic disease of the newborn by assisting the liver in prothrombin synthesis. (B) Vitamin K is needed for prothrombin synthesis by the liver. The supply is poor since the newborn's intestine is sterile at birth. (C) Vi-

tamin K is normally synthesized by the intestinal flora. (D) The primary function of vitamin K is to protect the newborn against hemorrhagic disease.

614. (C) Nursing process phase: implementation; client need: health promotion and maintenance; content area: pediatric nursing

Rationale

(A) Retracting the foreskin to the glans penis in infants is not recommended. Infants have tight foreskins, which can tear during retraction and lead to scarring. (B) The foreskin should be retracted gently as far as it will go during cleansing. (C) Good hygiene can be achieved with gentle retraction of the foreskin and then the return to a normal position. (D) The retracted foreskin will act to constrict blood flow to the glans penis.

615. (A) Nursing process phase: implementation; client need: physiological integrity; content area: pediatric nursing

Rationale

(A) Polycose is a carbohydrate supplement used to enhance caloric intake. (B) This is a protein supplement only with no carbohydrate content. (C) This is a medium-chain triglyceride source for fat intake only. (D) This is the name of a soybean-based formula.

616. (B) Nursing process phase: assessment; client need: physiological integrity; content area: pediatric nursing

Rationale

(A) Caput succedaneum has vague boundaries and extends beyond the bone margins. (B) Cephalohematoma is associated with forceps delivery. Blood vessels rupture and bleed between the bone and periosteum. However, bleeding and thus swelling does not extend beyond the margins of the bone. (C) A subgaleal hemorrhage extends beyond the bone margins and may be associated with severe blood loss and shock. (D) The use of forceps during vaginal deliveries has not been associated with parietal skull fractures.

617. (A) Nursing process phase: implementation; client need: physiological integrity; content area: pediatric nursing

Rationale

(A) Prior to the establishment of a milk supply, the newborn's intake of calories and fluid is poor. This fact is thought to cause breastfeeding jaundice. Thus, early introduction of feedings, nursing every 2 hours, and avoidance of supplementation will assist in establishing the milk supply and enhancing caloric and fluid intake. (B) The use of supplementation will decrease the infant's need to nurse. Decreased nursing will delay the establishment of the mother's milk supply. Thus, the infant will receive fewer calories and less fluid intake which may impair hepatic clearance of bilirubin. (C) Bottle-feeding is not an acceptable preventive measure for jaundice. (D) Newborns should be encouraged to nurse every 2 hours in order to establish the mother's milk supply and to receive an adequate caloric intake. Additionally, feeding on demand allows the newborn to sleep through many valuable feeding times.

618. (C) Nursing process phase: implementation; client need: safe, effective care environment; content area: pediatric nursing

Rationale

(A) The shunt tubing may kink, separate, or migrate. (B) Mechanical obstruction may occur when particulate matter from the ventricles flows through the shunt. Obstruction may also occur at the distal end from thrombosis. (C) Shunt infection is the most serious complication. The infection may result in septicemia, bacterial endocarditis, wound infection, meningitis, ventriculitis, or brain abscess. Shunt infections that involve the CNS are particularly grave since they often impact intellectual outcomes in these children. (D) This complication may occur initially with shunt placement when ICP is dramatically decreased along with cranial size.

619. (A) Nursing process phase: assessment; client need: physiological integrity; content area: pediatric nursing

Rationale

(A) A lowered or diminished LOC is one valuable indicator of increasing ICP. Other indicators that relate to the interaction with the environment may be indifference, decline in school performance, lethargy, memory loss, decreased motor response to command, and diminished response to painful stimuli. (B) Headache is a subjective indicator of ICP, but not as valuable as ICP changes. (C) Nausea and vomiting are associated with increased ICP, but may also reflect multiple other pediatric problems. (D) Diplopia and blurred vision may be found with increased ICP or other visual disturbances.

620. (C) Nursing process phase: implementation; client need: physiological integrity; content area: pediatric nursing

Rationale

(A) Sedation should not be requested since it may alter accurate neurological assessment of the infant. (B) The child may need NPO restriction, but this nursing action is not a priority. (C) Vomiting and irritability are signs of possible shunt failure or infection. The nurse must carefully assess the child's neurological status, surgical site, and vital signs. This assessment data should then be given to the neurosurgeon. (D) The infant's hydration status is of concern to the nurse because of the history of vomiting. However, the child's neurological status is of more priority.

621. (B) Nursing process phase: implementation; client need: physiological integrity; content area: pediatric nursing

Rationale

(A) This infant should be monitored closely in addition to notifying the physician. (B) The physician should be immediately notified since these symptoms are signs of possible tracheoesophageal fistula (TEF). (C) Unexplained episodes of cyanosis along with excessive frothy saliva in the mouth should signal possible TEF. The physician should be notified immediately. (D) Because of the risk of aspiration with TEF, feedings should be withheld until the physician is notified.

622. (A) Nursing process phase: implementation; client need: health promotion and maintenance; content area: pediatric nursing

Rationale

(A) FAS is a preventable birth defect. Any amount of alcohol consumed during pregnancy may cause this defect. (B) Any pregnant mother who consumes alcohol places her unborn child at risk for developing FAS. (C) Any amount of alcohol consumption may cause FAS. (D) At no time during pregnancy is alcohol consumption safe.

623. (B) Nursing process phase: implementation; client need: health promotion and maintenance; content area: pediatric nursing

Rationale
(A & B) Any infant with head lag present at 6 months of age should have a complete developmental and neurological evaluation. (C) At this time what the infant needs is further evaluation to identify any neurological deficits. (D) Client and family histories are an effective means of identifying pertinent data. However, the primary goal for this child is further evaluation.

624. (D) Nursing process phase: implementation; client need: health promotion and maintenance; content area: pediatric nursing

Rationale
(A) These activities are most appropriate for infants less than 1 month of age. (B) These activities are most appropriate for the 4- to 6-month-old infant. (C) These activities are most appropriate for the 6- to 9-month-old infant. (D) These activities are most appropriate for the 11-month-old infant.

625. (A) Nursing process phase: implementation; client need: health promotion and maintenance; content area: pediatric nursing

Rationale
(A) The early introduction of citrus fruits, meats, and eggs to infants (less than 6 months of age) has resulted in allergy development. (B) Vegetables need to be firmly cooked and offered by 8 to 9 months of age. Grapes are never appropriate for young infants and children because of the risk of aspiration. Also, cheese should be offered after 8 to 9 months of age. (C) Whole cow's milk cannot be digested by infants and should not be introduced until 1 year of age. (D) In large quantities these juices may cause abdominal pain, bloating, and diarrhea in infants.

626. (A) Nursing process phase: planning; client need: physiological integrity; content area: pediatric nursing

Rationale
(A) This disease is the result of inadequate caloric intake to stimulate growth and development. The priority nursing goal should be to increase the child's intake of calories. (B) This goal is valuable, but not highest in priority. (C) Some parents have difficulty forming attachments with their child and have learned negative parenting skills from their own parents. This certainly is a valuable goal, but not highest in priority. (D) This infant has developmental delays and needs intervention. However, developmental achievements can only be made when nutritional intake is adequate.

627. (B) Nursing process phase: implementation; client need: physiological integrity; content area: pediatric nursing

Rationale
(A) This intervention is important, but does not solve most of the problem. (B) Quickly changing the diaper when soiled eliminates the three factors causing dermatitis—skin wetness, increased pH, and fecal irritants. (C) Although effective, the interventions do not totally prevent or cure the dermatitis. (D) These diapers have been noted to decrease skin irritation in soiled diapers. However, timely diaper changes after soiling primarily prevents diaper dermatitis.

628. (B) Nursing process phase: implementation; client need: physiological integrity; content area: pediatric nursing

Rationale
(A) Gentle stimulation only should be used to initiate breathing. (B) Gentle stimulation will often initiate spontaneous breathing. (C) Changing the position may open the infant's airway and initiate spontaneous respirations. (D) CPR should be initiated after 15 to 30 seconds if stimulation remains ineffective.

629. (C) Nursing process phase: implementation; client need: health promotion and maintenance; content area: pediatric nursing

Rationale
(A) Offering rewards to children who are not physically or psychologically ready for toilet training will not impact their behavior. (B) Potty chairs give some children a sense of security. Placing the feet on the floor can assist with defecation. Since this child is still too young to train, he probably will only play with the potty chair. (C) Children generally are not ready to toilet train until 18 to 24 months of age. Sitting on the commode should be limited to 5 to 10 minutes. A parent should never force a child to sit on the commode. This strategy will only create a power struggle between the child and parent. (D) Both physiological and psychological readiness is not achieved until 18 to 24 months of age. In addition, the average age for training males is 2.5 years.

630. (A) Nursing process phase: assessment; client need: psychosocial integrity; content area: pediatric nursing

Rationale
(A) Toddlers have difficulty adjusting to changes in routine and parental attention brought about by a new sibling. The toddler's reaction to such changes brings about sibling rivalry. (B–D) Sibling rivalry seems to affect firstborns and younger children more dramatically.

631. (A) Nursing process phase: implementation; client need: health promotion and maintenance; content area: pediatric nursing

Rationale
(A–D) Currently, the only initial vaccination for newborns is hepatitis B.

632. (D) Nursing process phase: implementation; client need: health promotion and maintenance; content area: pediatric nursing

Rationale
(A–D) A second MMR will be needed when the child enters middle school or at 11 to 12 years of age.

633. (D) Nursing process phase: assessment; client need: health promotion and maintenance; content area: pediatric nursing

Rationale
(A) This type of abuse is relatively difficult to identify because few physical indicators exist. (B) Fewer incidents are reported because adults are typically less willing to believe these reports by children. (C) The physical signs and behaviors of children vary, making these children difficult to identify. (D) Sexually abused children may not possess more carnal knowledge, but may attach unusual affective responses to their explanation of sexual activity.

634. (B) Nursing process phase: implementation; client need: health promotion and maintenance; content area: pediatric nursing

Rationale

(A) This statement judges the mother's integrity and is likely to cause guilt or a defensive response. (B) These statements directly address the mother's need and provide a workable solution to her problem. (C) The nurse can assist the mother by providing a cheaper alternative. Referral to a social worker may be an additional strategy. (D) The mother needs an immediate solution for the problem. This question may be used as a secondary response to further identify barriers to the child's health care.

635. (A) Nursing process phase: implementation; client need: safe, effective care environment; content area: pediatric nursing

Rationale

(A) The child's medication should not be locked away in a distant area. The child's medication should always be stored in close proximity for his immediate use. (B) Locking medications in a closet limits the child's ability to receive medications that may save his life. (C) Once again, the child's ability to obtain life-saving medication is limited. (D) This action will limit the availability of medication when it is needed. The child's medication should be in the classroom, in his desk, or on the child.

636. (A) Nursing process phase: implementation; client need: safe, effective care environment; content area: pediatric nursing

Rationale

(A) These signs are all indicative of IV infiltration. (B) These subtle signs are usually more indicative of some ongoing generalized infection. (C) Movement may be restricted because of the amount of tape and placement on an arm board to secure the IV site. Pain may occur when tension is placed on the IV site or with infiltration. (D) Blood at the IV site or in the IV tubing is not a sign of infiltration.

637. (A) Nursing process phase: assessment; client need: safe, effective care environment; content area: pediatric nursing

Rationale

(A) These signs are early indicators of infection. (B) Signs of increased intracranial pressure would indicate hydrocephalus. (C) The presence of a myelomeningocele sac puts the infant at risk for infection, especially involving the CNS. (D) Genitourinary infection is possible. However, nuchal rigidity indicates CNS involvement.

638. (A) Nursing process phase: implementation; client need: safe, effective care environment; content area: pediatric nursing

Rationale

(A) True of the leg as an injection site. (B) True of the arm as an injection site. (C) True of the abdomen as an injection site. (D) True of the buttock as an injection site.

639. (A) Nursing process phase: assessment; client need: physiological integrity; content area: pediatric nursing

Rationale

(A) Severe colicky abdominal pain, vomiting, and currant

jellylike stools are classic signs and symptoms of intussusception. (B–D) These are not classic signs and symptoms of intussusception.

640. (C) Nursing process phase: implementation; client need: safe, effective care environment; content area: pediatric nursing

Rationale

(A) This nursing action is important, but is secondary to the need for a patient airway. (B) Privacy should be ensured after the child's airway is maintained. (C) Nursing actions that prevent aspiration and ensure a patent airway are the priority during a seizure episode. (D) The child's airway should be maintained and then call for help.

641. (A) Nursing process phase: implementation; client need: safe, effective care environment; content area: pediatric nursing

Rationale

(A) Directly administering diazepam into the vein or closest IV insertion site can prevent the drug from reacting with other drugs or IV fluids in the tubing. (B) Diazepam is not known to cause these side effect if given very slowly. (C) The development of aplastic anemia has not been associated with diazepam administration. (D) The drug has not been documented to cause further seizure activity.

642. (D) Nursing process phase: implementation; client need: safe, effective care environment; content area: pediatric nursing

Rationale

(A) With this action the nurse has prescribed the safe dosage and administered it without physician approval. The nurse can be held legally accountable. (B) During a seizure there is no time to retrieve other references. (C) The nurse willingly giving the incorrect dosage is legally accountable for wrongdoing. (D) Always alert the physician that the dosage ordered is above the recommended safe range.

643. (A) Nursing process phase: implementation; client need: health promotion and maintenance; content area: pediatric nursing

Rationale

(A) These daily choices represent the recommendations from the food pyramid. (B) Children need more servings of fruit and bread, but less meat. (C) Children need fewer servings of milk, meat, fruit, and vegetables. (D) Children need more servings of all fruit groups.

644. (A) Nursing process phase: assessment; client need: physiological integrity; content area: pediatric nursing

Rationale

(A) These signs and symptoms signal a possible urinary tract infection. (B) A febrile response is noted in infants from 1 month to 1 year. (C) Enuresis and pallor are symptoms noted in children aged 2 to 14 years. (D) Incontinence occurs in children who have been toilet trained.

645. (D) Nursing process phase: implementation; client need: health promotion and maintenance; content area: pediatric nursing

Rationale

(A) Diluted formula depletes the amount of calories required for effective growth. Concentrated formula may damage the infant's delicate gastrointestinal tract and cause electrolyte imbalance and possibly renal failure. (B) Microwaving bottles may cause burns from hot formula and exploding bottles. (C) The clean technique is appropriate when using a dishwasher and good hand washing. (D) Propping the bottle by parents should be discouraged. Infants should be held and cuddled when nippling to promote attachment and bonding.

646. (A) Nursing process phase: implementation; client need: health promotion and maintenance; content area: pediatric nursing

Rationale
(A) In 1992 the American Academy of Pediatrics recommended that healthy infants less than 6 months of age should be placed on their side or back in order to sleep. (B) Infants sleeping on soft bedding are three times more likely to die from SIDS. (C) These types of soft bedding increase the infant's risk for SIDS. (D) The incidence of SIDS in the United States has dramatically decreased since the use of side-lying and back positions for infant sleep.

647. (C) Nursing process phase: implementation; client need: health promotion and maintenance; content area: pediatric nursing

Rationale
(A) Bowel training is usually acquired before bladder training because it is more predictable. (B) Children may be so involved in their play activity that they ignore their body sensations. (C) Nighttime bladder training is usually achieved by 4 to 5 years of age. (D) Ten minutes is enough time to complete the elimination process. No child should be forced to sit on the toilet.

648. (A) Nursing process phase: assessment; client need: physiological integrity; content area: pediatric nursing

Rationale
(A) The consumption of lead paint chips by children is the number one cause of lead exposure in the United States. (B) Children's pets are not considered potential sources of lead. (C) The nurse should be concerned whether parents grow their own vegetables. (D) A child's eating habits alone would not identify potential sources of lead.

649. (B) Nursing process phase: assessment; client need: health promotion and maintenance; content area: pediatric nursing

Rationale
(A) Children may have a number of vague symptoms considered to be early warning signs. (B) Wheezing is not considered an early warning sign. (C) This notes airway restriction before overt signs and symptoms. (D) Trigger exposure should alert both the child and the parent that symptoms are likely to occur.

650. (A) Nursing process phase: implementation; client need: physiological integrity; content area: pediatric nursing

Rationale
(A) A child who is crying, talking, laughing, or moving may impair effective auscultation. (B) A child will react negatively to a cold stethoscope. For comfort, the stethoscope should be warm. (C) Firm contact with the chest will eliminate vibration and other unwanted sound transmission. (D) Avoid auscultation through clothing since this may create false adventitious sounds.

651. (D) Nursing process phase: assessment; client need: health promotion and maintenance; content area: pediatric nursing

Rationale
(A) Macrocephaly is not a feature of FAS. (B) These children experience poor coordination and motor retardation. (C) Prenatal and postnatal growth retardation is evident. (D) This option identifies some of the major features of FAS.

652. (A) Nursing process phase: analysis; client need: safe, effective care environment; content area: pediatric nursing

Rationale
(A) Parents who are abusive have not mastered the developmental task of trust. (B) Through role reversal with their children, abusive parents do receive some role gratification. (C) These parents are able to function outside the home; they just do not develop friendships easily. (D) Everyone has a value system.

653. (D) Nursing process phase: assessment; client need: physiological integrity; content area: pediatric nursing

Rationale
(A) Any person (including family and friends) who smokes in any room of the home must be identified as a potential trigger source. (B) This question only requires a yes or no answer. The extent of the pest control problem must be identified. Both decaying cockroaches and their fecal matter can become airborne allergens. (C) This question only requires a yes or no answer. (D) The mother must provide details regarding the child's room (i.e., carpet, bedding, curtains, stuffed animals) that may be potential triggers.

654. (B) Nursing process phase: implementation; client need: safe, effective care environment; content area: pediatric nursing

Rationale
(A) The recommended heparin flush ratio is 1:10 units per milliliter for children's devices. (B) This flush technique prevents clot formation in the catheter. (C) Saline is an acceptable flush if used with the positive-pressure technique on devices with larger than 24-gauge catheters. (D) The lock must be flushed with saline both before and after administering medication since heparin is incompatible with most medications.

655. (C) Nursing process phase: implementation; client need: health promotion and maintenance; content area: pediatric nursing

Rationale
(A) Prematurity does not imply a lack of love or desire by parents for a child. (B) A lack of prenatal care does not always result in prematurity. (C) Current research studies suggest that physical separation produces emotional separation, and thus inhibits the parent-infant attachment process. (D) The existence of prematurity does not necessarily suggest the presence of birth defects.

656. (A) Nursing process phase: assessment; client need: physiological integrity; content area: pediatric nursing

Rationale
(A) These signs all occur during the acute phase of neonatal narcotic withdrawal. (B) These infants experience little sleeping and are poor feeders. The remaining signs do not occur in neonatal narcotic withdrawal. (C) Sleepiness, lethargy, and hypotonicity are not signs of neonatal narcotic withdrawal. The infants experience little sleep and are hyperactive and hypertonic. The remaining signs do occur during withdrawal. (D) Constipation is not an acute sign. Instead, the infants experience diarrhea, along with the other listed signs.

657. **(D)** Nursing process phase: implementation; client need: safe, effective care environment; content area: pediatric nursing

Rationale
(A) Bright lights can trigger hyperactivity and irritability in these infants. Only dimmed lighting should be used to decrease environmental stimulation. (B) Infants should be wrapped snugly with a blanket. Wrapping the infant prevents possible self-stimulation using their arms and legs. (C) Group nursing activities to limit possible stimulation. (D) Nursing actions that decrease environmental stimulation are desirable. These infants are prone to hyperactivity and irritability often triggered by stimuli.

658. **(B)** Nursing process phase: implementation; client need: physiological integrity; content area: pediatric nursing

Rationale
(A) Only the prone position is recommended. In the prone position, less tension is placed on the sac. (B) The warmer or incubator aids the nude infant in maintaining body temperature. (C) Adherent dressings should be avoided since they increase the risk of tearing the sac when removed. (D) Vigorous cleansing of the sac may cause rupture or tearing and should be avoided.

659. **(C)** Nursing process phase: assessment; client need: health promotion and maintenance; content area: pediatric nursing

Rationale
(A) Phenytoin causes gum hyperplasia. (B) While on phenytoin, the tonsils and adenoids may enlarge, causing a snoring sound. (C) Phenytoin may negatively affect cognitive ability, school performance, and behavior. (D) Ataxia and rashes are not uncommon. These side effects diminish when drug dosages are decreased.

660. **(D)** Nursing process phase: assessment; client need: physiological integrity; content area: pediatric nursing

Rationale
(A–C) On a 3-year-old child, the anterior fontanelle would be closed. Thus, the anterior fontanelle and the head circumference on a 3-year-old child would not provide the nurse with information on dehydration. (D) All three assessment activities would provide the nurse with information regarding the child's hydration status.

661. **(D)** Nursing process phase: implementation; client need: health promotion and maintenance; content area: pediatric nursing

Rationale
(A) Toddlers do not have the cognitive ability to understand and assimilate the traffic rules for cycling. All tricycling should be done in an enclosed area away from automobile traffic. (B) Toddlers experience stranger anxiety. Rules for interacting with strangers are more helpful with older children. (C) All household cleaners should be stored in locked cabinets. Toddlers are curious and still place items in their mouths. Their curiosity can easily cause injury. (D) Serious burns have been caused by young children reaching for hot stove-top foods.

662. **(D)** Nursing process phase: implementation; client need: health promotion and maintenance; content area: pediatric nursing

Rationale
(A) A mild acute illness with or without fever is not a contraindication. (B) Taking antibiotic medications is not a contraindication. (C) Premature infants receive the same dosage and schedule as full-term infants. (D) Any anaphylactic reaction to a vaccine would prevent the child from receiving future doses of the vaccine.

663. **(C)** Nursing process phase: implementation; client need: health promotion and maintenance; content area: pediatric nursing

Rationale
(A) The infant should be fed smaller, but more frequent feedings. (B) The infant should be burped during and after feedings. (C) A change in the infant's environment may distract the infant from its colic pain. (D) An infant should be placed high on the shoulder to burp. This position enhances the child's ability to burp.

664. **(D)** Nursing process phase: implementation; client need: safe, effective care environment; content area: pediatric nursing

Rationale
(A) To ensure that feeding guidelines are followed, a limited number of staff nurses should be allowed to feed the infant. The limited number of nursing staff will also enable the nurses to learn the infant cues and respond appropriately. (B) The feeding environment should be calm and quiet to prevent distraction during mealtime. (C) New foods should be introduced very slowly to enhance the child's acceptance. (D) Only simple, easy-to-follow feeding instructions are communicated to the child. These instructions should be direct and maintain the child's focus on eating.

665. **(B)** Nursing process phase: implementation; client need: physiological integrity; content area: pediatric nursing

Rationale
(A) While under the bililight, eye shields should be worn at all times to prevent blindness. (B) Animal research studies suggest that covering the genitals during phototherapy may prevent any gonadal complications. No long-term studies exist that address gonadal function. Nurses should follow the protocol of their agency or institution. (C) The infant's temperature should be closely monitored. While receiving phototherapy, an infant may experience hypothermia or hyperthermia. (D) Once phototherapy is initiated, parents may remove the infant for short periods of time to feed and caress.

666. **(B)** Nursing process phase: planning; client need:

health promotion and maintenance; content area: pediatric nursing

Rationale
(A) Snellen's letter acuity charts are designed for school-age children who know their alphabet. This chart would not be suitable for preschool children who may or may not know some letters of the alphabet. (B) Occluders are needed to occlude a single eye during testing. (C) Penlights should be obtained rather than flashlights. Pupillary response to light is easily tested using a penlight. (D) A yardstick or wood or metal tape measure is more desirable than a foot ruler. This item is used to measure the appropriate footage a child must stand away from the vision charts.

667. **(B)** Nursing process phase: implementation; client need: health promotion and maintenance; content area: pediatric nursing

Rationale
(A) Breast milk has a natural laxative effect on the stool. (B) With its immunological benefits, breast milk assists the infant in fighting infection. (C) Vitamins A, B complex, C, D, E, and K are contained in breast milk. (D) Calcium and phosphorus are contained in breast milk.

668. **(D)** Nursing process phase: assessment; client need: physiological integrity; content area: pediatric nursing

Rationale
(A) Assessment findings indicative of an allergic reaction include uticaria, flushing, wheezing, and laryngeal edema. (B) Symptoms of an air embolism would include sudden difficulty in breathing, sharp pain in the chest, and apprehension. (C) Hemolytic reactions are manifested by chills, fever, nausea or vomiting, tightness in the chest, red or black urine, headache, flank pain, and progressive signs of shock or renal failure. (D) The listed assessment findings of precordial pain, dyspnea, distended neck veins, and a cough indicate circulatory overload.

Focus on Pediatric Drug Dosages

669. **(A)** Nursing process phase: implementation; client need: safe, effective care environment; content area: pediatric nursing

Rationale
80 mg : 1 tablet = 40 mg : x = 0.5 tablet
Math calculation explains incorrect answers.

670. **(C)** Nursing process phase: implementation; client need: safe, effective care environment; content area: pediatric nursing

Rationale
125 ml : 5 ml = 250 ml : x = 10 ml
Math calculation explains incorrect answers.

671. **(C)** Nursing process phase: implementation; client need: safe, effective care environment; content area: pediatric nursing

Rationale
15 mg/kg $\times$ 5 kg = 75 mg; 0.5 mg : 1 ml = 75 mg : x = 150 ml
Math calculation explains incorrect answers.

672. **(D)** Nursing process phase: implementation; client need: safe, effective care environment; content area: pediatric nursing

Rationale
500 mg : 5 ml = 500 mg : x = 5 ml
Math calculation explains incorrect answers.

673. **(A)** Nursing process phase: implementation; client need: safe, effective care environment; content area: pediatric nursing

Rationale
25 mg : 0.5 ml = 5 mg : x = 0.1 ml
Math calculation explains incorrect answers.

674. **(D)** Nursing process phase: implementation; client need: safe, effective care environment; content area: pediatric nursing

Rationale
1.3 m^2 divided by 1.7 m^2 $\times$ 60 mg = 46 mg
Math calculation explains incorrect answers.

675. **(D)** Nursing process phase: implementation; client need: safe, effective care environment; content area: pediatric nursing

Rationale
500 mg : 10 ml = 40 mg : x = 0.8 ml
Math calculation explains incorrect answers.

676. **(D)** Nursing process phase: implementation; client need: safe, effective care environment; content area: pediatric nursing

Rationale
20 mg : 2 ml = 24 mg : x = 2.4 ml
Math calculation explains incorrect answers.

677. **(B)** Nursing process phase: implementation; client need: safe, effective care environment; content area: pediatric nursing

Rationale
95 mg : 1 ml = 200 mg : x = 2 ml
Math calculation explains incorrect answers.

678. **(C)** Nursing process phase: implementation; client need: safe, effective care environment; content area: pediatric nursing

Rationale
100 mg : 2 ml = 40 mg : x = 0.8 ml
Math calculation explains incorrect answers.

679. **(C)** Nursing process phase: implementation; client need: safe, effective care environment; content area: pediatric nursing

Rationale
50 mg : 1 ml = 15 mg : x = 0.3 ml
Math calculation explains incorrect answers.

680. **(C)** Nursing process phase: implementation; client

need: safe, effective care environment; content area: pediatric nursing

Rationale
45.45 kg × 3.3 mg/kg = 150 mg
Math calculation explains incorrect answers.

681. (D) Nursing process phase: implementation; client need: safe, effective care environment; content area: pediatric nursing

Rationale
100 mg : 1 tablet = 300 mg : x = 3 tablets
Math calculation explains incorrect answers.

682. (C) Nursing process phase: implementation; client need: safe, effective care environment; content area: pediatric nursing

Rationale
100 mg : 1 tablet = 200 mg : x = 2 tablets
Math calculation explains incorrect answers.

683. (B) Nursing process phase: implementation; client need: safe, effective care environment; content area: pediatric nursing

Rationale
3.3 mg/m² × 1.7 m² = 5.6 mg
25 mg : 1 ml = 5.6 mg : x = 0.22 ml
Math calculation explains incorrect answers.

684. (A) Nursing process phase: implementation; client need: safe, effective care environment; content area: pediatric nursing

Rationale
50 mg : 1 tablet = 25 mg : x = ½ tablet
Math calculation explains incorrect answers.

685. (B) Nursing process phase: implementation; client need: safe, effective care environment; content area: pediatric nursing

Rationale
250 mg : 5 ml = 200 mg : x = 4 ml
Math calculation explains incorrect answers.

686. (B) Nursing process phase: implementation; client need: safe, effective care environment; content area: pediatric nursing

Rationale
50 mg : 1 ml = 8.5 mg : x = 0.2 ml
Math calculation explains incorrect answers.

687. (D) Nursing process phase: implementation; client need: safe, effective care environment; content area: pediatric nursing

Rationale
200 mg/kg × 10 kg = 2000 mg divided by 4 doses = 500 mg
Math calculation explains incorrect answers.

688. (B) Nursing process phase: implementation; client need: safe, effective care environment; content area: pediatric nursing

Rationale
250 mg : 1 ml = 290 mg : x = 1.2 ml
Math calculation explains incorrect answers.

689. (D) Nursing process phase: implementation; client need: safe, effective care environment; content area: pediatric nursing

Rationale
100 mg : 1 tablet = 184 mg : x = 2 tablets
Math calculation explains incorrect answers.

690. (C) Nursing process phase: implementation; client need: safe, effective care environment; content area: pediatric nursing

Rationale
262 mg : 15 ml = 300 mg : x = 17 ml
Math calculation explains incorrect answers.

691. (D) Nursing process phase: implementation; client need: safe, effective care environment; content area: pediatric nursing

Rationale
5 mg : 1 tablet = 10 mg : x = 2 tablets
Math calculation explains incorrect answers.

692. (A) Nursing process phase: implementation; client need: safe, effective care environment; content area: pediatric nursing

Rationale
4 mg : 1 tablet = 2 mg : x = ½ tablet
Math calculation explains incorrect answers.

693. (C) Nursing process phase: implementation; client need: safe, effective care environment; content area: pediatric nursing

Rationale
2 mg : 1 tablet = 6 mg : x = 3 tablets
Math calculation explains incorrect answers.

694. (D) Nursing process phase: implementation; client need: safe, effective care environment; content area: pediatric nursing

Rationale
50 mg : 1 ml = 690 mg : x = 13.8 ml
Math calculation explains incorrect answers.

695. (B) Nursing process phase: implementation; client need: safe, effective care environment; content area: pediatric nursing

Rationale
500 mg : 1 tablet = 500 mg : x = 1 tablet
Math calculation explains incorrect answers.

696. (C) Nursing process phase: implementation; client need: safe, effective care environment; content area: pediatric nursing

Rationale
250 mg : 5 ml = 150 mg : x = 3 ml
Math calculation explains incorrect answers.

697. (D) Nursing process phase: implementation; client need: safe, effective care environment; content area: pediatric nursing

Rationale
100 mg : 1 tablet = 400 mg : x = 4 tablets
Math calculation explains incorrect answers.

698. (D) Nursing process phase: implementation; client need: safe, effective care environment; content area: pediatric nursing

Rationale
0.62 ml : 1 capful = 5 ml : x = 8 capfuls
Math calculation explains incorrect answers.

699. (B) Nursing process phase: implementation; client need: safe, effective care environment; content area: pediatric nursing

Rationale
1000 mg : 1 ml = 540 mg : x = 0.54 ml
Math calculation explains incorrect answers.

700. (D) Nursing process phase: implementation; client need: safe, effective care environment; content area: pediatric nursing

Rationale
150 mg : 1 tablet = 300 mg : x = 2 tablets
Math calculation explains incorrect answers.

701. (D) Nursing process phase: implementation; client need: safe, effective care environment; content area: pediatric nursing

Rationale
450 mg : 5 ml = 5 ml : x = 450 mg
Math calculation explains incorrect answers.

702. (D) Nursing process phase: implementation; client need: safe, effective care environment; content area: pediatric nursing

Rationale
500 mg : 1 ml = 1000 mg : x = 2 ml
Math calculation explains incorrect answers.

703. (D) Nursing process phase: implementation; client need: safe, effective care environment; content area: pediatric nursing

Rationale
500 mg : 5 ml = 2500 mg : x = 25 ml
Math calculation explains incorrect answers.

704. (B) Nursing process phase: implementation; client need: safe, effective care environment; content area: pediatric nursing

Rationale
150 mg : 5 ml = 265 mg : x = 8.8 ml
Math calculation explains incorrect answers.

705. (A) Nursing process phase: implementation; client need: safe, effective care environment; content area: pediatric nursing

Rationale
10 mg : 1 tablet = 5 mg : x = ½ tablet
Math calculation explains incorrect answers.

706. (D) Nursing process phase: implementation; client need: safe, effective care environment; content area: pediatric nursing

Rationale
25 mg : 1 ml = 24 mg : x = 0.96 ml
Math calculation explains incorrect answers.

707. (C) Nursing process phase: implementation; client need: safe, effective care environment; content area: pediatric nursing

Rationale
50 mg : 1 ml = 115 mg : x = 2.3 ml
Math calculation explains incorrect answers.

708. (C) Nursing process phase: implementation; client need: safe, effective care environment; content area: pediatric nursing

Rationale
500 mg : 1 ml = 460 mg : x = 0.92 ml
Math calculation explains incorrect answers.

709. (D) Nursing process phase: implementation; client need: safe, effective care environment; content area: pediatric nursing

Rationale
25 mg : 1 ml = 50 mg : x = 2 ml
Math calculation explains incorrect answers.

710. (C) Nursing process phase: implementation; client need: safe, effective care environment; content area: pediatric nursing

Rationale
50 IU : 1 tablet = 75 IU : x = 1.5 tablets
Math calculation explains incorrect answers.

711. (C) Nursing process phase: implementation; client need: safe, effective care environment; content area: pediatric nursing

Rationale
50 mg : 1 ml = 171 mg : x = 3.4 ml
Math calculation explains incorrect answers.

712. (C) Nursing process phase: implementation; client need: safe, effective care environment; content area: pediatric nursing

Rationale
870 mg : 5 ml = 1000 mg : x = 6 ml
Math calculation explains incorrect answers.

713. (A) Nursing process phase: implementation; client need: safe, effective care environment; content area: pediatric nursing

Rationale
100 mg : 5 ml = 88 mg : x = 4.4 ml
Math calculation explains incorrect answers.

714. (B) Nursing process phase: implementation; client need: safe, effective care environment; content area: pediatric nursing

Rationale
200 mg : 1 tablet = 400 mg : x = 2 tablets
Math calculation explains incorrect answers.

715. (B) Nursing process phase: implementation; client need: safe, effective care environment; content area: pediatric nursing

Rationale
150 mg : 1 ml = 57 mg : x = 0.4 ml
Math calculation explains incorrect answers.

716. (A) Nursing process phase: implementation; client need: safe, effective care environment; content area: pediatric nursing

Rationale
20 mg : 1 ml = 10 mg : x = 0.5 ml
Math calculation explains incorrect answers.

717. (C) Nursing process phase: implementation; client need: safe, effective care environment; content area: pediatric nursing

Rationale
1 mg : 1 ml = 0.46 mg : x = 0.46 ml
Math calculation explains incorrect answers.

718. (C) Nursing process phase: implementation; client need: safe, effective care environment; content area: pediatric nursing

Rationale
25 mg/kg × 34 kg = 850 mg
Math calculation explains incorrect answers.

719. (A) Nursing process phase: implementation; client need: safe, effective care environment; content area: pediatric nursing

Rationale
100 mg : 1 ml = 50 mg : x = 0.5 ml
Math calculation explains incorrect answers.

720. (A) Nursing process phase: implementation; client need: safe, effective care environment; content area: pediatric nursing

Rationale
50 mg : 1 tablet = 25 mg : x = ½ tablet
Math calculation explains incorrect answers.

721. (B) Nursing process phase: implementation; client need: safe, effective care environment; content area: pediatric nursing

Rationale
20 mg : 1 ml = 17 mg : x = 0.85 ml
Math calculation explains incorrect answers.

722. (B) Nursing process phase: implementation; client need: safe, effective care environment; content area: pediatric nursing

Rationale
250 mg : 1 capsule = 500 mg : x = 2 capsules

chapter6

Medical/Surgical Nursing Q & A

by Ola Allen, Mary Martoff,
Bonnie Juvé Meeker, Louise Plaisance,
Lynn Ryan, Golden Tradewell, and
Alexandrea Weis

1. A 45-year-old male returned to his room an hour ago following a bronchoscopy. He is requesting some water. The nurse must:
   A. Keep the client NPO until an order is written.
   B. Check the vital signs first.
   C. Check the gag and swallowing reflexes.
   D. Encourage coughing and deep breathing.

2. A client is placed on seizure precautions. The nurse knows that an appropriate intervention for a grand mal seizure is:
   A. Insert a tongue blade between the teeth to prevent biting the tongue.
   B. Apply restraints to prevent injury to the self.
   C. Place the client in a supine position.
   D. Place the head in a lateral position.

3. A 15-year-old client fractured his tibia and several metatarsal bones. A cast has been applied; it extends from the knee to the toes. The nurse makes frequent assessments of which of the following:
   A. Quality of the popliteal and femoral pulses
   B. Color, temperature, and sensation in the toes
   C. Movement of the toes on both feet
   D. The pedal pulses in both lower extremities

4. A client is in traction for a fractured femur. Which of the following statements indicates understanding of the nurse's instruction:
   A. "The weights must hang freely at all times."
   B. "I'm free to move about in bed as I wish."
   C. "I'll be in a lot of pain and will need narcotics frequently."

D. "I won't have the time or energy to work on my paintings."

5. A 45-year-old client is receiving heparin sodium for a pulmonary embolus. The nurse evaluates which of the following laboratory reports of partial thromboplastin time as indicative of effective heparin therapy?
   A. Within normal range
   B. One to 1.5 times the control (normal) value
   C. Two to 2.5 times the control (normal) value
   D. Three times the control (normal) value

6. A client is on intravenous heparin therapy. The nurse would keep which of the following drugs available as an antidote?
   A. Vitamin K
   B. Protamine sulfate
   C. Epinephrine
   D. Norepinephrine

7. A client is taking warfarin (Coumadin) following placement of an artificial mitral valve. The nurse instructs this client to avoid taking the following commonly used drug:
   A. Maalox Plus
   B. Tylenol Cold and Flu Medication
   C. Sudafed
   D. Aspirin

8. During the evening following a partial gastrectomy, a client's oral temperature is 100°F. Other data include a blood pressure of 134/68, a pulse of 88, and a respiratory rate of 18. The nurse should:
   A. Notify the physician immediately.

B. Take the temperature every hour until it is normal.

C. Perform a thorough respiratory assessment.

D. Remove the dressing and check the operative site.

9. A client with insulin-dependent diabetes mellitus (IDDM) is being discharged. The nurse knows that the client has understood essential teaching when the following statement is heard:

A. "I need to cut my nails straight across."

B. "I can't make any substitutions in my diet."

C. "My insulin should be given into my arms."

D. "I should eat less before exercising."

10. A 45-year-old client has recently been told that she has acute myelocytic leukemia. She seems quite happy and laughs and jokes about everything. The nurse should:

A. Remind her of the seriousness of her diagnosis.

B. Encourage her to continue with her laughter and joking.

C. Wait and allow her to explore her feelings.

D. Reprimand her for not taking her treatment seriously.

11. A client is on chemotherapy for acute myelogenous leukemia. The nurse assesses the following laboratory test daily:

A. Complete blood count

B. Electrolyte panel

C. Prothrombin time

D. Blood urea nitrogen and creatinine

12. A client has developed depression of the bone marrow from antineoplastic drugs. The nurse states the nursing diagnosis of highest priority as:

A. Fluid volume deficit

B. High risk for aspiration

C. Ineffective thermoregulation

D. High risk for infection

13. Radioactive iodine is being used to treat a client with cancer of the thyroid gland. The nurse knows that the client has understood teaching about the treatment when the following statement is heard:

A. "Only my thyroid gland will be radioactive."

B. "I need not be concerned about radioactivity."

C. "My whole body will be radioactive."

D. "My body fluids will be radioactive for a short time."

14. A radioactive implant is being used to treat a client with cancer of the prostate. The implant is found on the floor near the patient. The nurse should:

A. Replace the implant, using forceps.

B. Place the implant in a radiation-proof container, using forceps.

C. Leave the implant for the radiation safety officer.

D. Place a lead shield between the nurse and the implant.

15. A nurse assesses an intravenous site of a client and finds it red, swollen, and painful; there is no blood return. The nurse should:

A. Remove the IV at once.

B. Watch to see if the swelling gets worse.

C. Report it to the physician.

D. Apply an antibiotic ointment to the site.

16. A client's total parenteral nutrition is 6 hours behind schedule. The nurse would:

A. Run the fluid at a rate to make up for the lost time.

B. Report the situation to the physician.

C. Run the IV at the prescribed site.

D. Check the blood glucose level.

17. A 44-year-old client is in acute congestive heart failure. The nurse and client establish a goal of highest priority as:

A. Rest mentally as well as physically.

B. Learn stress management.

C. Train for a less demanding job.

D. Prevent complications of immobility.

18. A 46-year-old client has just had a femoral-distal bypass. It would be most important for the nurse to assess:

A. Serum cholesterol levels

B. Popliteal pulses

C. Pedal pulses

D. Cardiac enzyme levels

19. A 33-year-old client is having a routine physical examination. The nurse evaluates which of the following data on a urinalysis report as normal?

A. Positive for ketones

B. Trace of protein

C. Positive for glucose

D. Cloudy

20. A client with chronic renal failure has an arteriovenous shunt in the left arm. The nurse makes which of the following assessments of the left arm each shift?

A. Blood pressure and pulse

B. Detection of a thrill and bruit

C. Venous and arterial distention

D. Skin turgor and skin integrity

21. A client diagnosed with insulin-dependent diabetes mellitus becomes irritable and confused; the skin is cool and clammy, and the pulse rate is 110. The first action of the nurse would be to:

A. Give a half-cup of orange juice.

B. Check the serum glucose.

C. Administer regular insulin.

D. Call the physician.

22. A client with IDDM is recovering from diabetic ketoacidosis. Information on the serum level of the following substance will be very important to the nurse:

A. Sodium

B. Calcium
C. Potassium
D. Magnesium

23. A 17-year-old client's mother has recently been diagnosed with pulmonary tuberculosis. The nurse would expect the doctor to order which of the following tests initially?
A. The Mantoux
B. An x-ray
C. A sputum culture
D. Gram stain of the sputum

24. The nurse injects 0.1 ml of purified protein derivative (PPD) intradermally into the inner aspect of the forearm of a client. This nurse will interpret the reaction to this test as positive when the following is seen:
A. Redness greater than 5 mm
B. Swelling greater than 7 mm
C. Induration greater than 10 mm
D. Exudate covering more than 12 mm

25. A client is receiving whole blood when she starts to shake with chills; her temperature is 101°F. The nurse should first:
A. Call the physician immediately.
B. Administer the PRN dose of aspirin.
C. Start another IV, running normal saline.
D. Stop the blood immediately.

26. A 66-year-old client with congestive heart failure takes both digoxin (Lanoxin) and furosemide (Lasix) daily. The nurse would want to know the results of the following laboratory test:
A. Complete blood count
B. Blood urea nitrogen and creatinine
C. Coagulation times
D. Electrolyte panel

27. A 29-year-old client has been taking prednisone 60 mg daily for an inflammatory condition for the past 6 months. The physician just wrote an order to discontinue the medication. The nurse should:
A. Stop the medication as ordered.
B. Continue the medication until the physician is available.
C. Call the physician and question the order.
D. Hold the medication until the physician is available.

28. A 49-year-old client with cancer of the lung just had a thoracentesis. The nurse would position the client:
A. On the affected side
B. Sitting
C. On the unaffected side
D. In Fowler's position

29. A 55-year-old client has a chest tube connected to a Pleur Evac system to remove blood from the pleural cavity. While turning the client, the nurse remembers to:

A. Keep the Pleur Evac below the level of the wound.
B. Remove the suction from the Pleur Evac.
C. Clamp the tubing connected to the Pleur Evac.
D. Drain the sterile water from the Pleur Evac.

30. A 26-year-old client is having a chest tube inserted into the left upper chest wall posteriorly. The nurse anticipates that which of the following will be used to cover the incision?
A. Sterile gauze
B. Kerlix
C. A sterile sealant
D. Sterile petrolatum (Vaseline) gauze

31. A client is recovering from a gastrectomy. Medications are to be given to this client through a nasogastric tube. Prior to giving the medications, the nurse will:
A. Irrigate the tube with saline.
B. Reposition the tube and reapply the tape.
C. Check the tube for placement.
D. Insert the tube 1 inch farther.

32. A client is to have a nasogastric tube removed. To prevent aspiration as the tube is pulled past the epiglottis, the nurse asks the client to:
A. Use a cascade cough.
B. Take a deep breath.
C. Exhale and hold it.
D. Use the Valsalva maneuver.

33. A 16-year-old client has nasal congestion, a temperature of 103°F, malaise, and aching muscles. A nurse recommends that the following medication be taken to lower the temperature:
A. Aspirin
B. Enteric-coated aspirin
C. Tylenol
D. Anacin

34. A 23-year-old client reports to the emergency room in status epilepticus. The nurse anticipates that the following drug will be needed:
A. Phenytoin (Dilantin)
B. Phenobarbital
C. Valproic acid
D. Diazepam (Valium)

35. A client has recently been told about a diagnosis of cancer. The nurse plans which of the following as priority actions:
A. A schedule of regular exercise
B. Activities for diversional therapy
C. Time for the client to share feelings
D. Social activities with a variety of people

36. A 34-year-old client has just had a uric acid stone removed from the ureter. The nurse teaches the client that prevention of another stone formation can be aided by forcing fluids and a diet that is:
A. High in vitamin C
B. Low in calcium

C. High in fiber

D. Low in purines

37. A 42-year-old client went home with a T-tube in place following an open cholecystectomy. She calls the clinic to report that she is experiencing nausea after meals. The nurse could suggest:
   A. Taking an antiemetic 1 hour before each meal.
   B. Reporting to the clinic to have the T-tube removed
   C. Irrigating the T-tube with sterile, normal saline
   D. Clamping the T-tube prior to each meal

38. A 72-year-old client just had a total replacement of the left hip joint. The nurse positions the client's legs in which of the following positions?
   A. Abducted at all times
   B. Flexed at the knees
   C. Internally rotated
   D. Adducted at all times

39. A 42-year-old client returned from the operating room 2 hours ago after having a lumbar diskectomy. The nurse would:
   A. Allow the client to remain in the same position.
   B. Encourage the client to turn himself.
   C. Obtain a trapeze to help the client turn himself.
   D. Turn the client every 2 hours by log-rolling him.

40. A 53-year-old client is scheduled for an arteriogram to evaluate a femoral-distal bypass in the right leg. In order to protect the kidneys from the effects of the iodine-based contrast medium to be used, the nurse should:
   A. Check for allergies to the contrast medium.
   B. See that the client gets a low protein diet prior to the test.
   C. Administer enemas until clear the evening before the test.
   D. See that the client is as well-hydrated as possible.

41. A 27-year-old client returns to the nursing unit following a barium enema. The nurse should see that the client:
   A. Has an order for a laxative
   B. Drinks plenty of fluids
   C. Has a dinner high in fiber
   D. Takes a sitz bath

42. A 17-year-old client has multiple fractures from a motor vehicle accident. Today the client is found confused and restless with dyspnea, a respiratory rate of 34, and a pulse of 144. The nurse assesses the client and recognizes that the highest priority is:
   A. Intravenous digoxin to help the heart beat more effectively
   B. Intravenous fluids to prevent hypovolemia and renal damage

C. Arterial blood gases to accurately assess pulmonary gas exchange

D. Oxygen by way of nasal cannula or Venturi mask

43. In planning for a client who has been diagnosed with leukemia and is about to begin antineoplastic therapy with drugs that cause alopecia, a nurse can:
   A. Arrange a fitting for a hair piece prior to the beginning of therapy.
   B. Obtain an order for the use of ice caps during therapy to prevent hair loss.
   C. Arrange an appointment with a cosmetologist for a perm during therapy.
   D. Set aside time for brushing the hair 100 strokes each day of therapy.

44. A 45-year-old client receiving antineoplastic therapy is experiencing fatigue and shortness of breath. The problems of fatigue and alteration in gas exchange could be related to the following effect of bone marrow depression: a decrease in
   A. Platelets
   B. Granulocytes
   C. Lymphocytes
   D. Erythrocytes

45. A client on antineoplastic therapy has a platelet count of 20,000/mm³. An appropriate intervention for the nurse to use would be:
   A. Administering vitamin K intramuscularly
   B. Massaging injection sites to aid absorption
   C. Encouraging use of firm toothbrushes and vigorous flossing
   D. Avoiding rectal temperatures and other rectal procedures

46. A client, who is receiving radiation to the abdomen for a malignant tumor, is having diarrhea. Which of the following statements would indicate to the nurse that the client has understood teaching about management of diarrhea?
   A. "I should eat foods rich in potassium."
   B. "I need a quart of milk a day or its equivalent."
   C. "I should drink liquid and eat a healthy diet."
   D. "I can have what I want of my favorite beverages."

47. A 35-year-old mother of three children has acute myelogenous leukemia and has recently completed the MOPP (mechlorethamine, Oncovin, procarbazine, and prednisone) protocol. The nurse recognizes that the highest priority for planning and educating the client is:
   A. Careful and frequent hand washing
   B. Vigorous brushing and flossing after meals
   C. Lots of fresh fruit and vegetables
   D. Frequent monitoring of rectal temperatures

48. A client has frequent nausea and vomiting following radiation therapy to the abdomen. An appropriate intervention for the nurse to use is:

A. Administer antiemetics with meals.
B. Monitor fluid intake and output.
C. Serve the diet while food is hot.
D. Provide music and conversation during meals.

49. A nurse notices an excessive amount of serous drainage coming from the surgical wound of a client who had the Whipple procedure 8 days ago. The nurse recognizes the excess drainage as an early sign of:
A. Infection
B. Eviscertion
C. Dehiscence
D. Hematoma formation

50. A client has been on morphine sulfate for several days and reports a pain rating of 9 (on a scale of 1 to 10) 1 hour following a dose of morphine. The nursing assessment also reveals constricted pupils. The nurse recognizes that the client is:
A. Becoming addicted
B. Developing tolerance
C. Malingering
D. Getting worse

51. A client started on amoxicillin (Amoxil) at 9 A.M. At 9:30 A.M., the blood pressure drops and the client is dyspneic. The nurse anticipates the need for:
A. Epinephrine
B. Glucagon
C. Cortisol
D. Aminophyllin

52. A client's blood pressure drops and he is gasping for air following an injection of penicillin. The nurse establishes her first priority as:
A. Effective heart beat
B. Effective tissue perfusion
C. Normal acid-base balance
D. Open airway

53. A client recovering from anaphylactic shock suddenly develops a stridor and hoarseness. The nurse prepares the client for:
A. Emergency surgery
B. Cardiopulmonary resuscitation
C. A tracheostomy
D. Insertion of an endotracheal tube

54. A 63-year-old client has narrow glaucoma. The nurse screens the client's medications for the following side effect:
A. Dilatation of the pupil
B. Constriction of the pupil
C. Constriction of blood vessels
D. Decreased heart rate

55. A nurse assumes responsibility for the care of a client at 7 A.M. NPH insulin is ordered for 7:30 A.M. Before giving the insulin, the nurse checks to see if the client will eat that day and for the:
A. Signs and symptoms of hypoglycemia
B. Previous sites of injection

C. Serum glucagon level
D. Serum glucose level

56. A client is taking sulfisoxazole 6 gms/day for a urinary tract infection. The nurse establishes an outcome of maintaining a:
A. Heart rate between 60 and 100 beats per minute
B. Respiratory rate between 12 and 20
C. Fluid intake of at least 2 L per day
D. Systolic blood pressure between 90 and 140 mm of Hg

57. Diazepam (Valium) is ordered for a client with a history of trait anxiety. Upon seeing the order, the nurse expresses a concern about:
A. Tolerance
B. Respiratory depression
C. Addiction
D. Anaphylaxis

58. A prescription for diazepam (Valium) is written for a client who is being discharged from the hospital. The nurse teaches the client to:
A. Avoid alcoholic drinks.
B. Take the pulse rate frequently.
C. Drive only in the daylight.
D. Decrease consumption of caffeine.

59. A client has both impaired gas exchange and anemia. The nurse is alert for signs of hypoxia and knows that one of the earliest signs is:
A. Cyanosis
B. Clubbing
C. Tachypnea
D. Restlessness

60. A nurse is teaching a client to observe for signs of hypoxia. The nurse explains that cyanosis is not a reliable indicator of the amount of oxygen that tissues are receiving because the blue color is caused by:
A. Reduced hemoglobin
B. A low partial pressure of oxygen in the blood
C. Inability of oxygen to enter the cell
D. Increased pH of the blood

61. A client has adult respiratory distress syndrome. The lowest fraction of inspired oxygen possible for optimizing gas exchange is used. The nurse explains to the family that the reason for this precaution is to:
A. Avoid respiratory depression
B. Prevent oxygen toxicity
C. Increase lung compliance
D. Promote production of surfactant

62. A nurse takes an order for a cough medication for her client who has pneumonia. This cough medication should contain a/an:
A. Mucolytic agent
B. Depressant for the cough reflex
C. Expectorant
D. Bronchiole relaxant

63. A client is being prepared for general surgery. The most important thing the nurse can do to help the client decrease anxiety is to:
    A. Explain everything that is going to happen.
    B. Take cues from the client and explain as needed.
    C. Teach the client relaxation exercises.
    D. Use humor to help the client relax.

64. A client who is recovering from a myocardial infarction demonstrates that teaching has been effective with the statement:
    A. "If my chest pain lasts more than 5 minutes, I should get myself to the emergency room."
    B. "I just need to avoid salty foods and not add salt to my food."
    C. "I need to avoid constipation and all activities that have caused me chest pain in the past."
    D. "I need to get to the drugstore to get some medicine for my cold."

65. When a client is taking an opiate, the nurse should plan for the possibility of the following nursing diagnosis:
    A. Diarrhea
    B. Urinary retention
    C. Impaired adjustment
    D. Constipation

66. The physician has left an order for a laxative PRN for a client. The nurse knows that this order should not be carried out for a client who is:
    A. Experiencing abdominal pain of unknown origin
    B. Recovering from an episode of congestive heart failure
    C. Showing signs of hepatic or renal failure
    D. Showing signs of fluid or electrolyte imbalance

67. A client is receiving digoxin (Lanoxin) daily. Prior to giving any preparation of digoxin, the nurse should assess the:
    A. Blood pressure
    B. Respirations
    C. Radial pulse
    D. Apical pulse

68. A neighbor calls to report that he has taken three nitroglycerin tablets sublingually in the last 15 minutes and that his chest pain is still not relieved. The nurse advises him to:
    A. Call his physician
    B. Rest and take his pain medicine
    C. Wait while she calls 911
    D. Drive to the nearest emergency room

69. A client is taking a nonselective beta-adrenergic agonist for asthma. The nurse checks the following organ for effects of the drug:
    A. Kidneys
    B. Stomach
    C. Liver
    D. Heart

70. A client is discharged on warfarin (Coumadin) therapy. Evidence that teaching related to this drug has been understood is provided, when the nurse hears the following statement:
    A. "I should have a partial thromboplastin time done regularly."
    B. "Protamine sulfate is the antidote for Coumadin."
    C. "I should avoid anything with aspirin in it."
    D. "My diet should be rich in foods with vitamin K."

71. A client is in acute congestive heart failure. The nurse explains that generalized arterial vasodilatation will help reduce the workload of the heart by decreasing:
    A. Preload
    B. Stroke volume
    C. Afterload
    D. Heart rate

72. A client is admitted to the hospital complaining of nervousness, heat intolerance, and muscle weakness. Her pulse rate is 118 and she has exophthalmos. An essential part of her assessment will be:
    A. Palpation of the thyroid gland
    B. Evaluation of fluid and electrolyte balance
    C. Evaluation of deep tendon reflexes
    D. Use of the Glasgow Coma Scale

73. A client is scheduled for a thyroidectomy. The nurse explains that propylthiouracil or an iodine preparation is given prior to surgery in order to:
    A. Increase the size of the thyroid gland
    B. Render the parathyroid glands visible
    C. Induce a euthyroid state in the body
    D. Separate the thyroid from the laryngeal nerve

74. A nurse explains to a client that it is difficult to anticipate the effect of exercise on serum glucose. Although it is usual for serum glucose to be lowered by cellular use of glucose to produce energy, exercise can also stimulate release of substances that actually elevate the serum glucose. These substances include glucagon, growth hormone, epinephrine, and:
    A. Norepinephrine
    B. Cortisol
    C. Acetylcholine
    D. Aldosterone

75. A client with systemic lupus erythematosus has just started on prednisone. The nurse explains that the serum levels of this drug will cause a decrease in:
    A. Epinephrine
    B. Norepinephrine
    C. Dopamine
    D. Cortisol

76. A client is scheduled for a thyroid scan. The nurse explains that:
    A. Thyroid medication should be continued.
    B. The radioactive iodine will not be dangerous.

C. Breakfast may be eaten as usual.

D. An enema will be needed following the test.

77. A client is being evaluated for the possibility of Graves' disease. The nurse teaches that the *best* laboratory test for evaluating whether a client has hypothyroidism or hyperthyroidism is the serum level of:

A. Thyroxine (T$_4$)

B. Triiodothyronine (T$_3$)

C. Thyroid-stimulating hormone (TSH)

D. Epinephrine

78. A client has just had a biopsy of the thyroid gland. The nurse will be alert for the following complication:

A. Hypocalcemia

B. Vomiting

C. Hoarseness

D. Respiratory difficulty

79. A nurse is preparing to receive a client from surgery following a total thyroidectomy. Emergency equipment that should be available for this client includes oxygen, a suction apparatus, a tracheostomy set, and:

A. Racemic epinephrine

B. Potassium chloride

C. Calcium gluconate

D. A suture removal set

80. The nurse is taking a client's blood pressure in the right arm the evening following a thyroidectomy. Following inflation of the cuff, the muscles in the right hand twitch and then contract. The reason for the contraction of the hand muscles is most likely to be:

A. Hypothyroidism

B. Hyperparathyroidism

C. Hypocalcemia

D. Nerve damage

81. A client asks how his autoimmune condition could have started. The nurse replies, "One theory holds that your white blood cells may have become sensitized to the thyroid gland and built antibodies to the receptors for thyroid-stimulating hormone. The antibodies would then bind to the receptors, stimulating growth and activity in the gland." The nurse is describing:

A. Graves' disease

B. Hashimoto's thyroiditis

C. Thyrotoxic crisis

D. Nontoxic goiter

82. A client is taking levothyroxine (Synthroid) for hypothyroidism. The nurse teaches the client to:

A. Monitor the pulse regularly.

B. Restrict sodium in the diet.

C. Take the drug with meals.

D. Measure urinary output.

83. A client has hyperparathyroidism. Which of the following statements (by the client) indicates understanding of the nurse's teaching:

A. "Calcium is the only electrolyte that is out of balance in my body."

B. "I will have to drink lots of fluids to keep stones from forming."

C. "The burning in my stomach is not related to hyperparathyroidism."

D. "The high levels of calcium in my blood should make my bones strong."

84. A client complains of slight polydipsia, polyphagia, and polyuria. The most specific, sensitive, and complete diagnostic test to rule out diabetes mellitus would be a:

A. Fasting blood sugar

B. Glucose tolerance test

C. Glycosylated hemoglobin test

D. C-peptide radioimmunoassay

85. A 56-year-old client takes estrogen and progesterone regularly. The nurse explains to the client that the major reason for taking these hormones is to:

A. Relieve the symptoms of menopause

B. Prevent cancer of the ovaries and breasts

C. Restore her usual sexual functioning

D. Prevent the occurrence of osteoporosis

86. A client with NIDDM is admitted to the hospital. The client is confused and has dry mucous membranes and poor skin turgor. The serum sodium is 149; the blood pressure 88/58; the pulse 118; and the serum glucose 465 mg/dl. The nurse anticipates that insulin and the following will be needed:

A. A potassium drip

B. Sodium bicarbonate

C. Intravenous fluids

D. Calcium gluconate

87. A hospitalized client is found in a coma. The skin is dry and flushed; Kussmaul respirations are noted and the smell of acetone is on the breath. The nurse prepares for the emergency treatment of:

A. Hyperosmolar hyperglycemic nonketotic syndrome

B. Diabetic ketoacidosis

C. Hypoglycemia

D. Dawn phenomenon

88. A client has requested pain medication. The order is for meperidine (Demerol) 75 mg and hydroxyzine (Vistaril) 50 mg intramuscularly. The nurse would:

A. Give the drugs separately.

B. Use the deltoid muscle.

C. Use the Z-track technique.

D. Rub vigorously afterward.

89. A nurse is teaching a diabetic client how to attain the optimal level of health. When assessing for other risk factors for stroke and heart attack, this nurse looks for:

A. Hypervolemia
B. Hypokalemia
C. Proteinuria
D. Hypertension

90. A client is receiving total parenteral nutrition (TPN), including a lipid emulsion, through a catheter inserted into the external jugular vein. When the nurse hangs a new bag of TPN, it is important to remember that the:
A. Clamp attached to the port must remain closed
B. Port must be flushed before the new bag of TPN is hung
C. Serum glucose must be checked prior to hanging the bag
D. Filter is placed between the port and the TPN solution

91. A 33-year-old client has burns involving the neck and upper extremities. The nurse will use the following intervention to prevent contractures:
A. Support the head with pillows.
B. Place a firm object in the hand so that the hand is grasping the object.
C. Allow the client to assume the most comfortable position.
D. Keep the arms in alignment close to the body.

92. A 55-year-old male reports seeing flashes and floaters on entering a darkened room. The nurse recommends that he:
A. Drive to the nearest emergency room.
B. Have a family member call his ophthalmologist.
C. Use the eye drop he is taking for glaucoma.
D. Remain calm because this is normal for a man his age.

93. A school nurse is teaching a class on prevention of HIV infection. The nurse knows that more instruction is needed when the students say:
A. "Social contact or even dry kissing will not spread the infection."
B. "Condoms are the best way to avoid the spread of infection."
C. "Babies may be infected with the virus when passing through the birth canal."
D. "Contact with any body fluid from an infected person is unsafe."

94. A 52-year-old client is being discharged following a laryngectomy for cancer of the larynx. Prior to discharge, the nurse assesses the following psychomotor skills:
A. Administering injections, changing dressings, and chest physical therapy
B. Taking the blood pressure and pulse rate, and monitoring serum glucose
C. Suctioning and caring for tracheostomies and tracheostomy tubes
D. Tube feedings, taking aerosol medications, and taking the temperature

95. A nurse stops at the sight of a motor vehicle accident to find a young woman slumped over the wheel. She is breathing with a regular rhythm at a rate of 22; ventilation efforts appear normal. Her pulse rate is 110. The nurse's next action would be to:
A. Check the level of consciousness.
B. Immobilize the spine.
C. Call the rescue squad.
D. Check for bleeding.

96. A 55-year-old client just had a myocardial infarction. The nurse places this client in the following position.
A. Supine with the head of the bed elevated 45 to 90 degrees
B. On the left side with slight elevation of the head
C. On the right side with slight elevation of the head
D. Supine with the head elevated on a pillow

97. A 55-year-old client is being prepared for discharge following a myocardial infarction. The nurse knows that her teaching has been understood when she hears:
A. "I guess my sex life is over."
B. "Depression is bad for me; I must stay happy and optimistic."
C. "The best way to know the amount of exercise I should take is to watch my pulse."
D. "The injured area will be replaced with new heart tissue."

98. An 86-year-old female complains of profound weakness and dyspnea. A nurse, who is a neighbor, finds that the temperature is 98.8°F, the pulse is 94, and respirations are 16 (with a normal rhythm). This nurse calls 911, and the client is later diagnosed with a myocardial infarction (MI). This nurse's actions were based on the fact that:
A. The client shows typical signs and symptoms of MI.
B. The vital signs taken support MI.
C. The nurse believed the problem to be respiratory in origin.
D. Atypical forms of disease are frequently seen in the elderly.

99. A 54-year-old client with insulin-dependent diabetes mellitus has a Foley catheter. Today her temperature is 101.5°F, and she complains of burning. A urine for culture and sensitivity is ordered. The nurse would obtain the specimen by:
A. Removing a sample from the collection bag
B. Cleaning the end of the catheter and allowing the urine to drip into a sterile container
C. Aspirating a sample from a port on the tubing, using aseptic technique
D. Aspirating a sample from the Foley, using aseptic technique

100. A client is scheduled for an intravenous pyelogram (IVP). The nurse should:
  A. Check for allergies to shellfish.
  B. Restrict fluids for 12 hours.
  C. Explain that a flushing sensation or salty taste are signs of danger.
  D. Inform the client that signing a consent form will not be necessary.

101. A client is receiving chemotherapy for breast cancer. She has a Foley catheter, and her urinary output for the last 6 hours was 150 ml. The nurse should:
  A. Increase the rate of her IV fluids.
  B. Report that she is voiding a sufficient amount.
  C. Report her urinary output to the physician.
  D. Increase he PO fluids.

102. A client is having a creatinine clearance test. The blood will be drawn, and the client will empty the bladder. The nurse should:
  A. Save this specimen and all other urine for 24 hours.
  B. Discard this specimen and then save urine for 24 hours.
  C. Send this specimen to the laboratory properly labeled.
  D. Send 30 ml of this specimen to the laboratory labeled.

103. A 35-year-old male is scheduled to start chemotherapy for advanced melanoma. The nurse would check the following objective data to be certain that the client has adequate renal function:
  A. Renal scan, cystogram, CT scan
  B. Daily weights, CBC, electrolytes
  C. Urinalysis, urine culture, renal angiogram
  D. BUN, creatinine, urinary output

104. A 55-year-old female visits her physician complaining of frequency of urination and dysuria. When the nurse assesses a report on the urinalysis, the following abnormality is discovered:
  A. pH 5.8
  B. Trace of protein
  C. Cloudy
  D. Occasional hyaline casts

105. A diabetic client is being evaluated for possible renal damage. The nurse collects a urine specimen for urinalysis. Half an hour later, the specimen still has not gone to the laboratory. The specimen should be:
  A. Refrigerated
  B. Discarded
  C. Ignored because the messenger will get it later
  D. Put in a special container with a preservative

106. A 34-year-old client has pyelonephritis. The client states that he must have developed this condition because he did not have treatment for a recent streptococcal infection of the throat. The nurse teaches this client about pyelonephritis and glo-merulonephritis. The following statement indicates that the client has understood the teaching:
  A. "Pyelonephritis is a sequela to untreated streptococcal infections."
  B. "Either disease could end in renal failure."
  C. "The urine usually appears like cola in pyelonephritis."
  D. "Nursing care for the two conditions is very different."

107. A 64-year-old client has a nephrostomy tube in the left kidney and a stent within the right ureter. The nurse would plan to:
  A. Maintain bedrest.
  B. Irrigate the stent and the nephrostomy tube PRN.
  C. Clamp the nephrostomy tube to facilitate transportation of the client.
  D. Record the output from the nephrostomy tube separately from the output from the bladder.

108. A 34-year-old female is being discharged after passing a urinary stone consisting mainly of uric acid. The nurse teaches prevention of stone formation, instructing the client to:
  A. Avoid scented feminine hygiene products.
  B. Take allopurinol daily.
  C. Force fluids and eat a low purine diet.
  D. Exercise daily and eat a low-fat diet.

109. A 42-year-old client has been admitted to the nursing unit with nausea and vomiting and complaining of acute flank pain. The medical diagnosis of nephrolithiasis is made. The nurse will plan to:
  A. Maintain bedrest.
  B. Restrict fluids.
  C. Strain the urine.
  D. Offer cranberry juice.

110. A 44-year-old client with a large stone blocking a ureter has a nephrostomy tube in place. When planning the care for this client, the nurse would plan to:
  A. Observe the condition of the skin around the tube.
  B. Restrict fluids until after the stone is removed.
  C. Restrict the amount of calcium in the diet.
  D. Irrigate with 25 ml of solution as ordered.

111. A 33-year-old client has a new ileal conduit following surgery for cancer of the bladder. The nurse would plan to:
  A. Observe the stoma frequently.
  B. Check the bowel sounds once a shift.
  C. Change the drainage bag every 2 hours.
  D. Report any signs of mucus in the urine.

112. An 87-year-old client is recovering from hip replacement surgery. Because of problems with mobility, she cannot get to the bathroom before voiding. The nurse would chart that the client has:
  A. Stress incontinence
  B. Functional incontinence

C. Urge incontinence
D. Reflex incontinence

113. A 45-year-old client had less than 400 ml of urinary output in the last 24 hours. The physician diagnoses acute renal failure. When planning for the care of this client, the nurse would plan to observe for signs and symptoms of the following:
    A. Hypercalcemia and hypomagnesemia
    B. Hyperchloremia and alkalosis
    C. Hyperkalemia and acidosis
    D. Hypernatremia and hypercalcemia

114. A 35-year-old client has just completed chemotherapy for acute myelogenous leukemia. During the last 24 hours, he has urinated only 360 ml. The physician says the client is in the oliguric phase of acute renal failure. When planning for this phase of the client's care, the nurse will plan for the client to receive an amount of fluid that is:
    A. Less than the loss during the previous 24 hours
    B. Equal to the loss during the previous 24 hours
    C. Greater than fluid lost during the previous 24 hours
    D. At least 2 to 3 L per 24-hour period

115. A 34-year-old client is in acute renal failure. In planning for his care, the nurse will be certain to include the following nursing diagnosis:
    A. Hopelessness
    B. Knowledge deficit
    C. Risk for impaired skin integrity
    D. Risk for infection

116. A client with acute lymphocytic leukemia is to receive 1 L of fluid over a 2-hour period prior to receiving a drug that is nephrotoxic. The nurse will perform the following assessment frequently during that 2-hour period in order to detect the first sign of hypervolemia:
    A. Take the vital signs.
    B. Check for jugular venous distention.
    C. Check skin turgor.
    D. Listen for rales in the lungs.

117. A 47-year-old diabetic asks the nurse how he can detect the first sign of renal damage from his disease. In response to this question, the nurse teaches him to:
    A. Test his urine for sodium.
    B. Do self-monitoring for glucose.
    C. Test the urine for protein.
    D. Palpate the kidney.

118. A client develops chronic renal failure after years of noncompliance with his medical regimen for diabetes mellitus. The nurse is encouraged that he may have learned something about chronic renal failure when the following statement is heard:
    A. "About the only thing I can eat plenty of is carbohydrates."
    B. "My red blood cells will increase to help me breathe better."

C. "My blood pressure won't get worse. Will it?"
D. "Ammonia will be changed to urea in my gut."

119. A 26-year-old client has been diagnosed with membranous proliferative glomerulonephritis. When planning the care for this client, the nurse writes an outcome to detect hypovolemia. The most appropriate outcome for such a purpose might be:
    A. The pulse rate will remain within normal limits.
    B. The blood pressure will remain within normal limits.
    C. No signs of edema will be present.
    D. Urine specific gravity will remain within normal limits.

120. A 56-year-old client has thrombophlebitis in the left leg. While being admitted to the nursing unit, she suddenly develops chest pain and becomes dyspneic and diaphoretic. The physician diagnoses a pulmonary embolus. The blood pressure is 134/76, and the pulse rate is 116. The first action of the nurse will be to:
    A. Do a complete respiratory assessment.
    B. Administer heparin.
    C. Give warfarin (Coumadin).
    D. Administer oxygen.

121. Which of the following would decrease client discomfort related to "the dumping syndrome" after surgery for peptic ulcer disease?
    A. Decreasing fat intake with meals
    B. Eating sugary snacks between meals
    C. Drinking large amounts of fluids with meals
    D. Eating small, frequent meals

122. A client has been hospitalized for a possible intestinal obstruction. He has increased bowel sounds, abdominal distention, and fecal vomiting. Which of the following would *not* be included as a nursing diagnosis for him?
    A. Altered comfort: acute pain related to hyperactive bowel sounds and abdominal distention
    B. Impaired verbal communication related to presence of nasogastric tube
    C. Fluid volume deficits related to vomiting
    D. Potential alteration in thought processes related to fluid and electrolyte imbalances

123. A client in respiratory failure has hypoxemia. The nurse knows that this can cause constriction of pulmonary vessels. Therefore, when planning this client's care, the nurse will include observation for:
    A. Pleural effusion
    B. Pneumothorax
    C. Subcutaneous emphysema
    D. Cor pulmonale

124. A client developed acute respiratory failure following abdominal surgery. The nurse would question an order for:
    A. Epidural catheter placement
    B. Epinephrine

C. Atropine

D. Neostigmine

125. A 42-year-old client developed acute respiratory distress syndrome (ARDS) following smoke inhalation from a fire in his home. He was placed on a ventilator, but his hemoglobin saturations have remained in the 70 to 80 percent range. Today positive end-expiratory pressure (PEEP) was initiated. When planning this client's care, the nurse will include observation for:

A. Pleural effusion

B. A pneumothorax

C. Cardiac tamponade

D. Signs of oxygen toxicity

126. A nurse practitioner is performing a pre-employment physical examination when a pulsating mass is palpated in the abdomen. The blood pressure is 162/96, and a bruit is heard over the aorta in the same area. The nurse would then assess:

A. Bowel sounds

B. The apical pulse

C. Pulses in the lower extremities

D. For jugular venous distention

127. A 16-year-old client has been diagnosed with sickle-cell anemia. The nurse would look for more data to support the nursing diagnoses of fatigue and:

A. Activity intolerance

B. Ineffective breathing pattern

C. Ineffective airway clearance

D. Impaired gas exchange

128. A 59-year-old client is being discharged following removal of two-thirds of the stomach. As part of the discharge planning, the nurse will incorporate plans to prevent the development of:

A. Pernicious anemia

B. Aplastic anemia

C. Thalassemia

D. Hypoproliferative anemia

129. A 62-year-old client has congestive heart failure, including 3+ edema over most of the body. When planning the care of this client, the nurse will want to include the following nurse diagnosis:

A. Body image disturbance

B. Risk for impaired skin integrity

C. Risk for infection

D. Sleep pattern disturbance

130. A 54-year-old client has periodic episodes of angina pectoris. While preparing him for discharge, the nurse teaches him that the major benefit of the vasodilator medication is:

A. Reduction of afterload

B. Increasing afterload

C. Increasing preload

D. Dilatation of coronary arteries

131. A client with insulin-dependent diabetes mellitus has just been admitted to the emergency room af-

ter hitting a telephone pole with her car. Bystanders said she acted as if she had been drinking. Her temperature is 37.4°C; pulse, 80; and respirations, 44 and deep. She complained of headache and acted confused. A fruity odor was noted on her breath. The ABG report read: pH = 7.32, $PaCO_2$ = 36 mm Hg, and bicarbonate = 18 mEq/L. The nurse prepared for treatment of:

A. Metabolic acidosis

B. Metabolic alkalosis

C. Respiratory acidosis

D. Respiratory alkalosis

132. A client is admitted to the intensive care unit in respiratory acidosis. He has an acute respiratory infection superimposed on emphysema. When planning for the care of this client, the nurse recognizes that compensation for respiratory acidosis will be made by the kidneys within:

A. Eight hours

B. Twenty-four hours

C. Two to three days

D. Four to five days

133. The mother of a 16-year-old client asks the nurse why it is important to prevent recurrence of rheumatic fever. The nurse replies that common sequelae to rheumatic fever include:

A. Kidney disease

B. Seizure activity

C. Liver trauma

D. Cardiac disease

134. A 33-year-old client has prolapse of the mitral valve with regurgitation. The nurse teaches this client that it is important to:

A. Take aspirin daily to prevent clotting.

B. Take antibiotics prior to dental or surgical procedures.

C. Drink at least 3 L of fluid daily.

D. Get at least 8 hours of sleep every night.

135. A client has chronic mitral regurgitation. The carotid pulses are brisk, and a third heart sound is heard with a murmur. When planning this client's care, the following nursing diagnosis will receive a high priority:

A. Activity intolerance

B. High risk for decreased cardiac output

C. High risk for fluid volume deficit

D. Impaired physical mobility

136. A client develops mitral stenosis following rheumatic fever. When planning the care of this client, the nurse includes regular assessments for tissue perfusion. This means that the extremities will be checked for neurovascular signs; the level of consciousness will be checked as well as:

A. Bowel sounds

B. Jugular venous distention

C. Urinary output

D. Breath sounds

137. A client has no bowel sounds and has been vomiting for the last hour. The nurse places a nasogastric tube (as ordered by the physician). In order to estimate the distance to the beginning of the esophagus, this nurse will measure the distance from the tip of the nose to the:
    A. Lower tip of the ear lobe
    B. Xiphoid process
    C. Thyroid gland
    D. Cricoid cartilage

138. A client is ready to have the nasogastric tube removed. As the nurse removes the tube, the client is asked to:
    A. Cough
    B. Breathe deeply
    C. Turn her head to the side
    D. Perform the Valsalva maneuver

139. A client has a nasogastric tube in place for continuous tube feedings, The nurse will:
    A. Irrigate the tube with normal saline every 4 hours.
    B. Insert the tube another inch every 2 hours.
    C. Check the tube for placement each shift.
    D. Remove the tape and check the nostril every shift.

140. A client has venous stasis ulcers. The nurse knows that the client has understood teaching about the condition when the following statement is heard:
    A. "I must check the pulses in my feet every day."
    B. "I should raise my feet whenever I am sitting."
    C. "I won't have to shave my legs as often; the hair will fall out."
    D. "If I don't take good care of my legs, they might have to be amputated."

141. A client has chronic arterial occlusive disease. The nurse recalls that a major difference between arterial disease and venous insufficiency is that the client with arterial disease should:
    A. Rest when pain is caused by exercise.
    B. Stop smoking.
    C. Keep the feet dependent when pain occurs.
    D. Keep the feet dependent whenever out of bed.

142. A nurse is performing a pre-employment physical examination on a client. When examining the liver, the nurse will ask the client to:
    A. Remain still.
    B. Take a deep breath and hold it.
    C. Exhale and hold it.
    D. Turn onto the right side.

143. A female client complains of dull abdominal discomfort. The client just became aware of the discomfort for the first time, and it is not related to meals, defecation, or any other factors. Bowel sounds are hypoactive, but the nurse detects rebound tenderness in the right lower quadrant. The tenderness is most likely caused by:
    A. Stool in the area where tenderness is palpated

B. An abdominal aneurysm
    C. Irritable bowel syndrome
    D. Peritoneal inflammation

144. A nurse is inspecting the mouth of an elderly neighbor. This nurse encourages the neighbor to seek medical attention for the following:
    A. Thickened white patches
    B. Cracking at angles of the mouth
    C. Red, slick tongue
    D. Bleeding gums

145. A client's bowel sounds are absent during a shift assessment. After confirming this finding, the nurse would:
    A. Document the absence.
    B. Administer the PRN laxative.
    C. Notify the physician.
    D. Reposition the nasogastric tube.

146. A client has obstruction of the common bile duct caused by cholelithiasis. The nurse would expect the stools to be:
    A. Dark brown and formed
    B. Black and liquid
    C. Light brown and formed
    D. Clay colored, fatty, and frothy

147. A client was admitted for evaluation of melena. Today this client returns to the hospital room following a barium enema. The nurse will be sure to:
    A. Obtain an order for a laxative.
    B. Check the vital signs frequently.
    C. Maintain NPO status until barium is passed.
    D. Evaluate lower extremities for neurovascular signs.

148. A client has severe pain in the umbilical area of the abdomen and complains of nausea and vomiting. A fasting blood sugar is 197. The client is admitted to the hospital to rule out cancer of the pancreas. An endoscopic retrograde cholangiopancreatogram is ordered. In planning for this procedure, the nurse includes the following:
    A. Provide a diet high in polyunsaturated fat the evening before the procedure.
    B. Assess the gag reflex following the procedure and the vital signs frequently.
    C. Observe for gastritis, a common complication of this procedure.
    D. Administer aspirin for pain as needed following the procedure.

149. A client is scheduled for a liver biopsy. When planning the nursing care for this procedure, the nurse will:
    A. Evaluate liver function tests prior to the procedure.
    B. Maintain NPO status for 8 hours prior to the procedure.
    C. Allow activity ad lib 8 hours following the procedure.

D. Keep the client on his or her right side for 2 hours after the procedure.

150. A client is to be started on tube feedings through a nasogastric tube. The nurse wishes to determine whether the end of the tube is located in the stomach or in the intestines. Placement could be determined by:
    A. Testing the pH of the drainage
    B. Injecting an air bubble and listening over the stomach
    C. Placing the tube in water and asking the client to cough
    D. Testing electrolyte content of the drainage

151. A client is receiving continuous tube feedings through a jejunostomy via a Keofeed tube. The nurse makes certain that:
    A. The container for the feeding does not run dry.
    B. The container for the feeding is never below the jejunum.
    C. The client is in high Fowler's position.
    D. The head of the bed remains elevated at 30 to 45 degrees.

152. A client is receiving continuous tube feedings through a nasogastric tube. The nurse will:
    A. Irrigate the tube with normal saline every 4 hours.
    B. Check for residual every 4 hours.
    C. Auscultate the lungs every 4 hours.
    D. Check bowel sounds every 4 hours.

153. A client is receiving continuous tube feedings through a Keofeed tube. The flow of the feeding is being controlled by a pump. The nurse should:
    A. Check the tube for kinks and dependent loops.
    B. Aspirate and flush the tube every 4 hours.
    C. Administer about 100 ml of water every 4 hours.
    D. Administer medications through the tube as needed.

154. A client becomes dyspneic and profusely diaphoretic following insertion of a catheter into the subclavian vein. The physician suspects an air embolism. The nurse would:
    A. Place the client in Trendelenburg position and on the left side.
    B. Raise the head of the bed and instruct the client to take a deep breath and hold it.
    C. Clamp a sterile petroleum jelly dressing over the site.
    D. Attempt to aspirate the air through the port in the catheter.

155. A 76-year-old neighbor has been diagnosed with osteoarthritis. The client states that it is her hips that bother her the most. The nurse teaches her about osteoarthritis but recognizes that more teaching is needed when the client makes the following statement:

A. "I should report any nausea, vomiting, or black stools to my doctor."
B. "I should rest my hips as much as possible."
C. "I can use moist heat, ice, or massage to relieve the pain."
D. "I should have my toilet seat elevated."

156. A client is recovering from the Whipple procedure and is receiving total parenteral nutrition (TPN). The nurse would change the IV tubing on the TPN solution:
    A. With each new bottle of solution
    B. Every 24 hours
    C. Every 48 hours
    D. Every 72 hours

157. A 34-year-old client is experiencing intractable nausea and vomiting following chemotherapy for advanced melanoma. He has a triple-lumen Hickman catheter and is receiving TPN with daily infusions of lipids, as well as several other IV medications. The lipids may be run:
    A. Into a port separate from the TPN solution
    B. In the same line as the TPN, between the filter and the port
    C. In the same line as the TPN, between the filter and TPN solution
    D. Using a special filter for lipids

158. A client with pancreatitis has an order to receive TPN, with lipid infusions three times a week. The first transfusion of lipids is started very slowly, but in a very few minutes, the client complains of back pain and becomes dyspneic. The nurse should:
    A. Take the vital signs.
    B. Stop the infusion of lipids and call the physician.
    C. Give the prn pain medication and the client's bronchodilator.
    D. Discontinue the IV.

159. A client with a small bowel obstruction has an order for TPN. Prior to hanging the TPN solution, the nurse is careful to leave the solution at room temperature a maximum of:
    A. Fifteen minutes
    B. Thirty minutes
    C. One hour
    D. Two hours

160. A client has just returned from surgery for repair of a mandibular fracture by intermaxillary fixation. When planning the care of this client, the nurse will most likely place highest priority on the following outcomes:
    A. Adequate nutrition and fluid balance
    B. Electrolyte balance and absence of infection
    C. Effective coping and prevention of aspiration
    D. Patent airway and effective communication

161. A client had a hemicolectomy 24 hours ago. When planning the care of this client, the nurse includes routine observation of bowel sounds and for any

signs of abdominal discomfort or pain, distention, constipation, or inability to pass gas. These signs and symptoms indicate that the nurse is observing for:

A. An impaired vomiting reflex
B. Paralytic ileus
C. Dehiscence
D. Evisceration

162. A client with amyotrophic lateral sclerosis (ALS) is receiving tube feedings and medications through a gastrotomy tube. The nurse initiates a feeding by aspirating gastric contents (for placement of the tube and for residual). Sixty milliliters are obtained. The nurse should handle the aspirate as follows:

A. Discard it.
B. Return it to the stomach.
C. Send it to the laboratory.
D. Add it to the feeding.

163. A client with ALS is receiving continuous feedings through a gastrotomy tube. Today he is sweating profusely and experiencing nausea, diarrhea, and borborygmi. His pulse rate is 112, and he says he feels nervous and jittery. The nurse aspirates for residual and gets 80 ml. The most likely explanation for the client's signs and symptoms is:

A. The tube feedings are hyperosmotic.
B. Paralytic ileus has occurred.
C. The tube has slipped into the small intestines.
D. The tube has slipped into the peritoneal cavity.

164. A client with breast cancer completed a round of chemotherapy several days ago. She has been nauseated and vomiting for the past 24 hours. The nurse will include the following intervention in the care of this client:

A. Teach distraction techniques.
B. Teach relaxation exercises.
C. Play music the client enjoys.
D. Minimize sensory stimuli.

165. A client demonstrates dampened deep-tendon reflexes (DTRs) during a neurological assessment. The nurse explains that the problem could be in the receptor, sensory nerve, motor nerve, muscle, or:

A. Brain stem
B. Spinal cord
C. Cerebellum
D. Cerebrum

166. A client recovering from a myocardial infarction asks why rectal temperatures are contraindicated. The nurse explains that:

A. The valsalva maneuver might be stimulated.
B. The vagus nerve might be stimulated and decrease heart rate.
C. The spinal accessory nerve might be stimulated and increase heart rate.
D. The decreased perfusion will make rectal temperatures less accurate.

167. A client with esophageal varices is brought to the emergency room bleeding profusely from the mouth. Immediately, the nurse will assist with the insertion of a central line and:

A. Hang packed red blood cells.
B. Insert a Foley catheter.
C. Insert a nasogastric tube through the nose.
D. Draw blood for the hemoglobin and hematocrit.

168. A client with bleeding esophageal varices is being treated in the emergency room. The nurse anticipates that the physicians will attempt to stop the bleeding by:

A. Insertion of a Sengstaken-Blakemore tube
B. Gastric lavage with iced saline
C. Endoscopic procedure
D. Local application of epinephrine

169. A client with gastrointestinal bleeding is started on oral neomycin. The nurse explains that the purpose of this drug is prevention of:

A. Infection
B. Stress ulcer
C. Constipation
D. Encephalopathy

170. A client has ascites caused by cirrhosis of the liver. Part of the care of this client includes measuring the abdomen daily. The nurse will:

A. Mark the place of measurement.
B. Measure the same time each day.
C. Have the client empty the bladder prior to measuring.
D. Use the same tape measure each time.

171. A 76-year-old client just had a total hip replacement. In order to detect the earliest sign of bleeding in this client, the nurse would check:

A. The dressing
B. Coagulation times
C. Hemoglobin and hematocrit
D. Liver function tests

172. A client was recently admitted following a motor vehicle accident The urine specific gravity has ranged between 1.25 and 1.030 for the last 24 hours. The nurse would assess for other defining characteristics of:

A. Fluid volume deficit
B. Fluid volume excess
C. Decreased cardiac output
D. Altered tissue perfusion

173. A client has been admitted to the hospital for treatment of gastric ulcers. The nurse assesses this client for risk factors. One such risk factor is:

A. Highly seasoned food
B. Alcoholic beverages
C. Acid ash diets
D. Nonsteroidal anti-inflammatory drugs

174. A 65-year-old client, diagnosed with peptic ulcer,

complains of severe upper abdominal pain that quickly radiates throughout the abdomen and to the shoulder. The nurse examines the client and finds a rigid abdomen, a pulse of 112, blood pressure 134/64, and respirations of 34. The nurse anticipates that medical treatment will be for:

A. Gastric outlet obstruction
B. Hemorrhage
C. Perforation
D. Gastrointestinal infarction

175. A client with peptic ulcers is taking amoxicillin, tamotidine (Pepcid), and Maalox. The nurse teaches the client to take the Maalox:

A. One to 2 hours before meals
B. One-half hour before meals
C. With meals
D. One or 2 hours after meals

176. The nurse teaches a client, who is taking Maalox for peptic ulcers, to always be aware of the electrolytes contained in an antacid. With Maalox, some magnesium may be absorbed with chronic use. Absorption of magnesium would be harmful only under the following condition:

A. Hepatic failure
B. Acidemia
C. Alkalemia
D. Renal insufficiency

177. A client with peptic ulcers is being discharged from the hospital on amoxicillin, cimetidine (Tagamet), and Maalox. The nurse knows that the client has understood the teaching about medications when the following statement is heard:

A. "I should not take the Maalox with the other medications."
B. "I might develop some diarrhea from taking the Maalox."
C. "The Maalox will make me constipated."
D. "I can increase the dose of Maalox if the pain is not relieved."

178. A client is admitted to the hospital with a small-bowel obstruction. When planning the care of this client, the nurse will include observation for signs and symptoms of:

A. Hemorrhage and mesenteric adenitis
B. Perforation and peritonitis
C. Electrolyte imbalance and fluid volume deficit
D. Volvulus and inflammatory bowel disease

179. A 44-year-old client returns from the postanesthesia suite after having an incisional cholecystectomy. When the nurse plans the care of this client, she will place most of the emphasis on prevention of the following postoperative complication:

A. Thrombophlebitis
B. Retention of urine
C. Hypostatic pneumonia
D. Hemorrhage

180. A client is being discharged from the hospital fol-

lowing an incisional cholecystectomy. A T tube is in place. The nurse teaches the following preparation for discharge:

A. The T tube should never be clamped.
B. Keep the bile drainage bag below the insertion site at all times.
C. Clean technique may be used when changing the dressing.
D. There are no restrictions on activity.

181. A client has a Jackson-Pratt drain in place following an incisional cholecystectomy. When planning the care of this client, the nurse will include:

A. Emptying the drain every 2 hours
B. Maintaining patency of the drain
C. Covering the drain with the sterile dressing
D. Observation of the skin around the drain for bile

182. A client returns from surgery for cancer of the colon with a colostomy in the left upper quadrant. The nurse will plan for care of the client's colostomy as follows:

A. Irrigate it to mimic the client's regular pattern of bowel movements.
B. Change the drainage bag each time the client has a stool.
C. Teach the client to maintain a low-residue diet.
D. Assess the skin around the stoma every 8 hours.

183. A client with a history of chronic hypertension comes to the emergency room complaining of severe abdominal pain. An abdominal aortic aneurysm is suspected. What would the nurse expect to find on abdominal examination?

A. A large pulsating mass
B. An absence of bowel sounds
C. A tight, rigid abdominal wall
D. Right upper quadrant pain

184. A client with varicose veins tells the nurse, "I am afraid they will burst while I am walking." Which response by the nurse would be the best?

A. "The only way to prevent rupture is to have surgery."
B. "You must find another job, one that requires less walking."
C. "If that happens, you could bleed to death."
D. "Rupture of varicose veins rarely occurs."

185. A client has a new ileostomy following surgery for ulcerative colitis. The nurse assesses the stoma and reports the following abnormality to the physician:

A. Moderate edema
B. Oozing of blood on touching the stoma
C. Dark red color
D. Pale color

186. A client with an ileostomy is being discharged from the hospital. The nurse would screen the client's medications and request that the physician change the following:

A. Liquid preparations
B. Time-released preparations
C. Oral antibiotics
D. Suppositories

187. A client is taking piperacillin for bacterial pneumonia. Today the client has diarrhea. The nurse would recommend:
A. Gatorade and a clear liquid diet
B. A low-fiber diet
C. Yogurt, cottage cheese, and buttermilk
D. Omitting milk products

188. A client is receiving gentamycin intravenously for treatment of gram-negative septicemia. When planning the care of this client, the nurse will plan routine assessments for:
A. Hepatic dysfunction and urticaria
B. Visual changes and dyspnea
C. Hypotension and vomiting
D. Hearing loss and renal damage

189. A client has been admitted to the hospital for evaluation of the etiology of jaundice. The total bilirubin is elevated but the direct (conjugated) is not. The nurse explains to the family (after the client has been informed by the physician) that the jaundice is caused by:
A. Hepatitis
B. Stones blocking the common bile duct
C. A hemolytic condition
D. Cholecystitis

190. A client has hepatitis. From knowledge of liver function, the nurse plans for routine assessments for:
A. Dehydration and cardiac arrhythmias
B. Edema and bleeding
C. Jugular venous distention and pleural effusion
D. Hypoactive bowel sounds and impaired skin integrity

191. A client is diagnosed with hepatitis, type A. The nurse teaches the client's significant others that they can prevent infection with the virus by:
A. Careful hand washing and good sanitation
B. Using fluid precautions around the client
C. Wearing a mask when entering the client's room
D. Using safe sexual practices

192. A 36-year-old has a colostomy because of cancer of the colon. The nurse can help this client best by:
A. Providing excellent colostomy care every day
B. Leaving some of the colostomy care for the client
C. Providing the opportunity for the client to socialize with others
D. Watching for cues that the client is ready to participate in colostomy care

193. A client just returned to the hospital room following a myelogram. The nurse will need to know the type of contrast medium used but will plan for the next few hours to:
A. Restrict fluid.
B. Offer several small meals.
C. Maintain bedrest.
D. Measure intake and output carefully.

194. A client is scheduled for a lumbar puncture. The nurse explains that the lumbar area will be cleaned with an antiseptic, a local anesthetic will be injected, and then a needle will be inserted into the:
A. Cauda equina
B. Root of the spinal nerve
C. Subdural space
D. Subarachnoid space

195. A client with heart block has a temporary pacemaker inserted as a precautionary measure. The nurse knows the client will now be especially susceptible to:
A. Pneumonia
B. Dysrhythmias
C. Electrical hazards
D. Digitalis drugs

196. A major risk factor associated with a myocardial infarction is:
A. Atherosclerosis
B. Strenuous excercise
C. The aging process
D. Environmental pollution

197. During a shift assessment of a client's eyes, the nurse finds that the client's gaze remains fixed straight ahead regardless of the position of the head. The nurse charts this finding as:
A. Fixed pupils
B. Midposition of the pupil
C. Doll's eyes
D. Nystagmus

198. A client asks why it is important to check the pupils. The nurse replies that changes in the pupils are a reflection of how well the following area of the nervous system is functioning:
A. Spinal cord
B. Brain stem
C. Midbrain
D. Cerebellum

199. A client is brought to the emergency room after being picked up by paramedics at the scene of a motor vehicle accident. The spine is hyperextended, and the teeth are clenched. The upper extremities are extended, adducted, and hyperpronated. The lower extremities are extended. The nurse would chart this position as:
A. Romberg's sign
B. Comatose
C. Decorticate
D. Decerebrate

200. A 22-year-old client is comatose following involvement in a motor vehicle accident. When planning the care of this client, the nurse will include the following outcome:

A. The environment will remain quiet.
B. The cornea will remain intact.
C. Score on the Glasgow Coma Scale will steadily decrease.
D. The head of the bed will remain flat.

201. A client sustained a head injury in a car accident recently. He has episodes of confusion and drowsiness. During these episodes the pupils react sluggishly, and breathing patterns change. The nurse assesses the vital signs. The blood pressure is 142/80; the pulse is 66. The nurse plans for the possibility of:

A. A seizure
B. Herniation of the brain
C. Increased intracranial pressure
D. A cerebral hemorrhage

202. The client's intracranial pressure is increasing. The blood pressure is now 164/80; the pulse is 60. The nurse helps the client to:

A. Hyperventilate
B. Assume the fetal position
C. Blow the nose
D. Pull up in bed

203. A client is on seizure precautions. The nurse would see that the client was on bedrest with side rails raised. Diazepam (Valium) or lorazepam (Ativan) would be available. An additional precaution would be:

A. Having a sitter at the bedside
B. Having a padded tongue blade available
C. Having an oral airway available
D. Padding the side rails

204. An 88-year-old client has been diagnosed Alzheimer's disease. This client has slurred speech and sometimes fails to recognize friends. Ambulation is difficult because of stiffness. The nurse makes the following recommendation to family members:

A. Use cues to help with orientation, such as clocks and calendars.
B. Provide socializing experiencing during mealtimes.
C. Plan walks or other forms of exercise for late afternoon.
D. Be an active listener and allow the client to take the lead in conversation.

205. A nurse is teaching a family about Alzheimer's disease. The nurse knows that the instructions have been understood when the following statement is heard:

A. "Restraints may be used as long as circulation is checked periodically."
B. "A variety of daily activities should be planned to prevent boredom."

C. "Alcohol and caffeine should be avoided."
D. "Naps should be discouraged to promote sleep during the night."

206. A 79-year-old client has been diagnosed with Parkinson's disease. The client has a tremor in the right hand. As the nurse assesses this client, it will be very important to obtain the following information:

A. Breath sounds
B. Peripheral pulses
C. Elimination patterns
D. Last dose of medication

207. A client has been experiencing progressive weakness with ambulation and some loss of strength in the upper extremities. The medical diagnosis of amyotrophic lateral sclerosis (ALS) has been made. The nurse is implementing a teaching plan for this client. This plan will include instructions to:

A. Conserve strength as much as possible by bedrest and sitting.
B. Use an incentive spirometer or similar device routinely.
C. Consume a balanced diet high in calcium.
D. Provide a calm and restful environment during mealtimes.

208. A client suddenly develops attacks during which he falls to the floor. He recovers quickly with no aftereffects. When the nurse is consulted, advice is given based on suspicion of the following:

A. Amyotrophic lateral sclerosis
B. Meniere's syndrome
C. Stroke
D. Transient ischemic attacks

209. A 34-year-old client has just been diagnosed with pulmonary tuberculosis. The community health nurse tests family members who have lived with the client during the past 6 months for tuberculosis. To administer the test, the nurse injects purified protein derivative intradermally. Feedback that the best technique was used for the intradermal injection will be shown at the site by:

A. Redness
B. Induration
C. A wheal
D. Swelling

210. A student nurse just received a Mantoux test to see whether she has been exposed to tuberculosis. How long after the intradermal injection of purified protein derivative should the results be read?

A. 12 to 24 hours
B. 24 to 48 hours
C. 48 to 72 hours
D. 4 to 5 days

211. A 65-year-old client complains of substernal chest pain radiating to the jaw. He takes three nitroglycerin tablets sublingually, but the pain is not relieved. He is sweating profusely. The vital signs in-

Handwritten notes at top of page:
- many on prioritizing/delegating to others
- → aminophylline - side effects
- Tricyclic antidepressants - side effects
- AIDS - many
- peds - mixed c̄ med/surg

clude a blood pressure of 182/92, a pulse of 118, and respirations of 24. A nurse calls 911 because the paramedics will be able to give the client a drug to help dissolve the clot and limit the size of a myocardial infarction. The name of this drugs is:

A. Heparin
B. Streptokinase
C. Urokinase
D. Alteplase

212. A 69-year-old client was recently admitted for a cerebral vascular accident (CVA) in the right hemisphere. He is alert and oriented to time and place. The nurse should assess for:

A. Confusion and impulsive action
B. Ratings on the Glasgow Coma Scale every hour
C. Receptive aphasia
D. Loss of memory

213. A client who recently had a CVA in the left hemisphere has damage to the optic tract posterior to the optic chiasm. This condition is recorded on the chart as homonymous hemianopsia. The nurse recognizes that this means loss of vision in the:

A. Temporal field of both eyes
B. Nasal field of both eyes
C. Temporal field of the left eye and nasal field of the right eye
D. Left eye only

214. A client is admitted to the nursing unit with a medical diagnosis of: rule out CVA. This client demonstrates positive Brudzinski's and Kernig's signs, nuchal rigidity, and restlessness. He complains of severe headache. The nurse recognizes these signs and symptoms as indicative of:

A. Meningeal irritation
B. Cerebral infarction
C. Subdural hematoma
D. Herniation of the brain stem

215. A client is comatose following a stroke. The nurse places this client in the most optimal position, which is:

A. Semi-Fowler's position
B. Supine with the head of the bed flat
C. On the side with head slightly elevated
D. Trendelenburg's position

216. A client is believed to have an intracranial aneurysm. The physician orders aneurysm precautions for the client. The nurse will carry out the following intervention(s):

A. Check rectal temperatures and other vital signs hourly.
B. Promote diversional activities of interest to the client.
C. Encourage turning, coughing, and deep breathing every 2 hours.
D. Monitor neurological signs hourly.

217. A 69-year-old client is in the acute phase of recovery from a CVA in the right hemisphere. This client has a history of atherosclerosis, and a CT scan revealed that the stroke was caused by a thrombus. The nurse plans the following intervention as a high priority:

A. Correcting impaired verbal communication
B. Administering antihypertensives to lower the blood pressure
C. Assisting the client at mealtimes
D. Initiating a program of rehabilitation

218. A client with aplastic anemia is to receive a transfusion of whole blood. Every precaution is taken to see that this client is properly matched for ABO groups and RH type. In addition, it will be very important for the nurse to:

A. Use an existing IV site.
B. Start the temperature and vital signs 15 minutes after the transfusion.
C. Run the blood at no more than 5 ml/min for the first 15 minutes.
D. Administer the blood over 6 to 8 hours.

219. A 45-year-old client is being seen in the clinic today for complaints of heartburn, indigestion, right upper quadrant pain, and nausea for 3 days. The physician suspects acute cholecystitis. The pain associated with acute cholecystitis is most likely to:

A. Begin in the lower left quadrant of the abdomen and radiate to the center of the back and down both legs
B. Begin in the lower right quadrant of the abdomen and radiate to the anterior chest and down the right arm
C. Begin in the right upper quadrant of the abdomen and radiate to the right shoulder and scapula
D. Begin in the left upper quadrant of the abdomen and radiate to the left scapula and shoulder

220. A 64-year-old client is admitted to the hospital with benign prostatic hypertrophy (BPH). He is scheduled to undergo a resection of the prostate. When recording this health history, the registered nurse asks about his chief complaint. The most serious symptoms that may accompany BPH is:

A. Acute urinary retention
B. Hesitancy in starting urination
C. Increased frequency of urination
D. Decreased force of the urinary stream

221. A 64-year-old client with the diagnosis of benign prostatic hyperplasia undergoes a transurethral resection of the prostate (TURP). He returns from surgery with a 3-way continuous Foley irrigation of normal saline in progress. The purpose of this bladder irrigation is to prevent:

A. Bladder spasms
B. Clot formation
C. Scrotal edema
D. Prostatic infection

222. Following a transurethral resection of the prostate

CHAPTER 6 • Medical/Surgical Nursing Q & A   **323**

(TURP), which of the following instructions would be appropriate for the nurse to give to a 60-year-old client to prevent or alleviate anxiety concerning the client's sexual functioning?
A. "You may resume sexual intercourse in 1 week."
B. "Many men experience impotence following TURP."
C. "A transurethral resection does not cause impotence."
D. "Check with your doctor about resuming sexual activity."

223. An 18-year-old client is in skeletal traction following a motor vehicle accident. Which pair of the following nursing assessments is most important to the safety of the client in skeletal traction?
A. Elimination and hydration
B. Nutrition and family relationships
C. Skin integrity and ability to sleep
D. Body alignment and neurovascular status

224. A 41-year-old male client sustained a head injury from an MVA. He has been unresponsive since his admission to the intensive care unit. On admission, the client's vital signs were stable. When assessing him 1 hour later, the nurse finds an increased blood pressure, decreased pulse, and decreased respirations. These findings would indicate which condition?
A. Ketoacidosis
B. Hypovolemic shock
C. Increased intracranial pressure
D. Respiratory alkalosis

225. Which of the following clinical findings is most important when assessing a 43-year-old client with a head injury who is unresponsive?
A. Noting pupillary changes
B. Noting urinary output
C. Noting the narrowing pulse pressure
D. Noting regular, shallow respirations

226. A 22-year-old client, who has a head injury and is unresponsive, is scheduled for a craniotomy today. The nurse knows that this procedure will best benefit the client by:
A. Assessing for ventricular size
B. Relieving increased intracranial pressure
C. Relieving pain
D. Assessing for trauma

227. A 43-year-old obese woman has been admitted to the medical/surgical unit with a diagnosis of cholecystitis and cholelithiasis. She complains of anorexia, nausea, and indigestion after eating fatty foods. The nurse recognizes that the best explanation for this discomfort is:
A. The liver is manufacturing inadequate amounts of bile.
B. Fatty foods are difficult to digest for most people.

C. There is inadequate bile in the small intestine for fat digestion.
D. Gastric hormones are not stimulating bile production by the gallbladder.

228. A 57-year-old client is 8 days' postoperative exploratory laparotomy. His midline abdominal incision is without redness, swelling, or discharges and has intact, well-approximated wound edges. The nurse recognizes that this is an example of healing by:
A. Primary intention
B. Secondary intention
C. Delayed primary intention
D. Tertiary intention

229. A 50-year-old second-day postoperative gastrectomy client is being monitored for possible electrolyte imbalance. The nurse knows that the normal serum sodium range for an adult is:
A. 2.5 to 5.2 mEq/L
B. 9.5 to 11.5 mEq/L
C. 125 to 135 mEq/L
D. 135 to 145 mEq/L

230. A 32-year-old client is being evaluated in the clinic today for possible Addison's disease. The nurse knows that the most common cause of Addison's disease is attributed to:
A. Autoimmune response
B. Blastomycosis
C. Disseminated tuberculosis
D. Diabetes mellitus

231. The nurse recognizes that which of the following medications is administered daily to achieve cortisol replacement in a client with Addison's disease?
A. 50 mg fludrocortisone q A.M.; 25 mg hs
B. 50 mg hydrocortisone q A.M.; 25 mg q afternoon
C. 100 mg fludrocortisone q A.M.; 10 mg hs
D. 20 hydrocortisone q A.M.; 10 mg q afternoon

232. The nurse knows that the recommended diet for a client with Addison's disease includes:
A. 1 gm Na
B. 3 gms Na
C. Low fat, low cholesterol
D. High potassium, high cholesterol

233. A 24-year-old female client is being evaluated in her doctor's office today for possible Cushing's syndrome. After the initial assessment and blood work, the nurse recognizes that which one of the following findings is present with Cushing's syndrome?
A. Weight gain
B. Hyperkalemia
C. Vitiligo
D. Hypotension

234. When giving dietary instructions to a client with

Cushing's disease, the nurse knows that this diet should be:
A. High calorie
B. Low sodium
C. Low potassium
D. Regular

235. A 36-year-old female client with a history of Cushing's disease is being seen in the emergency department for complaints of anorexia, vomiting, weakness, and muscle cramps for the past 24 hours. The nurse recognizes that these clinical findings are a result of:
A. Hypernatremia
B. Hypoglycemia
C. Hyperglycemia
D. Hypokalemia

236. The nurse recognizes that which of the following drugs would be avoided in the treatment of a client with Cushing's syndrome?
A. Spironolactone (Aldactone)
B. Hydrochlorothiazide (HydroDIURIL)
C. Triamterene (Dyrenium)
D. Amiloride (Midamor)

237. Included in the pharmacological treatment of a client with Cushing's syndrome, the nurse knows that which one of the following drugs would best benefit the client as an electrolyte and water-balance agent?
A. Hydrochlorothiazide (HydroDIURIL)
B. Furosemide (Lasix)
C. Spironolactone (Aldactone)
D. Trichlormethiazide (Diurese)

238. A 44-year-old female client who was recently diagnosed with primary hypothyroidism is being evaluated in the clinic today for treatment. The nurse recognizes that the treatment of choice is to:
A. Irradiate the gland.
B. Remove the diseased gland.
C. Withhold exogenous iodine.
D. Replace the missing hormone.

239. When caring for a 32-year-old hospitalized female client who is being treated for a thyroid malfunction, the nurse recognizes that a serious symptom often associated with myxedema is:
A. Hyperglycemia
B. Hypernatremia
C. Hypothermia
D. Hyperkinesis

240. The nurse recognizes that which one of the following is a symptom exhibited in a 36-year-old female client with myxedema?
A. Galactorrhea
B. Hypolipidemia
C. Polyuria
D. Increased fertility

241. The nurse recognizes that the clinical finding

commonly noted when assessing the client with Graves' disease is:
A. Anorexia
B. Intolerance to cold
C. Increased energy
D. Exophthalmos

242. A client with chronic hypoparathyroidism resulting from untreated or undertreated hypocalcemia may develop serious complications. The nurse recognizes that which of the following is reversible?
A. Papilledema
B. Bowing of the long bones
C. Defective tooth structure
D. Cataracts

243. The nurse recognizes that which clinical finding is assessed for in a client with possible hyperparathyroidism?
A. Restlessness
B. Weight gain
C. Increased deep-tendon reflexes
D. Kidney stones

244. When assessing a 40-year-old client with a possible parathyroid disorder, the nurse knows that which of the following is considered a positive Chvostek's sign?
A. The client experiences pain in the abdomen after deep palpation occurs.
B. Application of cuff pressure just above systolic pressure produces carpopedal spasm.
C. The facial muscles on one side of the face contract when that side is tapped.
D. The facial muscles on both sides of the face contract when one side is tapped.

245. After administering regular insulin to a 50-year-old diabetic client, the nurse explains to the client that the insulin would begin to work within:
A. ½ to 1 hour
B. 2 to 4 hours
C. 4 to 6 hours
D. 5 to 7 hours

246. Additional teaching to a newly diagnosed diabetic client related to effects of regular insulin is necessary when the client asks, "If I take my regular insulin at 8 A.M., when might I experience signs of a low blood sugar reaction?"
A. 8:30 A.M.
B. 11 A.M.
C. 1:30 P.M.
D. 4 P.M.

247. When teaching a client about home care related to outpatient corticosteroid therapy, the nurse emphasizes that side effects of corticosteroid therapy include:
A. Hyperglycemia and weight loss
B. Hyponatremia and hypotension
C. Hypoglycemia and gastric ulcers
D. Hyperglycemia and weight gain

248. A 24-hour urine collection is implemented for 17 ketosteroids. The test begins at 8 A.M. on Wednesday and is scheduled to end at 8 A.M. on Thursday. What should the nurse do with the specimen obtained at 8 A.M. on Wednesday?
   A. Measure the urine and discard it.
   B. Place it in the 24-hour collection container.
   C. Put the specimen in a separate container for urinalysis.
   D. Test the specimen for sugar, acetone, and osmolarity.

249. The nurse knows that a specimen of urine for a routine urinalysis should be:
   A. Sent the laboratory as a stat procedure
   B. At least 60 ml
   C. Put in a sterile container
   D. An early morning specimen

250. A 25-year-old white male client who had just been diagnosed with AIDS is being seen in the clinic today for treatment. The nurse recognizes that the transmission of AIDS is by:
   A. Airborne virus
   B. Cellular metabolistic
   C. Feces
   D. Bloodborne virus

251. The nurse is aware that the type of precaution indicated in caring for an AIDS client is:
   A. Strict isolation precautions
   B. Blood and body fluid precautions
   C. Acid-fast bacilli isolation precautions
   D. Enteric precautions

252. During the nursing assessment, which question by the nurse would be most beneficial in planning care for an AIDS client?
   A. "What is your sexual preference?"
   B. "Have you been sharing eating utensils with others?"
   C. "Can you tell me the types of food that you have eaten for the past week?"
   D. "Can you tell me about some of the behaviors of everyday living that you practiced before getting sick?"

253. A 25-year-old client is being treated in the clinic today for strep throat. The nurse recognizes that strep throat is:
   A. A self-limiting viral disease
   B. Associated with Epstein-Barr infections
   C. A result of neoplasms
   D. A bacterial infection which can result in rheumatic fever

254. A 79-year-old client is admitted to the hospital with a diagnosis of bacterial pneumonia. She has a temperature of 102.4°F, is coughing up tenacious purulent sputum, and is experiencing difficulty breathing. Which of the following nursing measures is most important in helping to liquefy these viscous secretions?
   A. Postural drainage
   B. Breathing humidified air
   C. Clapping and percussion over the affected lung
   D. Coughing and deep breathing exercises

255. A community health nurse is caring for a client with Hansen's disease. The nurse recognizes that which one of the following statements is most accurate about Hansen's disease?
   A. It is an infectious disease caused by *Staphylococcus saprophyticus*.
   B. Signs and symptoms include ecchymosis, diaphoresis, facial and scalp hair overgrowth, and frequent respiratory infections.
   C. There is more than one form of this disease.
   D. It is treated with cromolyn sodium, hydrocortisone, and prednisone.

256. A 45-year-old woman is seen in the clinic because she is concerned about being exposed to sexually transmitted diseases. She asks the nurse, "What method should I use to protect myself from AIDS?" The nurse's best reply is:
   A. "The practice of anal intercourse versus vaginal intercourse will help prevent sexual transmission of HIV."
   B. "The use of latex condoms with spermicide will help prevent sexual transmission of HIV."
   C. "Limiting sexual partners to 10 will eliminate the possibility of catching AIDS."
   D. "Avoiding deep kissing is the best way to prevent AIDS."

257. A 28-year-old female client states that she has recently noted some suspicious growths in the area of her perineum. She asks the nurse what herpes simplex looks like? Which of the following statements by the nurse would best explain this?
   A. Herpes consists of vesicles that form shallow, painful ulcers that often go away in about 2 weeks.
   B. Herpes causes a lot of itching and discharge in the perineal area, which results in bleeding and infection.
   C. A female is the carrier of this condition.
   D. The problem with herpes is that it creates a great deal of vaginal bleedings and discharges.

258. The nurse devises a teaching plan for a 28-year-old client with herpes simplex. Which of the following is most important to be included in this health teaching?
   A. Avoid wearing cotton underwear.
   B. Sexual contact can be practiced while lesions are present.
   C. Acyclovir (Zovirax) is most effective for recurrent and primary herpes.
   D. Sitz baths will irritate the genital lesions.

259. A 45-year-old client has just returned from the recovery room after a right middle lobe resection and a right mastectomy. A top priority in planning

her care is to minimize the pain she is experiencing and to maximize her breathing effort. The priority nursing diagnosis for this client is:
A. Ineffective airway clearance
B. Alteration in comfort: pain
C. Alteration in gas exchange
D. Potential for injury

260. When teaching a 45-year-old postoperative client about the best method for obtaining pain relief by means of analgesics, which of the following statements is most important for the nurse to emphasize initially?
A. "Pain medication may be habit forming."
B. "Pain medication will help in your recovery."
C. "Pain medication will be given when requested."
D. "Pain medication should be given at the onset of pain."

261. A 69-year-old client is leaving the country for a 3-month trip to Asia and Australia. He asks the nurse about being vaccinated for the flu. The nurse understands that the vaccine should be given to those at risk of developing infection. The nurse explains to the client that the following group would be considered to be at the highest risk:
A. Preadolescents
B. Children
C. People over 65
D. Nursing home residents

262. A 33-year-old client was involved in an automobile accident and is being seen in the ER. The x-ray film reveals several bone fragments at the distal end of the femur. The nurse recognizes that this type of fracture is an example of a(an):
A. Impacted fracture
B. Incomplete fracture
C. Comminuted fracture
D. Complicated fracture

263. A 21-year-old client was admitted with fractures sustained in an automobile accident. His fractures include compound fracture of right femur and closed fracture of pelvis and left humerus. His vital signs have been stable for the past 2 days. During morning assessment, the nurse notices that the client is confused and mildly agitated. His respirations are rapid, with diffuse crackles in both lung fields, and petechiae across his chest. Based on knowledge of his age, history of injury, and location of his fractures, which complication would the nurse suspect?
A. Aspiration pneumonia
B. Fat embolism
C. Emotional reaction to stress
D. Systemic reaction to analgesics

264. A 45-year-old obese woman has been admitted to the medical/surgical unit with a diagnosis of cholecystitis. She complains of anorexia, nausea, and indigestion, especially after eating fatty foods.

When the client asks what does cholecystitis mean, the nurse responds that it means:
A. Obstruction of the common bile duct by a stone
B. Inflammation of the bile ducts
C. Presence of gallstones in the gallbladder
D. Inflammation of the gallbladder due to obstruction or the inflammation process

265. The nurse is explaining to her 36-year-old female client which diagnostic studies would confirm the diagnosis of cholelithiasis-cholecystitis. The nurse recognizes that additional teaching is necessary when the client enquires whether she will have which of the following tests?
A. Ultrasonography
B. CBC (complete blood count)
C. Urinalysis
D. Electrocardiogram (EKG)

266. As the enlargement of the prostate occurs in the early stage of benign prostatic hyperplasia, increased pressure is exerted on the urethra and a symptom complex called prostatism is exhibited. Which one of the following symptoms occurs in the advanced stage of BPH?
A. Nocturia
B. Hesitancy in initiating voiding
C. An intermittent stream
D. Hematuria

267. When a 50-year-old client develops tissue breakdown under a cast, the nurse knows that which one of the following signs would be absent?
A. Pain under the cast
B. Drainage through the cast
C. Irritability or restlessness
D. Decreased body temperature

268. When caring for a 45-year-old male client in traction and lower leg splints, the nurse knows that which one of the following would least likely occur?
A. Renal calculi
B. Scoliosis
C. Constipation and impaction
D. Constrictive edema

269. When caring for a 27-year-old client in traction, the nurse recognizes that which one of the following situations would counteract the effectiveness of traction?
A. Traction force and direction are maintained.
B. All ropes are in the center tract of the pulley.
C. Traction weights are resting on the bed.
D. Clamps and bolts are tight.

270. In order to reduce or avoid potential complications such as inflammation or infection of the oral cavity when caring for a client with a nasogastric tube, which of the following nursing interventions would be of least benefit to the client?
A. Encourage frequent oral hygiene.

B. Change the anchor tape weekly.
C. Apply lubricant to the nostril where the tube is inserted.
D. Apply lip balm every 2 to 4 hours.

271. A 67-year-old client is scheduled for a transurethral resection of the prostate (TURP) today. The nurse knows that the major complication following TURP in the immediate postoperative period is:
    A. Hemorrhage
    B. Calculi
    C. Constipation
    D. Infection

272. The nurse knows that in describing communicable diseases, the correct term for the time frame when the infectious agent invades the host and establishes itself is:
    A. Constitutional period
    B. Incubation period
    C. Period of communicability
    D. Prodromal period

273. When teaching drug therapy to a 38-year-old client with tuberculosis, the nurse emphasizes that side effects most commonly associated with medications used in the treatment of tuberculosis include:
    A. Nephrotoxicity and hepatotoxicity
    B. Hepatotoxicity and ototoxicity
    C. Peripheral neuritis and nausea
    D. Neutropenia and nephrotoxicity

274. When caring for a client with a possible allergic reaction to a bee sting, the nurse recognizes that throughout the circulatory system there is massive vasodilation and increased capillary permeability, which leads to hypovolemia and vascular collapse. This reaction is seen in anaphylactic reactions and is caused by:
    A. Leukotrienes
    B. Heparin
    C. Histamine
    D. Tissue hypoxia

275. A 35-year-old client is being seen in the clinic today for possible systemic lupus erythematosus (SLE). When performing the assessment, the nurse knows that the most significant sign or symptom present in SLE is:
    A. Recurrent petechiae on the abdomen
    B. Recurrent low-grade afternoon fever
    C. Recurrent multiple ecchymoses over entire body
    D. Recurrent butterfly rash over cheeks and nose

276. A 23-year-old client developed rhinitis from exposure to pollen and dust. The local clinic suggested that a "natural" decongestant be taken with an antihistamine (Benadryl). The nurse explained to the client that which of the following over-the-counter (OTC) products would be the most effective and beneficial as a natural decongestant?
    A. Acetylsalicylic acid (ASA or aspirin)
    B. Alka-Seltzer
    C. Vitamin C tablets
    D. Mylanta

277. The nurse who is caring for a 19-year-old with several infected insect bites on his leg knows that which one of the following medications is most effective in the treatment of impetigo?
    A. Antihistamines (topical) (Benadryl)
    B. Analgesics (PO) (Tylenol)
    C. Steroids (topical) (cortisone)
    D. Antibiotics (PO) (penicillin)

278. The nurse is caring for a 60-year-old client with rheumatoid arthritis. She recognizes that the major goal of drug therapy in rheumatoid arthritis and other rheumatic conditions is to:
    A. Provide emotional support.
    B. Cure the underlying cause.
    C. Reduce inflammation of joints.
    D. Prepare the client for surgery.

279. When caring for a 33-year-old client with a urinary tract infection (UTI), the nurse knows that which of the following would be of least benefit in the care and treatment of UTI?
    A. Antibiotics usually used for UTI are Bactrim (trimethoprim-sulfamethoxazole), nitrofurantoin, ampicillin, and cephalosporin.
    B. Obtain a urine sample for culture and sensitivity before and after treatment with antibiotics.
    C. Increase fluid intake, empty bladder frequently, and teach importance of follow-up culture.
    D. Antibiotic therapy would be prescribed for a 3- to 5-day duration

280. Hand washing is crucial in preventing the spread of infection. The nurse recognizes that this practice is aimed at breaking the "chain of infection" during which phase of the cycle?
    A. Portal of entry to host
    B. Reservoir
    C. Method of transmission
    D. Portal of exit from source

281. The nurse is discussing various health issues with adults at a family practice health clinic. When asked about vaccinations, she emphasizes that which one of the following vaccines would manifest no side effects?
    A. Measles, mumps, and rubella (MMR)
    B. Diphtheria, polio, and tetanus (DPT)
    C. Tetanus toxoid
    D. Oral polio vaccine

282. As the nurse caring for a client in isolation to prevent transmission of infection related to feces, you recognize that this type of isolation is called:
    A. Blood and body fluids
    B. Contact
    C. Drainage and secretion
    D. Enteric

283. Surgical wound infections are the second most frequent type of nosocomial infection found in most hospitals. The nurse knows that she can best reduce these infections by:

A. Strictly adhering to the principles of effective hand washing

B. Always cleansing incisions from bottom to top—from the most contaminated to the least contaminated area

C. Leaving incisions open to air to promote healing

D. Using clean gloves as the protective barrier when changing dressings

284. A 57-year-old client has been experiencing anorexia, weight loss, and diarrhea and is admitted to the general surgery unit for diagnostic purposes. He has an order for enemas in preparation for a barium enema the next day. Which is the best nursing action related to correct enema administration procedure?

A. Insert tubing 1 to 2 inches with client lying in the left lateral position with right leg flexed.

B. Expel air from tubing, then lubricate and insert tip of tubing into the anus until resistance is felt. The client should be lying in the right lateral position with left leg flexed.

C. Insert tubing and open clamp to allow solution to flow moderately fast with container 20 inches above the client's anus.

D. Once tubing is inserted, allow the solution to flow slowly until the container is empty or until the client is unable to take anymore, then clamp the tubing and remove from anus.

285. After her cholecystectomy, a 50-year-old client has an incision site with a Penrose drain. When cleansing her wound, the best action by the nurse would be to:

A. Go over the wound several times with the same swab.

B. Use antiseptic solution followed by a normal saline rinse.

C. Cleanse from the outer regions of the wound toward the middle.

D. Start cleansing at the drain site and move outward.

286. When irrigating a wound, the nurse recognizes that the client should be positioned so that the solution will flow from one end of the wound toward the other end. The rationale for this action is to:

A. Direct the flow of liquid from least contaminated to most contaminated area.

B. Assist the nurse in proceeding in an organized fashion to complete the procedure.

C. Facilitate irrigating the wound as quickly as possible.

D. Enhance client comfort.

287. When caring for a 20-year-old client in ER with multiple trauma from a motor vehicle accident, the nurse recognizes that the grating sound that is heard or felt when ends of a broken bone are moved is known as:

A. Retraction

B. Rasping

C. Crepitus

D. Vibration

288. A 64-year-old client was admitted for diagnostic work-up associated with difficulty in urination. Benign prostatic hypertrophy (BPH) is suspected. When teaching the client about the signs and symptoms of this condition, the nurse emphasizes that which of the following would be absent in BPH?

A. Hesitancy in initiating urination

B. Decrease in the force of urination

C. Increase in the size of the urinary stream

D. Increase in bladder pressure

289. An 18-year-old male client sustained an open compound fracture of his left tibia while skiing and is being treated in the emergency room. The most important rationale for cleaning his wound using sterile technique is:

A. To help promote wound healing by removing any drainage

B. To remove any moisture that harbors organisms that may have collected

C. To prevent introduction of organisms into the wound

D. To prevent bacterial growth on surrounding tissues

290. The nurse recognizes that a frequent site and cause of a nosocomial infection is:

A. The urinary tract, related to placing the drainage bag above the bladder

B. The incision, related to use of aseptic technique when changing the dressing

C. The bloodstream, related to self-administration of insulin

D. The respiratory system, related to clients coughing without covering their mouth

291. The nurse recognizes which of the following as signs of early hypoxia?

A. Restlessness, yawning, and tachycardia

B. Hypotension, tachypnea, and lethargy

C. Confusion, bradycardia, and headache

D. Bradycardia, hypotension, and facial flushing

292. A 70-year-old client has a feeding tube in place. Before beginning his intermittent tube feeding, the best action by the nurse will be to:

A. Auscultate his bowel sounds with the instillation of 100 ml of air.

B. Auscultate his bowel sounds with the instillation of 10 ml of tap water.

C. Submerge the end of his tube in a glass of water.

D. Aspirate and reinstall his stomach contents.

293. What side effects would the nurse expect a 36-year-old client to experience when receiving external beam irradiation for esophageal cancer?
    A. Nausea, dysphagia, and bone marrow suppression
    B. Diarrhea, dysphagia, and bone marrow suppression
    C. Alopecia, nausea, and dysphagia
    D. Dysphagia, alopecia, and constipation

294. A 47-year-old female client is receiving external beam irradiation for squamous-cell cancer of the lung. After 2 weeks of treatment, her skin in the treatment field is red and warm to the touch. The nurse's most appropriate action would be to apply which of the following?
    A. Solarcaine, and notify the doctor
    B. A&D ointment, and notify the doctor
    C. Desitin, and notify the doctor
    D. nothing, but notify the doctor

295. Mrs. Brown, a 30-year-old Jehovah's Witness, was recently diagnosed with multiple myeloma. She presents with a hemoglobin (Hgb) of 6.3. Her doctor requests that she receive a transfusion of 4 units of RBCs. The client refuses. The nurse's most appropriate response would be to:
    A. Do nothing.
    B. Notify Mrs. Brown's doctor of her refusal.
    C. Convince Mrs. Brown to take the transfusion.
    D. Administer the transfusion as ordered.

296. Following a cholecystectomy, a 37-year-old female client develops jaundice. The nurse knows that this occurs as a result of:
    A. The development of an infection in the gallbladder
    B. Diminished synthesis of bile in the liver
    C. An inflammatory process in the hepatic duct
    D. Gallstones left in the common duct during surgery

297. A 68-year-old client has a new colostomy, and is being treated today at the clinic for diarrhea. When discussing diet with the client, the nurse explains to him that the one food that caused this problem was:
    A. Cabbage
    B. Eggs
    C. Tapioca
    D. Fried chicken

298. A 58-year-old client has a new colostomy and is being evaluated at the clinic today for colostomy obstruction. When discussing diet with the client, the nurse recognizes that which one of the following foods caused this problem?
    A. Mushrooms
    B. Baked beans
    C. Onions
    D. Cheese

299. A 22-year-old healthy male client has just returned to his room after a left inguinal hernia repair under spinal anesthesia. He moves his feet without difficulty and denies pain. The nurse knows that during the next 8 hours her priority nursing intervention will include assessing the client's ability to:
    A. Perform care of his incision
    B. Urinate
    C. Turn in bed without assistance
    D. Move arms and hands without difficulty

300. The nurse who is caring for a 77-year-old who is 3 days' postoperative colectomy recognizes that the most important risk factor to predispose the client to pneumonia in this case would be:
    A. He has a nasogastric (NG) tube and is NPO.
    B. He is out of bed to the chair twice a day.
    C. His abdominal incision is red and tender to touch.
    D. He had general anesthesia.

301. A 35-year-old male client who is being evaluated in the emergency department for possible nephrolithiasis is scheduled for an intravenous pyelogram (IVP). The most important nursing intervention following this procedure is:
    A. Observe closely for an allergic reaction.
    B. Encourage the client to drink at least 120 ml of water immediately after the procedure.
    C. Maintain the client's head elevated at 45 degrees for the next 10 hours.
    D. Keep the client NPO for 8 hours after the procedure.

302. A 60-year-old female client has just returned to the nursing unit after a renal biopsy. The nurse knows that the most important priority in the care of this client is:
    A. Using contact isolation precautions for the next 48 hours
    B. Keeping the client NPO for 8 hours postoperatively
    C. Monitoring for postoperative bleeding
    D. Encouraging the client to ambulate every 2 hours

303. When instructing a client to obtain a urine specimen at the clinic today, the best explanation by the nurse would be:
    A. Clean the area, start to urinate, and then catch the last few drops in the container.
    B. Clean the area and catch the entire amount of urine in the container.
    C. Clean the area and then catch the first 50 ml of urine in the container.
    D. Clean the area, start to urinate, catch the middle of the stream of urine in the container, and then finish urinating.

304. While caring for a 46-year-old male client with acute pancreatitis, the nurse knows that which one of the following is the most important priority?
    A. Prevent recurrence.

B. Administer pancreatic extracts.
C. Provide pain relief.
D. Promote nutrition.

305. Additional discharge teaching is necessary by the nurse when the client with acute pancreatitis makes the following statement:
A. "I need to eat less fat in my diet."
B. "Six small meals a day will make it easier for me to eat properly."
C. "I need to gradually increase activity and exercise to help regain strength."
D. "An occasional beer is OK with my meal."

306. The nurse is teaching a 52-year-old female client with rheumatoid arthritis (RA) how to relieve morning stiffness in joints. Which one of the following would be most beneficial for the client to use:
A. Isotonic exercises of weight-bearing joints
B. Firm mattress to support joints
C. Warm shower
D. Ice caps to the joints

307. You are the nurse caring for a 23-year-old male client who underwent an open reduction internal fixation of the mandible today because of injuries resulting from a motor vehicle accident. To prevent possible aspiration, you should instruct the client to:
A. Cough up secretions forcefully.
B. Keep the head of the bed up at least 45 degrees with wire cutters at the bedside.
C. Avoid using oral suction equipment because it can cause more damage to the fractured jaw.
D. Lie in the supine position and carefully turn your head to the side if you need to expectorate sputum or emesis.

308. A 72-year-old male client who has a diagnosis of peripheral vascular disease and renal hypertension is being prepared for arteriography of the lower extremities. The most important nursing intervention for this client is:
A. Explaining to the client to expect a warm sensation in the extremities when the dye is injected
B. Prepping the area that will be catheterized with an antiseptic solution
C. Documenting vital signs and pedal pulses in the client's medical record
D. Eliciting and documenting any allergy to contrast medication or iodine-containing substances

309. A 37-year-old male client is on the general surgery nursing unit and is being treated for possible nephrolithiasis. The physician orders a kidney, urethra, and bladder (KUB) study to confirm the diagnosis. The nurse would do which one of the following to prepare him for the procedure?
A. No special preparation is required for this procedure.

B. Instruct him that he is NPO.
C. Administer promethazine (Phenergan) 25 mg IM ½ hour before the procedure.
D. Give him a Fleet enema 1 hour before the procedure.

310. A 28-year-old male client is being seen in the emergency department for a large cut on his right lower leg and a back injury from a motor vehicle accident. When assessing the client, which one of the following would alert the nurse to a serious problem?
A. He sounds angry and frightened.
B. He is bleeding profusely from his right lower leg.
C. When asked to move his right leg, he responds, "I can't."
D. His breath smells of alcohol.

311. When caring for a 21-year-old client in the ER who has just been diagnosed with a C-6 spinal cord injury from a motor vehicle accident, the nurse recognizes that which of the following information is most important in planning his care?
A. He was drinking alcohol prior to the accident.
B. He last voided 6 hours ago.
C. He is a college football star.
D. He smokes one pack of cigarettes per week.

312. When caring for a 26-year old client with a spinal cord injury, the nurse recognizes that the most important priority of care when he begins to get out of bed into a chair is:
A. Encouraging him to discuss his progress and impending discharge home
B. Supporting normal actions by avoiding restraining devices
C. Helping him maintain bladder and bowel control
D. Monitoring his vital signs

313. The nurse is caring for a 44-year-old client who had a craniotomy for removal of a subdural hematoma. Included in this client's care, the nurse elevates the head of the bed 30 to 45 degrees. The rationale for this is to:
A. Increase oxygenation to the brain.
B. Reduce cerebral edema.
C. Promote respiratory function.
D. Prevent aspiration.

314. You are the nurse caring for a 55-year-old female client with chronic renal failure who is receiving dialysis today. Which one of the following would you expect to observe after dialysis treatment?
A. Increase in red blood cells
B. Increase in BUN level
C. Falling potassium level
D. Weight gain

315. The nurse is caring for a 68-year-old male client in the emergency department. He appears frightened and has a BP of 142/92, pulse of 100, and respirations of 38. He has the following blood gas val-

ues: pH, 7.52, $PaCO_2$, 30; HCO_3, 24. The priority nursing action is to:
A. Administer carbon dioxide by mask.
B. Administer oxygen at 2 L.
C. Prepare the client for intubation.
D. Have the client breathe into a paper bag.

316. The nurse who is caring for a 49-year-old client with pancreatitis recognizes that the most beneficial dinner menu for him would be:
A. Diced chicken, mashed potatoes, and peas
B. Steak, french fries, and creamed onions
C. Peanut butter sandwich, potato chips, and orange slices
D. Egg salad sandwich, sausage gumbo, and ice tea

317. The nurse is caring for a 51-year-old client who has a Sengstaken-Blakemore tube inserted for bleeding esophageal varices. The nurse recognizes that which position is most beneficial to the client?
A. Right lateral to promote comfort
B. Modified Trendelenburg to raise blood pressure
C. Alternating right and left sides to facilitate continued movements of the tube
D. Semi-Fowler's (head of bed [HOB] elevated at 30 to 45 degrees) to prevent aspiration

318. You are the nurse caring for a 51-year-old male client who is hospitalized for an exacerbation of ulcerative colitis. He has lost 25 pounds in the last 5 months and complains of frequent diarrhea, malaise, and anorexia. Total parenteral nutrition (TPN) is included in his orders. The nurse knows that the primary purpose of TPN for this client is to:
A. Correct electrolyte imbalances
B. Rest the bowel
C. Increase his weight
D. Prevent dehydration

319. When the nurse is evaluating the effect of a low-fat diet for a client recovering from cholecystectomy, which of the following is the desired outcome?
A. Absence of abdominal pain
B. Weight loss of 20 pounds
C. Decrease in cholesterol level
D. Decrease in peripheral edema

320. Due to impaired renal function, the nurse would expect an adult client with chronic renal failure (CRF) to have elevated serum blood urea nitrogen levels and:
A. Sodium 137 mEq/L, creatinine 1.5 mg/dl
B. Calcium 9.0 mg/dl, creatinine 1.5 mg/dl
C. Potassium 5.9 mEq/L, creatinine 4.5 mg/dl
D. Potassium 3.7 mEq/L, calcium 9.0 mg/dl

321. The development of acquired immune deficiency syndrome (AIDS) resulting from infection with the human immunodeficiency virus (HIV) has changed health-care practices. Universal blood and body fluid precautions are recommended for use with:
A. All clients cared for by health-care workers
B. All untested clients from high-risk population
C. All clients in high-risk categories for AIDS
D. All clients who are positive for HIV antibodies

322. Which statement indicates to the nurse that a 20-year-old, sexually active male understands basic measures to prevent contracting the human immunodeficiency virus (HIV)?
A. "I'll be sure to withdraw before I climax."
B. "I'll use a condom every time I have intercourse."
C. "I'll only have sex with people who are HIV negative."
D. "I'll make sure my partner uses a diaphragm each time."

323. A 52-year-old female underwent modified radical mastectomy for cancer of the breast. She is now receiving radiotherapy. The irritated area is slightly reddened and tender. Which suggestion should the nurse make to decrease the likelihood of complications?
A. "Report early signs of skin irritation."
B. "Apply mild lotion to the affected area."
C. "Gently apply talcum powder to the site."
D. "You may expect some ulceration to occur."

324. When assessing the client with pernicious anemia, the nurse identifies that the severe vitamin deficiency associated with pernicious anemia is often manifested by:
A. Jaundice and hyperactivity
B. Heartburn and palpitations
C. Constipation and weight gain
D. Neuropathy and loss of balance

325. When teaching clients about infection control, the nurse reinforces that currently the Centers for Disease Control recommends which of the following disinfectants in a 1:10 dilution for cleaning surfaces contaminated with blood or body fluids?
A. Bleach
B. Alcohol
C. Phenols
D. Peroxide

326. A 25-year-old male client is receiving TPN for severe malnutrition. As he begins to recover, he gains ¼ to ½ lb for several days in a row. The nurse should:
A. Determine whether the scale is functioning properly.
B. Suggest that the client's TPN rate be increased.
C. Record that the client is gaining weight satisfactorily.
D. Notify the doctor that the client is gaining weight too rapidly.

327. The nurse cares for a client with folic acid (FA) deficiency. The nurse recalls that one of the most frequent causes of folic acid deficiency is:

A. Poor nutritional intake due to alcoholism
B. Lack of absorption of the intrinsic factor
C. A diet that consists of vegetables only and no meat
D. A complicated pregnancy during the second trimester

328. A 90-year-old female is to be transfused with two units of packed red blood cells. Lasix (furosemide) 80 mg IVP has been ordered after the first unit of blood has infused. The client asks why she is getting Lasix IVP. The nurse replies that its purpose is to:
A. Prevent pulmonary emboli
B. Prevent circulatory overload
C. Decrease blood pressure
D. Counteract transfusion-induced hypercalcemia

329. A unit of packed red blood cells is ordered for a client with anemia. The nurse calculates the transfusion drip rate so that the transfusion will be infused within:
A. ½ hour
B. 1 hour
C. 4 hours
D. 6 hours

330. A 25-year-old male client with Hodgkin's disease is receiving MOPP chemotherapy. Which of the following observations is considered life threatening?
A. WBCs less than 1000/mm³
B. Pruritus relieved by diphenhydramine (Benadryl)
C. Platelets about 300,000/mm³
D. Intermittent vomiting for 3 days

331. When planning care for a client who is pancytopenic, the major goal should be:
A. Preventing hemorrhage and infection
B. Administering an oral iron preparation
C. Preventing fatigue and fluid overload
D. Encouraging consumption of a neutropenic diet

332. A client with iron-deficiency anemia develops an intolerance to oral iron therapy and is changed to parenteral iron injections. When giving this drug the nurse should:
A. Inject it into the client's arm.
B. Massage the site vigorously afterwards.
C. Inject it deeply using the "Z" track method.
D. Instruct the client to rest in bed afterward.

333. A 24-year-old is injured in a motor vehicle accident. A chest tube is inserted to relieve a pneumothorax. The Pleur-A-Vac is set at 20 cm H₂O pressure. When the nurse checks the chest tube, which observation indicates that the setup is working correctly?
A. The fluid in the water seal chamber fluctuates with respirations.
B. The fluid in the collection chamber bubbles continuously.

C. The fluid in the water seal chamber bubbles continuously.
D. The fluid in the suction chamber fluctuates with respirations.

334. A priority of nursing care following a bone marrow aspiration includes:
A. Ambulating the client to prevent emboli
B. Monitoring the puncture site for bleeding
C. Changing the dressing every 4 hours for 24 hours
D. Administering analgesia every 3 hours for pain

335. A 24-hour urine collection for 17-OHCS and ketosteroids is to be collected from 8 A.M. Monday to 8 A.M. Tuesday. What should the nurse do with the specimen voided at 8 A.M. Tuesday?
A. Put it in the 24-hour specimen container.
B. Put it in a separate urinary container.
C. Send it to the laboratory for culture.
D. Measure the urine and then discard it.

336. A client receives total parenteral nutrition (TPN) and has also begun receiving a fat emulsion solution (Intralipid) three times a week. The nurse explains to the client that the main reason fat emulsion solutions are given is to:
A. Increase the fluid intake.
B. Decrease serum lipid levels.
C. Restrict essential fatty acids.
D. Provide an extra source of calories.

337. The nurse identifies that a desirable outcome of TPN therapy for a 30-year-old man is:
A. Weight gain of ½ pound per day
B. Capillary blood glucose of 160 mg/dl
C. Serum sodium level of 127 mEq/L
D. Serum cholesterol level of 225 mg/dl

338. The nurse prepares to hang an infusion of total parenteral nutrition (TPN). Which of the following fluids can be given concurrently, through the same IV lines, as TPN?
A. Blood
B. Platelets
C. IVPB medications
D. Fat emulsion solutions

339. Health-care professionals including nurses are constantly exposed to hepatitis B. The best way to avoid contracting hepatitis B is to:
A. Double-bag soiled tissues.
B. Avoid needle stick injuries.
C. Obtain the appropriate immunization.
D. Protect clothing by wearing a gown.

340. A client asks how hepatitis A is usually transmitted. The nurse responds:
A. Sharing intravenous needles
B. Not washing hands prior to eating
C. Unprotected sex with multiple partners
D. Receiving multiple transfusions of blood

341. Hepatitis C is usually transmitted to others by:

A. Sexual intercourse
B. The fecal-oral route
C. Lack of hand-washing
D. The parenteral route

342. A client states, "I'm nearsighted." The nurse explains that is a lay term for:
A. Myopia
B. Presbyopia
C. Hypermetropia
D. Astigmatism

343. To monitor a client's inflammatory response, which laboratory value would the nurse most likely observe?
A. Increased erythrocyte sedimentation rate (ESR)
B. Decreased (ESR)
C. Decreased white blood cell count
D. Increased fibrinogen level

344. When caring for clients undergoing chemotherapy, the nurse identifies the most effective way to prevent infection in a neutropenic client is:
A. Meticulous hand-washing prior to client contact
B. Monitoring oral temperature every 4 hours
C. A sitz bath after each bowel movement
D. Encouraging a high-calorie, high-protein diet

345. When explaining what a malignant neoplasm means to a client's family, it would be essential for the nurse to know which of the statements best characterizes malignant neoplasms? They:
A. Grow very slowly
B. Appear as well-differentiated cells
C. Usually remain well encapsulated
D. Grow quickly and invade adjacent tissue

346. A client undergoes chemotherapy for lung cancer. Which cells are very susceptible to damage by antineoplastic drugs?
A. Bones
B. Muscles
C. Cartilage
D. Bone marrow

347. Which safety precaution should the nurse take during intravenous administration of vesicant chemotherapy drugs?
A. Assessing for nausea and vomiting
B. Checking for an adequate blood return
C. Weighing the client prior to drug administration
D. Apply heat to the injection site to facilitate drug absorption.

348. When explaining different effects of chemotherapy to students, the nurse correctly identifies which group of chemotherapy drugs that does not affect DNA synthesis to kill tumor cells?
A. Hormones
B. Plant alkaloids
C. Antimetabolites
D. Alkylating agents

349. A client is receiving vincristine (Oncovin) as part of combination chemotherapy for treatment of leukemia. Side effects that the nurse should assess for in this client include:
A. Neuropathy
B. Hypertension
C. Osteoporosis
D. Hyperglycemia

350. A female client undergoing chemotherapy develops stomatitis. To promote comfort, the nurse encourages her to eat:
A. Cherry Jell-O with banana bits
B. Barbecued chicken and green beans
C. Fried chicken and mashed potatoes
D. Homemade vegetable soup and crackers

351. A client with lung cancer develops superior vena cava syndrome (SVCS). To make the client more comfortable, the nurse should:
A. Encourage a fluid intake of 2 to 3 liters/day.
B. Do range-of-motion exercises to maintain muscle tone.
C. Weigh the client daily and restrict dietary sodium.
D. Position the client to decrease edema and promote ventilation.

352. The nurse reviews the histology report on a client with advanced lung cancer. The tumor "grading" listed on the report refers to:
A. The size of a primary tumor
B. Presence or absence of metastasis
C. Evidence of lymph node involvement
D. The degree of malignancy of the tumor

353. The nurse reviews the history and physical of a client with uterine cancer. Using the TNM classification system, the nurse recognizes that a primary tumor with no abnormal lymph node involvement and no metastasis would be designated as:
A. T2, N1, MI
B. T0, N0, MX
C. T1, N0, M0
D. TIS, NO, M0

354. To decrease the likelihood of diarrhea related to nasogastric tube feedings, the nurse plans to:
A. Dilute the strength of the tube feeding.
B. Decrease the temperature of the feeding.
C. Increase the concentration of the feeding.
D. Increase the height of the tube-feeding bag.

355. Upon assessment, one of the most frequently reported symptoms associated with the climacteric (menopause) includes:
A. Dry mouth
B. Constipation
C. Hot flashes
D. Skin rashes

356. The anesthesiologist has ordered atropine gr 1/150

as a preoperative medication. The purpose of anticholinergics preoperatively is to:

A. Decrease anxiety and provide sedation.

B. Decrease saliva and gastric juices.

C. Relieve pain and discomfort.

D. Prevent allergic reactions.

357. The surgical team approaches the sterile field for surgery. Which area of the scrubbed team's gowns is considered sterile?

A. 4 inches above front waist

B. 8 inches below front waist

C. 6 inches above the elbow

D. 4 inches above posterior chest

358. A client is scheduled to undergo a small bowel resection. The nurse teaches a client leg exercises that are to be done postoperatively. Postoperative instruction in leg exercises is intended to prevent which postoperative complication?

A. Infection

B. Cellulitis

C. Paralytic ileus

D. Phlebothrombosis

359. Tissue healing occurs in several ways. The most desirable outcome for surgical wound healing is by:

A. Primary intention

B. Secondary intention

C. Secondary suture

D. Third intention

360. A postoperative client in the postanesthesia care unit can be extubated when awake and reactive with normal blood gases. Prior to extubation, the nurse should also assess the client for the ability to:

A. Wiggle toes freely and speak

B. Grip a hand and wiggle toes

C. Blink eyes and raise the hand

D. Raise the head and grip one's hand

361. After a client experienced a severe coughing spasm, the nurse was notified that the client's abdominal surgical wound had eviscerated. Which nursing action is most appropriate at this time?

A. Apply moist, sterile dressings to the site.

B. Position the client in high Fowler's position.

C. Push the eviscerated organs back into the abdomen.

D. Administer a narcotic analgesic for pain.

362. When admitting a client to the postanesthesia care unit (PACU), which nursing assessment has highest priority?

A. IV patency

B. Vital signs

C. A patent airway

D. Surgical dressing

363. Clients who undergo hemodialysis must have small doses of heparin injected into their dialysis tubing to prevent clotting. The nurse monitoring the hemodialysis client must have the antagonist to heparin readily available. This medication is:

A. Protamine sulfate

B. Propoxyphene napsylate

C. Propanolol hydrochloride

D. Procarbazine hydrochloride

364. The nurse monitors the laboratory reports of a client with congestive heart failure. Which laboratory value indicates hyponatremia?

A. 60–100 mg/dl Na

B. 100–120 mg/dl Na

C. 125–134 mEq/L Na

D. 136–148 mEq/L Na

365. An acutely ill diabetic client has diabetic ketoacidosis with hyperkalemia. Which laboratory value indicates hyperkalemia?

A. 2.1–3.5 mEq/L K

B. 2.7–4.2 mEq/L K

C. 3.5–5.2 mEq/L K

D. 5.3–6.3 mEq/L K

366. Which clinical finding is commonly noted when the nurse is assessing a client with an anterior pituitary tumor?

A. Anorexia

B. Parasthesia

C. Dull headache

D. Nausea and vomiting

367. On assessment, one of the most prominent clinical findings associated with Addison's disease is:

A. Hyperglycemia

B. Hypokalemia

C. Hypernatremia

D. Hyperpigmentation

368. Client teaching regarding common side effects of corticosteroid therapy should include information about:

A. Hyperglycemia and weight gain

B. Hyperglycemia and weight loss

C. Hypoglycemia and gastric ulcers

D. Hyponatremia and poor wound healing

369. The recommended therapeutic diet for a client with Addison's disease is:

A. 1 gm Na, 2 gms K, fluids restricted to 1000 cc/day

B. 3 gms Na, 1 gm K, at least 3000 cc fluid per day

C. Low-fat, low-cholesterol, fluids restricted to 1000 cc/day

D. High-fiber, high-carbohydrate, at least 3000 cc fluid per day

370. Which clinical findings would the nurse most likely note during an addisonian crisis?

A. Serum potassium of 3.0 mEq/L, BP of 158/72

B. Serum potassium of 5.8 mEq/L, BP of 62/48

C. Serum sodium of 150 mEq/L, BP of 158/72

D. Serum sodium of 135 mEq/L, BP of 62/48

371. In emergency treatment of addisonian crisis, the nurse would prepare to administer IV saline and:

A. 20 units regular insulin

B. 60 mg furosemide (Lasix) intravenous pyelography (IVP)
C. 0.2 mg fludrocortisone (Florinef) IVP
D. 100 mg hydrocortisone (Solu-Cortef) IVP

372. Which outcome indicates that one of the goals for teaching a client with Addison's disease has been met? The client:
A. Has a BP of 76/58; serum sodium of 136 mEq/L
B. Has a BP of 142/82; serum potassium of 6.2 mEq/L
C. Takes glucocorticoid replacement therapy as needed
D. Wears a Medic Alert bracelet noting the health alteration

373. Upon nursing assessment, which clinical finding is often noted in Cushing's syndrome?
A. Weight loss
B. Hypertension
C. Serum glucose < 55 mg/dl
D. Serum sodium of 124 mEq/L

374. When teaching the client with Cushing's disease, which menu should the nurse discourage?
A. Broiled fish with green beans
B. Baked chicken with spinach salad
C. Ham sandwich and potato chips
D. Lettuce, tomato, and cucumber salad

375. Discharge client teaching for a client with pernicious anemia should include instructions to take this medication as prescribed:
A. 1.0 mg folic acid daily
B. 325 mg iron supplement daily
C. Vitamin B₁₂ injections monthly
D. Daily supplemental iron injections

376. The most likely symptoms that the nurse would note during an acute paroxysmal attack with pheochromocytoma are:
A. Dizziness, bradycardia, and hypertension
B. Tachycardia, weakness, and hypotension
C. Tachycardia, nervousness, and hypertension
D. Bradycardia, headache, and weakness

377. A client is hospitalized for acute glomerulonephritis. He has fever and periorbital edema; he complains of weakness and chills. The nurse assesses for a history of an infection caused by:
A. *Neisseria gonorrhoeae*
B. *Haemophilus influenzae*
C. *Pseudomonas aeruginosa*
D. Group A β-hemolytic streptococcus

378. The nurse develops a plan of care for a client with acute glomerulonephritis. Initially, these measures include:
A. Encouraging fluid intake
B. A planned exercise program
C. High-protein, low-fat diet
D. Administering penicillin as ordered

379. The nurse helps the client with acute glomeru-

lonephritis to select from a menu. Which choice is contraindicated for this client?
A. Hot apple pie
B. Rib eye steak
C. Waffles with butter and syrup
D. Buttered wheat toast with jelly

380. When explaining treatment to the glaucoma client, the nurse identifies the goal of treatment for chronic glaucoma is to:
A. Decrease intraocular pressure.
B. Rest the eye so that healing can occur.
C. Dilate the pupil to enhance outflow of aqueous humor.
D. Prevent complications such as retinal hemorrhage.

381. Medication is prescribed for a client with glaucoma. The nurse identifies the action of carbonic anhydrase inhibitors such as acetazolamide (Diamox) is to decrease intraocular pressure in acute glaucoma by:
A. Producing miosis
B. Producing mydriasis
C. Increasing outflow of aqueous humor
D. Decreasing aqueous humor production

382. On assessment, the nurse notes that which of the following symptoms is characteristic with hypoglycemia?
A. Polyuria
B. Pale, clammy skin
C. Dry mucous membranes
D. Kussmaul's respirations

383. When assessing laboratory values, the nurse knows which laboratory value falls within the range for a normal serum glucose level?
A. 38 mg/dl
B. 50 mg/dl
C. 102 mg/dl
D. 150 mg/dl

384. A desirable outcome for a client with diabetes is a:
A. Blood glucose level of 56 mg/dl
B. Blood glucose level of 110 mg/dl
C. Potassium level of 2.5 mEq/L
D. Potassium level of 5.4 mEq/L

385. The nurse evaluates the client's ability to self-monitor blood glucose levels at home. What information best indicates the average degree of diabetes control during the past 2 to 4 months?
A. Serum glycosylated hemoglobin
B. Postprandial blood glucose level
C. A written record of daily blood glucose levels
D. A written record of daily double-voided urine glucose levels

386. When assessing the feet of a diabetic client, which nursing observation is cause for concern?
A. Capillary refill less than 3 seconds
B. Bilateral dorsalis pedal pulses are 2+

C. No hair noted on either foot
D. A well-healed corn that is padded

387. Morphine 10 mg and promethazine (Phenergan) 25 mg IM have been ordered for postoperative pain. On hand is morphine 12 mg/cc and promethazine 50 mg/2 cc. How many total cubic centimeters will the nurse administer?
A. 0.8 cc
B. 1.0 cc
C. 1.8 cc
D. 2.2 cc

388. Which clinical symptom is most likely to be observed in a client in thyrotoxic crisis ("thyroid storm")?
A. WBC count of 8000
B. Blood glucose level of 84 mg/dl
C. Pulse rate of 140 to 160
D. Very warm, dry skin

389. A client has been diagnosed as in thyroid storm. The nurse recognizes that thyrotoxic crisis is most often precipitated by:
A. Insomnia and severe dehydration
B. Weight gain of more than 20 lb
C. Ingesting large amounts of protein
D. Infection and diabetic ketoacidosis

390. The priority nursing intervention for a client experiencing thyrotoxic crisis is:
A. Establishing a patent IV
B. Inserting a nasogastric tube
C. Maintaining a patent airway
D. Reducing the body temperature

391. The most appropriate nursing intervention to protect the eyes of a client with mild exophtalmos is to:
A. Administer methylcellulose eyedrops PRN
B. Tape the client's eyes shut at night
C. Restrict dietary sodium
D. Cover the client's eyes with saline-soaked gauze

392. Dietary teaching for a client with uncomplicated hyperthyroidism should encourage which diet?
A. Less protein, low fat, no caffeine
B. More protein, more calories, no caffeine
C. Less protein, less carbohydrate, moderate caffeine intake
D. More protein, less carbohydrate, moderate caffeine intake

393. Propranolol (Inderal) is commonly prescribed for clients with hyperthyroidism to:
A. Block formation of thyroid hormone
B. Decrease the vascularity of the thyroid
C. Inhibit peripheral conversion of T_4 to T_3
D. Decrease central nervous system stimulation

394. When performing a physical assessment of a client with hyperthyroidism, usually the nurse may find:
A. Intolerance to cold
B. Bradycardia with arrhythmias

C. Fluid retention and weight gain
D. Restlessness and decreased attention span

395. The nurse teaches safety measures to a client who is receiving radioactive iodine[131] for treatment of hyperthyroidism. What information should be taught to the client?
A. "Flush the toilet three to four times immediately after use."
B. "Decrease your intake of dietary sodium for the next 3 days."
C. "Close contact with pregnant women poses no threat to the fetus."
D. "If you vomit within 10 hours of ingesting the isotope, the dose must be readministered."

396. When assessing a client who is newly diagnosed with hypothyroidism, which symptom should the nurse expect?
A. Amenorrhea
B. Profound weight loss
C. Decreased tolerance to cold
D. "Moon facies" and hypernatremia

397. The nurse expects to find which of the most commonly altered laboratory findings in a client with hypothyroidism:
A. Hemoglobin level of 9.0 gm
B. Sodium level of 152 mEq/L
C. Cholesterol level of <200 mg
D. Serum amylase of 50 to 190 U/L

398. When planning care for the client with hypothyroidism, which nursing diagnosis should be included?
A. Altered nutrition: less than body requirements
B. Diarrhea related to increased metabolic rate
C. Activity intolerance
D. Fluid volume deficit

399. The priority nursing intervention for a client with hypothyroidism is:
A. A low sodium diet
B. Planned rest periods
C. Fluid intake of 3 L/day
D. Ambulating for 20 minutes tid

400. A client with long-standing hypoparathyroidism may exhibit serious complications. The nurse identifies which of the following symptoms as reversible?
A. Cataracts
B. Papilledema
C. Bowing of the long bones
D. Defective tooth structure

401. The desired outcome for a client with exophthalmos caused by Graves' disease is:
A. Absence of corneal abrasions
B. Minimal loss of visual acuity
C. BP within the 118/80 to 150/90 range
D. Weight loss of at least 10 to 20 percent

402. The most appropriate nursing diagnosis when

planning care for a client with the syndrome of inappropriate antidiuretic hormone (SIADH) is:
   A. Altered cardiac output
   B. Altered nutrition: less than body requirements
   C. Alteration in fluid balance: excess
   D. Alteration in fluid balance: deficit

403. A diabetic client is admitted to the ER with a blood sugar of 48 mg/dl. The client is pale, diaphoretic, and drowsy. Which medication will this client most likely receive?
   A. Glucagon 1.0 mg IM
   B. 500 cc of 5% dextrose in water (D_5W) @ 150 cc/hr
   C. Regular insulin 10 U IVP
   D. NPH insulin 10 U IVP

404. The nurse reviews the administration of Humulin Lente insulin with a newly diagnosed diabetic client. Which action indicates that the client understands how to self-administer insulin safely? The client:
   A. Attempts to substitute regular insulin for NPH
   B. Shakes the bottle vigorously prior to administration
   C. Rotates the bottle gently to disperse the precipitate
   D. Administers the injection at the same site every time

405. An IVPB of methyldopa (Aldomet) 500 mg in 50 cc D_5W is to infuse over 1 hour. If the administration set delivers 10 gtt/cc, at how many drops per minute should the IVPB be regulated?
   A. 8
   B. 11
   C. 12
   D. 16

406. The nurse notes that a client in chronic renal failure (CRF) is anemic. The main reason for the anemia is:
   A. Decreased absorption of vitamin B_{12} and folic acid
   B. Decreased production of erythropoietin by the kidney
   C. Damage to the red blood cells during hemodialysis
   D. Diminished transportation of iron to the tissues

407. A female client has recurring cystitis. When evaluating the effectiveness of client teaching to prevent recurring cystitis, teaching has been successful if the client verbalizes the need to:
   A. Wipe her perineal area from back to front after defecation.
   B. Drink at least 400 cc of cold water every day
   C. Empty her bladder immediately after sexual intercourse
   D. Void at least every 6 hours during waking hours

408. A client has been diagnosed with chronic hypertension. A care plan for chronic hypertension

would state which of the following as most accurate?
   A. Drink plenty of juice.
   B. Exercise vigorously three times a week.
   C. Avoid high-sodium foods.
   D. Avoid alcohol.

409. A 49-year-old client is discharged after a hospital stay for hypertensive crisis. The nurse is performing discharge instructions and the client is prescribed furosemide (Lasix). Which of the following statements would indicate the client needs further instruction?
   A. "I will not eat bananas or drink much juice because of the fluid pill."
   B. "I will avoid high-sodium foods such as potato chips."
   C. "I will take my medications at the same time daily."
   D. "I will try to do some regular exercise."

410. A 70-year-old female has had a lengthy hospital stay and is approaching discharge soon, after being diagnosed with a myocardial infarction. She states to you, "I know my cardiac condition isn't serious and I'm looking forward to resuming my former lifestyle." Which of the following grief stages would be most accurate?
   A. Depression
   B. Denial
   C. Acceptance
   D. Bargaining

411. A 62-year-old has been scheduled to be discharged soon after insertion of a permanent pacemaker. Which of the following would be most important for the nurse to teach during discharge instructions?
   A. "Do not be concerned if nonpurulent drainage from your incision occurs."
   B. "Take and record pulse daily and notify of any changes."
   C. "Avoid new-model microwave ovens."
   D. "Wear a medical alert bracelet."

412. A 55-year-old client is diagnosed with cellulitis. Which of the following body responses would the nurse expect to find?
   A. Diffuse inflammation and swelling of the affected area
   B. Eschar and fluid discharge of the affected area
   C. Petechiae and discoloration of the affected area
   D. Ecchymosis and bruising of the affected area

413. A 25-year-old male client diagnosed with AIDS seems angry. Which one of the following approaches by the nurse would be best?
   A. Ignore his behavior.
   B. Use open-ended questions.
   C. Call his physician.
   D. Call his family to visit.

414. A 25-year-old male is newly diagnosed with AIDS. The nurse would find which of the following most likely upon admission after interview?
    A. Acceptance by friends
    B. No family concerns
    C. A distant attitude
    D. Hostility toward staff

415. A 50-year-old client is admitted for hypertensive crisis. Which of the following information is most important for the nurse to obtain on admission?
    A. Neurological assessment
    B. Fluid retention assessment
    C. Laboratory profiles
    D. History

416. An 80-year-old female client is admitted with an uncomplicated myocardial infarction and chest pain. Her vital signs are BP 140/70, R 16, and P 78. Which of the following procedures with a doctor's order, if required, would the nurse expect to prepare for the client?
    A. Give nitroglycerin drip.
    B. Give dopamine drip.
    C. Give routine meds.
    D. Perform client or family teaching.

417. A 67-year-old client is admitted to the ICU with a BP of 220/150. He has a severe headache. Which of the following would the nurse identify as a level of care?
    A. Emergency immediate intervention
    B. Urgent intervention, requiring 15 minutes or more
    C. Priority intervention, requiring 30 minutes or more
    D. Observation, requiring frequent monitoring of the client

418. A 67-year-old is admitted to the ICU with hypertensive crisis. Which of the following drugs could the nurse anticipate the physician would order?
    A. Give diazepam.
    B. Give nitroprusside.
    C. Give hydrochlorothiazide.
    D. Give digoxin.

419. A 67-year-old client is admitted to the ICU with hypertensive crisis. Which of the following approaches by the nurse is best?
    A. Rest periods between activities
    B. Unrestricted visitors
    C. Encourage discussion of family problems.
    D. Encourage ventilation of frustrations.

420. A 51-year-old client is admitted to the hospital for a bone marrow aspiration. To prevent a hematoma, which of the following approaches would be best by the nurse?
    A. Cleanse the site as ordered.
    B. Apply pressure to the site.
    C. Dress the site.
    D. Turn the patient to the operative site.

421. A 65-year-old client is attending her clinic appointment after a hospitalization with severe anemia. In preparing to evaluate teaching, which of the following food choices by the client indicates the need for further teaching? "My diet will include lots of the following foods":
    A. Liver
    B. Beans
    C. Fish
    D. Green leafy vegetables

422. A client is prescribed ferrous sulfate tablets twice daily. She is a 40-year-old with iron-deficiency anemia. The nurse should teach the client which of the following?
    A. It will discolor her teeth.
    B. It will give her urine an odor.
    C. It will give her bad breath.
    D. It will darken her stools.

423. A 40-year-old client is diagnosed with iron-deficiency anemia. Which of the following laboratory reports would indicate the client's condition?
    A. Hemoglobin
    B. Hematocrit
    C. Erythrocyte indices
    D. CBC

424. A 50-year-old client is diagnosed with folic acid deficiency. He is to have a Schilling test to check his absorption of vitamin B_{12}. The nurse should teach the client which of the following?
    A. Drink a large quantity of water.
    B. Put on radiation precautions.
    C. Save all urine.
    D. Save all urine for 24 hours.

425. A 57-year-old client is admitted for cardiac symptoms and evaluation. A bruit is identified. Which of the following information would be important in assessing the client with a bruit?
    A. The client is experiencing orthostatic hypotension.
    B. The client has occluded blood vessels.
    C. The client has adequate peripheral circulation.
    D. There is turbulent blood flow through stenotic blood vessels.

426. A 67-year-old male client has arterial insufficiency in the legs. He is complaining of cold feet and has diabetes. Which of the following approaches by the nurse is best?
    A. Discourage exercise.
    B. Increase the room temperature.
    C. Apply heat to the client's feet.
    D. Remove socks.

427. A 70-year-old client is diagnosed with cardiac myopathy. The nurse should teach the client which of the following?
    A. To walk on a routine basis
    B. To continue smoking, but cut down

C. To ignore fat in the diet and count calories only

D. That shortness of breath is a minor symptom of a cardiac problem

428. A 70-year-old client is diagnosed with chronic congestive heart failure. The physician has ordered a strict low-sodium, high-potassium diet. The nurse should teach this client that her diet should include which of the following foods?
A. Smoked turkey sandwich, pickles, and skim milk
B. Low-sodium bread, salt-free eggs, and orange juice
C. Tea, chicken breast sandwich, and carrots
D. Coffee, chicken salad sandwich, and low-salt chips

429. A 45-year-old client has a history of chronic hypertension. He has a height of 5 feet 6 inches and weighs 200 pounds. The nurse should teach this client that his diet should include which of the following?
A. Canned and frozen foods
B. Avoidance of potassium-rich foods, if prescribed diuretics
C. High-calorie foods
D. Low-sodium, low-fat foods

430. A 72-year-old client in the CCU is diagnosed with left ventricular failure. The physician orders dopamine and nitroprusside IV drips. Which of the following approaches by the nurse is best?
A. Give a local anesthetic at the IV site to minimize local pain, by physician order.
B. Give the two drugs as ordered to maintain blood pressure.
C. Give the two drugs in the same IV site.
D. Give the drugs in the hand.

431. An 80-year-old client is diagnosed with respiratory failure. She is given an artificial airway via an endotracheal tube. What is the purpose of giving her the artificial airway?
A. Provide coughing stimulation.
B. Increase her lung capacity.
C. Remove lower lobe secretions.
D. Provide ventilation.

432. A 74-year-old client is diagnosed with tuberculosis. Which of the following laboratory reports would confirm the client's condition?
A. Chest x-ray
B. Creatinine clearance
C. Sputum for culture
D. CBC

433. A 74-year-old client is seen in the clinic with a confirmed diagnosis of TB. Which of the following symptoms would the nurse expect to observe?
A. Blood-streaked sputum and flank pain
B. Coughing up blood and an increase in body weight

C. Afternoon fever and thick mucus
D. Rash and night sweats

434. A 74-year-old client in a nursing home has a confirmed diagnosis of TB. He is put on respiratory isolation. When he asks why he is placed in isolation, the nurse explains: This helps to
A. Prevent transmission of TB via droplets
B. Promote rest by limiting visitors
C. Provide privacy for the client
D. Prevent transmission to others through close contact

435. A 30-year-old female in good health is scheduled for surgery. To prevent infection, the nurse should teach the client which of the following?
A. Shower the day of the surgical procedure.
B. Wash hair only after surgery.
C. An antibiotic will be given after surgery.
D. The incision site will be shaved prior to the surgery.

436. A 60-year-old known diabetic is found unconscious by the nurse. The client had a 60 blood glucose level. Which would be the best initial approach by the nurse?
A. Give dextrose by IVP.
B. Give prescribed insulin.
C. Initiate CPR.
D. Start an IV and give normal saline.

437. A 50-year-old client admitted with an onset of seizures. As the nurse observes the seizure, which is the most important nursing action?
A. Have the side rails padded.
B. Place a padded tongue blade in the mouth.
C. Document the client's level of consciousness.
D. Position client to maintain an open airway.

438. A 22-year-old is diagnosed with HIV. In the laboratory of the physician's office, the nurse is asked to draw blood. Which of the following approaches is best by the nurse?
A. Use universal precautions.
B. Isolate the patient.
C. Wear a gown to draw the blood.
D. Wear a face shield to draw the blood.

439. A 72-year-old client is being discharged from the hospital after a stay for COPD. The nurse's discharge teaching should include which of the following?
A. Combine activities.
B. Sleep flat.
C. Drink a lot of fluids.
D. Conserve on sodium.

440. A 20-year-old client is being discharged as a newly diagnosed diabetic. Which of the following statements by the nurse is most accurate when teaching the client about diabetes?
A. Test capillary blood glucose, as prescribed by physician.

B. Rotate injection sites for insulin only after all abdominal sites are used.

C. Eat three meals a day and a bedtime snack.

D. Eat prior to regular insulin administration.

441. A 20-year-old client is being discharged with a diagnosis of diabetes. The client states that after physical therapy she felt weak and that she had not eaten prior to her treatment. Which of the following statements would be most accurate when doing discharge teaching for the client?

A. Discuss that exercise increases the need for more glucose.

B. Eat candy to prevent weakness.

C. Take extra insulin when feeling badly.

D. Go off specified diet to increase calories.

442. A 60-year-old client has stable angina. He is on a telemetry unit and complains of chest pain. The nurse would expect to find which of the following pain descriptions?

A. Mild chest pain at night

B. Stabbing pain in the chest

C. Located on the left chest only

D. Squeezing pain in the chest

443. A 60-year-old client has stable angina. The physician prescribes nitroglycerin ointment. Which of the following approaches by the nurse is best?

A. Apply to upper chest or shoulders.

B. Massage or rub in ointment.

C. Remove if it becomes loose.

D. Rotate sites.

444. A 59-year-old client has cirrhosis of the liver with esophageal varices. The nurse should teach him to avoid actions that increase abdominal pressure. The nurse should teach which of the following actions?

A. Avoid straining at stool.

B. He may lift 5- to 10-pound objects only.

C. Wear antiembolism hose.

D. Increase sodium intake.

445. A 49-year-old female is admitted to your unit 1 week after an abdominal aneurysm repair. Her potassium is 8.0 mEq/L. Which of the following EKG changes would the nurse observe with this laboratory finding?

A. A broad QRS complex

B. A prominent U wave

C. No changes would be noted

D. A flattened T wave

446. A 78-year-old female is admitted on your unit with confusion and decreased urinary output (<30 ml/hr). The elderly are at risk for urinary infection. Which of the following factors may make it difficult to detect infections in an elderly client?

A. Fever may be present even though the temperature may not seem greatly elevated.

B. The client does not complain of pain or malaise lasting greater than 3 days.

C. Altered cognition makes it difficult to assess the elderly client's signs and symptoms.

D. The elderly normally have a decreased urine output due to decreased appetite and fluid intake.

447. A 60-year-old male is admitted to the unit in the intrarenal oliguric phase of renal dysfunction. Which of the following imbalances would the nurse expect to note in serum blood levels?

A. Elevated blood urea nitrogen

B. Decreased serum creatinine

C. Elevated hematocrit

D. Decreased potassium

448. A 60-year-old male is admitted on your unit with acute intrarenal dysfunction and he appears confused and drowsy. Which of the following is most likely to contribute to drowsiness and confusion in acute renal failure?

A. Hypomagnesemia

B. Respiratory acidosis

C. Hypoxia

D. Metabolic acidosis

449. A 43-year-old client is being evaluated for a renal transplant. When assessing the client, the nurse identifies that which of the following conditions is contraindicated for a renal transplant?

A. Anemia

B. Coronary artery disease

C. Diverticulosis

D. Hypothyroidism

450. A 50-year-old male is admitted to your unit with complaints of fever, chills, anorexia, drowsiness, and confusion. He is diagnosed in the anuric stage of acute renal failure. The nurse identifies which of the following to define an anuric urine output?

A. Less than 100 ml in 24 hours

B. Less than 200 ml in 24 hours

C. Less than 300 ml in 24 hours

D. Less than 400 ml in 24 hours

451. A 64-year-old male is admitted with anorexia, drowsiness, confusion, and a urine output of less than 400 ml in a 24-hour period. He has a repeated history of CHF. The physician orders two units of whole blood to improve his dangerously low hematocrit and hemoglobin. Because of the client's history, which of the following measures is critical in this client's care?

A. Measure and record intake and output of all fluids, including blood products.

B. Monitor all lab results, including electrolytes, hematocrit, and hemoglobin.

C. Monitor for possible GI bleeding by testing all stools for occult blood.

D. Question the doctor's order for whole blood products for this client.

452. A 39-year-old female is diagnosed as being in end-stage renal disease. She has been placed on the

waiting list of a kidney transplant. The nurse discusses some of the routine measures a transplant recipient must take after surgery. Which of the following statements would indicate the client needs further instruction?

A. "The steroid medication that I have to take may give me ulcers."

B. "I need to avoid being around people with colds and report any temperature above 98.6°F."

C. "Once I am feeling OK, I can stop taking my medication as long as I inform the doctor."

D. "I need to watch my weight and make sure I am not retaining fluid."

453. A 67-year-old female is admitted with recent changes in mental status reported by her daughter. The client is lethargic, has difficulty feeding herself, and has a 24-hour urine output of less than 150 ml. The doctor has ordered an intravenous pyelogram in the A.M. When assessing the client, the nurse identifies which of the following in the client's history that would contraindicate this procedure?

A. Long-term diuretic use

B. Allergy to shellfish

C. History of anemia

D. Recent myocardial infarction

454. A 50-year-old male is to be placed on hemodialysis. The physician has ordered surgery for the placement of an A-V fistula for dialysis access. Which of the following statements by this client would indicate an understanding of the purpose for this surgery?

A. "A tube is inserted into the artery in my neck and sewn into the skin. They will stick needles into this for my dialysis."

B. "A catheter is placed into my arm and then connected to the dialysis machine so they can clean my blood."

C. "They cut an opening into my arm to join a vein and an artery together. After the area has healed they will use the area to connect me to the dialysis machine."

D. "A tube is connected from your arm to your heart and sewn into the skin. The tube is then used to connect me to the dialysis machine."

455. A 59-year-old male is 2 days' postoperative for an A-V fistula placement for hemodialysis. Which of the following statements by the nurse to the client is correct about his A-V fistula home care?

A. "Carry clamps with you at all times in case of an emergency."

B. "The site will be ready for dialysis access in just a few days."

C. "Avoid wearing constrictive clothing on the arm with the fistula."

D. "Painful spasms can occur at the site during hemodialysis; this is normal."

456. A 36-year-old female has received multiple nephrotoxic antibiotics to treat a septic wound. As a result of her treatment, she has progressed into acute renal failure. The nurse identifies which of the following as the best description of this type of renal failure?

A. Anuric

B. Intrarenal

C. Prerenal

D. Postrenal

457. A 62-year-old male is admitted to the unit with a diagnosis of acute tubular necrosis. The nurse identifies which of the following to be the most life-threatening complication of this disorder?

A. Hyperkalemia

B. Hypochloremia

C. Hypermagnesemia

D. Hypernatremia

458. A 78-year-old female is admitted with a diagnosis of digitalis toxicity. The client is concerned about what has happened to her. The nurse realizes that education about drug administration is of great importance with this age group. Which of the following reasons makes the elderly more susceptible to drug-administration complications?

A. They consume nearly one-half of all prescribed medications.

B. They experience the same side effects from drugs as younger adults.

C. They are often taking a large amount of different medications for many different conditions.

D. They suffer from more confusion than younger adults and overdose more often on different medications.

459. A 58-year-old male has returned to the unit following a Quinton-Scribner shunt (catheter) placement for hemodialysis access. The catheter is located in the left subclavian vein. Which of the following are recommended nursing interventions for this type of access?

A. The catheter can be used for blood sampling, infusions, or hemodynamic monitoring.

B. A sign should be placed above the bed stating, "No sticks or blood pressures in left arm."

C. Apply pressure to the site with a sandbag for 8 hours and observe for hematoma formation.

D. Observe the site for drainage and hematoma formations and assess breath sounds frequently.

460. A 40-year-old female has been admitted in end-stage renal failure. She is scheduled for a kidney transplant. Which of the following is the most critical preoperative nursing intervention for this client?

A. Monitor for urinary retention.

B. Monitor for signs and symptoms of infection.

C. Monitor emotional response to impending surgery.

D. Monitor nutritional status and encourage fluids.

461. A 28-year-old female is hospitalized in an undetermined stage of renal failure. The nurse plans to teach the client about the test she will undergo. Which of the following is the best test to differentiate prerenal azotemia from intrarenal disease?
   A. Renal biopsy
   B. Renal ultrasound
   C. Creatinine clearance test
   D. Fluid challenge

462. A 56-year-old female in end-stage renal disease is receiving dialysis three times per week. During the dialysis one day she begins to exhibit signs of disequilibrium syndrome. Which of the following signs and symptoms would the nurse expect to see with this syndrome?
   A. Apprehension, hypotension, and thready pulse
   B. Headache, fever, nausea, and vomiting
   C. Vomiting, muscle twitching and cramps, and hypotension
   D. Hypotension, diaphoresis, dyspnea, and weak pulse

463. A 68-year-old male is admitted with chronic renal failure. Diet education needed by the chronic renal failure client would include which of the following?
   A. A high-sodium diet with limited protein
   B. Observe fluid restrictions and avoid high-potassium foods
   C. Encourage potassium-rich foods but monitor sodium intake
   D. Increase dietary bulk and fluid intake

464. A 26-year-old female is admitted after a motor vehicle accident (MVA) with a closed pneumothorax and low-pressure chest tube setup in place. A few hours later the client becomes agitated, diaphoretic, and hypotensive with increased respirations and heart rate. The nurse identifies that which of the following complications may be developing?
   A. Chest tube displacement
   B. Tissue hypoxia
   C. Air embolism
   D. Tension pneumothorax

465. A 65-year-old male is admitted with sudden abdominal pain and gastric fullness. He has a history of arteriosclerosis. Palpation of the abdomen reveals some tenderness over the upper quadrants. Auscultation of the abdomen reveals a systolic bruit. The client is scheduled for an abdominal ultrasound in the A.M. Which of the following changes would be important for the nurse to observe for in this client?
   A. Decreasing blood pressure
   B. Increasing blood pressure
   C. Decreasing pulse rate
   D. Cyanosis of the lips and gums

466. A 65-year-old thin male is admitted with a diagnosis of rule-out abdominal aortic aneurysm. Which of the following would the nurse expect to find in the assessment of a client with an abdominal aneurysm?
   A. A systolic bruit auscultated over the abdomen
   B. Decreased pedal pulses, bilaterally
   C. Decreased hair and shiny skin to lower legs
   D. History of heavy lifting or weight training

467. A 38-year-old male is admitted with a diagnosis of advanced AIDS. When assessing the client, the nurse might expect to find which of the following signs and symptoms as characteristics of this disease?
   A. Mouth ulcers present less than 1 week
   B. Increased T-cell count for over 1 month
   C. Lymphadenopathy in the neck for over 1 week
   D. Temperature greater than 100°F for more than 3 months

468. A 78-year-old female is admitted with confusion and unexplained weight loss. The client is cooperative but is disoriented to time, place, and person. In the nursing care plan, a diagnosis of altered thought process is developed. What other related nursing diagnosis could be used with this client?
   A. Impaired physical mobility
   B. High risk for violence
   C. High risk for injury
   D. Altered self-concept

469. A 36-year-old female is admitted in acute respiratory failure. She is now stable with a pulse oximetry reading of 98 percent on 2 L oxygen via nasal cannula. Which of the following would indicate to the nurse that the client is having respiratory difficulty or arrest?
   A. S_3
   B. Decreased pulse and increased BP
   C. ABG: pH = 7.56, $PaCO_2$ = 36, PaO_2 = 92, HCO_3 = 27
   D. Pulse oximetry reading of 76

470. A 40-year-old male is admitted to the unit with addisonian crisis. He has stabilized and is started on PO corticosteroid replacement therapy. Which of the following patient-teaching explanations given by the nurse would be most appropriate for this client?
   A. "Eat a healthy diet but monitor fat intake."
   B. "Use alcohol-free products on your skin."
   C. "Do not let your disease alter your lifestyle; stay active."
   D. "Muscle weakness and fatigue are not normal; see your doctor."

471. A 36-year-old male is admitted from ICU 3 days after an MVA. He has suffered multiple contusions and required three transfusions of blood and blood products. He begins to exhibit signs of tachypnea, tachycardia with frequent premature ventricular contractions, and a labile blood pres-

sure. He is increased from ventimask oxygen of 80 percent to 100 percent without relief. His pulse oximeter has remained steady at 80 percent despite the oxygen increase. Which of the following complications should the nurse be alert for in this client?

A. Fat embolus
B. Pneumonia
C. Adult respiratory distress syndrome (ARDS)
D. Pericarditis

472. A 76-year-old female has been admitted after surgery for a left hip replacement following a fall at home. The client has been recently diagnosed with Alzheimer's disease. Which of the following statements would indicate to the nurse that this client's family member needs further education about Alzheimer's disease?

A. "Mom will continue to progressively forget people and places."
B. "Mom is forgetful, but aren't most old people?"
C. "She will eventually need 24-hour-a-day care."
D. "There are community resources available for me and my family."

473. A 65-year-old male with a history of diabetes is admitted following a right below-the-knee amputation (BKA). Which of the following nursing measures is most appropriate for this client?

A. Tell the client to follow his diet to prevent further complications.
B. Keep the stump open to air to allow proper healing of the incision site.
C. Administer sedatives to keep the client quiet and still to prevent complications.
D. Elevate the stump on a pillow but keep the knee extended.

474. A 26-year-old female is 2 days' postoperative for a right wrist repair following a motor vehicle accident. She has a history of NKDA. Her doctor orders IVPB piperacillin 500 mg tid. During infusion of her antibiotic, the client becomes anxious, expresses feelings of doom, is diaphoretic, and has dyspnea and nasal pruritus. Which of the following actions should the nurse perform with this client?

A. Call the doctor
B. Take the client's vital signs.
C. Administer epinephrine IM, SQ, or IV.
D. Stop the infusion.

475. A 56-year-old male is scheduled for an angioplasty in the A.M. You review teaching for after the client has returned to the unit following the procedure. Which of the following statements would indicate to the nurse that the client understands about his care following the procedure?

A. "I can sit up in bed and eat as soon as I return to my room."

B. "I will be able to get out of bed as soon as I feel up to it."
C. "I will be paralyzed from the waist down for a few hours after the procedure."
D. "I will have to stay in bed and keep my leg with the incision straight to prevent bleeding."

476. A 22-year-old male is admitted following an acute asthma attack. Prior to this attack the client had no history of asthma. Which of the following would the nurse do to teach the client to prevent further attacks?

A. Instruct the client to carry oxygen with him at all times and use it if he feels an attack coming on.
B. Instruct the client to restrict fluid intake to, at most, 1500 cc per day.
C. Instruct the client to monitor caffeine, salt, and fat intake.
D. Instruct the client on deep breathing and encourage the client to cough up accumulated secretions every morning.

477. A 68-year-old male is admitted with an acute urinary tract infection. He also has a diagnosis of benign prostatic hyperplasia. In reviewing the client's admit orders, the nurse would question which of the following?

A. Insert a Foley catheter.
B. Monitor fluid intake and output.
C. Administer PO Valium 5mg q6.
D. Fluid restriction of less than 1000 cc/day

478. A 72-year-old female is admitted to same-day surgery for a left cataract removal. After the procedure, the nurse reviews home care instructions with the client. Which of the following would the nurse include with her instructions for this client?

A. Instruct the client not to bend or lift any heavy objects or cough vigorously.
B. Instruct the client that it is safe to return to her previous exercise regime, no matter how strenuous.
C. Inform the client that photophobia and red, watery eyes are normal for a time after this type of surgery.
D. Instruct the client to remove the eye patch over the affected eye when she gets home.

479. An obese 64-year-old woman with a history of diabetes is admitted to the unit. She is placed on a 1500-calorie ADA diet. She has gained 3 pounds in 2 days. When the nurse enters the client's room to take her vital signs, the nurse finds the client eating a hamburger and french fries brought to her by her family. Which of the following actions taken by the nurse would be appropriate?

A. Restrict visitors to the room and inspect all packages.
B. Reprimand the client for not following the physician's orders.

C. Inform the physician of the client's noncompliance and ask him to speak to the family.

D. Take the family aside and discuss with them the importance of helping the client follow her diet.

480. A 42-year-old female is starting chemotherapy for breast cancer. Before the first dose is to be given, the nurse reviews the client's chart. Which of the following has to be on a client's chart prior to starting chemotherapy?

A. A complete past medical history and drug history

B. Complete laboratory work-up, including CBC and SMA-20

C. A consent document signed by the client or the client's family member

D. A complete nursing care plan for managing the client's chemotherapy symptoms

481. A 58-year-old male is to return home 6 days after coronary artery bypass graft (CABG) surgery. Which of the following home care instructions given by the nurse would be appropriate for this client?

A. "Report any fever, sore throat, redness, or swelling to the doctor immediately."

B. "You may feel palpitations and your heart may be rapid and irregular during your recovery. This is normal."

C. "You can return to your regular diet at home, but no alcohol for at least 6 weeks."

D. "You can return to activities as tolerated; these include driving and yard work."

482. A 53-year-old male is admitted complaining of chest pain. The pain is reported by the client to be a 6 on a pain scale of 10, with 10 being intense, unbearable pain. Which of the following interventions would the nurse do first for this client?

A. Call the doctor.

B. Take the client's vital signs.

C. Call for stat EKG

D. Administer SL nitroglycerin.

483. A 37-year-old female is admitted with a diagnosis of Cushing's syndrome. Clients with Cushing's syndrome frequently develop which of the following complications?

A. Hypoglycemia and weight loss

B. Hypertension and dehydration

C. Osteoporosis and impaired wound healing

D. Sleep disturbances and muscle wasting

484. A 32-year-old female is admitted with a diagnosis of diabetes mellitus. She weighs 320 pounds and is 5 feet 1 inch in height. Sedatives are ordered around the clock to reduce anxiety. Which of the following would the nurse need to be aware of when administering sedatives to an obese client?

A. Obese clients take less time to fully recover from the effects of sedation.

B. Obese clients may require a lower dose of sedative medication.

C. Obese clients take more time to recover from the effects of sedation.

D. Obese clients should never be given sedative medication due to increased chance of injury.

485. A 28-year-old female has been diagnosed with systemic lupus erythematosus (SLE). Which of the following abnormal laboratory values would the nurse expect to see in the client with SLE?

A. Positive antinuclear antibody test

B. Abnormal alkaline phosphatase

C. Decreased sedimentation rate

D. Increased white blood cells

486. A 44-year-old male is admitted with a diagnosis of AIDS. The physician has ordered for the nurse to do frequent mouth and perianal care. Which of the following is the primary reason for this action?

A. These areas frequently become dry and crack in the immune-compromised client.

B. These areas are best for assessing for cyanosis and decreased perfusion.

C. These areas are frequently overlooked in caring for the immune-compromised client.

D. These areas are frequent sites of monilial infections in the immune-compromised client.

487. A 36-year-old female is admitted with acute gastric distress including nausea and vomiting. She has a history of systemic lupus erythematosus (SLE). She complains of continual gastric reflux and burning. The nurse is aware that which of the following drug therapies used with SLE can predispose a client to gastric distress?

A. Hydroxychloroquine therapy

B. NSAID therapy

C. Herbal therapy

D. Corticosteroid therapy

488. A 22-year-old male is admitted from the ER with multiple fractures to the ribs, a fractured pelvis, a fractured right femur, and a fractured right fibula, all the result of a motor vehicle accident. The nurse realizes which of these fractures has the greatest potential for increasing the client's risk for hemorrhage?

A. Femur

B. Ribs

C. Fibula

D. Pelvis

489. A 22-year-old male is admitted with multiple fractures to the skull, femur, ribs, and pelvis. The nurse notes the following changes in the client's assessment data on day two of his hospitalization: dyspnea, pulse rate of 132, BP 150/96, cyanosis to oral mucosa, and petechiae on thorax. Which of the following complications could be occurring with this client?

A. ARDS

B. Septic shock
C. Pneumothorax
D. Fat embolus

490. A 38-year-old male is admitted to the unit in the final stages of AIDS. He has no visitors and gets emotionally violent with all the staff. He begins to refuse all medications and treatment. He states, "I don't want anybody's help. The world has given up on me and I am giving up on it." Which of the following would be the best response by the nurse?
    A. "You sound very angry right now. Let me come back when you have calmed down."
    B. "Well, I agree, the world is a cold place. I don't blame you for how you feel."
    C. "You sound like you want to give up. You need to be strong right now."
    D. "You sound upset. Would you like to talk about it?"

491. A 58-year-old female has returned to the unit following a radical mastectomy of the right breast. She has two Jackson-Pratt drains, which are draining serosanguineous fluid. Which of the following nursing measures may help reduce a major complication of radical mastectomy surgery?
    A. Measure and record drainage every 8 hours.
    B. Monitor the dressing site for excess drainage.
    C. Elevate the right arm on a pillow.
    D. Administer pain medication as ordered.

492. An 80-year-old female is admitted with right lower lobe bacterial pneumonia. On her second day of hospitalization, she begins to complain of severe headaches and muscle stiffness and her temperature rises above 100°F. She also has a sore throat and photophobia. The nurse also observes that the client is disoriented to person and place. The nurse needs to monitor this client closely, because the elderly are at higher risk for developing which of the following complications?
    A. Cerebral infarctions
    B. Hearing loss
    C. Endocarditis
    D. Viral meningitis

493. A 76-year-old female with a history of right-sided cerebral vascular accident 7 years ago has been transferred to the unit from a nursing home. During the assessment, the nurse finds a 4 cm hole in the left heel that oozes a foul-smelling yellow fluid. The sore extends into the muscle and has developed a black crust around the edges. The ulcer is not painful to the client. The nurse would place this ulcer into which of the following stages of skin breakdown?
    A. I
    B. II
    C. III
    D. IV

494. A 72-year-old male is admitted with multiple fractures following a fall at home. He becomes confused and lethargic shortly after admission. The nurse recognizes this as the elderly client's response to stress. Which of the following is true regarding how the elderly respond to stress?
    A. Physiological responses to stress occur rapidly in the elderly.
    B. The elderly respond to stress the same as a 35-year-old.
    C. Stress levels return to normal rapidly in the elderly.
    D. Psychological responses to stress occur rapidly in the elderly.

495. A 42-year-old female is admitted with pneumonia. Her arterial blood gases (ABGs) on room air are as follows: pH=7.30, PCO_2=48, PO_2=60, HCO_3=22. The nurse realizes that these ABGs represent which of the following conditions?
    A. Respiratory alkalosis
    B. Respiratory acidosis
    C. Metabolic acidosis
    D. Metabolic alkalosis

496. A 36-year-old male is admitted with bacterial pneumonia. His admission arterial blood gases are PaO_2=80, pH=7.30, PCO_2=46, HCO_3=23 on room air. What would the nurse expect to see in order for the pH to return to normal?
    A. Decrease in HCO_3
    B. Increase in HCO_3
    C. Decrease in PCO_2
    D. Increase in PCO_2

497. A 38-year-old male is admitted with a diagnosis of respiratory acidosis. Four hours after admission, his arterial blood gases (ABGs) read: PaO_2=90 mm Hg, pH=7.37, PCO_2=60 mm Hg, HCO_3=38 mEq/dl. The nurses recognize these ABG readings to represent which of the following?
    A. Compensated metabolic alkalosis with respiratory acidosis
    B. Uncompensated respiratory acidosis
    C. Compensated respiratory acidosis with metabolic alkalosis
    D. Uncompensated metabolic acidosis

498. A 60-year-old female is admitted to the unit on a ventilator. A 7.0 endotracheal tube is taped to her left mouth. She is on an SIMV of 12. The nurse notes her chest is expanding unequally on inspiration. Which of the following should the nurse do first?
    A. Call for a chest x-ray.
    B. Reposition the tube.
    C. Call for ABGs.
    D. Auscultate breath sounds.

499. A 48-year-old female is receiving 5000 units of heparin SQ bid. Which of the following nursing actions is appropriate for a client receiving heparin?
    A. Encourage self-administration of heparin shots.

B. Monitor daily hematocrit and hemoglobin.
C. Monitor daily PTT results.
D. Monitor for changes in vital signs.

500. A 68-year-old female is admitted with congestive heart failure (CHF). The client states she delayed coming to the hospital because she did not realize she was sick. The nurse would instruct the client to monitor for which of the following early signs and symptoms of CHF?
A. Frothy sputum
B. Tachycardia
C. Activity intolerance
D. Loss of consciousness

501. A 32-year-old female is admitted to the unit with a diagnosis of supraventricular tachycardia (SVT). Her heart rate is now 76 and she is in a normal sinus rhythm. Which of the following signs would the nurse monitor for a return of SVT in this client?
A. Sudden increase in blood pressure
B. Sudden decrease in blood pressure
C. Decreased urine output
D. Change in consciousness

502. A 72-year-old female is admitted after falling down at home and breaking her hip. The client has stiffness and difficulty with her activities. The nurse is aware that these difficulties are associated with the most common illness found in the elderly. Which of the following diseases is the most common in this age group?
A. Arthritis
B. Depression
C. Hypertension
D. Osteoporosis

503. An 80-year-old female is admitted with a diagnosis of dehydration and malnutrition. The nurse observes during her assessment that the client has an exaggerated posterior curvature of the thoracic spine. Which of the following describes the condition observed by the nurse?
A. Kyphosis
B. Lordosis
C. Scoliosis
D. List

504. A 72-year-old male is admitted to the unit with increased confusion and agitation secondary to Alzheimer's disease. The nurse notes on her assessment the client's dorsalis pedis and posterior tibial pulses are difficult to palpate. The client's lower extremities are cool and pink, have shiny skin and very little hair, and the nailbeds of the toes are thick and rigid. Which of the following conditions would be considered appropriate for this client based on the nurse's observations?
A. Arterial insufficiency
B. Renal insufficiency
C. Normal changes of aging
D. Muscular dystrophy

505. An 82-year-old frail female is admitted with confusion and malnutrition. She has been found wandering around her neighborhood late at night. She sleeps intermittently in the hospital and always complains of feeling tired. The nurse is aware that which of the following is true regarding sleep in the elderly?
A. They require less sleep than the average adult.
B. They awaken more often during the night than the average adult.
C. They have fewer changes in their sleep-stage cycles than the average adult.
D. They often exhibit wandering tendencies during sleep.

506. A 42-year-old female is admitted to the unit after a modified mastectomy. On her third postoperative day, the nurse is to begin instructing the client on dressing changes for home care of her incision. The nurse enters the room to find the client despondent and depressed. Which of the following would be an appropriate action for the nurse?
A. Leave the client alone and come back later.
B. Approach the client and ask if she would like to talk.
C. Proceed with the teaching to get the client's mind off her troubles.
D. Call the doctor and recommend antidepressants.

507. A 34-year-old female is admitted with Bell's palsy to the left side of her face. She is recovering from a tooth abscess to her left lower molar. Which of the following would be important for the nurse to monitor in this client?
A. Weight loss
B. Aspiration
C. Pain
D. Elevated temperature

508. A 42-year-old female is admitted with an acute extrinsic asthma attack. Which of the following would the nurse identify as a cause of an extrinsic asthma attack?
A. Mold or dust
B. Stress
C. Fatigue
D. Elevated temperature

509. A 32-year-old is admitted with a diagnosis of a severe asthma attack. The nurse would monitor for which of the following signs associated with a severe asthma attack?
A. Brief wheezing, coughing, or dyspnea with activity
B. Marked wheezing or absent breath sounds
C. Marked coughing and wheezing
D. Impaired consciousness

510. A 30-year-old male was admitted 3 days ago with status asthmaticus. He is on theophylline therapy and has no further problems. Later in the shift the

client begins to complain of headache and nausea and has a productive cough. The nurse is alert for which of the following with this client?
A. Theophylline toxicity
B. Subtherapeutic theophylline levels
C. Dehydration
D. Pulmonary embolus

511. A 24-year-old female is admitted to the ER after fainting at her place of work. She has had a recent history of dramatic weight loss of greater than 20 pounds in the past 3 months. She is 15 percent below her ideal body weight. She complains of feeling cold and has not had a bowel movement in 5 days. She has not had a menstrual cycle in 3 months. Which of the following conditions would the nurse be alert for in this client?
A. Cachexia
B. Anorexia
C. Anorexia nervosa
D. Amenorrhea

512. A 40-year-old female is admitted with aplastic anemia. She is on oxygen via nasal cannula at 2 L and has received one unit pack of red blood cells. Her platelet count is 19,000/μL and WBCs are 38,000/μL. Which of the following nursing measures is appropriate for this client?
A. Administer IM injections instead of PO to avoid damage to mucous membranes.
B. Administer all medications PO to avoid hemorrhage at injection sites.
C. Encourage all visitors to wear masks and gowns to protect client from infection.
D. Monitor diet and encourage bulk fiber to promote regular bowel movements.

513. A 21-year-old male is admitted with suspected appendicitis. He is scheduled the next morning for an exploratory laparotomy. On his preoperative orders, the nurse notes an order for a Fleet Enema ×1 in the A.M. Which of the following would be an appropriate action for the nurse?
A. Administer the Fleets the night before surgery to allow more time for the enema to work.
B. Call the doctor and verify the order.
C. Administer the Fleets in the A.M. as ordered.
D. Ask the client if he has had a bowel movement today and hold the enema if he has.

514. A 30-year-old female was admitted 8 days ago for multiple fractures following a car accident. She has one-half normal saline (NS) at 50 ml per hour and is receiving narcotic analgesics every 4 hours for pain. She is on strict bedrest. She suddenly begins to complain of sharp pain radiating around the side of her back. The nurse is alarmed that the client may be developing which of the following complications?
A. Muscle contractures
B. Fat embolism

C. Hypovolemic shock
D. Renal calculi

515. A 70-year-old male is admitted with intermittent claudication of the calves on exertions, ischemic pain in the feet, leg pallor, and coolness with poor palpable pulses to the dorsalis pedis. The nurse would suspect an occlusive disease of which of the following arteries is creating the client's signs and symptoms?
A. Iliac artery
B. Aortic bifurcation
C. Mesenteric artery
D. Femoral and popliteal arteries

516. A 62-year-old male is admitted with intermittent claudication of his calves on exertion. He is scheduled for a femoral-popliteal bypass in 2 days. Which of the following would indicate to the nurse that this client's condition has deteriorated?
A. Peripheral pulses are +2 radial, +1 pedal
B. Urine output of 30 mL/h and falling
C. Lower extremities cool to the touch and blanching of bilateral feet upon elevation
D. Cramping of calf muscles and pain to lower extremities

517. A 46-year-old male is admitted with moderate second-degree burns on his body. The nurse would define second-degree burns as which of the following?
A. Damage is limited to the epidermis, causing erythema and pain.
B. Epidermis and part of the dermis are damaged, with blisters noted and mild edema.
C. Epidermis and dermis are damaged with blisters appearing, and thrombosed vessels are visible.
D. Damage extends through the subcutaneous tissue to the muscle and bone.

518. A 36-year-old male firefighter was admitted 2 days ago to the unit with minor third-degree burns to his arms and second-degree burns to his face and chest. Which of the following complications would the nurse monitor for in this client?
A. Impaired gas exchange
B. Anxiety
C. Fluid volume overload
D. Alteration in nutrition

519. A 42-year-old female is admitted to the unit with irritability, laryngospasms, convulsions, and painful muscle spasms. She has a history of hypoparathyroidism as a result of a congenital malfunction. Which of the following imbalances would the nurse expect to see in this client's laboratory work?
A. Hypercalcemia
B. Hypocalcemia
C. Hyperglycemia
D. Hypoglycemia

520. A 49-year-old male was admitted with signs and

symptoms of pulmonary embolus 1 week ago. He is to be started on Coumadin for long-term anticoagulation therapy. Which of the following would be appropriate for the nurse to teach the client about his home care?

A. "Monitor your skin for excess bruising."
B. "Limit your fluid intake to 1500 cc per day."
C. "You must get periodic PTT levels."
D. "You may get occasional nosebleeds; that's OK."

521. A 42-year-old female is admitted to the unit 3 days after craniotomy for the removal of a brain tumor. The nurse knows that which of the following causes brain tumors?

A. Excessive radiation exposure
B. Inappropriate diet
C. Drug abuse
D. Cause is unknown

522. A 30-year-old male is admitted following a motor vehicle accident. He has severe cerebral contusion with multiple scalp wounds. He is drowsy, confused, and his pupillary response is equal and brisk. Which of the following is essential to observe for in nursing this client?

A. Perform neurological checks every shift.
B. Observe input and output every shift.
C. Monitor vital signs every 8 hours.
D. Monitor for a halo sign.

523. A 40-year-old female presents to the emergency room with chest pain, nonradiating after eating fried chicken. She complains of belching, flatulence, indigestion, diaphoresis, and nausea. She is moderately overweight. Her EKG, vital signs, and blood work are normal. She is scheduled for surgery in the morning and has been transferred to your unit. The nurse understands these signs and symptoms represent which disorder?

A. MI
B. Cholecystitis
C. Pneumonia, bacterial
D. Duodenal ulcer

524. A 52-year-old female is admitted with chronic obstructive pulmonary disease (COPD). She has a history of repeat admissions for frequent respiratory infections, shortness of breath, and activity intolerance. The nurse understands which of the following is the leading cause of COPD?

A. Anemia
B. Recurrent infections
C. Smoking
D. Obesity

525. A 58-year-old male is admitted to the unit with a bladder obstruction. The Foley was very difficult to place and caused great discomfort to the client. His urine is blood tinged in the gravity bag. The nurse understands that the most frequent cause of bladder obstruction in a middle-aged male is which of the following?

A. Renal calculi
B. Prostatic hypertrophy
C. Bladder tumors
D. Urethral strictures

526. A 72-year-old male is admitted with hematuria and bladder pain after voiding. He complains of urinary frequency and nocturia. A cystoscope confirms a diagnosis of bladder cancer. He is scheduled for a cystectomy and urinary stoma placement in the morning. Which of the following actions taken by the nurse can help this client prepare for the changes this surgery can bring?

A. Encourage the client to discuss his feelings.
B. Allow the client to see and operate several stoma products.
C. Leave the client alone to have quiet time with family.
D. Allow the client to select a stoma site appropriate to his needs.

527. A 32-year-old female is admitted for allogenic bone marrow donation. Which of the following would the nurse teach the client following the procedure?

A. "Because your white blood cell count will be depleted, protect yourself from infections."
B. "Bleeding from your donor sites is normal for a few weeks postop."
C. "You will probably have pain for a few days from your donor sites."
D. "You will need to remain on bedrest for at least 1 week following the procedure."

528. A 26-year-old female is admitted with diverticulitis. She is scheduled for a bowel resection in the morning. The nurse needs to educate the client about which of the following anticipated postoperative care measures?

A. The client will awaken with a nasogastric tube to drain air and fluid from the intestinal tract.
B. The client will be on strict bedrest for 1 week until peristalsis returns.
C. The client will receive frequent enemas to remove fecal contents.
D. The client will wake up and be able to go home that afternoon.

529. A 36-year-old male returns to the unit following a bowel resection with anastomasis. Which of the following nursing measures should be performed in caring for this client?

A. Weigh every other day.
B. Change dressing to incision every day.
C. Take daily abdominal circumferences.
D. Administer tube feedings.

530. A 42-year-old female is admitted with weakness, dizziness, and fatigue. She has a history of a recent colostomy placement 4 months ago after the diagnosis of colon cancer. She is depressed and anxious. Which of the following complications related

to ostomy placement would the nurse suspect with this client?
- A. Hyperglycemia
- B. Depression
- C. Dehydration
- D. Cholecystitis

531. A 32-year-old female presents to her physician with complaints of persistent, extreme fatigue that does not resolve with bedrest. She is admitted for evaluation. All her blood work is normal, including her antinuclear antibody test. Her fatigue has been present for 6 months with low-grade temperatures, sore throats, myalgia, arthralgia without joint swelling, photophobia, and difficulty concentrating. The nurse realizes the client may be exhibiting signs of which disorder?
- A. Systemic lupus erythematosus (SLE)
- B. Anemia
- C. Hypothyroidism
- D. Chronic fatigue syndrome

532. A 42-year-old male is admitted with hepatic encephalopathy. The client undergoes continuing mental changes. He has a tremor that has progressed to asterixis. He has also begun to demonstrate signs of apraxia. The nurse identifies this client in which of the following phases of hepatic encephalopathy?
- A. Prodromal stage
- B. Impending stage
- C. Stuporous stage
- D. Comatose stage

533. A 50-year-old male is admitted with cirrhosis of the liver. He suffers from portal hypertension and hypoproteinemia. The nurse recognizes that the combination of these two symptoms increases the client's chances of developing which of the following conditions?
- A. Ascites
- B. Hypoglycemia
- C. Esophageal varices
- D. Hypovolemic shock

534. A 64-year-old male is admitted with cirrhosis of the liver. He has a history of chronic alcoholism and is extremely malnourished. The nurse realizes that alcohol-induced cirrhosis accounts for which amount of the cirrhosis cases in the United States?
- A. All the cases
- B. Less than half of the cases
- C. More than half of the cases
- D. About a third of the cases

535. A 56-year-old male with chronic cirrhosis of the liver has now developed the complication of portal hypertension. The nurse understands that which of the following cause portal hypertension in cirrhosis clients?
- A. Hyponatremia and hypoproteinemia
- B. Ecchymosis, edema, and jaundice
- C. Fibrotic tissue, from cell destruction
- D. Esophageal varices and hypoproteinemia

536. A 64-year-old male is admitted with cirrhosis of the liver. He has a history of chronic alcoholism and is extremely malnourished. The nurse identifies which of the four types of cirrhosis as most likely for this client?
- A. Laennec's
- B. Postnecrotic
- C. Biliary
- D. Cardiac

537. A 68-year-old obese female is admitted with complaints of heartburn 1 to 4 hours after meals, gastric reflux, substernal chest pain, and dysphagia for the past 6 months. She has no history of cardiac problems. Her EKG and laboratory work are normal. Which of the following would the nurse suspect the client is suffering from?
- A. Gastritis
- B. Esophageal varices
- C. Hirschsprung's disease
- D. Hiatal hernia

538. A 28-year-old male with no history of illness is admitted with sudden onset of severe lower abdominal pain and bilious vomiting. There is a history of bloody stools for 1 week. Abdominal inspection reveals distention and a palpable mass. There are no bowel sounds. His WBCs are 18,000/mm^3. The barium enema reveals a sigmoid "ace of spades" configuration. Which of the following would the nurse suspect with this client?
- A. Appendicitis
- B. Diverticulitis
- C. Volvulus
- D. Dumping syndrome

539. A 72-year-old male is admitted with severe abdominal pain and malnutrition. He is diagnosed with a epigastric ulcer. On his second day of hospitalization, he develops sudden, acute abdominal pain and his abdomen becomes rigid. He has no bowel sounds. Which of the following complications would the nurse suspect?
- A. Hemorrhage
- B. Perforation
- C. Gastritis
- D. None—these are classic ulcer symptoms.

540. A 40-year-old female client complains of gastric pain after eating meals. She is diagnosed with a hiatal hernia. The nurse would instruct this client to do which of the following?
- A. Eat large meals.
- B. Lie down and rest after meals.
- C. Eat small, frequent, spicy meals.
- D. Avoid alcohol and constrictive clothing.

541. A 68-year-old male is admitted with severe epigastric pain radiating to the back with nausea, vomiting, and weight loss. He has a history of chronic al-

cohol abuse. He is diagnosed with pancreatitis. The nurse would monitor this client's vital signs carefully for decreasing blood pressure and tachycardia. What is the nurse monitoring the client for?
A. Shock
B. Pancreatic abscess
C. Alcohol withdrawal
D. Pneumonia

542. A 43-year-old female has returned to the unit from a cholecystectomy and exploratory laparotomy. Twelve hours after surgery, she complains of severe abdominal pain, distention, and vomiting and appears in extreme distress. The client appears drowsy, is thirsty and aching, and has difficulty speaking. Bowel sounds are extremely hyperactive and can be heard without a stethoscope. Which of the following surgical complications may this client be developing?
A. Gastritis
B. Infection
C. Hypovolemia
D. Intestinal obstruction

543. A 63-year-old male is admitted after a right-sided cerebral vascular accident. He has inappropriate repetition of a vulgar set of words. The nurse is aware the client is demonstrating which of the following?
A. Scanning speech
B. Apraxia
C. Perseveration
D. Dementia

544. A 26-year-old female is admitted in status epilepticus. The nurse anticipates the physician will order which of the following as the drug of choice for this condition?
A. Thiamine
B. 50% dextrose
C. Diazepam
D. Digoxin

545. A 72-year-old female is admitted with multiple fractures suffered from a fall at home. While in the hospital, she is also diagnosed with Alzheimer's disease. The nurse understands that clients with early Alzheimer's disease can present with which of the following problems?
A. Forgetful of the past
B. Difficulty with activities of daily living
C. Loss of ability to speak and write
D. Forgetfulness of everyday objects

546. A 30-year-old female is admitted with a history of epilepsy. She is having recurring episodes of glossy stares, picking at her hospital gown, aimless wandering, lip smacking, and unintelligible speech. These seizures last for a few seconds to 20 minutes. Mental confusion seems to follow the episodes and the client has no memory of her activities. The nurse is aware that the client is exhibiting signs of which type of seizure?
A. Tonic-clonic
B. Akinetic
C. Simple partial
D. Complex partial

547. A 30-year-old female has just been diagnosed with epilepsy following a severe blow to the head. Which of the following would the nurse instruct the client to do to avoid seizure activity?
A. Exercise 7 days a week for 1 hour.
B. Eat foods high in fiber and protein.
C. Control stress and encourage loud music.
D. Avoid video games and flashing lights.

548. A 40-year-old male has returned to the unit from a craniotomy. The nurse is checking his intracranial pressure (ICP) every hour. The client's ICP reading has started to climb to a level of 10 mm Hg. He is also coughing a great deal. Which of the following signs of elevated ICP would be expected by the nurse?
A. Pupillary dilation to 7 cm
B. Increasing mental alertness
C. None, this ICP is WNL.
D. Nausea and vomiting

549. A 76-year-old male is admitted for pneumonia. He is stable, and during your initial assessment you note a large, bulging inguinal hernia. The physician confirms the finding and diagnoses the hernia as reducible. Which of the following options could the nurse recommend for relief of the hernia until the surgery is possible?
A. Bedrest
B. A truss
C. Proxyphene napsylate and acetaminophen (Darvocet = N 100) PO
D. No relief is needed.

550. A 32-year-old male is admitted after a motor vehicle accident. He is diagnosed with an inguinal hernia, but opts not to have surgery. The client is instructed by the nurse to watch for signs of incarceration or strangulation of the hernia. Which of the following should the nurse tell the client to watch for?
A. Headache, nosebleeds, and blurred vision
B. Nausea, vomiting, and shortness of breath
C. Muscle tremors, weakness, and fatigue
D. High fever, bloody stools, and severe pain

551. A 42-year-old female is being considered for an autologous bone marrow transplant. The nurse is aware that the client must meet a certain criterion to be considered for this procedure. Which of the following must the client have in order to be considered for this procedure?
A. A histocompatible donor
B. An identical twin
C. Aplastic anemia
D. Ability to endure prolonged myelosuppresion

552. A 36-year-old female is admitted following a splenectomy for chronic idiopathic thrombocytopenic purpura. Which of the following instructions for home care would the nurse give this client?
A. Avoid stress.
B. Avoid caffeine.
C. Avoid acetaminophen.
D. Avoid exercise.

553. A 32-year-old male is admitted with chest pain secondary to pneumonia. He has a triple-lumen catheter to his right subclavian. During a routine flush to the distal part, the nurse notices the flush is difficult to push. Which of the following would be an appropriate action for the nurse?
A. Call for a chest x-ray to check placement.
B. Call the doctor.
C. Stop the push, label the part "Do Not Use."
D. Push the flush through despite resistance.

554. A 62-year-old female diabetic is admitted for a below-the-knee amputation to the right leg. Following the surgery she is doing well. At 7 A.M., the nurse checks her blood sugar and gets a reading of 60. The client is arousable but groggy and received diphenhydramine (Benadryl) 50 mg IM at 6 A.M. At the bedside, her husband states that her blood sugar never goes that low but that diphenhydramine always makes her sleepy. Which of the following nursing interventions would be appropriate for this client?
A. Administer dextrose IVP.
B. Call the doctor.
C. Nothing, the client is groggy from the diphenhydramine.
D. Give orange juice with sugar.

555. After a blow to the head, a 28-year-old male is admitted for observation. He complains of seeing floating spots and recurrent light flashes in his right eye. He is also complaining of a decreased visual field or haziness in the same eye. In developing the client's care plan, the nurse uses the diagnosis of altered sensory perception. Which of the following could also be used in this client's care plan?
A. Altered thought processes
B. Anxiety
C. Impaired mobility
D. Altered self-concept

556. A 30-year-old female presents with severe abdominal pain, dark urine, jaundice, and low-grade fever. She has a history of sickle-cell disease from age 10. The nurse understands the client is experiencing which type of sickle-cell crisis?
A. Aplastic crisis
B. Neoplastic crisis
C. Vaso-occlusive crisis
D. Acute sequestration crisis

557. A 36-year-old male returns to the unit following a hernia repair. He received spinal anesthesia during the procedure. Which of the following would the nurse monitor for 24 hours following the use of spinal anesthesia?
A. Cushing's syndrome
B. Dysphagia
C. Distended bladder
D. Pneumonia

558. A 48-year-old female is admitted for a fever of unknown origin. She is receiving frequent vital signs and laboratory work. During lunch the client falls asleep over her meal. When questioned by the nurse, she complains of feeling tired and not getting enough sleep. Which of the following nursing interventions would benefit this client?
A. Administer prescribed sleep medication.
B. Allow appropriate, undisturbed rest periods.
C. Eliminate caffeine after 3 P.M.
D. Encourage activity to enhance sleep.

559. A 36-year-old male is admitted with a midline abdominal incision following an exploratory laparotomy. In developing a nursing care plan for this client, which of the following would the nurse include that might place the client at risk for delayed wound healing?
A. Age
B. Mobility
C. Anorexia
D. Pain

560. A 40-year-old female has an abdominal incision that exhibits endothelial budding and collagen synthesis. The nurse knows that the client is in which stage of wound healing?
A. Inflammation
B. Maturation
C. Resolution
D. Demarcation

561. A 32-year-old male is admitted with a history of severe alcohol and drug abuse. He has abdominal pain, nausea, vomiting, and chest pain. His blood pressure is 80/50 and he has reduced peripheral pulses. He is confused and combative. Which of the following would indicate to the nurse possible disseminated intravascular coagulation (DIC)?
A. Bleeding from three unrelated sites
B. Excessive nausea, vomiting
C. Bloody sputum and coughing
D. Hematuria in the urine collection bag

562. A 36-year-old male is admitted with *Klebsiella pneumoniae*. He has decreased cardiac output, peripheral vasoconstriction, and inadequate tissue perfusion. His skin is pale with mottled peripheral areas. He is obtunded. Respirations are rapid and shallow, and his urine output is less than 200 ml/hr. Which of the following complications indicates this client's condition?
A. Sepsis

B. Septic shock
C. Acute respiratory distress syndrome (ARDS)
D. Hypotension

563. A 30-year-old client is diagnosed as having sepsis secondary to a massive *Escherichia coli* infection. The nurse closely monitors this client for signs of septic shock. Which of the following describes the difference between septic shock and sepsis?
A. In septic shock there is delayed multiple organ dysfunction not seen in sepsis.
B. In sepsis there are bacterial cultures collected from the blood that are not present in septic shock.
C. In septic shock there is hypotension unresponsive to fluids. This is not seen in sepsis.
D. Sepsis only occurs in the elderly, whereas septic shock can occur in anyone.

564. A 50-year-old male is admitted with a right-sided cerebral vascular accident. In doing the assessment on this client, the nurse uses the Glasgow Coma Scale. Which of the following is the reason the Glasgow Coma Scale is used?
A. Assess intelligence
B. Assess motor ability
C. Assess level of consciousness
D. Assess cranial nerves

565. A 30-year-old male is admitted with a fracture of the C5 vertebra following an accident. The nurse needs to monitor the client closely for autonomic dysreflexia. Which of the following can stimulate autonomic dysreflexia in this client?
A. Hypertension
B. Muscle wasting
C. Diaphoresis
D. Distended bladder

566. A 23-year-old paraplegic is on the unit for rehabilitation following a car accident. The client suddenly becomes diaphoretic and hypertensive and has erythema above the level of the spinal injury. Below the level of injury, his extremities are cool and the skin looks pale. Which of the following is the drug of choice for this medical emergency?
A. Furosemide (Lasix)
B. Nitroglycerin
C. Hydralazine (Apresoline)
D. Digoxin

567. A 28-year-old male is admitted with hypoxemia following a drug overdose. The nurse understands which of the following causes of hypoxemia is responsible for this client's episode?
A. Mismatched ventilation-perfusion ratio
B. Alveolar hypoventilation
C. Pulmonary shunting
D. Low oxygen tension of inspired air

568. A 28-year-old female is admitted with chronic iron deficiency anemia. The nurse knows that which of the following sources of blood loss may lead to this condition?
A. Menstrual flow and chronic gastrointestinal bleeding
B. Polycythemia and chronic gastrointestinal bleeding
C. Massive trauma and surgical repair
D. Dehydration and hematuria

569. A 62-year-old female is admitted with respiratory distress. She is exhibiting deep and fast respirations, which then turn more shallow and slower with apneic periods. Which of the following would the nurse choose to define this type of breathing?
A. Kussmaul
B. Tachypnea
C. Cheyne-Stokes
D. Hyperventilation

570. A 23-year-old female is admitted with shingles secondary to a long-term respiratory infection. The nurse places the client on contact isolation. Which of the following agents is responsible for this disorder?
A. Varicella-zoster virus
B. Staphylococcus
C. A β-hemolytic streptococcus
D. *Rickettsia rickettsii*

571. A 30-year-old female is admitted with adrenal hypofunction. The nurse identifies which of the following to distinguish primary from secondary adrenal hypofunction?
A. Muscle weakness
B. GI disturbances
C. Weight loss
D. Hyperpigmentation

572. A 36-year-old female is admitted with Cushing's syndrome. She has a history of thrombocytopenia and has been taking corticosteroids for 7 years. She tells you that she has just recently separated from her husband and has a history of drug and alcohol abuse. The nurse realizes which of the following is the most common cause of Cushing's syndrome?
A. Drug and alcohol abuse
B. Sustained stress
C. Prolonged steroid use
D. Adrenal tumor

573. A 40-year-old male is admitted with diabetes insipidus secondary to a craniotomy for the removal of a tumor. The nurse knows which of the following medications is used in the treatment of diabetes insipidus?
A. Vasopressin
B. Regular insulin
C. Furosemide (Lasix)
D. Prednisone

574. A 56-year-old male is admitted with uncontrolled diabetes mellitus. He is on an every 6 hours blood

sugar check. His noon reading was 186 and he is on a sliding scale. The nurse knows which type of insulin is used with a sliding scale?
A. Humulin Lente
B. Humulin regular
C. Humulin NPH
D. Novolin Lente

575. A 50-year-old female has just returned from a colostomy placement for colon cancer. The nurse needs to teach the client how to care for her colostomy at home. The client frequently refers to her colostomy as "the thing." Which of the following situations would be the best time for the nurse to begin client teaching?
A. The client is crying and refuses to look at her colostomy bag.
B. The client is happy and her family is visiting in the room.
C. The client is angry and asks how she can possibly be expected to deal with "the thing."
D. The client is cooperative and has been medicated for pain.

576. A 48-year-old male has returned to the floor following abdominal surgery. He has a 20-year-old smoking habit of two packs per day. The nurse realizes that the client is at risk for developing which postoperative problem because of his preoperative lifestyle?
A. Skin breakdown
B. Impaired oxygen delivery
C. Delayed wound healing
D. Bleeding and hypovolemia

577. A 58-year-old male presents to the ER with chest pain and shortness of breath. Once admitted to the unit, the nurse assesses the client's heart sounds. The nurse hears an abnormal sound during diastole that sounds like vibration and occurred immediately after the closure of the semilunar valves was heard. Which of the following heart sounds did the nurse hear?
A. S_1
B. S_2
C. S_3
D. S_4

578. A 70-year-old male is admitted with right-sided weakness, rule out cerebrovascular accident (CVA). The nurse needs to assess the client's gag reflex before allowing him liquids or food. Which of the following is the correct technique for evaluating this reflex?
A. Place a tongue blade on the client's uvula.
B. Place the tongue blade in the middle of the tongue and have the client swallow.
C. Place the tongue blade on the anterior aspect of the tongue and have the client cough.
D. Place the tongue blade on the posterior aspect of the tongue.

579. A 62-year-old male is admitted to the unit following a head injury after an automobile accident. The nurse conducts frequent vital sign, neurological, and reflex checks. The nurse assesses the deep-tendon reflex and other reflexes of this client to monitor for which of the following conditions?
A. Muscle and skeletal damage
B. Spinal cord damage
C. Cranial nerve damage
D. Tendon and ligament damage

580. A 30-year-old female has a history of Crohn's disease. She reports to the nurse that she has been taking steroid medication for her condition for several years. How can steroid use affect this client's nutritional status?
A. It can lead to hypoglycemia.
B. It can lead to hyperkalemia.
C. It can lead to hypocalcemia.
D. It can lead to hyponatremia.

581. A 36-year-old female is diagnosed with folic acid deficiency. She is started on folic acid supplementation. The nurse would attribute this deficiency to which of the following medications?
A. Diuretics
B. Antihypertensives
C. Oral contraceptives
D. Monoamine oxidase (MAO) inhibitors

582. A 30-year-old female presents with a history of chronic alcoholism. She is sedated and monitored around the clock for signs and symptoms of withdrawal. The nurse realizes that a client with chronic alcoholism may have which of the following vitamin deficiencies?
A. Antioxidants
B. B complex
C. Vitamin E
D. Calcium

583. A 72-year-old female is admitted following a left hip fracture after a fall. Her status has placed her at high risk for a negative nitrogen balance. Which laboratory test would the nurse monitor to best assess the client's nutritional status?
A. Hemoglobin
B. Total protein
C. Glucose
D. Triglycerides

584. A 38-year-old female is admitted after an exploratory laparotomy. The nurse has orders to infuse 2 units of packed red blood cells (PRBCs) because of severe blood loss during the procedure. The nurse is to give the client home care teaching for iron deficiency anemia. Which of the following instructions would be appropriate for the nurse to give this client?
A. "You can resume all normal activities as soon as you get home."
B. "An adequate amount of iron to treat your con-

dition can be attained through a balanced diet."

C. "Even when you are feeling strong again, you must continue to take you supplements."

D. "It only takes about 6 weeks for your body to replace the lost iron into your system."

585. A 60-year-old male is admitted to the unit with chest pain. The client tells the nurse he is afraid of having a heart attack because he has poor eating habits. The nurse reviews the client's lipid profile. Which lipoprotein would place the client at high risk for coronary artery disease (CAD)?

A. High-density lipoproteins (HDLs)

B. Moderate-density lipoproteins

C. Low-density lipoproteins (LDLs)

D. All lipoproteins are associated with CAD.

586. A 72-year-old male is admitted to the long-term care unit following a feeding tube placement. After the tube has been cleared by the physician for use, the nurse begins to administer the medications through the tube. Which type of medication should the nurse administer through the feeding tube?

A. Enteric-coated tablets

B. Time-release compounds

C. Compressed tablets

D. Sublingual tablets

587. A 22-year-old female is admitted with a diagnosis of anorexia nervosa. She is extremely emaciated and very weak. She keeps her hospital room dimly lighted and complains of difficulty seeing when someone turns the lights up. The nurse recognizes that the client is suffering from night blindness. Which vitamin deficiency leads to night blindness?

A. Vitamin C

B. Vitamin D

C. Vitamin A

D. Vitamin E

588. A frail 72-year-old male with a history of Alzheimer's disease is diagnosed with a stage two ulcer to his sacrum. He is confused and incontinent. He eats less than a quarter of his meals, his hemoglobin is 10, and his hematocrit is 26. The physician has ordered a Clinitron bed and special skin-care products to be used on the client. Which of the following nursing interventions would help prevent further breakdown with this client?

A. Padding the client's body hollows with towels and soft blankets.

B. Assist the client with feedings and encourage calorie-rich snacks.

C. Monitor laboratory values for increasing WBCs and glucose levels.

D. Administer skin-care products as ordered and use adult incontinence briefs to keep bed dry.

589. A client's ECG shows evidence of an acute myocardial infarction. When telling him what to expect over the next few days, the nurse will base explanations on the knowledge that:

A. He will be unable to see his family.

B. He will soon feel much better.

C. He will need to rest to decrease the heart's workload.

D. He will be having frequent x-ray studies done.

590. A 70-year-old male is admitted with anorexia and weight loss. He has had several episodes of dizziness and complains of extreme fatigue. His laboratory values reveal hypokalemia and hypernatremia. Which of the following is a change associated with aging that can increase an elderly person's risk of nutritional problems?

A. Increased peristalsis and decreased enzyme secretion

B. Increased absorption time and increased saliva production

C. Decreased dentition and use of dentures

D. Increased sensitivity to salty and sweet foods

591. A 70-year-old female is admitted with fever of 98.7°F and confusion. Her WBC is elevated, and her urine is cloudy and amber colored. Her heart rate is 80 beats per minute, and her respirations are 22 per minute. The nurse caring for the elderly client is aware that which of the following is the most common source of infection in this age group?

A. Respiratory system

B. Urinary tract

C. Skin

D. Prostate

592. A 55-year-old male is admitted for a colonoscopy to rule out rectal cancer. In caring for this client, the nurse would look for which of following most common signs of rectal cancer?

A. Abdominal cramping, nausea, and diarrhea

B. Ribbonlike stool and abdominal pain

C. Rectal bleeding and tenesmus

D. Rectal bleeding with alternating diarrhea and constipation

593. A 44-year-old male is admitted with severe hemorrhoidal disease. He has rectal pain and bleeding. The nurse would include which of the following treatment measures in the plan of care for this client?

A. High-fiber diet

B. Fluid restrictions

C. Soft diet

D. High-protein diet

594. A 76-year-old female complains of having urinary incontinence when laughing. The nurse realizes that the client is suffering from stress incontinence. Which of the following can cause this disorder?

A. Weakening of the pelvic floor muscles

B. A chronically full bladder

C. Poor perfusion to the kidneys

D. Chronic urinary tract infections

595. A 68-year-old female is diagnosed with urge incontinence. The nurse would include which of the following bladder training interventions in this client's plan of care?
   A. Teach the client Kegel exercises
   B. Scheduled voiding trials
   C. Perform Credé's maneuver
   D. Perform the Valsalva maneuver

596. A 77-year-old female is found on the floor in her hospital room. In assessing the client, which of the following risk factors would the nurse associate with increased chance of falls in elderly clients?
   A. Dehydration
   B. Peptic ulcer disease
   C. Use of nonsteroidal anti-inflammatory drugs (NSAIDs)
   D. Chronic gout

597. A 54-year-old male is diagnosed with chronic gout to the left big toe. In teaching the client how to manage his disease, the nurse would include which of the following in the client's education?
   A. Eat large amounts of organ meats and shellfish.
   B. Work the affected joints as much as possible.
   C. Minimize the amount of alcohol in your diet.
   D. Avoid foods that are high in purines.

598. A 58-year-old male is admitted from ICU with a pneumonectomy of the left lung 3 days ago. The nurse realizes that pneumonectomy clients must be monitored closely for the development of which of the following conditions?
   A. Pleural effusion
   B. Hypoglycemia
   C. Hemothorax
   D. Congestive heart failure

599. A 26-year-old male is admitted for a scheduled surgery to remove a tumor from the pituitary. He complains of severe headaches, loss of visual acuity, and diaphoresis. Your assessment reveals an enlarged supraorbital ridge, thickened ears and nose, laryngeal hypertrophy, and thickening of the tongue. He is also easily irritable and hostile with the staff. The nurse knows that these signs and symptoms are indicative of which disease?
   A. Adrenal hypofunction
   B. Hypopituitary disease
   C. Acromegaly
   D. Hyperthyroidism

FOCUS ON GERONTOLOGICAL NURSING

600. A 79-year-old client with osteoarthritis is scheduled to have an arthroplasty (joint replacement) surgery to the right hip. The client has been active since retirement and is in good health. In the preoperative teaching, the nurse instructs the client that the physician will most likely begin ambulation on the third postoperative day. The rationale for early ambulation following joint replacement is:
   A. Prolonged inactivity in an older adult increases the chance of venous thrombosis.
   B. Prolonged bedrest increases the chance of developing decubitus ulcers.
   C. Late ambulation fosters dependence upon the nursing staff.
   D. Early ambulation ensures the client will return to the baseline functional status.

601. Preoperative instructions to arthroplasty clients include hip precaution measures. The nurse correctly instructs the client:
   A. Do not sit with your hips at a 90-degree or greater angle.
   B. Bend forward using correct body mechanics and use your knees.
   C. Do not bend to put on your shoes; use a long shoe horn.
   D. Do not keep pillows between legs when lying on your back.

602. Following hip replacement surgery (arthroplasty), the client is instructed in ambulating with a walker. The nurse correctly instructs the client to:
   A. Move the walker forward 12 inches and rest two of the four walker legs on the floor before stepping.
   B. Move the walker forward 12 inches and rest all four walker legs on the floor before stepping.
   C. Move the walker 6 inches and rest two of the four walker legs on the floor before stepping.
   D. Move the walker 6 inches and rest all four walker legs on the floor before stepping.

603. The client begins physical therapy for the first time on the third postoperative day. Although she has been resting for 30 minutes after the active physical therapy session, she continues to have elevated vital signs: blood pressure 160/94 and a pulse rate of 94. The most appropriate nursing action at this time is to:
   A. Do nothing and reevaluate her in an hour.
   B. Order a stat electrocardiogram (EKG).
   C. Call the physician.
   D. Call physical therapy and see if an error was made in therapy.

604. A nurse assigned to care for a 2-day postoperative arthroplasty client notices that she is experiencing some confusion regarding orientation to time. Although it is spring the client states, "I've got to go home and start my holiday cooking for Christmas." The nurse recognizes that the most likely cause of this confusion is:
   A. A normal aging change
   B. A reaction to the medications
   C. Early signs of dementia
   D. Separation from familiar surroundings

605. The physician writes an order to change the operative site dressing on a 72-hour postoperative arthroplasty client. The nursing staff correctly identifies that the most important goal in carrying out this physician's order is:
A. The need to prevent pain
B. The need to prevent infection
C. The need to be supportive
D. The need to explain the procedure to the client

606. A postoperative arthroplasty client successfully completes the physical therapy program and is scheduled for discharge. The most important area the nurse should assess before discharge is:
A. The ability to take medications as prescribed
B. The ability to manage activities of daily living
C. Support from family and friends
D. The ability to properly use the ambulatory aid (walker)

607. The arthroplasty client is discharged on a diet for weight control. The menu most reflective of the dietary needs of the older adult would be:
A. Broiled pork chop, green peas, and cantaloupe
B. Baked ham, spinach, and banana
C. Beef liver, carrots, and orange slices
D. Fried chicken, baked potato, and strawberries

608. An older adult has been discharged to a long-term care unit following arthroplasty surgery. The nurse recognizes that the most probable rationale for this discharge decision is:
A. To continue rehabilitation therapy
B. To reduce dependence on the family
C. To assist in maintaining activities of daily living
D. To prevent the client from resuming activity too soon

609. Normal age-related changes in vision could result in:
A. Difficulty in nighttime driving
B. Seeing halos around lights
C. The inability to see color with yellow tint
D. Increased numbers of floaters and tear production

610. An 85-year-old widower who has experienced recent dull eye pain is diagnosed with glaucoma. In planning care for this client, the most important initial nursing action is to:
A. Assess family history for glaucoma.
B. Assess former coping skills in crisis.
C. Assess for environmental safety hazards.
D. Assess the client's fine motor skills.

611. A nurse is planning care for the client with glaucoma. A priority nursing diagnosis identified by the nurse related to this client is:
A. Alteration in nutrition related to inability to prepare food

B. Sensory perceptual alteration related to increased peripheral vision
C. Potential for infection related to eye drop installation
D. Body image alteration related to thick-lensed eyeglasses

612. A 75-year-old client reports to the home health nurse that she has been having trouble sleeping. She reports going to bed at 9 P.M. most evenings, but always awakens at 4 A.M. She asks your advice on what she can do to sleep longer in the morning. The best response by the nurse based on knowledge of the older adult would be:
A. Have a protein-rich snack before going to bed.
B. Obtain a comprehensive physical examination.
C. Have a glass of milk and a sleeping pill at bedtime.
D. Do nothing, because this is not abnormal with age.

613. A general rule of thumb for nurses to remember when administering medications to an older adult is:
A. Drugs are given more frequently in the older adult.
B. Drugs are less effective in the older adult.
C. Most medications do more harm than good.
D. Most medications should be given in lower dosages.

614. A 75-year-old diabetic client is admitted with gangrene to the right leg. The physician discusses the need for an above-the-knee amputation (AKA) of the extremity. The initial approach by the nurse following this discussion is:
A. Spend time with the client and allow him to verbalize feelings.
B. Share with the client other persons who have had amputations.
C. Talk with the client's family about how to be supportive after surgery.
D. Explain the procedure for an above-the-knee amputation and answer questions.

615. One month following surgery, the nurse observes that the AKA wound is completely healed. The most appropriate action by the nurse following this observation is:
A. Discontinue wrapping the stump.
B. Provide a protective cushion to the stump.
C. Discuss the management of phantom pain.
D. Provide strengthening exercises to all limbs.

616. The client is being assessed for an artificial prosthesis to the right leg. In assessing the rehabilitation potential for an older adult, the nurse must:
A. Assess the ability to use unaffected extremities.
B. Assess the ability to follow instructions.
C. Assess the availability of support systems.
D. Assess whether the client will return home.

617. The client is fitted with prosthesis. He relates to the nurse that he is experiencing pain in the right leg, which was removed. The nurse recognizes this as phantom pain. The most appropriate intervention by the nurse is:
  A. Talk with the client about past experiences to get his mind off the pain.
  B. Delay ordering of the artificial limb until the pain subsides or improves.
  C. Call the doctor for pain medication and give it liberally during periods of pain.
  D. Expedite the order for an artificial limb and encourage strengthening exercises.

618. The client becomes short of breath shortly after beginning artificial limb walking. Based on the information, the nurse would modify the care plan to include:
  A. Provide crutches during the day to conserve energy.
  B. Provide a walker during the day to conserve energy.
  C. Encourage walking more frequently for shorter periods.
  D. Discontinue all activity and place on bedrest.

619. A diabetic client is to receive diabetic diet instructions prior to discharge. When working with the client in meal planning, the nurse allows the client to have occasional "forbidden foods" such as ice cream or other sweets. The rationale for this nursing action is:
  A. Knowledge that diabetics rarely follow dietary instructions to the letter
  B. Knowledge that rigid control of diet is less likely to promote compliance
  C. Knowledge that the new insulin therapy more easily maintains blood glucose levels
  D. Knowledge that clinicians occasionally need to assess clients' risk for hyperglycemia

620. An 87-year-old client attends a community health center during the week and receives a health screening monthly. Although he can walk with a three-prong cane, he often uses a wheelchair, especially when he is in a new environment. He is receiving a monthly screening by a nurse who is new to the center. The client relates to the nurse during the health screen that he has recently been troubled with impotence. The most appropriate nursing action at this time is:
  A. Listen and respond empathetically.
  B. Do nothing because this is normal.
  C. Do a complete health history including medications.
  D. Refer him to á physician.

621. A client complains of abdominal cramping shortly before lunch. The nurse questions the client to obtain data related to the abdominal pain and then palpates the abdomen for constipation. The action by the nurse was:

  A. Appropriate because constipation is a common problem for older adults
  B. Inappropriate because palpation in the gastrointestinal assessment is performed following percussion
  C. Inappropriate because the client did not complain of constipation
  D. Appropriate because abdominal pain is the first symptom of constipation

622. The nurse refers the client to his family physician because she fears he has an intestinal obstruction. The nurse bases this decision upon the following assessment data:
  A. Abdominal cramps and high-pitched bowel sounds
  B. Diffuse pain with low-grade temperature
  C. Absence of bowel sounds with hyperactivity
  D. Nausea with marked abdominal tenderness

623. The client is admitted to the hospital with a diagnosis of intestinal obstruction, and initial laboratory tests and x-rays are ordered. The night nurse notices that the client has been incontinent during the night. The most likely reason for the incontinence is:
  A. Frequency due to normal aging changes
  B. The inability to get to the bathroom in time
  C. Stress related to all the medical treatments
  D. Pressure from the intestinal obstruction

624. The nursing action most appropriate in assisting an incontinent client to remain dry during the night would be to:
  A. Use an absorbent garment such as an adult diaper.
  B. Provide a bedside commode and leave the night light on.
  C. Talk with the client to determine any life stressors.
  D. Insert a Foley catheter and maintain intake and output.

625. The client has surgery to relieve an intestinal obstruction. He returns to the unit with the following physician orders: meperidine (Demerol) 50 mg q 4 hrs PRN pain, diphenhydramine (Benadryl) 25 mg PO q HS PRN sleep, and gentamicin (Garamycin) 75 mg every 8 hours. The nurse notes that the client has a creatinine clearance value of 70 ml/min. The most appropriate action by the nurse would be:
  A. Give the medicines as scheduled.
  B. Do nothing because the values are within the normal limits.
  C. Hold the gentamicin and inform the doctor of creatinine results.
  D. Call the laboratory to see of this is in error.

626. The nurse recognizes that monitoring the creatinine clearance level is important because it is a diagnostic indicator of:

A. Respiratory function
B. Cardiovascular function
C. Renal function
D. Gastrointestinal function

627. A 68-year-old female is placed in the nursing home for rehabilitation following a cerebrovascular accident (CVA). She is to receive physical therapy to strengthen her left extremities. The client is receiving the following prescribed medications: carbamazepine (Tegretol) 300 mg twice daily and aspirin 325 mg once daily. The client has been in the nursing home for 3 weeks. She seems to be having more difficulty hearing a conversation and conversations must be repeated several times before she can hear them. The admission nursing history indicates the client was able to hear a watch ticking. The initial nursing action by the nurse would be to:
A. Talk louder so that she can hear you.
B. Inspect the ear canals for blockage.
C. Sit facing her so she can lip-read.
D. Call the physician and get an audiology exam.

628. The client is scheduled to receive carbamazepine (Tegretol) at 9 A.M. In checking the laboratory reports, the nurse notes that the client has a Tegretol level of 8 μg/ml. The action by the nurse is:
A. Administer the Tegretol as prescribed.
B. Call the physician before giving medications.
C. Give a reduced dose of Tegretol.
D. Withhold the Tegretol until the level returns to 3 μg/ml.

629. In planning nursing care for the client who has experienced a cerebrovascular accident, the nurse must keep in mind that clients with left hemisphere infarctions may have:
A. Dramatic mood swing
B. Impaired judgment
C. Labile affect
D. Aggressive potential

630. The nurse correctly identifies that the most important need for the client with left hemisphere infarction is:
A. Maintenance of nutritional status
B. Diversional activities
C. Prevention of injury
D. Psychological counseling

631. A nurse is planning care for a client with left hemisphere infarction. Which plan noted by the nurse best demonstrates her knowledge of caring for cerebrovascular accident clients?
A. Allow client to make decisions about his care.
B. Provide a clock and calendar to maintain orientation.
C. Encourage involvement and attendance at unit functions.
D. Provide a structured, consistent environment.

632. A cerebrovascular client becomes very apathetic and frequently refuses to attend scheduled therapies. The most important action by the nurse at this time is:
A. Perform a mental status for depression.
B. Do nothing because this behavior is normal.
C. Ask her family to make her attend therapy.
D. Call the physician and request his assistance.

633. The client is discharged following a CVA, but will continue with physical and speech therapy daily. Which statement by the family best demonstrates a supportive environment?
A. "I just don't know if we can manage Mother at home."
B. "We have widened the bathroom door for the wheelchair."
C. "We have a sitter who will be staying with Mother at night."
D. "Mother will be back to her old self once we get her home."

634. A 71-year-old client is admitted to the hospital following a fall from a ladder. Admission vital signs were BP 170/98, pulse 92, and respirations 22. In performing A.M. care for the client, the nurse notes a brown pigmentation around both ankles. The nurse correctly identifies this to be:
A. Suggestive of earlier abuse
B. Suggestive of skin change in aging
C. Suggestive of lymphatic disease
D. Suggestive of venous insufficiency

635. The client becomes extremely anxious when the physician tells him he wants to perform additional tests. The most appropriate action by the nurse at this time is:
A. Leave the room until his anxiety decreases.
B. Encourage him to verbalize his feelings.
C. Tell him there is nothing to worry about.
D. Inform the client that the doctor knows best.

636. A client is diagnosed with right-sided congestive heart failure and is placed on furosemide (Lasix) and digoxin. The symptom most reflective of right-sided congestive heart failure is:
A. Tachypnea
B. Pink frothy sputum
C. Korotkoff's sounds
D. Distended jugular veins

637. Which complaint by a client would alert the nurse to digoxin toxicity?
A. "I have to hold on to the wall to keep from falling."
B. "My ears are ringing."
C. "I can't see clearly and the lights have halos."
D. "I am itching all over."

638. Laboratory values reported this morning for the client include: serum digoxin level is 2.9 mg/ml and potassium 3.2 mEq/L. The most appropriate nursing action, based upon these laboratory values, by the nurse at this time is:

A. Give an additional dose of digoxin.
B. Do nothing because the digoxin level is within normal limits.
C. Give one-half the usual dose of digoxin.
D. Call the physician and inform him or her of the laboratory values.

639. In addition to potassium supplements, the nurse would encourage the client to choose which of the following menu items to increase potassium intake?
A. Boiled chicken, baked potato, and dried figs
B. Beef tips, rice, and banana
C. Roast beef, carrots, and fresh peach
D. Fried chicken, broccoli, and fresh pear

640. The nursing diagnosis identified for the client is hypokalemia. Early symptoms indicating hypokalemia include:
A. Muscle weakness and weak irregular pulse
B. Diminished deep tendon reflexes
C. Positive Trousseau's sign
D. Positive Chvostek's sign

641. The client's potassium level drops to 2.7 mEq/L. The physician orders potassium bicarbonate 80 mEq in 1000 ml of D5W intravenous over 8 hours. The most important nursing action related to intravenous potassium administration includes:
A. Monitor respiratory rate
B. Monitor urinary output
C. Monitor oral potassium intake
D. Monitor the intravenous site for edema

642. A client's medications upon discharge are potassium chloride (K-Dur) 20 mEq once daily and bumetaniade (Bumex) 1.0 mg once daily. The nurse prepares to teach the client about his medications and has prepared several handouts that describe the things he will need to know about each drug. Before beginning discharge teaching, the nurse needs to be aware of:
A. The client's attitude toward illness
B. The client's educational level
C. The client's past compliance to medications
D. The client's usual activities of daily living

643. The nurse recognizes the need to evaluate the client's understanding of his medications. Which response by the client best demonstrates to the nurse that the client has adequate knowledge?
A. "I will take K-Dur with my meals?"
B. "I will call the doctor immediately if I get a headache."
C. "I will have my cholesterol level checked every 3 months."
D. "I will take Bumex shortly before bedtime."

644. The client is scheduled for an appointment with the physician for a check-up. Which complaint by the client is most likely to be associated with an adverse reaction to potassium chloride (K-Dur)?
A. "I have had a headache for the past 2 days."
B. "I have trouble remembering things lately."

C. "I noticed my stools were dark and tarry this morning."
D. "I have trouble seeing things up close lately."

645. An 83-year-old female is admitted to the hospital to evaluate the cause of increasing memory loss, irritability, and decreasing interest in the family. Her son reports these symptoms have been present for about 2 years, but are slowly getting worse. He indicates to the nurse that he thinks this is just normal aging. The nurse correctly identifies that normal aging changes of the brain tissue of older adults include:
A. Increased concentration of acetylcholine
B. Increased gray and white matter
C. Increased lipofuscin deposits and neurofibrillary tangles
D. Increased monamine oxidase and transaminase

646. The client experiencing memory loss has lost weight. The most appropriate plan to encourage the Alzheimer's client to eat is:
A. Eliminate distractions from the environment.
B. Place him in the dining room for all meals.
C. Offer a variety of nourishing foods and allow him to select.
D. Serve hot foods to stimulate appetite.

647. The nursing assistant asks the nurse how to get the client to assist with her own personal hygiene. The nurse correctly informs the nursing assistant to:
A. Follow the procedure book when bathing.
B. Give her short, specific instructions for what to do next.
C. Provide written, step-by-step directions.
D. Explain ahead of time what you expect her to do.

648. The nursing assistant reports that the client has been incontinent twice during the shift. To assist the client to remain continent the nurse would:
A. Limit fluid intake to within 1000 ml daily.
B. Insert an indwelling catheter.
C. Set up a regular toileting schedule.
D. Label the bathroom door in large letters.

649. The most appropriate nursing action to ensure that a cognitively impaired client receives adequate nutrition is:
A. Weigh the client weekly and maintain a log.
B. Assign a staff member to feed her.
C. Offer high protein liquids between meals.
D. Provide several menus and allow the client to select.

650. The client is confused during the day, but this becomes much worse at night and often she calls "Mama" in a very loud voice. The most appropriate nursing action is:
A. Restrain her at night.
B. Close the door tightly to keep her from awakening the other clients.

C. Have the physician order a stronger sleeping medication.

D. Leave the lights on in the room.

651. The increasing irritability and anxiety experienced by dementia clients during the early evening hours is referred to as:
A. Agnosia
B. Apraxia
C. Sundowner's syndrome
D. Phase three dementia

652. The nurse talks with the son of a client with Alzheimer's disease about activities he might engage his mother in when they leave the hospital. Which response best demonstrates the family's understanding of Alzheimer's disease?
A. "We have a big yard and she can help us when we rake the leaves."
B. "She can prepare breakfast during the week for the children."
C. "She can write notes to all her friends."
D. "She can walk the dogs."

653. A 67-year-old retired engineer is diagnosed with Parkinson's disease. The nurse recognizes that this disease is:
A. Normal in persons over the age of 65 years
B. A neurological disorder
C. A musculoskeletal disorder
D. A reversible condition with medical management

654. The client is placed on carbidopa/levodopa therapy. In doing dietary counseling, the nurse correctly instructs the client to avoid:
A. Caffeine products
B. Foods high in fats
C. Foods high in calories
D. Foods containing vitamin B_6

655. In addition to carbidopa/levodopa, the client with Parkinson's disease also receives digoxin 125 mg daily, haloperidol (Haldol) 20 mg HS, and temazepam (Restoril) 25 mg HS. The client begins to experience involuntary rhythmic movements of his tongue, face, and extremities. The nurse correctly identifies that these behaviors are the result of:
A. Carbidopa/levodopa
B. Digoxin
C. Restoril
D. Haloperidol

656. A nursing diagnosis related to alteration in nutrition is developed for a client with Parkinson's disease. The plan of care most appropriate to assist the client with nutrition is:
A. Encourage liquids when chewing.
B. Allow the client to feed himself.
C. Place in an upright position for meals.
D. Ask the family to bring his favorite foods from home.

657. The client with Parkinson's disease is followed by home health nurses. The nurse finds the family willing to learn caregiving tasks although the wife is the primary caregiver. Which action by the nurse is important in assisting the client to remain at home?
A. Encourage him to perform activities of daily living for himself.
B. Assist him to communicate his needs both verbally and written.
C. Provide for physical and emotional needs of the caregiver.
D. Keep him actively involved in day-to-day household tasks.

658. Which response by the client's caregiver best indicates an understanding of the dietary restrictions for the client receiving levodopa that must be implemented in preparing daily meals?
A. "He should not eat nuts, bran, or whole grain cereal."
B. "He should drink skim rather than whole milk."
C. "He should drink juice rather than tea or coffee."
D. "Meats should be cut in very small pieces before serving."

659. A nurse at the local community health center is talking with a 74-year-old client who complains about a raised, dome-shaped, grayish black lesion located at the hairline. The nurse correctly informs the client to:
A. Not be alarmed because this is noninvasive and benign
B. Call his physician immediately and have it removed.
C. Use an antibiotic ointment until it is healed.
D. Apply a wart removal cream to the area to remove it.

660. A 52-year-old female regularly attends the center for hypertension. She shares with the nurse that she is concerned about osteoporosis. The nurse correctly informs the client that individuals most at risk for osteoporosis are:
A. Males who have taken steroid therapy
B. Obese females of Asian or Hispanic origin
C. Thin, underweight Caucasian males
D. Thin, postmenopausal Caucasian females

661. The physician prescribes estrogen therapy to decrease the amount of bone loss. The nurse correctly advises the client to:
A. Take the estrogen with meals.
B. Have a yearly mammography.
C. Have monthly fasting blood glucose.
D. Monitor blood pressure for hypotension.

662. The nurse instructs the client on the need for calcium for the prevention of osteoporosis. The client states "I drink at least three glasses of milk each day." The nurse correctly advises:

A. That 3 glasses of milk does not supply enough calcium

B. To supplement the milk with vitamin C to ensure absorption

C. That dietary intake of calcium is not utilized by the body

D. To increase daily oral phosphate as well as calcium

663. The nurse further instructs the client on the preventive therapies for osteoporosis. Which statement by the client best demonstrates understanding of osteoporosis prevention?
A. "I will include citrus juice in my breakfast menu."
B. "I will begin walking exercises three to five times weekly."
C. "I will decrease fat in my diet."
D. "I will start swimming as part of my daily exercise regimen."

664. A 65-year-old client is diagnosed with presbycusis. The nurse assesses the client for difficulty in:
A. Hearing high-pitched sounds
B. Ambulating without mechanical aids
C. Seeing objects at a distance
D. Distinguishing sweet and sour taste

665. Which of the following activities would the nurse suggest to assist the client with presbycusis to remain in his home and add to feelings of security?
A. Installation of a special chair to facilitate getting into and out of the bathtub
B. Installation of a special telephone that facilitates hearing consonant sounds
C. Installation of double thickness, double insulation, antiglare windows
D. Installation of antitheft burglar bars and alarms on all windows and doors

666. A 71-year-old client complains of blurred vision and difficulty in being outside on sunny days. The nurse correctly identifies this condition to be:
A. Caused by psychotropic drug therapy
B. An excuse to avoid exercise
C. A symptom of cataracts
D. Caused by diuretic therapy

667. The home health nurse visits an older adult in her home following discharge from the hospital. The client is found to have several bruises under her right breast. When questioned, the client says she doesn't know what caused the bruises. The most appropriate nursing action at this time would be:
A. Assess the family relationship to rule out abuse.
B. Question the family in the client's presence to determine the cause.
C. Review the medical record to provide information related to the bruise.
D. Do nothing because the client is calm and is not concerned.

668. The client's daughter discusses her fear that something is wrong with her mother because she has recently been short of breath on exertion and has begun sweating. She further states, "If she had chest pain during these episodes, I would think she is having a heart attack." The nurse correctly informs her that myocardial infarction in the elderly:
A. May not always be associated with chest pain
B. Seldom occurs in the absence of a history of cardiac disease
C. Is almost always fatal
D. Does not require oxygen therapy

669. The nurse suggests that the client might have an iron deficiency. Which assessment information exhibited by the client does the nurse base this decision on?
A. Paresthesia in the lower extremities
B. Spooning of the nails
C. Gingival hemorrhages
D. Carpopedal spasms

670. The client develops a stage two decubitus ulcer. What documentation, if made by the nurse correctly, reflects the diagnosis of a stage two decubitus ulcer?
A. A lesion appearing as a blister, which appears as a shallow crater
B. A lesion appearing as a large nonblanching erythema
C. A lesion that extends into the deeper subcutaneous tissue
D. A lesion that extends into the subcutaneous tissue with skin loss

671. A 75-year-old reports to a community nursing clinic for his annual flu injection. He appears tired and has a sad affect. He indicates that he is having difficulty sleeping, which results in trouble getting out of bed in the morning, and feeling tired and fatigued. He reports that he feels physically ill. What is the most important initial response of the nurse?
A. Take a complete medical history.
B. Refer him to his family physician.
C. Perform a complete physical examination.
D. Conduct a mental status examination.

672. The client tells the nurse that he has always been an avid golfer, but has stopped golfing with his friends because he feels so tired. The nurse correctly recognizes that this statement is an example of:
A. Anhedonia
B. Agnosia
C. Akathisia
D. Apraxia

673. The client is admitted to a geriatric psychiatric unit and is diagnosed as major unipolar depressive disorder. He is prescribed with trazodone (Desyrel) 25 mg tid and lithium carbonate 300 mg HS. The nurse correctly identifies unipolar depressive disorder being characterized as:

A. Depression with no manic or hypomanic episodes

B. Depression that is followed by mania

C. A first-time experience of depression

D. A left-brain alteration leading to depression

674. The client is scheduled to receive his first dose of lithium carbonate this HS. Which action by the nurse is essential before beginning lithium therapy?

A. Check thyroid function studies (TSH) results.

B. Check serum creatinine, blood urea nitrogen, and urinalysis results.

C. Check serum electrolytes results.

D. Check hemoglobin, hematocrit, and red blood cell count.

675. The client says to the nurse, "I feel so worthless, I'm not worth the air that I breathe." The most appropriate response by the nurse following this statement is:

A. "I understand, but I think you are a very worthy person."

B. "Don't be ridiculous, you were a successful person."

C. "Have you had thoughts of harming yourself."

D. "I don't understand; why do you feel this way?"

676. The client has received trazodone (Desyrel) for 12 days and the nurse notices little to no therapeutic results. The most appropriate action by the nurse at this time is:

A. Do nothing because therapeutic results may not be seen in this period of time.

B. Call the physician and ask him to prescribe another antidepressant medication.

C. Call the physician and ask him to discontinue the medication.

D. Observe the client at medication time to ensure he is not throwing it away.

677. The nurse instructs the client to return to the mental health clinic 1 month following discharge for follow-up examination. The follow-up examination will include having blood drawn for a lithium level. The nurse recognizes that the therapeutic lithium level for an older adult is:

A. 0.05 to 1 mEq/L

B. 0.5 to 1.5 mEq/L

C. 100 to 150 mEq/L

D. 500 to 1500 mEq/L

678. The nurse is assessing the client's forgetfulness to determine reversible and irreversible causes. Irreversible causes may be either Alzheimer's disease (DAT) or acquired immune deficiency syndrome (AIDS) dementia. The distinguishing characteristic between DAT and AIDS dementia is that in DAT:

A. The client experiences aphasia but no definite neurological findings.

B. The client experiences lethargy and a pronounced loss of weight.

C. The client experiences peripheral neuropathies in all extremities.

D. The client experiences leg weakness and tremors in all extremities.

679. A 76-year-old widower comes to the nursing clinic, complaining of headaches that have been occurring for about 2 months and are increasing in severity. The nurse notes his blood pressure is 180/102. He is diagnosed with severe hypertension and is placed on nadolol (Corgard) 40 mg PO daily. Which of the following assessment information is essential before treating hypertension with nadolol?

A. A history of chronic obstructive pulmonary disease

B. A history of hypothyroid illness in the family

C. A history of sinus tachycardia

D. A history of major depressive disorder

680. The nurse is preparing a care plan. A nursing diagnosis identified by the nurse is potential altered sexuality patterns. The rationale for this nursing diagnosis is:

A. The client is a widower and does not have an available sexual partner.

B. Altered sexual patterns are a normal physiological change that occur with age.

C. Altered sexual patterns could be a side effect of antihypertensive medication.

D. The client has a fear of having a heart attack during sexual activity.

681. A nursing diagnosis of potential altered sexuality patterns has been identified for a client taking nadolol (Corgard). The nurse is beginning to implement the plan of care. Based on the information the nurse has, which of the following nursing interventions would be most appropriate?

A. Instruct the client to notify his physician if any sexual problems occur.

B. Instruct the client on the need to use protection during sexual activity.

C. Instruct the client to rise slowly from a sitting or lying position.

D. Instruct the client to take a nitroglycerin tablet before sexual activity.

682. The evening charge nurse for a large nursing home facility reports to the director of nursing that two clients who have recently been admitted are displaying sexual expression and signs of intimacy to each other in public areas. Both clients are recovering from a hip fracture and are receiving physical therapy. What action by the director of nursing service is most important at this time?

A. Make arrangements for one of the clients to be moved to a different section of the nursing home.

B. Call the family members and inform them to talk with their relatives about this recent behavior change.

C. Perform a thorough sexual assessment on both clients including tests for sexually transmitted disease.

D. Call a nursing conference to discuss the feelings, attitudes, and concerns of the staff members.

683. A client complains to the nurse, "I am so embarrassed, my roommate was kissing all over that man last night, there must be something you can do to stop them from acting like that." The most appropriate action by the nurse is to:
A. Inform the client that you will have a talk with her roommate at once.
B. Inform the client that she should close her curtain if she is uncomfortable.
C. Provide the client's roommate with a privacy area to express intimacy.
D. Provide the client a private room so that she will stop complaining.

684. A 75-year-old, right-handed man suffered a cardiovascular accident (CVA) with right-sided hemiparesis and speech impairment 3 weeks ago. He is an adult-onset diabetic of 20 years and he has retinopathy and cataracts. The nurse is performing an assessment to determine the client's progress. The client responds to orientation questions with only his name. All responses to other orientation questions are, "da-da," "choo-choo," and "da-chee." The nurse recognizes these responses are:
A. Verbal paraphasia
B. Jargon
C. Perseverance
D. Literal paraphasia

685. The nurse notes that the client is unable to recite the days of the week and that naming of other objects is possible only with visual stimuli. These findings are indicative of:
A. Preserved automatic speech
B. Difficulty with word find
C. Fluent aphasia
D. Nonfluent aphasia

686. The client, following a cardiovascular accident (CVA), progresses in strength and is scheduled for discharge. During assessment, he answers orientation questions appropriately when he is wearing a hearing aid. The client is now able to name the days of the week and to recite the months of the year, but when shown a picture and asked to name the object, the response is correct only 50 percent of the time. The nurse correctly identifies that the client may be experiencing:
A. An organic brain syndrome
B. Impaired hearing acuity
C. Impaired verbal aphasia
D. Impaired visual acuity

687. The nurse is caring for an 80-year-old client who is

aphasic. The most common cause of aphasia in older adults is:
A. Malignant brain tumors
B. Cardiovascular accident (CVA)
C. Head trauma
D. Major depressive disorder

688. The nurse is caring for a client who has recently had a cardiovascular accident and has right-sided hemiparesis. The client has aphasia. The nurse recognizes that the most likely type of aphasia with right-sided hemiparesis is:
A. Broca's aphasia
B. Wernicke's aphasia
C. Conduction aphasia
D. Anomic aphasia

689. A 67-year-old female reports to the nurse that she is experiencing stress incontinence. The nurse recognizes that the most common cause of stress incontinence in females is the result of:
A. Stress brought on by menopause
B. Pelvic floor relaxation
C. Urinary tract infections
D. Normal aging changes

690. A client complains of difficulty voiding. The nurse correctly identifies that voiding is normally controlled by:
A. The central nervous system
B. The spinal cord
C. Sphincter pupillae
D. Detrusor muscle

691. The client reports feeling embarrassed by dampness due to stress incontinence. She reports that she wears a pad for protection, but always fears that others are aware of a smell. The client asks the nurse for information about treatment of stress incontinence. The nurse correctly informs the client that treatment for stress incontinence is:
A. Behavior modification and psychological counseling
B. Frequent change of pads and bathing twice a day
C. Elective and depends upon the severity of symptoms
D. A complex surgical procedure to restore bladder support

692. The client is placed on propantheline (Pro-Banthine) 15 mg tid. Before administration of this medication the nurse should assess:
A. Whether the client has urinary retention
B. Whether the client has diabetes mellitus
C. Whether the client has a urinary tract infection
D. Whether the client is currently on antibiotics

693. The nurse is providing instruction to the client regarding the side effects of propantheline (Pro-Banthine). Which problem should the client be instructed to report immediately to the physician?
A. Nasal draining with enlarged lymph nodes

B. Blurred vision with dilated pupils

C. Dizziness when rising from a sitting position

D. Inability to focus on near objects

694. Which statement made by the client would indicate to the nurse that the client has adequate knowledge of the cautions to be taken while on propantheline (Pro-Banthine)?
    A. "Even though I don't like green vegetables, I'll eat them."
    B. "I know I should not work in my garden on very hot days."
    C. "I know I should walk briskly for 30 minutes each day."
    D. "I know I should avoid caffeine, wine, and aged cheese."

695. A nurse is talking with a client who is being referred for a cystmetrogram (CMG). The nurse instructs the client that the purpose of this procedure is to assess:
    A. The ability of the bladder to empty effectively
    B. The ability of the urethral sphincters to contract
    C. The ability of the bladder to fill and store urine
    D. The ability of the renal system to filter waste

696. A 72-year-old client is diagnosed with functional incontinence. This disorder would most likely be a result of:
    A. A cognitive deficit
    B. A peripheral field deficit
    C. A cardiovascular accident (CVA)
    D. A trauma to the brain

697. During a home health visit, the nurse notes a large damp spot on the clothing of a 73-year-old client. She suspects the client may be experiencing incontinence. The client has never discussed this as a problem, but on questioning by the nurse indicates that these episodes have been occurring for 5 or 6 months. The nurse recognizes that the reason the client has not discussed the problem of incontinence is:
    A. The client is experiencing a mild cognitive impairment.
    B. The client feels discomfort and distress because of incontinence.
    C. The client feels this is a normal consequence of aging.
    D. The client fears placement in a long-term care facility.

698. The spouse of a 75-year-old client asks the nurse if biofeedback would be effective in treating functional incontinence. The most appropriate response by the nurse is:
    A. Biofeedback is most effective in incontinence brought about by structural causes.
    B. Biofeedback is most effective in incontinence brought about by physical causes.
    C. Biofeedback is most effective in incontinence brought about by major depression.
    D. Biofeedback is most effective in incontinence brought about by cognitive impairment.

699. The home health nurse is evaluating the progress of a client receiving continuous ambulatory peritoneal dialysis (CAPD). The client reports that following his last two treatments he has episodes of nausea, muscle weakness, and listlessness. The nurse recognizes that these symptoms indicate:
    A. Beginning congestive heart failure
    B. The CAPD is not effective in toxin removal
    C. Potassium depletion due to the dialysis
    D. Hypotension brought on by dialysis

700. The home health nurse is providing dietary teaching to a client with continuous ambulatory peritoneal dialysis (CAPD). The nurse instructs the client to:
    A. Limit potassium-rich foods such as fruits and vegetables.
    B. Limit sodium-rich foods such as kale and collard greens.
    C. Limit phosphorus-rich foods such as nuts and legumes.
    D. Limit protein-rich foods such as beef and chicken.

701. An 80-year-old female comes to the clinic with vague complaints of recent stomach discomfort, gas, and feelings of fullness. Following further assessment, the nurse immediately refers the client to a physician. The rationale for the nurse's action is:
    A. The nurse suspects the client has a fecal impaction.
    B. The nurse suspects the client has ovarian cancer.
    C. The nurse suspects the client is attention seeking.
    D. The nurse suspects the client has major depression.

702. A 70-year-old client reports to the nurse, "The American Cancer Society recommends that women undergo regular cervical smears between the ages of 20 and 65." The nurse correctly explains this recommendation to mean:
    A. Women over age 65 have very little chance for developing cervical cancer.
    B. Women over age 65 have less than 1 in 100 chance for cervical cancer.
    C. Cervical smears are based upon history and are at the discretion of the physician.
    D. Cervical smears will not detect cervical cancer in older women due to aging change.

703. A nursing home client is being seen by the nurse for vague complaints of constipation. The client relates numerous bouts of constipation and states, "I just don't seem to feel the urge to have a bowel move-

ment anymore." Based on this verbal statement by the client, the nurse would investigate further to identify the possible cause of constipation as:
A. An early-stage cognitive impairment
B. A sensory neurogenic dysfunction
C. A motor neurogenic dysfunction
D. An adverse reaction of a medication

704. The client is prescribed docusate sodium (Colace) for constipation. The nurse recognizes that this type of laxative acts by:
A. Retaining and increasing water content of feces by osmotic qualities
B. Absorbing water and increasing the volume of intestinal contents
C. Increasing peristalsis in the colon by irritating nerve endings in the mucosa
D. Dispersing wetting agents and producing a soft homogenous mixture

705. The nurse is preparing medications for a group of clients who are experiencing constipation. The physician has ordered milk of magnesia 15 ml at 8 A.M. For which of the following clients would the nurse question this order?
A. A client recovering from pneumonia
B. A client recovering from arthroplasty
C. A client with end-stage renal disease
D. A client with a history of fecal impaction

706. The nurse is evaluating the bowel management program that has been implemented for 3 months. Which of the following outcomes best indicates to the nurse that the program is successful?
A. Fecal impaction decreased by 50 percent.
B. Bowel accidents decreased by 50 percent.
C. Feces occurs regularly and is soft and well-formed.
D. Skin integrity is maintained and old decubitus ulcers are healed.

707. The nurse is caring for a client with neurogenic fecal incontinence. The most common cause of this dysfunction is:
A. Surgical trauma to the sphincter
B. Multiple sclerosis or spinal cord lesions
C. Psychiatric or behavioral disorders
D. Habitual use of laxatives or enemas

708. A home health nurse has been asked to see a client with end-stage renal disease for assessment of cachexia. If entered by the nurse, which documentation would correctly identify that the client is experiencing cachexia?
A. Unable to verbalize feelings or write important information
B. Unable to carry out activities of daily living without help
C. Involuntary muscular movements of the arms and legs
D. Emaciation, loss of subcutaneous fat, and lean body mass

709. The nurse completes the admission of the 80-year-old client admitted with a family report of a recent 16-pound weight loss. Repeat laboratory values for this client include: serum albumin 2 gms/dl, serum transferrin 100 mg/dl, and lymphocytes 750 cells/mm^3. Which action would be most appropriate for the nurse to initiate?
A. Prepare the client for a feeding tube.
B. Prepare the client for psychiatric transfer.
C. Monitor vital signs every 30 minutes.
D. Test all bowel movements for blood.

710. A nurse in the community has been asked for a resource for older adults to help them improve their driving skills. The most appropriate resource identified by the nurse is:
A. The local automobile insurance company
B. The local highway patrol driving program
C. The American Association of Retired Persons
D. The American Blindness Federation

711. A 70-year-old person is attending a senior citizen center. The client engages in conversation with others but refuses to participate in recreational or social events. The client's affect is appropriate and her appearance is well groomed. The initial action by the nurse based on this information is:
A. Assess the client for constipation.
B. Assess the client for pain.
C. Assess the client for depression.
D. Assess the client for cognitive impairment.

712. A geriatric nurse is caring for a 78-year-old client. The urinalysis for this client indicates a specific gravity of 1.03 and protein of 8.2/100 ml. The most important action by the nurse is:
A. Monitor the client for congestive heart failure.
B. Monitor the client for urinary tract infection.
C. Monitor the client for acute renal failure.
D. Do nothing because laboratory values are within normal limits.

713. A bedridden client with Alzheimer's disease with a stage IV decubitus ulcer is admitted to a long-term care facility. The client is incontinent of bowel and bladder. The nurse is preparing a care plan for this client. The most important nursing diagnosis identified by the nurse is:
A. Potential for social isolation
B. Potential for self-care deficit
C. Potential for injury
D. Potential for infection

714. The bedridden client with Alzheimer's disease is receiving decubitus ulcer care by the nurse. The nurse notes an increase in purulent wound drainage. Vital signs are temperature 99, pulse 78, respirations 18, and blood pressure 162/88. The most appropriate nursing action at this time is:
A. Administer the client a prescribed antipyretic medication.

B. Call the physician for an order for a white blood cell count.

C. Change the decubitus ulcer care treatment regimen more often.

D. Do nothing but continue to monitor vital signs.

715. A 79-year-old client is being admitted to the geriatrics unit of a large medical center. This is the first time the client has required hospitalization. A priority for this client at the beginning of hospitalization is:
A. Assessment of knowledge of prescription medications.
B. Assessment of knowledge of hospital procedures.
C. Assessment of baseline cognitive status.
D. Assessment of baseline functional status.

716. The nurse is preparing a community education program related to the needs of older adults for long-term care. The nurse correctly identifies:
A. That 25 percent of adults over the age of 85 are in institutional settings.
B. That 50 percent of adults over the age of 85 are in institutional settings.
C. That 5 percent of males over the age of 65 are in institutional settings.
D. That 5 percent of females over the age of 65 are in institutional settings.

717. During the presentation of a community program on the needs of long-term care insurance, the nurse correctly informs the audience that:
A. The trend is to send persons over the age of 85 years to institutional settings.
B. The trend is to provide more noninstitutional long-term care settings.
C. The trend is to provide more senior citizen centers for socialization.
D. The trend is to provide reimbursement to the family for providing care.

718. A guest speaker at a gerontological meeting relates to the audience that minority caregivers experience fewer negative consequences related to caregiving. The audience correctly questions the validity of this response because:
A. The speaker is not a doctorately prepared gerontological nurse researcher.
B. There has been little research related to the lived experience of caregiving.
C. Most caregiving research has been conducted with nonminority samples.
D. Most caregiving research has been conducted with predominantly minority samples.

719. A 70-year-old client at a free health screening was found to have a thyroid disorder. A nursing student assisting with the screening asks the instructor why the client had not sought medical attention for this disorder sooner. The instructor correctly informs the student that:
A. Older adults do not seek medical attention because they fear nursing home placement.
B. Older adults do not seek medical attention because of limited financial resources.
C. Older adults do not seek medical attention because they fear loss of independence.
D. Older adults do not seek medical attention because they exhibit few symptoms.

720. A nurse in a nursing clinic is approached by an older adult who says that the physician has diagnosed him with type II diabetes, but that he would be monitored for type I diabetes. The client asks, "What is the difference between type I and type II diabetes?" The nurse correctly responds:
A. "Type I diabetes has an absence of ketosis, which signifies insulin production."
B. "Type II diabetes has an absence of ketosis, which signifies insulin production."
C. "Type I diabetes has an absence of ketosis, which signifies no insulin is produced."
D. "Type II diabetes has an absence of ketosis, which signifies no insulin is produced."

721. An older adult who is diabetic calls the home health nurse and reports symptoms of a viral infection. The client indicates that she has no appetite and asks the nurse for suggestions. The most appropriate nursing action by the nurse would be to inform the client to:
A. Drink plenty of fluids and maintain carbohydrate intake.
B. Drink a high-protein nutritional supplement hourly.
C. Withhold your insulin until your fever returns to normal.
D. Report to the hospital emergency room immediately.

722. The nurse is giving dietary instruction to an older adult who is a newly diagnosed diabetic. The initial action of the nurse is to:
A. Determine the client's usual dietary habits.
B. Determine the client's ideal body weight.
C. Determine the client's compliance ability.
C. Determine the amount of insulin ordered.

723. The nurse conducts the dietary classes for newly diagnosed diabetics. The nurse correctly informs the members:
A. You should maintain an 1800-calorie diet with occasional sweets.
B. You should maintain an 1800-calorie low-fat diet with minimum sweets.
C. Your diet should contain 55 percent carbohydrates that are primarily complex.
D. Your diet should contain 25 percent carbohydrates that are primarily simple.

724. The nurse is presenting a nutrition class at a local

retirement center. The nurse discusses that before older adults begin diets for weight loss, they should know their ideal body weight. The nurse informs the group that ideal body weight for females over the age of 65 is:

A. 90 lb for the first 5 ft in height and 5 lb for each additional inch

B. 100 lb for the first 5 ft in height and 5 lb for each additional inch

C. 120 lb for the first 5 ft in height and 5 lb for each additional inch

D. 140 lb for the first 5 ft in height and 5 lb for each additional inch

725. While the nurse is presenting a nutrition class and is discussing ideal body weight for women, a gentleman asks "What is the ideal body weight for men?" The nurse correctly responds:

A. "There is not an ideal body weight for males because exercise determines fat burn."

B. "There is not an ideal body weight for males because they don't usually diet."

C. "Allow 106 lb for the first 5 ft and 6 lb for each additional inch."

D. "Allow 130 lb for the first 5 ft and 10 lb for each additional inch."

726. A 70-year-old insulin-dependent diabetic client shows the nurse an area on the leg where injections have been given. This area appears as an accumulation of subcutaneous fat. The nurse identifies this as lipohypertrophy. The initial action by the nurse is to:

A. Assess the client for signs and symptoms of infection.

B. Assess the client for signs and symptoms of cellulitis.

C. Assess the amount of insulin the client has been receiving.

D. Assess the injection rotation method the client uses.

727. The home health nurse has recommended biofeedback for the client who is experiencing incontinence. The following information is most important in evaluating the client for biofeedback as a treatment modality:

A. Medical factors and motivation

B. Medical factors and family support

C. Mental status and family support

D. Mental status and motivation

728. A newly diagnosed diabetic client is placed on tolbutamide (Orinase) 250 mg bid. The nurse reviews the medications that the client is currently taking for potential drug interactions. Which medication, if prescribed for the client and taken as prescribed, would the nurse inform the client is safe and does not need monitoring when administered with tolbutamide?

A. Propranolol

B. Acetaminophen

C. Salicylate

D. Furosemide

729. A newly diagnosed diabetic prescribed with tolbutamide (Orinase) questions the nurse about the rationale for the physician prescribing oral diabetic agents rather than insulin therapy. The nurse correctly informs the client:

A. "The goal is freedom from glycosuria with a fasting serum glucose of 125 mg."

B. "The goal is freedom from glycosuria with a fasting serum glucose of 180 mg."

C. "The doctor knows that many older adults are unable to maneuver injections."

D. "The doctor knows that many older adults are unable to read insulin syringes."

730. A 72-year-old female reports to the nurse that she has recently been experiencing vaginal dryness with dyspareunia and a diminished libido. The client indicates that she has been extremely worried about a son who has recently lost his job because of downsizing of his company. She reports that her husband had a heart attack 4 months ago and that their sex life has greatly decreased since that time. Six months ago her mother moved into the house because the mother was getting increasingly frail. In attending to the client's primary sexual concern, the nurse would initially assess:

A. The present relationship of the client with the mother

B. The present relationship of the husband and mother

C. The frequency with which the couple engage in sexual activity

D. The frequency with which the client and son communicate

731. The nurse completes the interview with the client who complains of dyspareunia, vaginal dryness, and diminished libido. The most appropriate action by the nurse is to:

A. Recommend that the client place her mother in a nearby nursing home.

B. Recommend that the client go for an appointment at a mental health center.

C. Recommend that the client go for an immediate gynecological examination.

D. Recommend to the client that intercourse continue at regular intervals.

732. A 73-year-old client with diabetes is admitted with gangrene of the right foot. The client is scheduled to have a right above-the-knee amputation. The client is 5 ft 9 inches tall and weights 195 lb. In determining the ideal body weight, the nurse must determine what the client's actual weight will be following the above-the-knee amputation. The nurse correctly identifies that the weight of this client would be approximately:

A. 165 lb

B. 160 lb

C. 175 lb
D. 185 lb

733. A client has a right below-the-knee amputation and recovers without incident. He returns to the geriatric orthopedic unit from the recovery room. The rehabilitation of this client includes returning home with a prothesis. The most important nursing action during the immediate and late postoperative period for this client is:
A. To prevent postoperative hemorrhage
B. To prevent secondary disabilities
C. To maintain comfort
D. To maintain vital signs

734. On the second postoperative day, the physician writes an order for physical therapy to assist with standing and balancing exercises on parallel bars progressing to ambulation. The rationale for this order for physical therapy is:
A. Early ambulation encourages socialization and prevents depression.
B. Early ambulation encourages hope and increases rehabilitation potential.
C. Early ambulation encourages activity and accelerates stump shrinkage.
D. Early ambulation encourages circulation and decreases calcium loss.

735. The client is gaining strength following the right below-the-knee amputation and has started stair-walking exercises. Which observation by the nurse would indicate that the client understands the correct procedure for stair walking?
A. The client places the left foot on the step and, holding the rail, moves the right foot.
B. The client places the right foot on the step and, holding the rail, moves the left foot.
C. The client uses a cane on the step, then moves the left foot followed by the right.
D. The client is able to climb stairs, but an elevator should be used if possible.

736. The nurse is instructing the client with a below-the-knee amputation in stump hygiene. The nurse correctly informs the client that when sleeping, the prosthesis should be removed. The rationale for this instruction is:
A. The client might roll over on the prosthesis and damage it.
B. The client might loosen the prosthesis during sleep and fall.
C. The prosthesis might cause personal body injury to the client.
D. The prosthesis might cause severe dermatitis resulting in loss of use.

737. While the nurse is assisting the client into the shower, mist from the shower head lands on the floor and the lower portion of the prosthesis, which is placed close to the shower door. The most appropriate action by the nurse is:

A. Take a hair dryer and dry the prosthesis before replacing.
B. Take a towel and carefully dry the prosthesis immediately.
C. Remind the client to be careful of falls when exiting the shower.
D. Remind the client to dry the prosthesis before putting it back on.

738. The client with the below-the-knee amputation returns to the community following completion of prosthetic rehabilitation. The nurse provides home-care instruction including the need for follow-up care. The nurse correctly informs the client:
A. You will need to return every 3 to 6 months for the next 2 years for follow-up.
B. You will need to return every year for the next 5 years for follow-up.
C. You will not need to return for follow-up unless you experience a problem.
D. You will need to make monthly appointments with your local physician.

739. The nurse is seeing the below-the-knee amputation client who has returned to the community following completion of the program for prosthetic rehabilitation. When the client returns for the follow-up appointment, which action by the nurse is essential?
A. Check the fasting blood sugar values for glucose level.
B. Check the circulatory status of the sound leg.
C. Check mental status and cognition level.
D. Check current family support systems.

740. The client reports to the nurse that he is experiencing pain in the stump. This pain is localized and tender to touch. The client describes the pain as going from mild to severe. The nurse correctly identifies this painful sensation as most likely caused by:
A. An ill-fitting prosthetic
B. Phantom pain
C. A spur formation
D. A circulation disorder

741. The nurse is evaluating the client's adjustment to the use of the prosthetic. Which statement, if made by the client, indicates that the client understands the correct use of the prosthetic and is using it correctly?
A. "I clean my prosthesis with a chlorine solution to prevent fungus."
B. "I inspect my stump with a mirror every month for damage."
C. "I use my wheelchair during the night to go to the bathroom."
D. "I continue to use my prosthesis even when it gets a little irritated."

742. A 76-year-old client is admitted to the emergency

room following a bout of chest pain while vigorously exercising at a local health fitness center. The client is a widower of 6 years. Two months ago the client began dating again after meeting a 64-year-old woman who is an aerobics instructor at the senior citizen center. The emergency room nurse identifies that the most probable reason for the chest pain experienced by this client is because of:
A. The stress of keeping up with a younger woman.
B. The stress incurred from too vigorous exercise.
C. Volume depletion caused by orthostatic hypotension.
D. A normal aging change of the cardiovascular system.

743. The client is admitted and is scheduled to have a stress test. The nurse explains to the client that the purpose of the stress test is to:
A. Identify a safe range for heart rate during exercise.
B. Identify daily stressors that the client encounters.
C. Identify appropriate cardiovascular training exercises.
D. Identify the reaction of the cardiopulmonary system to stress.

744. A nurse is discussing a home exercise plan with a client who has recently been hospitalized for depression. The plan includes a morning and evening walk for 20 minutes. The client is fearful of exercise and asks the nurse if the doctor should order a stress test. The most appropriate response by the nurse is:
A. "You will enjoy walking once you get started on the program and get used to it."
B. "Your fear of exercise is a part of your illness and you need to confront this fear."
C. "Stress testing without evidence of coronary disease is not necessary for walking."
D. "There is nothing physically wrong with you and a stress test will not help."

745. The nurse is designing an exercise program for a 70-year-old client who has been physically active until hospitalization for pneumonia. Which statement by the client would the nurse recognize as the need for further teaching regarding exercise?
A. "I hope to increase my endurance for exercise each day after discharge."
B. "I will warm up for 2 or 3 minutes with flexibility exercise."
C. "I will count my radial pulse rate for a full 10 seconds after exercising."
D. "I will exercise for 30 minutes each day when the weather permits."

746. A senior citizens group has asked the nurse to design and implement an exercise program that would be most suited for older adults. If carried out, which series of activities would be most effective in meeting the conditioning needs for older adults?
A. Walking, light jogging, and swimming
B. Walking, light jogging, and dancing
C. Walking, dancing, and swimming
D. Walking, biking, and swimming

747. The nurse is preparing individualized exercise programs for clients who are being discharged back to the community. For which of the following clients scheduled for discharge would the nurse provide a supervised exercise regimen?
A. A client with arthritis who has just had arthroplasty surgery
B. A client with a history of mitral and aortic valve murmurs
C. A client with acute respiratory distress with pneumonia
D. A client with a history of chronic organic brain disorder

748. A 73-year-old client is admitted to the cardiovascular unit. The physician orders daily electrocardiograms (EKGs) to assist in making a diagnosis. If present on the EKG, which condition would indicate a diagnosis of myocardial necrosis?
A. An abnormal Q wave
B. A depressed ST segment
C. An elevated ST segment
D. An inverted T wave

749. A client is scheduled for coronary artery bypass graft (CABG). The nurse is preparing the client for surgery and begins preoperative teaching. Which teaching by the nurse is essential prior to surgery?
A. The intensive care unit with ventilators, chest tubes, and IV lines
B. The cardiovascular unit with chest tubes, pain, and one-on-one nursing care
C. The need to turn, deep-breathe, and pain management through self-infusion
D. The need to resume an established exercise program and dietary modifications

750. The client has an internal mammary CABG graft and is returned to the nursing unit 3 days following surgery. The client complains of severe chest wall discomfort. The nurse recognizes that this discomfort is:
A. The result of postoperative complications
B. The result of nerve injury at the harvest site
C. The result of psychosomatic transference
D. The result of dependence on narcotic medication

751. The wife of a 75-year-old client being discharged following coronary artery bypass expresses concern for caring for her husband at home. She relates that prior to her husband's illness, they had been both physically and sexually active. She re-

lates fears that her husband will become excessively active following discharge and this will bring about further illness. The most appropriate response by the nurse is:
A. "There are no restrictions to resuming your sexual relations following discharge."
B. "There are some restrictions to sexual relations, but these are minor occurrences."
C. "Your husband may experience some impotence following surgery because of medications."
D. "Your husband may not be able to perform sexually for 6 months after discharge."

752. The client is discharged home following bypass surgery. Three weeks following discharge the client telephones the nurse to report left-sided muscle aching throughout the chest, upper back, shoulders, and neck. The most appropriate action by the nurse is:
A. Inform the client to call the physician immediately.
B. Inform the client to apply ice packs three times daily.
C. Inform the client to take muscle-relaxing medications.
D. Do nothing because muscle aches are expected following surgery.

753. A client with premature ventricular contractions has been receiving procainamide hydrochloride (Pronestyl) 500 mg four times per day for the past 8 months. Which symptom if experienced by the client would the nurse recognize as needing immediate investigation?
A. Constipation
B. Dizziness
C. Shivering
D. Diarrhea

754. The nurse is conducting an interview with a client who has bouts of paroxysmal atrial tachycardia and is placed on procainamide (Pronestyl) 500 mg qid. Which statement if made by the client indicates that teaching has been effective?
A. "If I miss taking my medication, I should discontinue it and call the doctor."
B. "This medication will have to be changed over time because of my body sensitivity."
C. "I should report any bruising or bleeding to my physician immediately."
D. "I should report any dizziness when rising from a sitting position to the nurse."

755. A nurse working in the cardiovascular unit is observing the EKG strips of newly admitted clients. The nurse observes one client who has a high pointed P wave. The best action of the nurse based on this observation is to:
A. Call the physician immediately for atrial fibrillation medication.
B. Call the nursing supervisor and order a cardiac arrest cart nearby.

C. Carefully assess and monitor the client for pulmonary disease.
D. Carefully assess and monitor the renal status and urinary output.

756. A 69-year-old client is scheduled to receive a demand pacemaker following a series of fainting spells. The nurse is preparing to teach the client about the pacemaker. The nurse correctly informs the client that the purpose of the pacemaker is to:
A. Sense the heart's electrical activity and permanently beat for the heart muscle.
B. Sense the heart's electrical activity and slow the heart rhythm.
C. Sense the heart's electrical activity and speed the heart rhythm.
D. Sense the heart's electrical activity and depolarize some portion of the heart muscle.

757. The client returns from surgery with a pacemaker in place. The nurse notes on the physician documentation that the pacemaker is in the VVI mode. The nurse correctly identifies that this mode indicates that:
A. The ventricle is sensed and paced and heartbeats are inhibited when natural heartbeats are frequent enough.
B. The ventricle is sensed and paced and heartbeats are triggered to set at 66 beats per minute.
C. The atrium and ventricle are sensed and heartbeats are triggered by the pacemaker when less than 66.
D. The ventricle is sensed and pacing of the heartbeat occurs when the heart rate is less than 60 plus 21.

758. The client is transferred to the recovery room following pacemaker implantation. The nurse caring for the client detects cardiac problems and calls a code. The physician responding to the code orders the nurse to defibrillate the client. The most appropriate action by the nurse is to:
A. Defibrillate, placing the paddles over the pacemaker.
B. Defibrillate, placing the paddles anteriorly and posteriorly.
C. Defibrillate, placing the paddles laterally over the chest.
D. Inform the physician that the client has a pacemaker.

759. The nurse is preparing the client for discharge after pacemaker implantation. Which of the following instructions should be started before surgery and continue throughout the hospital stay concerning potential problems?
A. The need for strict adherence to dietary regimen.
B. The need for strict adherence to exercise regimen.

C. The need to watch for infection at the implant site.

D. The need to carefully check pacemaker battery monthly.

760. The client with a pacemaker is ambulating in the room with the assistance of the nurse. The client reports feeling dizzy and short of breath. The nurse recognizes these symptoms are caused by:
A. Fatigue caused by prolonged bedrest.
B. Fear of pacemaker failure
C. Drop in cardiac output
D. Need for individualized attention

761. The client with a pacemaker is ambulating in the room with the assistance of the nurse. The client complains of dizziness and shortness of breath. The initial action by the nurse should be:
A. Reassure the client that you will stay with him.
B. Have him rest in bed immediately.
C. Monitor his vital signs every hour.
D. Do nothing because this is normal following surgery.

762. The client with a pacemaker is discharged home and is being followed by a home health nurse. The client reports to the nurse that he and his spouse enjoy traveling and have spent the last several years in Europe. The client questions the nurse regarding whether the pacemaker will interfere with their travels. Which instruction given by the nurse is most appropriate based on the needs for this client?
A. "You will need to have monthly follow-up evaluations, so your travel will be limited."
B. "You will need to show your pacemaker identification card to airport security."
C. "You will need to discuss your travel plans with your cardiologist before travel."
D. "You will be unable to travel for the first 3 years as your pacemaker is tested."

763. The client with a permanent pacemaker has returned home and is being seen by the home health nurse. The nurse notes an apical pulse rate of 50 and the rhythm is irregular. The client pacemaker code is set on 60. The client has no other symptoms and is not short of breath. The most appropriate action by the nurse is to:
A. Inform the hospital.
B. Inform his physician.
C. Obtain a 12-lead electrocardiogram.
D. Do nothing because pulse rate is within normal limits.

764. A client with a pacemaker is scheduled for a nuclear magnetic resonance (MRI) for undetermined back pain. Following the MRI, the physician indicates that the pacemaker will need to be reprogrammed and asks the nurse to ascertain the information to do this procedure. The nurse correctly obtains the following information needed for reprogramming:

A. The date of implementation and the physician
B. The date of implementation and the serial number
C. The model number and the name of the manufacturer
D. The model number and the serial number

765. An 80-year-old client presents with a blood pressure of 170/80 and reports dyspnea on minimal exertion. Pulse rate is 102. He also complains of a headache and dizziness. Based on this information, the most appropriate nursing action at this time is to:
A. Teach the client about postural hypotension.
B. Assess the client for isolated systolic hypotension.
C. Inform the client that this is a normal aging change.
D. Teach the client to eat a low-salt, low-fat diet.

766. A 71-year-old client is diagnosed with right-sided congestive heart failure (CHF). Which assessment by the nurse is most reflective of right-sided CHF?
A. Tachypnea
B. Pink, frothy sputum
C. Korotkoff's sounds
D. Distended jugular veins

767. The home health nurse visits a 98-year-old client who lives alone. The client is experiencing periods of forgetfulness and poor visual acuity. The client is currently taking the following medications: digoxin (Lanoxin) 0.125 mg bid; potassium chloride (K-Dur) 20 mEq daily; furosemide (Lasix) 40 mg daily; enalapril (Vasotec) 120 mg bid. The most appropriate nursing intervention for this client based on knowledge of pharmacology and drug interactions is:
A. Monitor for hypernatremia.
B. Monitor for hyperkalemia.
C. Monitor for postural hypotension.
D. Monitor for weight loss.

768. The nurse continues to visit with the client who is living alone and experiencing periods of forgetfulness and decreased visual acuity. The physician orders indicate that the client is to remain on his current medications until follow-up in 3 months. The most appropriate nursing action by the nurse to increase compliance with the medical regime is:
A. Teach the client the importance of follow-up medical appointments.
B. Teach the client about each medication and the need for compliance.
C. Prepare a prefilled medicine organizer each week with his medications.
D. Prepare a color-coded medication bottle for each medication prescribed.

769. A 70-year-old client is diagnosed with sleep apnea. The nurse begins teaching the client about this condition and therapeutic approaches to dealing

with sleep apnea. The nurse correctly teaches the client to:
A. Drink a small glass of sherry before retiring for bed.
B. Avoid any alcoholic beverage during the daytime.
C. Take an over-the-counter stimulant during the daytime.
D. Eat a high-calorie, protein-rich food right before bedtime.

770. A nurse working in staff development is presenting a program about older adults and prescription drug use. The nurse tells the audience, "Persons over the age of 65 make up 11 percent of the population, yet they take 25 percent of all prescription drugs sold in the United States." The nurse attributes this statement related to prescription drugs to:
A. Persons over the age of 65 complain about aches and pains more than younger people.
B. Persons over the age of 65 are entitled to Medicare, therefore they visit the physician more often.
C. Persons over the age of 65 have more chronic, long-term illness than do younger people.
D. Persons who are advancing in age have physiological changes that bring about physical disabilities.

771. A 66-year-old client is seen by the home health nurse. The client reports insomnia with periods of hyperactivity accompanied by sluggishness, depression, cold intolerance, decreased appetite, and generalized aching all over. The physician notes that the client is receiving the following prescriptions medications: paroxetine (Paxil) 20 mg at bedtime (HS); multiple vitamin with ginseng bid; Amvien 10 mg PRN insomnia. The client questions why she is experiencing hyperactivity when she feels depressed. The most appropriate response by the nurse is:
A. "Many times depression is accompanied by anxiety."
B. "Paroxetine may cause sluggishness and anxiety in some people."
C. "Insomnia can be caused by depression and anxiety."
D. "This may be caused by your medication or by hypothyroidism."

772. An 85-year-old client is attending a senior citizen center where the nurse is conducting blood pressure screening. The client tells the nurse that she has recently had problems with constipation. The nurse knows that the client has a history of colon cancer about 14 years ago and had surgery but no metastasis. The most appropriate nursing action at this time is:
A. Tell the client to increase fruits, fiber, and fluids in the diet.

B. Tell the client that constipation is to be expected sometimes.
C. Tell the client to take an over-the-counter stool softener.
D. Tell the client to see her physician for an evaluation.

773. A 78-year-old with increasing mental confusion is admitted to the emergency room from the nursing home. The client has been a nursing home resident for 3 months following the death of her spouse. The client had previously been alert and able to feed herself and respond appropriately to simple questions. She has been receiving the following medications: furosemide (Lasix) 40 mg daily; digoxin 0.025 mg daily; captopril (Capoten) 25 mg tid. On admission to the emergency room, initial assessment reveals a temperature of 99°F, pulse 68, respirations 24, and blood pressure 90/60. The nurse notes that the client has dry skin with poor skin turgor, and the lips and oral mucous membranes are dry. The nurse recognizes that the client is most likely experiencing:
A. A reaction to the medications
B. A normal grief reaction for the spouse
C. Symptoms of acute dehydration
D. Symptoms of an infectious process

774. The home health nurse is admitting a 66-year-old who is newly diagnosed as having insulin-dependent diabetes mellitus. The client lives alone in a low-income apartment. The nurse notes that the client has no cognitive impairment but does have some difficulty learning. The primary nursing goal for this client is:
A. Encourage family involvement to promote compliance.
B. Refer to social services to gain financial assistance.
C. Provide educational materials to decrease knowledge deficit.
D. Assist with lifestyle change to adjust to current health concerns.

775. A 72-year-old client with bipolar disorder has been taking lithium 300 mg bid for the last 3 years to control the symptoms of mental illness. He reports to a family physician for an annual check-up. The physician has been monitoring the client for hypertension, which he has been able to control with regular exercise and diet. Today the client has vital signs of temperature 98°F, pulse 92, respiration 20, and blood pressure 170/92. The physician orders captopril (Capoten) 6.25 mg tid for hypertension and sends the office nurse in to teach the client about this medication. The most appropriate action by the nurse is:
A. Instruct the client to take the medication orally 1 hour after meals.
B. Instruct the client to be careful when rising to a standing position.

C. Inform the physician of the potential for lithium toxicity with this drug.

D. Inform the physician that the client will not be compliant because mental illness.

776. A 67-year-old adult is admitted to an acute care unit with the diagnosis of intestinal obstruction. Routine laboratory tests and x-rays were ordered. On reviewing laboratory results, the nurse noted a blood sugar of 200. The nurse questions the client who indicates to the nurse that he ate approximately 2 hours prior to blood being drawn for laboratory work. The initial action by the nurse is:

A. Order the client a regular diet immediately.

B. Do nothing but continue to monitor the client status.

C. Inform the physician of the client's elevated blood sugar.

D. Call the laboratory and ask for a re-evaluation of the results.

777. A community health nurse is preparing a program on hearing loss for a senior citizen group. Which statement by the nurse is correct related to hearing in older adults?

A. Only about 30 percent of older adults who need hearing aids have them.

B. Only about 30 percent of nursing home residents have hearing impairment.

C. Hearing loss is a normal aging change and hearing aids will not help.

D. Hearing loss that occurs with age cannot be corrected with aids.

778. A nurse is evaluating a client for conductive hearing loss. If experienced by the client, which of the manifestations would the nurse correctly identify as associated with conductive hearing loss?

A. The client speaks in an excessively loud voice in many situations.

B. The client speaks in a relatively quiet voice that is difficult to hear.

C. The client may be sensitive to loud intensities of sound.

D. The client has scarring and sclerotic changes in the middle ear.

779. The nurse discusses the common cause of conductive hearing deficits with an older adult group. The nurse correctly informs the group that the most common cause of conductive deficits in older adults is:

A. Scarring and sclerotic changes in the middle ear

B. Normal aging changes to the acoustic nerve

C. Bilateral damage of high-frequency nerve endings

D. Total occlusion of the external canal by cerumen

780. A 74-year-old client has been evaluated for hearing loss and is being fitted for a hearing aid. The nurse correctly instructs the client that the hearing aid:

A. Can be ordered for a 2- to 4-week trial period

B. Can be purchased and reimbursed by Medicare

C. Can only be purchased by his physician

D. Cannot be returned to the vendor

781. The client receives the new hearing aid and is being fitted by the nurse. The client has a moderate loss of hearing in the left ear and a mild hearing loss in the right ear. The nurse correctly inserts the hearing aid:

A. In the ear having the mild loss of hearing

B. In the ear having the moderate loss of hearing

C. In the ear that the client requests

D. In bilateral hearing loss, the location is unimportant.

782. The nurse is instructing the client on the wearing of the new hearing aid. The nurse correctly informs the client to:

A. Wear the hearing aid 24 hours a day for the first week.

B. Wear the hearing aid during the day and remove at night.

C. Wear the hearing aid 4 hours a day at first and progress.

D. Wear the hearing aid when watching television or visiting.

783. If made by the client, which statement would indicate to the nurse that teaching related to hearing aid care has been effective?

A. "I will clean the ear mold with an alcohol and water solution."

B. "I should not be concerned if I don't hear a whistle set at loud volume."

C. "I should have to change the batteries every 10 to 14 days."

D. "I should have the hearing aid checked yearly for maintenance."

784. The nurse continues teaching the client about the hearing aid. Which statement by the nurse might be most important to assist the client in adapting to wearing a hearing aid?

A. "You may feel tense and nervous initially because of the sudden noise."

B. "You may need to ask for assistance from friends when adjusting your aid."

C. "You will be able to change your batteries after a few practice sessions."

D. "You will be able to hear only the voices of persons speaking to you."

785. A 79-year-old living in a retirement community had a routine audiological screening at a senior citizens' center. Her prescribed medications include digoxin, furosemide (Lasix), and potassium supplement. She also takes 5 to 10 aspirin daily for arthritic pain. The client is noted to have impaired hearing manifested by a 38-decibel (dB) threshold in the right ear and a 50-dB threshold in the left

ear. The client is referred for a complete audiological evaluation, which does not reveal any external or middle ear disease. The client asks the nurse what could have caused her to have problems hearing during the screening. The most appropriate response by the nurse is:
A. "The audiologist has more sensitive equipment to test hearing loss."
B. "You may have been apprehensive during the screening at the center."
C. "You probably had an accumulation of earwax during the screening."
D. "You might have listened better during the testing since it was expensive."

786. Three months after the hearing screen, the 79-year-old client is seen by her primary-care physician for a routine visit to assess her chronic congestive heart failure, poststatus myocardial infarction, and osteoarthritis. Her prescribed medications include digoxin, furosemide (Lasix), and potassium supplement. She also takes 5 to 10 aspirin daily for arthritic pain. The nurse notes considerable difficulty in communication. Her hearing loss seems to be markedly worse and tinnitus is present bilaterally; however, she has no vomiting or vertigo. The client is inattentive and dozes off in the chair. The nurse correctly identifies that this dramatic drop in hearing acuity may be attributed to:
A. A normal progression of hearing loss in the aging process
B. A normal build-up of cerumen occurring in the inner ear
C. An abnormal response to undiagnosed Meniere's disease
D. An ototoxicity to the prescribed medications being taken

787. An older adult is talking with the nurse about the visual difficulties presently being experienced. From the symptoms described by the client, the nurse thinks this might be an irreversible blindness. The leading cause of irreversible blindness in older adults is:
A. Cataracts
B. Macular degeneration
C. Chronic blepharitis
D. Diabetic retinopathy

788. The community health nurse has been asked to speak to a local group of older adults about hypertension. The nurse is presenting information about normal aging changes and hypertension. The nurse correctly reports that as age increases:
A. Systolic blood pressure increases, while diastolic pressure is unchanged.
B. Systolic blood pressure is unchanged and diastolic pressure increases.
C. Both systolic and diastolic blood pressure are increased.
C. Neither systolic nor diastolic blood pressure is changed.

789. An older adult reports to the nurse that she has been on a low-salt diet to control blood pressure. She indicates to the nurse that her blood pressure is still slightly elevated and that she is thinking of curtailing her salt intake even more drastically. The best action by the nurse is to:
A. Inform the client that salt intake will not affect hypertension.
B. Inform the client that the minimal salt intake should be 500 mg.
C. Inform the client that the minimal salt intake should be 2000 mg.
D. Inform the client to decrease salt intake to 200 mg and eat fruits.

790. The nurse is assessing a newly admitted client to the nursing home. When performing an eye examination, the nurse observes that the lower lid margin of the eye is no longer in contact with the globe. The nurse correctly identifies this condition as:
A. Trichiasis
B. Entropion
C. Ectropion
D. Xanthelasma

791. A nurse is discussing theories of aging. A theory which indicates that each individual must learn specific developmental tasks and that successful achievement contributes to the individual's happiness and feelings of success is described. The developmental tasks arise from physical maturation, cultural expectations of society, and personal values and aspirations. Developed by Havighurst, this theory is known as:
A. Developmental Task Theory
B. Theory of Generativity vs. Stagnation
C. Wear-and-Tear Theory
D. Ego Transcendence Theory

792. The nurse is conducting a community program about Medicare and Medicaid issues. The nurse correctly informs the audience that these programs:
A. Were enacted as part of the Older Americans Act in 1964
B. Were enacted as part of the National Insurance Act in 1964
C. Were enacted as part of the Omnibus Budget Reconciliation Act
D. Were enacted as part of the Social Security Amendments of 1965

793. A nursing home director is orienting a new graduate on the provision of care requirements outlined by the Omnibus Budget Reconciliation Act (OBRA). The director states that under this requirement, residents must be assessed to identify medical problems, describe their capacity to perform daily functions, and note any significant impairments in functional status. The form to conduct this assessment is:

A. The instrumental activity-of-daily-living scale
B. The functional status inventory
C. The minimum data set
D. The quality-of-life scale

794. The nurse is discussing hypertension and aging at a community program. The audience asks the nurse if treatment of hypertension for older adults is effective in preventing death. The nurse correctly reports that treatment of diastolic hypertension resulted in decreased mortality for:
A. African-American males and white males, but not females
B. African-American females and white females, but not males
C. African-American males and females and white males
D. African-American males and females and white females

795. A 72-year-old client is admitted to the emergency room after being found at home by his daughter. When found, he was on the floor and was unconscious. Physical examination reveals a blood pressure of 200/120. The physician tells the daughter her father has had a stroke. The daughter asks the nurse providing care to the client about her father's prognosis. The most appropriate response by the nurse is:
A. "Your father has an excellent chance of recovery with proper treatment."
B. "Your father has a very poor prognosis because of his hypertension."
C. "Your father's condition is uncertain during this early stage of stroke."
D. "You will have to ask the physician about your father's condition."

796. A 73-year-old client presents with a 3-cm nodule to the left neck in the thyroid area. The client reports to the nurse that the nodule has recently increased in size, and is hard but not tender. The client indicates that hoarseness is the only other symptom associated with this nodule. The client asks the nurse if this nodule could be cancerous. The nurse correctly indicates to the client that if the nodule is a thyroid malignancy, it is most likely to be:
A. A lymphoma of the thyroid gland
B. A follicular carcinoma
C. A papillary carcinoma
D. A noninvasive carcinoma

797. A 79-year-old is being seen by the nurse. The client has a history of recurrent depression and hypothyroidism. The client reports to the nurse symptoms of increasing fatigue, muscle aches, cramps, and sleepiness. The nurse notes that the client is withdrawn and appears depressed, and moves and speaks slowly. Present weight is 132 lb (a loss of about 5 lb in the last few weeks); vital signs are blood pressure 160/60, pulse 64, temperature 97.6°F, and respirations 18. On physical examination, the nurse notes puffiness around the eyelids and pigmentation in the palmar creases, the thyroid gland is not palpable, and the biceps reflex is delayed. The nurse suspects that the client may be experiencing symptoms of hypothyroidism. What laboratory data would the nurse use to confirm this diagnosis?
A. The T_4 of radioimmunoassay (RIA) with a T_3 resin uptake
B. The T_2 of radioimmunoassay (RIA) with a T_3 resin uptake
C. The T_3 of radioimmunoassay (RIA) with a T_4 resin uptake
D. The T_3 and T_4 of radioimmunoassay (RIA) with iodine uptake

798. A 69-year-old client reports to a nursing clinic. The client reports recently meeting a very significant other and wants to lose some weight to be more attractive and to maintain longevity. The weight for the client is within the normal limits for age and height. The most appropriate response by the nurse is:
A. "You can't lose more than 5 more pounds or you'll look sickly."
B. "You can take an appetite suppressant and drink a dietary supplement."
C. "Your weight is normal for your age and height."
D. "You should consult a dietician trained in nutritional needs of older adults."

799. A 70-year-old client has been seeing the nurse for 4 months for a weight-loss program. The client reports to the nurse a complaint of pain in the abdomen for which the physician prescribed cimetidine (Tagamet) and antacid. The client has a history of peptic ulcers. The client is unable to communicate his dietary regimen with the nurse and appears confused. The most appropriate action by the nurse is:
A. Call the physician and get an order to discontinue cimetidine.
B. Call the physician and get an order for magnetic resonance imaging (MRI).
C. Call the physician and get an order for a mental evaluation.
D. Call the physician and get an order for immediate hospital admission.

800. The nurse is seeing a 74-year-old at a community health screening. The nurse notes that the client has a heavy plaque build-up and suggests to the client that a visit with the dentist is needed. The client questions how often a dental examination is needed for older adults. The most appropriate response by the nurse is:
A. "You should visit the dentist at least once a year."
B. "You should visit the dentist at least every 6 months."

C. "You should visit the dentist at least every 3 months."

D. "You should visit the dentist when you get plaque buildup."

801. The director of nursing in a local nursing home is teaching a class to a group of newly employed nursing staff. The director of nursing indicates that an oral examination is to be performed on each resident monthly. The most appropriate rationale for monthly oral examinations is:
A. The federal government mandates a monthly oral assessment.
B. The majority of nursing home residents have significant dental problems.
C. The majority of nursing home residents continue to have their own teeth.
D. The institutional facility requires comprehensive monthly assessments.

802. A 74-year-old client is being examined by the nurse. The client's denture contained fractured areas and poor oral hygiene is noted. On removing the client's dentures, the nurse notes a yellowish-white lesion on the palate, which is not removed by wiping with a swab. The most appropriate action by the nurse based on this assessment is:
A. Take a culture of the lesion and call the physician for a nystatin rinse.
B. Take a biopsy of the lesion and call the physician for a hospital admission.
C. Take a culture of the lesion and call the physician for an antibiotic.
D. Do nothing because this is a normal finding caused by poor oral hygiene.

803. The nurse is caring for a client with organic brain syndrome. The client is going for a diagnostic test. The client is extremely agitated prior to the procedure. The nurse calls the physician concerning the client. If prescribed by the physician, which order would the nurse question for this client?
A. Chlorpromazine (Thorazine) 25 mg IM
B. Thiothixene (Navane) 2 mg IM
C. Meperidine (Demerol) 50 mg PO
D. Haloperidol (Haldol) 1 mg PO

804. An older adult is scheduled to go to the dentist for a thorough examination and cleaning. The client has a history of rheumatic heart disease, which has caused valvular damage. Which nursing action is most appropriate for this client?
A. Monitor the vital signs before and hourly for 3 hours after the procedure.
B. Call the dentist for an order for penicillin.
C. Administer a mild antianxiety medication to reduce the client's stress.
D. Do nothing because this is not a stressful procedure for an older adult.

805. An 81-year-old client is being seen in a foot-care clinic. The client has a large toenail that is over-grown and is yellow-brown in color. All the other toenails are overgrown, but are not discolored. The client complains of pain in the large toenail area, especially when wearing shoes. The nurse correctly identifies that the client has:
A. Beginning gangrene of the toe
B. A fungal infection of the toe
C. Arterial insufficiency of the toe
D. Deep-vein thrombosis of the toe

806. The nurse is treating a client in the foot-care clinic for calluses. In teaching related to calluses, the nurse correctly instructs the client to:
A. Wear properly fitted shoes.
B. Maintain proper weight-bearing and balance.
C. Avoid walking without shoes.
D. Have monthly podiatrist treatment.

807. A staff nurse asks a gerontological nurse to explain the difference between gerontology and geriatrics. The nurse correctly responds that gerontology is the study that examines diverse aspects of aging while geriatrics focuses on:
A. The theoretical nature of aging
B. The normal aging processes
C. The clinical aspects of aging
D. The developmental aspects of aging

808. The nurse is presenting a program to a group of senior citizen about normal aging changes. The nurse correctly informs the audience that according to census data since 1980, sex differences in life expectancy have:
A. Increased, with women having a much greater life expectancy
B. Remained almost constant for the past 20 years
C. Increased, with men having a much greater life expectancy
D. Declined, with women having a small gain in life expectancy

809. A nurse researcher wants to conduct a study to explore the attitudes of older adults toward the current health-care reform issues. She conducts 100 interviews with people born in 1930 and 1940. She plans to interview these same individuals 5 years from the date of the original interview. The nurse correctly identifies this type of research design as:
A. Time-dimensional longitudinal design
B. Time-sequential design
C. Cross-sequential design
D. Cohort-sequential design

810. A nurse researcher is studying the health-care needs to ethnic-minority older adults and contacts the local chapter of the American Association of Retired Persons (AARP) to obtain a list of potential subjects. The president of this organization responds that the group will not be able to assist in accomplishing the purpose of this research. The most appropriate rationale for the president's response is:

A. The AARP is a private agency and does not assist with nursing research.

B. The AARP members are all retired and do not like to be research subjects.

C. The AARP members are generally too ill to answer questions or surveys.

D. The AARP members are generally financially secure and nonminorities.

811. The nurse is conducting a community program on normal aging changes and wants to address the social theories of aging. The nurse correctly informs the audience that nursing uses social theories to learn about:

A. How older people adapt to aging

B. How older people engage in socialization

C. How older people interact with family

D. How physiological changes affect society

812. The nurse is preparing a program on the theoretical nature of aging. One aspect of this program will be on society's values of work and productivity. The most appropriate theory used by the nurse to address this concept is:

A. The activity theory

B. The learned-helplessness theory

C. The generativity versus despair theory

D. The disengagement theory

813. The nurse is conducting a class on normal aging changes and the effects on sexuality. The nurse correctly informs the group that aging alters men's sexual functioning by:

A. Increasing the likelihood of impotence and decreased sexual desire

B. Reducing the time between the excitement phase and the erection

C. Increasing the time between orgasm and subsequent erections

D. Increasing the need for increased erotic materials for arousal

814. A group of community planners are developing programs for older adults. Which of the following programs indicates these planners are following the Healthy People 2000 report?

A. Programs related to Medicare services

B. Programs related to health promotion activities

C. Programs related to long-term care services

D. Programs related to advanced directives

815. The nurse at a senior citizen center is preparing a program on exercise and aging. The rationale for the nurse presenting this program is:

A. Common chronic illnesses are related to lifestyle behaviors.

B. Older persons do not get enough regularly scheduled exercise.

C. With normal aging, there is an increased amount of body fat.

D. Problems with mobility are a major concern of older adults.

816. According to the current demographic census trends, the largest ethnic group of the future is:

A. African-Americans

B. Whites

C. Hispanics

D. Native Americans

FOCUS ON MEDICAL/SURGICAL DRUG DOSAGE CALCULATION

817. A 65-year-old client was being prepared for an exploratory laparotomy. To prepare the client for surgery, the physician ordered cefazolin (Ancef) 250 mg prophylactically. Using a 1 gm/ml vial, how many milliliters did the nurse administer?

A. 0.25 ml

B. 0.50 ml

C. 0.75 ml

D. 1.0 ml

818. A 75-year-old client was seen in the local ER with severe ventricular tachycardia. The physician ordered amiodarone (Cordarone) 1000 mg PO. In stock were 200 mg tablets. How many tablets did the nurse administer?

A. 2 tablets

B. 3 tablets

C. 4 tablets

D. 5 tablets

819. A 27-year-old rape victim was seen in the local ER. The physician ordered tetracycline (Achromycin) 500 mg qid times 7 days PO to prevent infection. On hand were 250 mg tablets. The nurse instructed the client to take how many tablets?

A. ½ tablet

B. 1 tablet

C. 1½ tablets

D. 2 tablets

820. A 47-year-old client was seen in the local ambulatory care center with BP of 180/100. The physician ordered nifedipine (Adalat) 10 mg tid. The pharmacist dispensed 10 mg capsules. The nurse instructed the client to take how many capsules?

A. 1 capsule

B. 2 capsules

C. 3 capsules

D. 4 capsules

821. A 35-year-old was seen in the local physician's office with severe rhinitis. The physician prescribed flunisolide (AeroBid) aerosol spray and instructed the client to instill two sprays in each nostril bid. Each spray contains 25 μg of medication. How many micrograms will the client receive?

A. 25 μg

B. 50 μg

C. 75 μg
D. 1.0 μg

822. An 89-year old nursing home resident developed rheumatoid arthritis. The physician ordered auranofin 6 mg every day. The nurse administered how many 3 mg tablets?
A. ½ tablet
B. 1 tablet
C. 1½ tablets
D. 2 tablets

823. A 30-year-old was admitted to the hospital for recurring urinary tract infections. The physician ordered cefamandole (Mandol) 500 mg every 8 hours. Using a 1 g/ml vial, how many milliliters did the nurse administer?
A. 0.5 ml
B. 1.0 ml
C. 1.5 ml
C. 2.0 ml

824. A 45-year-old client was readmitted for clots that developed in the grafts used for a popliteal bypass. The physician ordered alteplase (Activase) 100 mg IV with 60 mg over first hour, 20 mg over second hour, and 20 mg over third hour. Using a 50 mg/ml vial, how many milliliters did the nurse administer?
A. 0.5 ml
B. 1.0 ml
C. 1.5 ml
C. 2.0 ml

825. A 47-year-old was admitted to the local ER with ascites secondary to cirrhosis of the liver. The physician ordered spironolactone (Aldactone) 100 mg every day. The pharmacist dispensed 50 mg tablets. The nurse instructed the client to take how many tablets?
A. ½ tablet
B. 1 tablet
C. 1½ tablets
D. 2 tablets

826. A 50-year-old client was diagnosed with type 1 Gaucher's disease. He weighed 50 kg. The physician ordered alglucerase (Ceredase) 60 units/kg (3000 units) diluted in 100 ml of 0.9% normal saline. Using an 80 unit/ml vial, how many milliliters did the nurse add to the IV solution?
A. 17.5 ml
B. 27.5 ml
C. 37.5 ml
D. 47.5 ml

827. A 25-year-old client was discharged from the hospital after passing kidney stones that were composed of phosphate crystals. The physician ordered aluminum hydroxide (Basaljel) 10 ml PRN to prevent future development of these crystals. Using a 400 mg/5 ml elixir, how many milligrams did the nurse instruct the client to take?

A. 200 mg
B. 400 mg
C. 600 mg
D. 800 mg

828. An AIDS client developed a respiratory tract infection. The physician ordered amantadine 100 mg bid. The nurse instructed the client to take how many 100 mg tablets?
A. ½ tablet
B. 1 tablet
C. 1½ tablets
D. 2 tablets

829. A 32-year-old client was seen at the physician's office with a urinary tract infection. The physician ordered amikacin 250 mg bid. Using a 250 mg/ml vial, how many milliliters did the nurse administer intramuscularly (IM)?
A. 0.5 ml
B. 1.0 ml
C. 1.5 ml
D. 2.0 ml

830. A 25-year-old client with hemophilia was hospitalized for bleeding. The physician ordered aminocaproic acid (Amicar) 5 gms IV loading dose. Using a 250 mg/ml vial, how many milliliters did the nurse add to the IV solution?
A. 5 ml
B. 10 ml
C. 15 ml
D. 20 ml

831. A 78-year-old client was admitted with severe flatulence and dyspepsia. The physician ordered activated charcoal (Charcotabs) 975 mg after meals. On hand were 325 mg tablets. How many tablets did the nurse administer?
A. 1 tablet
B. 2 tablets
C. 3 tablets
D. 4 tablets

832. A 28-year-old renal failure client's laboratory work revealed hyperphosphatemia. The physician ordered aluminum hydroxide (Amphojel) 500 mg. Using a 600 mg/5 ml suspension, how many milliliters did the nurse administer?
A. 2.2 ml
B. 3.2 ml
C. 4.2 ml
D. 5.2 ml

833. A 28-year-old client developed a urinary tract infection with *Escherichia coli* as the causative organism. The physician ordered tetracycline 500 mg qid. Using a 125 mg/5 ml elixir, how many milliliters did the nurse administer?
A. 5.0 ml
B. 10 ml
C. 15 ml
D. 20 ml

834. A 46 kg woman was admitted to the local ER with seizure activity. The physician ordered valproic acid 15 mg/kg (345 mg) bid IM. Using a 250 mg/5 ml vial, how many milliliters did the nurse administer?
A. 1.0 ml
B. 1.2 ml
C. 1.4 ml
D. 1.6 ml

835. An 88-year-old client was admitted for symptoms of transient ischemic attacks. The physician sent the client home with a prescription for aspirin (Ecotrin) 650 mg qid. The nurse instructed the client to take how many 325 mg chewable tablets?
A. ½ tablet
B. 1 tablet
C. 1½ tablets
D. 2 tablets

836. A 54-year-old client developed an adrenocortical carcinoma. The physician ordered mitotane (Lysodren) 3 gms tid. The pharmacist dispensed 500 mg tablets. The nurse instructed the client to take how many tablets?
A. 2 tablets
B. 4 tablets
C. 6 tablets
D. 8 tablets

837. A 12-year-old client was being treated with rifampin 600 mg PO 1 hour before meals as a prevention for TB. The client's father was receiving isoniazid for an active case of TB. The nurse instructed the client to take how many 300 mg tablets?
A. ½ tablet
B. 1 tablet
C. 1½ tablets
D. 2 tablets

838. A 27-year-old client developed a respiratory infection secondary to a tuberculin lung. The physician ordered streptomycin 1 gm every day IM to be given along with antituberculin drugs. Using a 1 gm/ml vial, how many milliliters did the nurse administer IM?
A. 0.5 ml
B. 1.0 ml
C. 1.5 ml
D. 2.0 ml

839. A 25-year-old client with renal failure developed severe polyneuritis. The physician ordered riboflavin (Riobin-50) 25 mg every day. The nurse instructed the client to take how many 50 mg tablets?
A. ½ tablet
B. 1 tablet
C. 1½ tablets
D. 2 tablets

840. A 79-year-old nursing home resident was diagnosed with Parkinson's disease. The physician ordered levodopa 500 mg bid with meals. The nurse administered how many 250 mg tablets?
A. ½ tablet
B. 1 tablet
C. 1½ tablets
D. 2 tablets

841. A 37-year-old head injury client continued to have partial seizures. The physician ordered felbamate (Felbatol) 400 mg tid. Using a 600 mg/5 ml elixir, how many milliliters did the nurse administer?
A. 1.3 ml
B. 2.3 ml
C. 3.3 ml
D. 4.3 ml

842. A 65-year-old client developed dizziness not associated with movement. The physician ordered meclizine (Antivert) 50 mg daily. How many 25 mg chewable tablets must the client take?
A. ½ tablet
B. 1 tablet
C. 1½ tablets
D. 2 tablets

843. A 70-year-old client developed cutaneous larva migrans (creeping eruptions) on the skin. The client weighed 68 kg. The physician ordered thiabendazole (Mintezol) 25 mg/kg (1700 mg). Using a 500 mg/5 ml elixir, how many milliliters did the nurse administer?
A. 15 ml
B. 16 ml
C. 17 ml
D. 18 ml

844. A 30-year-old tuberculin client developed a vitamin B_6 deficiency secondary to ioniazid therapy. The physician ordered pyridoxine 15 mg every day PO. The nurse instructed the client to take how many 10 mg tablets?
A. ½ tablet
B. 1 tablet
C. 1½ tablets
D. 2 tablets

845. A 77-year-old client was diagnosed with pernicious anemia. The physician ordered Betalin 12, 150 μg IM every day times 2 weeks. Using a 120 μg/ml vial, how many milliliters did the nurse administer IM?
A. 0.5 ml
B. 1.0 ml
C. 1.25 ml
D. 1.50 ml

846. A 78-year-old Parkinson's client was given selegiline (Eldepryl) 5 mg at breakfast and lunch as adjunct management of the symptoms. The nurse instructed the client to take how many 5 mg tablets?
A. ½ tablet
B. 1 tablet

C. 1½ tablets
D. 2 tablets

847. A 27-year-old client developed extrapyramidal symptoms secondary to neuroleptic drug therapy. The physician ordered biperiden 2 mg IV. Using a 5 mg/ml vial, how many milliliters did the nurse administer?
A. 0.2 ml
B. 0.4 ml
C. 0.6 ml
D. 0.8 ml

848. The physician ordered theophylline (Bronkodyl) 500 mg every 6 to 8 hours to a 72-year-old client with COPD. The nurse instructed the family members to give how many 250 mg tablets?
A. ½ tablet
B. 1 tablet
C. 1½ tablets
D. 2 tablets

849. A 75-year-old home health client developed acute gouty arthritis. The physician ordered phenylbutazone (Butazolidin) 400 mg PO every 8 hours. The home health nurse instructed the client to take how many 100 mg tablets?
A. 2 tablets
B. 4 tablets
C. 6 tablets
D. 8 tablets

850. A 68-year-old client was admitted with atrial fibrillation. The physician ordered quinidine 200 mg every 2 to 3 hours PO. The nurse administered how many 100 mg tablets?
A. ½ tablet
B. 1 tablet
C. 1½ tablets
D. 2 tablets

851. A 69-year-old client was diagnosed with angina pectoris caused by coronary insufficiency. The physician ordered diltiazem (Cardizem) 30 mg qid PO. How many 60 mg tablets did the nurse administer?
A. ½ tablet
B. 1 tablet
C. 1½ tablets
D. 2 tablets

852. A 28-year-old client was seen in the local ambulatory center with seasonal rhinitis. The physician ordered Claritin 10 mg every day. The nurse instructed the client to take how many 10 mg tablets?
A. ½ tablet
B. 1 tablet
C. 1½ tablets
D. 2 tablets

853. A 90-year-old nursing home resident developed a severe cough that was accompanied by pleurisy pain. The physician treated the cough with hydromorphone (Dilaudid) cough syrup 1 mg PRN. Using a 1 mg/5 ml elixir, how many milliliters did the nurse administer?
A. 2 ml
B. 3 ml
C. 4 ml
D. 5 ml

854. A 72-year-old client with congestive heart failure was admitted to the local ER. The physician ordered furosemide (Lasix) 80 mg IV. Using a 10 mg/ml vial, how many milliliters did the nurse administer?
A. 2 ml
B. 4 ml
C. 6 ml
D. 8 ml

855. A 27-year-old client developed severe allergy symptoms. The physician ordered astemizole (Hismanal) 10 mg every day. The nurse instructed the client to take how many 10 mg tablets?
A. ½ tablet
B. 1 tablet
C. 1½ tablets
D. 2 tablets

856. A 75-year-old nursing home resident developed osteoarthritis. The physician ordered piroxicam (Feldene) 10 mg bid. How many 20 mg tablets did the nurse administer?
A. ½ tablet
B. 1 tablet
C. 1½ tablets
D. 2 tablets

857. A 70-year-old was admitted with congestive heart failure. The physician ordered hydrochlorothiazide (Esidrex) 75 mg daily IM. Using a 100 mg/ml vial, how many milliliters did the nurse administer?
A. 0.55 ml
B. 0.65 ml
C. 0.75 ml
D. 0.85 ml

858. A 37-year-old client was admitted with ulcerative colitis. The physician ordered mesalamine 800 mg tid. How many 400 mg tablets did the nurse administer?
A. ½ tablet
B. 1 tablet
C. 1½ tablets
D. 2 tablets

859. Your client, age 68, is a newly diagnosed non-insulin-dependent diabetic. The physician ordered chlorpropamide (Diabinese) 150 mg PO bid. The pharmacy sent Diabinese 0.1 gm tablets. The nurse will administer how many tablets to the client?
A. 1
B. 1.5

C. 2

D. 2.5

860. The client has undergone a popliteal femoral bypass. Postoperative orders read "Heparin 5,000 units subcutaneously daily." The pharmacy sends a vial containing heparin sodium 10,000 units/ml. How much will the nurse draw up to administer the required dosage?

A. 0.1 cc

B. 0.2 cc

C. 0.5 cc

D. 1.0 cc

861. The client was receiving furosemide (Lasix) 40 mEq for symptoms of congestive heart failure. To replace potassium, the physician ordered potassium chloride (Slow-K) 16 mEq PO bid. The dosage on hand was Slow-K 8 mEq tablets. How many tablets will the client receive?

A. 0.5

B. 1

C. 1.5

D. 2

862. A client developed a dry hacky cough during her hospital stay. She had no history of respiratory problems. The physician ordered promethazine (Phenergan) with codeine gr 1/6 PO every 4 to 6 hours PRN cough. The pharmacy sent Phenergan with codeine solution 10 mg/5 ml. How many cc's (ml) are required to deliver Phenergan with codeine gr 1/6?

A. 1 ml

B. 2 ml

C. 5 ml

D. 10 ml

863. A client, age 18, was undergoing oral surgery to have her wisdom teeth removed. The physician placed her on penicillin V (Pen•Vee) 1 gm PO 1 hour before surgery. The client requested to have the medication in elixir form instead of pill form. The nurse had on hand Pen•Vee K oral suspension 250 mg (400,000 Units) per 5 ml. How many milliliters did the nurse administer to the client?

A. 20 ml

B. 15 ml

C. 10 ml

D. 5 ml

864. The nurse has to administer lactulose 20 gms via a gastric tube. On hand is lactulose syrup 10 gms/15 ml. How much will the nurse give?

A. 1 ml

B. 10 ml

C. 20 ml

D. 30 ml

865. The client was admitted for peptic ulcer. The physician ordered Maalox Plus 30 ml 30 minutes after meals and hour of sleep. How many contain-

ers will be needed from pharmacy for a 24-hour schedule? (Each container holds 30 cc.)

A. 1

B. 4

C. 5

D. 10

866. The client was admitted for severe respiratory distress secondary to acute bronchitis. The physician ordered prednisone 10 mg PO tid. The stock tablets of Prednisone were labeled 2.5 mg. How many tablets would the nurse give?

A. 4

B. 3

C. 2

D. 1

867. A client, age 75, was admitted with left-sided heart failure. The physician ordered digoxin 0.25 mg PO every day. The stock supply contained digoxin 0.5 mg. How many tablets would the nurse have to give?

A. ½

B. 1

C. 1½

D. 2

868. The client had a urinary tract infection. The physician ordered cephalexin (Cephalex) in oral suspension 0.35 gm PO every 6 hours to be given via the gastrostomy tube. The liquid on hand was labeled 125 mg/5 ml. How many milliliters does the nurse have to administer?

A. 10 ml

B. 14 ml

C. 15 ml

D. 20 ml

869. Your client was diagnosed as having hypothyroidism. The physician placed her on levothyroxine (Synthroid) 0.3 mg PO every day. The tablets are labeled 300 μg. How many tablets must the client take?

A. ½

B. 1

C. 2

D. 3

870. The client was having grand mal seizures. The physician ordered phenytoin (Dilantin) suspension 150 mg PO tid to be given via the nasogastric tube. The stock supply was labeled 75 mg/7.5 ml. How many milliliters need to be given to fulfill the order?

A. 7.5

B. 10

C. 15

D. 20

871. The client was admitted for cardiac arrthymias. The physician ordered procainamide hydrochloride 50 mg/kg of body weight PO every day given in equally divided doses every 6 hours. He weighs

185 lb. How much will the client receive for each dose?
A. 1050 mg
B. 900 mg
C. 800 mg
D. 700 mg

872. The client was admitted with a severe vitamin K deficiency secondary to long-term warfarin (Coumadin) therapy. The physician orders vitamin K 150 mg. The oral dose is supplied in 50 mg. How many tablets must the nurse give to deliver 150 mg?
A. 1
B. 2
C. 3
D. 4

873. The client was diagnosed with Parkinson's disease. The physician ordered levodopa (L-dopa) 750 mg tid. What is the total 24-hour dose for this client?
A. 1500 mg
B. 2000 mg
C. 2200 mg
D. 2250 mg

874. The client was having pruritus secondary to severe anxiety. The physician ordered diphenhydramine (Benadryl) 75 mg. Available is Benadryl injection 25 mg/ml in a 10 ml multiple-dose vial. How many milliliters should be administered to the client?
A. ½ ml
B. 1 ml
C. 1½ ml
D. 3 ml

875. A child, age 5, was to be given an injection of penicillin V (V-Cillin K). The dosage was in a 2 ml syringe. What is the maximum dosage to be administered per intramuscular injection to a child 5 years of age?
A. 1 ml
B. 2 ml
C. 3 ml
D. 4 ml

876. A client was receiving morphine sulfate 3–5 mg IV for pain. The physician ordered the morphine to be titrated. The morphine was supplied in a 10 mg/ml single-dose vial. The nurse needed to titrate the morphine with how much normal saline in order to deliver 1 mg/ml?
A. 1 ml
B. 5 ml
C. 7.5 ml
D. 9 ml

877. The client was receiving clindamycin (Cleocin) 150 mg implementation every 12 hours for a wound infection. On hand is Cleocin 300 mg/2 ml. How many milliliters are required to deliver each of the two doses?
A. 1

B. 2
C. 3
D. 4

878. The client, age 5, was having her tonsils removed. The physician ordered atropine sulfate 0.15 mg subcutaneously. Atropine sulfate 0.4 mg/ml is on hand. How much should the nurse draw up?
A. 0.38 ml
B. 0.50 ml
C. 0.75 ml
D. 1 ml

879. The client was diagnosed with strep throat. The physician ordered benzathine penicillin G (Bicillin) 2,400,000 Units implementation stat. The pharmacy sent a 10 ml vial of Bicillin containing 600,000 Units/ml. How many milliliters need to be given?
A. 1 ml
B. 2 ml
C. 3 ml
D. 4 ml

880. The client was admitted for severe nausea and vomiting. The physician ordered trimethobenzamide (Tigan) 200 mg stat, then 100 mg every 6 hours PRN for nausea. The pharmacy dispensed a 2 ml ampule of Tigan containing 100 mg/ml. How many milliliters are given for the stat dose?
A. 1 ml
B. 2 ml
C. 3 ml
D. 4 ml

881. During an emergency situation, the nurse used a tuberculin syringe to draw up 30 units of Humulin R Regular U-100 insulin. How much did the nurse draw up?
A. 0.10 ml
B. 0.20 ml
C. 0.30 ml
D. 0.40 ml

882. The client was undergoing a cholecystectomy in the morning. The physician ordered lorazepam (Ativan) 2.4 mg IM at hour of sleep. On hand was lorazepam 4 mg/ml. How much did the nurse give?
A. 0.3 ml
B. 0.4 ml
C. 0.5 ml
D. 0.6 ml

883. The client was admitted for simple linear cerebral fracture. The physician ordered ticarcillin (Ticar) 500 mg IM every 6 hours. Ticarcillin disodiumma 6 gm vial was available. The instructions read, "For IM use, add 12 diluent to the 6 gm vial and each 2.6 ml of solution will contain 1 gm of drug." How many milliliters will be needed to administer 500 mg?
A. 0.5 ml

B. 1.0 ml

C. 1.3 ml

D. 1.5 ml

884. The client was admitted for a severe urinary tract infection. The physician ordered oxacillin (Prostaphlin) 500 mg IM every 4 hours. The directions on the single unit dose read to dilute the solution with 1.4 ml of diluent. This will reconstitute to provide 250 mg/1.5 ml. How many milliliters are needed to deliver 500 mg?
A. 1.0 ml
B. 1.5 ml
C. 2.5 ml
D. 3.0 ml

885. The client was experiencing severe pain secondary to a migraine headache. The physician's orders read: "Give morphine sulfate 12 mg IM stat for pain." On hand was morphine 15 mg/ml. How many milliliters will the nurse draw up?
A. 0.2 ml
B. 0.4 ml
C. 0.6 ml
D. 0.8 ml

886. The physician ordered carbenicillin disodium 1 gm IM every 6 hours The stock vial of powder was 5 gm. To reconstitute the 5 gm vial, the nurse needed to add 7.0 ml of diluent. Each 2 ml will deliver 1 gm of medication. How many milliliters will the nurse need to draw from the 5 gm vial?
A. 1.0 ml
B. 2.0 ml
C. 2.5 ml
D. 4.0 ml

887. The client was admitted isotonic dehydration. The physician ordered 1000 ml of Ringer's lactate IV to infuse in 12 hours. The nurse placed the solution on an infusion pump. How fast did she set the rate?
A. 50 ml/hr
B. 73 ml/hr
C. 80 ml/hr
D. 83 ml/hr

888. The client was admitted with generalized edema. The physician wanted to limit fluid intake by placing the patient NPO and using 500 ml of normal saline IV to infuse in 4 hours. There was no pump on hand, so the nurse used a tubing that delivered 20 gtt/ml. How many drops per minute are needed to deliver this infusion in 4 hours?
A. 25 gtt/min
B. 30 gtt/min
C. 42 gtt/min
D. 45 gtt/min

889. The order read, "Give 1000 ml D$_5$W in 2 hours. The nurse noticed on the chart that at 0900, the IV was regulated to flow at 125 gtt/min; at 0930, the nurse noted that there was 450 ml left in the bag.

The administration tubing delivers 15 gtt/min. How fast should the flow rate be to finish delivering the required amount?
A. 50 gtt/min
B. 60 gtt/min
C. 70 gtt/min
D. 75 gtt/min

890. The client was experiencing acute renal failure. The physician ordered 500 ml Ringer's lactate IV every day to run in 4 hours. The nurse used a Buretrol with a microdrip administration tubing. How fast will the nurse set the rate?
A. 100 gtt/min
B. 125 gtt/min
C. 130 gtt/min
D. 150 gtt/min

891. Your client was receiving ampicillin 500 mg IV in 50 ml 5% dextrose and ½ normal saline in 30 minutes by an infusion pump. How fast would the nurse set the infusion pump to deliver this medication?
A. 50 ml/hr
B. 100 ml/hr
C. 150 ml/hr
D. 200 ml/hr

892. An 85-year-old client was admitted with isotonic dehydration from the local nursing home. The physician ordered 1800 ml normal saline IV to infuse in 15 hours by controller. How fast would the nurse set the rate?
A. 50 ml/hr
B. 75 ml/hr
C. 100 ml/hr
D. 120 ml/hr

893. The nurse was calculating the IV flow rate for 1200 ml of normal saline to be infused in 6 hours. The infusion set is calibrated for a drop factor of 15 gtt/ml. How fast will the nurse set the rate?
A. 50 gtt/min
B. 100 gtt/min
C. 150 gtt/min
D. 200 gtt/min

894. The postoperative patient returned from surgery with the following orders: "Infuse 3000 ml D$_5$W IV over 24 hours." The nurse noted that the IV tubing delivered 10 gtt/ml. How fast should the rate be set?
A. 10 gtt/min
B. 15 gtt/min
C. 20 gtt/min
D. 21 gtt/min

895. The client was receiving ampicillin 250 mg in 100 ml of normal saline. The physician ordered the IV piggyback to infuse in 40 min. The IV tubing delivers 20 gtt/min. How fast should the rate be set?
A. 15 gtt/min
B. 20 gtt/min

C. 30 gtt/min
D. 50 gtt/min

896. A 78-year-old client was receiving D_5W ½ normal saline IV with 20 mEq potassium chloride (KCl) per liter to infuse at 25 ml/hr. The IV tubing delivered 60 gtt/ml. How fast should the rate be set?
A. 25 gtt/min
B. 50 gtt/min
C. 75 gtt/min
D. 100 gtt/min

897. A 28-year-old cancer patient was admitted to receive two 500-cc units of whole blood in 4 hours. The Y tubing delivers 20 gtt/min. How fast should the rate be set?
A. 63 gtt/min
B. 73 gtt/min
C. 83 gtt/min
D. 93 gtt/min

898. Hyperalimentation solution is ordered for 1500 ml to infuse in 12 hours using an infusion set with tubing calibrated for 20 gtt/min. How fast should the rate be set?
A. 30 gtt/min
B. 32 gtt/min
C. 40 gtt/min
D. 42 gtt/min

899. The physician ordered cefazolin (Kefzol) 0.5 gm in 100 ml D_5W IV piggyback to run over 30 minutes. The piggyback was to be infused as a secondary IV on a controller. How fast should the rate be set to deliver milliliters per hour?
A. 100 ml
B. 150 ml
C. 200 ml
D. 250 ml

900. Cefazolin (Ancef) 1 gm in 100 cc D_5W IVPB was ordered to infuse in 45 minutes. The primary tubing delivers 60 gtt/min. How fast should the rate be set?
A. 123 gtt/min
B. 133 gtt/min
C. 143 gtt/min
D. 153 gtt/min

901. The physician ordered cefazolin (Ancef) 1 gm in 100 cc normal saline to infuse IVPB by an automatic controller in 30 min. How fast should the rate be set?
A. 50 ml/hr
B. 100 ml/hr
C. 150 ml/hr
D. 200 ml/hr

902. The physician ordered carbenicillin disodium (Geopen) 2 gm IVPB diluted in 50 ml D_5W to infuse in 15 minutes. The IV tubing delivers 15 gtt/ml. How fast should the rate be set?
A. 15 gtt/min

B. 20 gtt/min
C. 30 gtt/min
D. 50 gtt/min

903. The nurse decided to place the carbenicillin disodium 2 gms diluted in 50 ml of D_5W on an electronic infusion pump. The physician ordered the medication to go in 15 minutes. The flow rate will be:
A. 100 ml/hr
B. 200 ml/hr
C. 300 ml/hr
D. 400 ml/hr

904. The physician ordered 2000 ml normal saline to be infused on a diabetic client for 12 hours. The IV tubing delivers 10 gtt/ml. After 8 hours, the nurse found that there was 750 ml remaining. The flow rate needs to be adjusted to deliver how much?
A. 25 gtt/min
B. 31 gtt/min
C. 40 gtt/min
D. 42 gtt/min

905. At the beginning of the shift, the nurse added 1000 ml D_5W to the IV and set the rate to infuse in 8 hours. The tubing delivered 20 gtt/ml. After 4 hours, there was 800 ml remaining. The nurse adjusted the flow rate to:
A. 37 gtt/min
B. 47 gtt/min
C. 57 gtt/min
D. 67 gtt/min

906. The physician ordered 1500 ml D_5 lactated Ringer's IV to run KVO (keep vein open) for 24 hours. The IV tubing delivers 60 gtt/ml. The flow rate will be set on:
A. 50 gtt/min
B. 52 gtt/min
C. 60 gtt/min
D. 62 gtt/min

907. The physician ordered 500 ml D_5W IV every 4 hours. The order was written at 1515 and the IV was started at 1530. At 1800, the IV was significantly behind schedule. The nurse decided to place the IV on an electronic controller to better regulate the flow rate. The physician wanted 500 ml to infuse in 4 hours. The nurse set the controller at a rate of:
A. 75 cc/hr
B. 100 cc/hr
C. 125 cc/hr
D. 150 cc/hr

908. The physician orders amoxicillin 250 mg in 50 ml D_5W IVPB to infuse in 30 minutes qid. The client was on an electronic controller. The nurse set the rate to deliver:
A. 50 ml/hr

B. 75 ml/hr
C. 100 ml/hr
D. 150 ml/hr

909. At the beginning of the 7 to 3 shift, the nurse noted that an IV bag of D_5W was infusing at the rate of 25 gtt/min. The infusion set is calibrated for a drop factor of 15 gtt/ml. How much can you anticipate the client to receive during this 8-hour shift?
A. 500 ml/8 hr
B. 600 ml/8 hr
C. 700 ml/8 hr
D. 800 ml/8 hr

910. The physician ordered 80 ml D_5W IV at 20 micro-drops per minute. The drop factor is 60 gtt/ml. How long will the IV infuse?
A. 1 hour
B. 2 hours
C. 3 hours
D. 4 hours

911. A 72-year-old client was admitted for lung biopsy to rule out cancer. In order to facilitate the endotracheal intubation, the physician ordered succinylcholine (Anectine) 25 mg IV slowly. Using a 20 mg/ml vial, how many milliliters did the nurse administer?
A. 0.5 ml
B. 1.0 ml
C. 1.25 ml
D. 1.50 ml

Answers

1. (C) Nursing process phase: implementation; client need: safe, effective care environment; content area: medical/surgical nursing

Rationale
(A) It is not necessary for the client to be NPO if his gag and swallowing reflexes are intact. (B) The vital signs should have been checked frequently during the past hour; it is more important to be certain that the client can swallow without aspirating. (C) If the gag and swallowing reflexes are not intact, the client is in danger of aspirating. (D) Coughing and deep breathing could initiate hemorrhage immediately following a bronchoscopy.

2. (D) Nursing process phase: implementation; client need: safe, effective care environment; content area: medical/surgical nursing

Rationale
(A) The client could be injured more by inserting a tongue blade into the mouth. (B) A client who is restrained and thrashing about in a grand mal seizure could sustain body injury. (C) An unconscious client should not be on his back unless the client is intubated. (D) This action helps to maintain an open airway and allows drainage of secretions.

3. (B) Nursing process phase: assessment; client need: physiological integrity; content area: medical/surgical nursing

Rationale
(A) The femoral and popliteal pulses are between the heart and the cast; therefore, they do not require frequent assessment. (B) The cast could interfere with circulation or nerve supply to the toes. (C) No data have been provided to indicate that the toes may be moved. A physician must approve any movement in a fractured extremity. (D) The pedal pulses are covered by the cast in the affected extremity.

4. (A) Nursing process phase: evaluation; client need: safe, effective care environment; content area: medical/surgical nursing

Rationale
(A) If the weights are resting on any object, the purpose of the traction is defeated. (B) The body must remain in proper alignment; some positions are contraindicated. (C) Only mild discomfort should be experienced when the muscle spasms cease. (D) Clients in traction need a lot of diversional activity.

5. (C) Nursing process phase: evaluation; client need: safe, effective care environment; content area: medical/surgical nursing

Rationale
(A) A normal value for the partial thromboplastin time (PTT) does not indicate that the therapy is being effective. (B) A PTT only 1 to 1.5 times normal indicates that the therapy is not as effective as it could be. (C) The best indicator that heparin therapy is being effective is a PTT of 2 to 2.5 times normal. (D) If the PTT is three times the control, the client is in danger of hemorrhaging.

6. (B) Nursing process phase: planning; client need: physiological integrity; content area: medical/surgical nursing

Rationale
(A) Vitamin K is an antidote for warfarin but not heparin. (B) Protamine sulfate neutralizes heparin. (C) Epinephrine is used only to arrest local bleeding. (D) Norepinephrine is not used to treat bleeding disorders.

7. (D) Nursing process phase: implementation; client need: safe, effective care environment; content area: medical/surgical nursing

Rationale
(A) Maalox Plus does not interact with Coumadin. (B) Tylenol does not interact with Coumadin. (C) Sudafed does not interact with Coumadin. (D) Aspirin prevents aggregation of platelets; therefore, the client's risk of bleeding would be much greater.

8. (B) Nursing process phase: analysis; client need: health promotion and maintenance; content area: medical/surgical nursing

Rationale
(A) The physician does not need to be notified because all vital signs are normal except the temperature. A slight elevation of temperature can be caused by the inflammatory process resulting from the surgery. (B) The temperature does need to be observed frequently to rule out some cause other than the in-

flammatory process. (C) A thorough respiratory assessment is not indicated at this time. (D) Most physicians want to make the first dressing change themselves. Until they have an order for a dressing change, nurses should only reinforce dressings.

9. **(A)** Nursing process phase: evaluation; client need: health promotion and maintenance; content area: medical/surgical nursing

Rationale

(A) This way of cutting helps prevent ingrown nails, which could become the site of an infection for a diabetic. (B) Substitutions may be made within an exchange in the diet developed by the American Diabetes Association and the American Dietetic Association. (C) Injection sites should be rotated according to a regular schedule. (D) More calories from carbohydrates are needed prior to exercise in order to keep the serum glucose within normal limits.

10. **(C)** Nursing process phase: analysis; client need: psychosocial integrity; content area: medical/surgical nursing

Rationale

(A) The client needs to face the seriousness of her diagnosis when she is ready. (B) Encouraging her would be offering false hope. (C) The client needs to face reality and deal with her feelings when she is ready. (D) Denial is a stage in the grieving process; a reprimand would not be appropriate.

11. **(A)** Nursing process phase: assessment; client need: health promotion and maintenance; content area: medical/surgical nursing

Rationale

(A) Most protocols in chemotherapy contain drugs that depress the bone marrow. Bone marrow depression would be revealed in the complete blood count. (B) The most serious complication of chemotherapy is depression of bone marrow. (C) The prothrombin time is not usually affected by chemotherapy. (D) These tests are not usually done daily.

12. **(D)** Nursing process phase: analysis; client need: safe, effective care environment; content area: medical/surgical nursing

Rationale

(A) Fluid-volume deficit is not caused directly by bone marrow depression. (B) Aspiration does not usually result from bone marrow depression. (C) This nursing diagnosis might be appropriate after the client developed an infection. (D) White cells are almost always depressed with depression of bone marrow. A decrease in the number of white cells places a client at high risk for infection.

13. **(D)** Nursing process phase: evaluation; client need: safe, effective care environment; content area: medical/surgical nursing

Rationale

(A) The statement is not accurate. (B) Radioactivity is a concern for clients receiving treatment with radioactive isotopes. (C) The entire body will not be radioactive. (D) Body fluids will be radioactive until the isotope has been eliminated from the body.

14. **(B)** Nursing process phase: implementation; client need: safe, effective care environment; content area: medical/surgical nursing

Rationale

(A) Only a physician can replace the implant. (B) This is the recommended way to handle the situation. (C) The patient and others would be exposed to radiation unnecessarily. (D) Lead shields do not stop radiation from all isotopes.

15. **(A)** Nursing process phase: implementation; client need: safe, effective care environment; content area: medical/surgical nursing

Rationale

(A) The IV is infiltrated and should be removed. (B) This would result in injury to the client. (C) This action would cause a delay and injury to the client. (D) This action would not correct the problem.

16. **(D)** Nursing process phase: implementation; client need: safe, effective care environment; content area: medical/surgical nursing

Rationale

(A) Hyperglycemia would probably result. (B) Notifying the physician is not necessary at this time. (C) The client could be hypoglycemic. (D) The level of serum glucose needs to be known prior to taking further action.

17. **(A)** Nursing process phase: planning; client need: safe, effective care environment; content area: medical/surgical nursing

Rationale

(A) Decreasing the workload on the heart is the highest priority for someone in acute congestive heart failure. (B) The client needs both physical and mental rest. (C) The data do not indicate that the client is ready to train for a new job. (D) Decreasing the workload on the heart takes a higher priority at this time.

18. **(C)** Nursing process phase: assessment; client need: physiological integrity; content area: medical/surgical nursing

Rationale

(A) Serum cholesterol levels do not need frequent assessment. (B) The popliteal pulses do not reflect full assessment of the graft. (C) The presence of pedal pulses indicates that the graft is functioning. (D) Cardiac enzyme levels are not indicated.

19. **(B)** Nursing process phase: analysis; client need: health promotion and maintenance; content area: medical/surgical nursing

Rationale

(A) Ketones would be an abnormal finding. (B) A trace of protein in urine is normal. (C) No glucose should be found in urine. (D) Cloudy urine indicates that infection is present.

20. **(B)** Nursing process phase: assessment; client need: safe, effective care environment; content area: medical/surgical nursing

Rationale

(A) Blood pressure should never be taken in an arm where a shunt is located. (B) Palpation of a thrill and hearing a bruit indicate that the shunt is open. (C) This assessment is not indicated. (D) The arm is not a good place to assess for skin turgor.

21. **(A)** Nursing process phase: implementation; client need:

safe, effective care environment; content area: medical/surgical nursing

Rationale
(A) The signs of hypoglycemia should be evident and prompt action is needed before the blood glucose level goes lower. (B) The serum glucose could continue to drop while the serum glucose is being checked. (C) Insulin would lower the blood glucose level even more. (D) This action also would cause delay; therefore, it should not be the first action to be taken. If brain cells are deprived of glucose, brain damage results.

22. **(C)** Nursing process phase: assessment; client need: physiological integrity; content area: medical/surgical nursing

Rationale
(A) The risk of a sodium imbalance is not as great as the risk for a potassium imbalance. (B) Calcium imbalance is not usually associated with diabetic ketoacidosis. (C) During the acidotic phase, potassium left the cells in exchange for hydrogen ions and was subsequently lost from the body. (D) The risk of a magnesium imbalance is not as great as the risk of a potassium imbalance.

23. **(A)** Nursing process phase: assessment; client need: health promotion and maintenance; content area: medical/surgical nursing

Rationale
(A) The Mantoux may be read in 3 days and will reveal whether the tubercle bacillus has entered the client's body. (B) An x-ray will expose the client to radiation. (C) The client could have tuberculosis with a sputum negative for acid-fast bacilli. (D) Gram stain is only a quick method of ruling out acid-fast bacilli in the sputum.

24. **(C)** Nursing process phase: evaluation; client need: health promotion and maintenance; content area: medical/surgical nursing

Rationale
(A & C) A positive reading for the Mantoux test is an induration greater than 10 mm. (B) Swelling does not indicate a positive reaction. (D) An exudate does not indicate a positive reaction to the PPD.

25. **(D)** Nursing process phase: evaluation; client need: health promotion and maintenance; content area: medical/surgical nursing

Rationale
(A) Calling the physician first would delay time in stopping the blood. (B) Giving aspirin would delay discontinuing the blood. (C) The client does not need another IV access. (D) The client is having a reaction to the blood; it should be stopped immediately.

26. **(D)** Nursing process phase: assessment; client need: physiological integrity; content area: medical/surgical nursing

Rationale
(A) The cells of the blood are not usually affected by the drugs being taken. (B) The data do not indicate that kidney function is compromised. (C) Blood coagulation should not be affected, nor will it affect the medications. (D) Electrolyte imbalances may be caused by Lasix; such imbalances can cause

digoxin toxicity even when serum levels of digoxin are within normal range.

27. **(C)** Nursing process phase: implementation; client need: physiological integrity; content area: medical/surgical nursing

Rationale
(A) The client would probably develop adrenal insufficiency if this were done. (B) If this were done, the client would receive too much prednisone. (C) This action should be taken in order to decrease the dosage gradually so that adrenocorticotropic hormone (ACTH) could build up again and stimulate the adrenal gland to function. (D) Adrenal insufficiency could develop.

28. **(C)** Nursing process phase: implementation; client need: physiological integrity; content area: medical/surgical nursing

Rationale
(A) It is more important to allow the punctured side to heal initially by positioning the client on the unaffected side. (B) The client is usually positioned in a sitting position prior to the procedure to allow fluid to pool in the base of the pleural space. (C) Placing the client on the unaffected side allows the puncture site to close. (D) Positioning the client in Fowler's position is not necessary after the procedure, but may provide comfort to the client.

29. **(A)** Nursing process phase: implementation; client need: physiological integrity; content area: medical/surgical nursing

Rationale
(A) The Pleur Evac must be kept below the level of the wound to prevent backward flow of drainage due to gravity. (B) The suction should not be removed for turning. (C) This is not recommended because blood could continue to collect in the pleural cavity and collapse the lung. (D) The sterile water should not be drained from the Pleur Evac.

30. **(D)** Nursing process phase: implementation; client need: physiological integrity; content area: medical/surgical nursing

Rationale
(A) Sterile gauze would not put a seal around the catheter. (B) Kerlix would not provide a seal. (C) This would not be necessary. (D) This dressing provides sterility and a seal around the catheter.

31. **(C)** Nursing process phase: implementation; client need: physiological integrity; content area: medical/surgical nursing

Rationale
(A) Nasogastric tubes should be checked for placement before anything is put into them. (B) Clients with nasogastric tubes following a gastrectomy should not have the tubes repositioned. (C) Nasogastric tubes should be checked for placement, usually by x-ray. (D) These tubes should not be inserted farther after placement has been verified (usually by x-ray).

32. **(D)** Nursing process phase: implementation; client need: physiological integrity; content area: medical/surgical nursing

Rationale

(A) This would open the respiratory tract. (B) The respiratory tract would be open. (C) Aspiration could result. (D) The epiglottis would be covering the respiratory tract.

33. **(C)** Nursing process phase: implementation; client need: physiological integrity; content area: medical/surgical nursing

Rationale

(A) If aspirin is given to anyone who has influenza and who is under the age of 18, Reye's syndrome could result. (B) Enteric-coated aspirin would not prevent Reye's syndrome. (C) Tylenol could be given safely to lower the temperature. (D) All products containing aspirin must also be avoided.

34. **(D)** Nursing process phase: implementation; client need: physiological integrity; content area: medical/surgical nursing

Rationale

(A & B) This drug is given to control seizure activity on a daily basis. (C) This drug is used for absence seizures. (D) Valium is the drug of choice to terminate the seizures of status epilepticus.

35. **(C)** Nursing process phase: implementation; client need: psychosocial integrity; content area: medical/surgical nursing

Rationale

(A) Exercise is important but not the most immediate concern. (B) Diversion will help, but handling feelings is a more immediate concern. (C) One manages feelings by talking about them; time should be planned for the client to explore and share feelings. (D) The client may not want to socialize with different people until after feelings are managed.

36. **(D)** Nursing process phase: planning; client need: health promotion and maintenance; content area: medical/surgical nursing

Rationale

(A) Vitamin C would help render the urine acid; therefore, it would not help prevent formation of another uric acid stone. (B) Low calcium would not help prevent a uric acid stone. (C) Fiber is not known to be helpful in preventing stones. (D) An end product of purine metabolism is uric acid. A low-purine diet would help prevent formation of another uric acid stone.

37. **(D)** Nursing process phase: implementation; client need: safe, effective care environment; content area: medical/surgical nursing

Rationale

(A) Antiemetics often have serious side effects. (B) The T-tube should not be removed yet. (C) Physicians irrigate T-tubes. (D) A few days following surgery, T-tubes may be clamped for meals to aid in digestion of fat.

38. **(A)** Nursing process phase: implementation; client need: safe, effective care environment; content area: medical/surgical nursing

Rationale

(A) Abduction of the legs will maintain the left hip in proper alignment. (B) The knees may be flexed, but this is not necessary. (C) Internal rotation would throw the left hip out of

alignment. (D) Adduction would throw the left hip out of alignment.

39. **(D)** Nursing process phase: implementation; client need: safe, effective care environment; content area: medical/surgical nursing

Rationale

(A) Postoperative complications from immobility would result. (B) Turning himself could result in injury to the spine. (C) Injury to the spine would be likely. (D) Log-rolling every 2 hours is safe and helps prevent postoperative complications.

40. **(D)** Nursing process phase: implementation; client need: safe, effective care environment; content area: medical/surgical nursing

Rationale

(A) Checking for allergies would be important, but is not the best action to take to protect the kidneys. (B) A low protein diet is not necessary. (C) Enemas would make the patient less hydrated. (D) The contrast medium is potentially nephrotoxic; it should be diluted as much as possible to prevent damage to renal tubules.

41. **(A)** Nursing process phase: implementation; client need: safe, effective care environment; content area: medical/surgical nursing

Rationale

(A) A laxative is needed to clean the barium out of the gastrointestinal system. (B) The barium needs to be cleaned out of the body. (C) High fiber would not be sufficient to clean out the barium. (D) A sitz bath would not remove the barium from the body.

42. **(D)** Nursing process phase: implementation; client need: safe, effective care environment; content area: medical/surgical nursing

Rationale

(A) The heart is not the source of the problem. (B) Fluid volume is not the source of the problem. (C) Obtaining arterial blood gases first would delay the administration of oxygen, the highest priority for the client at this time. (D) The signs and symptoms indicate that the client has a fat embolism. Oxygen and supportive therapy are needed to prevent death.

43. **(A)** Nursing process phase: planning; client need: safe, effective care environment; content area: medical/surgical nursing

Rationale

(A) Use of a hair piece is an appropriate solution to the problem of alopecia. (B) Ice caps could prevent the drugs from reaching all areas of the circulatory system, and some malignant cells could escape destruction. (C) Perms will contribute to the loss of hair. (D) Brushing will contribute to the loss of hair.

44. **(D)** Nursing process phase: analysis; client need: physiological integrity; content area: medical/surgical nursing

Rationale

(A) A decrease in platelets could cause bleeding, not fatigue. (B) Decreased granulocytes would not cause these problems. (C) Decreased lymphocytes would not cause these problems. (D) A decrease in erythrocytes could cause fatigue and impaired gas exchange due to the decreased ability of the blood to carry oxygen.

45. **(D)** Nursing process phase: implementation; client need: safe, effective care environment; content area: medical/surgical nursing

Rationale
(A) Intramuscular injections could initiate hemorrhage. (B) Massaging injection sites would encourage bleeding. (C) Firm toothbrushes and vigorous flossing could cause bleeding. (D) Rectal procedures could initiate hemorrhage.

46. **(A)** Nursing process phase: evaluation; client need: health promotion and maintenance; content area: medical/surgical nursing

Rationale
(A) Potassium will be lost in the stools and should be replaced. (B) Many people with diarrhea are allergic to lactose in milk or milk products. (C) A healthy diet is rich in fiber. People with diarrhea should have a low-residue diet, which is low in fiber. (D) Drinks containing caffeine could make diarrhea worse.

47. **(A)** Nursing process phase: implementation; client need: safe, effective care environment; content area: medical/surgical nursing

Rationale
(A) Careful and frequent hand washing is most important in prevention of infection. Both the disease and therapy are placing this client at high risk for infection. (B) The antineoplastic drugs could cause thrombocytopenia; therefore, vigorous brushing and flossing would be contraindicated. (C) Fresh fruits and vegetables carry bacteria. (D) Rectal procedures could be a source of infection.

48. **(B)** Nursing process phase: implementation; client need: safe, effective care environment; content area: medical/surgical nursing

Rationale
(A) Antiemetics should be administered 30 minutes before meals to give them a chance to take effect. (B) Fluid imbalance could easily result from nausea and vomiting. (C) Foods cold or at room temperature are usually better tolerated. (D) Stimuli should be minimized in order to decrease the chances of stimulating the center for nausea and vomiting.

49. **(C)** Nursing process phase: analysis; client need: physiological integrity; content area: medical/surgical nursing

Rationale
(A) Infection would produce purulent drainage. (B) Dehiscence would occur prior to evisceration. (C) Excessive serous drainage is a sign that dehiscence could occur. (D) A hematoma would cause swelling at the site; no data exist to suggest swelling.

50. **(B)** Nursing process phase: analysis; client need: safe, effective care environment; content area: medical/surgical nursing

Rationale
(A) The data do not support addiction. (B) Tolerance can develop to the pain-relieving effects of morphine. However, tolerance does not develop to the side effect of pupil con-

striction. (C) Data do not exist to support malingering; therefore, the client should be considered the authority on the pain. (D) The data are insufficient to support this answer.

51. **(A)** Nursing process phase: analysis; client need: physiological integrity; content area: medical/surgical nursing

Rationale
(A) Epinephrine is the drug of choice for anaphylactic shock; a nurse should recognize the signs and be prepared to assist the physician. (B) Treatment for anaphylaxis would be delayed. (C) Cortisol is not the drug of choice for anaphylaxis. (D) Aminophyllin is not the drug of choice for anaphylactic shock.

52. **(D)** Nursing process phase: analysis; client need: physiological integrity; content area: medical/surgical nursing

Rationale
(A–D) An open airway is the highest priority in anaphylactic shock because brain cells will die within 6 minutes of anoxia.

53. **(D)** Nursing process phase: analysis; client need: physiological integrity; content area: medical/surgical nursing

Rationale
(A) Emergency surgery is not necessary and would delay the needed treatment. (B) Effective treatment should prevent respiratory arrest. (C) A tracheostomy is not indicated. (D) The data indicate laryngeal edema and a need for an endotracheal tube to maintain an open airway.

54. **(A)** Nursing process phase: analysis; client need: physiological integrity; content area: medical/surgical nursing

Rationale
(A) Dilatation of the pupil is contraindicated because the canal of Schlemm could be blocked. Blockage of this canal would lead to even greater pressure in the eye. (B) Constriction of the pupil would not close the route of drainage from the eye. (C) Constriction of blood vessels to the eye would help decrease the pressure in the eye. (D) A decreased heart rate could lead to a decreased blood pressure; this might help decrease pressure in the eye.

55. **(D)** Nursing process phase: assessment; client need: safe, effective care environment; content area: medical/surgical nursing

Rationale
(A) This is not the best answer; the serum glucose will give more accurate information. (B) It is more important to check the serum glucose. If injection sites are not rotated, a local reaction in the tissues is the worst thing that could happen. (C) The serum glucose level does not give the information needed. (D) If insulin is given when the serum glucose is too low, hypoglycemic coma could result.

56. **(C)** Nursing process phase: planning; client need: safe, effective care environment; content area: medical/surgical nursing

Rationale
(A) This drug does not affect the heart. (B) The drug does not affect respirations. (C) Fluids must be forced to prevent

crystalluria and renal damage. (D) Blood pressure is not affected by the drug.

57. **(C)** Nursing process phase: analysis; client need: safe, effective care environment; content area: medical/surgical nursing

Rationale
(A) Although tolerance does develop to Valium, addiction to the drug is a bigger problem. (B) Respiratory depression does not usually occur with normal doses of the drug. (C) More people become addicted to this drug than any other drug. (D) Anaphylaxis does not usually occur when this drug is given.

58. **(A)** Nursing process phase: implementation; client need: safe, effective care environment; content area: medical/surgical nursing

Rationale
(A) Alcohol is a central nervous system depressant that can potentiate the effects of other central nervous system depressants. It could cause death if combined with another depressant of the central nervous system. (B) Taking the pulse rate is not part of the standard procedure for clients on central nervous system depressants. (C) Clients should not drive at all while taking central nervous system depressants. (D) Tolerance develops to the effects of caffeine; it is not necessary to decrease consumption.

59. **(D)** Nursing process phase: analysis; client need: physiological integrity; content area: medical/surgical nursing

Rationale
(A) Cyanosis would not occur until a sufficient amount of hemoglobin was reduced to produce the color. (B) Structural changes in the body must occur before clubbing would appear. (C) Tachypnea would not be seen until compensation for hypoxia occurred. (D) Restlessness can occur when the blood supply to the brain decreases; it is one of the earliest signs of hypoxia.

60. **(A)** Nursing process phase: analysis; client need: physiological integrity; content area: medical/surgical nursing

Rationale
(A) Reduced hemoglobin causes the color of cyanosis. (B) Sufficient hemoglobin must be reduced before cyanosis appears. (C) Diffusion of oxygen into the cell is not blocked. (D) A change in the pH of the blood does not cause cyanosis.

61. **(B)** Nursing process phase: implementation; client need: safe, effective care environment; content area: medical/surgical nursing

Rationale
(A) Clients with adult respiratory distress syndrome do not have carbon dioxide narcosis, a condition in which a low concentration of oxygen is the only drive for breathing. (B) Avoiding the complications caused by oxygen toxicity is the reason for giving the lowest concentration of oxygen possible. (C) Lung compliance is not increased by low concentrations of oxygen. (D) Surfactant production is not increased by low concentrations of inspired oxygen.

62. **(C)** Nursing process phase: implementation; client

need: safe, effective care environment; content area: medical/surgical nursing

Rationale
(A) Cough medications do not usually contain a mucolytic agent. (B) Depressing the cough reflex does not help remove infectious material from the lungs. (C) An expectorant is needed to promote removal of secretions from the lungs. (D) Relaxing the bronchioles would not promote removal of secretions.

63. **(B)** Nursing process phase: implementation; client need: psychosocial integrity; content area: medical/surgical nursing

Rationale
(A) Some clients do not want to know everything. (B) The nurse knows which explanations are needed but should take cues from the client about how much information to give. (C) The client may be too anxious to learn relaxation exercises. (D) The client may not be in a mood for humor.

64. **(C)** Nursing process phase: evaluation; client need: safe, effective care environment; content area: medical/surgical nursing

Rationale
(A) The client should rest and take medication for 15 minutes to see if the chest pain goes away. Under no circumstances should the client drive to an emergency room. (B) The client also needs to consume a diet low in saturated fat. (C) This statement is true. Constipation could lead to use of the Valsalva maneuver, which is contraindicated for clients following myocardial infarction. (D) The client should not take over-the-counter medication without the physician's approval.

65. **(D)** Nursing process phase: analysis; client need: safe, effective care environment; content area: medical/surgical nursing

Rationale
(A) A side effect of opiates is not diarrhea. (B) Urinary retention is not a side effect of opiates. (C) Opiates do not usually impair adjustment. (D) Constipation is a common side effect of opiates.

66. **(A)** Nursing process phase: implementation; client need: physiological integrity; content area: medical/surgical nursing

Rationale
(A) Because the origin of the pain is not known, it is not safe to give a laxative. A complication of the pain, such as a ruptured appendix, could occur. (B) The data do not support a contraindication for a laxative. (C) Laxatives are not contraindicated for either renal or hepatic failure. (D) Fluid and electrolyte balance might be affected by a laxative, but abdominal pain would be a better answer.

67. **(D)** Nursing process phase: assessment; client need: safe, effective care environment; content area: medical/surgical nursing

Rationale
(A) A change in blood pressure is not an early sign of digoxin toxicity. (B) A change in respirations is not an early sign of digoxin toxicity. (C) The radial pulse is not the most accurate reflection of cardiac activity. (D) The apical pulse is the most accurate way to assess for an arrhythmia.

68. (C) Nursing process phase: implementation; client need: physiological integrity; content area: medical/surgical nursing

Rationale

(A & C) The client may be having a myocardial infarction. The rescue squad can probably be reached sooner and should have emergency equipment available. (B) The client should receive emergency care immediately because he may be having a myocardial infarction. (D) If the client has a myocardial infarction, he could endanger himself and others.

69. (D) Nursing process phase: analysis; client need: safe, effective care environment; content area: medical/surgical nursing

Rationale

(A) Beta-adrenergic receptors are not located in the kidneys. (B) Beta-adrenergic receptors are not located in the stomach. (C) Beta-adrenergic receptors are not located in the liver. (D) Beta-adrenergic receptors are located on both the airways and the heart. A nonselective agonist would affect all beta receptors.

70. (C) Nursing process phase: evaluation; client need: safe, effective care environment; content area: medical/surgical nursing

Rationale

(A) The prothrombin time is the test used to follow Coumadin therapy. (B) The antidote for Coumadin is vitamin K. (C) Aspirin prevents the aggregation of platelets; therefore, it would place the client at higher risk for bleeding. (C) Consuming large quantities of vitamin K could antagonize the anticoagulant effects of Coumadin.

71. (C) Nursing process phase: planning; client need: safe, effective care environment; content area: medical/surgical nursing

Rationale

(A) Arterial vasodilatation would not decrease preload. (B) Arterial vasodilatation would not decrease stroke volume. (C) Arterial vasodilatation would decrease afterload, thus reducing the workload on the heart. (D) Arterial vasodilatation would not decrease heart rate.

72. (A) Nursing process phase: analysis; client need: health promotion and maintenance; content area: medical/surgical nursing

Rationale

(A) The signs and symptoms may all be related to hyperthyroidism; the thyroid gland is usually enlarged with this condition. (B) The signs and symptoms do not point to a fluid or electrolyte imbalance. (C) The data do not support a problem in the nervous system. (D) The data do not indicate that the problem is in the nervous system.

73. (C) Nursing process phase: planning; client need: safe, effective care environment; content area: medical/surgical nursing

Rationale

(A) The thyroid will be reduced in size and vascularity as a result of this medication. (B) The medication will not have this effect. (C) One reason for giving this medication is to induce a euthyroid state. (D) The medication will not have this effect.

74. (B) Nursing process phase: planning; client need: safe, effective care environment; content area: medical/surgical nursing

Rationale

(A) Norepinephrine is not one of the counter-regulatory agents that oppose the actions of insulin. (B) Cortisol is one of the counter-regulatory hormones. (C) Acetylcholine does not oppose the actions of insulin. (D) Aldosterone does not oppose the actions of insulin.

75. (D) Nursing process phase: planning; client need: safe, effective care environment; content area: medical/surgical nursing

Rationale

(A) Prednisone does not decrease epinephrine. (B) Prednisone does not decrease norepinephrine. (C) Prednisone does not decrease dopamine. (D) Prednisone does decrease release of cortisol by way of a negative feedback loop on ACTH and corticotropin-releasing factor. All clients on this drug should understand this in order to prevent adrenal insufficiency.

76. (B) Nursing process phase: implementation; client need: safe, effective care environment; content area: medical/surgical nursing

Rationale

(A) Thyroid medication is discontinued 4 to 6 weeks before a scan. (B) The dose of radioactive material will not be dangerous to the client or to others. (C) The client should fast after midnight. (D) Thyroid scans do not require an enema afterward.

77. (A) Nursing process phase: analysis; client need: safe, effective care environment; content area: medical/surgical nursing

Rationale

(A) The serum level of thyroxine (the major thyroid hormone) is the best basic screening tool and is used to monitor response to treatment. (B) Thyroxine is converted to T_3 in the tissues; therefore, T_4 is a better indicator of thyroid activity. (C) TSH levels do not indicate thyroid activity. (D) Epinephrine levels are influenced by many factors.

78. (D) Nursing process phase: assessment; client need: safe, effective care environment; content area: medical/surgical nursing

Rationale

(A) It would be most unlikely that all four parathyroid glands would have been removed by a biopsy. (B) Vomiting is not a usual complication of thyroid biopsy. (C) Damage to the laryngeal nerve, the usual cause of hoarseness, would not be likely. (D) Bleeding and/or edema are possible; both could lead to respiratory difficulty.

79. (C) Nursing process phase: implementation; client need: safe, effective care environment; content area: medical/surgical nursing

Rationale

(A) Epinephrine is not usually required following a thyroidectomy. (B) Potassium is not usually required following a thyroidectomy. (C) An intravenous preparation of calcium does need to be available to treat possible hypocalcemia resulting from removal of the parathyroid glands. (D) A suture removal set is not part of the emergency equipment that needs to be available following a thyroidectomy.

80. (C) Nursing process phase: analysis; client need: physiological integrity; content area: medical/surgical nursing

Rationale

(A) The data support only hypocalcemia. (B) Hyperparathyroidism would be most unusual following a thyroidectomy. (C) Trousseau's sign is a sign of hypocalcemia, a possible complication of a thyroidectomy. (D) Nerve damage would be unusual.

81. (A) Nursing process phase: analysis; client need: physiological integrity; content area: medical/surgical nursing

Rationale

(A) The data describe the theoretical physiology of Graves' disease. (B) Hashimoto's thyroiditis causes hypothyroidism. (C) The data do not support a situation that is an emergency. Thyrotoxic crisis is an emergency. (D) Most patients with nontoxic goiter are euthyroid.

82. (A) Nursing process phase: implementation; client need: physiological integrity; content area: medical/ surgical nursing

Rationale

(A) Tachycardia would be one of the first signs of overdose. (B) The data do not indicate a need for sodium restriction. (C) Synthroid should be taken on an empty stomach. (D) The data do not support a need to measure urinary output.

83. (B) Nursing process phase: evaluation; client need: health promotion and maintenance; content area: medical/surgical nursing

Rationale

(A) Hypercalcemia will cause the kidneys to eliminate more phosphate. (B) The statement is true. Calcium can crystallize in the kidneys and damage the tubules. Stones may also form from calcium. Both the crystals and the stones can lead to renal failure. (C) Chronic hypercalcemia may act as a stimulus for release of gastrin, which can cause peptic ulcer. (D) Excess parathormone increases bone resorption, leading to osteoporosis and cyst formation in the bones.

84. (B) Nursing process phase: assessment; client need: physiological integrity; content area: medical/surgical nursing

Rationale

(A) This test is not as sensitive as the glucose tolerance test. (B) This is the most sensitive test for diabetes mellitus. Diabetics cannot tolerate a standard dose of glucose; the serum glucose level will rise abnormally and remain elevated much longer in a diabetic. (C) This test is best at monitoring long-term glucose control in someone who has been a diabetic for some time. (D) This test reflects endogenous insulin secretion; it tells little or nothing about resistance to insulin.

85. (D) Nursing process phase: planning; client need: safe, effective care environment; content area: medical/surgical nursing

Rationale

(A) Symptoms of menopause would be relieved. However, re-lieving these symptoms would probably not justify using these drugs, which have some dangerous side effects. (B) These drugs may actually increase the risk of cancer of the breast. (C) This is not an expected outcome of the therapy. (D) Preventing osteoporosis is the major reason these drugs are taken.

86. (C) Nursing process phase: planning; client need: physiological integrity; content area: medical/surgical nursing

Rationale

(A & C) The data indicate that the client has hyperosmolar, hyperglycemic, nonketotic syndrome (HHNK). The highest priority for such a client would be intravenous fluid and insulin to correct the hyperosmolar state. (B) Metabolic acidosis should not be a problem with HHNK. (D) The data do not indicate hypocalcemia.

87. (B) Nursing process phase: analysis; client need: physiological integrity; content area: medical/surgical nursing

Rationale

(A) The data do not support a problem of HHNK. (B) All of the data are consistent with the complication of diabetic ketoacidosis. (C) The data do not support hypoglycemia. (D) The data are more consistent with the problem of diabetic ketoacidosis.

88. (C) Nursing process phase: implementation; client need: safe, effective care environment; content area: medical/surgical nursing

Rationale

(A) The drugs are compatible; therefore, two separate injections would cause unnecessary discomfort. (B) The deltoid is too small for an irritating drug such as Vistaril. (C) The Z-track is the best technique to use when injecting an irritating drug such as Vistaril. (D) Rubbing vigorously would help to distribute the irritating drug throughout the tissues and, thus, increase the client's discomfort.

89. (D) Nursing process phase: implementation; client need: health promotion and maintenance; content area: medical/surgical nursing

Rationale

(A) Hypervolemia is not a risk factor for atherosclerosis. (B) Hypokalemia is not a risk factor for atherosclerosis. (C) Proteinuria is not a risk factor for atherosclerosis. (D) Hypertension is a risk factor for atherosclerosis.

90. (A) Nursing process phase: implementation; client need: safe, effective care environment; content area: medical/surgical nursing

Rationale

(A) The clamp to the port must be clamped to prevent air from entering the jugular vein when the lumen of the intravenous catheter is exposed to atmospheric pressure. (B) It is not necessary to flush the port between bags of TPN solution. (C) The serum glucose is checked at regular intervals; therefore, it does not need to be checked prior to hanging a new bag of TPN solution. (D) If lipids are administered, they should not be filtered.

91. (B) Nursing process phase: implementation; client

need: health promotion and maintenance; content area: medical/surgical nursing

Rationale
(A) Pillows will place the head in a position for development of a contracture. (B) The grasping position is the most functional position for the hand. A firm object prevents stimulation of a reflex that would cause the hand to assume another, less functional position. (C) Positions of comfort can be positions promoting development of contractures. (D) The arms should be in their most functional positions, that is, at 90-degree angles to the body.

92. **(B)** Nursing process phase: implementation; client need: physiological integrity; content area: medical/surgical nursing

Rationale
(A) This advice should not be given because the client could have an accident. (B) The symptoms are indicative of retinal detachment, which is treated by hospitalization, bedrest, and then surgery. (C) The symptoms are indicative of retinal detachment. (D) The symptoms may indicate a retinal detachment and require immediate evaluation by an ophthalmologist.

93. **(B)** Nursing process phase: implementation; client need: health promotion and maintenance; content area: medical/surgical nursing

Rationale
(A) This statement is true. (B) This statement is false. The best method is abstinence. Accidents may occur even when latex condoms are used with 5% nonoxynol 9. (C) This statement is true. (D) This statement is true.

94. **(C)** Nursing process phase: evaluation; client need: health promotion and maintenance; content area: medical/surgical nursing

Rationale
(A) Changing dressings is the only psychomotor skill required by the data provided. (B) The data do not indicate a need for these psychomotor skills. (C) The client should return demonstration on suctioning and caring for tracheostomies and tracheostomy tubes. (D) The data do not indicate a need for these psychomotor skills.

95. **(D)** Nursing process phase: implementation; client need: physiological integrity; content area: medical/surgical nursing

Rationale
(A) Two other actions would take priority over checking the level of consciousness. (B) The spine would need to be immobilized following a quick check for bleeding. (C) Bleeding should be arrested and the spine immobilized prior to making a call for help. (D) Preventing shock is next to an open airway in priority.

96. **(A)** Nursing process phase: implementation; client need: physiological integrity; content area: medical/surgical nursing

Rationale
(A) The supine position with elevation of the head would be best for decreasing the work of breathing and reducing venous return to the heart. (B) The side position would not facilitate the work of breathing nor reduce venous return to the

heart. (C) This is not the best answer for the same reason as stated above. (D) The head would be too flat to decrease the work of breathing and reduce venous return to the heart.

97. **(C)** Nursing process phase: evaluation; client need: health promotion and maintenance; content area: medical/surgical nursing

Rationale
(A) Guidelines for resumption of sexual activity should have been given to the client. (B) The client needs to work through emotionally to realistic acceptance of the condition. Staying happy and optimistic all of the time could delay this process. However, excessive depression should be treated. (C) Monitoring the pulse rate is the best way to determine the amount of exercise a client can have. (D) Cardiac tissue does not regenerate.

98. **(D)** Nursing process phase: analysis; client need: physiological integrity; content area: medical/surgical nursing

Rationale
(A) The signs and symptoms are not typical of MI. (B) The vital signs taken are all normal. (C) The data do not support such an assumption. (D) The sympathetic response to physiological stress is dampened in the elderly. For this reason and others, the elderly often have atypical signs and symptoms of a disease or condition.

99. **(C)** Nursing process phase: implementation; client need: safe, effective care environment; content area: medical/surgical nursing

Rationale
(A) The urine has been collecting in the bag for some time, and the technique would be poor. (B) The technique would be poor aseptic technique. (C) This is the correct way to collect the urine specimen. (D) The Foley does not contain a special port for aspiration, and an opening would be left in the catheter.

100. **(A)** Nursing process phase: implementation; client need: safe, effective care environment; content area: medical/surgical nursing

Rationale
(A) An iodine contrast medium will be used for the test. An allergy to shellfish could imply an allergy to iodine. (B) Hydration is very important to dilute the toxic effects of iodine on the renal tubules. Restricting fluids for more time than is necessary would be hazardous to the client. (C) These sensations are normal reactions to the dye. (D) Consent forms are required when contrast media are used.

101. **(C)** Nursing process phase: analysis; client need: physiological integrity; content area: medical/surgical nursing

Rationale
(A) The physician should make the decision about the required action for the low urinary output. (B) The client is not voiding a quantity sufficient, which would be a minimum of 30 ml/hr. (C) The reason has been stated under part A. (D) The physician needs to evaluate the situation.

102. **(B)** Nursing process phase: implementation; client need: safe, effective care environment; content area: medical/surgical nursing

Rationale

(A) The first specimen should be discarded when collecting a 24-hour urine. (B) This is the correct way to save urine for 24 hours because you are starting the collection with an empty bladder. (C) A 24-hour urine is needed for a creatinine clearance test. (D) A 24-hour urine is needed.

103. **(D)** Nursing process phase: assessment; client need: safe, effective care environment; content area: medical/surgical nursing

Rationale

(A) These tests are not the best tests to evaluate renal function. (B) The CBC would give little help in assessment of renal function. (C) The renal angiogram is a more definitive test to be used when the physician suspects disease involving renal blood vessels. (D) Results of the BUN and creatinine would show renal ability to eliminate metabolic wastes. The urinary output shows the ability of the kidneys to filter blood and eliminate urine. Results of all three tests would give the best picture of renal functioning.

104. **(C)** Nursing process phase: analysis; client need: safe, effective care environment; content area: medical/surgical nursing

Rationale

(A) The pH is normal for urine. (B) A trace of protein is considered normal. (C) Cloudy urine is abnormal and usually indicates urinary tract infection. (D) Occasional hyaline casts are considered normal.

105. **(A)** Nursing process phase: implementation; client need: safe, effective care environment; content area: medical/surgical nursing

Rationale

(A) Refrigeration will help prevent multiplication of bacteria and evaporation of water. (B) The client would have to provide another specimen. (C) Valid results would not be obtained from a specimen that has been kept at room temperature too long. (D) A preservative could distort the results of the test.

106. **(B)** Nursing process phase: evaluation; client need: safe, effective care environment; content area: medical/surgical nursing

Rationale

(A) Glomerulonephritis is the sequela to untreated streptococcal infections. (B) The statement is true; both diseases (if not treated properly) could end in renal failure. (C) Cola-colored urine is a sign of glomerulonephritis. Blood may enter Bowman's capsule and eventually become part of the urine in this condition. Blood lost from the glomerulus will turn urine the color of cola. (D) Nursing care for the two conditions includes far more similarities than differences.

107. **(D)** Nursing process phase: planning; client need: physiological integrity; content area: medical/surgical nursing

Rationale

(A) Bedrest would not be required unless hematuria were present. (B) Both the stent and the nephrostomy tube should not be irrigated without a physician's order. If either were ordered to be irrigated, strict aseptic technique would be required, and no more than 10 ml of solution could be used.

(C) Nephrostomy tubes should never be clamped; hydronephrosis could develop. (D) The entire stent would be located in the ureter. Output from the nephrostomy tube should be recorded separately from output through the stent.

108. **(C)** Nursing process phase: implementation; client need: health promotion and maintenance; content area: medical/surgical nursing

Rationale

(A) This practice might help prevent urinary tract infections but would only indirectly affect formation of stones. (B) This action would be too drastic and would be beyond the scope of most nurses. (C) Forcing fluids and eating a low-purine diet would help decrease the formation of uric acid stones. (D) Exercise would help, but a low-fat diet is not known to prevent formation of stones in the urinary tract.

109. **(C)** Nursing process phase: implementation; client need: safe, effective care environment; content area: medical/surgical nursing

Rationale

(A) The data do not indicate a need for bedrest. (B) Fluids should be forced to aid in removal of the stone. (C) The urine must be strained so that the stone or stones may be analyzed for content. (D) The data do not indicate a need for cranberry juice.

110. **(A)** Nursing process phase: planning; client need: safe, effective care environment; content area: medical/surgical nursing

Rationale

(A) Assessing the skin around the tube would be necessary in order to maintain skin integrity. (B) Fluids should be forced in order to dilute bacteria and minerals in the urine. (C) Recent data have indicated that a diet high in calcium may decrease renal excretion of oxalate, a common ingredient in several types of stones. (D) Such a large amount of solution would be contraindicated.

111. **(A)** Nursing process phase: planning; client need: safe, effective care environment; content area: medical/surgical nursing

Rationale

(A) The stoma should be observed frequently for prolapse, bleeding, necrosis, or stenosis. (B) The bowel sounds should be checked more frequently because ileus could develop. (C) Such frequent changes would be contraindicated because the skin surrounding the stoma would probably be damaged. (D) It is normal for the segment of ileum to secrete mucus postoperatively.

112. **(B)** Nursing process phase: analysis; client need: safe, effective care environment; content area: medical/surgical nursing

Rationale

(A) Urine would be lost with any increase in intra-abdominal pressure. (B) The client has functional incontinence because she cannot get to an appropriate place to empty her bladder in time, even though her bladder and sphincter are normal. (C) The urge to void would be very brief and followed by a loss of a large volume of urine. (D) Urine would be lost without any warning or urge.

113. **(C)** Nursing process phase: planning; client need: physiological integrity; content area: medical/surgical nursing

Rationale

(A) Hypercalcemia and hypomagnesemia are not usually seen in acute renal failure. (B) Hyperchloremia and alkalosis are unusual with acute renal failure. (C) Potassium would be released from cells (because of acidosis), and the kidneys would retain potassium. Excretion of acid products of metabolism would be compromised in acute renal failure. (D) The kidneys do not usually retain sodium in renal failure. Phosphate would be retained, and calcium has an inverse relationship to phosphate.

114. **(B)** Nursing process phase: planning; client need: physiological integrity; content area: medical/surgical nursing

Rationale

(A) The kidneys would probably be damaged more with less fluid. (B) Fluid replacement equal to loss during the previous 24 hours is standard practice during the oliguric phase of acute renal failure. (C & D) An amount of fluid greater than that lost (sensible and insensible) during the previous 24 hours could cause hypervolemia, pulmonary edema, and other problems.

115. **(D)** Nursing process phase: planning; client need: safe, effective care environment; content area: medical/surgical nursing

Rationale

(A) Acute renal failure is reversible in many cases. (B) This nursing diagnosis would not be appropriate at this time; the client is probably too ill to learn. (C) The risk is not as great as the risk for infection. (D) The leading cause of death for clients in acute renal failure is infection because the immune response is altered.

116. **(D)** Nursing process phase: planning; client need: physiological integrity; content area: medical/surgical nursing

Rationale

(A–D) The first sign of hypervolemia is usually rales because fluid will leave the low-pressure pulmonary system immediately. This can be detected by the presence of rales.

117. **(C)** Nursing process phase: implementation; client need: health promotion and maintenance; content area: medical/surgical nursing

Rationale

(A) Urine sodium would not provide evidence for the start of diabetic nephropathy. (B) Controlling serum glucose is the best way to prevent diabetic nephropathy but would not help the client detect the first signs of this condition. (C) Diabetic nephropathy begins with the loss of protein in the urine; more than a trace of protein would indicate renal involvement. (D) Palpation of the kidney would not help the client detect the first signs of diabetic nephropathy.

118. **(A)** Nursing process phase: implementation; client need: health promotion and maintenance; content area: medical/surgical nursing

Rationale

(A) Protein, fat, fluid, sodium, and potassium should be restricted in the diet of a client with chronic renal failure. (B)

The red blood cells will decrease because of a lack of erythropoietin. (C) Chronic renal failure will cause the client's hypertension to get worse. (D) Urea will be changed to ammonia in the gastrointestinal system.

119. **(B)** Nursing process phase: planning; client need: physiological integrity; content area: medical/surgical nursing

Rationale

(A) The pulse rate would not detect hypovolemia, decreased volume in the plasma compartment, first; the pulse would change following response of the sympathetic nervous system. (B) A change in blood pressure, whether in the compensatory stage of shock or following compensation, would probably be the first sign that fluid was being lost from the plasma compartment. (C) Although edema could occur if fluid were to shift from the plasma compartment into the interstitial spaces, a drop in blood pressure would occur whether hypovolemia were caused by a shift of fluid into another compartment or by loss from the body. (D) A drop in blood pressure would probably be the best detector of fluid loss from the plasma compartments. The specific gravity of urine usually denotes the fluid status of the entire body and might not change with fluid shifts.

120. **(D)** Nursing process phase: implementation; client need: physiological integrity; content area: medical/surgical nursing

Rationale

(A) The situation is an emergency; a complete respiratory assessment would not be the highest priority. (B) Oxygen would be a higher priority than heparin. (C) The onset of action for warfarin (Coumadin) is several hours; it will be used later in the treatment for a pulmonary embolism. (D) Oxygen administration is the highest priority to prevent hemoglobin saturation from dropping to levels incompatible with life.

121. **(D)** Nursing process phase: analysis; client need: physiological integrity; content area: medical/surgical nursing

Rationale

(A) High-fat meals decrease discomfort. (B) Low-carbohydrate meals are helpful. (C) Avoiding fluids with meals is encouraged. (D) The "dumping syndrome" can be helped by eating small, frequent meals.

122. **(B)** Nursing process phase: analysis; client need: physiological integrity; content area: medical/surgical nursing

Rationale

(A) Hyperactive bowel and abdominal distention result in pain and discomfort. (B) The client will still be able to verbally communicate with a nasogastric tube in place. This is not an appropriate nursing diagnosis. (C) Fluid and electrolytes are lost with vomiting, resulting in fluid volume deficits. (D) Alterations in sensorium may occur if the fluid and electrolyte imbalance is severe.

123. **(D)** Nursing process phase: planning; client need: physiological integrity; content area: medical/surgical nursing

Rationale

(A) Constriction of pulmonary vessels does not usually cause pleural effusion. (B) The data do not indicate that the client is in danger of a pneumothorax. (C) Constriction of pulmonary vessels does not cause subcutaneous emphysema. (D) Constriction of pulmonary vessels could lead to cor pulmonale.

124. **(D)** Nursing process phase: implementation; client need: safe, effective care environment; content area: medical/surgical nursing

Rationale

(A) An epidural catheter would be desirable to control pain and minimize the risk of further respiratory depression. (B) One action of epinephrine is bronchodilatation, an effect that would help the client in respiratory depression. No data exist to suggest that epinephrine would be contraindicated. (C) Atropine is an anticholinergic drug; it would dilate the bronchioles and help dry up airway secretions. The data do not suggest a contraindication for this drug. (D) Neostigmine should not be given; it is a cholinergic drug, causing airway constriction.

125. **(B)** Nursing process phase: planning; client need: physiological integrity; content area: medical/surgical nursing

Rationale

(A) The data do not indicate a need to observe for pleural effusion. (B) A pneumothorax could occur in response to PEEP. (C) The data do not indicate a need to observe for cardiac tamponade. (D) The data do not indicate that oxygen toxicity has developed, and the initiation of PEEP will decrease the client's risk of developing oxygen toxicity.

126. **(C)** Nursing process phase: analysis; client need: physiological integrity; content area: medical/surgical nursing

Rationale

(A) The data indicate that the client has an abdominal aneurysm. Bowel sounds would not provide data to support such a problem, which, if present, should be reported to a physician immediately. (B) The apical pulse would not provide the additional data the nurse is seeking. (C) Data on pulses in the lower extremities would be helpful in validating the nurse's decision to make a referral immediately. (D) The data are not related to an aortic aneurysm.

127. **(D)** Nursing process phase: analysis; client need: safe, effective care environment; content area: medical/surgical nursing

Rationale

(A) Most interventions for this nursing diagnosis could be included under fatigue. (B) The data do not provide a cue in support of this nursing diagnosis. (C) The data do not provide a cue in support of this nursing diagnosis. (D) Anemia means that insufficient hemoglobin is available to pick up oxygen that is diffused into the blood. This will impair gas exchange.

128. **(A)** Nursing process phase: planning; client need: health promotion and maintenance; content area: medical/surgical nursing

Rationale

(A) Intrinsic factor, secreted by the parietal cells of the stomach, is essential to the absorption of vitamin B_{12}. A deficiency of this vitamin causes pernicious anemia. (B) This type of anemia is related to depression of bone marrow. (C) Thalassemia is a genetic disorder and is not related to the stomach. (D) Hypoproliferative anemias are related to chronic disease but are not directly related to the stomach.

129. **(B)** Nursing process phase: planning; client need: safe, effective care environment; content area: medical/surgical nursing

Rationale

(A) This would be a possible nursing diagnosis but not as important as high risk for impaired skin integrity. (B) Edema implies a high risk for breaks in the skin. (C) As long as the skin remains intact, the risk of infection is not a major problem. (D) The data do not include a cue for this nursing diagnosis.

130. **(A)** Nursing process phase: implementation; client need: safe, effective care environment; content area: medical/surgical nursing

Rationale

(A) Reduction of afterload decreases the work of the heart and is believed to be the major benefit of vasodilators in treating angina pectoris. (B) Afterload would not be increased. (C) Preload would not be increased. (D) This effect is believed to be less helpful than reduction of afterload.

131. **(A)** Nursing process phase: analysis; client need: physiological integrity; content area: medical/surgical nursing

Rationale

(A) The client is acidic, and the bicarbonate is low. These data plus the other information point to metabolic acidosis. (B) The client is not alkalotic. (C) The client does not have respiratory acidosis because the carbon dioxide is within normal limits. (D) The client is not alkalotic.

132. **(C)** Nursing process phase: planning; client need: physiological integrity; content area: medical/surgical nursing

Rationale

(A–D) The kidneys compensate for respiratory acidosis by eliminating hydrogen ions and conserving bicarbonate, but it takes 2 to 3 days.

133. **(D)** Nursing process phase: implementation; client need: health promotion and maintenance; content area: medical/surgical nursing

Rationale

(A) Kidney disease is not a sequela to rheumatic fever. (B) Seizure activity is not a sequela to rheumatic fever. (C) Rheumatic fever is not followed by liver trauma. (D) Cardiac disease is a sequela of rheumatic fever.

134. **(B)** Nursing process phase: implementation; client need: health promotion and maintenance; content area: medical/surgical nursing

Rationale

(A) Anticoagulant therapy would probably be used if needed. (B) Prophylactic antibiotic treatment prior to dental or surgical procedures is important to prevent endocarditis. (C) It would be important to avoid hypervolemia (excess stress on the heart). (D) Rest would not be as important as prophylactic antibiotic treatment.

135. (B) Nursing process phase: planning; client need: physiological integrity; content area: medical/surgical nursing

Rationale
(A) The data do not indicate that the client has a problem tolerating the regurgitation. (B) The left ventricle will be strained by chronic mitral regurgitation. The client should be aware of the signs and symptoms of decreased cardiac output so that help could be obtained if they should appear. Such signs and symptoms might include a weak pulse; alterations in pulse rate; arrhythmias; fatigue; distention of the jugular vein; cyanosis; pallor; decreased urinary output; cold, clammy skin; rales or dyspnea. (C) Preventing retention of fluid is a greater concern. (D) Impaired physical mobility is not appropriate for the data provided.

136. (C) Nursing process phase: analysis; client need: physiological integrity; content area: medical/surgical nursing

Rationale
(A) Bowel sounds are not an effective check for tissue perfusion. (B) Level of consciousness would tell more about perfusion to the brain. (C) Perfusion of kidneys is essential to maintaining renal function and should be evaluated when checking tissue perfusion. (D) Breath sounds do not provide a lot of information on tissue perfusion.

137. (A) Nursing process phase: implementation; client need: safe, effective care environment; content area: medical/surgical nursing

Rationale
(A, C, & D) The distance from the nose to the tip of the ear lobe is equivalent to the distance from the nose to the area where the epiglottis covers the respiratory tract and the esophagus begins. (B) The distance from the tip of the nose to the xiphoid process would not be a good estimate.

138. (D) Nursing process phase: implementation; client need: safe, effective care environment; content area: medical/surgical nursing

Rationale
(A) The epiglottis would be open with coughing. (B) The opening into the respiratory tract would be open, and aspiration could occur. (C) Removal of the tube would be more complicated. (D) The Valsalva maneuver would close the epiglottis and prevent aspiration.

139. (C) Nursing process phase: implementation; client need: safe, effective care environment; content area: medical/surgical nursing

Rationale
(A) Too much irrigation would wash out electrolytes. (B) The tube should stay in position unless otherwise ordered by the physician. (C) Placement is checked each shift to be sure it is not in the respiratory tract. (D) The tape should be removed only as necessary.

140. (B) Nursing process phase: evaluation; client need: safe, effective care environment; content area: medical/surgical nursing

Rationale
(A) Pedal pulses would not need to be checked daily with venous insufficiency. (B) The statement is true; the legs should be elevated to promote venous return. (C) Hair is not lost with venous insufficiency. (D) Amputation is usually done for gangrene; gangrene is rare with venous insufficiency.

141. (C) Nursing process phase: implementation; client need: safe, effective care environment; content area: medical/surgical nursing

Rationale
(A) Clients with arterial as well as venous insufficiency should rest when pain is present. Rest will promote arterial perfusion with arterial conditions and help prevent accumulation of fluid with venous disorders. (B) Clients with both arterial and venous insufficiency should stop smoking, although smoking affects arteries much more than veins. (C) The client with arterial disease would keep the feet dependent when pain occurs to promote arterial perfusion. The client with venous problems would elevate the feet to encourage return of venous blood to the heart. (D) Keeping the feet dependent whenever the client was out of bed would promote venous stasis and make the problem worse.

142. (B) Nursing process phase: assessment; client need: health promotion and maintenance; content area: medical/surgical nursing

Rationale
(A) The normal liver cannot be palpated unless the client takes a deep breath and holds it. (B) The client should take a deep breath and hold it as explained above. (C) The normal liver could not be palpated if the client exhaled. (D) The client should be in supine position.

143. (D) Nursing process phase: analysis; client need: safe, effective care environment; content area: medical/surgical nursing

Rationale
(A) Rebound tenderness indicates pathology. A large, formed stool might be palpable but should not cause tenderness. (B) Abnormal pulsations should be detected if an aneurysm were present. (C) The data do not suggest irritable bowel syndrome; diarrhea would be present. (D) Rebound tenderness does indicate peritoneal inflammation. Other signs and symptoms might include abdominal distention, fever, nausea, vomiting, altered bowel habits, tachycardia, or tachypnea.

144. (A) Nursing process phase: analysis; client need: health promotion and maintenance; content area: medical/surgical nursing

Rationale
(A) Leukoplakia is a premalignant lesion. (B) Cracking at the corners of the mouth could probably be corrected with riboflavin. The nurse could provide a list of foods rich in riboflavin. (C) A red, slick tongue may be caused by a deficiency of vitamin B_{12}. (D) The neighbor should be referred to the dentist for bleeding gums.

145. (C) Nursing process phase: assessment; client need: physiological integrity; content area: medical/surgical nursing

Rationale
(A) The physician should be notified at once. (B) A laxative

should never be given when bowel sounds are absent, because obstruction, ileus, or peritonitis is likely. (C) The physician should be notified because the absence is most likely because of ileus, obstruction, or peritonitis. (D) A physician needs to evaluate the client for the reasons explained above.

146. (D) Nursing process phase: analysis; client need: safe, effective care environment; content area: medical/surgical nursing

Rationale
(A) The stools would be lacking stercobilinogen and would contain undigested fat. (B) Black stools would be indicative of bleeding. (C) The stools would contain undigested fat. (D) The stools should be clay-colored, fatty, frothy, and foul-smelling because they lack stercobilinogen and contain undigested fat.

147. (A) Nursing process phase: implementation; client need: safe, effective care environment; content area: medical/surgical nursing

Rationale
(A) A laxative is needed to clean the barium out of the gastrointestinal tract. (B) A frequent check of vital signs will not be necessary. (C) Fluids should be forced to help eliminate the barium, and the client should eat. (D) Evaluation of lower extremities for neurovascular signs would not be necessary.

148. (B) Nursing process phase: assessment; client need: safe, effective care environment; content area: medical/surgical nursing

Rationale
(A) A diet high in polyunsaturated fat would not be necessary. (B) The gag reflex should be checked because the throat will probably be anesthetized. The vital signs should be checked to look for perforation. (C) Pancreatitis, not gastritis, is a frequent complication of the procedure. (D) Aspirin would be contraindicated because it prevents aggregation of platelets and would mask signs of infection. Observing for perforation and infection are important following this procedure.

149. (D) Nursing process phase: planning; client need: physiological integrity; content area: medical/surgical nursing

Rationale
(A) Evaluation of liver function tests would not be necessary. Evaluation of coagulation studies would. (B) The client does not need to be NPO. (C) The client must be in bed in a flat position for 12 to 14 hours following the procedure. (D) The client must remain on the right side for 2 hours to provide pressure on the puncture site.

150. (A) Nursing process phase: implementation; client need: safe, effective care environment; content area: medical/surgical nursing

Rationale
(A) The most accurate way to determine location of the end of the tube would be to test pH of the drainage. Drainage coming from the stomach would be acidic; drainage coming from the intestines would be alkaline. (B) Injecting an air bubble would not be an effective method of differentiating the stomach from the intestines. (C) No bubbling would mean that the tube was not in the respiratory tract. The loca-

tion of the tube in the gastrointestinal tract could not be determined. (D) Testing the electrolyte content of drainage would not be practical.

151. (D) Nursing process phase: implementation; client need: safe, effective care environment; content area: medical/surgical nursing

Rationale
(A) It is not necessary to keep the container filled at all times. (B) No damage would be done if the container for the feeding were below the jejunum. (C) The client might be uncomfortable in high Fowler's position. (D) The head of the bed must remain elevated 30 to 45 degrees at all times to prevent aspiration.

152. (B) Nursing process phase: implementation; client need: safe, effective care environment; content area: medical/surgical nursing

Rationale
(A) Irrigating the tube will probably not be necessary with continuous feedings. (B) The residual will need to be checked about every 4 hours to make certain that the client is not receiving liquid faster than it can be absorbed. Aspiration or other complications could occur. (C) The lungs would not need to be examined so frequently. (D) The bowel sounds could be checked once a shift.

153. (C) Nursing process phase: implementation; client need: safe, effective care environment; content area: medical/surgical nursing

Rationale
(A) The pump would alarm if occlusion occurred. (B) Aspirating and flushing a Keofeed tube would be difficult because of the size of the bore. (C) Water is necessary to prevent dehydration caused by osmotic diuresis. Most tube feedings have a high osmolarity. (D) Unless medications were in liquid form, they would probably clog the tube.

154. (A) Nursing process phase: implementation; client need: physiological integrity; content area: medical/surgical nursing

Rationale
(A) The Trendelenburg position on the left side would help to trap air in the right atrium. (B) Raising the head of the bed and instructing the client to use the Valsalva maneuver would not help. (C) Clamping sterile petroleum jelly (Vaseline) gauze over the site would not help. (D) Aspirating the embolism would probably be impossible because of the rapid movement of blood in the subclavian vein.

155. (B) Nursing process phase: implementation; client need: safe, effective care environment; content area: medical/surgical nursing

Rationale
(A) The statement is correct. Gastrointestinal irritation is a side effect of both salicylates and nonsteroidal anti-inflammatory drugs; both groups of drugs are used for treatment of arthritic pain. (B) Aerobic exercise has been shown to improve osteoarthritis; therefore, the statement is false. (C) Heat, ice, and massage are all recommended treatments for arthritic pain. (D) The toilet seat should be elevated to avoid extreme flexion of the hips.

156. (A) Nursing process phase: implementation; client need: safe, effective care environment; content area: medical/surgical nursing

Rationale
(A) TPN provides an excellent medium for bacterial growth, so the tubing should be changed with each new bottle of solution. (B) The tubing should be changed more frequently than every 24 hours for the reason stated above. (C) The tubing should not be changed every 48 hours as explained above. (D) The tubing needs to be changed more frequently as explained above.

157. (B) Nursing process phase: implementation; client need: safe, effective care environment; content area: medical/surgical nursing

Rationale
(A) Lipids may be run into the same line as TPN. (B) Lipids should be run below the filter to prevent essential elements from being removed. (C) Essential elements of the lipids would be removed by the filter. (D) Lipids should not be run through a filter.

158. (B) Nursing process phase: implementation; client need: physiological integrity; content area: medical/surgical nursing

Rationale
(A) The situation could be life-threatening. The vital signs may be checked after the lipids have been stopped and the physician has been notified. (B) The infusion of lipids should be stopped, and the physician should be notified. The client is having a reaction to the lipids. (C) The nurse should not attempt to treat the reaction; this reaction requires medical attention. (D) The IV line should be kept open.

159. (B) Nursing process phase: implementation; client need: safe, effective care environment; content area: medical/surgical nursing

Rationale
(A) Fifteen minutes would not allow sufficient time for warm-up. (B) The solution should not be removed from the refrigerator more than 30 minutes prior to hanging because it provides an excellent medium for bacterial growth. (C) One hour would allow too much bacterial growth. (D) Two hours would be too long.

160. (D) Nursing process phase: planning; client need: safe, effective care environment; content area: medical/surgical nursing

Rationale
(A–D) The highest priority should be on a patent airway and effective communication because the jaws have been wired shut. If these outcomes are not achieved, the client could die.

161. (B) Nursing process phase: planning; client need: safe, effective care environment; content area: medical/surgical nursing

Rationale
(A) The vomiting reflex should not be impaired following a hemicolectomy. (B) Paralytic ileus is a postoperative complication the nurse would want to detect following a hemicolectomy. Manipulation of the intestines during surgery is a common cause of this complication. (C) The data do not indicate that dehiscence, opening of the wound, is likely. (D) The

data do not indicate that evisceration, removal of viscera from the abdominal cavity, is likely.

162. (B) Nursing process phase: implementation; client need: effective care environment; content area: medical/surgical nursing

Rationale
(A) The aspirate should not be discarded because electrolytes would be wasted. (B) The aspirate should be returned to the stomach to preserve electrolyte balance. (C) The data do not indicate that a specimen should be sent to the laboratory. (D) The aspirate should not be added to the feeding because bacterial growth would be enhanced.

163. (C) Nursing process phase: implementation; client need: safe, effective care environment; content area: medical/surgical nursing

Rationale
(A) The tube feedings are probably hyperosmotic, but this alone would not account for the signs and symptoms the client is experiencing. (B) Paralytic ileus could not be present with borborygmi. (C & D) The opening of the gastrostomy tube has probably slipped into the duodenum or jejunum, producing the signs and symptoms of dumping syndrome the client is experiencing.

164. (D) Nursing process phase: implementation; client need: safe, effective care environment; content area: medical/surgical nursing

Rationale
(A) All sensory stimuli should be minimized as much as possible to avoid stimulation of the vomiting center in the brain stem. (B) Relaxation would help, but probably not as much as absence of stimuli. (C & D) Minimizing stimuli reduces the chance of stimulating the vomiting center in the brain stem.

165. (B) Nursing process phase: analysis; client need: safe, effective care environment; content area: medical/surgical nursing

Rationale
(A) The spinal cord is the best answer (B) The spinal cord provides the synapse network for completion of the reflex. (C) The spinal cord is the best answer (D) The cerebrum is not involved in a reflex.

166. (B) Nursing process phase: implementation; client need: physiological integrity; content area: medical/surgical nursing

Rationale
(A) Taking the temperature rectally will not stimulate the Valsalva maneuver. (B) The vagus supplies the heart and abdominal viscera. Stimulation could slow heart rate. (C) The spinal accessory does not supply the rectum. (D) The statement is not true.

167. (B) Nursing process phase: implementation; client need: physiological integrity; content area: medical/surgical nursing

Rationale
(A) Packed cells would not contain coagulation factors. (B) A Foley catheter would be inserted so that the urinary output could be measured every hour to prevent renal failure. (C) A large tube would be needed for gastric lavage, and a large

tube could more easily be inserted through the mouth. (D) It would be more important to insert the Foley; it would take time for the effect of the hemorrhage to show up in the values of the hemoglobin and hematocrit.

168. **(C)** Nursing process phase: implementation; client need: safe, effective care environment; content area: medical/surgical nursing

Rationale
(A) Various procedures administered through an endoscope are the preferred method of treating varices today. However, the Sengstaken-Blakemore could be used to apply pressure to the varices. (B) Gastric lavage with saline could be used, but procedures administered through an endoscope are usually more effective. (C) Direct visualization of the varices makes it easier for the physicians to arrest the hemorrhage. A variety of methods may be tried. (D) A sclerosing agent would most likely be used.

169. **(D)** Nursing process phase: implementation; client need: safe, effective care environment; content area: medical/surgical nursing

Rationale
(A) Neomycin would do little to help prevent infection because it is poorly absorbed from the gastrointestinal tract. (B) Stress ulcers would not be prevented. (C) Neomycin would not prevent constipation. (D) The drug would reduce bacterial flora in the gastrointestinal tract and, thus, decrease the production of ammonia. Such ammonia would be absorbed into the blood stream. High levels of serum ammonia produce encephalopathy.

170. **(A)** Nursing process phase: assessment; client need: safe, effective care environment; content area: medical/surgical nursing

Rationale
(A) In order to standardize measurement of an irregularly shaped object such as the abdomen, it would be necessary to measure in the same place each day. Accurate measurement would be important in assessing the status of ascites. (B) If the client were eating, the time of day might be important but would not be as important as a standard place for measurement. (C) The amount of fluid in the bladder should not affect the measurement of the abdomen, unless the measurements were being taken directly over the bladder. Measuring over the symphysis pubis would not be a good location for assessing ascites. (D) Tape measures are standard.

171. **(C)** Nursing process phase: assessment; client need: physiological integrity; content area: medical/surgical nursing

Rationale
(A) Internal bleeding might not show up on the dressing. (B) Coagulation could be normal, but bleeding could occur because of a ruptured blood vessel. (C) A drop in hemoglobin or hematocrit would be one of the fastest ways to detect bleeding. Data from these laboratory reports would be combined with data from assessment of the vital signs for the quickest detection. (D) Evaluation of liver function tests would be neither effective nor practical.

172. **(A)** Nursing process phase: analysis; client need: physiological integrity; content area: medical/surgical nursing

Rationale
(A) A consistently high urine specific gravity indicates fluid volume deficit. (B) High specific gravity of the urine does not indicate fluid volume excess. (C) Cardiac output could be decreased, but the etiology of the problem would be fluid volume deficit. (D) Tissue perfusion could be altered, but the etiology of the problem would be fluid volume deficit.

173. **(D)** Nursing process phase: assessment; client need: safe, effective care environment; content area: medical/surgical nursing

Rationale
(A) No evidence exists that highly seasoned foods cause ulcers. (B) Alcoholic beverages in moderation probably do not cause ulcers. (C) Acid ash diets do not cause ulcers. (D) Nonsteroidal anti-inflammatory drugs are an identified risk factor for gastric ulcers. They inhibit prostaglandins, which help to form a protective barrier on the gastric mucosa.

174. **(C)** Nursing process phase: planning; client need: physiological integrity; content area: medical/surgical nursing

Rationale
(A) The signs and symptoms are classical for perforation. Pain throughout the abdomen and contraction of abdominal muscles indicate pathology involving the entire peritoneal cavity. (B) Hemorrhage without perforation would occur into the gastrointestinal tract. The data do not support such an occurrence. (C) The signs and symptoms are classical for perforation. The nurse should prepare the client for surgery and insert a nasogastric tube (with an order from the physician). (D) The data do not support gastrointestinal infarction.

175. **(D)** Nursing process phase: implementation; client need: safe, effective care environment; content area: medical/surgical nursing

Rationale
(A) Antacids on an empty stomach are passed through the gastrointestinal tract without coming into contact with much acid. (B–D) To be most effective, antacids should be given to coincide with gastric secretion; they are most effective when given 1 to 2 hours following a meal.

176. **(D)** Nursing process phase: implementation; client need: safe, effective care environment; content area: medical/surgical nursing

Rationale
(A) Maalox is not detoxified by the liver prior to elimination. (B) Excess magnesium would be eliminated by the kidneys, even under acid conditions of the blood. (C) Excess magnesium would be eliminated by the kidneys, even under alkaline conditions of the blood. (D) The client could develop toxicity to magnesium if renal insufficiency developed.

177. **(A)** Nursing process phase: implementation; client need: safe, effective care environment; content area: medical/surgical nursing

Rationale
(A) The statement is true. Maalox could interfere with proper absorption of the other drugs. (B) Aluminum and magnesium have been combined to prevent both diarrhea and constipation. (C) The magnesium will help prevent constipation. (D) The statement is incorrect. Increasing the dosage of Maalox could lead to dangerous side effects.

178. (C) Nursing process phase: assessment; client need: physiological integrity; content area: medical/surgical nursing

Rationale
(A) Hemorrhage and mesenteric adenitis would not be as likely to occur as hypovolemia and electrolyte imbalance. (B) Perforation and peritonitis are not very likely to occur. (C) The increased pressure in the lumen of the intestine (proximal to the obstruction) will force fluid and electrolytes from the capillaries in the intestinal wall into the peritoneal cavity. Fluid volume deficit and electrolyte imbalances are likely to occur unless the obstruction is treated. (D) Volvulus would be possible but not as likely as hypovolemia and electrolyte imbalances.

179. (C) Nursing process phase: planning; client need: physiological integrity; content area: medical/surgical nursing

Rationale
(A) A client with an incisional cholecystectomy has no more than the usual risk of developing thrombophlebitis. (B) The risk of urinary retention would be the same as for any other surgical client. (C) The risk of hypostatic pneumonia would be greater because the incision is located just below the rib cage, and it is extremely painful for the client to cough. (D) The risk of hemorrhage would be the same as for any postoperative client.

180. (B) Nursing process phase: implementation; client need: physiological integrity; content area: medical/surgical nursing

Rationale
(A) The T tube can be clamped for meals to allow bile into the duodenum to digest fat. (B) The bile drainage bag should be kept below the insertion site at all times to prevent back flow of bile into the common bile duct. (C) Sterile technique should be used to dress a cholecystectomy incision. (D) The client should not lift anything heavy for 4 to 6 weeks to prevent wound dehiscence. Sexual activity might also be restricted.

181. (D) Nursing process phase: implementation; client need: safe, effective care environment; content area: medical/surgical nursing

Rationale
(A) The Jackson-Pratt drain is emptied once per shift and as needed. (B) The drain is removed by the surgeon when it is no longer draining. (C) The dressing would need to be removed each time the drain was emptied. (D) Bile could drain through the insertion site for the drain or into the drain itself. If this happened, the surgeon would need to be notified. Bile located in tissues where it is not ordinarily found can be damaging to the tissues.

182. (D) Nursing process phase: planning; client need: safe, effective care environment; content area: medical/surgical nursing

Rationale
(A) The colostomy will not be irrigated unless the physician orders an irrigation. (B) The skin around the stoma would become excoriated very quickly if the drainage bag were changed with each stool. (C) A normal diet can be tolerated by most clients with a colostomy. The client should start with low-residue foods and then add other foods, one at a time to see which foods can be tolerated. (D) The skin around the stoma should be assessed every 8 hours.

183. (A) Nursing process phase: assessment; client need: physiological integrity; content area: medical/surgical nursing

Rationale
(A) A large abdominal aneurysm can be palpated. A bruit would be heard over the aneurysm during auscultation. (B–D) These assessments would not be found with an abdominal aneurysm.

184. (D) Nursing process phase: implementation; client need: health promotion and maintenance; content area: medical/surgical nursing

Rationale
(A) Varicose veins rarely rupture and this would not be the purpose of surgery. (B) Walking is not related to varicose veins. (C) If a vein ruptures, it is not a life-threatening emergency, because venous pressure is low. (D) This statement is true.

185. (C) Nursing process phase: analysis; client need: physiological integrity; content area: medical/surgical nursing

Rationale
(A) Moderate edema is normal for the first few days after surgery. (B) The stoma is very vascular; oozing of blood on touching it would be normal. (C) Dark red color would indicate a problem with blood supply; this should be reported at once. (D) Pale color could indicate anemia.

186. (B) Nursing process phase: implementation; client need: safe, effective care environment; content area: medical/surgical nursing

Rationale
(A) The data do not indicate a need to change liquid preparations because they would be absorbed in the small intestines. (B) Time-released preparations would need to be changed because of possible problems with absorption. (C) The data do not indicate a need to change oral antibiotics. (D) Suppositories to stimulate bowel elimination would not be used (or ordered), but other medications via the rectum would be possible.

187. (C) Nursing process phase: implementation; client need: safe, effective care environment; content area: medical/surgical nursing

Rationale
(A) The bacterial flora of the intestines need to be restored. (B) A low-residue diet will not restore the bacterial flora in the intestines. (C) Yogurt, cottage cheese, and buttermilk contain the lactobacillus acidophilous, which helps to restore the normal bacterial flora in the intestines. This restoration will help restore the stool to its normal consistency. (D) The data do not indicate lactose intolerance, so omitting milk products would not help.

188. (D) Nursing process phase: assessment; client need: physiological integrity; content area: medical/surgical nursing

Rationale
(A) Hypersensitivity is a possibility, but the risk for a hyper-

sensitive reaction is not as great as the risk for renal and hearing damage. (B) Dyspnea is a sign of anaphylactic shock, which could happen but is not very likely. Visual changes are neither a side effect nor a sign of toxic reaction. (C) Vomiting would be unusual. Hypotension is a sign of anaphylactic shock, which is possible but not likely. (D) The aminoglycosides are nephrotoxic and may damage hearing. These are the most common toxic reactions to this family of drugs to which gentamycin belongs.

189. **(C)** Nursing process phase: implementation; client need: safe, effective care environment; content area: medical/surgical nursing

Rationale
(A) With hepatitis, both the direct and indirect bilirubin are usually elevated. (B) The direct bilirubin would be elevated with stones obstructing the common bile duct. (C) Elevation of indirect bilirubin but normal direct bilirubin usually indicates excessive destruction of red blood cells. (D) Indirect bilirubin should not be elevated with cholecystitis.

190. **(B)** Nursing process phase: assessment; client need: safe, effective care environment; content area: medical/surgical nursing

Rationale
(A) Dehydration is possible, but cardiac arrhythmias would be unexpected. (B) The liver makes albumin, the major protein in the blood, and clotting factors. When hepatocytes are destroyed, as in hepatitis, liver function would be compromised. With less albumin, the osmolality of the blood would decrease, and edema would be possible. With a decrease in clotting factors, bleeding could occur. (C) Jugular venous distention and pleural effusion would be unlikely. (D) Hypoactive bowel sounds would not be expected. Impaired skin integrity is a possibility but not as likely as edema and bleeding.

191. **(A)** Nursing process phase: implementation; client health promotion and maintenance; content area: medical/surgical nursing

Rationale
(A) Hepatitis A is spread through feces, contaminated water, or contaminated food. (B) The virus is not spread through body fluids. (C) The virus is not spread via the respiratory tract. (D) It would be most unusual to spread the virus through sex.

192. **(D)** Nursing process phase: implementation; client need: psychosocial integrity; content area: medical/surgical nursing

Rationale
(A) The client needs to accept the colostomy and start to become independent in self-care. (B) The client should be allowed to face the problem when ready and not forced into an emotional adjustment. (C) The client may not be ready to socialize with others. (D) Watching for cues that the client is ready to participate in colostomy care allows for individual coping skills and is probably the most efficient way to promote self-care.

193. **(C)** Nursing process phase: implementation; client need: safe, effective care environment; content area: medical/surgical nursing

Rationale
(A) Fluids should be forced after the myelogram. (B) The usual diet is not resumed until the following day. (C) Maintaining bedrest for several hours is crucial following all myelograms. The amount of time for bedrest and the position of the bed will vary with the type of contrast medium used. Bedrest is necessary to prevent herniation of the brain through the opening in the skull. (D) The data do not indicate a need for measurement of intake and output.

194. **(D)** Nursing process phase: implementation; client need: safe, effective care environment; content area: medical/surgical nursing

Rationale
(A) The needle will be inserted into the subarachnoid space during a lumbar puncture. (B–D) The subarachnoid space is the only answer.

195. **(C)** Nursing process phase: planning; client need: safe, effective environment; content area: medical surgical nursing

Rationale
(A, B, & D) These are not conditions that someone with a temporary pacemaker would be susceptible to. (C) The pacemaker electrode provides a direct pathway for the conduction of stray electricity to the heart muscle. This is not a danger for permanent pacemakers because the pacemaker itself, as well as the electrode, is placed under the skin.

196. **(A)** Nursing process phase: analysis; client need: physiological integrity; content area: medical/surgical nursing

Rationale
(A) The buildup of atherosclerotic plaque in the coronary arteries narrows the lumen. The narrowed lumen results in diminished blood flow to the myocardium. When this tissue is oxygen-deprived for a long period, tissue damage (myocardial infarction) results. (B–D) These are not major risk factors associated with a myocardial infarction.

197. **(C)** Nursing process phase: analysis; client need: physiological integrity; content area: medical/surgical nursing

Rationale
(A) The data do not indicate that the pupils are fixed. (B) Doll's eyes would be a more appropriate description. (C) The phenomenon is called doll's eyes. (D) The data do not indicate that nystagmus is present.

198. **(B)** Nursing process phase: analysis; client need: safe, effective care environment; content area: medical/surgical nursing

Rationale
(A) The pupils indicate how well the brain stem is functioning. (B) The pupils reflect brain-stem functioning. (C) The pupils are a reflection of brain-stem functioning. (D) The pupils do not reflect functioning of the cerebellum.

199. **(D)** Nursing process phase: analysis; client need: physiological integrity; content area: medical/surgical nursing

Rationale
(A) Romberg's sign is an indication of a loss of the sense of position. The client loses balance when standing erect, with feet

together and eyes closed. (B) Comatose would not describe the condition at the appropriate level of specificity. A comatose condition is characterized by the absence of spontaneous eye movements and speaking; the client in coma does not respond to painful stimuli. (C) A decorticate posture is characterized by flexion of the upper extremities at the elbows and wrists. The legs may also be flexed. This posture indicates a lesion in the mesencephalic region of the brain and may be elicited in response to painful stimuli in the comatose client. (D) The position is decerebrate. This posture indicates compression of the lower brain stem.

200. (B) Nursing process phase: planning; client need: safe, effective care environment; content area: medical/surgical nursing

Rationale
(A) The environment should be quiet, but the client also needs sensory stimulation. (B) The cornea does need regular care to prevent ulceration; the client does not have a blink reflex. (C) Score on the Glasgow Coma Scale should steadily increase (D) If the head of the bed is flat, intracranial pressure could increase.

201. (C) Nursing process phase: assessment; client need: physiological integrity; content area: medical/surgical nursing

Rationale
(A, C, & D) The subtle signs are those seen in the early stages of increasing intracranial pressure. (B) Intracranial pressure would have to increase before herniation occurred.

202. (A) Nursing process phase: implementation; client need: physiological integrity; content area: medical/surgical nursing

Rationale
(A) Hyperventilation produces vasoconstriction and reduction of blood volume in the brain. (B) The fetal position would be contraindicated because venous drainage from the skull would be impeded. (C) Blowing the nose would increase intracranial pressure. (D) Pulling up in bed could also increase intracranial pressure.

203. (D) Nursing process phase: implementation; client need: physiological integrity; content area: medical/surgical nursing

Rationale
(A) Having a sitter at the bedside would not be necessary. (B) A padded tongue blade is no longer recommended because more damage is usually done when inserting it during a seizure. (C) An oral airway is not recommended for the same reason the tongue blade is not recommended. (D) The side rails should be padded to prevent injury during a seizure.

204. (A) Nursing process phase: implementation; client need: safe, effective care environment; content area: medical/surgical nursing

Rationale
(A) Cues will help orient the client to the present. (B) The client should have privacy and a restful environment during mealtimes. Use of hands may be necessary to encourage independence. Dysphagia may also be a problem for the client. (C) Fatiguing activities should be planned for early in the day to avoid agitation. Sundowning might also occur at the end of

the day. (D) The client will need orientation cues during conversation. The family should listen actively but provide cues to the client periodically.

205. (C) Nursing process phase: implementation; client need: safe, effective care environment; content area: medical/surgical nursing

Rationale
(A) Restraints are likely to increase frustration and should be used only when all other safety measures have failed. (B) Routine helps to optimize existing skills. (C) Stimulants may increase agitation. (D) Rest helps to foster cooperation. Frequent rest periods should be planned.

206. (D) Nursing process phase: analysis; client need: safe, effective care environment; content area: medical/surgical nursing

Rationale
(A & D) Breath sounds are important but not as important as information on the last dose of medication. Medication will affect motor performance, the most important area for assessment in the client with Parkinson's disease. (B) Assessment of perfusion is important but not as important as information on the last dose of medication. (C) Elimination patterns would be important but not as important as information about medication.

207. (B) Nursing process phase: implementation; client need: safe, effective care environment; content area: medical/surgical nursing

Rationale
(A) The upright position and exercise should be encouraged to promote bone integrity and independence. (B) Use of an incentive spirometer would be helpful to strengthen muscles of inspiration so that independent respirations may be maintained as long as possible. (C) Dysphagia may become a problem. A diet high in calcium would be likely to contain milk products, and food stimulating secretion of mucus would make the dysphagia worse. (D) The client with ALS and the family need social activities. In addition, the Heimlich maneuver might be needed if dysphagia becomes a problem.

208. (D) Nursing process phase: analysis; client need: safe, effective care environment; content area: medical/surgical nursing

Rationale
(A) Amyotrophic lateral sclerosis is progressive, not sudden in onset. (B) Vertigo and tinnitus would be more symptomatic of Meniere's syndrome. (C) Quick recovery would rule out stroke. (D) Drop attacks are symptomatic of transient ischemic attacks.

209. (C) Nursing process phase: evaluation; client need: safe, effective care environment; content area: medical/surgical nursing

Rationale
(A) A successful intradermal injection of purified protein derivative is marked by a wheal. (B) A wheal should be produced. (C) The solution should collect as a wheal between the layers of skin. (D) A wheal is the best answer.

210. (C) Nursing process phase: analysis; client need: safe, effective care environment; content area: medical/surgical nursing

Rationale

(A) The results of the intradermal injection of purified protein derivative should not be read in 12 to 24 hours. The hypersensitivity reaction may not have had time to take place. (B) The results should not be read in 24 to 48 hours because it is still too soon. (C) Results of the test should be read in 48 to 72 hours because the T lymphocytes and macrophages will have had time to produce the hypersensitivity reaction. (D) The hypersensitivity reaction would have faded or disappeared in 4 to 5 days.

211. **(D)** Nursing process phase: implementation; client need: physiological integrity; content area: medical/surgical nursing

Rationale

(A) Heparin will not dissolve clots. (B) Streptokinase is not used to reduce the size of an infarct immediately following a myocardial infarction. (C) Urokinase is not used to reduce the size of an infarct immediately following a myocardial infarction. (D) Alteplase binds to fibrin in clots and stimulates conversion of plasminogen (in the clot) to plasmin, helping to dissolve the clot and reduce the size of the infarct. It is given immediately following a myocardial infarction for this purpose.

212. **(A)** Nursing process phase: assessment; client need: safe, effective care environment; content area: medical/surgical nursing

Rationale

(A) Confusion and/or impulsive behavior could result from perceptual and spatial disabilities caused by damage to the right hemisphere. This confusion and/or impulsive behavior are likely to cause the client major problems. (B) Using the Glasgow Coma Scale every hour would not be necessary. (C) Receptive aphasia is seen in left-sided lesions. (D) Assessing loss of memory would not be as important as assessing for confusion and impulsive behavior.

213. **(C)** Nursing process phase: analysis; client need: safe, effective care environment; content area: medical/surgical nursing

Rationale

(A) A lesion on the left side of the brain would not affect the temporal field of the right eye because nerves supplying the temporal field of the right eye are found only on the right side of the brain. (B) The lesion described could not possibly affect the nasal fields of both eyes because nerves supplying the nasal fields of the eyes (from the retina) cross at the optic chiasm. (C) Because the fibers supplying the nasal halves of the eyes cross at the optic chiasm, a lesion on the left side of the brain posterior to the chiasm would affect the temporal field of the left eye and the nasal field of the right eye. (D) Anatomy of the optic tract is such that only choice C is the correct answer.

214. **(A)** Nursing process phase: analysis; client need: physiological integrity; content area: medical/surgical nursing

Rationale

(A) The signs and symptoms are classical for meningeal irritation because of blood in the subarachnoid space. (B) The signs and symptoms are due to blood in the subarachnoid space. The problem is probably caused by hemorrhage rather than infarction. (C) The data do not support a subdural hematoma. (D) The data do not support herniation of the brain stem.

215. **(C)** Nursing process phase: implementation; client need: safe, effective care environment; content area: medical/surgical nursing

Rationale

(A) The best position for drainage of oral secretions would be on the side with the head of the bed slightly elevated. Maintaining a patent airway would be the highest priority for this comatose client. In addition, a semi-Fowler's position would affect intracranial pressure. (B) A supine position would not be the optimal position for drainage of oral secretions. Keeping the head of the bed flat would cause an increase in intracranial pressure. (C) A side position with the head of the bed slightly elevated would be the optimal position for drainage of oral secretions and preventing changes in intracranial pressure. (D) The client could choke on oral secretions in the Trendelenburg position, and cerebral perfusion would be increased.

216. **(D)** Nursing process phase: implementation; client need: physiological integrity; content area: medical/surgical nursing

Rationale

(A) Rectal procedures would be contraindicated in order to avoid stimulation of the vagus nerve. (B) The client must remain as quiet as possible to avoid rupture of the aneurysm. (C) Coughing could cause the aneurysm to rupture. (D) Neurological signs should be monitored hourly in order to detect any change in the client's status so that immediate treatment could be given.

217. **(C)** Nursing process phase: implementation; client need: safe, effective care environment; content area: medical/surgical nursing

Rationale

(A) The nurse needs to establish an environment in which the client feels safe to make mistakes in communication. (B) The nurse's goal will be to maintain normal cerebral blood flow. Antihypertensives would be administered so as to maintain this normal flow without any dramatic changes. A dramatic decrease in blood pressure could lead to further ischemia. (C) Assisting and staying with the client at mealtimes would be a high priority in order to prevent aspiration. (D) Rehabilitation is not usually initiated until after the acute phase has passed and the client's physiological status has stabilized.

218. **(C)** Nursing process phase: implementation; client need: physiological integrity; content area: medical/surgical nursing

Rationale

(A) The needle needs to be at least 19 gauge in size to avoid hemolysis of red blood cells. (B) Baseline temperature and vital signs will be needed for comparison. Therefore, the temperature and vital signs should be started before the transfusion is started. (C) The blood should be run at no more than 5 ml/min for the first 15 minutes so that the nurse can catch the first sign of a reaction to the blood. (D) Blood should be administered within 4 hours to prevent multiplication of bacteria at room temperature.

219. **(C)** Nursing process phase: assessment; client need: physiological integrity; content area: medical/surgical nursing

Rationale
(A) Pain in lower left quadrant denotes dysfunction associated with ovaries, testes, spleen, colon, etc. not gallbladder. (B) Pain in the lower right quadrant denotes dysfunction associated with ovaries, testes, colon, appendix, etc., not gallbladder. (C) Pain associated with cholecystitis begins in the right upper quadrant of the abdomen and radiates to the right shoulder and scapula. (D) Pain in the left upper quadrant denotes dysfunction related to the stomach, esophagus, transverse colon, heart, etc., not gallbladder.

220. (A) Nursing process phase: assessment; client need: physiological integrity; content area: medical/surgical nursing

Rationale
(A) BPH is a progressive enlargement of the prostate that results in bladder outlet obstruction due to compression of the prostatic urethral lumen. As enlargement of the prostate continues, increased pressure is exhibited on the urethra and leads to inability to empty the bladder completely. Retained urine in the bladder is the most serious symptom of BPH because it can lead to the complication of urinary tract infection and kidney damage. (B) With BPH, enlargement of the prostate continues and begins to exert more pressure on the urethra. This results in a symptom complex called prostatism in which there is hesitancy in starting urination. Even though this occurs in the early to middle stages of BPH, it is not the most serious symptom. (C) With BPH, enlargement of the prostate progresses and begins to exert more pressure on the urethra. This results in inadequate emptying of the bladder and bladder pressure. Bladder pressure leads to discomfort and therefore can result in more frequent attempts to empty the bladder and relieve pressure and discomfort. Even though this symptom occurs in the early to middle stages of BPH, it is not the most serious symptom listed. (D) In BPH, as enlargement of the prostate progresses, increased pressure is exerted on the urethra. This results in decreased force of the urinary stream, which occurs in the early to middle stages of BPH. This is not the most serious symptom that can occur with BPH.

221. (B) Nursing process phase: implementation; client need: safe, effective care environment; content area: medical/surgical nursing

Rationale
(A) Normal saline Foley irrigation would not prevent bladder spasms. Bladder spasms are common after a TURP and are treated with B & O suppositories or oxybutynin (Ditropan). (B) Foley irrigation with normal saline or sterile water is prescribed postoperatively to prevent blood clots from blocking the catheter, thereby causing bladder distention, possibly fresh bleeding, and pain. (C) Foley irrigation with normal saline would irrigate the bladder, and therefore does not cause scrotal edema after a TURP. (D) Foley irrigation is used to irrigate the bladder. TURP removes prostate tissue that is outside the bladder, not inside, and therefore is not used to prevent an infection.

222. (C) Nursing process phase: evaluation; client need: health promotion and maintenance; content area: medical/surgical nursing

Rationale
(A) Sexual activity is delayed for at least 3 to 4 weeks or as directed by the physician to ensure adequate healing of tissue, nerve, and blood supply sources to this area. (B) This type of

surgery can cause sterility from retrograde ejaculation, but not impotence. (C) A transurethral resection procedure does not cause impotence. (D) Sexual dysfunction can occur and should be discussed related to actual or anticipated changes in sexual function after surgery.

223. (D) Nursing process phase: assessment; client need: safe, effective care environment; content area: medical/surgical nursing

Rationale
(A) Elimination and hydration are important in the care of a client in traction and are monitored daily. This gives adequate time for the nurse to intervene and prevent any complications that may occur. (B) Proper nutrition and family relationships are monitored by the nurse in a daily manner and can easily be adjusted as the need arises. Although necessary, these are not the most important or immediate assessments. (C) Assessment of skin integrity and rest or sleep are necessary in the care of a client in skeletal traction. However, daily monitoring by nurses can prevent complications by frequent turning, good skin care, quiet environment, and pharmacological interventions to promote client comfort. (D) Body alignment assessment is extremely important and urgent as a safety factor when caring for a client in skeletal traction because within minutes the client can develop severe pain or muscle spasms from improper body alignment. Also, assessment of the client's neurovascular status is most important to detect changes of circulatory compromise and subsequent tissue damage. These two assessments are most important because they can cause severe, unreversible complications within a short time.

224. (C) Nursing process phase: assessment; client need: physiological integrity; content area: medical/surgical nursing

Rationale
(A) Signs and symptoms of ketoacidosis includes decreased blood pressure, increased pulse, and increased respirations. (B) Signs and symptoms of hypovolemic shock include decreased blood pressure, increased pulse, and increased respirations. (C) Signs and symptoms of ICP include initial hypotension and then rapid hypertension, increased pulse, and increased respirations. (D) Signs and symptoms of respiratory alkalosis include decreased blood pressure, increased pulse, and increased respirations.

225. (A) Nursing process phase: assessment; client need: physiological integrity; content area: medical/surgical nursing

Rationale
(A) Pupillary changes are very important in the assessment of a client with a head injury. Dilated, unequal, pinpoint, nonresponsive, and ovoid pupillary findings indicate increased ICP. (B) Head injury with potential increased ICP may lead to urinary incontinence, but urine production is not affected unless there is trauma of renal and GU structures. In unresponsive clients, a Foley catheter is used to monitor urinary output. (C) Increased ICP causes increased blood pressure with a widened pulse pressure and bradycardia. (D) Increased ICP can manifest in irregular respiration patterns that include Cheyne-Stokes, central neurogenic hyperventilation, apneustic breathing, cluster breathing, and ataxic breathing.

226. (B) Nursing process phase: implementation; client

need: health promotion and maintenance; content area: medical/surgical nursing

Rationale
(A) Assessment for ventricular size is done with CT scan and not the surgical procedure craniotomy. (B) A craniotomy is indicated in this case to relieve increased ICP, evacuate a subdural or epidural hematoma, or remove necrotic or temporal lobe tissue. (C) The purpose of performing a craniotomy in this case is not to relieve pain. Pain will be managed by other interventions. (D) Assessment of trauma is done by physical assessment, blood work, and diagnostic studies (i.e., CT scan). The problem will be identified and in this case a surgical intervention is indicated.

227. **(C)** Nursing process phase: analysis; client need: physiological integrity; content area: medical/surgical nursing

Rationale
(A) The symptoms of anorexia, nausea, and indigestion after eating fatty foods are the result of digestion of food with chemical reaction with bile and are not the result of bile production. (B) Excessively fatty foods may cause periodic digestive disturbances, but clients who have symptoms of gallbladder disease experience increased difficulty digesting fatty foods due to inadequate release of bile by gallbladder (due to inflammation or blockage of the bile duct by stones) to aid in fat digestion. (C) Inadequate bile in the small intestine for fat digestion is due to inflammation or blockage of the bile duct by stones and will cause symptoms of anorexia, nausea, and indigestion. (D) Bile is produced by the liver and stored in the gallbladder. Ingestion of food stimulates the gallbladder to contact and release bile into the common bile duct (not the duodenum) to mix with food and aid in fat digestion.

228. **(A)** Nursing process phase: assessment; client need: physiological integrity; content area: medical/surgical nursing

Rationale
(A) Healing by primary (first) intention occurs in clean wounds in which the edges of the wound are well approximated and there is limited erythema, edema, or exudate due to minimal cell damage at the injury site. (B) Healing by secondary intention occurs when tissue is lost through trauma, infection, or other conditions that cause wound edges to be uneven and not well approximated. Also, increased edema, erythema, and exudate are present due to infection or trauma at the site. (C) Closure of the wound, ulcer, or cavity is delayed due to contamination and infection. The wound is later sutured after the infection has cleared. (D) This is also called delayed primary intention in which the wound is sutured after infection is cleared.

229. **(D)** Nursing process phase: analysis; client need: physiological integrity; content area: medical/surgical nursing

Rationale
(A–C) These values are below the normal serum sodium range for an adult. (D) The normal serum sodium range for an adult is approximately 135 to 148 mEq/L.

230. **(A)** Nursing process phase: analysis; client need: physiological integrity; content area: medical/surgical nursing

Rationale
(A) The most common cause of Addison's disease (80%) is an autoimmune process. (B) This granulomatous disease has a history of being a rare cause of Addison's disease and is not common. (C) This was associated with the cause of Addison's disease prior to 1950, but is not considered the primary cause today. (D) A small percent (40%) of persons with Addison's disease have a family history or relatives with an idiopathic disorder, that is, pernicious anemia, vitiligo, and insulin-dependent diabetes mellitus, but DM is not known to cause Addison's.

231. **(D)** Nursing process phase: implementation; client need: health promotion and maintenance; content area: medical/surgical nursing

Rationale
(A) Fludrocortisone is prescribed as 0.1 mg 3 times/week to 0.2 mg/day PO for adrenocortical insufficiency and 0.1–0.2 mg/day PO for salt-losing adrenogenital syndrome. Therefore; 75 mg is an overdose. (B) Hydrocortisone is prescribed as 15–20 mg PO q A.M. and 10 mg PO q afternoon; therefore, 75 mg is an overdose. (C) Fludrocortisone is prescribed PO up to 6.2 mg/day; therefore, 110 mg/day is an overdose. (D) This is the correct dose of hydrocortisone prescribed for the client with Addison's disease. Dosages are adjusted according to the client's blood pressure, physical appearance, sense of well-being, and various stressors.

232. **(B)** Nursing process phase: planning; client need: health promotion and maintenance; content area: medical/surgical nursing

Rationale
(A) This is an inadequate amount of sodium intake for treatment of a client with Addison's disease. (B) All clients with Addison's disease need to maintain a high salt intake (a minimum of 150 mEq/day or 3 grams sodium). Sodium (Na) intake would be increased if the client experiences profuse perspiration or develops diarrhea. (C) The client will be on a regular diet with increased sodium intake of 3 grams. A diet low in fat and cholesterol is not the prescribed diet. (D) The client will be on a regular diet with increased sodium intake of 3 grams. A diet high in potassium and cholesterol is not the prescribed diet.

233. **(A)** Nursing process phase: assessment; client need: physiological integrity; content area: medical/surgical nursing

Rationale
(A) Weight gain is common in Cushing's syndrome, with increased deposits of fat on the trunk (truncal), neck, and face. "Buffalo hump" and "moon face" are characteristic of Cushing's syndrome. (B) In Cushing's syndrome there is an excess in cortisol production, resulting in an electrolyte imbalance because of altered cation exchange in the renal tubule. As a result, there is an increased potassium excretion, which leads to hypokalemia. (C) Vitiligo is an acquired cutaneous condition characterized by milk-white patches on the skin. It is associated with hyperthyroidism, diabetes mellitus, and Addison's disease. With Cushing's syndrome, the client develops ecchymosis; purplish red striae on the abdomen, breasts, shoulders, and buttocks; and acne in women. (D) In Cushing's syndrome, the electrolyte imbalances of hypokalemia and hypernatremia result in fluid retention and hypertension.

234. (B) Nursing process phase: planning; client need: health promotion and maintenance; content area: medical/surgical nursing

Rationale
(A) To discourage further weight gain, a low-calorie diet is prescribed for clients with Cushing's syndrome. (B) A low-sodium diet is prescribed for a client with Cushing's disease to decrease sodium retention, which leads to fluid retention and hypertension. (C) Clients with Cushing's disease experience increased potassium excretion because of an electrolyte imbalance. Therefore, the diet must be rich in potassium to prevent hypokalemia. (D) Clients with Cushing's disease are prescribed a low-calorie, low-sodium, potassium-rich, and diabetic diet in order to prevent complications of hypokalemia, hyperglycemia, edema, and hypertension.

235. (D) Nursing process phase: analysis; client need: physiological integrity; content area: medical/surgical nursing

Rationale
(A) Hypernatremia causes edema and hypertension, and not specifically anorexia, nausea, vomiting, weakness, and muscle cramps. (B) Hypoglycemia causes sweating, headache, anxiety, hunger, blurred vision, and palpations. (C) Although clients with Cushing's syndrome can develop hyperglycemia, signs and symptoms include polyuria, polydipsia, polyphagia, and acetone breath. (D) Clients with Cushing's syndrome can often develop hypokalemia because of increased potassium secretion. Signs and symptoms of hypokalemia include weakness, muscle cramps, EKG changes, anorexia, nausea, vomiting, and altered level of consciousness.

236. (B) Nursing process phase: implementation; client need: safe, effective care environment; content area: medical/surgical nursing

Rationale
(A) Aldactone is a potassium-sparing diuretic and would be used in the treatment of Cushing's syndrome. (B) HydroDIURIL is a potassium-depleting diuretic and would not be used in the treatment of a client with Cushing's syndrome because potassium depletion is a serious problem associated with Cushing's syndrome. Therefore, this drug would be harmful. (C) Dyrenium is a potassium-sparing diuretic and would be used in the treatment of Cushing's syndrome. (D) Midamor is a potassium-sparing diuretic and would be used in the treatment of Cushing's syndrome.

237. (C) Nursing process phase: implementation; client need: health promotion and maintenance; content area: medical/surgical nursing

Rationale
(A) Clients with Cushing's syndrome can experience severe, life-threatening hypokalemia. Therefore, a potassium-sparing diuretic is prescribed. HydroDIURIL is a potassium-depleting diuretic and would be harmful to the client. (B) Lasix is a potassium-depleting diuretic and can result in severe hypokalemia, which is a problem for a client with Cushing's syndrome. A potassium-sparing diuretic would be prescribed. (C) A potassium-sparing diuretic is prescribed for a client with Cushing's syndrome to prevent hypokalemia, which is severe and life threatening. (D) A potassium-depleting diuretic would be harmful to a client with Cushing's syndrome because it can cause severe, life-threatening hypokalemia. A potassium-sparing diuretic would benefit the client.

238. (D) Nursing process phase: planning; client need: health promotion and maintenance; content area: medical/surgical nursing

Rationale
(A) Thyroid replacement is indicated in the treatment and not radiation therapy. (B) Thyroid replacement is indicated in the primary treatment and not surgical removal of the gland. (C) Treatment will include exogenous iodine therapy to restore the client to a euthyroid state. (D) Treatment includes restoring the client to a euthyroid state by replacing the missing thyroid hormone.

239. (C) Nursing process phase: analysis; client need: physiological integrity; content area: medical/surgical nursing

Rationale
(A) A serious symptom often associated with myxedema is hypoglycemia, not hyperglycemia. (B) A serious symptom often associated with myxedema is hyponatremia, which results from delay in excretion of water load, and development of dilutional hyponatremia. (C) Along with a decrease in basal metabolic rate and cold intolerance, a client with myxedema experiences hypothermia. (D) A serious symptom often associated with myxedema is hypokinesis in which the client exhibits decreased motor action to stimuli.

240. (A) Nursing process phase: assessment; client need: physiological integrity; content area: medical/surgical nursing

Rationale
(A) Due to an increase in prolactin secretion, this can cause galactorrhea in female clients with myxedema. (B) Myxedema can cause reduced synthesis and rate of lipid breakdown. This results in hyperlipidemia. (C) Due to reduced renal blood flow that leads to decreased glomerular filtration rate (GFR), there is a reduction in urine output (anuria) and not polyuria. (D) Myxedema is associated with reduced progesterone secretion and altered pituitary function; therefore, this causes decreased fertility.

241. (D) Nursing process phase: assessment; client need: physiological integrity; content area: medial/surgical nursing

Rationale
(A) A common clinical finding noted in clients with Graves' disease is increased appetite and not anorexia. (B) A common clinical finding noted with Graves' disease is heat intolerance and not cold intolerance. (C) Common clinical findings noted with Graves' disease are fatigue and weakness, not increased energy. (D) A common clinical finding noted in clients with Graves' disease is exophthalmos.

242. (A) Nursing process phase: planning; client need: health promotion and maintenance; content area: medical/surgical nursing

Rationale
(A) This complication is caused by hypocalcemia. It is reversible when the calcium serum level is returned to normal with calcium therapy. (B) This is a major long-term complication of hypocalcemia and is irreversible. (C) This is a major long-term complication of hypocalcemia and results in irreversible defective tooth structure of various extent. (D) This is a major long-term complication of hypocalcemia. Once de-

veloped, cataracts will not regress when the client is restored to the normocalcemic state.

243. (D) Nursing process phase: assessment; client need: physiological integrity; content area: medical/surgical nursing

Rationale
(A) A client with hyperparathyroidism exhibits drowsiness and fatigue, not restlessness. (B) A client with hyperparathyroidism exhibits weight loss, not weight gain. (C) A clinical finding with hyperparathyroidism is a decrease in deep-tendon reflexes, not increased deep-tendon reflexes. (D) A clinical finding with hyperparathyroidism is renal calculi due to increased serum calcium.

244. (C) Nursing process phase: assessment; client need: safe, effective care environment; content area: medical/surgical nursing

Rationale
(A) This pain experience is associated with rebound tenderness related to findings of appendicitis or Murphy's sign related to findings of acute cholecystitis. (B) Carpopedal spasm is referred to as Trousseau's sign. (C) Chvostek's sign is elicited when the facial nerve on one side of the face it tapped and the facial muscles contract on that side of the face only. It is considered positive in clients with hypoparathyroidism (hypocalcemia). (D) Chvostek's sign involves contraction of facial muscles on only one side of the face when tapped, not both sides.

245. (A) Nursing process phase: planning; client need: psychosocial integrity; content area: medical/surgical nursing

Rationale
(A) The onset of action of regular insulin is ½ to 1 hour. (B) This is within the peak time of insulin or when it reaches the ultimate effect. (C & D) These ranges are within the duration of regular insulin within the body. The onset is ½ to 1 hour after administration.

246. (B) Nursing process phase: implementation; client need: health promotion and maintenance; content area: medical/surgical nursing

Rationale
(A) This time frame is specific to the onset of action of regular insulin and not the peak in which a hypoglycemic reaction can occur. (B) The peak of regular insulin is within 2 to 4 hours after administration. This is when regular insulin is at its most potent effect and decreases the serum blood sugar (hypoglycemia). Clients may experience fatigue, restlessness, irritability, and weakness. (C) This time frame is specific to the duration of regular insulin in the body, not peak. (D) This time frame is after the total duration time of regular insulin in the body, not peak.

247. (D) Nursing process phase: planning; client need: psychosocial integrity; content area: medical/surgical nursing

Rationale
(A) Although corticosteroid therapy causes an increase in serum blood sugar, it causes an increase in appetite that leads to weight gain and not weight loss. (B) Corticosteroid therapy causes hypernatremia and hypertension. (C) Although corticosteroid therapy can aggravate gastric ulceration, it causes an increase in serum blood sugar. (D) Corticosteroid therapy causes hyperglycemia and an increase in appetite that leads to weight gain

248. (A) Nursing process phase: implementation; client need: safe, effective care environment; content area: medical/surgical nursing

Rationale
(A) To begin the 24-hour urine collection, the client voids and discards the first specimen so that the urine from the previous night is not included. Thereafter, all the urine is saved for the next 24 hours in a large collection bottle. (B) The first voided early morning specimen is discarded because it accumulated in the bladder from the previous night and is not considered part of the 24-hour collection. (C) A urinalysis is not considered a part of this laboratory test. (D) In this test, sugar, acetone, and osmolarity are not indicated as part of the urine analysis procedure.

249. (D) Nursing process phase: implementation; client need: safe, effective care environment; content area: medical/surgical nursing

Rationale
(A) A routine urinalysis is not considered a stat procedure unless specifically ordered by the physician. The urine specimen needs to be sent to the laboratory to be examined within 2 hours, otherwise it will become alkaline unless refrigerated. (B) For a routine urinalysis, the laboratory needs at least 10 ml of urine. (C) A routine urinalysis does not require being in a sterile container. Any small clean container is appropriate. A sterile container is required for a urine culture and sensitivity. (D) The first voided specimen in the morning is best for a routine urinalysis because the urine is concentrated and any abnormalities will become more evident in the screening procedure.

250. (D) Nursing process phase: analysis; client need: physiological integrity; content area: medical/surgical nursing

Rationale
(A) AIDS is not an airborne virus. (B) AIDS is not considered cellular metabolistic. (C) Transmission of AIDS is not by feces. (D) AIDS is a bloodborne disease and is transmitted through sexual contact, exposure to infected blood or blood components, and from mother to neonate.

251. (B) Nursing process phase: planning; client need: psychosocial integrity; content area: medical/surgical nursing

Rationale
(A) Strict isolation is specifically used to prevent highly contagious infections spread by direct contact or airborne routes, such as, smallpox, chickenpox, shingles, and diphtheria. (B) This type of isolation is indicated to prevent the transmission of infection in blood or body fluids, such as AIDS, hepatitis, and syphilis. (C) This type of isolation is indicated to prevent the transmission of pulmonary tuberculosis (TBC) in clients with a positive sputum smear or positive chest x-ray for TBC. (D) This type of isolation is indicated to prevent the transmission of infections in feces.

252. (D) Nursing process phase: assessment; client need: safe, effective care environment; content area: medical/surgical nursing

Rationale
(A) Even though AIDS is transmitted through sexual contact, sexual preference is not a concern when planning the care for this client. (B) AIDS is not transmitted by sharing eating utensils, but by sexual contact, infected blood or blood products, and from mother to neonate. (C) AIDS is not transmitted through consumption of various foods. (D) This type of verbal assessment elicits specific information that supports the clinical findings of this client with AIDS diagnosis.

253. (D) Nursing process phase: analysis; client need: physiological integrity; content area: medical/surgical nursing

Rationale
(A) Strep throat is caused by bacteria, not a virus. (B) Epstein-Barr infections are associated with viral pharyngitis, which is not bacterial as strep throat is. (C) Neoplasms cause general inflammation of the pharynx (pharyngitis) and are not related to strep throat. (D) Strep throat is caused by bacteria and can lead to the complication of rheumatic fever in clients who are untreated or did not complete a full course of prescribed antibiotics.

254. (B) Nursing process phase: implementation; client need: physiological integrity; content area: medical/surgical nursing

Rationale
(A) Postural drainage assists the client in expectorating the secretions, not liquefying them. (B) Breathing humidified air helps to liquefy secretions for easy removal. (C) This intervention helps loosen secretions for expectoration, not liquefy them. (D) These exercises help the client to expectorate secretions and expand the lungs, not liquefy secretions.

255. (C) Nursing process phase: analysis; client need: psychosocial integrity; content area: medical/surgical nursing

Rationale
(A) Hansen's disease (leprosy) is caused by *Mycobacterium leprae*. *Staphylococcus saprophyticus* is a newly recognized staph species that can cause urinary tract infections. (B) The signs and symptoms of Hansen's disease include sensory loss, loss of sweating ability, loss of facial hair (especially eyebrows), skin lesions, and corneal abrasions. Ecchymosis and frequent respiratory infections are not associated with Hansen's disease. (C) There is more than one form of Hansen's disease. The two principal forms are lepromatous and tuberculoid. (D) These are anti-inflammatory drugs and are not used to treat leprosy. Antileprosy agents include clofazimine, dapsone, ethionamide, and rifampin.

256. (B) Nursing process phase: planning; client need: health promotion and maintenance; content area: medical/surgical nursing

Rationale
(A) AIDS is transmitted by sexual contact and the practice of anal intercourse will not protect persons from AIDS. (B) Using latex condoms with a spermicide will help prevent sexual transmission of HIV, although the only safe method is abstinence. (C) An increase in the number of sexual partners increases the possibility of acquiring STD, especially AIDS. (D) HIV has been found in saliva and avoiding deep throat kissing will not prevent a person from contracting AIDS.

257. (A) Nursing process phase: assessment; client need: health promotion and maintenance; content area: medical/surgical nursing

Rationale
(A) This statement describes the herpes simplex appearance. (B) This statement does not describe what herpes simplex looks like, but rather some possible associated complications. (C) This statement does not describe what herpes simplex looks like, but rather a method of transmission. (D) This statement does not describe what herpes looks like, but describes possible complications for females.

258. (C) Nursing process phase: planning; client need: safe, effective care environment; content area: medical/surgical nursing

Rationale
(A) Cotton underwear is encouraged to help keep the genital area clean and dry for longer periods of time. (B) Clients are advised to avoid sexual activity when lesions are present. (C) Acyclovir (Zovirax) is effective for both primary (initial) and recurrent herpes simplex virus (HSV-1 and HSV-2). (D) Sitz baths are encouraged three to four times a day to provide increased comfort and good genital hygiene.

259. (A) Nursing process phase: planning; client need: safe, effective care environment; content area: medical/surgical nursing

Rationale
(A) The immediate postoperative period is crucial for airway clearance because of secretions and effects of anesthesia. (B) This is important, but not the priority problem in the immediate postoperative period. (C) This is important, but airway clearance is crucial so that normal gas exchange can be achieved. (D) All postoperative clients are at risk for potential for injury because of surgical incisions and effects from anesthesia, but it is not the priority problem in the immediate postoperative period.

260. (D) Nursing process phase: planning; client need: physiological integrity; content area: medical/surgical nursing

Rationale
(A) Although pain medication can be habit forming if taken consistently over a period of time, it is most therapeutic if used briefly for postoperative pain. (B) The use of pain medication will help in the recovery process, but if it is not taken at the onset of pain, stress and anxiety can increase and can lead to a longer recovery period. (C) Pain medication should be encouraged at short (3–4 hr) intervals during the immediate postoperative period (first 24 hours) to maintain optimum comfort. It can often be ineffective if given after pain is present for a while because the client often has severe pain by the time there is a verbal request for pain medication. (D) This is the best response because pain medication is most effective when given at the onset of pain experience, therefore resulting in increased comfort and decreased anxiety and stress. This can lead to a quicker recovery.

261. (C) Nursing process phase: analysis; client need: physiological integrity; content area: medical/surgical nursing

Rationale
(A) Healthy preadolescents are not the age group requiring

the flu vaccination because of their optimum immune function during those years. (B) Healthy children are not the age group requiring the flu vaccine because of their optimum immune function during this time. (C) The elderly are the population with the greatest risk for infections and, therefore, it is recommended that they get the flu vaccine. Because of the aging process, the immune system cannot respond to fight infection and, therefore, medication is necessary to assist the process. (D) The elderly are at risk, but nursing home residents are not going on a trip out of the country.

262. (C) Nursing process phase: analysis; client need: physiological integrity; content area: medical/surgical nursing

Rationale
(A) An impacted fracture would result in a crushing of one bone into another and usually involves a joint (i.e., ankle, wrist, shoulder, etc.). (B) An incomplete fracture is where part of the bone is still intact and is not completely detached from the other part. (C) A comminuted fracture involves several bone fragments that have clearly broken off of the main bone, as described with this injury. (D) Although some fractures may have varying degrees of complication, this is not an example of a fracture type, but rather a degree or extent of injury.

263. (B) Nursing process phase: analysis; client need: physiological integrity; content area: medical/surgical nursing

Rationale
(A) The clinical findings present in clients with pneumonia include rales, rhonchi, wheezes, and bronchial breath sounds, not diffuse crackles. Agitation and chest petechiae are not clinical findings in clients with pneumonia. (B) These clinical findings are specific in clients who develop fat emboli. (C) Clients with emotional reaction to stress may exhibit anxiety, not agitation, crackles in lung fields, or chest petechiae. (D) Systemic reaction to analgesics does not exhibit these findings, but can cause dyspnea, rash, and itching.

264. (D) Nursing process phase: assessment; safe, effective care environment; content area: medical/surgical nursing

Rationale
(A) The term for this description is choledocholithiasis. (B) The term for this condition is choledochitis. (C) The term for this condition is cholelithiasis. (D) Cholecystitis refers to inflammation of the gallbladder due to obstruction from stones or bile and related to inflammation or infection.

265. (C) Nursing process phase: planning; health promotion and maintenance; content area: medical/surgical nursing

Rationale
(A) Ultrasonography is used as a diagnostic measure to confirm cholelithiasis-cholecystitis, because it determines whether there are stones and where they are located. (B) A CBS is used as a diagnostic measure to confirm cholelithiasis-cholecystitis, because there will be an elevated WBC with this condition and the blood test will reveal this finding. (C) A urinalysis will not reveal the presence of stones or inflammation in the gallbladder. (D) An EKG is used as a diagnostic measure to confirm cholelithiasis-cholecystitis because clients often have epigastric chest pain, which can suggest cardiac involvement, therefore an EKG is done to rule out a myocardial infarction (MI).

266. (D) Nursing process phase: assessment; client need: safe, effective care environment; content area: medical/surgical nursing

Rationale
(A) Nocturia begins to occur in the early stage of BPH and results from pressure exerted on the urethra, causing incomplete emptying of the bladder; therefore, the client gets up often at night to urinate. It is one of the first symptoms reported by the client. (B) Hesitancy in initiating the urinary stream occurs in the early to middle stages of BPH as enlargement of the prostate progresses. Pressure is exerted on the urethra and causes the urinary flow to be decreased; initial urination is actually droplets or dribbling. It is not considered a more advanced symptom of BPH. (C) Intermittent urinary stream occurs in the early to middle stages of BPH due to progressive enlargement of the prostate. This occurs simultaneously with hesitancy, nocturia, dribbling, and decreased size and force of the urinary stream. Because it occurs early, it is not considered a symptom that would begin in the later or advanced stage of BPH. (D) As hyperplasia of the prostate progresses into the advanced stage of BPH, the client develops hematuria. This is caused by the rupture of dilated veins over the prostate surface, mucosal irritation, or renal damage. When hematuria occurs, the client usually recognizes that this is more serious than other earlier symptoms and will seek medical attention.

267. (D) Nursing process phase: assessment; client need: safe, effective care environment; content area: medical/surgical nursing

Rationale
(A) Pain under a cast is a warning sign of tissue breakdown under the cast and needs immediate attention. (B) Drainage through a cast is a warning sign of tissue breakdown under the cast and needs immediate attention. (C) Irritability or restlessness is a warning sign of many problems including tissue breakdown under a cast. (D) If there is tissue breakdown under a cast, it usually leads to infection and pain. The symptoms would include an elevated body temperature due to infection and not a decreased body temperature.

268. (B) Nursing process phase: analysis; client need: physiological integrity; content area: medical/surgical nursing

Rationale
(A) Renal calculi is a complication of traction and splint therapy caused by immobility; they increase during concentration because of altered elimination patterns. (B) Scoliosis is a congenital anomaly and is not a complication of traction and splint therapy. (C) Constipation-impaction is a common complication of traction and splint therapy caused by immobility. (D) Constrictive edema can occur because of too tight a cast, but not with traction or splints, which do not constrict tissue and muscles of extremities.

269. (C) Nursing process phase: evaluation; client need: physiological integrity; content area: medical/surgical nursing

Rationale
(A) When traction force and direction are maintained, traction would be effective. (B) When all ropes are in the center tract of the pulley, traction is effective (C) When traction weights rest on the bed, this is not effective and counteracts the ultimate goal of traction. (D) When clamps and bolts are secure on the traction apparatus, then traction is effective.

270. (B) Nursing process phase: implementation; client need: health promotion and maintenance; content area: medical/surgical nursing

Rationale
(A) Frequent oral hygiene (every 1 to 2 hours) would greatly benefit the client with an NG tube because it will control halitosis and prevent oral irritation and infection. (B) Changing the anchor tape weekly would lead to nasal irritation and infection. The anchor tape needs to be changed daily or sooner if soiled. (C) Lubricant on the nostril where the tube is inserted will decrease irritation and skin breakdown. This action is appropriate and will make the client more comfortable. (D) It is beneficial to the client for lip balm to be applied every 2 to 4 hours or more often if necessary. This will prevent cracking of the lips leading to pain and infection.

271. (A) Nursing process phase: analysis; client need: physiological integrity; content area: medical/surgical nursing

Rationale
(A) Hemorrhage is the major complication in the immediate postoperative period because of the surgical procedure, which involves cutting tissue in a well-supplied vascular area (prostate-urethra). (B) Calculi may develop from other renal-urinary problems, but they are not the major complication after a TURP. (C) Constipation may develop in postoperative clients for varied reasons, but it is not common in clients post-TURP and is not a major concern during the immediate postoperative period. (D) Infection can develop in clients postoperatively with TURP, but it does not occur during the immediate postoperative period and therefore is not the major complication.

272. (B) Nursing process phase: analysis; client need: physiological integrity; content area: medical/surgical nursing

Rationale
(A) Constitutional period is another term for the acute phase in which there is an interaction between the host and infectious organisms that results in actual symptoms of an acute illness. (B) The incubation period is when the infectious agent invades the host and establishes itself. (C) The period of communicability is immediately prior to incubation in which the prospective host is exposed to the infectious agent. (D) The prodromal period is the initial stage of the communicable disease process, the interval between the earliest symptoms and the appearance of a rash or fever.

273. (A) Nursing process phase: implementation; client need: health promotion and maintenance; content area: medical/surgical nursing

Rationale
(A) Common medications used to treat TB will cause serious side effects of both nephrotoxicity and hepatotoxicity. (B) Common drugs used to treat TB are toxic to the liver, but are not ototoxic. (C) Common drugs used to treat TB normally do not cause peripheral neuritis and nausea (occasional). (D) Common drugs used to treat TB do not cause neutropenia, but are toxic to the liver.

274. (C) Nursing process phase: analysis; client need: physiological integrity; content area: medical/surgical nursing

Rationale
(A) This is not the substance that causes an anaphylactic reaction. It is a group of chemical mediators of inflammation and plays a role in asthma. (B) This is not the substance that causes an anaphylactic reaction. Heparin is an anticoagulant. (C) The release of histamine causes an anaphylactic reaction as described in this situation. (D) Tissue hypoxia does not cause an anaphylactic reaction.

275. (D) Nursing process phase: assessment; client need: health promotion and maintenance; content area: medical/surgical nursing

Rationale
(A) Petechiae on the abdomen are not a clinical finding of SLE. (B) Low-grade afternoon fever is not a clinical finding of SLE. (C) Multiple ecchymoses of the body are not clinical findings in clients with SLE. (D) A recurrent butterfly rash of the face is a distinct clinical finding of clients with SLE.

276. (C) Nursing process phase: implementation; client need: health promotion and maintenance; content area: medical/surgical nursing

Rationale
(A) Aspirin is an antipyretic that reduces fever and promotes comfort, not natural decongestant action. (B) Alka-Seltzer has antacid actions and is not a decongestant. (C) Vitamin C has antihistamine actions and reduces the response to histamines that cause nasal congestion and rhinitis. (D) Mylanta is an antacid, not a decongestant.

277. (D) Nursing process phase: planning; client need: health promotion and maintenance; content area: medical/surgical nursing

Rationale
(A) Since impetigo is an infection, Benadryl would provide comfort by preventing itching, not antibiotic action. (B) Tylenol would provide comfort, not antibiotic action. (C) Cortisone would reduce inflammation and promote comfort, but would not destroy the staphylococcal or streptococcal infection. (D) Appropriate systemic broad-spectrum antibiotics, such as a cephalexin (Keflex), ampicillin, or tetracycline, are common examples of the drugs of choice. These antibiotics destroy the staphylococcal and streptococcal organisms that caused the infection.

278. (C) Nursing process phase: planning; client need: psychosocial integrity; content area: medical/surgical nursing

Rationale
(A) Emotional support is necessary in the treatment of rheumatoid arthritis (RA), but it is not the major goal of drug therapy. (B) The major goal of drug therapy in RA to reduce inflammation in joints and promote comfort. Drug therapy does not cure RA. (C) The major goal of drug therapy in RA is to reduce inflammation in joints and promote comfort. (D) Drug therapy in RA treatment is not directed to prepare the client for surgery. Drug therapy reduces inflammation in joints and promotes comfort.

279. (D) Nursing process phase: planning; client need: health promotion and maintenance; content area: medical/surgical nursing

Rationale

(A) The antibiotics listed here are the drugs of choice and are most commonly used to treat a UTI. (B) A urine for culture and sensitivity is performed before and after treatment of a UTI and therefore is used in the treatment. (C) Increasing fluids, emptying the bladder frequently, and follow-up teaching are included in the care and treatment of a UTI. These interventions will reduce the risk of a recurrent infection. (D) Treatment for a UTI would include antibiotics for a 10-day duration. If it is stopped before that, there is an increased chance of re-occurrence of the UTI, which could lead to renal damage.

280. (C) Nursing process phase: implementation; client need: safe, effective care environment; content area: medical/surgical nursing

Rationale

(A) The portal of entry to host is a source of acquiring an infection—not a practice to break the "chain of infection." (B) The reservoir is a host for infection—not a method to transfer infection from one source to another and therefore not a practice to break the "chain of infection." (C) The method of transmission of infection is the phase in which hand washing before and after various tasks can break the "chain of infection" and lead to safe, effective client care. (D) The portal of exit from host refers to blood, wound drainage, feces, and urine, which can transmit disease because of improper handling and improper hand-washing technique.

281. (D) Nursing process phase: planning; client need: health promotion and maintenance; content area: medical/surgical nursing

Rationale

(A) Measles, mumps, and rubella (MMR) vaccine is given intramuscularly and usually causes localized soreness of the muscle area, low-grade fever, and irritability. (B) Diphtheria, polio, and tetanus (DPT) vaccine is given intramuscularly and usually causes localized soreness of the muscle area, low-grade fever, and irritability. (C) Tetanus toxoid is given intramuscularly and often causes soreness of the muscle area and irritability. (D) Oral polio vaccine (OPV) is given by mouth and does not cause any side effects.

282. (D) Nursing process phase: implementation; client need: safe, effective care environment; content area: medical/surgical nursing

Rationale

(A) Isolation specific to preventing transmission of infection related to feces is not blood and body fluids. (B) Isolation specific to preventing transmission of infection related to feces is not contact isolation. (C) Drainage and secretion isolation is used with clients for protection of wound drainage, not specifically for infection related to feces. (D) Enteric isolation is specifically used to prevent the transmission of infection related to feces.

283. (A) Nursing process phase: implementation; client need: safe, effective environment; content area: medical/surgical nursing

Rationale

(A) Hand washing is considered one of the most effective ways to prevent the spread of infection because of the constant contact of nurses with infectious materials. Various other options listed here may help to prevent infection of wounds, but the best prevention is basic hand washing. (B) Incisions are cleansed from top to bottom, which includes cleaning from the least contaminated to the most contaminated area. (C) Although this intervention would help prevent wound infection in some cases, it is not the best action by the nurse in this situation. (D) Although this practice may help prevent the transmission of infections, hand washing before and after is the safest and most effective method of preventing the spread of infection.

284. (B) Nursing process phase: implementation; client need: safe, effective care environment; content area: medical/surgical nursing

Rationale

(A) The tip of the tubing has to be lubricated for easier insertion and must be inserted approximately 3 to 4 inches into the rectum past the internal sphincter. Inserting the tube 1 to 2 inches is not far enough because it is still in the anal canal and needs to be further beyond the internal sphincter. (B) The tube is inserted 3 to 4 inches into the rectum. Further insertion may damage intestinal mucous membrane. Also, the client needs to be in the left lateral position with the right leg flexed to promote comfort while the solution is introduced into the intestine. (C) The solution should be introduced slowly over a period of 5 to 10 minutes to prevent rapid distention of the intestine and a desire to defecate. The container should not be higher than 18 inches above the anus, or this will increase the rate and cause rapid bowel distention. (D) Fluid should flow slowly. The client should take as much as possible of the amount ordered. The tubing should be clamped before removing it from the anus to prevent leakage. The tip is lubricated, and the left lateral position with right leg flexed facilitates accurate fluid distribution in the intestine and minimizes discomfort from cramping.

285. (D) Nursing process phase: implementation; client need: safe, effective care environment; content area: medical/surgical nursing

Rationale

(A) Once a swab or gauze has been used, it is considered contaminated and should be discarded, and then a new one should be used. (B) Wound care with an antiseptic solution requires a physician's order. (C) This method introduces organisms back into the wound for recontamination. (D) The wound or incision should be cleansed from the area of least contamination to the area of greater contamination.

286. (A) Nursing process phase: implementation; client need: safe, effective care environment; content area: medical/surgical nursing

Rationale

(A) This method prevents further contamination of the wound and reduces the chance of infection. (B) This does not describe the correct rationale for irrigating a wound and does not guarantee organization by the nurse to complete the procedure. (C) This is not the correct rationale for the direction of fluid flow to irrigate a wound. (D) Irrigation of a wound with the client in various positions does not always enhance comfort.

287. (C) Nursing process phase: analysis; client need: physiological integrity; content area: medical/surgical nursing

Rationale
(A) This term does not describe a grating sound, but a backward movement. (B) This term does not describe a grating sound from a broken bone, but a breath or lung sound. (C) This term describes the grating sound that is heard or felt when the ends of a broken bone are moved. (D) This term describes what is felt over air-filled cavities on the body, that is, lungs and trachea, after percussion or verbal sounds are done.

288. (C) Nursing process phase: assessment; client need: health promotion and maintenance; content area: medical/surgical nursing

Rationale
(A) This is not the correct response. Because of overgrowth of the prostate gland, the urethra becomes narrowed and results in several problems with urination, especially difficulty in starting the urinary stream. (B) This is not the correct response. Overgrowth of the prostate gland around the urethra causes a decrease in the force of urination. (C) This is the correct response. Because of overgrowth of the prostate gland around the urethra, there would be a decrease in the size and force of the urinary stream—not an increase. (D) This condition causes pressure or narrowing of the urethra and not bladder pressure. An inability to empty the bladder may lead to infection and urinary frequency, but the client can still urinate in small amounts.

289. (C) Nursing process phase: implementation; client need: safe, effective care environment; content area: medical/surgical nursing

Rationale
(A) Sterile technique will promote wound healing, but even though the excess drainage is removed, there will be continuous drainage. Cleaning the wound every few hours using sterile technique is necessary to prevent infection. (B) Although moisture is removed, it is part of the healing process to have moisture on the wound for at least 72 hours. (C) Wounds are cleaned from the least contaminated to the more contaminated area to prevent introduction of organisms back into the wound. This is the most important rationale for using sterile technique. (D) Sterile technique aids in removing bacteria from the wound and surrounding tissues, but does not stop or prevent normal bacterial growth on surrounding tissues.

290. (A) Nursing process phase: implementation; client need: safe, effective care environment; content area: medical/surgical nursing

Rationale
(A) A nosocomial infection is one that results from the delivery of health services in a health-care facility. The urinary tract is a prime site; placing the urinary drainage bag above the level of the bladder allows a reflux of urine in the catheter or bag (which could be contaminated) to re-enter the bladder and become a source of infection. (B) Aseptic technique would help prevent an infection at the incision site, but a UTI is the most common nosocomial infection. (C) Self-administration of insulin would not cause a nosocomial infection. (D) Spreading germs by not covering the mouth is not an example of a nosocomial infection.

291. (A) Nursing process phase: assessment; client need: physiological integrity; content area: medical/surgical nursing

Rationale
(A) Restlessness, yawning, tachycardia, and hypertension are all early signs of hypoxia. (B) Although tachypnea is an early sign of hypoxia, the client exhibits hypertension and restlessness, not hypotension and lethargy. (C) As the oxygen deprivation continues, confusion occurs. Tachycardia is a sign of early hypoxia, not bradycardia. Headaches occur in chronic hypoxia—not in the acute stage. (D) Early signs of hypoxia include tachycardia, hypertension, and paleness, which are opposite of the signs listed here.

292. (D) Nursing process phase: assessment; client need: safe, effective care environment; content area: medical/surgical nursing

Rationale
(A) Although instillation of air assists in placement assessment, it does not provide the nurse with residual volume data. (B) Auscultating the bowel sounds with the use of 10 ml of tap water is not a safe intervention because the fluid can be aspirated into the lungs and only air should be instilled to ensure accurate tube placement. (C) Although submerging the end of a feeding tube in a glass of water can indicate correct tube placement, aspirating the contents is the safest and most accurate nursing intervention in this situation. (D) It is best for the nurse to aspirate the stomach contents in order to ascertain tube position as well as the client's absorption of the tube feedings. The gastric contents are reinstilled to prevent electrolyte imbalance.

293. (A) Nursing process phase: assessment; client need: physiological integrity; content area: medical/surgical nursing

Rationale
(A) Because radiation therapy affects fast-growing cells, the hemopoietic and GI systems would be affected. Because the treatment field incorporates the throat, esophagus, and stomach, the GI symptoms most commonly seen would include nausea and dysphagia. (B) Bone marrow suppression would occur, because the treatment field includes the sternum. Diarrhea would not be seen because the small bowel is not included in the treatment field. (C) Alopecia is observed only in brain irradiation. (D) Radiation therapy does not cause constipation.

294. (D) Nursing process phase: intervention; client need: safe, effective care environment; content area: medical/surgical nursing

Rationale
(A–C) The nurse should never apply any OTC medications to a radiation treatment field. Because most of these products contain petroleum derivatives or metallic fragments, they may actually intensify the burning process. (D) The nurse should notify the physician and obtain orders for a water-based emollient such as Aquaphor. Most OTC products contain petroleum derivatives and may intensify the burning process; therefore, nothing should be applied until the doctor is notified.

295. (B) Nursing process phase: intervention; client need: safe, effective care environment; content area: medical/surgical nursing

Rationale
(A) Because of the serious nature of the problem (a low Hgb), it would not be safe and correct standards of nursing care to do nothing. (B) Jehovah's Witnesses are opposed to blood

transfusions and organ donations. Because the client's refusal may be life-threatening, the nurse should notify the client's physician. (C) It is not appropriate for the nurse to try to convince the client to go against religious practices and accept the transfusion. (D) The nurse should not administer the blood without the client's consent.

296. (D) Nursing process phase: analysis; client need: physiological integrity; content area: medical/surgical nursing

Rationale

(A) The client had the gallbladder removed (cholecystectomy); therefore, infection within the gallbladder could not occur postoperatively. (B) Bile is produced by the liver and stored in the gallbladder. Synthesis of bile would not cause postoperative jaundice. (C) An inflammatory process would cause pain, localized tenderness, and fever, not jaundice. (D) The major cause of postoperative jaundice is one or more retained stones in the common bile duct. Retained stones are not detected and removed at the time of surgery and occur in 1 to 3 percent of clients postoperatively.

297. (D) Nursing process phase: evaluation; client need: health promotion and maintenance; content area: medial/surgical nursing

Rationale

(A) Cabbage produces odor and flatus, not diarrhea. (B) Eggs produce odor, not diarrhea. (C) Rice and tapioca cause constipation, not diarrhea. (D) Fried, greasy foods cause diarrhea and should be consumed with caution.

298. (A) Nursing process phase: evaluation; client need: health promotion and maintenance; content area: medical/surgical nursing

Rationale

(A) Mushrooms, raw vegetables, peelings, and seeds are not digested well and therefore often cause colostomy obstruction. (B) Baked beans cause diarrhea, not obstruction. (C) Onions cause odor and flatus, not obstruction. (D) Cheese causes odor and flatus, not obstruction.

299. (B) Nursing process phase: assessment; client need: physiological integrity; content area: medical/surgical nursing

Rationale

(A) The client will be instructed to do this procedure within the next 24 hours prior to his discharge home. It is not an immediate priority. (B) Because of the effects of general anesthesia on the genitourinary system, the ability to urinate is the priority concern within the next 8 hours postoperatively. The nurse will be assessing for bladder distention and discomfort reported by the client. (C) Within a short time after spinal anesthesia and while in the recovery room, the client is assessed for movement of extremities. So when the client is returned to the nursing unit after the hernia repair, it has been validated that voluntary movement of all extremities is confirmed. Therefore, this occurs before an 8-hour interval. (D) Spinal anesthesia involves depressed motor function of the lower extremities, so the nurse would be concerned about voluntary movement of the lower extremities, not upper.

300. (D) Nursing process phase: analysis; client need: physiological integrity; content area: medical/surgical nursing

Rationale

(A) The NG tube will decompress the bowel to prevent nausea and vomiting. This promotes normal gastrointestinal functioning postoperatively—not respiratory function. (B) Getting out of bed, especially twice a day, promotes improved circulatory and respiratory function, resulting in a quicker recovery and decreased pulmonary complications. (C) Signs and symptoms of wound infection as described here relate to the skin and surrounding tissue structures—not pulmonary complications such as pneumonia. (D) An elderly client who had general anesthesia for a surgical intervention is at risk for the development of pneumonia because of increased secretions accumulating in the lungs during surgery. Immediately postoperatively, this client should be instructed to cough and deep-breath every 1 to 2 hours while awake to remove secretions and promote adequate lung expansion so that complications may be prevented.

301. (A) Nursing process phase: implementation; client need: physiological integrity; content area: medical/surgical nursing

Rationale

(A) Immediately following an IVP, the client should be monitored closely for signs of an allergic reaction to the dye (iodine) used during the procedure. (B) The client will be encouraged to drink fluids after the procedure to minimize potential renal deterioration. However, fluids will be introduced in small amounts orally after signs of nausea have subsided. IV fluids will be administered until the client can tolerate oral fluids. (C) An IVP does not require the client to be on bedrest with the head elevated for 10 hours. The client will be ambulatory as tolerated. (D) Following an IVP, the client returns to a normal diet and fluids unless nausea is present, or surgery is indicated.

302. (C) Nursing process phase: implementation; client need: physiological integrity; content area: medical/surgical nursing

Rationale

(A) Contact isolation precautions are not indicated after this procedure. They would be indicated 24 to 72 hours later if a wound infection develops. (B) The client would resume the previous diet immediately after biopsy unless nausea is present or additional surgical interventions are indicated. (C) Monitoring for postbiopsy bleeding is the most important and immediate priority nursing intervention. Nursing care would include monitoring vital signs and observing for excessive bleeding at the biopsy site. These interventions would help prevent the complication of hypovolemic shock. (D) This is not the most important priority immediately after biopsy. Ambulation will be encouraged often, after the incidence of potential postbiopsy bleeding has subsided.

303. (D) Nursing process phase: implementation; client need: safe, effective care environment; content area: medical/surgical nursing

Rationale

(A) Catching the midstream of urine will provide the most accurate urinalysis. Also, the laboratory needs at least 10 ml of urine for proper analysis. (B) If all urine is collected in the container, there is a greater chance of contamination of the urine from bacteria and cleaning solution collected with the specimen. (C) The first 50 ml of urine may be contaminated with bacteria and cleansing solution. The midstream provides the most accurate urinalysis. (D) The midstream of urine provides minimal or no contamination by bacteria or cleansing solution and therefore provides the best specimen for an accurate urinalysis.

304. (C) Nursing process phase: implementation; client need: physiological integrity; content area: medical/surgical nursing

Rationale

(A) Various measures can be encouraged to prevent recurrence, but this is not the most important nursing priority in this situation. (B) Pancreatic extracts such as pancrelipase (Cotazym, Pancrease, or Ilozyme), which contain 30,000 to 50,000 units of lipase, are given with meals to improve malabsorption in clients with chronic pancreatitis. During acute pancreatitis, the client is usually NPO to avoid pancreatic stimulation and therefore receives nutrition by TPN. (C) Because of the extent of inflammation, clients with pancreatitis are in a great deal of pain; therefore, pain relief is the most important priority. (D) The client with acute pancreatitis is usually NPO to avoid pancreatic stimulation. Oral feedings are usually resumed when the client's serum amylase returns to normal and appetite has returned.

305. (D) Nursing process phase: planning; client need: psychosocial integrity; content area: medical/surgical nursing

Rationale

(A) This statement supports the treatment of pancreatitis since fat aggravates the condition. This statement by the client indicates understanding of treatment. (B) Frequent small meals will ensure proper nutrition and increase tolerance by the client with pancreatitis. This statement indicates the client's understanding of the condition and treatment. (C) The client with pancreatitis does need to gradually increase exercise and activity to promote strength and stimulate appetite. This statement indicates good understanding of treatment by the client. (D) Additional teaching is necessary here because the client needs to abstain from alcohol to prevent further pain attacks and extension of inflammation and pancreatic insufficiency.

306. (C) Nursing process phase: planning; client need: health promotion and maintenance; content area: medical/surgical nursing

Rationale

(A) In RA, exercises are necessary to reduce pain and increase joint mobility and strength; however, exercises do not relieve morning stiffness. (B) A firm mattress helps to support joints, but does not prevent morning stiffness. (C) Heat application (showers, baths, etc.) increases blood flow to the joints and therefore decreases pain and stiffness by increasing mobility. (D) Ice application will decrease blood flow to the joints, thereby increasing stiffness and pain.

307. (B) Nursing process phase: planning; client need: safe, effective care environment; content area: medical/surgical nursing

Rationale

(A) If the client coughs forcefully, further damage to the operative area and wiring apparatus will be damaged. The client should be instructed to cough normally. (B) The client should maintain a semi-Fowler's position or higher to facilitate adequate swallowing and promote good respiratory function. Wire cutters should be at the bedside so that wires can be cut if the client develops difficulty swallowing or breathing. (C) Oral suction equipment is beneficial because it facilitates removal of excess secretions and gives the client security that the secretions can be evacuated from the oral cavity within seconds to prevent aspiration. (D) The supine position is too low to facilitate adequate swallowing and respiratory function. The client should be instructed to maintain the Fowler's position with the head of the bed at least 45 degrees.

308. (D) Nursing process phase: implementation; client need: physiological integrity; content area: medical/surgical nursing

Rationale

(A) It is true that a warm sensation is felt when the contrast dye is injected, but it is not the most important intervention in this situation. (B) The area is scrubbed and prepped for the procedure, but it is not the most important nursing intervention in this situation. (C) Documentation of vital signs and pedal pulses is necessary nursing care before this procedure, but it is not the most important nursing action in this situation. (D) Assessing for an allergy to contrast medium and iodine is the most crucial nursing intervention before this procedure, because it can cause a reaction and result in harm or death to the client.

309. (A) Nursing process phase: implementation; client need: safe, effective care environment; content area: medical/surgical nursing

Rationale

(A) A KUB is an x-ray that visualizes the kidney, urethra, and bladder structures, and requires no preparation. (B) A KUB is an x-ray and does not require the client to be NPO. (C) A KUB is an x-ray and does not require any medication. If the client experiences nausea and vomiting, then an antiemetic such as promethazine may be ordered. There were no reports of nausea experienced by this client. (D) A KUB is a general x-ray procedure and does not require bowel preparation.

310. (C) Nursing process phase: assessment; client need: safe, effective care environment; content area: medical/surgical nursing

Rationale

(A) It is common to appear angry and frightened after an incident such as this, but it is not the most serious problem in this situation. (B) Profuse bleeding from the lower extremity is serious and needs attention, but it is not the most serious concern at this time. (C) Since he sustained a back injury and states "I can't move," this suggests a spinal cord injury and requires careful handling. (D) The smell of alcohol on his breath is a problem that can be addressed later, but the fact that he cannot move is more serious. He is angry, but cannot move and, therefore, is not dangerous.

311. (B) Nursing process phase: analysis; client need: physiological integrity; content area: medical/surgical nursing

Rationale

(A) Consumption of alcohol prior to the accident is of concern because of the possibility of withdrawal. However, it is not the most important assessment in this situation. (B) In the initial period following a spinal cord injury (spinal shock), the bladder will not empty because of absent reflexes. It continues to fill and distend, which requires careful monitoring and immediate attention. (C) This identity problem will be a long-term concern, and not the most immediate concern by the nurse. (D) Smoking may predispose the client to respiratory complications, but it is not the most immediate concern in planning his care.

312. (D) Nursing process phase: planning; client need: physiological integrity; content area: medical/surgical nursing

Rationale

(A) It is important to encourage or assist the client to recognize progress, but physiological needs are most important in this case. (B) Safety issues are always important when the client has motor and sensory deficits; therefore, restraining devices can be used to provide safety in this situation, but are not a priority. Restraints either physical or chemical should be used only after all other safety measures are instituted. (C) Even though establishing bladder and bowel control or function for a client with a spinal cord injury is an important part of care, it can be a long-term goal. Meanwhile, as the client begins to sit out of bed, incontinence of urine and/or feces may occur. Therefore, the use of protective pads or diapers when the client is out of bed and in a chair is a common nursing practice. (D) Clients with spinal cord injuries are highly susceptible to hypotension and bradycardia when their position is changed; therefore, monitoring vital signs is the most important priority in this case.

313. (B) Nursing process phase: analysis; client need: safe, effective care environment; content area: medical/surgical nursing

Rationale

(A) This position will put excess pressure on brain structures and prevent adequate oxygenation to the brain because of edema. (B) A 30- to 45-degree head-of-bed elevation promotes venous drainage, which helps to prevent edema without putting excess pressure on brain structures. (C) A 30- to 45-degree head-of-bed elevation may help to promote respiratory function, but it is not the best rationale for this position in a client who is at risk for increased intracranial pressure. (D) A 30- to 45-degree head-of-bed elevation does not necessarily prevent aspiration.

314. (B) Nursing process phase: analysis; client need: physiological integrity; content area: medical/surgical nursing

Rationale

(A) Dialysis will not stimulate production of erythropoietin by the kidneys to increase the number of red blood cells. (B) Dialysis will remove nitrogen from the blood and therefore cause the BUN to decrease, not increase. (C) Potassium is removed during dialysis. (D) Since fluid is removed with dialysis, weight loss should be evident.

315. (D) Nursing process phase: implementation; client need: physiological integrity; content area: medical/surgical nursing

Rationale

(A) Carbon dioxide by mask is inappropriate and not available. Carbon dioxide needs to be rebreathed by using a paper bag. (B) Oxygen is contraindicated. The client needs carbon dioxide, not oxygen. (C) There is no evidence given that would suggest the client needs an endotracheal tube. (D) The client's blood gases conform to respiratory alkalosis, probably secondary to anxiety. The most appropriate nursing intervention is to have the client rebreathe carbon dioxide to a safe level.

316. (A) Nursing process phase: implementation; client need: physiological integrity; content area: medical/surgical nursing

Rationale

(A) This client needs a diet with high-carbohydrate, low-fat protein. Chicken is a low-fat protein; mashed potatoes and peas add needed calories. (B) Steak is a high-fat protein. French fries and creamed onions are high-fat foods. (C) Peanut butter is an incomplete protein (from vegetables). This client needs complete protein (from animal sources). (D) Eggs are high in fat and protein. Sausage is high in fat.

317. (D) Nursing process phase: analysis; client need: physiological integrity; content area: medical/surgical nursing

Rationale

(A) It is not beneficial for the client to be flat. (B) Even though the client has had blood loss, the client should not be flat. (C) This would be appropriate for a client following passage of an intestinal tube, that is, a Miller-Abbott or a Cantor tube, not a Sengstaken-Blakemore. (D) This position would best benefit the client because it would facilitate easier swallowing of secretions, which is difficult with this condition.

318. (C) Nursing process phase: analysis; client need: physiological integrity; content area: medical/surgical nursing

Rationale

(A) Although electrolytes can be added to TPN, this is not the primary purpose. Electrolytes can be corrected in IV fluids. (B) The client may or may not be NPO during this time. The purpose of TPN is to provide nutrients and calories even if the client is receiving IV fluids and/or food. Therefore, TPN is not specifically ordered to rest the bowel. (C) TPN has the nutrients and calories that regular IV fluids do not have; therefore, it will help the client gain weight. (D) TPN is not ordered to prevent dehydration; IV fluids can do this.

319. (A) Nursing process phase: evaluation; client need: health promotion and maintenance; content area: medical/surgical nursing

Rationale

(A) The post-cholecystectomy client should not experience pain or abdominal cramping or fullness on a low-fat diet. (B) Weight loss may not be desirable in some clients. Low-fat diet is prescribed if fat is poorly tolerated, not necessarily for weight loss. (C) Although a low-fat diet may reduce serum cholesterol, this is not the most desirable outcome. (D) The post-cholecystectomy client does not usually have peripheral edema related to cholelithiasis.

320. (C) Nursing process phase: assessment; client need: physiological integrity; content area: medical/surgical nursing

Rationale

(A, B, & D) These levels are within normal limits (WNL); they would be out of range in the client with CRF. (C) Potassium and creatinine levels are usually elevated in the undialyzed client with CRF. Calcium levels are decreased in the CRF client.

321. (A) Nursing process phase: implementation; client need: health promotion and maintenance; content area: medical/surgical nursing

Rationale
(A) When the health-care worker is at risk of being directly exposed to any client's blood or body secretions, universal precautions are mandated. (B) The health-care worker often has no way of knowing which clients have been tested or are at risk for HIV infection. (C) The health-care worker often does not know which clients are members of high-risk groups; therefore, universal precautions are necessary for all client contact where risk is involved. (D) Universal precautions are necessary for all client contact where risk of blood/or body fluid exposure is possible.

322. (B) Nursing process phase: evaluation; client need: health promotion and maintenance; content area: medical/surgical nursing

Rationale
(A) This behavior will not reduce risk of exposure to potentially infectious secretions. (B) Barrier methods such as latex condoms greatly reduce risk of exposure to HIV during sexual intercourse. (C) The client has no way of knowing who is definitely HIV negative. (D) Barrier methods such as diaphragms do not provide adequate protection against exposure to HIV during sexual intercourse.

323. (A) Nursing process phase: intervention; client need: health promotion and maintenance; content area: medical/surgical nursing

Rationale
(A) The irritated area should be monitored for signs of irritation to ensure prompt intervention. (B) Lotions should not be applied to the irritated area unless advised by the radiologist. (C) Powder should not be applied to the irritated area unless recommended by the radiologist. (D) Ulceration is not an expected side effect of radiotherapy; it can usually be prevented.

324. (D) Nursing process phase: analysis; client need: physiological integrity; content area: medical/surgical nursing

Rationale
(A–C) These symptoms are not associated with pernicious anemia. (D) In addition to general symptoms of anemia, vitamin B_{12} deficiency may be manifested by peripheral neuropathy and loss of balance resulting from a subacute degeneration of the spinal cord.

325. (A) Nursing process phase: analysis; client need: safe, effective care environment; content area: medical/surgical nursing

Rationale
(A) Freshly prepared solutions of sodium hypochlorite (bleach) in a 1:10 dilution are effective disinfectants. (B–D) Sodium hypochlorite (bleach) is the most effective disinfectant for cleaning up blood and body fluid spills.

326. (C) Nursing process phase: evaluation; client need: physiological integrity; content area: medical/surgical nursing

Rationale
(A) If the client is consistently gaining weight, the scale is probably not faulty. (B) There is no reason to suggest this.

(C) Successful TPN therapy is evidenced by consistent weight gain, about ¼–½ lb/day. (D) There is no reason to do this because therapy is successful.

327. (A) Nursing process phase: analysis; client need: physiological integrity; content area: medical/surgical nursing

Rationale
(A) Alcoholism is a leading cause of FA deficiency. (B) Lack of intrinsic factor absorption causes vitamin B_{12} deficiency or pernicious anemia. (C) FA deficiency rarely occurs in people who eat lots of vegetables. (D) Folic acid (FA) requirements are increased during the second and third trimesters, but FA deficiency does not result from pregnancy complications.

328. (B) Nursing process phase: implementation; client need: health promotion and maintenance; content area: medical/surgical nursing

Rationale
(A) Lasix is not indicated for this purpose. (B) Diuretics such as Lasix may be administered to prevent or correct transfusion-induced circulatory overload. (C) Lasix may decrease the client's blood pressure, but this is not the reason it is administered to this client. (D) Lasix is not given for this reason.

329. (C) Nursing process phase: planning; client need: safe, effective care environment and physiological integrity; content area: medical/surgical nursing

Rationale
(A & B) Rapid transfusion of blood in nonemergency situations could cause circulatory overload. (C) Blood transfusions should not exceed 4 hours because of the risk of bacterial proliferation. (D) A blood transfusion should be concluded within 4 hours of initiation.

330. (A) Nursing process phase: analysis; client need: safe, effective care environment; content area: medical/surgical nursing

Rationale
(A) This WBC is greatly diminished. Daily monitoring of laboratory work is essential because of the risk of infection. (B) Pruritus is common in Hodgkin's disease and it is not life threatening. Other measures may be needed to decrease itching. (C) This platelet count is WNL. (D) Intermittent vomiting is probably not life threatening; many antiemetics are available to control this problem.

331. (A) Nursing process phase: planning; client need: health promotion and maintenance; content area: medical/surgical nursing

Rationale
(A) A greatly diminished platelet and WBC count leaves the client prone to hemorrhage and infection, a leading cause of death in aplastic anemia. (B) Iron supplements will be given, but it is not the priority goal. (C) Fatigue will be present, but prevention of fatigue and fluid overload is not the priority. (D) A neutropenic diet may be indicated, but it is not the priority goal.

332. (C) Nursing process phase: implementation; client need: safe, effective care environment; content area: medical/surgical nursing

Rationale

(A) Parenteral iron should be given deep intramuscular, not in the deltoid. (B) Massage could cause leakage and staining of the skin. (C) This is the correct method for parenteral iron therapy in order to avoid staining of the skin and decrease the potential for fat necrosis. (D) Bedrest is not necessary after iron injection.

333. **(A)** Nursing process phase: evaluation; client need: safe, effective care environment; content area: medical/surgical nursing

Rationale

(A) Fluid level should rise and fall with respirations; if it does not, either the chest tube is clogged or the lung has re-expanded. (B) This should not happen unless there is an air leak. (C) If the water seal chamber bubbles continuously, an air leak is present. (D) Fluid in the suction control chamber will bubble continuously to indicate that it is working properly; the fluid level will not fluctuate.

334. **(B)** Nursing process phase: implementation; client need: safe, effective care environment; content area: medical/surgical nursing

Rationale

(A) Embolization is not a risk usually associated with bone marrow aspiration. (B) Although bleeding is usually minimal, the site should be monitored for bleeding. (C) A pressure dressing is applied over the puncture site to stop the minimal bleeding that usually occurs. (D) Analgesia may be administered PRN, but it is not as high a priority as answer B.

335. **(A)** Nursing process phase: implementation; client need: safe, effective care environment; content area: medical/surgical nursing

Rationale

(A) The first specimen collected at 8 A.M. Monday is discarded; all urine voided till 8 A.M. Tuesday is collected. (B & C) There is no need to do these. (D) Discarding the urine would invalidate the results of the test.

336. **(D)** Nursing process phase: implementation; client need: physiological integrity; content area: medical/surgical nursing

Rationale

(A) The volume of fat emulsions given will not increase fluid intake appreciably. (B) Fat emulsions will increase serum lipid levels. (C) Fat emulsions supply essential fatty acids. (D) Fat emulsions supply high-calorie essential fatty acids in a relatively small volume of fluid.

337. **(A)** Nursing process phase: planning; client need: health promotion and maintenance; content area: medical/surgical nursing

Rationale

(A) Nutritional status should improve with TPN, as evidenced by consistent weight gain. (B) Capillary blood glucose levels should be within normal limits (60–120 mg/dl). (C) This value indicates hyponatremia. (D) This cholesterol value is elevated for a 30-year-old man.

338. **(D)** Nursing process phase: implementation; client need: safe, effective care environment; content area: medical/surgical nursing

Rationale

(A & B) Blood and blood products should not be given through the same line with TPN because they could coat the inner lumen of the catheter, thus restricting the flow of TPN. (C) Medications are not routinely administered concurrently with TPN because they could be incompatible. (D) Fat emulsions (Intralipid) are administered concurrently with TPN, usually three times a week.

339. **(C)** Nursing process phase: implementation; client need: safe, effective care environment; content area: medical/surgical nursing

Rationale

(A, B, & D) These actions are not the best way to prevent contracting hepatitis B. (C) Immunization with the hepatitis B vaccine is the best way to prevent infection with the hepatitis B virus.

340. **(B)** Nursing process phase: implementation; client need: health promotion and maintenance; content area: medical/surgical nursing

Rationale

(A & D) The bloodborne route is not the way that hepatitis A is transmitted. (B) The fecal-oral route is the main way hepatitis A is transmitted; poor hand-washing practices enhance transmission of hepatitis A. (C) This behavior is not the main method of transmitting hepatitis A, although hepatitis A can be transmitted via oral-genital intercourse.

341. **(D)** Nursing process phase: analysis; client need: physiological integrity; content area: medical/surgical nursing

Rationale

(A–C) Hepatitis C is not transmitted by these routes. (D) Hepatitis C is usually transmitted by the parenteral route, following administration of blood or blood products or IV drug use.

342. **(A)** Nursing process phase: implementation; client need: health promotion and maintenance; content area: medical/surgical nursing

Rationale

(A) In myopia, the eyeball is elongated and the light comes into focus in front of the retina, resulting in nearsightedness. (B) Presbyopia is changes in the eye stemming from the aging process. (C) In hypermetropia, the eyeball is shortened and the light comes into focus behind the retina, resulting in farsightedness. (D) Astigmatism is an asymmetric curvature of the cornea causing blurred vision.

343. **(A)** Nursing process phase: analysis; client need: physiological integrity; content area: medical/surgical nursing

Rationale

(A) Moderate to severe inflammatory responses can produce an increase in ESR. (B) ESR would rise, not decrease. (C) The WBC count would rise in inflammatory conditions, not fall. (D) Fibrinogen level would not necessarily rise.

344. **(A)** Nursing process phase: analysis; client need: physiological integrity and health promotion and maintenance; content area: medical/surgical nursing

Rationale

(A) This measure is the best way to prevent infection. (B)

Measuring temperature does not prevent infection; it indicates presence of infection. (C & D) These measures are helpful in preventing infection, but meticulous hand-washing is more effective.

345. (D) Nursing process phase: analysis; client need: physiological integrity; content area: medical/surgical nursing

Rationale
(A) Malignant neoplasms tend to grow rapidly. (B) Malignant neoplasms usually consist of anaplastic, poorly differentiated cells. (C) Although benign neoplasms remain well encapsulated, malignant neoplasms tend to invade adjacent tissue. (D) Malignant neoplasms are usually rapid growing and they quickly invade adjacent tissue.

346. (D) Nursing process phase: analysis; client need: physiological integrity; content area: medical/surgical nursing

Rationale
(A–C) Toxicities to antineoplastic drugs are drug specific and not all body cells are affected. (D) Body sites most often affected by antineoplastic drugs are the bone marrow, hair follicles, and the GI tract because these sites contain rapidly dividing cells.

347. (B) Nursing process phase: implementation; client need: physiological integrity; content area: medical/surgical nursing

Rationale
(A) Although nausea and vomiting may occur at this time, many clients are premedicated with an antiemetic. Premedicating for nausea and vomiting is a comfort measure, not a safety measure. (B) Checking for adequate blood return is necessary to prevent infiltration (extravasation), with resulting tissue necrosis. (C) Although the client's weight may be obtained, it is not the priority safety measure during administration of a vesicant drug. (D) This intervention is not appropriate.

348. (A) Nursing process phase: analysis; client need: safe, effective care environment; content area: medical/surgical nursing

Rationale
(A) Hormonal chemotherapy agents are cytostatic, not cytotoxic. Hormonal treatment involves making the client's normal environment unsuitable for a hormone-dependent tumor. (B) Plant alkaloids interfere with the M phase of the cell during mitotic spindle formation. (C) Antimetabolites act specifically during the S phase of the cell cycle by inserting the antimetabolite into the DNA during DNA synthesis. (D) Alkylating agents produce breakage and cross-linkage in the DNA, thus preventing all replication.

349. (A) Nursing process phase: assessment; client need: safe, effective care environment; content area: medical/surgical nursing

Rationale
(A) Severe paresthesias, jaw drop, loss of deep tendon reflexes, atoxia, and foot drop are neurotoxic side effects of vincristine that must be prevented. (B–D) These side effects are not observed with administration of vincristine.

350. (A) Nursing process phase: implementation; client need: health promotion and maintenance; content area: medical/surgical nursing

Rationale
(A) A soft, bland diet containing cool foods is indicated for clients with stomatitis. (B) Spicy foods will aggravate stomatitis. (C) Crunchy foods will aggravate stomatitis. (D) Both spicy and crunchy foods irritate the mucosa in stomatitis.

351. (D) Nursing process phase: implementation; client need: physiological integrity; content area: medical/surgical nursing

Rationale
(A) Fluids are monitored closely to minimize edema. (B) This measure is not indicated. (C) Although these measures usually help to monitor or reduce edema, they cannot correct the underlying condition causing SCVS. (D) The client is positioned to minimize progressive shortness of breath and edema.

352. (D) Nursing process phase: analysis; client need: physiological integrity; content area: medical/surgical nursing

Rationale
(A–C) The information would be reflected in tumor staging, such as the TNM classification system. (D) Tumor grading, or the degree of malignancy, is based on histological examination of the lesion.

353. (D) Nursing process phase: assessment; client need: physiological integrity; content area: medical/surgical nursing

Rationale
(A) Indicates progressive increase in tumor size, abnormal lymph nodes with distant metastasis. (B) Indicates no evidence of primary tumor, no lymph node involvement with no assessment for metastasis. (C) Indicates progressive increase in tumor size, normal lymph nodes, and no distant metastasis. (D) Indicates a tumor in situ, normal regional lymph nodes, with no known metastasis.

354. (A) Nursing process phase: planning; client need: safe, effective care environment; content area: medical/surgical nursing

Rationale
(A) Hyperosmolar feedings may cause diarrhea; diluting the strength may decrease diarrhea. (B) Administering cold tube feedings stimulates peristalsis. (C) Hyperosmolar feedings may cause diarrhea. (D) Increasing the height of the bag will increase the rate of infusion, causing an increase in peristalsis.

355. (C) Nursing process phase: assessment; client need: physiological integrity; content area: medical/surgical nursing

Rationale
(A, B, & D) These symptoms are not usually noted by women experiencing menopause. (C) Hot flashes are reported by a majority of women experiencing menopause.

356. (B) Nursing process phase: analysis; client need: safe, effective care environment; content area: medical/surgical nursing

Rationale

(A) Sedatives or antianxiety agents are given preoperatively for this reason. (B) One of the effects of anticholinergics is drying of the mouth and other secretions, thereby decreasing risk of postoperative aspiration. (C) Narcotics would be given preoperatively for this reason. (D) Antihistamines would be given preoperatively to prevent this.

357. (A) Nursing process phase: implementation; client need: safe, effective care environment; content area: medical/surgical nursing

Rationale

(A) Only a small part of the scrubbed person's body is considered sterile: from the waist to the shoulder area, forearm, and gloves. (B) The scrub gown below the waist is not considered sterile. (C) The scrub gown above the elbow is not considered sterile. (D) The back of one's scrub gown is not considered sterile.

358. (D) Nursing process phase: implementation; client need: health promotion and maintenance; content area: medical/surgical nursing

Rationale

(A & B) Leg exercises will not prevent these postoperative complications. (C) Adequate fluid and food intake, along with ambulation, may prevent paralytic ileus; leg exercises will not. (D) Leg exercises will increase circulation, thereby decreasing the likelihood of phlebothrombosis.

359. (A) Nursing process phase: evaluation; client need: physiological integrity; content area: medical/surgical nursing

Rationale

(A) Surgical wounds should heal with little tissue reaction and minimal scar tissue by first intention. (B) Healing by second intention occurs after abscess formation; the wound heals more slowly. (C & D) Secondary suture and third intention healing are the same. Resuturing a wound is not desirable.

360. (D) Nursing process phase: assessment; client need: safe, effective care environment; content area: medical/surgical nursing

Rationale

(A) The client will be unable to speak when intubated. (B & C) These observations indicate that neurological, rather than respiratory function, is intact.. (D) The actions indicate that function has returned to the diaphragmatic muscles and that ventilation should be adequate if the client is extubated.

361. (A) Nursing process phase: implementation; client need: safe, effective care environment; content area: medical/surgical nursing

Rationale

(A) Sterile, moistened saline dressings are kept in place until the surgeon arrives. (B) High Fowler's position would place more tension on the wound and could exacerbate the evisceration. (C) This action could cause infection or trauma to the eviscerated intestines. (D) Although evisceration causes pain that requires analgesia, this is not the priority intervention.

362. (C) Nursing process phase: analysis; client need: physiological integrity and safe, effective care environment; content area: medical/surgical nursing

Rationale

(A) Assessing IV patency is important, but not the priority. (B) Assessing vital signs is important, but a patent airway is the priority. (C) Airway patency and respiratory function are always assessed first when a client is transferred to the PACU. (D) Assessing postoperative surgical dressings is important, but not the priority.

363. (A) Nursing process phase: planning; client need: safe, effective care environment; content area: medical/surgical nursing

Rationale

(A) This drug forms a physiologically inert complex when it combines with heparin. (B) This drug (Darvocet-N) is an analgesic, not an antidote for heparin. (C) This drug (Inderal) is a beta-adrenergic blocking agent, not an antidote for heparin. (D) This drug (Matulane) is an antibiotic antineoplastic agent, not an antidote for heparin.

364. (C) Nursing process phase: assessment and analysis; client need: physiological integrity; content area: medical/surgical nursing

Rationale

(A & B) Extracellular concentration of sodium is expressed in mEq/L and these are not the normal range for sodium. (C) This range is below the normal sodium level. (D) This is the normal range for sodium level.

365. (D) Nursing process phase: assessment and analysis; client need: physiological integrity; content area: medical/surgical nursing

Rationale

(A & B) These ranges represent severe hypokalemia. (C) This is the normal extracellular potassium level. (D) This range is elevated above the normal extracellular potassium level.

366. (C) Nursing process phase: assessment; client need: physiological integrity; content area: medical/surgical nursing

Rationale

(A, B, & D) These symptoms are not associated with development of an anterior pituitary tumor. (C) Neurological findings associated with this tumor usually include complaint of a dull, aching headache that is unaffected by position and is not accompanied by visual changes or nausea.

367. (D) Nursing process phase: assessment; client need: health promotion and maintenance; content area: medical/surgical nursing

Rationale

(A–C) Cortisol deficiency causes hypoglycemia because of decreased hepatic gluconeogenesis. Aldosterone deficiency causes increased sodium loss and increased potassium reabsorption. (D) Hyperpigmentation is often present because of elevated adrenocorticotropic hormone (ACTH) and melanocyte-stimulating hormone (MSH) levels.

368. (A) Nursing process phase: implementation; client need: health promotion and maintenance; content area: medical/surgical nursing

Rationale

(A) Prolonged use of steroids causes sodium retention and

edema; hyperglycemia is often noted. (B–D) Corticosteroid use is not associated with weight loss, hypoglycemia, or hyponatremia.

369. **(B)** Nursing process phase: implementation; client need: health promotion and maintenance; content area: medical/surgical nursing

Rationale
(A & C) Fluid intake should not be restricted in the client with Addison's disease. (B) A diet of at least 3 gm Na and 3 L fluid per day is desired to prevent hypotension. (D) While a high-fiber, high-carbohydrate diet is desirable for many clients, it does not specify the amount of sodium necessary for replacement and the degree of potassium restriction.

370. **(B)** Nursing process phase: assessment; client need: physiological integrity; content area: medical/surgical nursing

Rationale
(A & C) Vascular collapse occurs during addisonian crisis; these values may be normotensive in adults. (B) The serum potassium is elevated and sodium levels and BP are profoundly decreased in addisonian crisis. (D) The sodium level is within normal limits (WNL).

371. **(D)** Nursing process phase: implementation; client need: physiological integrity; content area: medical/surgical nursing

Rationale
(A) The client may be hypoglycemic during this crisis; insulin will potentiate the hypoglycemia. (B) The client is dehydrated and hypotensive; furosemide will potentiate the fluid loss. (C) Fludrocortisone is used orally in conjunction with hydrocortisone in adrenal insufficiency. It has a potent mineralocorticoid effect; it has little glucocorticoid effect with the daily 0.1 or 0.2 mg tablet dose. (D) Corticosteroids and fluid replacement are necessary to restore normal vascular volume during addisonian crisis.

372. **(D)** Nursing process phase: evaluation; client need: health promotion and maintenance; content area: medical/surgical nursing

Rationale
(A) This client is hypotensive, although the sodium level is WNL. (B) Although the BP is WNL, this value indicates severe hyperkalemia. (C) Glucocorticoid replacement therapy must be taken as prescribed, not prn. (D) Clients with any serious health alteration should wear or use Medic Alert bracelets or cards.

373. **(B)** Nursing process phase: assessment; client need: physiological integrity; content area: medical/surgical nursing

Rationale
(A) Obesity is common in Cushing's syndrome. (B) Sodium retention, along with hypertension and weight gain, is usually noted in Cushing's syndrome. (C) Increased glucose levels are noted in Cushing's syndrome. Diabetes mellitus may develop. (D) Sodium retention (hypernatremia), rather than hyponatremia, is noted in Cushing's syndrome.

374. **(C)** Nursing process phase: implementation; client need: health promotion and maintenance; content area: medical/surgical nursing

Rationale
(A, B, & D) These foods are relatively low in sodium and high in potassium. (C) These foods should be discouraged because they are high in sodium.

375. **(C)** Nursing process phase: implementation; client need: health promotion and maintenance; content area: medical/surgical nursing

Rationale
(A, B, & D) Oral or parenteral iron preparations or folic acid will not correct pernicious anemia. (C) Pernicious anemia is initially treated with vitamin B_{12} injections of 100 μg three times a week until hemoglobin values are WNL. Thereafter, the client will require lifelong monthly vitamin B_{12} injections.

376. **(C)** Nursing process phase: assessment; client need: physiological integrity; content area: medical/surgical nursing

Rationale
(A, B, & D) Bradycardia and hypotension would not usually be noted in a client with pheochromocytoma. (C) Catecholamine production is increased in pheochromocytoma, resulting in an increased basal metabolic rate. Clinical symptoms that are often noted include hypertension, tachycardia, anxiety, and weight loss.

377. **(D)** Nursing process phase: analysis; client need: safe, effective care environment; content area: medical/surgical nursing

Rationale
(A–C) These organisms do not cause glomerulonephritis. (D) Group β-hemolytic strep causes an antigen-antibody reaction in the body, resulting in glomerulonephritis.

378. **(D)** Nursing process phase: implementation; client need: safe, effective care environment; content area: medical/surgical nursing

Rationale
(A) Initially, fluid intake will be restricted to counteract fluid overload. (B) The client will be placed on bedrest. Activity may cause proteinuria and hematuria at this time. (C) Dietary protein will be restricted to decrease nitrogen retention and the BUN. (D) Clients with acute glomerulonephritis are treated with penicillin; treatment may continue for several months to prevent a reoccurrence of the strep infection.

379. **(B)** Nursing process phase: implementation; client need: physiological integrity; content area: medical/surgical nursing

Rationale
(A, C, & D) These foods are mainly carbohydrates and fats; they are appropriate for the client in acute glomerulonephritis. (B) This food is mainly protein which is restricted in acute glomerulonephritis to lower proteinuria and the BUN.

380. **(A)** Nursing process phase: planning; client need: physiological integrity; content area: medical/surgical nursing

Rationale
(A) This is the goal of treatment, in order to prevent further damage to the intraocular structures, to decrease and control the intraocular pressure. (B) Rest may relieve the "tired eye" feeling that accompanies glaucoma; it will not reverse in-

traocular damage. (C) Medications are given to produce miosis (pupillary constriction), thus permitting drainage of aqueous humor. Pupillary dilation is contraindicated. (D) Damage resulting from increased intraocular pressure, not retinal hemorrhage, is the usual complication of glaucoma.

381. **(D)** Nursing process phase: analysis; client need: physiological integrity; content area: medical/surgical nursing

Rationale
(A–C) Acetazolamide does not decrease intraocular pressure in this way. (D) Acetazolamide blocks carbonic anhydrase and promotes renal excretion of sodium, potassium, bicarbonate, and water. It also decreases aqueous humor production in the eyes.

382. **(B)** Nursing process phase: assessment; client need: physiological integrity; content area: medical/surgical nursing

Rationale
(A, C, & D) This symptom will be present in hyperglycemia. (B) Diaphoresis in hypoglycemic clients results from stimulation of the autonomic nervous system.

383. **(C)** Nursing process phase: analysis; client need: physiological integrity; content area: medical/surgical nursing

Rationale
(A & B) This value indicates hypoglycemia in adults. (C) This serum glucose value is WNL. (D) This value indicates hyperglycemia.

384. **(B)** Nursing process phase: evaluation; client need: physiological integrity; content area: medical/surgical nursing

Rationale
(A) The serum glucose level is not desirable because it is too low and indicates hypoglycemia. (B) This serum glucose level is WNL and is therefore desirable. (C) This value indicates hypokalemia. Hypokalemia, which is not desirable, may occur after diabetic ketoacidosis (DKA) is corrected. (D) This value indicates hyperkalemia, which often occurs in DKA.

385. **(A)** Nursing process phase: evaluation; client need: health promotion and maintenance; content area: medical/surgical nursing

Rationale
(A) The life span of an RBC is about 120 days, and glycosylated hemoglobin measurements are time-averaged values for blood glucose over the past 2 to 4 months. (B) This is an isolated measure of serum glucose. (C & D) While many clients keep accurate records of blood and urine glucose levels, these records can be falsified.

386. **(C)** Nursing process phase: assessment; client need: physiological integrity; content area: medical/surgical nursing

Rationale
(A & B) This is normal and desirable. (C) Foot pain at rest is a symptom of impaired circulation; so is absence of hair in the lower extremities. (D) This is not cause for concern. Well-healed corns in diabetics should be padded to decrease pressure.

387. **(C)** Nursing process phase: analysis; client need: safe, effective care environment; content area: medical/surgical nursing

Rationale
(A–D) Morphine   Promethazine

$$\frac{10\ mg}{x} = \frac{12\ mg}{1\ cc} \qquad\qquad \frac{50\ mg}{2\ cc} = \frac{25\ mg}{x}$$

$$\frac{12x}{12} = \frac{10\ cc}{12} \qquad\qquad \frac{50\ cc}{12} = \frac{25\ mg}{50}$$

$$x = 0.83\ cc\ or\ 0.8\ cc \qquad 1\ cc = x$$

$$0.8\ cc$$
$$Total = +\ \underline{1.0cc}$$
$$1.8\ cc$$

388. **(C)** Nursing process phase: assessment; client need: physiological integrity; content area: medical/surgical nursing

Rationale
(A) This WBC is WNL. Infection is a major cause of thyrotoxic crisis. (B) This blood glucose level is WNL. Diabetic ketacidosis is a major precipitating factor in thyrotoxic crisis. (C) Severe tachycardia leading to high-output heart failure is often noted in this condition. (D) Extreme diaphoresis is noted in thyrotoxic crisis.

389. **(D)** Nursing process phase: analysis; client need: physiological integrity; content area: medical/surgical nursing

Rationale
(A–C) Insomnia, weight gain, and protein ingestion do not cause this condition. Severe dehydration may be present because of diabetic ketoacidosis, a precipitating factor in thyroid storm. (D) These conditions are commonly known to precipitate thyrotoxic crisis.

390. **(C)** Nursing process phase: implementation; client need: safe, effective care environment; content area: medical/surgical nursing

Rationale
(A) Establishing an IV to treat dehydration and electrolyte imbalance and to administer IV medication will probably be indicated; however, it is not the priority intervention. (B) While a nasogastric tube may be needed to administer medications, it is not the priority intervention. (C) The client may have a depressed gag reflex. Maintaining a patent airway is always the main priority in any life-threatening crisis. (D) Reducing the temperature with prescribed acetaminophen and cooling devices will be necessary, but they are not the priority interventions.

391. **(A)** Nursing process phase: implementation; client need: physiological integrity; content area: medical/surgical nursing

Rationale
(A) The use of physiological eye drops is indicated to counteract dryness. (B) This action is unnecessary unless the exophthalmos is severe and the client's eyes do not close completely. (C) This action may decrease periorbital edema; it will not protect the client's eyes. (D) This action will not protect the client's eye from injury.

392. **(B)** Nursing process phase: implementation; client need: health promotion and maintenance; content area: medical/surgical nursing

Rationale

(A) Protein should not be restricted. (B) A high-protein, high-calorie diet is recommended; caffeine should be avoided. (C & D) Protein and carbohydrates should not be restricted; caffeine should be avoided.

393. **(D)** Nursing process phase: analysis; client need: physiological integrity; content area: medical/surgical nursing

Rationale

(A) Propranolol does not block thyroid hormone formation. (B) Propranolol does not decrease the thyroid's vascularity. (C) Propranolol does not have this effect. (D) An adrenergic blocker such as propranolol may increase the hyperthyroid client's comfort by controlling the tremors, tachycardia, and anxiety resulting from excessive sympathetic nervous system function.

394. **(D)** Nursing process phase: assessment; client need: physiological integrity; content area: medical/surgical nursing

Rationale

(A–C) This observation will be noted in hypothyroidism. (D) Thyroid hormone excess is most often manifested as a generalized acceleration of body processes, resulting in restlessness and distractibility.

395. **(A)** Nursing process phase: implementation; client need: safe, effective care environment; content area: medical/surgical nursing

Rationale

(A) Flushing the toilet several times after use minimizes the risk of family exposure to the isotope. (B) This measure is unnecessary. (C) Clients undergoing I^{131} therapy should avoid close contact with pregnant women for 24 hours after treatment. (D) Clients should be observed for 2 to 4 hours for vomiting after ingesting the isotope.

396. **(C)** Nursing process phase: assessment; client need: physiological integrity; content area: medical/surgical nursing

Rationale

(A) Menorrhagia is relatively common in hypothyroidism. (B) Modest weight gain (about 10 lb) and edema are common in hypothyroidism. (C) This is a common complaint in hypothyroidism, possibly because of a decreased metabolic rate. (D) "Moon facies," or cushingoid effect, is not present. Hyponatremia may be present because of increased inappropriate ADH secretion.

397. **(A)** Nursing process phase: assessment; client need: physiological integrity; content area: medical/surgical nursing

Rationale

(A) Anemia often results in hypothyroidism because of menorrhagia, decreased oxygen demand by the tissues, and decreased erythropoietin production. (B) Hyponatremia may be present because of increased inappropriate ADH secretion. (C) Hypercholesterolemia is often noted in hyperthyroidism. (D) Pancreatic function is usually unaffected in hypothyroidism.

398. **(C)** Nursing process phase: planning; client need: physiological integrity; content area: medical/surgical nursing

Rationale

(A) The metabolic rate is decreased; nutritional needs are lessened. (B) Constipation is a common complaint because of decreased activity level and lowered metabolic rate. (C) Activity intolerance and complaint of fatigue are common because of muscle weakness and lowered metabolic rate. (D) This is not a typical finding.

399. **(B)** Nursing process phase: planning; client need: physiological integrity; content area: medical/surgical nursing

Rationale

(A) A diet low in calories, cholesterol, and saturated fat is recommended. (B) Frequent rest periods are a priority because of the extreme fatigue that is present. (C) Fluids should be encouraged, but not increased because of the risk of congestive heart failure. (D) Rest is essential until the client responds to hormone replacement therapy.

400. **(B)** Nursing process phase: analysis; client need: physiological integrity; content area: medical/surgical nursing

Rationale

(A, C, & D) While this complication may arise from chronic hypoparathyroidism, it is not reversible. (B) The papilledema resulting from chronic hypoparathyroidism will resolve when calcium levels are once again WNL, after treatment.

401. **(A)** Nursing process phase: evaluation; client need: health promotion and maintenance; content area: medical/surgical nursing

Rationale

(A) Nursing interventions are aimed at protecting the client's eyes. (B) Any loss of visual acuity is not a desirable goal. (C) While this is a desirable outcome for most clients, this is not the priority outcome. (D) Clients in the acute stage of Graves' disease exhibit weight loss despite hyperphagia; further weight loss is not desirable.

402. **(C)** Nursing process phase: planning; client need: physiological integrity; content area: medical/surgical nursing

Rationale

(A, B, & D) This nursing diagnosis is not typically associated with SIADH. (C) ADH-induced antidiuresis causes fluid volume expansion, which inhibits adrenocortical secretion of aldosterone, causing salt loss in the urine and decreased reabsorption of sodium in the renal tubules. Plasma osmolarity is decreased; ADH continues to be secreted, causing water intoxication, hyponatremia, and cellular swelling.

403. **(A)** Nursing process phase: implementation; client need: safe, effective care environment; content area: medical/surgical nursing

Rationale

(A) Hypoglycemic clients who cannot swallow should be given glucagon to increase the blood sugar. (B) While an IV of D_5W may be started, the client will respond to glucagon more quickly. (C & D) Insulin is not given to hypoglycemic clients; this would potentiate the hypoglycemia.

404. **(C)** Nursing process phase: evaluation; client need: health promotion and maintenance; content area: medical/surgical nursing

Rationale

(A) Regular insulin should never be substituted for NPH insulin. (B) "Cloudy" insulins should not be shaken prior to withdrawal from the bottle. Shaking creates bubbles, which can displace insulin in the syringe, thus causing inaccurate dosing. (D) "Cloudy" insulins should be gently rotated before preparing the injection. (D) The site of insulin injections should be rotated to prevent lipodystrophies.

405. (A) Nursing process phase: analysis; client need: safe, effective care environment; content area: medical/surgical nursing

Rationale

$$\frac{\text{Total volume} \times \text{gtt factor}}{\text{No. of minutes}}$$

or

$$\frac{50 \text{ ml} \times 10 \text{ gtt/ml}}{60 \text{ min}} = \frac{500 \text{ gtt}}{60 \text{ min}} = 8 \text{ gtt/min}$$

406. (B) Nursing process phase: analysis; client need: physiological integrity; content area: medical/surgical nursing

Rationale

(A) Anemia in CRF is not due to this cause. (B) One of the functions of the kidney is to produce erythropoietin. Diminished secretion of erythorpoietin leads to anemia. (C) While minimal damage to the RBCs may occur during hemodialysis, this not the main reason for the anemia in CRF. (D) This is not the cause of anemia in CRF.

407. (C) Nursing process phase: evaluation; client need: health promotion and maintenance; content area: medical/surgical nursing

Rationale

(A) Females should wipe from front to back after defecation. (B) A fluid intake of 400 cc/day is too low and will not flush bacteria from the bladder. (C) The client should verbalize the importance of urinating before and immediately after sexual intercourse to flush bacteria from the bladder. (D) Voiding only every 6 hours is too infrequent and may contribute to recurring cystitis.

408. (C) Nursing process phase: planning; client need: health promotion and maintenance; content area: medical/surgical nursing

Rationale

(A) Diuretics are often used in hypertension. The client with CHF may have a fluid limitation. (B) Exercise can lower blood pressure, but vigorous exercise could be contraindicated. (C) Sodium reduction would be the most accurate treatment for hypertension and can be done without physician orders. (D) Avoiding alcohol would be recommended but would be dependent on the prescribed medication regime.

409. (A) Nursing process phase: implementation; client need: health promotion and maintenance; content area: medical/surgical nursing

Rationale

(A) Foods high in potassium should be consumed if client is not on a potassium-sparing diuretic. (B) Foods high in sodium should be avoided. (C) Medication should be taken at the same time daily to maintain blood levels and compliance. (D) Regular exercise can improve peripheral resistance.

410. (B) Nursing process phase: planning; client need: psychosocial integrity; content area: medical/surgical nursing

Rationale

(A) Depression would occur earlier in the hospital stay. (B) Denial would be the first reaction to a life-threatening disease and often returns as the client begins to feel better. (C) Acceptance would be the final stage of grieving. (D) Bargaining would occur prior to acceptance.

411. (B) Nursing process phase: implementation; client need: safe, effective care environment; content area: medical/surgical nursing

Rationale

(A) The client should report incisional drainage and be taught the signs and symptoms of inflammation and infection. (B) Pulse should be taken and recorded daily and any increases or decreases should be reported, because changes in pulse rate could indicate a pacemaker malfunction. (C) New models of microwaves should not be of danger. (D) A medical alert bracelet should be worn, but reporting a change in pulse would be the most important instruction.

412. (A) nursing process phase: assessment; client need, physiological integrity; content area: medical/surgical nursing

Rationale

(A) Cellulitis is inflammation of the skin and connective tissue. (B) Eschar and fluid would occur with cell death. (C) Petechiae and discoloration would not be a sign of cellulitis. (D) Ecchymosis and bruising would not be a sign of cellulitis.

413. (B) Nursing process phase: implementation; client need: psychosocial integrity; content area: medical/surgical nursing

Rationale

(A) Ignoring his behavior may promote aggression. (B) Open-ended questions would allow him to participate and could stimulate a response. (C) Documentation of his behavior would be appropriate. (D) He may not desire visitors and this would be an inappropriate action by a nurse.

414. (D) Nursing process phase: assessment; client need: psychosocial integrity; content area: medical/surgical nursing

Rationale

(A) AIDS patients often feel rejected by their friends. (B) AIDS patients often have mixed feelings toward family. (C) AIDS patients feel isolated. (D) Hostility toward staff is seen in AIDS patients during the anger phase of coping with death and dying.

415. (A) Nursing process phase: assessment; client need: safe, effective care environment; content area: medical/surgical nursing

Rationale

(A) An abnormal neurological assessment would be indicative of hypertensive encephalopathy, with increased vascular resistance and cerebral edema. (B) Fluid retention would not be the most critical assessment and would be present in other diseases. (C) Laboratory values would be examined after an admission assessment. (D) History would reveal risk factors, medications, and history of similar events, but would be taken after the neurological assessment.

416. (A) Nursing process phase: implementation; client need: physiological integrity; content area: medical/surgical nursing

Rationale
(A) Nitroglycerin would be given as a vasodilator to decrease chest pain. (B) Dopamine would be given for low blood pressure. Her blood pressure is within normal limits. (C) Routine meds would not be the best approach since they might not help the chest pain. (D) Client or family teaching would not be the best approach initially.

417. (A) Nursing process phase: assessment; client need: safe, effective care environment; content area: medical/surgical nursing

Rationale
(A) Emergency intervention is correct with hypertensive crisis, requiring immediate care. (B) Urgent intervention would be a lower level of care than emergency and not rapid enough for hypertensive crisis, with an initiation time of 15 minutes or more. (C) Priority intervention would be a lower level of care than urgent and not rapid enough for hypertensive crisis, with an initiation time of 30 minutes or more. (D) Observation would not be appropriate until after intervention and the patient is stable.

418. (B) Nursing process phase: analysis and planning; client need: safe, effective care environment; content area: medical/surgical nursing

Rationale
(A) Sedative action would not be the best intervention, because it could mask neurological symptoms. (B) Antihypertensives would be the best intervention to cause vasodilation and reduce blood pressure. (C) Diuretic action would not be the best intervention, but would be used to augment antihypertensives to decrease fluid volume and reduce blood pressure. (D) Digoxin action would be a cardiac intervention and would not be used as an immediate treatment in hypertensive crisis.

419. (A) Nursing process phase: implementation; client need: safe, effective care environment; content area: medical/surgical nursing

Rationale
(A) Scheduled rest periods would allow the client to rest between activities to prevent fatigue and provide opportunities to relax. (B) Unrestricted visitors would not be conducive to rest. (C) Exploring family problems would not be appropriate until hypertensive crisis has been resolved. (D) Encouraging ventilation of frustrations would not be appropriate until hypertensive crisis has been resolved.

420. (B) Nursing process phase: implementation; client need: physiological integrity; content area: medical/surgical nursing

Rationale
(A) Cleansing of the site would not prevent hematoma and should be done prior to the procedure. (B) Applying pressure would cause vasoconstriction and help to prevent accumulation of blood. (C) The site should require only a small bandage and this would not prevent hematoma. (D) Turning the patient to the operative site would not prevent hematoma.

421. (C) Nursing process phase: implementation; client need: health promotion and maintenance; content area: medical/surgical nursing

Rationale
(A) Liver is rich in iron. (B) Beans would not be as rich in iron as liver. (C) Fish is not rich in iron. (D) Green leafy vegetables contain iron.

422. (D) Nursing process phase: implementation; client need: health promotion and maintenance; content area: medical/surgical nursing

Rationale
(A) Ferrous sulfate tablets would not stain teeth. (B) Urine would not be affected; the iron is absorbed in the intestines. (C) Breath would not be affected. (D) Stool would turn black or green because only 50 percent of the iron is absorbed and the rest excreted in the stool.

423. (C) Nursing process phase: evaluation; client need: safe, effective care environment; content area: medical/surgical nursing

Rationale
(A) This measures the hemoglobin, the oxygen content in the blood. (B) Hematocrit measures the hydration state of the body. (C) Erythrocyte indices measures the size and hemoglobin content of erythrocytes, or red blood cells. (D) CBC would show the hemoglobin, hematocrit, and RBCs, but not the size of the RBCs.

424. (D) Nursing process phase: implementation; client need: safe, effective care environment; content area: medical/surgical nursing

Rationale
(A) Dilute urine would alter the results. (B) The small amount of radiation would not require isolation. (C) Urine for 24 hours only would be needed. (D) Urine is saved for 24 hours, except for the first voided specimens after the test has begun. The test would measure the amount of vitamin B_{12} excreted in the urine after ingestion of a radioactive vitamin is given.

425. (D) Nursing process phase: assessment; client need: physiological integrity; content area: medical/surgical nursing

Rationale
(A) Bruits are not associated with hypotension. (B) Bruits are not associated with occluded blood vessels. (C) Collateral circulation development would result from cardiac insufficiency, not from the presence of a bruit. (D) The sound auscultated is caused by turbulent blood flow through stenotic blood vessels.

426. (B) Nursing process phase: implementation; client need: safe, effective care environment; content area: medical/surgical nursing

Rationale
(A) Exercise would improve circulation. (B) This would be correct in increasing warmth. (C) Do not apply heat to im-

paired circulation. (D) Leaving the client's socks on would improve warmth to the feet.

427. **(A)** Nursing process phase: implementation; client need: health promotion and maintenance; content area: medical/surgical nursing

Rationale

(A) Walking would improve cardiovascular function. (B) The client should cease smoking. (C) A low-fat, decreased caloric intake should be followed if weight loss is indicated. (D) Shortness of breath should be reported and evaluated immediately by a physician.

428. **(B)** Nursing process phase: implementation; client need: health promotion and maintenance; content area: medical/surgical nursing

Rationale

(A) Smoked turkey and pickles contain high levels of sodium. (B) Low-sodium bread, salt-free eggs, and orange juice would be low in sodium and high in potassium. (C) Chicken breast and bread would have to be salt free. (D) Chicken salad and chips would contain high levels of sodium.

429. **(D)** Nursing process phase: implementation; client need: health promotion and maintenance; content area: medical/surgical nursing

Rationale

(A) Canned and frozen foods are high in sodium and promote fluid retention and increase blood pressure to increase glomerular filtration rate to excrete sodium. (B) If non-potassium-sparing diuretic therapy is prescribed, foods high in potassium should be taken. (C) Weight reduction or maintenance is necessary in chronic hypertension and high-calorie foods would promote weight gain. (D) Low-sodium and low-fat foods would be the correct dietary regime for chronic hypertension.

430. **(B)** Nursing process phase: implementation; client need: physiological integrity; content area: medical/surgical nursing

Rationale

(A) The drugs should not cause pain if given in a large vein. (B) The two drugs are compatible and are given together to maintain blood pressure. Dopamine is a vasopressor and nitroprusside is a vasodilator and may be given to dilate coronary vessels. The drugs should be administered through a large vein. The drugs should be given through separate sites. (C) The drugs should be given in separate sites. (D) The drugs should be given in large veins only.

431. **(D)** Nursing process phase: analysis and planning: client need: physiological integrity; content area: medical/surgical nursing

Rationale

(A) An artificial airway would not be indicated to promote a cough reflex. (B) Artificial airway induction would not increase lung capacity. (C) Lower lobe secretions would be removed by postural drainage and bronchodilators. (D) The endotracheal tube would provide ventilation as an artificial airway.

432. **(C)** Nursing process phase: analysis and planning; client need: safe, effective care environment; content area: medical/surgical nursing

Rationale

(A) Chest x-ray would show lung changes, but does not confirm TB. (B) Creatinine clearance indicates urological function. (C) Sputum for tubercle bacilli would indicate a confirmed diagnosis of TB. (D) CBC would not be an indicator of TB.

433. **(C)** Nursing process phase: assessment; client need: safe, effective care environment; content area: medical/surgical nursing

Rationale

(A) Flank pain would not indicate TB. (B) Weight loss would be seen in TB. (C) Productive cough and afternoon temperature elevation are symptoms of TB. (D) Rash would not be a symptom of TB.

434. **(A)** Nursing process phase: implementation; client need: safe, effective care environment; content area: medical/surgical nursing

Rationale

(A) TB is transmitted via droplets from coughing, sneezing, and talking. Droplets can be inhaled and some may dry and remain in the air for long periods of time, requiring respiratory isolation. (B) Visitor restriction would be by the request of the patient, physicians, or family. Respiratory isolation would not require limited visitors. (C) Respiratory isolation is not to provide privacy. Privacy is provided through limiting visitors and phone calls. (D) TB does not require close contact; the infected droplets are airborne.

435. **(D)** Nursing process phase: implementation; client need: safe, effective care environment; content area: medical/surgical nursing

Rationale

(A) The client may shower the day of surgery, but this is not known to prevent infection. (B) The client may wash hair prior to surgery, but this is not known to prevent infection. (C) Antibiotics may not be prescribed after surgery, depending on the procedure. This may prevent resistant bacteria and an overgrowth of healthy bacteria. (D) Shaving of the surgery site is known to prevent infection because the body hair may retain bacteria from the skin.

436. **(A)** Nursing process phase: implementation; client need: physiological integrity; content area: medical/surgical nursing

Rationale

(A) The nurse should give 50% glucose to raise the blood glucose level and to prevent neurological complications. (B) Insulin would lower the blood sugar. (C) If the patient has a pulse and respiration, CPR would not be indicated. (D) Normal saline would be administered, if hyperglycemia were known to be the cause.

437. **(D)** Nursing process phase: implementation; client need: physiological integrity; content area: medical/surgical nursing

Rationale

(A) This would be helpful in decreasing injury to the client, but would not be a priority. (B) Placing a padded tongue blade in the mouth might injure the jaw or break the teeth. (C) This would be a necessity after the occurrence of the seizure. (D) Maintenance of the airway through positioning would be the priority.

438. (A) Nursing process phase: implementation; client need: safe, effective care environment; content area: medical/surgical nursing

Rationale
(A) Universal precautions, which include gloving and correct disposal of sharps, would be used with all patients. (B) Isolation of the patient would not be necessary for blood drawing. (C) Drawing a routine blood sample would not require gowning. (D) Wearing a face shield would not be necessary during routine blood drawing.

439. (C) Nursing process phase: implementation; client need: safe, effective care environment; content area: medical/surgical nursing

Rationale
(A) Activities should be spaced to provide rest periods. (B) A slightly elevated position would improve lung expansion. (C) Increase in fluids would be the appropriate point to emphasize in discharge teaching to prevent dehydration and loosen secretions. This would be ordered by the physician. (D) Sodium restriction would not be necessary, unless another disease warrants the restriction.

440. (D) Nursing process phase: implementation; client need: safe, effective care environment; content area: medical/surgical nursing

Rationale
(A) Capillary blood glucose should be checked daily. (B) Arms and thighs should be utilized for subcutaneous injections. (C) This is appropriate, but not the most accurate instruction. (D) Food intake prior to insulin injection is the most accurate point to teach because insulin acts within 30 minutes.

441. (A) Nursing process phase: implementation; client need: safe, effective care environment; content area: medical/surgical nursing

Rationale
(A) This would be the most accurate point to emphasize with the patient. (B) Candy should not be taken; it could result in hyperglycemia. (C) Extra insulin would decrease blood sugar, resulting in hypoglycemia. (D) Specified diet should be maintained to deliver glucose load calculated for the client.

442. (D) Nursing process phase: assessment; client need: physiological integrity; content area: medical/surgical nursing

Rationale
(A) Stable angina does not produce nocturnal pain. (B) Stable angina does not produce stabbing chest pain. (C) Stable angina migrates and does not remain in one spot. (D) Stable angina produces a squeezing pain, like heartburn or indigestion.

443. (D) Nursing process phase: implementation; client need: safe, effective care environment; content area: medical/surgical nursing

Rationale
(A) The ointment can be applied to nonhairy areas of skin such as the chest, abdomen, or thighs but avoiding distal extremities. (B) This increases absorption and interferes with

sustained action. (C) Ointment should remain on for prescribed time; secure the ointment application by applying an occlusive dressing. If the first application falls off or becomes loose, apply a new dosage unit. (D) Sites should be rotated to prevent skin irritation.

444. (A) Nursing process phase: implementation; client need: safe, effective care environment; content area: medical/surgical nursing

Rationale
(A) Straining at stool would increase abdominal pressure and could rupture esophageal varices. (B) Lifting should be avoided to minimize the risk of increasing abdominal pressure. (C) Antiembolism hose would not increase abdominal pressure. (D) Sodium restriction would be necessary to decrease ascites.

445. (A) Nursing process phase: assessment; client need: physiological integrity; content area: medical/surgical nursing

Rationale
(A) A broad QRS complex is seen in hyperkalemia. (B) A prominent U wave is an indicator of hypokalemia (<3.5 mEq/L) and would not be expected in this case. (C) Changes would be expected in a client with such a high potassium level. (D) A flattened T wave is seen in a client with hypokalemia or a serum potassium level of less than 3.5 mEq/L.

446. (A) Nursing process phase: assessment; client need: physiological integrity; content area: medical/surgical nursing

Rationale
(A) Many elderly clients are normally hypothermic and a temperature that appears within the normal range may in fact be elevated for this client. (B) The usual signs and symptoms of infection may not be present in elderly clients, and they may not complain of the usual discomforts associated with an infection. (C) Altered cognition may be one of the first signs that an elderly client has an infection. The nurse would not consider this a hindrance to his or her assessment. (D) The elderly client does have a slightly decreased urinary output, but this output is too low.

447. (A) Nursing process phase: assessment; client need: physiological integrity; content area: medical/surgical nursing

Rationale
(A) Serum blood urea nitrogen becomes elevated (>20 mg/dl) in acute renal failure. (B) Serum creatinine levels are elevated during the acute renal phase, not decreased (0.8 to 1.2 mg/dl). (C) Hematocrit is usually decreased in acute renal failure. (D) Potassium levels are usually elevated during acute renal failure.

448. (D) Nursing process phase: assessment; client need: physiological integrity; content area: medical/surgical nursing

Rationale
(A) A client in acute renal failure would have hypermagnesemia, although hypomagnesemia could result in mood changes and confusion. (B) Respiratory acidosis would not be seen in a client with acute renal failure. This occurs as a compensatory mechanism in clients with chronic metabolic

alkalosis. (C) Hypoxia is seen when there is a low PaO$_2$ level. It is accompanied by cyanosis, restlessness, and tachycardia. These symptoms are not observed with this client. (D) Metabolic acidosis in acute renal failure occurs when an underexcretion of acids or the inability to conserve base bicarbonate results in excess acid accumulation in the bloodstream. Changes in level of consciousness are noted from lethargy and drowsiness to confusion.

449. (B) Nursing process phase: analysis; client need: physiological integrity; content area: medical/surgical nursing

Rationale

(A) Anemia is a reversible condition and is not contraindicated in transplants. (B) Coronary artery disease is not a reversible condition. It can lead to postoperative complications that can damage the new kidney and increase the client's chances of having complications. (C) Diverticulosis is a nonsymptomatic disorder and, although the client will need to be monitored to avoid advancement of the condition to diverticulitis, the condition does not contraindicate a renal transplant. (D) Hypothyroidism is a slowing of the metabolic process as a result of deficiency in the production of T$_3$ and T$_4$. This disorder can be controlled with medication and will not affect a transplant client's outcome.

450. (A) Nursing process phase: assessment; client need: physiological integrity; content area: medical/surgical nursing

Rationale

(A) Less than 100 ml in a 24-hour period is an anuric urine output. (B–D) These would be considered oliguric outputs, of less than 400 ml in a 24-hour period.

451. (D) Nursing process phase: analysis; client need: physiological integrity; content area: medical/surgical nursing

Rationale

(A–C) These are proper nursing measures for this client; however, they are not the most critical for this client at this time. (D) A client in acute renal failure with a history of congestive heart failure should never receive whole blood products. The client will not be able to tolerate the excess fluid.

452. (C) Nursing process phase: evaluation; client need: health promotion and maintenance; content area: medical/surgical nursing

Rationale

(A) This statement is correct and the client understands the ramifications of her medication therapy. (B) The client is correct and understands the ramifications of long-term immunosuppressive therapy. (C) The client is incorrect and needs further explanation on the importance of lifelong immunosuppressive therapy and why she will not be able to discontinue the medication. (D) The client is correct and understands the need for continued monitoring of weight for fluid volume overload.

453. (B) Nursing process phase: analysis; client need: safe, effective care environment; content area: medical/surgical nursing

Rationale

(A) Long-term diuretic therapy, although harmful to the kidneys, does not contraindicate this procedure. (B) An allergy to shellfish does contraindicate this procedure because radiated iodine is used during the procedure. An allergy to shellfish contraindicates any procedure using iodine. (C) A history of anemia would not interfere with the procedure or its accuracy. (D) A client with recent MI would be at risk for other complications with this diagnosis, but this factor would not contraindicate this procedure.

454. (C) Nursing process phase: evaluation; client need: health promotion and maintenance; content area: medical/surgical nursing

Rationale

(A, B, & D) The client does not understand the surgery and needs further education. (C) The client has a clear understanding of what is involved with this procedure.

455. (C) Nursing process phase: implementation; client need: health promotion and maintenance; content area: medical/surgical nursing

Rationale

(A) The client does not need to carry clamps for emergencies. This is incorrect information to give this client. (B) The site may take weeks to months before it can develop sufficient blood flow for hemodialysis. (C) The client needs to avoid constrictive clothing around his fistula site to promote adequate perfusion. (D) Painful spasms are not normal and need to be reported to the dialysis nurse.

456. (B) Nursing process phase: analysis; client need: physiological integrity; content area: medical/surgical nursing

Rationale

(A) Anuric is a type of urine output, not a classification of renal failure. (B) Intrarenal is correct. Damage to the kidneys in this classification of renal failure is brought on by nephrotoxic medications. (C) Prerenal failure is the result of cardiovascular disorders, hypovolemia, peripheral vasodilation, or renovascular obstruction. (D) Postrenal failure results from an obstruction of urine flow either from bladder, ureter, or urethral obstruction.

457. (A) Nursing process phase: analysis; client need: physiological integrity; content area: medical/surgical nursing

Rationale

(A) This is the most life-threatening complication of acute renal failure. Hyperkalemia can lead to muscle weakness, flaccid paralysis, and cardiac arrest. (B) Hyperchloremia results from decreased chloride intake or absorption and is not seen in acute tubular necrosis. (C) Hypermagnesemia is more common in chronic renal failure, the overuse of magnesium-containing antacids, or with severe dehydration. (D) Hypernatremia is seen in patients with extreme fluid shifts, such as burns, fever, acute diabetes insipidus, or Cushing's syndrome.

458. (C) Nursing process phase: analysis; client need: health promotion and maintenance; content area: medical/surgical nursing

Rationale

(A) The elderly consume one-third, not one-half, of all prescribed medications in this country. (B) The elderly experience different effects from drugs than do younger adults. (C)

The elderly are often taking a large number of medications for a variety of chronic or acute conditions. Drug interactions need to be checked carefully. (D) The elderly do not overdose on medications due to confusion more than younger adults.

459. (D) Nursing process phase: implementation; client need: safe, effective care environment; content area: medical/surgical nursing

Rationale
(A) The catheter should be used for hemodialysis access only, unless otherwise ordered by the physician. (B) A sign like this should only be used for a client following a A-V fistula surgery. This is not necessary for Quinton-Scribner catheter placement. (C) This is the protocol used for a client returning from an angiogram and should not be followed for clients returning from a subclavian Quinton-Scribner catheter placement. (D) The nurse should follow these actions to monitor for hemorrhage or pneumothorax.

460. (B) Nursing process phase: implementation; client need: physiological integrity; content area: medical/surgical nursing

Rationale
(A) Monitoring urinary retention in a client with end-stage renal failure is not necessary because the client probably has no output. (B) Monitoring for signs and symptoms of infection is critical, because development of any infection can delay surgery. (C) This is not the most critical nursing intervention for this client. (D) This is not the most critical nursing intervention; however, it is important to make sure the client is as strong as she can be prior to the surgery.

461. (D) Nursing process phase: analysis; client need: physiological integrity; content area: medical/surgical nursing

Rationale
(A) A renal biopsy allows only for identification of underlying pathology and does not evaluate kidney function. (B) A renal ultrasound can determine the cause of renal failure but it cannot evaluate the functional capability of the kidneys. (C) A creatinine clearance study only indicates the amount of protein cleared through the kidneys in 24 hours. It is not a procedure for helping to identify functional capability. (D) A fluid challenge is the most reliable test for differentiating between prerenal and intrarenal disease.

462. (C) Nursing process phase: assessment; client need: safe, effective care environment; content area: medical/surgical nursing

Rationale
(A) These symptoms are indicative of internal bleeding. (B) These symptoms are indicative of possible infection from pathogens in the dialysis equipment. (C) These are the symptoms of disequilibrium syndrome. It is caused by rapid fluid removal and electrolyte changes. (D) These are symptoms of an air embolism, which is a potentially fatal complication.

463. (B) Nursing process phase: implementation; client need: health promotion and maintenance; content area: medical/surgical nursing

Rationale
(A) The client needs to limit both protein and sodium intake to avoid fluid retention. (B) The client needs to observe fluid restrictions and avoid high-potassium foods. (C) The client needs to limit both potassium and sodium intake. (D) The client can benefit from increasing dietary bulk, but he must observe fluid restrictions.

464. (D) Nursing process phase: analysis; client need: physiological integrity; content area: medical/surgical nursing

Rationale
(A) Chest tube dislodgement can lead to a tension pneumothorax, a potentially fatal complication. (B) Tissue hypoxia is indicate by cyanosis, increased respirations, tachycardia, and a changing mental status. (C) An air embolism would present with severe chest pain, increased heart rate, decreased blood pressure, increased respirations, and blood-tinged sputum. (D) A tension pneumothorax is a complication associated with chest tube placement. Air trapped in the pleural space is under high pressure and can cause the lung to collapse. Continued pressure increases in the chest can cause a shift of the vital organs to the unaffected side.

465. (A) Nursing process phase: analysis; client need: safe, effective care environment; content area: medical/surgical nursing

Rationale
(A) Decreasing blood pressure would indicate a rapid change in fluid volume, primarily acute blood loss as a result of aneurysm rupture. (B) An increasing blood pressure would not be seen with a rupturing abdominal aneurysm. (C) A decreasing pulse rate would be a late sign of blood loss and a late indicator of the client's condition. (D) Cyanosis is a late sign of oxygen or blood loss.

466. (A) Nursing process phase: assessment; client need: physiological integrity; content area: medical/surgical nursing

Rationale
(A) The bruit could be auscultated in a person who is thin, and a pulsating mass in the periumbilical area may also be palpated. (B) Pedal pulses would not be affected by the aneurysm unless the mass has ruptured, which would be an emergency situation. (C) Decreased hair to lower legs and shiny skin are indicative of decreased peripheral perfusion. (D) Abdominal aneurysms develop slowly and are the result of arteriosclerosis and not weight training or heavy lifting.

467. (D) Nursing process phase: assessment; client need: safe, effective care environment; content area: medical/surgical nursing

Rationale
(A) Mouth ulcers of a herpes simplex nature greater than 1 month's duration are characteristic of advanced AIDS. (B) A decreased, not increased, T-cell count is seen with advanced AIDS. (C) Lymphadenopathy can be seen in the early stages of the disease within 3 to 6 weeks of initial exposure. (D) A temperature greater than 100°F for 3 months is indicative of an advanced disease condition due to multiple infections.

468. (C) Nursing process phase: planning; client need: safe, effective care environment; content area: medical/surgical nursing

Rationale
(A) The client does not have a problem with mobility and this would not be an appropriate diagnosis for this client. (B) The

client has exhibited no violent tendencies and is reported to be cooperative. This would not be an appropriate diagnosis. (C) This would be an appropriate diagnosis because the client could injure herself as the result of her confusion. (D) This would be a difficult diagnosis to assess because the client is confused and it would be difficult to tell the level of her self-concept.

469. **(D)** Nursing process phase: analysis; client need: safe, effective care environment; content area: medical/surgical nursing

Rationale

(A) An auscultated S_3 would not indicate that the client is in respiratory arrest. (B) An increased pulse and decreased blood pressure would indicate oncoming arrest or respiratory problems. (C) These are normal ABGs and would not be expected in a client experiencing respiratory difficulty. (D) A pulse oximetry reading of less than 90 indicates a severe loss of oxygen to the tissues. This would indicate a deterioration in the respiratory status of the client.

470. **(B)** Nursing process phase: implementation; client need: health promotion and maintenance; content area: medical/surgical nursing

Rationale

(A) A diet that monitors sodium and potassium intake and provides adequate protein is essential for these clients. This is not correct information for this client. (B) Skin care is crucial for the client with Addison's disease. Alcohol-free products can reduce skin drying and irritation. (C) Staying active is appropriate; however, you also need to inform the client to provide adequate rest periods to avoid fatigue. (D) Muscle weakness and fatigue are normal for this disease. However, the nurse needs to counsel the client on how to manage his energy and to provide frequent rest periods to avoid fatigue.

471. **(C)** Nursing process phase: analysis; client need: physiological integrity; content area: medical/surgical nursing

Rationale

(A) A client with a fat embolus would also have wheezing, confusion, restlessness, disorientation, and possible chest pain. They may also have pink-tinged sputum not seen here. (B) Pneumonia would present with a low-grade fever, chest pain, and productive cough. The pulse oximeter reading would also be higher than with this client. (C) The hallmark of ARDS is continued hypoxia despite increased supplemental oxygen. (D) Pericarditis presents with chest pain that may radiate to the extremities and the pain increases on inspiration. There is hypotension, neck vein distention, and pallor.

472. **(B)** Nursing process phase: evaluation; client need: health promotion and maintenance; content area: medical/surgical nursing

Rationale

(A) This family member understands the progress of the disease. (B) This family member does not understand the progress of Alzheimer's disease and needs further education. (C) This family member is prepared for the progress of the disease and understands what to expect. (D) This family member understands that resources are available.

473. **(D)** Nursing process phase: implementation; client need: safe, effective care environment; content area: medical/surgical nursing

Rationale

(A) This is not the immediate need for this client. (B) A new BKA needs to be properly wrapped to apply compression needed to mold the stump for prosthesis placement. (C) The client should be encouraged to turn to prevent atelectasis, to stretch the flexor muscles, and prevent complications. (D) This is the correct action for this client. This will prevent hamstring contracture and reduce edema.

474. **(D)** Nursing process phase: implementation; client need: safe, effective care environment; content area: medical/surgical nursing

Rationale

(A) You would not leave the client alone and in distress to call the doctor. There is a more appropriate nursing action. (B) This not the most immediate nursing measure that you can do for this client. (C) You need a doctor's order to give this medication. There is a more appropriate nursing action for this client. (D) Stop the infusion; take the client's vital signs; call the doctor, leaving someone to watch the client; and then, once ordered, administer the epinephrine.

475. **(D)** Nursing process phase: evaluation; client need: physiological integrity; content area: medical/surgical nursing

Rationale

(A) The client does not understand his instructions, according to this statement, and needs further education about the procedure. (B) The client needs further instructions and does not understand the procedure. (C) The client needs further instruction about the procedure. (D) The client demonstrates an understanding of the procedure and care following the procedure.

476. **(D)** Nursing process phase: implementation; client need: health promotion and maintenance; content area: medical/surgical nursing

Rationale

(A) The client needs to carry an oral inhaler, not oxygen, to east attacks. (B) The client needs to increase his fluid intake to at least eight glasses of water a day to help mobilize secretions. (C) Instruct the client to eat a well-balanced diet, but there are no dietary restrictions with an asthma client unless there are food allergies at the root of the asthma attacks. (D) This will help to avoid secretions from accumulating and to keep the airway clear.

477. **(C)** Nursing process phase: analysis; client need: safe, effective care environment; content area: medical/surgical nursing

Rationale

(A) A Foley catheter would be an appropriate intervention for this client, to monitor output and ease bladder emptying. (B) Monitoring intake and output would be an appropriate intervention for this client to monitor for dehydration. (C) Administration of any tranquilizers can worsen the obstruction in a client with benign prostatic hyperplasia. The nurse would question the use of diazepam (Valium). (D) This is an appropriate intervention for this client.

478. **(A)** Nursing process phase: implementation; client need: health promotion and maintenance; content area: medical/surgical nursing

Rationale

(A) The client should avoid activities that increase intraocular pressure on the affected eye. (B) The client should refrain from any strenuous activity for 6 to 10 weeks. (C) The client should be instructed to call the doctor immediately if any of these symptoms occur. (D) The client should be instructed to wear the eye patch during sleep for several weeks.

479. **(D)** Nursing process phase: implementation; client need: health promotion and maintenance; content area: medical/surgical nursing

Rationale

(A) This is not an appropriate action because you would not want to deny the client access to her support systems. (B) This is not appropriate in any situation with a client. (C) This is a nursing action and it is up to the nurse to deal with the situation and help the client. (D) Speaking to the family in a gentle and reassuring manner may help them to help their family member change her habits.

480. **(C)** Nursing process phase: implementation; client need: safe, effective care environment; content area: medical/surgical nursing

Rationale

(A) This does need to be on the client's chart, but this is not a legal document that is required before a treatment can be started. (B) Laboratory work should be on the client's chart but it is not legally required. (C) A consent form is a legal document that needs to be on a client's chart and signed by the client or an appropriate family member before the procedure or treatment can be initiated. (D) A nursing care plan can accompany the chart but it is not legally required.

481. **(A)** Nursing process phase: implementation; client need: health maintenance and promotion; content area: medical/surgical nursing

Rationale

(A) The client needs to report any of these signs of infection as soon as possible. (B) The client should not experience any irregular heartbeats or a rapid pulse. The client should report these signs to the physician as soon as possible. (C) The client should return home on a low-sodium and low-cholesterol diet, or one prescribed by the physician. (D) The client should be instructed to do only light activity, until his doctor gives him clearance to increase his activities.

482. **(B)** Nursing process phase: implementation; client need: safe, effective care environment; content area: medical/surgical nursing

Rationale

(A) You do not leave the client's bedside to call the doctor. There is a more appropriate nursing intervention for this client. (B) This is the correct intervention. You would want to assess the client's vital signs in order to evaluate the client's status. (C & D) These would not be the first appropriate actions to take with this client.

483. **(C)** Nursing process phase: assessment; client need: physiological integrity; content area: medical/surgical nursing

Rationale

(A) These are not complications of the disorder, but are signs and symptoms. (B) These are not complications of Cushing's

syndrome, but are symptoms of the disease. (C) Osteoporosis and impaired wound healing are potential complications that can result from Cushing's syndrome. (D) These are not complications of this syndrome but are considered signs and symptoms.

484. **(C)** Nursing process phase: analysis; client need: safe, effective care environment; content area: medical/surgical nursing

Rationale

(A, B, & D) These are not true for the obese client. (C) Many sedatives can deposit in the adipose tissue and take longer to clear the system.

485. **(A)** Nursing process phase: assessment; client need: safe, effective care environment; content area: medical/surgical nursing

Rationale

(A) A positive or elevated antinuclear antibody test is expected in a large percentage of SLE clients. (B) An alkaline phosphatase test would be normal in clients with SLE. (C) The sedimentation rate is usually elevated in clients with SLE. (D) The white blood cell count is usually decreased in clients with active SLE.

486. **(D)** Nursing process area: assessment; client need: physiological integrity; content area: medical/surgical nursing

Rationale

(A) This is not the primary reason for this action in caring for the immune-compromised client. (B) These are not the best areas for assessing cyanosis and that is not the reason for this action. (C) This is not the primary reason for this action in caring for the immune-compromised client. (D) The primary reason for checking these areas is searching for secondary infections, such as yeast, in the immune-compromised client.

487. **(B)** Nursing process phase: analysis; client need: physiological integrity; content area: medical/surgical nursing

Rationale

(A) Hydroxychloroquine is an antimalarial treatment that is successful with SLE clients. It does not predispose the client to gastric distress. (B) Nonsteroidal anti-inflammatory drugs are used primarily with this group to control joint pain. The major side effect with these drugs is their ability to irritate the stomach lining. (C) This is not considered a drug therapy utilized with this group of clients. (D) Steroids can cause gastric distress but they are not the drugs used primarily with SLE.

488. **(D)** Nursing process phase: analysis; client need: safe, effective care environment; content area: medical/surgical nursing

Rationale

(A) The femur has a small amount of venous innervation and would not place the client at risk for hemorrhage. (B) The ribs have some venous innervation but are not the greatest potential risk to this client. (C) The fibula does have some venous innervation, but it is not the greatest potential risk for this client. (D) The pelvis has the largest amount of venous innervation of all the bones and if fractured can lead to massive hemorrhage.

489. (D) Nursing process phase: assessment; client need: physiological integrity; content area: medical/surgical nursing

Rationale

(A) ARDS presents with dyspnea, increased BP initially then decreasing BP, a productive cough, tachycardia, and possibly cyanotic skin. There is no presence of petechiae on the chest walls with ARDS. This is also a condition not expected in a 22-year-old with multiple fractures. (B) Septic shock would be seen in a septic client. It is characterized by a decreasing blood pressure that is unresponsive to intravenous fluids. (C) A pneumothorax would present with increased respirations, BP, and heart rate. There would be sudden, sharp pain exacerbated by breathing, chest movement, or coughing. (D) The most common complication of multiple fracture is a fat embolus. Petechiae on the chest wall is an important diagnostic indicator.

490. (D) Nursing process phase: implementation; client need: psychosocial integrity; content area: medical/surgical nursing

Rationale

(A) This is not the proper response. You do not leave a client feeling hurt or angry and facing the unknown. You need to listen to the client more and allow him to express his anger. (B) This is not a therapeutic technique. You have just ignored what the client is trying to express to you. You need to listen more to your client and not express your opinion or pass judgment. (C) This is sympathy. The client needs someone to listen to him and not be judgmental. He needs to express his feelings to someone with empathy. (D) Allow your client the opportunity to express his feelings and speak openly about his fears in a nonjudgmental environment. With this statement, you are saying to the client that you are there for him and willing to listen.

491. (C) Nursing process phase: implementation; client need: safe, effective care environment; content area: medical/surgical nursing

Rationale

(A & B) These are appropriate nursing actions for this client, but they are not nursing actions that can help prevent one of the major complications of radical mastectomy surgery. (C) Lymphedema is the major complication of a radical mastectomy, and this nursing action can help prevent edema to the right extremity. (D) This action can help to reduce pain, but it is not related to any major complication with this type of surgery.

492. (D) Nursing process phase: analysis; client need: safe, effective care environment; content area: medical/surgical nursing

Rationale

(A) A cerebral infarction can be a complication associated with age; however, this client is at risk for another type of complication due to her depressed immune system. (B) This is not a complication that the elderly are at high risk of developing. (C) Endocarditis is not the complication that this elderly client is at high risk of developing. (D) The elderly and the very young are at higher risk of developing viral meningitis as a result of secondary infection related to the limited immune response.

493. (C) Nursing process phase: assessment; client need: physiological integrity; content area: medical/surgical nursing

Rationale

(A) Stage I is when the skin is red and unbroken and the sore is reversible if the pressure is removed. (B) Stage II appears as a break in the skin and discoloration may occur. This stage penetrates to the subcutaneous fat layer and is very painful. (C) In Stage III, the wound penetrates to the muscle, the client may or may not have pain, and necrosis can set in. (D) Stage IV is where the wound penetrates to the bone and can only be corrected with surgical treatment.

494. (D) Nursing process phase: assessment; client need: safe, effective care environment; content area: medical/surgical nursing

Rationale

(A) The physiological response to stress in the elderly client can occur at a much slower rate and be more detrimental to the client's condition. (B) The elderly respond differently to stress due to their depressed immune systems and various psychosocial factors not faced by a 35-year-old adult. (C) Stress levels in the elderly take longer to return to prestress or normal levels due to the physiological changes associated with aging. (D) Psychological responses to stress in the elderly occur rapidly and can be caused by changes in a familiar environment. Changes noted, such as confusion, can be seen before physiological symptoms develop.

495. (B) Nursing process phase: analysis; client need: physiological integrity; content area: medical/surgical nursing

Rationale

(A) The pH level is too low to indicate alkalosis; a PCO_2 level less than 35 mm Hg would indicate alkalosis. (B) A PCO_2 above 35 indicates acidosis and the pH is acidotic. (C) The HCO_3 reflects the metabolic state in the client with a normal range from 22 to 26 mEq/dl. The reading above is within normal limits and indicates there is no metabolic disorder. (D) The HCO_3 is within normal limits, indicating there is not a metabolic disorder.

496. (B) Nursing process phase: analysis; client need: physiological integrity; content area: medical/surgical nursing

Rationale

(A) To return the acidotic pH to a more normal level an increase, not a decrease, in base (HCO_3) is needed. (B) By increasing the amount of base (HCO_3) the body is compensating to return the pH level to normal. (C) An increase in PCO_2 would increase the client's respiratory acidosis to a dangerous level. (D) A decrease in the PCO_2 would not help change the pH level. Base needs to be added to the system to counteract the effects of the acidosis. This would place the client in a compensating metabolic alkalosis.

497. (C) Nursing process phase: analysis; client need: physiological integrity; content area: medical/surgical nursing

Rationale

(A) This is respiratory acidosis. The PCO_2 is greater than 45, which is compensated; however, this started out as a respiratory acidosis that was compensated, not a metabolic alkalosis. (B) This is a compensated reading because of the elevated PCO_2 and the elevated HCO_3. (C) The pH is within normal limits while the PCO_2 is elevated, indicating respiratory acidosis. The HCO_3 is also elevated as a result of base being released to lower the pH and this brought on the metabolic alkalosis. (D) This is not a metabolic acidosis. The HCO_3, which indicates metabolic status, is greater than 26, which indicates a metabolic alkalosis.

498. **(D)** Nursing process phase: assessment; client need: safe, effective care environment; content area: medical/surgical nursing

Rationale
(A) You need to do an assessment of the client first to be better able to report your findings to the doctor when you call to get orders for a chest x-ray. (B) You never reposition the tube. This is done by respiratory therapy or the M.D. You could dislodge the tube, damage the chest wall, or cut off the client's airway. (C) You need to assess your client first before you call to get physician orders for ABGs. (D) If you suspect anything is wrong with the client's ventilation, check the client's breath sounds, saturations, and respiratory rate.

499. **(C)** Nursing process phase: evaluation; client need: physiological integrity; content area: medical/surgical nursing

Rationale
(A) You do not allow a client to administer his or her own SQ injections unless ordered to do so or if the client needs to practice before going home on SQ medication. (B) Hematocrit and hemoglobin will not evaluate the effectiveness of heparin therapy on this client. (C) The nurse needs to monitor the daily PTT levels of the client to evaluate whether the client is receiving the adequate amount of medication. (D) You should always monitor the client's vital signs, but there is a more effective means presented here to monitor the client's status with heparin therapy.

500. **(C)** Nursing process phase: implementation; client need: health promotion and maintenance; content area: medical/surgical nursing

Rationale
(A) Frothy sputum is a late sign of CHF. This indicates that the fluid has accumulated in the lungs to dangerous levels. (B) Tachycardia is a late sign of CHF due to decreased oxygen levels in the blood. (C) Activity intolerance, as evidenced by shortness of breath and fatigue, is an early warning sign of fluid accumulation in the lungs. (D) Loss of consciousness would be a very late sign indicating the brain is not getting enough oxygen.

501. **(B)** Nursing process phase: assessment; client need: safe, effective care environment; content area: medical/surgical nursing

Rationale
(A) A sudden increase in blood pressure is not associated with SVT. The heart rate soars over 120 bpm and there is decreased filling time in the atriums and ventricles. (B) The heart is beating too fast for adequate perfusion to maintain adequate blood pressure. (C) Urine output would be a late indicator of SVT. The peripheral circulation would have to be reduced to have a decreased urine output. (D) There would be a change in consciousness in a client with SVT, but this would be a late indicator of decreased peripheral perfusion to the brain.

502. **(A)** Nursing process phase: analysis; client need: physiological integrity; content area: medical/surgical nursing

Rationale
(A) Arthritis, or osteoarthritis, is a disease of the movable, weight-bearing joints. It affects 50 percent of persons in their 60s and 85 percent of those over the age of 75. It is a phenomenon associated with aging. (B) It is a common misconception that the elderly are depressed. Depression appears much less frequently than in young adults. It is, however, the most common psychiatric problem among the elderly population. (C) Hypertension in the elderly is the persistent elevation of the arterial blood pressure to levels greater than 95 mm Hg diastolic and 160 mm Hg systolic. (D) Osteoporosis is directly responsible for hip fractures and other dependent fractures in the elderly. It is one of the most common metabolic bone disorders of aging. It is dependent on diet, sex, race, and exercise. It is more common in women and the second most common disorder found in the elderly.

503. **(A)** Nursing process phase: assessment; client need: physiological integrity; content area: medical/surgical nursing

Rationale
(A) Kyphosis is an exaggerated posterior curvature of the thoracic spine usually associated with aging. (B) Lordosis is when the normal lumbar concavity of the spine is further accentuated as usually seen in pregnancy. (C) Scoliosis is a lateral S-shaped curvature of the spine. It is more prevalent in adolescent females and can be corrected with surgery in acute presentations. (D) List is a condition in which the spine tilts to one side and is usually associated with pressure on a spinal nerve root from a herniated disc.

504. **(C)** Nursing process phase: assessment; client need: safe, effective care environment; content area: medical/surgical nursing

Rationale
(A) The nurse would suspect arterial insufficiency in a younger client if he or she presented with these findings; however, for this client, due to his age, this is considered normal. (B) You have no justification or data from this assessment to support this condition. (C) These are normal changes associated with aging due to loss of skin elasticity, decreased perfusion, and decreased cardiac output. (D) This not a consideration in your client. Muscular dystrophy is a disease commonly found in children.

505. **(B)** Nursing process phase: analysis; client need: safe, effective care environment; content area: medical/surgical nursing

Rationale
(A) Because of changes in metabolism and sleep cycles, the elderly person may spend more time in bed and require naps throughout the day. The elderly person spends more time trying to rest and sleep than the average adult. (B) The elderly client awakens more during the night due to reductions in the time spent in REM or stage IV sleep. (C) The elderly spend 50 percent less time in REM or stage IV sleep. This time is replaced by stage II and III sleep, which are less restful. (D) This is not true of healthy elderly persons or the elderly in general.

506. **(B)** Nursing process phase: implementation; client need: psychosocial integrity; content area: medical/surgical nursing

Rationale

(A) Never leave a client alone when she is obviously in emotional distress. The client needs help adjusting to her change in body image. (B) The nurse needs to address the problem and help the client to explore the feelings that are distressing her. (C) The client is not in a frame of mind that is conducive to teaching. Teaching should be postponed until the client is ready to receive the information. (D) This is not an appropriate nursing action. The client does not have a psychological problem, but is exhibiting a normal response to her circumstances.

507. (B) Nursing process phase: planning; client need: safe, effective care environment; content area: medical/surgical nursing

Rationale

(A) Weight loss is an important factor to monitor with this client. However, it is not the most important factor related to the client's safety. (B) The client with Bell's palsy will have left-sided weakness in her mouth and throat, which can affect her ability to eat and swallow. The client is at risk for aspiration of her food and needs to be watched. (C) Pain is a concern for all clients in the hospital, but it is not the most important concern for this client. (D) An elevated temperature can indicate an infection, which the client is recovering from. Because infections can bring about Bell's palsy in adults, the client needs to be followed up and treated for her molar abscess.

508. (A) Nursing process phase: analysis; client need: physiological integrity; content area: medical/surgical nursing

Rationale

(A) Mold or dust are considered extrinsic factors associated with causing asthma. Other extrinsic factors are pollen, animal hair, feathers, or food additives. (B) Stress is usually identified as an intrinsic factor associated with certain types of asthma. (C) Fatigue is usually identified as an intrinsic factor. (D) An elevated temperature related to infection can also be considered an intrinsic factor that can predispose a client to an asthma attack.

509. (B) Nursing process phase: assessment; client need: physiological integrity; content area: medical/surgical nursing

Rationale

(A) These are signs associated with a mild asthma attack. (B) These are signs of a severe asthma attack. It is marked by respiratory distress because there is no air exchange in the lungs. (C) These are signs associated with a moderate asthma attack. The respiratory distress is mild and there is moderate air exchange in the lungs. (D) This is a sign of respiratory failure, in which the brain is not receiving enough oxygen.

510. (A) Nursing process phase: analysis; client need: safe, effective care environment; content area: medical/surgical nursing

Rationale

(A) Nausea, vomiting, and headache are signs of theophylline toxicity. (B) Wheezing and respiratory distress would be signs of subtherapeutic levels of theophylline. The client has a productive cough as a result of his asthma. He is not in respiratory distress. (C) Dehydration would not present with a productive cough. The client would have tachycardia, feel hot, appear flushed, and have increased respirations. (D) The client would exhibit signs of severe chest pain, have elevated blood pressure and pulse, and would appear in extreme distress.

511. (C) Nursing process phase: assessment; client need: physiological integrity; content area: medical/surgical nursing

Rationale

(A) Cachexia is marked by general malnutrition, weakness, and emaciation usually associated with a serious disease, such as tuberculosis or cancer. (B) Anorexia is the lack or loss of appetite resulting from an inability to eat. It can be related to a variety of physiological and psychological causes. (C) This condition is marked by a weight loss leading to a body weight 15 percent below the ideal body weight. Amenorrhea for 3 consecutive months and a distorted body image are signs related to this disorder. (D) Amenorrhea in this case is a symptom of a much more serious condition.

512. (B) Nursing process phase: implementation; client need: physiological integrity; content area: medical/surgical nursing

Rationale

(A) With a client's platelet count as low as $19,000/\mu L$, the nurse would want to avoid IM injections for this client. (B) You would want to monitor the client for bleeding and avoid trauma to the skin, such as IM injections, that could promote bleeding. (C) This intervention is not necessary for this client. (D) This client needs to use stool softeners to decrease the chances of trauma to the rectal mucosa and possible bleeding.

513. (B) Nursing process phase: implementation; client need: safe, effective care environment; content area: medical/surgical nursing

Rationale

(A) You would administer any medication as ordered unless a problem developed with your client or he refused the medication. However, this situation is different. (B) You never administer enemas to a client with suspected appendicitis because you can rupture the appendix. You would call and question the doctor about this order. (C) You would never administer an enema to a client with suspected appendicitis. (D) The purpose of the enema is to clear the intestines of any matter prior to surgery. Whether or not the client has had a bowel movement, in this situation, is not relevant.

514. (D) Nursing process phase: analysis; client need: physiological integrity; content area: medical/surgical nursing

Rationale

(A) Muscle contractures would be present in a client with decreased range of motion to an extremity and prolonged bedrest, greater than 2 weeks. The client's pain is related to another problem. (B) A fat embolus is an emergency condition in which the client would be anxious, short of breath, diaphoretic, and complain of extreme chest pain if located in the lungs. If the embolus were located in an extremity, there would be coolness and decreased pulses to that extremity. (C) Hypovolemic shock is suspected when the client has a rapid pulse, decreased blood pressure, pallor, and cool skin. These are not the signs exhibited by this client. (D) Prolonged immobility can produce renal calculi from decalcification of the bones. In this client's case this is further complicated by multiple fractures, which can increase bone decalcification. Renal pain can be in the middle to lower back and can radiate to the client's flank.

515. (D) Nursing process phase: assessment: client need: physiological integrity; content area: medical/surgical nursing

Rationale

(A) The iliac artery occlusion would present with intermittent claudication to the lower back, buttocks, and thighs. (B) An occlusion of the aortic bifurcation can produce muscle weakness, numbness, paralysis, and signs of ischemia in both legs. (C) The mesenteric artery, when occluded, will cause bowel ischemia, abdominal pain, nausea, and vomiting. (D) Femoral and popliteal occlusion would produce all of the signs and symptoms exhibited by this client.

516. (B) Nursing process phase: assessment; client need: physiological integrity; content area: medical/surgical nursing

Rationale

(A, C, & D) These would be expected findings in a client with reduced peripheral perfusion and are not indicators that the client's condition is deteriorating. (B) A urine output of 30 mL or less per hour is a serious indicator that the client has decreased renal perfusion, which could cause kidney damage.

517. (B) Nursing process phase: assessment; client need: physiological integrity; content area: medical/surgical nursing

Rationale

(A) This is the definition of a first-degree burn. (B) This is the definition of a second-degree burn. (C) This is the definition of a third-degree burn. (D) This is the definition of a fourth-degree burn.

518. (A) Nursing process phase: analysis; client need: safe, effective care environment; content area: medical/surgical nursing

Rationale

(A) Gas exchange may be impaired because of restricted respiratory expansion due to chest burns and probable smoke inhalation. (B) Anxiety would not be a primary complication for this client at this time. (C) Fluid volume deficit, not overload, would be a complication expected with a burn victim. (D) Alteration in nutrition would be a complication for this client, but not at this time. Keeping his airway open and his lungs clear is more important.

519. (B) Nursing process phase: analysis; client need: physiological integrity; content area: medical/surgical nursing

Rationale

(A) Hypoparathyroidism results in a decrease in parathyroid hormone (PTH) production, which is necessary for calcium absorption. The client would not have increased calcium levels. (B) The client would have decreased calcium levels due to decreased production of parathyroid hormone. (C) This is an increase in blood sugar and would not be expected in this disorder. (D) This is a decrease in blood sugar and would not be expected in this client.

520. (A) Nursing process phase: implementation; client need: health promotion and maintenance; content area: medical/surgical nursing

Rationale

(A) It is important to teach the client to monitor for excess bleeding by checking his skin for bruising, petechiae, hematuria, and bleeding gums. (B) The client needs to maintain adequate hydration and the nurse should encourage fluid intake, not a fluid restriction. (C) The client does not need to be concerned about the blood test at this time. This is a medical maintenance problem and the tests need to be ordered by the physician, usually when the client has visited the physician or has been visited by a home health nurse. (D) This is the wrong information. The client needs to be instructed to seek medical assistance as soon as possible for any signs of excess bleeding, such as nosebleeds.

521. (D) Nursing process phase: assessment; client need: physiological integrity; content area: medical/surgical nursing

Rationale

(A) Excessive radiation exposure through x-ray or other devices has not been proved to cause brain tumors. (B) Inappropriate diet has not been proved to cause brain tumors. (C) Drug abuse has not been proved to cause brain tumors. (D) This is correct. The actual cause of brain tumors is unknown.

522. (D) Nursing process phase: implementation; client need: physiological integrity; content area: medical/surgical nursing

Rationale

(A) Neurological checks should be performed more frequently in this client than every shift. Every 1 to 4 hours would be more appropriate. (B) This is not a priority since input and output would be expected to be affected by this client's injuries. (C) Vital signs should be monitored more frequently in this client's case. The nurse would want to observe for changes in pulse and respiratory status. (D) This is correct. A halo sign is the lighter ring surrounding a drop of blood of serosanguinous drainage from the nares or ears. It indicates leaking cerebrospinal fluid and is a critical indicator.

523. (B) Nursing process phase: analysis; client need: safe, effective care environment; content area: medical/surgical nursing

Rationale

(A) A myocardial infarction (MI) would present with different signs and changes in her vital signs and EKG. (B) This is correct. The client is within the characteristic 40, female, flatulent, and overweight categories associated with this disorder. Pain usually occurs after ingestion of fatty foods. (C) Pneumonia would not correlate with this client's signs and symptoms. She would be short of breath and have abnormal blood work (elevated WBCs) and increased temperature. (D) A duodenal ulcer would be a possibility except for the pain starting after eating a meal. Ulcer pain is eased with food and aggravated when the stomach is empty.

524. (C) Nursing process phase: analysis; client need: physiological integrity; content area: medical/surgical nursing

Rationale

(A) Anemia is not a cause of COPD; however, the presence of this disorder can aggravate the client's condition. (B) Recurrent pulmonary infections can predispose an individual to COPD, but it is not the leading cause of COPD. (C) Smoking is the leading cause of this disorder. It causes increased mucus production, inflammation of the airway, and it impairs ciliary action and destroys alveolar space. (D) Obesity does not predispose a client to COPD; however, it can aggravate this condition by increasing oxygen demand of the muscles.

525. (B) Nursing process phase: analysis; client need: safe, effective care environment; content area: medical/surgical nursing

Rationale
(A) Renal calculi would not cause obstruction of the urethra. (B) Prostatic hypertrophy is the most common cause of bladder obstruction in the middle- and older-aged males. (C) Bladder tumors are not the most common cause of bladder obstruction. (D) Urethral strictures are not the most common cause of bladder obstructions.

526. (B) Nursing process phase: implementation; client need: psychosocial integrity; content area: medical/surgical nursing

Rationale
(A) Allowing the client to discuss his feelings is an appropriate action; however, it will not help the client prepare for the changes this type of surgery will bring. (B) This is correct. Allowing the client to visualize and handle the products used can help generate questions and can allow the opportunity for the client to discuss his feelings about the impending body image change. (C) Never leave a client or the client's family alone. They need information from an informed individual about the surgery and his illness. (D) This is not up to the client. It is based on his diagnosis, degree of cancer, and products selected and is up to the surgeon. The surgeon will try to select a site accessible to the client to ensure ease of use.

527. (C) Nursing process phase: implementation; client need: health promotion and maintenance; content area: medical/surgical nursing

Rationale
(A) The client receiving the donor marrow will be suffering from immunosuppression and needs to avoid infections. (B) Bleeding for a few weeks postoperatively is abnormal, so the client needs to see a physician. (C) The client will have pain for a few days postoperatively, so this is the correct statement. (D) The client will not need to remain on bedrest, so this statement is incorrect.

528. (A) Nursing process phase: implementation; client need: physiological integrity; content area: medical/surgical nursing

Rationale
(A) This is correct. The client will awaken with an NG tube and needs to be prepared for it. (B) The client will ambulate the first day after surgery to promote the return of peristalsis. Peristalsis returns in 2 to 3 days. (C) The client will receive enemas before the surgery to remove fecal contents. (D) The client will remain in the hospital for a few days. This is not an outpatient procedure, yet.

529. (C) Nursing process phase: implementation; client need: safe, effective care environment; content area: medical/surgical nursing

Rationale
(A) Daily weights, not every other day, should be done to monitor intake and output and developing fluid retention. (B) Dressing changes to the incision should be done twice a day or every shift to monitor the site and to check drainage and for signs of infection, especially with abdominal wounds. (C) This is correct. Daily abdominal circumferences are used to monitor the abdomen for distention or rigidity caused by obstruction of the bowel. (D) Until peristalsis returns, tube feedings should not be given and the client should remain NPO.

530. (C) Nursing process phase: analysis; client need: physiological integrity; content area: medical/surgical nursing

Rationale
(A) Hyperglycemia is not a complication related to colostomy placement. (B) Depression related to the client's change in body image can result from the placement of a colostomy. However, although it is a problem, it is not a complication. (C) This is correct. Dehydration caused by excessive drainage from the stoma is a complication of ostomy placement and needs medical attention. (D) Cholecystitis is not a complication associated with colostomy placement.

531. (D) Nursing process phase: analysis; client need: safe, effective care environment; content area: medical/surgical nursing

Rationale
(A) Clients with SLE have elevated antinuclear antibody tests. SLE clients usually suffer from alopecia, sun-induced rashes, malar rashes, and fatigue. However, they do not suffer from chronic flu symptoms as seen here. (B) Anemia would not explain the low-grade temperatures, sore throats, or joint pain. (C) Hypothyroid clients also suffer from weight gain and skin disorders. They do not suffer from fevers, sore throats, or severe fatigue. (D) This is correct. The precise cause of chronic fatigue syndrome is unknown. It is marked by extreme fatigue of at least 6 months' duration. There is no definitive treatment for this disorder.

532. (B) Nursing process phase: assessment; client need: physiological integrity; content area: medical/surgical nursing

Rationale
(A) Prodromal stage is marked by early symptoms such as slight personality changes, agitation, belligerence, disorientation, and difficulty concentrating. (B) This is correct. The impending stage is marked by continuing mental changes and the appearance of asterixis. (C) The stuporous stage is when the client shows marked mental changes and confusion. He may appear drowsy, but when aroused is noisy and abusive. (D) The comatose stage is when the client cannot be aroused, is obtunded, and may experience seizures. Reflexes are hyperactive and there is a positive Babinski's reflex.

533. (A) Nursing process phase: analysis; client need: physiological integrity; content area: medical/surgical nursing

Rationale
(A) This is correct. Ascites can result from the combination of portal hypertension and hypoproteinemia. This is caused by electrolyte imbalances and the back-up of blood into the spleen and collateral channels; fluid pools in the abdominal cavity, and paracentesis may be required to relieve abdominal pressure. (B) Hypoglycemia would not result from the combination of these two factors in a client with cirrhosis. (C)

Esophageal varices result from portal hypertension and are not affected by hypoproteinemia. (D) Hypovolemic shock can develop in cirrhosis, but it is the result of several compounding factors and not just the combination of portal hypertension and hypoproteinemia. Hypovolemic shock results from massive hematemesis that quickly results in heavy hemorrhage leading to shock.

534. (C) Nursing process phase: analysis; client need: safe, effective care environment; content area: medical/surgical nursing

Rationale
(A) Alcohol does not account for all the cases of cirrhosis in the United States. (B) Alcohol accounts for more than half the cases of cirrhosis in the United States. (C) This is correct. Alcohol accounts for more than half of all the cases of cirrhosis in the United States. (D) Alcohol accounts for more than a third of all the cases of cirrhosis in the United States.

535. (C) Nursing process phase: analysis; client need: physiological integrity; content area: medical/surgical nursing

Rationale
(A) Hyponatremia and hypoproteinemia are often found in cirrhosis clients but do not cause portal hypertension. (B) These are signs and symptoms of cirrhosis and do not cause portal hypertension. (C) This is correct. Fibrotic tissue accumulation as a result of hepatic cell destruction causes increased resistance of blood flow and portal hypertension. (D) Esophageal varices are the result of portal hypertension and do not cause it. Neither does hypoproteinemia.

536. (A) Nursing process phase: assessment; client need: physiological integrity; focus area: medical/surgical nursing

Rationale
(A) Laennec's is seen mostly in males who are chronic alcoholics and malnourished. (B) Postnecrotic cirrhosis is more common in women and results from complications of viral hepatitis. It may also occur after exposure to live toxins. (C) Biliary cirrhosis results from prolonged biliary tract obstruction or inflammation. (D) Cardiac cirrhosis is associated with protected venous congestion in the liver caused by right ventricular failure.

537. (D) Nursing process phase: assessment; client need: safe, effective care environment; content area: medical/surgical nursing

Rationale
(A) Gastritis occurs after the client has ingested an irritating substance or food. The client complains of cramping, indigestion, nausea, and vomiting that last for a few hours or days. (B) Esophageal varices are related to the portal hypertension seen in cirrhosis of the liver. The client with this disorder would not present with GI disturbances. (C) Hirschsprung's disease is a congenital disorder of the large intestines. This disorder causes severe constipation in an infant. (D) This is correct. Hiatal hernia incidence is higher in women than men. It is a defect in the diaphragm that permits a portion of the stomach to pass through the diaphragmatic opening into the chest.

538. (C) Nursing process phase: analysis; client need: physiological integrity; content area: medical/surgical nursing

Rationale
(A) Pain in appendicitis would be localized to the right lower abdomen. Clients with appendicitis will have normal bowel sounds. Palpation reveals no abnormal findings except for tenderness. (B) Diverticulitis is a disorder where the diverticula in the GI wall are pushed through the mucosal lining through the surrounding muscle and become inflamed. The client with diverticulitis has a history of diverticulosis. There is left lower quadrant pain, which is dull and steady. Palpation reveals rebound tenderness. A rectal examination may disclose a tender mass. (C) This is correct. This is a twisting of the bowel on itself. The client presents with the above symptoms and has the classic "ace of spades" configuration on x-ray. (D) Dumping syndrome is characterized by cramps, diarrhea, nausea, and weakness an hour after eating because of rapid gastric emptying after a gastrectomy.

539. (B) Nursing process phase: analysis; client need: physiological integrity; content area: medical/surgical nursing

Rationale
(A) A client with a bleeding ulcer or hemorrhage would report black, tarry stools, but his bowel sounds would be present. (B) Perforation is correct. This is an emergency situation where the client's stomach lining has been eaten away through to the peritoneal cavity. (C) Gastritis would present with nausea, vomiting, and diarrhea brought on by a specific food or substance. Bowel sounds would be present. (D) This is an abnormal situation—these are not classic ulcer symptoms.

540. (C) Nursing process phase: implementation; client need: health promotion and maintenance; content area: medical/surgical nursing

Rationale
(A) Do not instruct the client to eat large meals. This increases stomach bulk and acid secretion, causing greater discomfort. (B) Do not instruct the client to lie down after meals. Instruct the client to keep her head elevated for at least 2 hours after eating. (C) The client should eat small, frequent meals but bland, not spicy, food is recommended. (D) This is correct. The client should avoid alcohol and constrictive clothing. Both factors can aggravate the hiatal hernia and cause discomfort.

541. (A) Nursing process phase: implementation; client need: physiological integrity; content area: medical/surgical nursing

Rationale
(A) This is correct. Shock can result from massive hemorrhage and total destruction of the pancreas. This is an emergency situation. (B) A pancreatic abscess would present with pain, fever, elevated blood pressure, and pulse. This is a complication of pancreatitis but not for this client. (C) Alcohol withdrawal would present with changes in behavior and sensorium. (D) Pneumonia would present with dyspnea, fever, changes in blood pressure, and tachycardia.

542. (D) Nursing process phase: analysis; client need: physiological integrity; content area: medical/surgical nursing

Rationale
(A) Gastritis would not be a complication of this surgery and can relate to viral causes. (B) It is too early to detect whether the client has an infection or not. We would suspect this 2 to 3 days' postoperatively. (C) Hypovolemia can be an effect of

abdominal surgery; however, this is not the complication exhibited by this client. (D) The client is exhibiting the signs of a simple intestinal obstruction, which can be a complication of this type of surgery.

543. (C) Nursing process phase: analysis; client need: safe, effective care environment; content area: medical/surgical nursing

Rationale
(A) Scanning speech is alternating slowness and explosiveness in speech. (B) Apraxia is the inability to carry out learned movements. (C) Perseveration is correct. This is the inappropriate repetition of words or actions. (D) Dementia is characterized by deterioration of mental functions.

544. (C) Nursing process phase: analysis; client need: physiological integrity; content area: medical/surgical nursing

Rationale
(A) Thiamine would be given if seizure activity were related to chronic alcoholism or withdrawal. (B) 50% dextrose would be given if the seizure activity were related to hypoglycemia. (C) This is correct. Diazepam would be the drug of choice to give to this client to ease seizures. (D) Digoxin is used to increase cardiac contractility and is not used in this condition.

545. (D) Nursing process phase: assessment; client need: safe, effective care environment; content area: medical/surgical nursing

Rationale
(A) The early stages of Alzheimer's are characterized by forgetfulness of recent events, not the past. (B) Difficulty with activities of daily living is seen in advanced stages, not early stages of the disease. (C) Loss of ability to speak and write is seen in late stages of Alzheimer's. (D) This is correct. Early Alzheimer's is marked by forgetfulness of recent events. Clients often misplace keys and other everyday objects.

546. (D) Nursing process phase: assessment; client need: safe, effective care environment; content area: medical/surgical nursing

Rationale
(A) Tonic-clonic seizures begin with a cry, followed by the client falling to the ground and losing consciousness. The body stiffens (tonic phase) and then alternates between muscle spasm and relaxation (clonic phase). (B) Akinetic seizures are characterized by general loss of muscle tone and a temporary loss of consciousness. (C) Simple partial seizures are characterized by a jerking or tingling sensation in one limb. (D) This is correct. Complex partial seizures are characterized by the signs given by this client. They are also called psychomotor temporal lobe seizures.

547. (D) Nursing process phase: implementation; client need: health promotion and maintenance; content area: medical/surgical nursing

Rationale
(A) Instruct the client to exercise moderately for 3 to 4 days a week for half an hour. Excessive exercise can increase stress to the body and decrease glucose, predisposing the client to seizures. (B) Balanced, regular meals should be stressed. No changes in diet are needed, unless certain food items trigger seizures. (C) The client does need to control stress levels; however, loud music should be discouraged. (D) This is cor-

rect. Bright, flashing lights as seen in video games can cause seizures in epileptic clients.

548. (C) Nursing process phase: analysis; client need: safe, effective care environment; content area: medical/surgical nursing

Rationale
(A) Pupillary changes are indicative of increasing ICP, but this is not the situation with this client. (B) Increasing mental alertness is not a sign of increasing ICP. Decreasing mental alertness indicates increasing ICP. (C) This is correct. This ICP is within normal range of 0 to 10 mm Hg. (D) Nausea and vomiting are signs of increasing ICP, but this is not the situation with this client.

549. (B) Nursing process phase: implementation; client need: health promotion and maintenance; content area: medical/surgical nursing

Rationale
(A) Bedrest is not needed to relieve a reducible hernia. There is a better option. (B) A truss is correct. This garment is a firm pad placed over a belt, which can be worn by the client to keep the hernia reduced. It provides temporary relief until the client is well enough to withstand surgery. (C) Unless this medication is ordered PRN for pain, medication for the client is usually not needed for a hernia. (D) Relief may be needed by this client because his pneumonia and productive cough are placing stress on the herniated area, which can cause enlargement of the hernia.

550. (D) Nursing process phase: implementation; client need: health promotion and maintenance; content area: medical/surgical nursing

Rationale
(A) Headache, nose bleeds, and blurred vision are not signs of abdominal incarceration or strangulation. (B) Nausea, vomiting, and shortness of breath combined are not signs of abdominal incarceration or strangulation; however, nausea and vomiting are signs of problems. (C) Muscle tremors, weakness, and fatigue are signs that the nurse would note. (D) High fever, bloody stools, and severe pain are symptoms of complete obstruction of the bowel and developing strangulation.

551. (D) Nursing process phase: planning; client need: physiological integrity; content area: medical/surgical nursing

Rationale
(A) A histocompatible donor is used for an allogenic, not an autologous, transplant. (B) An identical twin is used in a syngeneic, not an autologous, transplant. (C) Aplastic anemia means the client's bone marrow is depressed and would not meet the criteria for an autologous procedure. (D) This is correct. Autologous transplants are where the client donates his or her own bone marrow before beginning chemotherapy and radiation. The client must be able to withstand several weeks of myelosuppression in order to be considered for this procedure.

552. (A) Nursing process phase: implementation; client need: health promotion and maintenance; content area: medical/surgical nursing

Rationale
(A) This is correct. Instruct the client to avoid stressful situa-

tions that can deplete resistance and increase chance of infection. (B) The client does not need to avoid caffeine. (C) The client does not need to avoid acetaminophen but should avoid aspirin products, which can increase bleeding time. (D) The client should be encouraged to exercise moderately since this can help strengthen the immune system.

553. (C) Nursing process phase: implementation; client need: safe, effective care environment; content area: medical/surgical nursing

Rationale
(A) This is only done once a catheter has been placed by the physician to check for placement and possible pneumothorax. (B) Calling the doctor is not an appropriate nursing action here. (C) This is correct. If the nurse feels resistance to the flush, she must stop and label the part "Clotted Off" or "Do Not Use." (D) This is wrong. Never push fluid through a triple-lumen catheter if you feel resistance. You could dislodge a clot and the catheter tip and cause an embolus for your client.

554. (D) Nursing process phase: implementation; client need: safe, effective care environment; content area: medical/surgical nursing

Rationale
(A) Dextrose is only given with a doctor's order for a client with a blood sugar below 50. (B) This is not an appropriate action. The blood sugar is low for this client and can be managed without calling the doctor. (C) The nurse does need to do something for the client because it is difficult to detect whether the client is groggy because of low blood sugar or diphenhydramine. If you left her alone, her blood sugar may fall even lower. (D) This is correct. Giving orange juice with sugar helps determine the origin of the client's grogginess.

555. (B) Nursing process phase: planning; client need: safe, effective care environment; content area: medical/surgical nursing

Rationale
(A) The client is not experiencing altered thought processes. This is not appropriate. (B) This is correct. The client may experience anxiety because of visual changes and/or hospitalization. (C) This is not an appropriate diagnosis for this client. (D) This is not the best diagnosis for this client.

556. (C) Nursing process phase: analysis; client need: physiological integrity; content area: medical/surgical nursing

Rationale
(A) Aplastic crisis is associated with an infection (usually viral) and results from bone marrow depression. The client experiences pallor, lethargy, sleepiness, dyspnea, and possible coma. (B) There is no such thing as a neoplastic crisis. (C) This is correct. The client is experiencing a vaso-occlusive crisis, which is the most common crisis and the hallmark of this disease. (D) An acute sequestration crisis occurs in infants between the ages of 8 months and 2 years. This crisis causes massive entrapment of RBCs in the spleen and liver.

557. (C) Nursing process phase: planning; client need: safe, effective care environment; content area: medical/surgical nursing

Rationale
(A) This would not be a complication seen following spinal

anesthesia. This is a disorder of glucocorticoid excess. (B) Dysphagia would not be a complication seen following spinal anesthesia. This is seen in clients following cerebral vascular accidents with paralysis. (C) This is correct. The client may have difficulty urinating because of decreased sensation. (D) Pneumonia is a potential postsurgical complication 24 to 48 hours following general anesthesia surgery.

558. (B) Nursing process phase: implementation; client need: safe, effective care environment; content area: medical/surgical nursing

Rationale
(A) Sleep medications would not help the client rest since these medications do not help the client achieve needed rapid eye movement (REM) sleep to produce rest. (B) This is correct. Allow the client time to rest. Coordinate scheduled laboratory and vital signs to allow for uninterrupted sleep. (C) Caffeine could be eliminated before bedtime; however, there is a more appropriate choice. (D) Activity for a fatigued client can be dangerous and increase her risk for injury.

559. (C) Nursing process phase: planning; client need: safe, effective care environment; content area: medical/surgical nursing

Rationale
(A) A client over the age of 65 would be at risk for impaired wound healing because of a decreased immune system. This is not appropriate for this client. (B) Mobility would not be a factor placing this client at risk for delayed wound healing. (C) This is correct. Anorexia would place this client at risk because nutrition is needed to promote cell growth and healing. (D) Pain would not place this client at risk; however, it could promote anorexia, which would place him at risk.

560. (C) Nursing process phase: assessment; client need: physiological integrity; content area: medical/surgical nursing

Rationale
(A) The inflammation phase is marked by edema, migration of monocytes, increased vascular permeability, and migration of neutrophils. (B) The maturation phase is marked by myofibroblast contraction and remodeling of collagen fibers. (C) This is correct. Resolution is marked by the synthesis of collagen, endothelial budding, and epithelialization. (D) This is not a phase in wound healing.

561. (A) Nursing process phase: analysis; client need: physiological integrity; content area: medical/surgical nursing

Rationale
(A) Bleeding from three unrelated sites is a key indicator for DIC, a disorder of abnormal bleeding. (B) Excessive nausea and vomiting would not cause the nurse to suspect DIC. (C) Bloody sputum in addition to two other sites of bleeding would indicate DIC, but not on its own. (D) Hematuria in combination with bleeding from two other sites would indicate DIC, but not by itself.

562. (B) Nursing process phase: assessment; client need: physiological integrity; content area: medical/surgical nursing

Rationale
(A) The client is septic, but he has progressed to a dangerous complication of bacterial infection. This is not the best

choice. (B) This is correct. The client is in the progressive phase of septic shock. (C) The client is not exhibiting an indication of ARDS. This is not the best choice. (D) The client is hypotensive, but there is a better choice to explain why his condition is this way.

563. (C) Nursing process phase: analysis; client need: safe, effective care environment; content area: medical/surgical nursing

Rationale

(A) In sepsis and septic shock, you can see delayed multiple organ dysfunction. (B) In sepsis and septic shock, you can collect bacterial cultures from the blood. (C) This is correct. Septic shock only has unresponsive hypotension—not sepsis. (D) This is incorrect. Both sepsis and septic shock can occur in the elderly and in anyone with a compromised immune system.

564. (C) Nursing process phase: assessment; client need: safe, effective care environment; content area: medical/surgical nursing

Rationale

(A) This test does not assess intelligence. (B) It is not used to assess motor ability. (C) This is correct. The Glasgow Coma Scale is an indicator of level of consciousness. A fully alert, normal person has a score of 15, whereas a score of 7 or less reflects coma. (D) There are different assessment measures to evaluate cranial nerves.

565. (D) Nursing process phase: analysis; client need: safe, effective care environment; content area: medial/surgical nursing

Rationale

(A) Hypotension cannot cause autonomic dysreflexia, but it is usually a result of this neurological emergency. The client becomes extremely hypertensive. (B) Muscle wasting is not a stimulant for autonomic dysreflexia. (C) Diaphoresis above the level of injury is usually an indicator of autonomic dysreflexia. (D) This is correct. A client with a distended bladder can send excessive stimuli to the spinal cord, causing increasing blood pressure and diaphoresis above the level of injury with cool skin and falling pressure below the injury. This is a medical emergency.

566. (C) Nursing process phase: planning; client need: safe, effective care environment; content area: medical/surgical nursing

Rationale

(A) Furosemide is a diuretic and would not be beneficial to the client with autonomic dysreflexia. (B) Nitroglycerin is not the drug of choice. It is used as an antianginal and is not appropriate for a hypertensive crisis. (C) This is correct. Hydralazine is the drug of choice for a hypertensive crisis. (D) Digoxin is an antiarrythmic and would not be beneficial in a hypertensive crisis.

567. (B) Nursing process phase: analysis; client need: physiological integrity; content area: medical/surgical nursing

Rationale

(A) A ventilation-perfusion mismatch would be seen in more obstructive disorders such as asthma and COPD. The client is unable to ventilate adequately to perfuse the tissues. (B) This is correct. Alveolar hypoventilation is seen when there is mechanical difficulty ventilating air to the lungs. Ruptured diaphragm, muscle fatigue, or pain contribute to this type of hypoxemia. (C) Pulmonary shunting is seen in cases where there is decreased alveolar space to accommodate perfusion. (D) Low oxygen tension of inspired air is related to environmental factors such as smoke-filled rooms during a fire or high altitudes. Here, enough oxygen is not available for perfusion because of a lack of oxygen in the environment.

568. (A) Nursing process phase: analysis; client need: safe, effective care environment; content area: medical/surgical nursing

Rationale

(A) This is correct. Menstrual flow and chronic gastrointestinal bleeding are the major sources of chronic anemia. (B) Polycythemia is a factor that leads to an increased hematocrit. Chronic gastrointestinal bleeding does lead to chronic anemia. (C) Massive trauma and surgical repair would be factors associated with acute blood loss or acute anemia. (D) Dehydration can lead to an increased hematocrit, whereas surgery can lead to a decreased hematocrit and blood loss.

569. (C) Nursing process phase: assessment; client need: physiological integrity; content area: medical/surgical nursing

Rationale

(A) Kussmaul respirations are deep, regular sighing breathing that may be associated with a slow or fast rate. (B) Tachypnea is an increased rate and increased depth of respirations. (C) This is correct. Cheyne-Stokes breathing is characterized by a period of apnea as the ventilation declines. (D) Hyperventilation is characterized by an increased rate and depth of respirations, usually associated with anxiety.

570. (A) Nursing process phase: analysis; client need: physiological integrity; content area: medical/surgical nursing

Rationale

(A) Shingles is caused by varicella-zoster virus, a virus similar to herpes-zoster. This is a condition seen in clients with depressed immune systems or as the result of increased stress. (B) Staphylococcus is responsible for a large number of skin disorders from rashes to furuncles. It is not the cause of shingles. (C) A β-hemolytic streptococcus is responsible for a large number of skin disorders including impetigo, seen in children. (D) *Rickettsia rickettsii* is the organism responsible for Rocky Mountain spotted fever.

571. (D) Nursing process phase: analysis; client need: physiological integrity; content area: medical/surgical nursing

Rationale

(A) Muscle weakness is seen in both primary and secondary adrenal hypofunction. (B) GI disturbances are seen in both primary and secondary adrenal hypofunction. (C) Weight loss is seen in both primary and secondary adrenal hypofunction. (D) Hyperpigmentation is the only characteristic seen in primary adrenal hypofunction and not secondary. This is caused by the lower corticotropin and MSH levels in secondary hypofunction.

572. (C) Nursing process phase: analysis; client need: physiological integrity; content area: medical/surgical nursing

Rationale
(A) Drug and alcohol abuse are not a cause of Cushing's syndrome. (B) Sustained stress is not a cause of Cushing's syndrome. (C) Prolonged steroid use is attributed to about 70 percent of Cushing's syndrome cases. (D) Adrenal tumors only account for less than 30 percent of the Cushing's syndrome cases diagnosed.

573. **(A)** Nursing process phase: implementation; client need: safe, effective care environment; content area: medical/surgical nursing

Rationale
(A) Vasopressin is used to control fluid balance and prevent dehydration. (B) Insulin, regular or otherwise, is not used as a treatment in diabetes insipidus. (C) Furosemide is a diuretic, and your client already has dehydration because of excessive output. Lasix is not a treatment for diabetes insipidus. (D) Prednisone is a corticosteroid, which would not be effective in treating diabetes insipidus.

574. **(B)** Nursing process phase: analysis; client need: safe, effective care environment; content area: medical/surgical nursing

Rationale
(A) Lente is an intermediate-acting insulin modified with zinc chloride. Its peak duration is 7 to 15 hours. It is not the most rapid acting insulin used for sliding scales. (B) This is correct. Humulin regular insulin is used with all sliding scales, unless otherwise ordered. (C) Humulin NPH is an intermediate-acting insulin with a peak duration of up to 12 to 24 hours. (D) Novolin Lente is the same intermediate-acting insulin as Humulin Lente.

575. **(C)** Nursing process phase: implementation; client need: health promotion and maintenance; content area: medical/surgical nursing

Rationale
(A) The client is not ready for teaching and is having difficulty dealing with the change in her body image. (B) The client has visitors, and this would not be a good time to send the visitors out of the room or the client is not ready to reveal her ostomy or receive teaching in front of her family. The client needs as much emotional support as possible at this time. Allow the client time with her family. (C) This is correct. The client is asking for help and has opened up to the nurse that she is ready to learn, even though she may appear angry. (D) The client will not be ready for teaching because the pain medication will affect her ability to retain information.

576. **(B)** Nursing process phase: analysis; client need: physiological integrity; content area: medical/surgical nursing

Rationale
(A) Skin breakdown would be expected in a client who is extremely thin with bony prominences or who is elderly and/or who has a compromised immune system. (B) This is correct. The client who smokes would be at risk for respiratory infection—especially a client who has had abdominal surgery and may have difficulty deep breathing and coughing. (C) Delayed wound healing would not be a postoperative complication as long as the client eats a well-balanced diet with extra protein to promote healing. (D) Bleeding and hypovolemia could be a postoperative problem if the client develops complications or has been taking aspirin prior to his surgery. Aspirin increases clotting time and promotes bleeding.

577. **(C)** Nursing process phase: assessment; client need: safe, effective care environment; content area: medical/surgical nursing

Rationale
(A) S_1 occurs with closure of the AV valves and signals the beginning of systole. This is a normal heart sound. (B) S_2 occurs with the closure of the semilunar valves and signals the end of systole. This is a normal heart sound. (C) S_3 is correct. This is an abnormal heart sound that occurs during diastole and is created by the vibrations caused by ventricular filling, when the ventricles are resistant to filling during the early rapid filling phase of the heart. (D) S_4 is an abnormal heart sound that occurs at the end of diastole just before S_1. It is caused by the atria contracting and forcing blood into a noncompliant ventricle.

578. **(D)** Nursing process phase: assessment; client need: safe, effective care environment; content area: medical/surgical nursing

Rationale
(A & B) This is not the correct way to assess the gag reflex. (C) This would be one method of looking at a client's throat, but you would have them say "ah" and not cough. (D) This is correct. This action of placing the tongue blade on the posterior aspect of the tongue elicits the gag reflex.

579. **(B)** Nursing process phase: assessment; client need: safe, effective care environment; content area: medical/surgical nursing

Rationale
(A) If the nurse suspected muscle or skeletal damage, the nurse would not test the reflexes. This would cause pain and perhaps further damage to the client. (B) This is correct. Reflex assessment helps evaluate whether specific cervical, thoracic, lumbar, and sacral spinal segments are intact. (C) Cranial nerve reflexes are tested on the eyes, mouth, tongue, and neck of the client. They are not tested on the extremities. (D) If the nurse suspected any tendon or ligament damage, the nurse would not test for reflexes. This could cause the client pain and perhaps cause further damage to the area affected.

580. **(C)** Nursing process phase: analysis; client need: physiological integrity; content area: medical/surgical nursing

Rationale
(A) Long-term steroid use cannot lead to hypoglycemia in this client. There is another condition that can affect this client's nutritional status. (B) Long-term steroid use can lead to hypokalemia, not hyperkalemia, because of fluid retention and electrolyte imbalances. (C) This is correct. Steroids can produce adverse changes in a client's nutritional status, causing calcium depletion. Long-term hypocalcemia can lead to osteoporosis. (D) Steroid use can cause hypernatremia, or sodium retention, not hyponatremia.

581. **(C)** Nursing process phase: analysis; client need: physiological integrity; content area: medical/surgical nursing

Rationale
(A) The client taking diuretics would not be at risk for folic acid deficiency. The client taking diuretics can have fluid and electrolyte imbalances. (B) The client taking antihyperten-

sives would not be at risk for folic acid deficiency. The client on hypertensive medication can have calcium, selenium, and essential amino acid deficiencies. (C) This is correct. Oral contraceptive use can increase the need for folic acid in the diet of women. The oral contraceptive seems to affect the body's ability to absorb folic acid from the diet. Oral contraceptives also deplete the body of vitamins C, D, E, and other B complex vitamins. (D) A client taking MAO inhibitors would not be at risk for folic acid deficiency. MAO inhibitors may cause vitamin C deficiencies.

582. (B) Nursing process phase: analysis; client need: safe, effective care environment; content area: medical/surgical nursing

Rationale

(A) The client with chronic alcoholism can have a vitamin deficiency caused by chronic malnutrition, which is common with this disorder. Antioxidant deficiency (A,C,E) could be seen in advanced stages of malnutrition; however, there is a more appropriate answer for this situation. (B) This is correct. Alcoholics are usually deficient in most B complex vitamins, especially B_1. These vitamins are water-soluble and not stored in the body, and deficiencies can occur quickly. (C) Vitamin E is an antioxidant and a fat-soluble vitamin. The body can store certain levels of this vitamin to prevent deficiency. As long as there is an adequate diet to constantly replenish stores, deficiency is rare. (D) Calcium deficiencies are not usually seen in young chronic alcoholics. This tendency changes with the age.

583. (B) Nursing process phase: analysis; client need: safe, effective care environment; content area: medical/surgical nursing

Rationale

(A) Hemoglobin aids in diagnosing a client with anemia and would not assess the client's nutritional status as well as another test option given. (B) This is correct. A negative nitrogen balance results from inadequate protein intake and can be detected by a total protein test. (C) Glucose aids in the diagnosis of diabetes mellitus and would not assess the client's nutritional status related to her negative nitrogen balance. (D) Triglycerides determine the client's risk for coronary artery disease (CAD) and do not assess the client's nutritional status.

584. (C) Nursing process phase: implementation; client need: health promotion and maintenance; content area: medical/surgical nursing

Rationale

(A) The client should be encouraged to provide adequate rest and to avoid stress until the body has replenished the lost iron to the system. The immune system can be compromised by iron deficiency anemia. Activity can lead to shortness of breath and palpitations. The client should be encouraged to return to activities slowly. (B) The client cannot take in enough iron through a balanced diet to treat iron-deficient anemia. Supplementation is required. An average-sized adult would have to eat 10 lb of steak a day to receive therapeutic amounts of iron. (C) This is correct. The nurse must encourage the client to continue with all supplementation therapy until the physician tells the client to stop. (D) It can take up to 6 months, not 6 weeks, for the body to replace lost iron stores in cases of severe anemia.

585. (C) Nursing process phase: analysis; client need: safe,

effective care environment; content area: medical/surgical nursing

Rationale

(A) HDLs are associated with decreased risk of CAD. These HDLs may help remove excess cholesterol from the arteries. (B) There are no such lipoproteins as moderate-density lipoproteins. (C) This is correct. LDLs are associated with having a higher incidence of CAD. LDLs help cause build-up of cholesterol in the arteries. (D) There are two types of lipoproteins, high-density and low-density.

586. (C) Nursing process phase: implementation; client need: safe effective care environment; content area: medical/surgical nursing

Rationale

(A) Enteric-coated capsules and tablets are made to protect the lining of the stomach from aggravation by the drug. Enteric pills should never be crushed, and if the medication arrives with this type of coating, the nurse should call the pharmacy to try to get a liquid form of the medication for administration down the feeding tube. (B) Time-released compounds should never be crushed to place down a feeding tube. The pills are made to be released slowly into the system, and crushing the medication will negate this effect. A liquid form of the medication should be requested if a time-release form of the medication arrives from pharmacy. (C) This is correct. These are the only type of pill medication that should be crushed for administration into a feeding tube. (D) Sublingual medication, such as nitroglycerin, is meant to be placed under the tongue for slow absorption. This type of medication is not to be crushed and placed into a feeding tube.

587. (C) Nursing process phase: assessment; client need: physiological integrity; content area: medical/surgical nursing

Rationale

(A) A deficiency in vitamin C is called scurvy and is characterized by a breakdown of collagen. Loss of appetite, growth cessation, tenderness to touch, weakness, and gum bleeding all are symptoms of this condition. (B) Vitamin D deficiency is called rickets in children and osteomalacia in adults. It is characterized by bending of the spine and "bowing" of the legs. (C) This is correct. Vitamin A deficiency initially presents in early stages with night blindness. Later symptoms can include keratinization and xerosis (drying) of the eye, eventually leading to blindness. (D) Vitamin E deficiency is rare. However, erythrocyte hemolysis is seen in premature babies when the vitamin is not transferred by the mother to the infant. The baby's red blood cells rupture causing severe anemia.

588. (B) Nursing process phase: implementation; client need: physiological integrity; content area: medical/surgical nursing

Rationale

(A) Clintron beds are not to be packed with pillows or blankets. This keeps the bed from circulating air between the bed and the client's skin. This can also promote sweating by the client, which can aggravate the skin and cause breakdown. (B) This is correct. The client is anemic and frail. A depressed immune system compounded by malnourishment can increase the client's susceptibility to breakdown. Increasing calorie intake and providing protein can help the client fight infection and prevent further breakdown. (C) Monitoring the client for infection and further skin breakdown is important and can be reflected in these laboratory values. However, this is not an intervention that will help prevent further breakdown. (D) You would administer skin-care products ordered by the physician. However, you would not place adult briefs on the client. These would maintain moisture close to the skin and promote breakdown.

589. **(C)** Nursing process phase: implementation; client need: physiological integrity; content area: medical/surgical nursing

Rationale
(A) This situation does not warrant limiting family visits. Support from family may actually decrease anxiety for the client. (B) This is giving false reassurance. (C) Physical and emotional rest to decrease the workload of the heart is the major priority in this situation. (D) Frequent x-ray studies are not indicated for this client.

590. **(C)** Nursing process phase: analysis; client need: safe, effective care environment; content area: medical/surgical nursing

Rationale
(A) The elderly have decreased peristalsis and decreased enzyme production. (B) The elderly have decreased peristalsis, which does increase the time needed to absorb nutrients. The elderly, however, have decreased saliva production, not increased. (C) This is correct. Because of tooth loss and the use of dentures, the elderly are at higher risk for malnutrition. Ill-fitting dentures can cause pain, and elderly with this problem often suffer from some form of malnutrition. (D) The elderly have decreased sensitivity to sweet and salty food because of a reduction in taste buds and decreased saliva production.

591. **(B)** Nursing process phase: assessment; client need: physiological integrity; content area: medical/surgical nursing

Rationale
(A) Respiratory infections are the second most common cause of infections, and pneumonia is one of the leading causes of death in the frail elderly (over 85). (B) This is correct. The most common infection found in the elderly is urinary tract infections. It is sometimes difficult to diagnose with this age group because it can present with only signs of confusion and vital signs within normal limits. The nurse working with this age group has to be aware of her client's status and watch for changes in mental status, usually the first indicator of infection. (C) Skin infections are caused by the elderly client's reduced immune system. Breakdown and infection of broken skin are not the most common forms of infection in this age group; however, they are a problem. (D) This infection would not be a concern for this client. Prostate infections are not as common as the other forms of infection listed.

592. **(C)** Nursing process phase: assessment; client need: safe, effective care environment; content area: medical/surgical nursing

Rationale
(A) Abdominal cramping, nausea, and diarrhea could be a sign of any of a number of abdominal problems. These could be signs and symptoms of right-sided colon cancer. There are more obvious signs associated with this disorder. (B) The client with ribbon-looking stool and abdominal pain could be suffering from left-sided colon cancer. (C) This is correct.

The client with rectal cancer would have rectal bleeding, a mucouslike discharge, and persistent rectal spasms. (D) The client with alternating constipation and diarrhea could be suffering from left-sided colon cancer. Rectal bleeding could also be associated with this disorder.

593. **(C)** Nursing process phase: implementation; client need: safe, effective care environment; content area: medical/surgical nursing

Rationale
(A) The client with severe hemorrhoids needs comfort-care measures to reduce irritation to the rectal mucosa. A high-fiber diet would produce frequent bowel movements and would produce firm stools that would cause the client pain. (B) The client with severe hemorrhoids needs frequent fluids to prevent constipation and aggravation to the rectal mucosa. (C) This is correct. A client with severe hemorrhoids would require a soft diet to promote soft-formed stools and decrease the risk of aggravation to the rectal mucosa and pain for the client. (D) A high-protein diet would increase the client's risk of constipation, especially if given in conjunction with decreased fluid intake.

594. **(A)** Nursing process phase: assessment; client need: physiological integrity; content area: medical/surgical nursing

Rationale
(A) This is correct. The female abdominal muscles weaken because of gravity and increased childbirth. There is decreased urethral resistance because of the weakening of the pubococcygeus muscle. (B) A chronically full bladder would not be prone to stress incontinence unless the pelvic floor or pubococcygeus muscle were in a weakened condition. (C) Poor perfusion to the kidneys would affect the type and amount of urine produced. It would not affect the way the urine is expelled. (D) Chronic urinary tract infections would not increase a client's risk of stress incontinence.

595. **(B)** Nursing process phase: implementation; client need: safe, effective care environment; content area: medical/surgical nursing

Rationale
(A) The Kegel exercises would be taught to the client with stress incontinence to increase the strength of the pelvic floor muscles. (B) This is correct. Urge incontinence is when the client has an immediate urge to void with immediate urine loss. The client would need to practice scheduled voiding trials. This would include having the client void every 2 hours and gradually increasing the time between voiding to increase bladder capacity. (C & D) This maneuver would be performed with clients with stress incontinence—not urge incontinence.

596. **(A)** Nursing process phase: assessment; client need: safe, effective care environment; content area: medical/surgical nursing

Rationale
(A) This is correct. The client is suffering from dehydration metabolic imbalances, which can lead to confusion, dizziness, and other conditions, which can increase the client's risk for falls. (B) Peptic ulcer disease does not increase the client's risk of falls. (C) The use of NSAIDs does not increase the client's risk for falls, unless the use of these medications is associated with increased GI bleeding. This could lead to possi-

ble confusion and fatigue from blood loss. (D) The client with chronic gout would not be at increased risk for falls unless the gout had flared up, causing the client pain in an extremity and decreased movement of that extremity.

597. **(D)** Nursing process phase: implementation; client need: health promotion and maintenance; content area: medical/surgical nursing

Rationale

(A) All of these foods are high in purines, which the client with chronic gout should avoid. (B) The client should be instructed to rest the extremity affected during periods of increased pain and stiffness. Increasing mobility to the joint will cause undue stress and pain to the client. (C) The client should be instructed to avoid all alcohol in the diet. Alcohol can increase the side effects of medication and can aggravate his condition. (D) This is correct. Purines seem to aggravate gout, so the client would avoid all foods high in purines, such as shellfish, organ meats, and preserved fish (anchovies).

598. **(D)** Nursing process phase: analysis; client need: safe, effective care environment; content area: medical/surgical nursing

Rationale

(A) A pleural effusion can result from fluid build-up in the pleural spaces. A pneumonectomy can lead to congestive heart failure, not a pleural effusion. (B) Hypoglycemia, or low blood sugar, cannot develop as the result of a pneumonectomy. (C) A hemothorax is blood entering the pleural cavity as a result of chest trauma. In a pneumonectomy, the lung has been removed. (D) This is correct. Congestive heart failure (CHF) can develop from a pneumonectomy caused by the fact that the client has lost 50 percent of the functional lung surface. This increases the workload of the other lung and can cause fluid accumulation around the heart.

599. **(C)** Nursing process phase: assessment: client need: physiological integrity; content area: medical/surgical nursing

Rationale

(A) Adrenal hypofunction is Addison's disease, which does not present with these signs and symptoms. (B) Hypopituitary disease produces infantile facial features and is associated with dwarfism as the result of inadequate human growth hormone. (C) This is correct. Acromegaly is excessive secretion of growth hormone after normal completion of body growth. It produces the signs and symptoms seen with this client. (D) Hyperthyroidism does not produce these symptoms.

FOCUS ON GERONTOLOGICAL NURSING

600. **(A)** Nursing process phase: analysis; client need: health promotion and maintenance; content area: medical/surgical—gerontological nursing

Rationale

(A) Immobilization or even a relatively sedentary existence favors stasis of blood in the veins and predisposes the elderly client to thrombosis. (B) Although prolonged bedrest does increase the chance of developing decubitus ulcers, this is not the rationale for early ambulation following a hip replacement. (C) There is no evidence to support the statement that late ambulation fosters dependence. (D) Although this is a nursing goal, there is no assurance that early ambulation will return the client to baseline functional status.

601. **(C)** Nursing process phase: implementation; client need: physiological integrity; content area: medical/surgical—gerontological nursing

Rationale

(A) Hip precaution teaching includes instructions to maintain the hip in a position of abduction and neutral rotation. Sitting with the hips at a 90-degree or greater angle is necessary to maintain the hips in this position. (B) Although use of correct body mechanics is usually a proper instruction to clients, arthroplasty clients should not bend forward more than 90 degrees. (C) Use of a long shoe horn will assist the client to continue to do activities of daily living such as putting on shoes and prevent the necessity of bending forward greater than 90 degrees. (D) Use of pillows between the legs while in bed will assist in maintaining abduction to the hips.

602. **(D)** Nursing process phase: implementation; client need: safe, effective care environment; content area: medical/surgical—gerontological nursing

Rationale

(A & C) All four legs of the walker should be on the floor before the feet are moved up to the walker. (B) The walker is moved up only 6 inches in front of the body as the feet are moved up to the walker. (D) The walker is moved up 6 inches in front before moving both feet to the front of the walker. The walker must always rest on all four legs.

603. **(A)** Nursing process phase: implementation; client need: health promotion and maintenance; content area: medical/surgical—gerontological nursing

Rationale

(A) Exercise increases the body's need for oxygen and requires the cardiovascular and respiratory systems to increase the workload to meet this demand. Because of the rigidity of the vessels and the loss of elasticity, the older adult requires a longer amount of time to regain homeostasis. (B–D) Normal aging changes in the cardiovascular and respiratory systems require a longer period of time to regain hemostasis. Because the client has no other symptoms associated with increased blood pressure, these choices are not the most appropriate.

604. **(B)** Nursing process phase: analysis; client need: safe, effective care environment; content area: medical/surgical—gerontological nursing

Rationale

(A) Confusion is not a normal aging change. (B) Drugs prescribed by physicians or purchased over the counter are among the most common causes of confusional states in the older adult. Arthroplasty clients should receive narcotic analgesics during the first 48 hours postoperatively on a regular basis. (C) Although clients with dementia do have confusion, confusion is most likely reversible in this situation and does not indicate early signs of dementia. (D) Separation from familiar environment is a possible cause, but because the client has been hospitalized for at least 4 days in this situation, it is less likely than drug therapy.

605. (B) Nursing process phase: planning; client need: physiological integrity; content area: medical/surgical—gerontological nursing

Rationale

(A) Pain is not of primary concern at this time because the client is several days' postoperative and pain should be diminishing. (B) The skin is the first line of defense in the prevention of infection. The defense is broken due to an opening from the operative site and provides a medium for the entry of bacteria. Infection is a primary concern because this could be dangerous to the client. (C) A supportive environment is an important component of care, but the matter is not life threatening. (D) Explanation of procedures is an important component of care, but the matter is not life threatening.

606. (D) Nursing process phase: implementation; client need: health promotion and maintenance; content area: medical/surgical—gerontological nursing

Rationale

(A) The ability to take medications as prescribed is an important assessment item, but is not as important in terms of safety and prevention of injury in ambulating. (B) The ability to manage activities of daily living is an important assessment item, but is not as important in terms of safety and prevention of injury in ambulating. (C) Support from family and friends is an important assessment item, but is not as important in terms of safety and prevention of injury in ambulating. (D) Prosthetic implants require strict adherence to partial weight bearing for at least 2 months. The older adult usually begins with a walker to achieve the partial weight bearing and then progresses to a cane. Weight bearing can cause injury to the joint and require hospitalization to repair.

607. (A) Nursing process phase: analysis; client need: health promotion and maintenance; content area: medical/surgical—gerontological nursing

Rationale

(A) Diet plans for the elderly should focus on increasing vitamins and minerals and decreasing caloric intake. Broiled pork chop is high in the B vitamins and reduces the fat through the broiling process. Cantaloupe is higher in vitamin C than orange slices or strawberries. (B) Ham is high in sodium and both spinach and banana are lower in vitamins and minerals, particularly vitamins B and C, that the older adult requires. (C) Liver as a menu choice may not be the best selection because many people do not like the taste of liver and unless prepared properly it may be difficult for an older adult to chew. Both carrots and orange slices are lower in vitamins B and C, which the older adult requires (D) Fried foods are not recommended for older adults because these increase calories and fats.

608. (A) Nursing process phase: analysis; client need: health promotion and maintenance; content area: medical/surgical—gerontological nursing

Rationale

(A) With diagnosis-related groups and shorter hospital stays, older clients may need to have continued rehabilitation therapy and may require a brief stay in a long-term care unit that provides these services. (B) Older clients having arthroplasty surgery may need assistance with some activities of daily living, but there is no evidence to support dependence upon family following joint replacement surgery. (C) Arthroplasty surgery clients may need assistance to maintain some activities of daily

living, but this assistance can be given by home health nurses or family and does not require long-term care. (D) With proper preoperative and postoperative instructions, the client should be able to resume activities as tolerated upon discharge.

609. (A) Nursing process phase: analysis; client need: health promotion and maintenance; content area: medical/surgical—gerontological nursing

Rationale

(A) Changes in both the lens and vitreous result in increased scattering of light in the ocular media, especially at night or in low levels of illumination. Thus, it is not unusual for the older adult to complain of the glare of oncoming headlights while driving at night. (B) Halos around lights may represent adverse effects from medications such as digitalis preparations. (C) The yellowing of the lens seen in aging results in difficulty identifying cool colors such as blue, green, and violet. (D) Floaters are normal and harmless but may be a sign of a more serious condition. Tear production decreases, not increases, with age.

610. (D) Nursing process phase: assessment; client need: health promotion and maintenance; content area: medical/surgical—gerontological nursing

Rationale

(A) Family history of glaucoma is important prior to diagnosis, not after diagnosis. (B) Assessment of coping skills is important because vision loss may be an outcome of glaucoma. However, coping skills are not the primary concern for this client initially and may need to be assessed over time. (C) An environmental assessment is important to visually impaired older adults, but is not the initial concern for this client and may be ongoing. (D) Glaucoma requires lifelong medical treatment with medication that must be instilled into the eye. Assessment of fine motor skills and hand-eye coordination is necessary because these may be beyond the manual dexterity of some older adults.

611. (C) Nursing process phase: planning; client need: health promotion and maintenance; content area: medical/surgical—gerontological nursing

Rationale

(A) There is no information given that indicates the client is unable to prepare food. (B) Sensory perceptual alteration is an appropriate nursing diagnosis for a client with glaucoma. Glaucoma, however, results in decreased peripheral vision, not an increase. (C) Clients with glaucoma will be on lifelong medications that must be instilled into the eye daily. For this reason, a nursing diagnosis of potential eye infection related to eye drop instillation must be a priority in planning care. (D) Body image is important, but a sight-threatening infection is a priority.

612. (D) Nursing process phase: analysis; client need: safe, effective care environment; content area: medical/surgical—gerontological nursing

Rationale

(A) A protein-rich snack before bedtime would be filling, but the fullness might interfere with sleep. (B) There is no evidence at this time that a comprehensive physical examination is warranted, and, unless the client verbalizes additional complaints, it should not be done. (C) Milk is an effective sedative source at bedtime; however, sleeping pills are not recommended for the elderly. (D) Sleep problems are common in older adults, who report spending increased time in bed not sleeping, frequent nocturnal arousals, shortened nocturnal sleep time, and prolonged time falling asleep.

613. **(D)** Nursing process phase: planning; client need: safe, effective care environment; content area: medical/surgical—gerontological nursing

Rationale
(A) Drugs given more frequently would result in a greater amount of the medication to the client. Greater amounts of medication place the client at high risk for toxicity because of the decreased renal function that is a normal aging change. (B) Administering medications more frequently places the client at high risk for toxicity because of the decreased renal function that is a normal aging change. (C) Medications, when administered properly and individualized to client needs, are seldom harmful. (D) In clinical practice, the doses of many drugs that are excreted primarily by the kidneys are routinely adjusted for older adults to compensate for alteration in renal function.

614. **(A)** Nursing process phase: implementation; client need: psychosocial integrity; content area: medical/surgical—gerontological nursing

Rationale
(A) Knowledge that one is about to lose a limb, no matter what age, is anxiety producing. Spending time with the client and allowing him to verbalize feelings is important to decrease anxiety and to increase coping and acceptance. (B) Allowing the client to interact with persons who have similar conditions may be helpful during rehabilitation; however, it minimizes the feelings of the client and decreases verbalization initially. (C) Although the family should be included in the plan of care for this client, this action by the nurse initially negates nursing responsibility and may potentially decrease successful coping that can be explored. (D) Explanation of the surgical procedure is an important nursing action, but is not the primary concern for the client initially. This action does little to assist the client in resolving emotional issues.

615. **(D)** Nursing process phase: implementation; client need: health promotion and maintenance; content area: medical/surgical—gerontological nursing

Rationale
(A) Stump wrapping is continued until the client is fitted with a prosthesis. (B) Protective cushioning prevents the stump from becoming hard and firmly shaped and is contraindicated. (C) Phantom pain should be discussed prior to surgery because the sensation usually occurs early on and disappears over a period of weeks or months. (D) Before a prosthesis is prescribed, the client's general strength must be improved through general conditioning and resistive exercises.

616. **(B)** Nursing process phase: assessment; client need: physiological integrity; content area: medical/surgical—gerontological nursing

Rationale
(A) Although assessment of the ability to use unaffected extremities is important, passive therapy can be given to strengthen unaffected extremities if the client is unable to do so initially. (B) For rehabilitation to be effective for an older adult, active participation is necessary. If a client is unable to follow directions, active participation is not possible. (C) Al-

though assessment of support systems may enhance rehabilitation in an older adult, it is not necessary for rehabilitation to be effective. (D) Clients may benefit from rehabilitation even if not returning to the community or home setting. Often, long-term care is necessary for rehabilitation to continue.

617. **(D)** Nursing process phase: implementation; client need: psychosocial integrity; content area: medical/surgical—gerontological nursing

Rationale
(A) Talking with the client about past experiences, unless therapeutic communication is utilized, does little to help increase the psychological adjustment to the loss of a limb. (B) Delaying the use of a prosthesis until phantom pain is diminished or disappears hampers the rehabilitation of the client and may promote phantom sensations. (C) The liberal use of analgesics is usually not helpful in phantom pain and may impair rehabilitation due to side effects, confusion, or sedation. (D) Increased stimuli to the stump area relieves phantom pain. Wearing the prosthesis provides stimulation and decreases pain.

618. **(C)** Nursing process phase: evaluation; client need: physiological integrity; content area: medical/surgical—gerontological nursing

Rationale
(A) Walking with crutches would consume more energy because the client would have to manipulate the crutches and his body. (B) Walking with a walker requires energy to pick up the appliance and to move it forward. Both feet must be brought forward, requiring more energy consumption. (C) Encouraging walking with the prosthesis more frequently for shorter periods of time will require less energy and will allow the client to increase endurance. (D) Strict bedrest is not warranted in this situation and would actually interfere with rehabilitation and return to homeostasis.

619. **(B)** Nursing process phase: analysis; client need: health promotion and maintenance; content area: medical/surgical—gerontological nursing

Rationale
(A) This statement is a generalization and is stereotypical. This statement does not provide nursing action based on knowledge. (B) Through careful meal planning, older adults who are diabetic may occasionally have sweets or alcoholic beverages. A reasonable, collaborative approach in diabetic teaching is much more likely to result in compliance than rigid control. (C) The goal of insulin therapy is to maintain blood glucose levels within normal parameters, but often a great deal of adjustment is required to achieve a balance. (D) Many clinicians allow more flexibility in blood sugar levels and allow them to rise above normal to determine that the client is not at risk for hypoglycemia, not hyperglycemia.

620. **(C)** Nursing process phase: assessment; client need: psychosocial integrity; content area: medical/surgical—gerontological nursing

Rationale
(A) Listening to the client is therapeutic, but should follow data collection that is to assist in finding the cause. (B) Impotence is related to physiological or psychological causes and is not a normal aging change. (C) A sexual history, with emphasis on current sexual function, should be part of the general medical evaluation of an older person. When a problem

exists, evaluation of drugs being taken, psychological testing, and surgery may be necessary. (D) Although the nurse might refer the client to the physician, this would not be done until the nurse has completed assessment data to identify the problem. These data will guide the nurse and client to mutually seek the most effective solution.

621. **(B)** Nursing process phase: assessment; client need: safe, effective care environment; content area: medical/ surgical—gerontological nursing

Rationale
(A) Constipation is a common experience of older adults, but this question refers to the technique of doing physical examination of the gastrointestinal system. The technique used by the nurse is inappropriate. (B) Because of the bowel activity that can be initiated by the use of palpation, the correct assessment technique sequence in the gastrointestinal examination includes: inspection, auscultation, and percussion, following lastly by palpation. (C & D) The question refers to the technique used by the nurse in performing physical examination of the gastrointestinal system. The technique used by the nurse is inappropriate.

622. **(A)** Nursing process phase: implementation; client need: physiological integrity; content area: medical/ surgical—gerontological nursing

Rationale
(A) Acute intestinal obstruction is characterized by rapid onset of abdominal cramping, vomiting, and distention. Cramps are associated with high-pitched bowel sounds due to peristalsis. (B) Diffuse pain and low-grade temperature are symptoms of appendicitis. (C) Hyperactivity is associated with bowel sounds and is not present in the absence of bowel sounds. (D) Nausea and marked abdominal tenderness are symptoms of cholecystitis.

623. **(B)** Nursing process phase: analysis; client need: safe, effective care environment; content area: medical/surgical—gerontological nursing

Rationale
(A) Incontinence is caused by neurological or muscular impairments and is not a normal aging change. (B) Functional incontinence is observed in clients with normal bladder and urethral function. Too often, the diagnosis of functional incontinence is made inappropriately when the real problem is due to the client's restricted mobility and failure to get to the bathroom in time. (C) Stress incontinence is the involuntary loss of urine during physical exertion. (D) There is no evidence to suggest that there is pressure causing the incontinence.

624. **(B)** Nursing process phase: implementation; client need: safe, effective care environment; content area: medical/surgical—gerontological nursing

Rationale
(A) Absorbent pads do assist in keeping the client dry, but are demoralizing to the client who has cognitive awareness and should not be used unless other approaches prove unsatisfactory. (B) Because the client is only incontinent at night, the use of toilet supplements such as bedside commode, urinal, or bedpan can assist in remaining continence. The use of a night light also assists the client to orient himself to a new environment more quickly and reduce the chance of accidents. (C) Stress is not known to cause incontinence at night. (D) A Fo-

ley catheter allows for the introduction of bacteria and predisposes the client to urinary tract infection.

625. **(C)** Nursing process phase: implementation; client need: safe, effective care environment; content area: medical/surgical—gerontological nursing

Rationale
(A & C) Gentamicin is excreted by the kidneys. For men, normal creatinine clearance ranges from 85 to 125 ml/minute; values of 70 ml/minute indicate decreased renal function. Continuing to give the gentamicin could result in accumulation and untoward pharamacological effects. (B) Normal creatinine clearance ranges from 85 to 125 ml/minute; values of 70 ml/minute indicate decreased renal function. (D) Calling the laboratory to see if this is in error is not an appropriate answer in terms of safety in medication administration.

626. **(C)** Nursing process phase: analysis; client need: physiological integrity; content area: medical/surgical—gerontological nursing

Rationale
(A) Creatinine clearance is not an indicator of respiratory function. (B) Creatinine clearance is not an indicator of cardiovascular function. (C) An excellent diagnostic indicator of renal function, the creatinine clearance test determines how efficiently the kidneys are clearing creatinine from the blood. (D) Creatinine clearance is not an indicator of gastrointestinal function.

627. **(B)** Nursing process phase: assessment; client need: safe, effective care environment; content area: medical/surgical—gerontological nursing

Rationale
(A) Talking louder may increase the pitch of the voice; normal hearing changes affect the hearing of high-pitched noise. (B) Accumulation of cerumen may be rock hard and cause the client to complain of hearing loss and a feeling of fullness in the ear. Obstruction of the external canal is obvious on examination. (C) To sit facing the client so she can lip-read is an appropriate nursing action, but because the client is having more difficulty hearing than normal since admission, finding the cause is most important. (D) There is no need to have an audiology exam until a thorough assessment is complete.

628 **(A)** Nursing process phase: implementation; client need: safe, effective care environment; content area: medical/surgical—gerontological nursing

Rationale
(A) Tegretol is slowly and incompletely absorbed from the gastrointestinal tract. Therapeutic serum levels are between 4 and 12 µg/ml. This is within the therapeutic level and the medication should be given as prescribed. (B) Therapeutic serum levels are between 4 and 12 µg/ml. This is within the therapeutic level and there is no reason to call the physician. (C & D) Therapeutic serum levels are between 4 and 12 µg/ml. This is within the therapeutic level and the medication should be given as prescribed.

629. **(B)** Nursing process phase: planning; client need: safe, effective care environment; content area: medical/surgical—gerontological nursing

Rationale
(A) Cerebrovascular accident clients do have dramatic mood

swings; however, safety is the most important need for the client at this time. (B) Clients with left hemisphere infarctions tend to have poor judgment and to overestimate physical abilities. In addition, they react quickly and impulsively and are at high risk for injury. Because there is the potential for injury, this is a safety need and thus is a priority plan. (C) Cerebrovascular accident clients do have labile affect; however, safety is the most important need for the client at this time. (D) Aggression would be individualized and is not necessarily a problem with cerebrovascular accident clients.

630. **(C)** Nursing process phase: planning; client need: safe, effective care environment; content area: medical/surgical—gerontological nursing

Rationale

(A) Although it is important to maintain nutritional status, impaired judgment makes safety the most important need for the client with left hemisphere infarction. (B) Although diversional activity is important, safety is the most important need for the left hemisphere infarction client. (C) Clients with left hemisphere infarctions have poor judgment, overestimate physical abilities, and react quickly and impulsively. These behaviors make them a high risk for injury. (D) Although psychological counseling may be part of the treatment plan for the client, impaired judgment makes safety the most important need.

631. **(D)** Nursing process phase: planning; client need: physiological integrity; content area: medical/surgical—gerontological nursing

Rationale

(A) Making decisions about care is important to emotional health, but does not demonstrate knowledge specific to care of the cerebrovascular accident client. (B) The use of clock and calendar for orientation purposes is important, but there is no evidence that the client is experiencing disorientation. (C) Attending unit functions is important in social isolation diagnosis, but there is no evidence to suggest that the client is socially isolated. (D) Both left and right hemiplegic clients cope better in a structured, consistent environment.

632. **(A)** Nursing process phase: implementation; client need: psychosocial integrity; content area: medical/surgical—gerontological nursing

Rationale

(A) Depression, characterized by apathy and withdrawal, is common following cerebrovascular accidents. (B) Apathy and withdrawal are common following CVA, but with effective nursing intervention it is possible to restore psychological integrity. (C) Asking the family to make her attend therapy would not help the client and might further lower self-esteem. (D) Calling the physician for assistance in this problem does not allow the nurse to be creative in dealing with a challenge and is not appropriate. A team conference would be a more appropriate solution.

633. **(B)** Nursing process phase: evaluation; client need: psychosocial integrity; content area: medical/surgical—gerontological nursing

Rationale

(A) This response casts doubt on the ability of the family to function and places feelings of burden on the loved one. (B) This response indicates acceptance of the change in the loved one and changing the environment so that she can function more easily within the home. (C) This response may be supportive but shows no indication of family interaction. (D) This response may indicate unrealistic expectations that may not be reachable.

634. **(D)** Nursing process phase: assessment; client need: physiological integrity; content area: medical/surgical—gerontological nursing

Rationale

(A) Brown pigmentation is not a characteristic symptom of earlier elder abuse. (B) Brown pigmentation is not a characteristic skin change in normal aging. (C) Brown pigmentation around the eyes and nose, not the ankles, is characteristic of lymphatic disease. (D) Chronic venous insufficiency is common in the elderly and is evidenced by distended tortuous veins, hair loss, brown pigmentation around the ankles, cool skin, and pedal edema that worsens during the day.

635. **(B)** Nursing process phase: implementation; client need: psychosocial integrity; content area: medical/surgical—gerontological nursing

Rationale

(A) Leaving the room is only appropriate when the anxiety level is escalating quickly and allows the client to regain control. (B) The nurse should use a calm voice to aid in decreasing the anxiety level while encouraging verbalization of feelings. The nurse should try to identify the cause of the anxiety and to find measures to help the client cope more effectively with the anxiety. (C) Telling him there is nothing to worry about is false assurance, which is nontherapeutic. (D) Telling the client that the doctor knows best does little to assist in managing the anxiety or finding its source.

636. **(D)** Nursing process phase: assessment; client need: physiological integrity; content area: medical/surgical—gerontological nursing

Rationale

(A) Tachypnea is a symptom of left-sided congestive failure. (B) Pink frothy sputum indicates pulmonary edema. (C) Korotkoff's sounds is a symptom of left-sided congestive failure. (D) Symptoms of right-sided congestive heart failure include orthostatic hypotension, edema, distended jugular veins, liver enlargement, and S_3 gallop.

637. **(C)** Nursing process phase: analysis; client need: safe, effective care environment; content area: medical/surgical—gerontological nursing

Rationale

(A) Holding onto the wall may indicate dizziness, which is not a sign of digoxin toxicity in older adults. (B) Ringing of the ears is usually a result of aspirin toxicity, not digoxin. (C) The clinical manifestations of digitalis toxicity are different in the elderly. Gastrointestinal disturbances, disorientation, agitation, hallucinations, color vision changes such as halos around lights, and changes in behavior are frequently seen. (D) Itching can be an adverse reaction to a medication, but is not a symptom of digoxin toxicity.

638. **(D)** Nursing process phase: implementation; client need: physiological integrity; content area: medical/surgical—gerontological nursing

Rationale

(A) Normal serum digoxin level is 0.5 to 2.0 mg/ml. Giving an additional dose of digoxin is not a nursing decision and the client could quickly become digoxin toxic. (B) The value given is above the normal serum digoxin level of 0.5 to 2.0 mg/ml. (C) The value given is above the normal serum digoxin level of 0.5 to 2.0 mg/ml. Giving one-half the dose of digoxin is not a nursing decision and the client could quickly become digoxin toxic. (D) The value given is above the normal serum digoxin level of 0.5 to 2.0 mg/ml. Hypokalemia further disposes the client to digoxin toxicity and the physician should be notified.

639. (A) Nursing process phase: planning; client need: health promotion and maintenance; content area: medical/surgical—gerontological nursing

Rationale
(A–C) Chicken is higher in potassium than beef products. The baked potato and figs are both higher in potassium than any of the other menu selections. (D) Fried foods are not appropriate for the cardiovascular client.

640. (A) Nursing process phase: analysis; client need: physiological integrity; content area: medical/surgical—gerontological nursing

Rationale
(A) Weakness, muscle fatigue, decreased muscle tone, and weak irregular pulse are early symptoms of hypokalemia. (B) Diminished deep tendon reflexes indicate hypermagnesemia. (C) A positive Trousseau's sign is a symptom of hypocalcemia. (D) A positive Chvostek's sign is a symptom of hypocalcemia.

641. (B) Nursing process phase: implementation; client need: physiological integrity; content area: medical/surgical—gerontological nursing

Rationale
(A) Monitoring respiratory rate is important but is not critical in providing care to the client. (B) Monitoring urinary output is critical when administering intravenous potassium because diminished urine flow can rapidly lead to hyperkalemia. (C) Monitoring oral potassium intake is important but is not critical at this time. (D) Monitoring the intravenous site for edema is important but is not critical at this time.

642. (B) Nursing process phase: assessment; client need: health promotion and maintenance; content area: medical/surgical—gerontological nursing

Rationale
(A) Attitude toward illness is important for the nurse to be aware of but is not a key ingredient in the teaching process. (B) Because the nurse has prepared written information regarding his medication, these instructions should be reflective of the client's educational level. (C) Past compliance with medical regimen is important information but may be due to numerous causes. Past compliance is not a key ingredient to the teaching plan, but will require follow-up. (D) The client's usual activities of daily living are not important in looking at medications ordered as a daily dose. Daily dose schedule allows flexibility in administration.

643. (A) Nursing process phase: evaluation; client need: health promotion and maintenance; content area: medical/surgical—gerontological nursing

Rationale
(A) Potassium chloride (K-Dur) should not be taken on an empty stomach because of its potential for gastric irritation. (B) Headache may be important to monitor but is not associated with the discharge medications ordered for the client. (C) Cholesterol may be important to monitor but is not associated with the discharge medications ordered for the client. (D) Bumetanide (Bumex) is a rapid-acting diuretic and should be taken during awakening hours.

644. (C) Nursing process phase: analysis; client need: physiological integrity; content area: medical/surgical—gerontological nursing

Rationale
(A) Headaches are not a normal occurrence but are not indicative of adverse reactions to K-Dur. (B) Impairment in cognition is not a normal occurrence but is not indicative of adverse reactions to K-Dur. (C) Tarry stools may indicate gastrointestinal bleeding from gastric irritation and an adverse reaction to K-Dur. (D) Difficulty seeing things close up (presbyopia) is a normal aging change.

645. (C) Nursing process phase: assessment; client need: health promotion and maintenance; content area: medical/surgical—gerontological nursing

Rationale
(A) Decreased concentrations of acetylcholine are found normally in the aging brain. (B) There is a decrease in both gray and white matter in the aging brain. (C) Lipofuscin deposits are normal findings in both cardiac and brain tissue of the older adult. Neurofibrillary tangles are formed in the normal aging brain, but in Alzheimer's disease there is increased accumulation of both lipofuscin deposits and neurofibrillary tangles. (D) Increased MAO is indicative of depression.

646. (A) Nursing process phase: planning; client need: safe, effective care environment; content area: medical/surgical—gerontological nursing

Rationale
(A) A quiet environment with no more than one or two people is necessary to reduce distraction and allow the client to complete a task. (B) The dining room will be filled with distractions that will further increase the client's frustration and irritability. (C) Offering a choice of items may produce frustration because the client may be unable to make decisions. (D) Hot foods may produce a burn if dropped or thrown.

647. (B) Nursing process phase: implementation; client need: psychosocial integrity; content area: medical/surgical—gerontological nursing

Rationale
(A) Following hospital procedure for bathing is appropriate for nursing staff to remember, but does little to get the client involved in personal hygiene. (B) Giving the client short, specific instructions of what to do allows the client to process the information and aids in following directions. (C) Written, step-by-step instructions may be difficult for the client to comprehend and produce frustration. (D) Explaining what is expected ahead of time requires increased cognitive ability and will not assist to get the client involved in personal hygiene.

648. (C) Nursing process phase: planning; client need: safe, effective care environment; content area: medical/surgical—gerontological nursing

Rationale

(A) Limiting fluids to 1000 ml daily could cause the client to be at risk for electrolyte imbalance, dehydration, and infections. (B) An indwelling catheter provides a medium for urinary tract infections and is not appropriate for incontinence associated with dementia. (C) A regular, consistent schedule of toileting provides an environment that decreases anxiety and frustration. (D) Although labeling the door may help the client to find the bathroom, there is no assurance that this will increase continence.

649. **(A)** Nursing process phase: implementation; client need: physiological integrity; content area: medical/surgical—gerontological nursing

Rationale

(A) Weighing the client weekly will provide data that best indicate whether the client is receiving adequate nutrition. (B) Having the staff feed her decreases the ability of the client to perform self-care. While this may be easier than allowing the client to feed herself, it will not provide a measure by which nutritional status can be consistently measured. (C) Selection of a menu requires cognitive ability and may increase the client's frustration. (D) Providing high protein liquids is an appropriate nursing action, but will not provide a measure by which nutritional status can be consistently measured.

650. **(D)** Nursing process phase: implementation; client need: physiological integrity; content area: medical/surgical—gerontological nursing

Rationale

(A) The use of restraints is not recommended for clients with dementia because they are attributed to complications such as increased confusion and injury. (B) Closing the door may help the other residents to rest but do little to help the client and may increase agitation as she tries to gain orientation in an unfamiliar environment. (C) Strong medications for sleep are not recommended for dementia clients because they are attributed to complications such as increased confusion and injury. (D) Leaving the lights on assists the client to gain orientation to the environment and research suggests that light decreases irritability seen later in the evening hours.

651. **(C)** Nursing process phase: analysis; client need: psychological integrity; content area: medical/surgical—gerontological nursing

Rationale

(A) Agnosia is a disturbance in the recognition of objects. (B) Apraxia is the inability to carry out a learned movement voluntarily. (C) Sundowner's syndrome is a condition that is seen in dementia clients in the early evening hours and is characterized by insomnia, restlessness, agitation, wandering, and increased confusion. (D) Irritability is not seen in stage or phase three dementia. This phase is characterized by emaciation and the client is often bedridden.

652. **(A)** Nursing process phase: evaluation; client need: health promotion and maintenance; content area: medical/surgical—gerontological nursing

Rationale

(A) Raking leaves is a repetitive, nonthreatening activity that allows both exercise and range of motion to the extremities. (B) Cooking might be a dangerous activity if the stove is not turned off and she could be burned if cooking utensils are not used appropriately. (C) Writing notes to friends requires cog-

nitive ability and could increase frustration if she is unable to complete the task. (D) The mother might become lost when walking the dog, even in a familiar neighborhood.

653. **(B)** Nursing process phase: assessment; client need: physiological integrity; content area: medical/surgical—gerontological nursing

Rationale

(A) Parkinson's disease is a progressive, degenerative process of the nerve cells in the extrapyramidal system. Although many persons over the age of 65 are affected, it is not a normal aging change. (B) Parkinson's disease is a progressive, degenerative process of the nerve cells in the extrapyramidal system, neurological in nature, and irreversible. (C) Although the musculoskeletal system is affected, the cause is neurological. (D) Parkinson's disease is progressive and is not reversible.

654. **(D)** Nursing process phase: implementation; client need: physiological integrity; content area: medical/surgical—gerontological nursing

Rationale

(A) Caffeine products may not be a therapeutic dietary need in the older adult, but they do not affect the drug therapy. (B) Foods high in fat are not recommended for the older adult, but they do not affect the drug therapy. (C) Foods high in calories are not recommended for the older adult, but do not affect the drug therapy. (D) Vitamin B_6 encourages the conversion of levodopa to dopamine, thereby inhibiting the effects of levodopa. Even with increased calories, the client with Parkinson's disease may lose weight, so extra calories are not a problem.

655. **(D)** Nursing process phase: analysis; client need: physiological integrity; content area: medical/surgical—gerontological nursing

Rationale

(A) These behaviors are extrapyramidal symptoms and are not the result of carbidopa/levodopa. (B) These behaviors are extrapyramidal symptoms and are not the result of digoxin. (C) These behaviors are extrapyramidal symptoms and are not the result of Restoril. (D) These behaviors are extrapyramidal symptoms and are brought on as a result of haloperidol.

656. **(C)** Nursing process phase: planning; client need: safe, effective care environment; content area: medical/surgical—gerontological nursing

Rationale

(A) Adding liquids while chewing might cause the client to aspirate. (B) Allowing the client to feed himself may increase the desire to eat and contribute to psychological well-being, but does little for the difficulty in swallowing experienced by the Parkinson's disease client. (C) Placing the client in an upright position minimizes facial and pharyngeal muscle rigidity. (D) Having the family bring favorite foods from home may stimulate the appetite and taste better than institutionally prepared menus, but does little for the difficulty in swallowing experienced by the client with Parkinson's disease.

657. **(C)** Nursing process phase: implementation; client need: psychosocial integrity; content area: medical/surgical—gerontological nursing

Rationale

(A) Encouraging the client to perform activities of daily living for himself is important, but is not the most important action in keeping the client in his home. (B) Finding ways for the client to communicate his needs may decrease some frustration, but communication is not essential for the client to remain at home. (C) Attending to the physical and emotional needs of the caregiver is the most important nursing intervention in keeping the client at home. Providing for these needs decreases frustration, burnout, and feelings of social isolation, all of which contribute to physical illness of the caregiver and may make it necessary for institutionalization of the client. (D) Keeping the client active may not be possible as the disease progresses and is not a key factor in his remaining in the home.

658. (A) Nursing process phase: evaluation; client need: health promotion and maintenance; content area: medical/surgical—gerontological nursing

Rationale

(A) Foods high in vitamin B_6 include nuts, bran, and whole grain cereals. These foods should be avoided when taking levodopa. (B) Drinking skim milk is correct therapeutically for older adults but is not necessary in the Parkinson's disease clients. Milk is also high in vitamin B_6, the dietary restriction when taking levodopa. (D) Drinking juice rather than tea or coffee decreases caffeine in the diet but is not restricted when on levodopa therapy. (D) Meats may be cut in small pieces to aid in eating, but are not a dietary restriction indicated by levodopa therapy.

659. (A) Nursing process phase: assessment; client need: physiological integrity; content area: medical/surgical—gerontological nursing

Rationale

(A) The lesion described is a seborrheic keratosis, a black or brownish gray wartlike lesion usually found at the hairline. (B) Although the physician might be seen to confirm diagnosis, removal is not indicated unless malignant. (C) Antibiotic ointments are not suggested by the nurse for skin lesions. (D) Wart removal creams are not suggested for skin lesions.

660. (D) Nursing process phase: analysis; client need: health promotion and maintenance; content area: medical/surgical—gerontological nursing

Rationale

(A) Males are at lower risk for osteoporosis than are females. Steroid therapy does not interfere with bone processes. (B) Thin Caucasian females are more at risk than obese Asian or Hispanic females. (C) Males are at lower risk for osteoporosis than are females. (D) Persons at high risk for osteoporosis are thin, sedentary, Caucasian females who are experiencing estrogen loss as a result of menopause.

661. (B) Nursing process phase: analysis; client need: health promotion and maintenance; content area: medical/surgical—gerontological nursing

Rationale

(A) There is no evidence of the need to take the drug with meals. (B) It is especially important that women receiving estrogen therapy undergo yearly mammography because estrogen increases the risk of breast cancer. (C) Estrogen has not been associated with glucose tolerance. (D) Estrogen has not been associated with hypotension.

662. (A) Nursing process phase: implementation; client need: physiological integrity; content area: medical/surgical—gerontological nursing

Rationale

(A) Recommended calcium intake for premenopausal women is 1000 mg per day. Each glass of milk contains about 300 mg of calcium. (B) Vitamin D, not vitamin C, is necessary for calcium absorption. (C) Dietary calcium intake is utilized by the body; however, the average dietary intake of calcium is less than half what is recommended. (D) Oral phosphate has not been proved to reduce osteoporosis.

663. (B) Nursing process phase: evaluation; client need: health promotion and maintenance; content area: medical/surgical—gerontological nursing

Rationale

(A) Foods containing vitamin C and decreasing fat in the diet are not attributed to preventive measures for osteoporosis. (B) A regimen of moderate weight-bearing exercise 45 to 60 minutes three to five times per week is effective in the prevention of osteoporosis due to enhanced calcium absorption. (C) Elimination of fat in the diet is therapeutic but is not effective in the prevention of osteoporosis. (D) Swimming, although good exercise, is not weight bearing and is not beneficial to calcium absorption.

664. (A) Nursing process phase: assessment; client need: physiological integrity; content area: medical/surgical—gerontological nursing

Rationale

(A) Presbycusis is a bilateral symmetric, sensorineural hearing loss affecting very high frequencies. (B) Presbycusis is not difficulty in ambulating without mechanical aids. (C) Inability to see objects at close distance is presbyopia. (D) Although the ability to taste sweet and sour is diminished in the older adult, it is not known as presbycusis.

665. (B) Nursing process phase: planning; client need: psychosocial integrity; content area: medical/surgical—gerontological nursing

Rationale

(A) A special chair to facilitate getting into and out of the bathtub might benefit the client, but there is no evidence that he has need of a special chair at this time. (B) Presbycusis causes difficulty hearing high-pitched consonant sounds such as "ch" and "st." Telephones that facilitate the hearing of these sounds allow the person to remain independent in the home because a sense of security is maintained by reaching assistance and in communication of needs. (C) Antiglare devices are necessary for presbyopia, but can be accomplished by blinds and less expensive means than antiglare windows. (D) Burglar bars may add to feelings of security, but may also serve as a potential for injury if a fire occurred and the client could not get out quickly.

666. (C) Nursing process phase: analysis; client need: health promotion and maintenance; content area: medical/surgical—gerontological nursing

Rationale

(A) Psychotropic drug therapy may cause dizziness, but is not associated as a general rule with vision disturbance. (B) There is no evidence to suggest that the client is using visual disturbance as an excuse to avoid exercise. (C) An early symptom of posterior subcapsular cataracts is the complaint of glare from bright lights during the day or at night as a result of rays of light being scattered by the opacities. (D) Diuretic therapy may cause dizziness, but is not associated as a general rule with vision disturbance.

667. **(A)** Nursing process phase: assessment; client need: psychosocial integrity; content area: medical/surgical—gerontological nursing

Rationale
(A) Assessment of family relationship and communication patterns will provide the nurse with insight into the potential pattern for abuse. (B) When assessing for potential abuse, the client and family member are always questioned separately to pick up discrepancies in what occurred. (C) Review of the medical record is timely and may not provide the insight into the present condition. (D) Further assessment is necessary because physical and emotional safety are a primary goal of nursing and professional accountability calls for immediate action.

668. **(A)** Nursing process phase: analysis; client need: physiological integrity; content area: medical/surgical—gerontological nursing

Rationale
(A) Myocardial infarction (MI) in the elderly may present as dyspnea, syncope, weakness, vomiting, or confusion, rather than as chest pain. Myocardinal infarctions are often silent in the elderly. (B) Generally, a diagnosis of myocardial infarction may be confirmed with family history or prior history of cardiac disease. (C) Myocardial infarction does not have to be fatal if treatment can be initiated early. (D) Treatment for myocardial infarction does include the use of oxygen, although the amount may be reduced to accommodate for the impaired ventilation system of the older adult.

669. **(B)** Nursing process phase: assessment; client need: health promotion and maintenance; content area: medical/surgical—gerontological nursing

Rationale
(A) Paresthesia in the lower extremities is indicative of vitamin B_{12} deficiency. (B) Spooning of the nails should alert the practitioner to an iron deficiency. (C) Gingival hemorrhage reflects a vitamin C deficiency. (D) Carpopedal spasms indicate a magnesium deficiency.

670. **(A)** Nursing process phase: assessment; client need: physiological integrity; content area: medical/surgical—gerontological nursing

Rationale
(A) A stage two decubitus ulcer appears as a superficial ulcer that may be a blister, abrasion, or shallow crater. (B) A stage one decubitus ulcer is a nonblanching erythema. (C) A stage three decubitus ulcer formation extends into the deeper subcutaneous tissue. (D) A stage four decubitus ulcer extends into the deep subcutaneous tissue and ends in full-thickness skin loss.

671. **(D)** Nursing process phase: assessment; client need: psychosocial integrity; content area: medical/surgical—gerontological nursing

Rationale
(A) A complete medical history is important, but the symp-

toms being expressed, even the somatic symptoms of feeling physically ill, are indicators of depression in older adults. The nurse should conduct a mental status examination first, before following up with a medical history and physical examination. (B) The nurse must perform a complete assessment of the client to obtain information about his mental and physical health before accurate referral can be made. (C) A complete physical examination is not warranted until the mental status examination and a medical history are completed. (D) The client is presenting with signs and symptoms of depression. Conducting a complete mental status examination will assist the nurse to intervene appropriately.

672. **(A)** Nursing process phase: analysis; client need: psychosocial integrity; content area: medical/surgical—gerontological nursing

Rationale
(A) Anhedonia is the loss of pleasure and interest in activities previously enjoyed. (B) Agnosia is the loss of comprehension of auditory, visual, or other sensation. (C) Akathisia is motor restlessness brought on by dopamine-blocking drugs. (D) Apraxia is the loss of ability to carry out purposeful movements.

673. **(A)** Nursing process phase: analysis; client need: psychosocial integrity; content area: medical/surgical—gerontological nursing

Rationale
(A) Unipolar depression is characterized by only episodes of depression with no manic or hypomanic episodes. (B) Depression associated with mania is a bipolar disorder. (C) Unipolar depression may occur more than one time. (D) Altered neurotransmission, not the brain side, is one of the biological theories of depression.

674. **(B)** Nursing process phase: analysis; client need: physiological integrity; content area: medical/surgical—gerontological nursing

Rationale
(A) Thyroid function studies, serum thyroxine, and thyroid-stimulating hormone (TSH) should be evaluated at baseline because lithium may predispose the older adult to hypothyroidism, but measurement of renal function also is essential before beginning lithium therapy. (B) Renal insufficiency may delay excretion of lithium and lead to toxicity. Blood urea nitrogen, serum creatinine, and urinalysis must be performed prior to beginning lithium therapy to determine hydration status, renal flow, and presence of renal defects. (C) Checking serum electrolytes is recommended prior to initiating lithium therapy but is not an essential nursing action. (D) White blood cell counts, total and differential, not red blood cell studies, are checked prior to administering lithium.

675. **(C)** Nursing process phase: assessment; client need: psychosocial integrity; content area: medical/surgical—gerontological nursing

Rationale
(A) This response does little to assist the client to verbalize feelings and may prevent further communication. (B) This response minimizes the feelings of the client and puts focus on the past rather than the here and now. (C) Feelings of worthlessness are common in major depression and may lead to suicidal ideation. Observation for behaviors or statements that may be indicators of self-harm may signal suicidal

thoughts or intent and should be assessed. (D) "Why" questions are not considered therapeutic responses. This response does little to explore the feelings being expressed and may change the focus of the conversation.

676. (A) Nursing process phase: evaluation; client need: psychosocial integrity; content area: medical/surgical—gerontological nursing

Rationale
(A) Significant therapeutic results occur after 2 weeks of therapy in 75 percent of clients receiving the medication, but may require 2 to 4 weeks before noticeable improvement is seen. (B) Requesting a new antidepressant at this time would hinder the therapeutic regime and could result in prolonging depressive symptoms. (C) Discontinuing the medication unless there are adverse effects noted is not warranted. (D) There is nothing to suggest that the client is throwing the medication away. Although the nurse may monitor for this, it is not the most appropriate action at 12 days.

677. (B) Nursing process phase: analysis; client need: physiological integrity; content area: medical/surgical—gerontological nursing

Rationale
(A) Lithium levels in this range would be too low. The normal therapeutic range for an older adult is 0.5 to 1.5 mEq/L. (B) The therapeutic range for clients receiving lithium should be 0.5 to 1.5 mEq/L. (C & D) Lithium levels in these ranges would be too high. The normal therapeutic range for an older adult is 0.5 to 1.5 mEq/L.

678. (A) Nursing process phase: analysis; client need: physiological integrity; content area: medical/surgical—gerontological nursing

Rationale
(A) Although AIDS dementia and DAT have similar presenting symptoms, aphasia often accompanies DAT but is rarely seen in AIDS dementia. In addition, in early Alzheimer's disease there are no definite neurological findings; ataxia, leg weakness, tremors, and peripheral neuropathies may be present with AIDS dementia. (B) Lethargy and a pronounced loss of weight are symptoms of AIDS dementia and are not seen until the later stages of DAT. (C) Peripheral neuropathies are not usually seen in DAT until the later stages although they may be present in early AIDS dementia. (D) Leg weakness and tremors may be present in AIDS dementia, but are rarely seen in DAT until the later stages.

679. (A) Nursing process phase: assessment; client need: safe, effective care environment; content area: medical/surgical—gerontological nursing

Rationale
(A) Nadolol (Corgard) is contraindicated in clients who have bronchial asthma or chronic obstructive pulmonary disease. (B) Nadolol (Corgard) is used with caution in clients who have a history of hyperthyroidism, not hypothyrodism. (C) Nadolol (Corgard) is contraindicated in clients with sinus bradycardia, not sinus tachycardia. (D) Nadolol (Corgard) use may be monitored with antidepressant medication, but is not contraindicated.

680. (C) Nursing process phase: planning; client need: physiological integrity; content area: medical/surgical—gerontological nursing

Rationale
(A) There is no evidence to suggest that because the client is a widower, he does not have an available sexual partner. (B) Altered sexuality patterns are defined as the state in which a client expresses concern about sexuality. This diagnosis is appropriate when the older adult has experienced a life change causing a new impediment to sexual functioning. Although there may be some slowing of sexual performance; alteration in sexual activity or in sexual performance is not a normal physiological aging change. (C) Altered sexuality patterns are defined as the state in which a client expresses concern about sexuality. This diagnosis is appropriate when the older adult has experienced a life change causing a new impediment to sexual functioning. Beta-blocking antihypertensive medications may cause impotence and interfere with sexual performance. (D) Although clients who have had myocardial infarctions may fear a heart attack during sexual performance, there is nothing to suggest to the nurse that this client has had a heart attack and there is nothing to suggest that this client fears having a heart attack.

681. (A) Nursing process phase: implementation; client need: physiological integrity; content area: medical/surgical—gerontological nursing

Rationale
(A) The client is taking nadolol (Corgard), a beta-adrenergic blocker, which may cause impotence or other sexual problems. Instructing the client to report any sexual problems to the physician is important for the nursing diagnosis of altered sexual patterns. (B) Use of condoms for protection during sexual activity is important for older adults, but is not appropriate for this client because there is nothing in the assessment information to suggest fear of pregnancy or of acquiring a sexually transmitted disease. (C) Instructing the client to rise slowly from a sitting or lying position is important for this client due to the osthostatic hypotension potential. This instruction does not fit the nursing diagnosis for potential altered sexuality pattern. (D) This information may be given to a client who is resuming sexual activity following myocardial infarction, but there is nothing to support the need for nitroglycerin with this client.

682. (D) Nursing process phase: implementation; client need: safe, effective care environment; content area: medical/surgical—gerontological nursing

Rationale
(A) Moving one client to another section of the nursing home facility will not assist with the behavior being noted in these two cognitively aware individuals. (B) Calling family members is not warranted because both of the clients are cognitively aware and have the right to make decisions related to expressions of sexuality and intimacy. (C) Performing a thorough sexual assessment on both clients including tests for sexually transmitted disease is appropriate nursing action; however, it is not the most important action for the director to take at this time. The feelings, attitudes, and concerns of the staff must be taken into account before further interventions are planned. (D) The feelings, attitudes, and concerns of the staff must be known before appropriate nursing interventions can be implemented. Calling a nursing conference will give the staff an opportunity to verbalize any concerns and to plan for the intimacy needs of these two individuals.

683. (C) Nursing process phase: implementation; client

need: psychosocial integrity; content area: medical/surgical—gerontological nursing

Rationale

(A) Informing the client that you will have a talk with the roommate at once does little to solve the need for privacy to express feelings of intimacy. (B) If the client is uncomfortable with the open display of affection and intimacy, closing the curtain may prevent visualization but does not ensure privacy for display of affection. (C) Providing the roommate with a private area to express intimacy and display of affection is important and prevents the concerns of uncomfortableness being expressed by the client. (D) Moving the client to a private room may be unfeasible and costly. Providing a private area for the expression of intimacy is an important issue in long-term care facilities and should be addressed by the nursing staff.

684. **(B)** Nursing process phase: analysis; client need: physiological integrity; content area: medical/surgical—gerontological nursing

Rationale

(A) Verbal paraphasia is the substitution of an inappropriate word during an effort to say a word with another word, such as saying rubber for eraser or comb for brush. (B) Jargon is the unintelligible verbal output in communication in response to questions. (C) Perseverance is the persistent repeating of words over and over again, such as "mama, mama, mama." (D) Literal paraphasia is the substitution of a similar-sounding word for another, such as "pone" from phone.

685. **(B)** Nursing process phase: analysis; client need: safe, effective care environment; content area: medical/surgical—gerontological nursing

Rationale

(A) Automatic speech is the repetition of overlearned sequences, such as counting from 1 to 10 or reciting the days of the week. (B) The client needs visual and verbal cues in order to name objects and is clearly having difficulty with word find. (C) Fluent aphasia is marked by verbal output of words and neologisms or meaningless words. (D) Nonfluent aphasia is marked by restricted speech with awkward articulation and limited vocabulary.

686. **(D)** Nursing process phase: assessment; client need: safe, effective care environment; content area: medical/surgical—gerontological nursing

Rationale

(A) Organic brain syndrome would interfere with the client's ability to answer orientation information. (B) The client may be experiencing impaired hearing acuity, but is wearing a hearing aid and is able to hear well enough to provide answers to orientation questions. This makes it unlikely that this is the reason for the inability to name visual objects. (C) Aphasia is the loss of previously acquired language facility and results from cerebral dysfunction. Because the client is able to verbalize the days of the week and the months, impaired verbal aphasia is unlikely. (D) Undetected poor visual acuity may be affecting the client's ability to read or to see the objects that the nurse is asking to be named.

687. **(B)** Nursing process phase: analysis; client need: physiological integrity; content area: medical/surgical—gerontological nursing

Rationale

(A) Malignant brain tumors are sometimes experienced by older adults, but are primarily seen in younger clients. (B) Cardiovascular accidents (CVA) are the most common cause of aphasia in the older adult. (C) Head trauma may cause aphasia in older adults but is not the most likely cause of aphasia. (D) Major depressive disorder may interfere with the ability of the older adult to communicate, but does not cause aphasia.

688. **(A)** Nursing process phase: analysis; client need: physiological integrity; content area: medical/surgical—gerontological nursing

Rationale

(A) Approximately 80 percent of clients with Broca's aphasia have right-sided hemiparesis. (B) Wernicke's aphasia results from a posterior lesion in the temporal gyrus. (C) Conduction aphasia is a fluent type of aphasia that results from a posterior lesion of the dominant speech hemisphere. (D) Anomic aphasia is more likely to occur with diffuse disease and may be difficult to localize.

689. **(B)** Nursing process phase: analysis; client need: physiological integrity; content area: medical/surgical—gerontological nursing

Rationale

(A) Many postmenopausal women have voiding difficulty; however, stress incontinence is not due to stress brought on by menopause. (B) Stress incontinence is due to loss of structural support to the bladder neck and is caused by pelvic floor relaxation. (C) Urinary tract infections may bring about a feeling of need to urinate frequently, but do not usually bring about an involuntary loss of urine from the bladder. (D) Incontinence is not a normal aging change.

690. **(A)** Nursing process phase: analysis; client need: physiological integrity; content area: medical/surgical—gerontological nursing

Rationale

(A) The central nervous system controls normal micturition. Afferent innervation proceeds from the bladder through the pelvic and hypogastric nerves into the dorsal horn of the spinal cord, and continues into complex connections that transmit impulses which permit voluntary control of the bladder. (B) Originally, it was thought that the spinal cord was the operating and coordinating center of bladder function. The sacral cord can generate reflex contraction of the bladder, but not the complex process of micturition. (C) The sphincter pupillae is a muscle that expands the iris, narrowing the diameter of the pupil of the eye. (D) The detrusor muscle is a complex of longitudinal fibers that form the external layer of the muscular coat of the bladder and controls the storage of urine.

691. **(C)** Nursing process phase: implementation; client need: safe, effective care environment; content area: medical/surgical—gerontological nursing

Rationale

(A) Behavior modification and psychological counseling may be implemented to treat sensory incontinence, but do not assist with incontinence that occurs as a result of pelvic floor relaxation. (B) Although this recommendation to the client may be made, this is not the only treatment for stress incontinence. Frequent change of pads and bathing twice a day may not be feasible for this client, who is experiencing embarrassment due to the incontinence. (C) All treatment for stress is elective and depends upon the severity of symptoms and the degree of concern and interference with lifestyle. (D) Surgical procedures are used as a form of treatment for stress incontinence, but may not be complex. Surgical procedures are not used for all clients with stress incontinence.

692. (A) Nursing process phase: assessment; client need: safe, effective care environment; content area: medical/surgical—gerontological nursing

Rationale
(A) Propantheline (Pro-Banthine) should be used with caution in clients with urinary retention. (B) Propantheline (Pro-Banthine) should be used with caution in clients with heart disease, kidney disease, liver disease, and lung disease but is not contraindicated in clients with diabetes mellitus. (C) Propantheline (Pro-Banthine) should be used with caution in clients with heart disease, kidney disease, liver disease, and lung disease but is not contraindicated in clients with a urinary tract infection. (D) Propantheline (Pro-Banthine) should be used with caution with drugs with anticholinergic effects, but is not contraindicated with antibiotics.

693. (B) Nursing process phase: implementation; client need: physiological integrity; content area: medical/surgical—gerontological nursing

Rationale
(A) Enlarged lymph nodes may be a result of an infectious process but are not related to the side effects of propantheline (Pro-Banthine). It is doubtful that the client would experience nasal drainage due to the drying properties of propantheline (Pro-Banthine). (B) Side effects of propantheline (Pro-Banthine) include dry mouth, dry eyes, blurred vision, increased intraocular pressure, and constipation. Blurred vision with dilated pupils may indicate increased intraocular pressure and acute glaucoma. If left untreated, acute glaucoma results in complete and permanent blindness within 2 to 5 days. (C) Orthostatic hypotension is a side effect of propantheline (Pro-Banthine) but is not life threatening or indicative of a more serious problem. Blurred vision with dilated pupils may indicate increased intraocular pressure and acute glaucoma. If left untreated, acute glaucoma results in complete and permanent blindness within 2 to 5 days. (D) Presbyopia, the inability to focus on near objects, is a normal aging change and is expected to be found in older adults.

694. (B) Nursing process phase: evaluation; client need: safe, effective care environment; content area: medical/surgical—gerontological nursing

Rationale
(A) Even though constipation may be a side effect of propantheline (Pro-Banthine) and eating green vegetables is encouraged to increase fiber in the diet, the anticholinergic action of the drug may decrease sweat and heat release from the body and working in the garden on a very hot day could be more problematic for the client. (B) The anticholinergic action of the drug may decrease sweat and heat release from the body and clients should be cautioned to avoid activities such as hot baths, hot showers, saunas, and strenuous activities during hot weather. Working in the garden on a very hot day could be problematic for the client. (C) Even though constipation may be a side effect of propantheline (Pro-Banthine) and exercise is encouraged to prevent constipation, the anti-

cholinergic action of the drug may decrease sweat and heat release from the body and working in the garden on a very hot day could be more problematic for the client. (D) Caffeine, red wine, and aged cheese are to be avoided with MAO inhibitors, not with propantheline (Pro-Banthine).

695. (C) Nursing process phase: implementation; client need: safe, effective care environment; content area: medical/surgical—gerontological nursing

Rationale
(A–D) A cystometrogram (CMG) is a graphic representation of bladder pressure and provides assessment information regarding the ability of the bladder to fill and store urine.

696. (A) Nursing process phase: analysis; client need: psychosocial integrity; content area: medical/surgical—gerontological nursing

Rationale
(A & D) According to the North American Nursing Diagnosis Association (NANDA), functional incontinence is urinary leakage caused by environmental or functional factors. It is not associated with any pathological condition of the urinary system or voiding mechanism and is usually associated with cognitive deficits or motivational disorders. (B) A peripheral field deficit may cause the client to not be able to discriminate heights and to impair vision from the side view but is not a likely cause of functional incontinence. (C) While CVA may bring about incontinence because of immobility changes, this would likely be associated with a pathological condition. According to NANDA, functional incontinence is urinary leakage caused by environmental or functional factors. It is not associated with any pathological condition of the urinary system or voiding mechanism and is usually associated with cognitive deficits or motivational disorders.

697. (C) Nursing process phase: assessment; client need: safe, effective care environment; content area: medical/surgical—gerontological nursing

Rationale
(A) Cognitive impairment is a cause of incontinence but does not prevent the client from discussing the problem of incontinence. Research studies indicate that the majority of individuals (particularly females) believe that incontinence is a normal result of aging. (B) While incontinence does bring about feelings of embarrassment and distress, research studies indicate that the majority of individuals (particularly females) believe that incontinence is a normal result of aging. (C) Research studies indicate that the majority of individuals (particularly females) believe that incontinence is a normal result of aging. (D) Incontinence is a major factor in making a decision for long-term care; however, this does not prevent the client to discuss incontinence as a problem. Research studies indicate that the majority of individuals (particularly females) believe that incontinence is a normal result of aging.

698. (A) Nursing process phase: analysis; client need: safe, effective care environment; content area: medical/surgical—gerontological nursing

Rationale
(A) Biofeedback is most effective in stress and urge incontinence, both of which are caused by structural problems of the bladder or sphincter musculature. (B) Biofeedback is not effective with incontinence brought about by physical causes such as spinal cord injuries or head trauma. (C)

Biofeedback requires that the client must be cognitively intact and have a motivation to learn bladder inhibition and sphincter contraction activities. Clients with major depression may not have the energy or the desire to participate in biofeedback treatment modalities. (D) Biofeedback requires that the client must be cognitively intact and have a motivation to learn bladder inhibition and sphincter contraction activities. Clients with cognitive impairment may not have the cognition required to participate in biofeedback treatment modalities.

699. (C) Nursing process phase: evaluation; client need: physiological integrity; content area: medial/surgical—gerontological nursing

Rationale
(A) Symptoms of left-sided congestive heart failure include dyspnea, tachycardia, fatigue, muscle weakness, and restlessness. Symptoms of right-sided congestive heart failure include dependent edema, anorexia, nausea, and vague abdominal pain. The symptoms reported by the client are indicators of potassium depletion as a result of the dialysis and perhaps inadequate dietary intake of potassium. (B) Symptoms of nitrogenous toxin include mental status changes, fatigue, neurological disorders, hypertension, nausea and vomiting with pruritus. The symptoms reported by the client are indicators of potassium depletion as a result of the dialysis and perhaps inadequate dietary intake of potassium. (C) The symptoms reported by the client are indicators of potassium depletion as a result of the dialysis and perhaps inadequate dietary intake of potassium. (D) Symptoms of hypotension include dizziness and blood pressure levels not adequate for normal perfusion. Hypotension in dialysis may occur as a result of sodium depletion.

700. (C) Nursing process phase: implementation; client need: safe, effective care environment; content area: medical/surgical—gerontological nursing

Rationale
(A) Clients on CAPD need to increase potassium intake by eating a wide variety of fruits and vegetables each day. (B) Sodium restriction is not necessary with CAPD clients, and both kale and collard greens contain potassium, which should be increased. (C) Nutritionists recommend a dietary regimen that limits phosphorus intake to 1200 mg/day. Foods such as nuts and legumes are phosphorous-rich. (D) Protein intake is increased to provide 1.2 to 1.5 g/kg body weight.

701. (B) Nursing process phase: implementation; client need: physiological integrity; content area: medical/surgical—gerontological nursing

Rationale
(A) Clients with a fecal impaction may have similar symptoms, but the nursing action would not warrant referral to a physician. (B) Ovarian cancer is often "silent," with the most common sign being enlargement of the abdomen caused by accumulation of fluid. In women over age 40, vague digestive complaints such as stomach discomfort, gas, or distention that persists and cannot be explained by any other cause should be thoroughly investigated. (C) Although older adults often complain of numerous complaints, this does not indicate attention-seeking behavior. Attention seeking would not require referral to a physician. (D) Older adults with depression will most probably have symptoms that imitate dementia, with difficulty with memory and concentration.

702. (C) Nursing process phase: analysis; client need: safe, effective care environment; content area: medical/surgical—gerontological nursing

Rationale
(A & B) Older women in the United States have been found to have two to three times the percentage of abnormal smears compared with women less than age 65. (B) The American College of Obstetricians and Gynecologists recommends that women be screened annually, and that after a woman has had three or more consecutive satisfactory examinations with normal findings, the interval may be less frequent and at the discretion of her physician. (D) Cervical cytology is effective in detecting preinvasive disease, although the false-negative rate may be higher in elderly women.

703. (B) Nursing process phase: assessment; client need: safe, effective care environment; content area: medical/surgical—gerontological nursing

Rationale
(A) The early stage of cognitive impairment is not characterized by numerous complaints of constipation, and there is no evidence to suggest that this client is experiencing impaired cognition. (B) Sensory neurogenic dysfunction is damage to the sensory components of the rectal reflex arc or the sensory components of the central nervous system that takes the message of stool in the rectum to the cerebral cortex. The motor components are intact, but the individual is not aware of stool in the rectum. (C) Motor neurogenic dysfunction is damage to the motor components of the central nervous system or the motor components of the rectal reflex arc. The individual feels the stool in the rectum, but is unable to evacuate the stool. (D) Constipation is a common adverse drug reaction; however, in this situation there is nothing to suggest that this client is receiving a medication.

704. (D) Nursing process phase: analysis; client need: safe, effective care environment; content area: medical/surgical—gerontological nursing

Rationale
(A) The action described in this situation is the action of a saline laxative. Saline laxatives act by retaining and increasing water content of feces by osmotic qualities. (B) The action described in this situation is the action of a bulk laxative. Bulk laxatives act by absorbing water and increasing the volume of intestinal contents. (C) The action described in this situation is the action of a hyperosmotic agent. Hyperosmotic agents act by retaining and increasing water content of feces by osmotic qualities. (D) Docusate sodium (Colace) is an emollient or fecal softening agent. It acts by dispersing wetting agents, facilitating mixture of water and fatty substances within the fecal mass; when a homogenous mixture is produced, the feces becomes soft.

705. (C) Nursing process phase: implementation; client need: safe, effective care environment; content area: medical/surgical—gerontological nursing

Rationale
(A–C) Milk of magnesia is a saline laxative and is contraindicated in cardiac clients or those with renal impairments. (D) Milk of magnesia is a saline laxative and is contraindicated in cardiac clients or those with renal impairments. It is a laxative of choice for fecal impaction if these conditions are not present.

706. (A) Nursing process phase: evaluation; client need:

physiological integrity; content area: medical/surgical—gerontological nursing

Rationale

(A & C) The goal of a bowel management program is soft, well-formed stool that are regular on the planned day and within 1 hour of the planned time. (B) The goal of a bowel management program is soft, well-formed stools that are regular on the planned day and within 1 hour of the planned time. Accidents do happen, and when they do, the nurse should evaluate the cause. (D) Skin integrity is not an appropriate evaluation criterion for a bowel management program. The goal of a bowel management program is soft, well-formed stools that are regular on the planned day and within 1 hour of the planned time.

707. **(B)** Nursing process phase: analysis; client need: safe, effective care environment; content area: medical/surgical—gerontological nursing

Rationale

(A) Injuries caused by surgical damage may result in disruption of the sphincter musculature or pudendal or sacral nerve branches, but are not neurogenic in nature. (B) Fecal incontinence caused by neurological disorders such as multiple sclerosis or spinal cord lesions are classified as neurological incontinence. (C) Psychiatric or behavioral disorders rarely cause fecal incontinence in older adults. (D) Fecal incontinence may be a result of habitual use of laxatives or enemas, but this would diminish muscle tone and would not be neurogenic in nature.

708. **(D)** Nursing process phase: implementation; client need: physiological integrity; content area: medical/surgical—gerontological nursing

Rationale

(A) The inability to speak or write is expressive aphasia or Broca's aphasia. (B & D) Cachexia is manifested by emaciation, loss of subcutaneous fat and lean body mass, brittleness of the hair, ridged or banded nails, and dermatosis of the lower legs. (C) Involuntary muscular movements of the arms and legs is an extrapyramidal symptoms known as dystonia.

709. **(A)** Nursing process phase: implementation; client need: physiological integrity; content area: medical/surgical—gerontological nursing

Rationale

(A) Clients with severe malnutrition may be too weak to swallow, and a variety of enteral or parenteral routes may be employed if oral feedings are not adequate. (B) There is no reason to believe that transfer to a psychiatric unit is necessary for this client. (C) Monitoring of vital signs may be important with this client, but monitoring every 30 minutes is not necessary based on the information given. (D) Hematesting of bowel movements may be initiated if cancer is suspect; however, the client is manifesting symptoms of severe malnutrition and the nurse would need to initially intervene into the alteration in nutrition.

710. **(C)** Nursing process phase: implementation; client need: safe, effective care environment; content area: medical/surgical—gerontological nursing

Rationale

(A) Some auto insurance companies provide premium reductions to graduates of the American Association of Retired Persons (AARP) Mature Driver/55 Alive Program. (B) The local highway patrol does not usually have a driving program geared to older adults. (C) The AARP Mature Driver/55 Alive Program helps older drivers improve their skills and prevent traffic accidents by covering age-related physical changes, declining perceptual skills, rules of the road, and local driving problems. (D) The American Blindness Federation is a resource for audiovisual material for visually impaired persons.

711. **(B)** Nursing process phase: assessment; client need: psychosocial integrity; content area: medical/surgical—gerontological nursing

Rationale

(A) Constipation is not known to inhibit participation in recreational or social events. (B) Pain can influence participation in recreational and social events, ambulation, posture, appetite, memory, dressing, grooming, and sleep patterns. (C) Depression may inhibit participation in recreational and social events, but the client is engaging in conversation that would make depression a less likely cause of this behavior. (D) There is nothing to suggest that this client has a cognitive impairment.

712. **(B)** Nursing process phase: implementation; client need: physiological integrity; content area: medical/surgical—gerontological nursing

Rationale

(A) The values reported are not characteristic urinalysis values of clients with congestive heart failure. (B & D) In older adults, proteinuria is commonly found and may not be of any clinical significance. Its presence, however, does warrant investigation to rule out urinary tract infection or kidney disease. (C) The older adult with acute renal disease usually has a sudden decline in urinary output and an increase in both blood urea nitrogen (BUN) and creatinine levels.

713. **(D)** Nursing process phase: planning; client need: physiological integrity; content area: medical/surgical—gerontological nursing

Rationale

(A) The client with Alzheimer's disease that has progressed to the immobilized state may have social isolation, but this would not be life-threatening. (B) The client with Alzheimer's disease that has progressed to the immobilized state has existing, not potential, self-care deficit. (C) While there is a potential for injury because of the bedridden status of the client, this potential is not as great as infection. (D) Osteomyelitis, an infection of the bone caused by bacteria entering through the blood supply and entering the bone, is seen most often as a complication of stage IV decubitus ulcer.

714. **(B)** Nursing process phase: implementation; client need: physiological integrity; content area: medical/surgical—gerontological nursing

Rationale

(A) Administering the prescribed antipyretic medication is not warranted with a temperature of 99°F. (B & D) These are symptoms of osteomyelitis, and it is necessary for this condition to be diagnosed and treated early. If the condition progresses to the sepsis stage, prognosis is poor. (C) There is nothing to indicate a need for the change in the decubitus care treatment regimen.

715. (D) Nursing process phase: assessment; client need: safe, effective care environment; content area: medical/surgical—gerontological nursing

Rationale
(A) Assessment of knowledge of prescription medications is important, but at this point the nurse has no evidence to suggest that the client is on medication. (B) Older adults need to be given instruction in small units. The nurse must continuously assess the client's knowledge of hospital procedures. (C) Assessment of baseline cognitive status is important and must be completed on the client shortly after admission. A priority at the beginning of every hospital admission for the older adult is the assessment of baseline functional status in order to develop an individual plan of care within the acute-care setting. (D) A priority at the beginning of every hospital admission for the older adult is the assessment of baseline functional status in order to develop an individual plan of care within the acute-care setting.

716. (A) Nursing process phase: analysis; client need: health promotion and maintenance; content area: medical/surgical—gerontological nursing

Rationale
(A) The largest group of older adults in institutional settings is the 85-year-old and older group. Only 5 percent of the population over age 65 resides in institutional settings, but this percentage increases with age from 1 percent of people aged 65 to 74, to 5 percent of people 74 to 84, and 25 percent of people aged 85 and older. (B–D) Only 5 percent of the population over age 65 resides in institutional settings, but this percentage increases with age from 1 percent of people aged 65 to 74, to 5 percent of people 74 to 84, and 25 percent of people aged 85 and older.

717. (B) Nursing process phase: analysis; client need: health promotion and maintenance; content area: medical/surgical—gerontological nursing

Rationale
(A) There is growing awareness that institutional settings are not the ideal or preferred setting for older adults, and there is a trend toward the provision of more noninstitutional long-term care services. (B) The trend is to provide more noninstitutional long-term care settings. There is growing awareness that institutional settings are not the ideal or preferred setting for older adults, and there is a trend toward the provision of more noninstitutional long-term care services. (C) Funding for senior citizen centers is primarily through the Older Americans Act and United Way and is used primarily for active older adults. (D) There is no mechanism in place to reimburse family members for caring for older adults.

718. (C) Nursing process phase: evaluation; client need: health promotion and maintenance; content area: medical/surgical—gerontological nursing

Rationale
(A) There is no information in this situation on which to base this answer. (B) There is ample research related to care giving, but most studies have been conducted with predominantly nonminority populations. (C & D) There is ample research related to care giving, but most studies have been conducted with predominantly nonminority populations, so there is little understanding about the dynamics of care giving in other racial and ethnic groups.

719. (D) Nursing process phase: analysis; client need: health promotion and maintenance; content area: medical/surgical—gerontological nursing

Rationale
(A) While older adults may fear nursing home placement, the reason they do not seek medical care for thyroid disorders is because they exhibit few of the classic symptoms of the disease. (B) While older adults may have limited financial resources, the reason they do not seek medical care for thyroid disorders is because they exhibit few of the classic symptoms of the disease. (C) While older adults may fear loss of independence, the reason they do not seek medical care for thyroid disorders is because they exhibit few of the classic symptoms of the disease. (D) The reason they do not seek medical care for thyroid disorders is because they exhibit few of the classic symptoms of the disease.

720. (B) Nursing process phase: analysis; client need: safe, effective care environment; content area: medical/surgical—gerontological nursing

Rationale
(A & C) Type I diabetes is characterized by ketosis, signifying a lack of effective insulin. (B & D) Type II diabetes is distinguished by the absence of ketosis, signifying the presence of at least some effective insulin.

721. (A) Nursing process phase: implementation; client need: health promotion and maintenance; content area: medical/surgical—gerontological nursing

Rationale
(A) The elderly person with a viral infection is very susceptible to dehydration. It is important that clients maintain their fluid and carbohydrate intake. Toast and crackers can be used to maintain energy levels. (B) The elderly person with a viral infection is very susceptible to dehydration. It is important that clients maintain their fluid and carbohydrate intake. Toast and crackers can be used to maintain energy levels. Nutritional supplements may make the client nauseated and encourage vomiting. (C) The elderly person should contact the physician and ask about adjustments in type or amount of insulin that may be indicated based on blood and urine sugar levels. (D) While the physician may need to be notified of this condition and asked about adjustments in type or amount of insulin that may be indicated based on blood and urine sugar levels, there is nothing to suggest that emergency room care is needed immediately.

722. (B) Nursing process phase: implementation; client need: safe, effective care environment; content area: medical/surgical—gerontological nursing

Rationale
(A) While the client's usual dietary habits are important, in diabetic teaching, the first step is to determine the client's ideal body weight. (B) The first step in teaching diabetic dietary needs is to determine the client's ideal body weight. (C) While the client's compliance ability is important to assess, the first step in teaching diabetic dietary needs is to determine the client's ideal body weight. (D) Once the food plan is agreed on, the insulin dosage is adjusted to the prescribed diet, not vice versa.

723. (C) Nursing process phase: analysis; client need: health promotion and maintenance; content area: medical/surgical—gerontological nursing

Rationale
(A & B) The number of calories an individual needs is based on the ideal body weight, the age, and the physical activity level. (C & D) Diabetic diets would contain about 55 percent carbohydrates, with 35 to 45 percent derived from complex and 10 to 20 percent from simple carbohydrates.

724. **(B)** Nursing process phase: analysis; client need: health promotion and maintenance; content area: medical/surgical—gerontological nursing

Rationale
(A & B) A simple approach for women is to assign 100 lb for the first 5 ft of height and 5 lb for each additional inch. (C) A simple approach for women is to assign 100 lb for the first 5 ft of height and 5 lb for each additional inch. A 5 ft 5 inch woman could easily weigh 145 lb based on this formula. (D) A simple approach for women is to assign 100 lb for the first 5 ft of height and 5 lb for each additional inch. A 5 ft 5 inch woman could easily weigh 165 lb based on this formula.

725. **(C)** Nursing process phase: analysis; client need: health promotion and maintenance; content area: medical/surgical—gerontological nursing

Rationale
(A) Exercise is important in planning the number of calories, but a simple approach to determining ideal body weight is to allow 106 lb for the first 5 ft and 6 lb for each additional inch. (B) Men are concerned with body appearance just as females are. This statement is a generalization and is not based on fact. (C) For males, a simple approach to determine ideal body weight is to allow 106 lb for the first 5 ft and 6 lb for each additional inch. (D) For males, a simple approach to determine ideal body weight is to allow 106 lb for the first 5 ft and 6 lb for each additional inch. With this formula, a male who is 5 ft 8 inches would have an ideal body weight of 210 lb.

726. **(D)** Nursing process phase: assessment; client need: physiological integrity; content area: medical/surgical—gerontological nursing

Rationale
(A & B) Lipohypertrophy is an accumulation of subcutaneous fat, which occurs with repeated injections at the same site. Rotation of the injection site must be encouraged. (C & D) Lipohypertrophy is an accumulation of subcutaneous fat, which occurs with repeated injections at the same site. Injections in these sites may be less uncomfortable and therefore rotation of the injection site must be encouraged.

727. **(D)** Nursing process phase: evaluation; client need: safe, effective care environment; content area: medical/surgical—gerontological nursing

Rationale
(A–C) While medical factors and family support are important in the assessment for incontinence, biofeedback requires that the client be cognitively intact and motivated to learn bladder inhibition and sphincter contraction. (D) Biofeedback requires that the client be cognitively intact and motivated to learn bladder inhibition and sphincter contraction.

728. **(B)** Nursing process phase: implementation; client need: safe, effective care environment; content area: medical/surgical—gerontological nursing

Rationale
(A, C, & D) Drugs frequently used by the elderly that either intensify or weaken the effects of sulfonamide are glucocorticoid, thiazide, furosemide, nicotinic acid, alcohol, beta blockers (propranolol), and the salicylates. (B) When taken as prescribed, acetaminophen is not known to have any potential drug interactions.

729. **(A)** Nursing process phase: evaluation; client need: physiological integrity; content area: medical/surgical—gerontological nursing

Rationale
(A & B) The major goal in the use of oral diabetic agents is freedom from glycosuria in addition to attaining fasting serum glucose levels of around 120 to 125 mg/dl. (C) While many older adults may have difficulty maneuvering the equipment necessary to give an injection, this is not the reason a physician prescribes an oral diabetic agent. (D) While many older adults may have difficulty reading the small figures on an insulin syringe, this is not the reason a physician prescribes an oral diabetic agent.

730. **(C)** Nursing process phase: assessment; client need: health promotion and maintenance; content area: medical/surgical—gerontological nursing

Rationale
(A) The relationship of the client and the mother is important, but she does not indicate that the problem occurred 6 months ago, so the nurse would assess for changes that would bring about the symptoms, particularly a change in sexual activity. (B) The present relationship of the husband and the mother may be important, but there is nothing to suggest that the relationship may contribute to the sexual discomfort experienced by the client. (C) Periods of abstinence are more likely to be associated with stenosis and discomfort with sexual activity. Because the client indicates that the sexual activity has slowed since the husband's recent heart attack, this would be the initial starting point of assessment. (D) The amount of time the client and son spend in communication may have little or nothing to do with the symptoms being experienced by the client.

731. **(D)** Nursing process phase: implementation; client need: psychosocial integrity; content area: medical/surgical—gerontological nursing

Rationale
(A) Placing the mother in a nearby nursing home will do little to correct the problem experienced by the client and is not warranted based on the information. (B) There is no evidence to suggest that the client is not coping with the situations being presented, so mental health center services are not warranted until other causes have been ruled out. (C) From the situation presented, the nurse may ascertain that the change in sexual frequency may be the cause of the symptoms being described by the client. Referral is appropriate following a complete assessment by the nurse. (D) These symptoms are less likely if intercourse continues on a regular basis because periods of abstinence are more likely to be associated with these symptoms.

732. **(C)** Nursing process phase: analysis; client need: health promotion and maintenance; content area: medical/surgical—gerontological nursing

Rationale
(A–D) When calculating the actual body weight of a client

with an amputation, the calculation is about 10 percent of actual body weight for an above-the-knee amputation. Because this client weighs 195 pounds, 19.5 pounds would be deducted for the amputation; therefore, the weight of the client would approximately be 175 to 176 pounds.

733. **(B)** Nursing process phase: implementation; client need: health promotion and maintenance; content area: medical/surgical—gerontological nursing

Rationale
(A) Prevention of postoperative hemorrhage is important for the nurse to monitor, but the most important aim during the immediate and late postoperative period is to prevent secondary disabilities, especially contracture. Flexion contracture of the hip or knee would make prosthetic fitting difficult—if not impossible. (B) The most important aim during the immediate and late postoperative period is to prevent secondary disabilities, especially contracture. Flexion contracture of the hip or knee would make prosthetic fitting difficult—if not impossible. (C) Maintaining comfort is an important nursing action, but the most important aim during the immediate and late postoperative period is to prevent secondary disabilities, especially contracture. Flexion contracture of the hip or knee would make prosthetic fitting difficult—if not impossible. (D) Maintaining an accurate accounting of the vital signs for the elderly postoperative client is important, but the most important aim during the immediate and late postoperative period is to prevent secondary disabilities, especially contracture. Flexion contracture of the hip or knee would make prosthetic fitting difficult—if not impossible.

734. **(C)** Nursing process phase: evaluation; client need: health promotion and maintenance; content area: medical/surgical—gerontological nursing

Rationale
(A) There is no assurance that physical therapy will encourage socialization or prevent depression in this client. (B) There is no assurance that early ambulation encourages hope and increases rehabilitation potential. (C) The elderly amputee should begin standing and balancing exercises on parallel bars as early as possible. Early ambulation makes the amputee active and accelerates stump shrinkage. (D) While early ambulation will encourage circulation and decrease calcium loss, the reason for the order for physical therapy with this client is to make the amputee active and to accelerate stump shrinkage.

735. **(C)** Nursing process phase: evaluation; client need: safe, effective care environment; content area: medical/surgical—gerontological nursing

Rationale
(A–C) Especially when ascending or descending stairs, an elderly amputee should always use an ambulation aid such as crutches or a cane. (D) Elderly clients are able to climb stairs safely. However, especially when ascending or descending stairs, an elderly amputee should always use an ambulation aid such as crutches or a cane.

736. **(D)** Nursing process phase: implementation; client need: health promotion and maintenance; content area: medical/surgical—gerontological nursing

Rationale
(A–D) Because a lower-extremity prosthesis is a device only for ambulation, an amputee should never wear it while sleeping; otherwise severe dermatitis may develop and result in prolonged loss of use of the prosthesis.

737. **(B)** Nursing process phase: implementation; client need: safe, effective care environment; content area: medical/surgical—gerontological nursing

Rationale
(A) Although this action is important if the floor and surrounding area is wet, a prosthesis is neither waterproof nor water-resistant. Therefore, if even a part of the prosthesis becomes wet, it must be dried immediately and thoroughly. Heat should never be used. (B & D) A prosthesis is neither waterproof nor water-resistant. Therefore, if even a part of the prosthesis becomes wet, it must be dried immediately and thoroughly. Heat should never be used. (C) This action by the nurse does not care for the prosthetic device or the safety of the client.

738. **(A)** Nursing process phase: implementation; client need: physiological integrity; content area: medical/surgical—gerontological nursing

Rationale
(A–D) A client who successfully completes the program of prosthetic rehabilitation and returns to the community should be followed every 3 to 6 months for the first 2 years.

739. **(B)** Nursing process phase: implementation; client need: physiological integrity; content area: medical/surgical—gerontological nursing

Rationale
(A) If the client were diabetic, this would be an important action, but not as important as checking the circulatory status of the sound leg. (B) The circulatory status of the sound leg should be examined at follow-up, because this leg should be kept intact as long as possible. Any areas of concern for the circulatory status of the sound leg should be addressed at follow-up. (C) There is nothing to suggest that this client might be experiencing mental status or cognitive difficulties. Although this might be an important action, the circulatory status of the sound leg should be examined at follow-up, because this leg should be kept intact as long as possible. (D) There is nothing to suggest that this client might need family or other support systems. Although this might be an important action, the circulatory status of the sound leg should be examined at follow-up, because this leg should be kept intact as long as possible.

740. **(A)** Nursing process phase: assessment; client need: health promotion and maintenance; content area: medical/surgical—gerontological nursing

Rationale
(A) The most common complaint is pain in the stump, and the most common causes of a painful stump are either a painful amputation neuroma or spur formation at the amputated end of the bone. While an ill-fitting socket may be the cause, phantom pain and amputation neuroma or spur formation should be ruled out. (B) Phantom pain is not localized because the sensation is frequently incomplete since many clients sense this only in the foot area. (C & D) The most common complaint is pain in the stump, and the most common causes of a painful stump are either a painful amputation neuroma or spur formation at the amputated end of the bone.

741. (C) Nursing process phase: evaluation; client need: safe, effective care environment; content area: medical/surgical—gerontological nursing

Rationale
(A) To prevent fungal growth and subsequent infection of the stump, mild soap may be used for cleaning the inside of the socket, but not chlorine solution. (B) The stump should be inspected daily with a mirror, not monthly. (C) During the night, it is too bothersome to put on a prosthesis and using crutches without a prosthesis may be unsafe. Using the wheelchair would be a safe practice at night. (D) If there is an opening on the skin, the prosthesis should not be used until the wound has healed.

742. (B) Nursing process phase: evaluation; client need: health promotion and maintenance; content area: medical/surgical—gerontological nursing

Rationale
(A) While the client is dating a woman 12 years his junior, the chest pain is caused by the cardiovascular response to exercise, not from the interpersonal relationship. (B) The goals of exercise in those over 75 years of age should be on maintenance of flexibility, strength, coordination, and on balance—but not on aerobic training. In those 75-year-olds who have remained physically active, exercise may include moderate aerobic conditioning. (C) There is nothing to indicate that this client experienced orthostatic hypotension. (D) There are normal aging changes in the cardiovascular system of older adults that influence the amount of exercise and the outcomes of this exercise. The chest pain experienced by the client is not a result of normal aging.

743. (A) Nursing process phase: analysis; client need: safe, effective care environment; content area: medical/surgical—gerontological nursing

Rationale
(A) The purpose of stress testing is to identify a safe range for heart rate during exercise, regardless of the presence or absence of coronary artery disease. (B) The purpose of stress testing is to identify a safe range for heart rate during exercise, regardless of the presence or absence of coronary artery disease. (C) The results of the stress tests will be used by the physician and the health team to determine appropriate exercise protocol, but the purpose is to identify a safe range for heart rate during exercise, regardless of the presence or absence of coronary artery disease. (D) The purpose of stress testing is to identify a safe range for heart rate during exercise, regardless of the presence or absence of coronary artery disease.

744. (C) Nursing process phase: implementation; client need: psychosocial integrity; content area: medical/surgical—gerontological nursing

Rationale
(A) There is no assurance that the client will enjoy walking once a walking program is established. (B) Individuals who experience depression may not have the motivation to exercise, but this does not indicate a fear of exercise. Confrontation of fears might be more appropriate for clients experiencing a phobia. (C) Clients without evidence of coronary artery or other cardiovascular disease do not require stress testing if the planned exercise program consists only of walking. (D) The client does have a mental health diagnosis of de-

pression; however, this is not the reason that a stress test is not required for the walking program planned by the nurse.

745. (B) Nursing process phase: evaluation; client need: physiological integrity; content area: medical/surgical—gerontological nursing

Rationale
(A) This is an appropriate statement and indicates that the client has an understanding of the exercise regimen. (B) All exercise sessions should begin with 5 to 10 minutes of gentle stretching and flexibility exercises of the neck, trunk, and limbs. Only 2 or 3 minutes of exercise might place the client at high risk for musculoskeletal complications and myocardial ischemia. (C) Individuals should palpate the radial pulse in the first 10 seconds after ceasing activity and multiply by 6 to calculate their exercise heart rate. (D) Most studies show that an optimal training effect results from a 30-minute period of increased heart rate 3 to 4 times a week.

746. (C) Nursing process phase: implementation; client need: health promotion and maintenance; content area: medical/surgical—gerontological nursing

Rationale
(A) Walking and swimming are appropriate activities for older adults; however, jogging is inappropriate for older persons not already accustomed to this activity. (B) Walking and dancing are appropriate activities for older adults; however, jogging is inappropriate for older persons not already accustomed to this activity. (C) Walking, dancing, and swimming all provide excellent conditioning with less stress on the lower back and lower extremities. (D) While all these activities provide excellent conditioning for older adults, biking may increase muscle fatigue before an adequate heart rate is reached.

747. (D) Nursing process phase: implementation; client need: safe, effective care environment; content area: medical/surgical—gerontological nursing

Rationale
(A) The client with arthritis who is postarthroplasty surgery should be able to continue with an unsupervised exercise regimen that has been individualized for this condition. Very frail elderly persons and those with cognitive impairments precluding reliable self-monitoring should increase activity only under supervision. (B) Clients with history of mitral and aortic valve murmurs should be able to continue with an unsupervised exercise regimen that has been individualized for this condition. Very frail elderly persons and those with cognitive impairments precluding reliable self-monitoring should increase activity only under supervision. (C) A client with acute respiratory distress with pneumonia should be able to continue with an unsupervised exercise regimen that has been individualized for this condition. Very frail elderly persons and those with cognitive impairments precluding reliable self-monitoring should increase activity only under supervision. (D) Supervised exercise programs are recommended for very frail elderly persons and those with cognitive impairments precluding reliable self-monitoring.

748. (A) Nursing process phase: assessment; client need: physiological integrity; content area: medical/surgical—gerontological nursing

Rationale
(A) The Q wave, the first negative deflection on the EKG, is

not always seen. When seen, it may be normal or it may indicate myocardial infarction (necrosis). An abnormal Q wave appears 1 to 3 days after a transmural infarction. (B) A depressed ST segment suggests ischemia and/or injury to the inner or endocardial surface of the heart, which may be the result of angina. (C) An elevated ST segment reflects injury to the outer surface of the heart, the epicardium. (D) The T wave represents ventricular repolarization and is usually upright. Ischemia delays repolarization and causes the T wave to be inverted.

749. (A) Nursing process phase: implementation; client need: safe, effective care environment; content area: medical/surgical—gerontological nursing

Rationale
(A) A preoperative explanation of the recovery experience is a must. The client should first be introduced to the intensive care environment and to the equipment that will be necessary following surgery: the ventilator, a chest tube, an electrocardiogram monitor, and intravenous lines. A full explanation will prevent shocking the client and the family, who may not be expecting this experience. (B) Rarely is there a time when coronary artery bypass graft clients receive one-on-one nursing care. (C) Nursing care will include turning and deep-breathing, but pain management in the intensive care unit is not usually achieved through self-infusion. (D) This teaching is started preoperatively with the client and the family, but this teaching can continue throughout hospitalization. The essential teaching is that of the intensive care environment and expectations.

750. (B) Nursing process phase: analysis; client need: health promotion and maintenance; content area: medical/surgical—gerontological nursing

Rationale
(A) The two most common postoperative complications of coronary artery bypass graft surgery is reduced mobility and infection. Pain from the incision is to be expected. Mammary grafts may have longer and more severe chest-wall discomfort related to nerve injury at the harvesting site. (B) Pain from the incision is to be expected. Mammary grafts may have longer and more severe chest-wall discomfort related to nerve injury at the harvesting site. (C) There is nothing to suggest that the client who is 3 days' postoperative is having psychosomatic pain. (D) There is nothing to suggest that the client is becoming dependent on narcotic medication.

751. (A) Nursing process phase: implementation; client need: psychosocial integrity; content area: medical/surgical—gerontological nursing

Rationale
(A, B, & D) There are no restrictions to resuming marital relations following rehabilitation from bypass surgery. The exertion is often compared to climbing a flight of stairs and can be resumed when the client is so inclined. (C) Impotence is not an expected result of bypass surgery and may be a psychological response and should be followed up.

752. (B) Nursing process phase: implementation; client need: health promotion and maintenance; content area: medical/surgical—gerontological nursing

Rationale
(A) It is very common to experience muscle aches throughout the chest, upper back, shoulders, and neck. There is no rea-

son to call the physician for this occurrence. (B) It is very common to experience muscle aches throughout the chest, upper back, shoulders, and neck. An ice pack can be placed on the muscle for 15 minutes and reapplied three times a day as necessary. (C) It is very common to experience muscle aches throughout the chest, upper back, shoulders, and neck. An ice pack can be placed on the muscle for 15 minutes and reapplied three times a day as necessary. Medication is not recommended unless the spasms persist. (D) While muscle aches are common, they are uncomfortable, so the nurse should suggest placing an ice pack on the area for 15 minutes three times a day as necessary.

753. (C) Nursing process phase: assessment; client need: safe, effective care environment; content area: medical/surgical—gerontological nursing

Rationale
(A) Constipation may occur with procainamide, but is not life-threatening. (B) Dizziness may occur with procainamide, especially with older adults, but is not life-threatening. (C) Investigate even a vague change such as shivering or fever because these may signal agranulocytosis. (D) Procainamide produces gastrointestinal irritation in some individuals. To lessen the irritation, the drug may be taken with or after meals. This side effect is not life-threatening.

754. (C) Nursing process phase: evaluation; client need: physiological integrity; content area: medical/surgical—gerontological nursing

Rationale
(A) The client should not take a missed dose of medication, but should be cautioned to take the next regularly prescribed dose at the appropriate time. (B) Procainamide can be given as a long-term therapy as long as the client does not have adverse drug reactions or inappropriate blood values. Sensitivity to this drug is not suggested. (C) Any symptoms of unusual bleeding or bruising should be reported immediately. (D) Dizziness is an expected side effect of procainamide, and the client should be taught to be careful when rising from a sitting to a standing position. This side effect however is not as crucial as bleeding.

755. (C) Nursing process phase: implementation; client need: health promotion and maintenance; content area: medical/surgical—gerontological nursing

Rationale
(A & C) The first wave (P) represents atrial depolarization. High-pointed P waves occur with pulmonary disease. (B) High-pointed P waves occur with pulmonary disease and do not necessitate having a cardiac arrest cart nearby. (D) While the kidneys may try to regulate fluid and electrolyte imbalance, the high-pointed P waves indicate pulmonary disease, so the nurse should assess and monitor pulmonary status.

756. (D) Nursing process phase: analysis; client need: safe, effective care environment; content area: medical/surgical—gerontological nursing

Rationale
(A & D) The purpose of the pacemaker is to sense and to pace. In sensing, the device detects the heart's own electrical activity. The pacemaker is programmed to allow no heart rate lower than 60 beats per minute. If the heart depolarizes spontaneously and contracts unaided, the pacemaker will reset itself. Therefore, the heart is allowed to beat and contract on its

own before the pacemaker performs this action. (B & C) The standard permanent pacemaker will not speed or slow the rhythm of the heart—its only mission is to prevent bradycardia.

757. (A) Nursing process phase: analysis; client need: safe, effective care environment; content area: medical/surgical—gerontological nursing

Rationale
(A) A pacemaker that can sense and pace in the ventricle and is inhibited by the client's own ventricular depolarization is said to be in the VVI mode. (B) A pacemaker that is triggered will be followed by a T or a D, which indicates the device's response to the sensing of natural heart depolarization: T for triggered, I for inhibited, or D for dual. (C & D) A pacemaker that is sensed in the atrium and the ventricles will be coded D for dual. This will be followed by a T or a D, which indicates the device's response to the sensing of natural heart depolarization, T for triggered, I for inhibited, or D for dual.

758. (B) Nursing process phase: implementation; client need: physiological integrity; content area: medical/surgical—gerontological nursing

Rationale
(A & C) The best paddle position is anterior-posterior. Care should be taken to avoid placing a paddle on, or within a few inches of, the pacemaker since the defibrillator's discharge may damage it. (B) The best paddle position when a client must be defibrillated is the anterior-posterior position. (D) The information given to the physician is not important if the client needs defibrillation.

759. (C) Nursing process phase: planning; client need: safe, effective care environment; content area: medical/surgical—gerontological nursing

Rationale
(A) There is little need for adherence to a dietary regimen following pacemaker implant. (B) While exercise is important, there is little need for adherence to a strict exercise regimen following pacemaker implant. (C) Client should be instructed early on to watch for and monitor signs of infection at the implant site, including pain or tenderness, local heat or erythema, drainage, or wound dehiscence. (D) Follow-up checks are important, but the client is not able to check pacemaker batteries. Follow-up examinations are usually at 3-month intervals.

760. (C) Nursing process phase: assessment; client need: physiological integrity; content area: medical/surgical—gerontological nursing

Rationale
(A) Pacemaker implant does not result in prolonged bedrest. Undue fatigue, dizziness, syncope, and dyspnea may signal a drop in cardiac output. (B) The client may have a fear of pacemaker failure; however, undue fatigue, dizziness, syncope, and dyspnea may signal a drop in cardiac output. (C) Undue fatigue, dizziness, syncope, and dyspnea may signal a drop in cardiac output. (D) There is nothing to suggest that these symptoms are psychosomatic or that the client needs individualized attention from the nurse.

761. (B) Nursing process phase: implementation; client need: physiological integrity; content area: medical/surgical—gerontological nursing

Rationale
(A) Dizziness and shortness of breath may indicate a drop in cardiac output. The initial action by the nurse should be to place the client in bed and have him rest immediately to reduce the need for more cardiac output. Reassurance may assist the client emotionally, but does little to decrease the need for cardiac output. (B & D) Dizziness and shortness of breath may indicate a drop in cardiac output. The initial action by the nurse should be to place the client in bed and have him rest immediately to reduce the need for more cardiac output. (C) Dizziness and shortness of breath may indicate a drop in cardiac output. The initial action by the nurse should be to place the client in bed and have him rest immediately to reduce the need for more cardiac output. Thereafter, the vital signs should be monitored every 15 minutes, not hourly.

762. (B) Nursing process phase: implementation; client need: psychosocial integrity; content area: medical/surgical—gerontological nursing

Rationale
(A) There will be follow-up examinations, but these can be done by phone every 3 months or so using a telephone transmitter supplied by the physician. (B) Because pacemakers will trigger alarms in metal detectors, the client should be advised to show his pacemaker identification card to airport security personnel before passing through the detector. (C & D) Once the client is dismissed from the hospital, the client is free to resume regular activities of daily living and is encouraged to do so.

763. (B) Nursing process phase: implementation; client need: physiological integrity; content area: medical/surgical—gerontological nursing

Rationale
(A) Informing the hospital is not appropriate because the client is in need of supervision from the cardiologist. (B & D) Significant pulse deficits are often the first indication that the pacemaker is not working correctly. Reporting this to the physician might remedy the situation early on. (C) The initial action by the nurse is to call the physician, who in turn may want an EKG run to determine the amount of pacing and capturing.

764. (D) Nursing process phase: analysis; client need: health promotion and maintenance; content area: medical/surgical—gerontological nursing

Rationale
(A & D) Both the model number and the serial number are needed to reprogram a pacemaker. (B & C) The information needed to reprogram a pacemaker is the model number and the serial number.

765. (B) Nursing process phase: implementation; client need: safe, effective care environment; content area: medical/surgical—gerontological nursing

Rationale
(A) There is nothing to suggest that the client is taking a medication that causes postural hypotension. The symptoms exhibited by the client are indicative of isolated systolic hypotension. (B) Symptoms of isolated systolic hypotension include headache, dizziness, and increased vital signs. (C) These are not normal aging changes. (D) The client may need dietary consultation and teaching; however, this condi-

tion should be carefully assessed by the nurse and followed up with a physician to determine the treatment of choice.

766. (D) Nursing process phase: assessment; client need: physiological integrity; content area: medical/surgical—gerontological nursing

Rationale
(A) Tachypnea is a symptom of left-sided CHF. (B) Pink, frothy sputum indicates pulmonary edema. (C) Korotkoff's sounds are a symptom of left-sided CHF. (D) Symptoms of right-sided CHF include orthostatic hypotension, edema, distended jugular veins, liver enlargement, and S_3 gallops.

767. (B) Nursing process phase: implementation; client need: health promotion and maintenance; content area: medical/surgical—gerontological nursing

Rationale
(A) While furosemide does place the client at high risk for postural hypotension, the client is getting a potassium supplement in combination with enalapril, an angiotensin converting enzyme inhibitor (ACE). ACE inhibitors may increase potassium levels, and even though this has been prescribed by the physician, the nurse must be aware of the potential for a drug interaction. (B) The client is getting a potassium supplement in combination with enalapril, an angiotensin converting enzyme inhibitor (ACE). ACE inhibitors may increase potassium levels, and even though this has been prescribed by the physician, the nurse must be aware of the potential for drug interaction. (C) While postural hypotension is an important aspect of care and should be included in client teaching, the potential for hyperkalemia is more serious and therefore is essential for the nurse to monitor. (D) The medications prescribed for this client are not associated with anorexia or decreased appetite and weight loss should not occur.

768. (C) Nursing process phase: implementation; client need: safe, effective care environment; content area: medical/surgical—gerontological nursing

Rationale
(A) While this action is important, the client has 3 months before being seen by the physician; however, medications present a daily problem for the client with decreased visual acuity and forgetfulness. (B) While this action is important, the client is experiencing periods of forgetfulness. Teaching about the need for compliance does not assure it, nor does it deal with the problems that the client has—forgetfulness, decreased visual acuity, and medications. (C) Preparing a prefilled medication organizer weekly will assist the client to know if the medication has been taken and allows the nurse to monitor compliance. (D) Color coding the medication bottles may not be the best action for a client who has decreased visual acuity.

769. (B) Nursing process phase: implementation; client need: health promotion and maintenance; content area: medical/surgical—gerontological nursing

Rationale
(A & B) Alcohol interferes with REM sleep and should be avoided when possible. (C) The client with sleep apnea is encouraged to avoid any medication that might interfere with sleep, including stimulants, sedatives, or hypnotics. (D) Clients with sleep apnea are encouraged to join in weight-loss programs. A high-calorie, protein-rich food right before bedtime is not appropriate for weight loss.

770. (C) Nursing process phase: analysis; client need: health promotion and maintenance; content area: medical/surgical—gerontological nursing

Rationale
(A) There is nothing to suggest that complaints of aches and pains in older adults occur more often than in younger populations or that it leads to an increase in prescription drug use. (B) Not all people qualify for Medicare, and this is not a justified rationale for the increase in prescription drug use. (C) Eighty percent of older adults suffer from one or more chronic long-term illness, which necessitate the use of prescription drug use. (D) Advancing age may bring about some physical disabilities; however, most prescription drugs are for chronic long-term conditions.

771. (D) Nursing process phase: analysis; client need: health promotion and maintenance; content area: medical/surgical—gerontological nursing

Rationale
(A) While a depressed client may experience anxiety, this is not the rationale for the hyperactivity experienced by the client. (B) Paroxetine may cause somnolence, sweating, tremors, and fatigue, but anxiety is not associated with paroxetine. (C) Insomnia can be caused by anxiety and depression, but this response by the nurse does not answer the question of the hyperactivity experienced by the client. (D) The client does have symptoms of hypothyroidism and drug interaction, so this should be assessed by the physician and the nurse.

772. (D) Nursing process phase: implementation; client need: health promotion and maintenance; content area: medical/surgical—gerontological nursing

Rationale
(A) While increasing fruits, fiber, and fluids is an appropriate nursing action with the client history of previous cancer of the colon and the recent change in bowel habit, this should be evaluated by a physician. (B) Any recent change is bowel habit should be carefully assessed. Constipation is not a normal aging change. (C) Taking an over-the-counter stool softener may mask the symptoms exhibited by the client and make diagnoses difficult. (D) With the client's history of previous cancer of the colon and the recent change in bowel habit, this should be evaluated by a physician.

773. (C) Nursing process phase: analysis; client need: physiological integrity; content area: medical/surgical—gerontological nursing

Rationale
(A) These are not signs and symptoms expected as a reaction to the medications being taken by the client. (B) These are not normal symptoms of a normal grief reaction for the spouse. (C) The nurse correctly identifies that these responses are most likely symptoms of dehydration because the client is receiving diuretic therapy and may not have an adequate intake of fluid. (D) These are not symptoms of an infectious process other than elevated temperature.

774. (D) Nursing process phase: planning; client need: health promotion and maintenance; content area: medical/surgical—gerontological nursing

Rationale
(A) There is nothing noted in this situation that the client has family or that the family would be willing or able to assist. Also,

there is no assurance that with family involvement, compliance would be the outcome. (B) While the client lives in low-income housing, there is nothing to suggest that this client has a need for financial assistance. (C) If the client has some difficulty with learning, the educational level might be such that educational reading materials would be helpful to the client. (D) A newly diagnosed older adult with diabetes will have to learn new lifestyle behaviors. The nurse should prepare a carefully structured individualized plan to assist the client to learn new lifestyle behaviors and to implement these changes in daily living.

775. (C) Nursing process phase: implementation; client need: safe, effective care environment; content area: medical/surgical—gerontological nursing

Rationale
(A) This medication is usually prescribed to be taken 1 hour prior to meals—not 1 hour after meals. (B) While this is a concern with clients who have CHF heart failure and who are prescribed this drug, the potential interaction with lithium is a more serious concern. (C) Captopril may increase lithium concentrations and lead to toxicity. (D) There is nothing to suggest that this client with a bipolar disorder is unable to maintain compliance because of the mental illness.

776. (B) Nursing process phase: implementation; client need: physiological integrity; content area: medical/surgical—gerontological nursing

Rationale
(A) This may be important, but the client has a normal blood sugar for an older adult. (B & D) A 2-hour blood glucose of 200 is normal and requires only to be monitored by the nurse. (C) This is not a priority because this is normal for older adults.

777. (A) Nursing process phase: analysis; client need: health promotion and maintenance; content area: medical/surgical—gerontological nursing

Rationale
(A) Despite the high prevalence of hearing loss among the elderly, only about 30 percent of those who need hearing aids actually have them. (B) Impaired hearing is common in older adults and at least 90 percent of the elderly living in nursing homes are affected by hearing loss. (C) Hearing loss is not a normal aging change. (D) Most hearing impairments occurring in older adults can be helped with the assistance of hearing devices.

778. (B) Nursing process phase: assessment; client need: safe, effective care environment; content area: medical/surgical—gerontological nursing

Rationale
(A) A client with sensorineural hearing loss may speak in an excessively loud voice in many situations where a loud voice is inappropriate. (B) The client with a conductive hearing loss usually speaks in a relatively quiet voice, making it difficult to hear him. (C) A client with sensorineural hearing loss may be sensitive to loud intensities of sound and hear better in a quiet environment. (D) While the tympanic membrane may appear sclerotic and scarred in the older adult, these changes do not usually affect hearing.

779. (D) Nursing process phase: analysis; client need: health

promotion and maintenance; content area: medical/surgical—gerontological nursing

Rationale
(A) While the tympanic membrane may appear sclerotic and scarred in the older adult, these changes do not usually affect hearing. (B) Sensorineural hearing loss is caused by changes around the foramina of the acoustic nerve. (C) Presbycusis is the general term used to denote the gradual, progressive, permanent bilateral loss of hearing of high-frequency tones, caused by degenerative changes throughout the auditory system. (D) The total occlusion of the external canal by cerumen is the most common cause of a conductive deficit in the older adult.

780. (A) Nursing process phase: implementation; client need: health promotion and maintenance; content area: medical/surgical—gerontological nursing

Rationale
(A & D) A hearing aid can be ordered from the hearing aid vendor for a 2- to 4-week trial. If for any reason the client cannot adjust to amplification, the hearing aid can be returned to the vendor within 4 weeks, which is allowed by law. (B) Medicare reimbursement does not include hearing aids. (C) The Food and Drug Administration requires an examination by a physician prior to dispensing a hearing aid, but does not require the physician to purchase the aid.

781. (B) Nursing process phase: implementation; client need: safe, effective care environment; content area: medical/surgical—gerontological nursing

Rationale
(A, B, & D) If the poorer ear has a moderate loss of hearing and the better ear a mild loss, fit the poorer ear to enable the better ear to participate in communication situations. (C) If the poorer ear has a moderate loss of hearing and the better ear a mild loss, fit the poorer ear to enable the better ear to participate in communication situations. If the client requests the other ear, then the nurse should explain the rationale for inserting the hearing aid in the poorer ear.

782. (C) Nursing process phase: implementation; client need: health promotion and maintenance; content area: medical/surgical—gerontological nursing

Rationale
(A–D) The client should be instructed to wear the hearing aid 4 to 5 hours at first and for a longer period of time each day, removing the aid for bed, bathing, or showering.

783. (C) Nursing process phase: evaluation; client need: psychosocial integrity; content area: medical/surgical—gerontological nursing

Rationale
(A) The ear mold should be cleaned once a week with a cloth dampened with mild, soapy water. (B) If a whistle (feedback) is not heard when the volume control is fully on, change the battery and the whistle should be heard; if not, there is a problem with the aid. (C) Hearing aid batteries are changed every 10 days to 2 weeks. (D) There is no set maintenance schedule for a hearing aid.

784. (A) Nursing process phase: implementation; client need: psychosocial integrity; content area: medical/surgical—gerontological nursing

Rationale
(A) After living in a quiet world, suddenly hearing loud voices and noises can cause the client to become tense and nervous. Informing the client of this will assist the client in adapting to the hearing aid. (B) Adjusting the hearing aid in public or asking for assistance can be traumatic and embarrassing to the client. (C) Some clients may have physical impairments that make manipulation of the hearing aid batteries difficult or impossible, so the assistance of family members may be needed. (D) The hearing aid not only makes the speaker's voice louder, but it also amplifies everyone's speech and other noises in the room.

785. **(B)** Nursing process phase: implementation; client need: psychosocial integrity; content area: medical/surgical—gerontological nursing

Rationale
(A) The screening indicated the client had an impairment in hearing, while the audiologist evaluation did not. More sensitive equipment would be more likely to indicate impairment, not the opposite. (B) Anxiety might have affected the client's ability to hear and comprehend and therefore may have produced the results noted in the screening at the center. (C) While cerumen may have caused the difficulty in hearing, it is unlikely that it resolved itself without intervention. (D) Fee-induced medical services are not known to contribute to the attention and concentration of the older adult.

786. **(D)** Nursing process phase: analysis; client need: physiological integrity; content area: medical/surgical—gerontological nursing

Rationale
(A) This is not the result of a normal progression of hearing loss as a result of aging. (B) Cerumen causes a conductive hearing loss, while the symptoms are more characteristic of sensorineural loss. (C) The clinical picture is not consistent with Meniere's disease because of the lack of nausea and vertigo. (D) Medications may be a possibility for the hearing loss because ototoxic drugs affect hearing and vestibular function.

787. **(B)** Nursing process phase: analysis; client need: safe, effective care environment; content area: medical/surgical—gerontological nursing

Rationale
(A) While cataracts do cause visual difficulties, cataracts are corrected by surgery. (B) While this condition does not cause total blindness, macular degeneration is the leading cause of irreversible blindness in older adults. (C) Chronic blepharitis is a common ophthalmic problem in older adults and is the result of poor facial hygiene, lack of stimulation of the lid tissue, and secretion accumulation. This does not lead to blindness. (D) Diabetic retinopathy is not a common cause of irreversible blindness in older adults because clients with severe diabetes with proliferative retinopathy usually do not live to older adulthood.

788. **(C)** Nursing process phase: analysis; client need: safe, effective care environment; content area: medical/surgical—gerontological nursing

Rationale
(A–D) Because of the normal aging changes in the cardiovascular system, both the systolic and the diastolic pressure are increased with age.

789. **(B)** Nursing process phase: implementation; client need: health promotion and maintenance; content area: medical/surgical—gerontological nursing

Rationale
(A) Exercise and watching the intake of sodium are both recommended for the control of blood pressure. (B & C) The minimal daily adult intake of salt is 500 mg. (D) While eating fruits may be beneficial to the client, the minimal daily adult intake of salt is 500 mg.

790. **(C)** Nursing process phase: analysis; client need: safe, effective care environment; content area: medical/surgical—gerontological nursing

Rationale
(A) Trichiasis is a condition caused by scarring of the cornea and conjunctiva brought about by entropion. (B) Entropion is the inward turn of the lower lid, bringing the eyelashes at the lid margin in contact with the eyeball. (C) Ectropion occurs if the lower lid margin is no longer in contact with the globe, resulting in the inability of tears to drain properly. (D) Xanthelasma is a raised, yellowish, well-circumscribed plaque typically appearing along the nasal portion of the eyelids.

791. **(A)** Nursing process phase: analysis; client need: psychosocial integrity; content area: medical/surgical—gerontological nursing

Rationale
(A) The Developmental Task Theory developed by Havighurst in 1972 indicates that each individual must learn specific developmental tasks and that successful achievement contributes to the individual's happiness and feelings of success. (B) This is the eighth stage described by Erickson in which the individual feels that life has been successful or non-successful; achievement of this stage results in individuals feeling that they have been productive, successful individuals and thus are progressing toward healthy aging. (C) The wear-and-tear theory was developed by Selye, who states that the body systems wear out because of stress. (D) Ego transcendence is one of Peck's three developmental stages—not a theory.

792. **(D)** Nursing process phase: analysis; client need: safe, effective care environment; content area: medical/surgical—gerontological nursing

Rationale
(A–D) Medicare and Medicaid programs were enacted as part of the Social Security Amendments of 1965.

793. **(C)** Nursing process phase: analysis; client need: safe, effective care environment; content area: medical/surgical—gerontological nursing

Rationale
(A–D) Under the provision-of-care requirements, residents must be assessed to identify medical problems, describe their capacity to perform daily functions, and note any significant impairments in functional status. A state-specified instrument, the minimum data set (MDS) must be used to conduct this assessment.

794. **(C)** Nursing process phase: analysis; client need: health promotion and maintenance; content area: medical/surgical—gerontological nursing

Rationale
(A–D) According to research findings, decreased mortality re-

sulted from treatment of African-American males and females and white males aged 60 to 74 years whose diastolic pressures were in the range of 90 to 104 mm HG prior to treatment. There was no decrease in mortality in white women.

795. (C) Nursing process phase: implementation; client need: safe, effective care environment; content area: medical/surgical—gerontological nursing

Rationale
(A–C) Immediately after a stroke, the client can die from complications or neurological causes. Neither a medical nor a rehabilitation prognosis can be given during the first 48 hours following a stroke. (D) The nurse should have the knowledge that immediately after a stroke, the client can die from complications or neurological causes. Neither a medical nor a rehabilitation prognosis can be given during the first 48 hours, and the nurse can explain this to the family.

796. (B) Nursing process phase: analysis; client need: health promotion and maintenance; content area: medical/surgical—gerontological nursing

Rationale
(A–D) The most common malignancy of the thyroid in older adults is a follicular carcinoma.

797. (A) Nursing process phase: assessment; client need: health promotion and maintenance; content area: medical/surgical—gerontological nursing

Rationale
(A–D) The T_4 by RIA is the best screening test for hypothyroidism and should be performed along with a T_3 resin uptake.

798. (C) Nursing process phase: implementation; client need: physiological integrity; content area: medical/surgical—gerontological nursing

Rationale
(A) If the client's weight is within normal limits, encouraging an additional 5-pound weight loss would be inappropriate. (B) Appetite suppressants are not recommended for older adults. Because the client' weight is within normal limits, the nurse should encourage adherence to the present dietary regimen. (C) Because the client's weight is within the normal limits, the nurse should encourage adherence to the present dietary regimen and inform the client that there is no evidence that less than normal weight is more healthy. (D) This might be an appropriate action if the nurse recognizes the need for dietary information; however, the client's weight is within the normal limits. If the client continues to be concerned with weight following this information, dietary consultation may be recommended.

799. (A) Nursing process phase: implementation; client need: safe, effective care environment; content area: medical/surgical—gerontological nursing

Rationale
(A) The confusion experienced by the client may be caused by the cimetidine. Discontinuing this medication is the first action to evaluate the cause of confusion. (B) There is little need at this point to evaluate for physiological causes of confusion until the nurse has ruled out the obvious causes. (C) A mental evaluation for dementia is not warranted at this time. (D) The mental confusion experienced by the client is a nor-

mal drug interaction with cimetidine and does not require hospitalization to correct.

800. (B) Nursing process phase: implementation; client need: health promotion and maintenance; content area: medical/surgical—gerontological nursing

Rationale
(A & B) Because of the vulnerability of the teeth and soft tissues in the mouth of older adults, a dental evaluation is recommended every 6 months. (C) Because of the vulnerability of the teeth and soft tissues in the mouth of older adults, a dental evaluation is recommended every 6 months. Every 3 months would be necessary only if a problem is discovered. (D) Because of the vulnerability of the teeth and soft tissues in the mouth of older adults, a dental evaluation is recommended every 6 months. Because of decreased visual acuity, the older adult may be unaware of excess plaque buildup.

801. (B) Nursing process phase: assessment; client need: safe, effective care environment; content area: medical/surgical—gerontological nursing

Rationale
(A) While federal regulations do mandate oral assessment, the most appropriate reason for conducting monthly oral examinations is to identify dental problems, which occur with increasing frequency as one ages. (B) Of the 30 percent of persons with natural teeth, 90 percent demonstrate significant periodontal (gingival) disease, loss of alveolar bone, and dental decay. Monthly oral examinations will assist the nurse to identify dental problems early and to seek intervention. (C) Only about 30 percent of nursing home residents are dentulous. (D) The institution may require monthly oral examinations, but this is not the most appropriate rationale for performing this assessment.

802. (A) Nursing process phase: implementation; client need: physiological integrity; content area: medical/surgical—gerontological nursing

Rationale
(A) This lesion is probably candidiasis and is best diagnosed by a culture. The nystatin rinse is the treatment most often used for this condition. (B) There is no reason for a biopsy of this area, because the characteristics contraindicate biopsy or malignancy. (C) Antibiotics are not effective for fungal infections such as candidiasis, which fits the description of this lesion. (D) Any lesion on the palate should require intervention because this is not normal and may not be the result of poor oral hygiene.

803. (C) Nursing process phase: implementation; client need: safe, effective care environment; content area: medical/surgical—gerontological nursing

Rationale
(A) Because it decreases anxiety, this would be an appropriate dosage of this medication for a client with organic brain syndrome who is agitated prior to a diagnostic procedure. (B) Because it decreases anxiety with its sedative effect, this would be an appropriate dosage of this medication for a client with organic brain syndrome who is agitated prior to a diagnostic procedure. (C) Narcotics are not recommended for older adults because of the hypotension and other side effects that might increase symptoms. (D) Because it decreases anxiety and is used to control aggressive behavior in cognitively impaired clients, this would be an appropriate dosage of this

medication for a client with organic brain syndrome who is agitated prior to a diagnostic procedure.

804. (B) Nursing process phase: implementation; client need: health promotion and maintenance; content area: medical/surgical—gerontological nursing

Rationale

(A) There is no need for the vital signs to be monitored either before or after for a dental examination and cleaning. (B & D) The American Dental Association recommends that a client who has a history of rheumatic heart disease should be treated with penicillin therapy at least 1 hour prior to the cleaning and every 6 hours thereafter for eight doses to prevent further damage to the vessels. (C) There is little need for an antianxiety medication for an older adult who is having a dental examination.

805. (B) Nursing process phase: assessment; client need: health promotion and maintenance; content area: medical/surgical—gerontological nursing

Rationale

(A) Beginning gangrenous conditions include impaired circulation, resulting in death to the tissues. The extremity will have a deep blue to black appearance. Pain may or may not be present. (B) Onychomycosis is a fungal infection of the nail that appears discolored, ranging from yellow-brown to green in appearance. Inflammation surrounding the nail may be a complicating factor and result in cellulitis. (C) Arterial insufficiency may present a blueness to the extremity and make the older adult prone to ulcers. There is decreased temperature and sensation. (D) The signs and symptoms of deep-vein thrombosis include warmness to the extremity, shiny reddened appearance, and tenderness to touch.

806. (B) Nursing process phase: implementation; client need: physiological integrity; content area: medical/surgical—gerontological nursing

Rationale

(A) Clients often blame foot problems on improperly fitted shoes, and although this may contribute to the discomfort and irritation, it is not the primary cause of the callus. (B) Contributing to the development of hyperkeratotic lesions are factors such as weight-bearing imbalances, vascular disease, diabetes mellitus, and soft-tissue disease. (C) Walking without shoes is not a contributing factor in weight-bearing imbalances. (D) A podiatrist may be used to assist with disorders of the feet, but this does not contribute to the cause of calluses.

807. (C) Nursing process phase: analysis; client need: safe, effective care environment; content area: medical/surgical—gerontological nursing

Rationale

(A–D) Gerontology is the study of the biological, sociological, and psychological aspects of aging. Geriatrics is focused on how to prevent or manage the diseases of aging.

808. (D) Nursing process phase: analysis; client need: health promotion and maintenance; content area: medical/surgical—gerontological nursing

Rationale

(A–D) Sex differences in life expectancy have declined since 1980 when females born that year could expect to live 7.4 years more than men.

809. (C) Nursing process phase: implementation; client need: safe, effective care environment; content area: medical/surgical—gerontological nursing

Rationale

(A) A time-dimensional longitudinal design measures the attitudes of one group over a period of time. (B) A time-sequential design measures the changes between two or more groups over two or more periods of time. Persons who are 60 years old today are compared to persons who will be 60 years old in 10 years, for example. (C) With the cross-sequential design, the researcher compares the attitudes of people who were age 50 in 1960 and again in 1970 when they are 60. (D) This design measures the attitudes of one group of people with the attitudes of another group of people. These are followed over a period of years.

810. (D) Nursing process phase: evaluation; client need: safe, effective care environment; content area: medical/surgical—gerontological nursing

Rationale

(A–D) Although the AARP is a organization made up of older adults, healthy, more financially secure members are overrepresented. This population would not be representative of the needs of ethnic minorities.

811. (A) Nursing process phase: analysis; client need: psychosocial integrity; content area: medical/surgical—gerontological nursing

Rationale

(A) Social theories attempt to answer questions of how people adapt to the changes characteristically associated with aging. (B & C) While this might be one aspect of social theory, social theories attempt to answer questions of how people adapt to the changes characteristically associated with aging. (D) Social theories might look at how physiological changes affect the social and psychological nature of the individual, but not the effects of these changes on society.

812. (A) Nursing process phase: implementation; client need: psychosocial integrity; content area: medical/surgical—gerontological nursing

Rationale

(A) The activity theory presumes that a person's self-concept is validated through participation in life, such as keeping busy and remaining active. It is consistent with our society's value system, which emphasizes work and productivity. (B) The learned-helplessness theory is a theory related to depression. The individual is confronted with a negative life event and feels that control is lost. The person loses motivation and becomes depressed. (C) The generativity versus despair theory is a life stage outlined by Erikson. In this stage, the successful person feels he or she has accomplished life's goals and is able to prepare for death. The person who feels that the accomplishment of life's goals has not been met will have feelings of despair. (D) The disengagement theory suggests that older people decrease their activity and seek more passive roles, finally withdrawing from society in preparing for death. This is a mutual process.

813. (C) Nursing process phase: implementation; client need: physiological integrity; content area: medical/surgical—gerontological nursing

Rationale

(A–D) Normal physiological changes alter sexual response.

These changes include a slower response to sexual stimulation, with a longer time needed to obtain an erection; less full erections; decreased volume and force of ejaculation; occasional lack of orgasm during intercourse; and increased length of time between orgasm and subsequent erections.

814. **(B)** Nursing process phase: analysis; client need: health promotion and maintenance; content area: medical/surgical—gerontological nursing

Rationale
(A) Although Medicare services may be of interest, Healthy People 2000 indicates that attention should be given to the health promotion and disease prevention needs of older people. (B–D) In the Surgeon General's latest report, Healthy People 2000, major attention is given to the health promotion and disease prevention needs of older people.

815. **(A)** Nursing process phase: implementation; client need: health promotion and maintenance; content area: medical/surgical—gerontological nursing

Rationale
(A) Three of the four most common causes of death among older adults—heart disease, cancer, and stroke—are the result of an unhealthy lifestyle. (B) While some older adults do not get enough regularly scheduled exercise, this is not the reason a nurse would present a program on exercise. (C) This is a true statement, but it is not the rationale for a program on exercise. Three of the four most common causes of death among older adults—heart disease, cancer, and stroke—are the result of an unhealthy lifestyle. (D) Mobility problems are a concern to some older adults, but the rationale for an exercise program is for a change in lifestyle behavior.

816. **(C)** Nursing process phase: analysis; client need: health promotion and maintenance; content area: medical/surgical—gerontological nursing

Rationale
(A, B, & D) Hispanic whites will be the largest ethnic group in the future because of the group's high birth rates and large percentage of younger women. (C) Current 1990 census data estimate the population makeup as 8 percent Hispanic with a growth rate of 44 percent. Hispanic whites will be the largest ethnic group in the future because of the group's high birth rates and younger women.

FOCUS ON MEDICAL/SURGICAL DRUG DOSAGES

817. **(A)** Nursing process phase: implementation; client need: safe, effective care environment; content area: medical/surgical nursing—dosage calculation

Rationale
1000 mg : 1 ml = 250 mg : x = 0.25 ml
Math calculation explains incorrect answers.

818. **(D)** Nursing process phase: implementation; client need: safe, effective care environment; content area: medical/surgical nursing—dosage calculation

Rationale
200 mg : 1 tablet = 1000 mg : x = 5 tablets

819. **(D)** Nursing process phase: implementation; client need: safe, effective care environment; content area: medical/surgical nursing—dosage calculation

Rationale
250 mg : 1 tablet = 500 mg : x = 2 tablets
Math calculation explains incorrect answers.

820. **(A)** Nursing process phase: implementation; client need: safe, effective care environment; content area: medical/surgical nursing—dosage calculation

Rationale
10 mg : 1 capsule = 10 mg : x = 1 capsule
Math calculation explains incorrect answers.

821. **(B)** Nursing process phase: implementation; client need: safe, effective care environment; content area: medical/surgical nursing—dosage calculation

Rationale
25 μg/spray × 2 sprays = 50 μg
Math calculation explains incorrect answers.

822. **(D)** Nursing process phase: implementation; client need: safe, effective care environment; content area: medical/surgical nursing—dosage calculation

Rationale
3 mg : 1 tablet = 6 mg : x = 2 tablets
Math calculation explains incorrect answers.

823. **(A)** Nursing process phase: implementation; client need: safe, effective care environment; content area: medical/surgical nursing—dosage calculation

Rationale
1000 mg : 1 ml = 500 mg : x = 0.5 ml
Math calculation explains incorrect answers.

824. **(D)** Nursing process phase: implementation; client need: safe, effective care environment; content area: medical/surgical nursing—dosage calculation

Rationale
50 mg : 1 ml = 100 mg : x = 2.0 ml
Math calculation explains incorrect answers.

825. **(D)** Nursing process phase: implementation; client need: safe, effective care environment; content area: medical/surgical nursing—dosage calculation

Rationale
50 mg : 1 tablet = 100 mg : x = 2 tablets
Math calculation explains incorrect answers.

826. **(C)** Nursing process phase: implementation; client need: safe, effective care environment; content area: medical/surgical nursing—dosage calculation

Rationale
80 units : 1 ml = 300 units : x = 37.5 ml
Math calculation explains incorrect answers.

827. **(D)** Nursing process phase: implementation; client need: safe, effective care environment; content area: medical/surgical nursing—dosage calculation

Rationale
400 mg : 5 ml = x : 10 ml = 800 mg
Math calculation explains incorrect answers.

828. **(B)** Nursing process phase: implementation; client need: safe, effective care environment; content area: medical/surgical nursing—dosage calculation

Rationale
100 mg : 1 tablet = 100 mg : x = 1 tablet
Math calculation explains incorrect answers.

829. **(B)** Nursing process phase: implementation; client need: safe, effective care environment; content area: medical/surgical nursing—dosage calculation

Rationale
250 mg : 1 ml = 250 mg : x = 1 ml
Math calculation explains incorrect answers.

830. **(D)** Nursing process phase: implementation; client need: safe, effective care environment; content area: medical/surgical nursing—dosage calculation

Rationale
250 mg : 1 ml = 5000 mg : x = 20 ml
Math calculation explains incorrect answers.

831. **(C)** Nursing process phase: implementation; client need: safe, effective care environment; content area: medical/surgical nursing—dosage calculation

Rationale
325 mg : 1 tablet = 975 mg : x = 3 tablets
Math calculation explains incorrect answers.

832. **(C)** Nursing process phase: implementation; client need: safe, effective care environment; content area: medical/surgical nursing—dosage calculation

Rationale
600 mg : 5 ml = 500 mg: : x = 4.2 ml
Math calculation explains incorrect answers.

833. **(D)** Nursing process phase: implementation; client need: safe, effective care environment; content area: medical/surgical nursing—dosage calculation

Rationale
125 mg : 5 ml = 500 mg : x = 20 ml
Math calculation explains incorrect answers.

834. **(C)** Nursing process phase: implementation; client need: safe, effective care environment; content area: medical/surgical nursing—dosage calculation

Rationale
250 mg : 5 ml = 345 mg : x = 1.4 ml
Math calculation explains incorrect answers.

835. **(D)** Nursing process phase: implementation; client need: safe, effective care environment; content area: medical/surgical nursing—dosage calculation

Rationale
325 mg : 1 tablet = 650 mg : x = 2 tablets
Math calculation explains incorrect answers.

836. **(C)** Nursing process phase: implementation; client need: safe, effective care environment; content area: medical/surgical nursing—dosage calculation

Rationale
500 mg : 1 tablet = 3000 mg : x = 6 tablets
Math calculation explains incorrect answers.

837. **(D)** Nursing process phase: implementation; client need: safe, effective care environment; content area: medical/surgical nursing—dosage calculation

Rationale
300 mg : 1 tablet = 600 mg : x = 2 tablets
Math calculation explains incorrect answers.

838. **(B)** Nursing process phase: implementation; client need: safe, effective care environment; content area: medical/surgical nursing—dosage calculation

Rationale
1 gm : 1 ml = 1 gm : x = 1 ml
Math calculation explains incorrect answers.

839. **(A)** Nursing process phase: implementation; client need: safe, effective care environment; content area: medical/surgical nursing—dosage calculation

Rationale
50 mg : 1 tablet = 25 mg : x = ½ tablet
Math calculation explains incorrect answers.

840. **(D)** Nursing process phase: implementation; client need: safe, effective care environment; content area: medical/surgical nursing—dosage calculation

Rationale
250 mg : 1 tablet = 500 mg : x = 2 tablets
Math calculation explains incorrect answers.

841. **(C)** Nursing process phase: implementation; client need: safe, effective care environment; content area: medical/surgical nursing—dosage calculation

Rationale
600 mg : 5 ml = 400 mg : x = 3.3 ml
Math calculation explains incorrect answers.

842. **(D)** Nursing process phase: implementation; client need: safe, effective care environment; content area: medical/surgical nursing—dosage calculation

Rationale
25 mg : 1 chewable tablet = 50 mg : x = 2 chewable tablets
Math calculation explains incorrect answers.

843. **(C)** Nursing process phase: implementation; client need: safe, effective care environment; content area: medical/surgical nursing—dosage calculation

Rationale
500 mg : 5 ml = 1700 mg : x = 17 ml
Math calculation explains incorrect answers.

844. **(C)** Nursing process phase: implementation; client need: safe, effective care environment; content area: medical/surgical nursing—dosage calculation

Rationale
10 mg : 1 tablet = 15 mg : x = 1½ tablet
Math calculation explains incorrect answers.

845. (C) Nursing process phase: implementation; client need: safe, effective care environment; content area: medical/surgical nursing—dosage calculation

Rationale
$$120 \ \mu g : 1 \ ml = 150 \ \mu g : x = 1.25 \ ml$$
Math calculation explains incorrect answers.

846. (B) Nursing process phase: implementation; client need: safe, effective care environment; content area: medical/surgical nursing—dosage calculation

Rationale
$$5 \ mg : 1 \ tablet = 5 \ mg : x = 1 \ tablet$$
Math calculation explains incorrect answers.

847. (B) Nursing process phase: implementation; client need: safe, effective care environment; content area: medical/surgical nursing—dosage calculation

Rationale
$$5 \ mg : 1 \ ml = 2 \ mg : x = 0.4 \ ml$$
Math calculation explains incorrect answers.

848. (D) Nursing process phase: implementation; client need: safe, effective care environment; content area: medical/surgical nursing—dosage calculation

Rationale
$$250 \ mg : 1 \ tablet = 500 \ mg : x = 2 \ tablets$$
Math calculation explains incorrect answers.

849. (B) Nursing process phase: implementation; client need: safe, effective care environment; content area: medical/surgical nursing—dosage calculation

Rationale
$$100 \ mg : 1 \ tablet = 400 \ mg : x = 4 \ tablets$$
Math calculation explains incorrect answers.

850. (D) Nursing process phase: implementation; client need: safe, effective care environment; content area: medical/surgical nursing—dosage calculation

Rationale
$$100 \ mg : 1 \ tablet = 200 \ mg : x = 2 \ tablets$$
Math calculation explains incorrect answers.

851. (A) Nursing process phase: implementation; client need: safe, effective care environment; content area: medical/surgical nursing—dosage calculation

Rationale
$$60 \ mg : 1 \ tablet = 30 \ mg : x = \tfrac{1}{2} \ tablet$$
Math calculation explains incorrect answers.

852. (B) Nursing process phase: implementation; client need: safe, effective care environment; content area: medical/surgical nursing—dosage calculation

Rationale
$$10 \ mg : 1 \ tablet = 10 \ mg : x = 1 \ tablet$$
Math calculation explains incorrect answers.

853. (D) Nursing process phase: implementation; client need: safe, effective care environment; content area: medical/surgical nursing—dosage calculation

Rationale
$$1 \ mg : 5 \ ml = 1 \ mg : x = 5 \ ml$$
Math calculation explains incorrect answers.

854. (D) Nursing process phase: implementation; client need: safe, effective care environment; content area: medical/surgical nursing—dosage calculation

Rationale
$$10 \ mg : 1 \ ml = 80 \ mg : x = 8 \ ml$$
Math calculation explains incorrect answers.

855. (B) Nursing process phase: implementation; client need: safe, effective care environment; content area: medical/surgical nursing—dosage calculation

Rationale
$$10 \ mg : 1 \ tablet = 10 \ mg : x = 1 \ tablet$$
Math calculation explains incorrect answers.

856. (A) Nursing process phase: implementation; client need: safe, effective care environment; content area: medical/surgical nursing—dosage calculation

Rationale
$$20 \ mg : 1 \ tablet = 10 \ mg : x = \tfrac{1}{2} \ tablet$$
Math calculation explains incorrect answers.

857. (C) Nursing process phase: implementation; client need: safe, effective care environment; content area: medical/surgical nursing—dosage calculation

Rationale
$$100 \ mg : 1 \ ml = 75 \ mg : x = 0.75 \ ml$$
Math calculation explains incorrect answers.

858. (D) Nursing process phase: implementation; client need: safe, effective care environment; content area: medical/surgical nursing—dosage calculation

Rationale
$$400 \ mg : 1 \ tablet = 800 \ mg : x = 2 \ tablets$$
Math calculation explains incorrect answers.

859. (B) Nursing process phase: implementation; client need: safe, effective care environment; content area: medical/surgical nursing—dosage calculation

Rationale
$$150 \ mg \ \text{divided by} \ 100 \ mg \times 1 \ tablet = 1.5 \ tablets$$
Math calculation explains incorrect answers.

860. (C) Nursing process phase: implementation; client need: safe, effective care environment; content area: medical/surgical nursing—dosage calculation

Rationale
$$5{,}000 \ \text{units divided by} \ 10{,}000 \ \text{units} \times 1 \ ml = 0.5 \ ml$$
Math calculation explains incorrect answers.

861. (D) Nursing process phase: implementation; client need: safe, effective care environment; content area: medical/surgical nursing—dosage calculation

Rationale
$$16 \ mEq \ \text{divided by} \ 8 \ mEq \times 1 \ tablet = 2 \ tablets$$
Math calculation explains incorrect answers.

862. (C) Nursing process phase: implementation; client need: safe, effective care environment; content area: medical/surgical nursing—dosage calculation

Rationale
$$1 \ gr : 60 \ mg = \tfrac{1}{6} \ gr : x = 10 \ mg$$
$$10 \ mg : 5 \ ml = 10 \ mg : x = 5 \ ml$$
Math calculation explains incorrect answers.

863. (A) Nursing process phase: implementation; client need: safe, effective care environment; content area: medical/surgical nursing—dosage calculation

Rationale
        1000 mg divided by 250 mg × 5 ml = 20 ml
Math calculation explains incorrect answers.

864. (D) Nursing process phase: implementation; client need: safe, effective care environment; content area: medical/surgical nursing—dosage calculation

Rationale
        20 gms divided by 10 gms × 15 ml = 30 ml
Math calculation explains incorrect answers.

865. (B) Nursing process phase: implementation; client need: safe, effective care environment; content area: medical/surgical nursing—dosage calculation

Rationale
        A dose after each meal = 3 doses, plus 1 dose at bedtime makes a total of 4 containers needed.
Math calculation explains incorrect answers.

866. (A) Nursing process phase: implementation; client need: safe, effective care environment; content area: medical/surgical nursing—dosage calculation

Rationale
        10 mg divided by 2.5 mg × 1 tablet = 4 tablets
Math calculation explains incorrect answers.

867. (A) Nursing process phase: implementation; client need: safe, effective care environment; content area: medical/surgical nursing—dosage calculation

Rationale
        0.25 mg divided by 0.5 mg × 1 tablet = 0.5 tablet
Math calculation explains incorrect answers.

868. (B) Nursing process phase: implementation; client need: safe, effective care environment; content area: medical/surgical nursing—dosage calculation

Rationale
        350 mg divided by 125 mg × 5 ml = 14 ml
Math calculation explains incorrect answers.

869. (B) Nursing process phase: implementation; client need: safe, effective care environment; content area: medical/surgical nursing—dosage calculation

Rationale
        0.3 mg = 300 μg = 1 tablet
Math calculation explains incorrect answers.

870. (C) Nursing process phase: implementation; client need: safe, effective care environment; content area: medical/surgical nursing—dosage calculation

Rationale
        150 mg divided by 75 mg × 7.5 ml = 15 ml
Math calculation explains incorrect answers.

871. (A) Nursing process phase: implementation; client need: safe, effective care environment; content area: medical/surgical nursing—dosage calculation

Rationale
        84 kg × 50 mg = 4200 mg divided by 4 doses = 1050 mg
Math calculation explains incorrect answers.

872. (C) Nursing process phase: implementation; client need: safe, effective care environment; content area: medical/surgical nursing—dosage calculation

Rationale
        150 mg divided by 50 mg × 1 tablet = 3 tablets
Math calculation explains incorrect answers.

873. (D) Nursing process phase: implementation; client need: safe, effective care environment; content area: medical/surgical nursing—dosage calculation

Rationale
        750 mg × 3 doses = 2250 mg
Math calculation explains incorrect answers.

874. (D) Nursing process phase: implementation; client need: safe, effective care environment; content area: medical/surgical nursing—dosage calculation

Rationale
        75 mg divided by 25 mg × 1 ml = 3 ml
Math calculation explains incorrect answers.

875. (A) Nursing process phase: implementation; client need: safe, effective care environment; content area: medical/surgical nursing—dosage calculation

Rationale
The muscle of a 5-year-old can absorb only 1 cc of medication.

876. (D) Nursing process phase: implementation; client need: safe, effective care environment; content area: medical/surgical nursing—dosage calculation

Rationale
It takes 9 ml of normal saline to be mixed with 1 ml of morphine sulfate (10 mg) to deliver 1 mg/ml.

877. (A) Nursing process phase: implementation; client need: safe, effective care environment; content area: medical/surgical nursing—dosage calculation

Rationale
        150 mg divided by 300 mg × 2 ml = 1 ml
Math calculation explains incorrect answers.

878. (A) Nursing process phase: implementation; client need: safe, effective care environment; content area: medical/surgical nursing—dosage calculation

Rationale
        0.15 mg divided by 0.4 mg × 1 ml = 0.38 ml
Math calculation explains incorrect answers.

879. (D) Nursing process phase: implementation; client need: safe, effective care environment; content area: medical/surgical nursing—dosage calculation

Rationale
    2,400,000 units divided by 600,000 units × 1 ml = 4 ml
Math calculation explains incorrect answers.

880. (B) Nursing process phase: implementation; client need: safe, effective care environment; content area: medical/surgical nursing—dosage calculation

Rationale

200 mg divided by 100 mg $\times$ 1 ml = 2 ml
Math calculation explains incorrect answers.

881. **(C)** Nursing process phase: implementation; client need: safe, effective care environment; content area: medical/surgical nursing—dosage calculation

Rationale

30 units divided by 100 units $\times$ 1 ml = 0.30 ml
Math calculation explains incorrect answers.

882. **(D)** Nursing process phase: implementation; client need: safe, effective care environment; content area: medical/surgical nursing—dosage calculation

Rationale

2.4 mg divided by 4 mg $\times$ 1 ml = 0.6 ml
Math calculation explains incorrect answers.

883. **(C)** Nursing process phase: implementation; client need: safe, effective care environment; content area: medical/surgical nursing—dosage calculation

Rationale

500 mg divided by 1000 mg $\times$ 2.6 ml = 1.3 ml
Math calculation explains incorrect answers.

884. **(D)** Nursing process phase: implementation; client need: safe, effective care environment; content area: medical/surgical nursing—dosage calculation

Rationale

500 mg divided by 250 mg $\times$ 1.5 ml = 3.0 ml
Math calculation explains incorrect answers.

885. **(D)** Nursing process phase: implementation; client need: safe, effective care environment; content area: medical/surgical nursing—dosage calculation

Rationale

12 mg divided by 15 mg $\times$ 1 ml = 0.8 ml
Math calculation explains incorrect answers.

886. **(B)** Nursing process phase: implementation; client need: safe, effective care environment; content area: medical/surgical nursing—dosage calculation

Rationale

2.0 ml will deliver 1 gm of medication.
Math calculation explains incorrect answers.

887. **(D)** Nursing process phase: implementation; client need: safe, effective care environment; content area: medical/surgical nursing—dosage calculation

Rationale

1000 ml divided by 720 minutes = 83 ml/hr
Math calculation explains incorrect answers.

888. **(C)** Nursing process phase: implementation; client need: safe, effective care environment; content area: medical/surgical nursing—dosage calculation

Rationale

It will take 42 gtt/min to deliver 500 cc of fluid.
Math calculation explains incorrect answers.

889. **(D)** Nursing process phase: implementation; client need: safe, effective care environment; content area: medical/surgical nursing—dosage calculation

Rationale

450 ml divided by 90 minutes $\times$ 15 gtt/min = 75 gtt/min
Math calculation explains incorrect answers.

890. **(B)** Nursing process phase: implementation; client need: safe, effective care environment; content area: medical/surgical nursing—dosage calculation

Rationale

500 ml divided by 240 minutes $\times$ 60 gtt/min = 125 gtt/min
Math calculation explains incorrect answers.

891. **(B)** Nursing process phase: implementation; client need: safe, effective care environment; content area: medical/surgical nursing—dosage calculation

Rationale

50 ml : 30 min : x : 60 min = 100 ml/hr
Math calculation explains incorrect answers.

892. **(D)** Nursing process phase: implementation; client need: safe, effective care environment; content area: medical/surgical nursing—dosage calculation

Rationale

1800 ml divided by 15 hours = 120 ml/hr
Math calculation explains incorrect answers.

893. **(A)** Nursing process phase: implementation; client need: safe, effective care environment; content area: medical/surgical nursing—dosage calculation

Rationale

1200 ml divided by 360 minutes $\times$ 15 gtt/min = 50 gtt/min
Math calculation explains incorrect answers.

894. **(D)** Nursing process phase: implementation; client need: safe, effective care environment; content area: medical/surgical nursing—dosage calculation

Rationale

3000 ml divided by 24 hours = 125 ml divided by 60 min $\times$ 10 gtt/min = 21 gtt/min
Math calculation explains incorrect answers.

895. **(D)** Nursing process phase: implementation; client need: safe, effective care environment; content area: medical/surgical nursing—dosage calculation

Rationale

100 ml divided by 40 min $\times$ 20 gtt/min = 50 gtt/min
Math calculation explains incorrect answers.

896. **(A)** Nursing process phase: implementation; client need: safe, effective care environment; content area: medical/surgical nursing—dosage calculation

Rationale

25 ml divided by 60 min $\times$ 60 gtt/min = 25 gtt/min
Math calculation explains incorrect answers.

897. **(C)** Nursing process phase: implementation; client need: safe, effective care environment; content area: medical/surgical nursing—dosage calculation

Rationale

1000 ml divided by 240 min $\times$ 20 gtt/min = 83 gtt/min
Math calculation explains incorrect answers.

898. **(D)** Nursing process phase: implementation; client need: safe, effective care environment; content area: medical/surgical nursing—dosage calculation

Rationale

1500 ml divided by 12 hours = 125 ml divided by 60 min $\times$ 20 gtt/min = 42 gtt/min

Math calculation explains incorrect answers.

899. **(C)** Nursing process phase: implementation; client need: safe, effective care environment; content area: medical/surgical nursing—dosage calculation

Rationale

100 ml : 30 min : x : 60 min = 200 ml/hr

Math calculation explains incorrect answers.

900. **(B)** Nursing process phase: implementation; client need: safe, effective care environment; content area: medical/surgical nursing—dosage calculation

Rationale

100 ml divided by 45 min $\times$ 60 gtt/min = 133 gtt/min

Math calculation explains incorrect answers.

901. **(D)** Nursing process phase: implementation; client need: safe, effective care environment; content area: medical/surgical nursing—dosage calculation

Rationale

100 ml : 30 min : x : 60 min = 200 ml/hr

Math calculation explains incorrect answers.

902. **(D)** Nursing process phase: implementation; client need: safe, effective care environment; content area: medical/surgical nursing—dosage calculation

Rationale

50 ml divided by 15 min $\times$ 15 gtt/ml = 50 gtt/min

Math calculation explains incorrect answers.

903. **(B)** Nursing process phase: implementation; client need: safe, effective care environment; content area: medical/surgical nursing—dosage calculation

Rationale

50 ml : 15 min : x : 60 min = 200 ml/hr

Math calculation explains incorrect answers.

904. **(B)** Nursing process phase: implementation; client need: safe, effective care environment; content area: medical/surgical nursing—dosage calculation

Rationale

750 ml divided by 240 minutes $\times$ 10 gtt/min = 31 gtt/min

Math calculation explains incorrect answers.

905. **(D)** Nursing process phase: implementation; client need: safe, effective care environment; content area: medical/surgical nursing—dosage calculation

Rationale

800 ml divided by 240 min $\times$ 20 gtt/min = 67 gtt/min

Math calculation explains incorrect answers.

906. **(D)** Nursing process phase: implementation; client need: safe, effective care environment; content area: medical/surgical nursing—dosage calculation

Rationale

1500 ml divided by 24 hours = 62.5 ml divided by 60 min $\times$ 60 gtt/ml = 62 gtt/min

Math calculation explains incorrect answers.

907. **(C)** Nursing process phase: implementation; client need: safe, effective care environment; content area: medical/surgical nursing—dosage calculation

Rationale

500 ml divided by 4 hr = 125 ml/hr

Math calculation explains incorrect answers.

908. **(C)** Nursing process phase: implementation; client need: safe, effective care environment; content area: medical/surgical nursing—dosage calculation

Rationale

50 ml : 30 min : x : 60 min = 100 ml/hr

Math calculation explains incorrect answers.

909. **(D)** Nursing process phase: implementation; client need: safe, effective care environment; content area: medical/surgical nursing—dosage calculation

Rationale

25 gtt/min $\times$ 480 min/8 hr = 12,000 gtt/8 hr divided by 15 gtt/ml = 800 ml/8 hr

Math calculation explains incorrect answers.

910. **(D)** Nursing process phase: implementation; client need: safe, effective care environment; content area: medical/surgical nursing—dosage calculation

Rationale

80 ml $\times$ 60 gtt/ml = 4800 gtt divided by 20 micro-drops/min = 240 min = 4 hours

Math calculation explains incorrect answers.

911. **(C)** Nursing process phase: implementation; client need: safe, effective care environment; content area: medical/surgical nursing—dosage calculation

Rationale

20 mg : 1 ml = 25 mg : x = 1.25 ml

Math calculation explains incorrect answers.

chapter 7

Psychiatric Nursing
Q & A

*by Eileen W. Keefe, Pauline F. Bohannon,
and Golden Tradewell*

1. Nursing care for the substance abuse client experiencing alcohol withdrawal delirium includes:
   A. Maintaining seizure precautions
   B. Restricting fluid intake
   C. Increasing sensory stimuli
   D. Applying ankle and wrist restraints

2. The nurse, in working with the severely mentally ill, should be aware that:
   A. All severely mentally ill clients require long-term hospitalization.
   B. Some severely mentally ill clients do not require hospitalization.
   C. Most severely mentally ill clients do not return to their families.
   D. Large public mental institutions house the majority of the severely mentally ill clients.

3. The nurse is aware that many clients admitted to a psychiatric unit are concerned about:
   A. Confidentiality
   B. Anonymity
   C. Insanity defense
   D. Moral distress

4. The distraught parents of a 14-year-old male escorted their son to the emergency room because of his disrespectful and bizarre behavior. The client was admitted to the adolescent unit. During the assessment interview, he cursed the nurse and spit in her face. The best response by the nurse would be:
   A. "You are an ugly young man. You need to behave yourself."
   B. "I understand that you are angry. I will not tolerate this behavior."

   C. "No wonder your parents brought you here."
   D. "You're very sad. I think you should pay more attention to your behavior."

5. Many clients have difficulty expressing anger. Which one of the following nursing interventions would assist a client with expressing anger appropriately?
   A. Isolate from others.
   B. Encourage acting out.
   C. Encourage verbalization.
   D. Introduce self-care improvement.

6. The client says to the nurse, "I'm physically and emotionally healthy." Which response by the nurse would support the client's thinking?
   A. "That statement is cause for concern."
   B. "I have observed that you accept yourself as a person."
   C. "That statement is not based on sound judgment."
   D. "What makes you think that you are emotionally healthy?"

7. A college student experiences disabling interferences related to social relationships, occupational pursuits, and sexual adjustments that are alien to the student's personality. The nurse would recognize this form of personality disturbance as:
   A. Psychosis
   B. A character disorder
   C. Neurosis
   D. A psychophysiological disorder

8. A hostile client is admitted with very little insight, disorganized speech, poor contact with reality, and severe personality decompensation. This be-

havior is most suggestive of which of the following disorders?

A. Personality disorder
B. Psychosis
C. Neurosis
D. Psychophysiological disorder

9. The client reported to the nurse that the therapy session was a failure and a waste of time. The client then remarked, "The next time, I'll just sit there and be a nonparticipant." What defense mechanism is the client demonstrating?

A. Compensation
B. Identification
C. Rationalization
D. Projection

10. During the initial interview, the client tells the nurse that he grew up on the "wrong side of the tracks." He feels rejected by family, socially unacceptable, and works hard to become the meanest fighter in his block. Which of the following defense mechanisms is the client exhibiting?

A. Projection
B. Compensation
C. Reaction formation
D. Rationalization

11. A 10-year-old boy was hospitalized because he was underweight. He imagined that he was strong and could conquer the school bully, thus making him the superhero. The nurse would recognize this defense mechanism as:

A. Rationalization
B. Compensation
C. Identification
D. Fantasy

12. A 10-year-old girl hit a playmate with a baseball bat. The school nurse intervened in the incident. The girl shouted, "He hit me. He hit me. He hit me." Which of the following defense mechanisms is the girl exhibiting?

A. Displacement
B. Projection
C. Rationalization
D. Sublimation

13. A nurse on the obstetrical unit was preparing a client for discharge after the birth of a son. The client suddenly developed blindness. After an extensive work-up, no physical problems were evident. Which of the following defense mechanisms was the client using?

A. Regression
B. Repression
C. Reaction formation
D. Conversion reaction

14. A client angrily explained to the nurse that her admission to the hospital for adjustment to her antipsychotic medication was a mistake. She says to the nurse, "I've been taking the medication for 5 years without a problem. I don't need it anymore. My thinking is OK." The nurse is aware that this is an example of:

A. Regression
B. Rationalization
C. Sublimation
D. Denial

15. An angry, hostile client complained to the therapist that his promotion was denied, but stated he did not complain to his employer. When he returned home he beat his wife because of her inability to keep the house clean. Which defense mechanism is exhibited?

A. Displacement
B. Projection
C. Reaction formation
D. Sublimation

16. A 20-year-old client was sexually abused by a family member. The patient is unable to recall the incident and has periods of muteness. The nurse recognizes this defense mechanism as:

A. Displacement
B. Projection
C. Reaction formation
D. Repression

17. A 30-year-old lady, after the death of her mother, assumed many of her mother's characteristics. Which defense mechanism is demonstrated in this situation?

A. Rationalization
B. Fantasy
C. Introjection
D. Compensation

18. A salesman hoards all personal receipts, junk mail, news clippings, and restaurant napkins. He tells the nurse that he has no control over his behavior. What is the most appropriate nursing intervention?

A. Form a therapeutic alliance with the client.
B. Assist the client to prevent the ritualistic behaviors.
C. Encourage the client to rationalize his irrational behaviors.
D. Refer the client for hypnosis.

19. A 3-year-old girl was excited about having a new brother and welcomed him home with a hug and a kiss. After a few days, she started wetting her pants and told her mother that she wanted a diaper. This is most suggestive of:

A. Regression
B. Undoing
C. Repression
D. Reaction formation

20. The nurse is caring for a client with strong aggressive impulses. He tells the nurse that he is a star basketball player. This is an example of which of the following defense mechanisms?

A. Sublimation
B. Reaction formation
C. Displacement
D. Conversion reaction

21. The nurse is assessing a client who is a substance abuser. During the interview, the client minimizes the problem when he says to the nurse, "I use every day, but it rarely interferes with my work." The client is using which defense mechanism?
A. Projection
B. Displacement
C. Reaction formation
D. Denial

22. The clinic nurse assisted a client who just had a magnetic resonance imaging test of the abdomen. Because of the family history, the physician suggested other tests to rule out cancer. The client said to the nurse, "There is nothing wrong and I refuse to accept any more tests and any medical treatment." Which of the following defense mechanisms is the client using?
A. Undoing
B. Rationalization
C. Denial
D. Sublimation

23. A healthy 24-year-old man who was gainfully employed, engaged to be married, and actively involved in church activities attempted to get out of bed one morning and discovered that he could not walk. The client is using which defense mechanism?
A. Reaction formation
B. Somatization disorder
C. Conversion reaction
D. Fantasy

24. A 40-year-old male is admitted for treatment of alcoholism and depression. He tells the nurse that he has been depressed all of his life but does not mention a drinking problem. When the client was questioned about alcoholism, he reported that he was a social drinker. Which defense mechanism is the client using?
A. Regression
B. Reaction formation
C. Denial
D. Projection

25. An 8-year-old client admires his soccer coach and takes on the mannerisms and values of the coach. Which of the following defense mechanisms is the client using?
A. Introjection
B. Fantasy
C. Repression
D. Projection

26. A 30-year-old client was given 5 mg of haloperidol (Haldol) for agitation. The client's chart was clearly stamped "Allergic HALDOL." The client

suffered anaphylactic shock and died. The family sued for:
A. Intentional tort
B. Negligence
C. An overdose of Haldol
D. Assault

27. A psychiatric nurse was instructed by the attending psychiatrist to administer 10 mg of haloperidol (Haldol) to a severely dysfunctional client. The client refused all medications. Which was the best nursing action?
A. Restrain the client and give the medication IM.
B. Accept the client's decision.
C. Plead with the client to reconsider.
D. Obtain a discharge order for noncompliance.

28. On admission to a psychiatric unit, a 22-year-old male client signed a voluntary admission form. After a period of 12 hours, the client informs the nurse of his desire to leave by yelling, "I don't need to be here. Let me out." What is the best response by the nurse?
A. "You can't leave this hospital."
B. "Think about staying for 1 week."
C. "Please sign this legal form indicating your intentions and wait 24 hours."
D. "Ask your doctor about discharge so he can start legal procedures."

29. A 27-year-old female client, who slashed both wrists, was admitted to the psychiatric unit under a physician's emergency certificate (PEC). She requested an immediate discharge. Which is the best response by the nurse?
A. "I understand that you are self-destructive. I cannot let you leave."
B. "You must sign this legal document, which indicates that you are leaving the hospital against medical advice (AMA)."
C. "Discuss the issue with your physician."
D. "I will notify your minister."

30. Disclosure of information, beyond members of the multidisciplinary team, without the consent of the client is a breach of:
A. Anonymity
B. Confidentiality
C. Duty
D. Habeas corpus

31. A 25-year-old male with a history of homicidal ideation toward his ex-wife left the mental health clinic in a rage. It was feared that he would harm her. The ex-wife was notified about the event. The nurse's responsibility is to:
A. Maintain confidentiality.
B. Protect the client's rights.
C. Assume the client will return.
D. Warn the potential victim.

32. A 27-year-old client diagnosed as having borderline personality disorder called her attorney, re-

porting client abuse and that the institution was holding her hostage. The nurse is aware that this is an example of:
A. Breach of confidentiality
B. Privileged communication
C. Right of confidentiality
D. Failure to comply with telephone rules

33. A 60-year-old, severely depressed client was admitted to a psychiatric unit under an involuntary commitment. The nurse understands that all of the following are incorrect except:
A. The client loses all civil rights.
B. The client may at any time sign a voluntary admission.
C. The client loses the right to vote.
D. The client loses the right to marry.

34. The activity therapist informs the nurse that she will be helping supervise a 15-person outing scheduled for early afternoon. The nurse would be correct in telling the therapist that:
A. "It's a good idea for the clients to participate in an outing."
B. "That is not a safe practice. A 2:15 ratio is too many clients."
C. "I will be glad to participate."
D. "Have you requested additional help?"

35. A 32-year-old client lost control of her behavior. She threatened staff and other clients and broke several windows. She was escorted to the seclusion room and put in four-point restraints. Which statement is most correct when explaining the situation to the client?
A. "This is a form of punishment for losing control."
B. "This is a means of providing safety for you and everyone else on the unit."
C. "The length of time is undetermined."
D. "The staff will do periodic checks."

36. Psychiatric clients have a right to refuse treatment. When persuasion and manipulation are used to get the client engaged in treatment, the nurse is aware that:
A. The client has no fundamental right to refuse treatment.
B. There is a responsibility to complete treatment once it is started.
C. Paternalism is operating.
D. Constitutional rights are abused.

37. Which of the following ethical guidelines do not relate to client rights?
A. Informed consent
B. Treatment
C. Refusal of treatment
D. Judicial commitment

38. A 29-year-old male client admitted himself for psychiatric treatment. The nurse determines that this admission is:

A. Voluntary
B. Judicial
C. Informal
D. Involuntary

39. A 30-year-old client who frequently suffers from sweaty palms, palpitations, shortness of breath, and dizziness told the nurse practitioner that he has had these feelings for the past year and that they interfere with his ability to function. After a diagnostic work-up, there was no evidence of a physical disorder. The nurse would recognize the behavior as moderate anxiety, which is a sensation triggered by:
A. Physiological changes
B. Psychosocial impairment
C. A perceived threat
D. Perpetual certainty

40. The most effective nursing intervention to assist a client who is experiencing moderate anxiety is to:
A. Focus on anxiety reduction.
B. Probe the cause.
C. Investigate decompensation behaviors.
D. Accept the level of anxiety.

41. A 34-year-old female client suffering from numbness of the extremities, trembling, and dyspnea is admitted with a diagnosis of severe anxiety disorder. An initial nursing intervention should be to:
A. Discuss functional coping measures.
B. Determine the source of the problem.
C. Quickly administer an anxiolytic medication.
D. Provide safety and comfort.

42. A 50-year-old male client discussed his pending divorce. He told the nurse that he has been married for 30 years and doesn't want the divorce. During the assessment, the nurse learns that the client is suffering from insomnia, anorexia, feels insecure, and has a history of suicidal gestures. Which statement by the nurse is most appropriate?
A. "Why are you so upset?"
B. "I can see that you are upset. This is a difficult time for you."
C. "Tell me about the suicidal gestures?"
D. "Thirty years of marriage! You have been a successful person."

43. At the time of admission, a female client suffered from insomnia, shortness of breath, and a rapid pulse. The client was agitated and stated that she was going crazy and losing control. The diagnosis was panic disorder. The nursing plan of care should include:
A. Large doses of antianxiety medications
B. Family education
C. The etiology and management of panic disorders
D. Cognitive restructuring

44. A 42-year-old male client experienced a severe psychic trauma 1 month ago. He developed paralysis

of the lower extremities. Which of the following is the best nursing intervention?
- A. Encourage the client to talk about his feelings.
- B. Assess the client for organic causes of paralysis.
- C. Provide range of motion (ROM) to the lower extremities.
- D. Encourage discussion of future goals.

45. After a complete diagnostic work-up for a client with neurobiological changes, it was determined that the client was experiencing post-traumatic stress disorder (PTSD). In planning care for the client, the nurse should be aware that:
- A. The symptoms are a mechanism that help him cope with an unacceptable situation.
- B. The symptoms are a mechanism that help him cope and support his dependence.
- C. The symptoms are a means to manipulate others.
- D. The symptoms develop from a nonspecific psychic event.

46. A 35-year-old client has a history of multiple somatic complaints involving several organ systems. Diagnostic studies revealed no organic or physiological causes. In planning nursing care, it is important that the nurse understand that the client is suffering from:
- A. Psychosis
- B. Depression
- C. Somatization disorder
- D. Delusional disorder

47. A 25-year-old female client tells the clinical nurse specialist that she has an irrational fear of spiders and goes out of her way to avoid them. In planning care for the client, it is important for the nurse to know that:
- A. The client has displaced a conscious conflict to an object symbolically related to the conflict.
- B. The anxiety is free-floating.
- C. The client accepts the source of distress.
- D. The behavioral style of phobic clients is avoidance.

48. During the multidisciplinary team conference, the client explained that she was terrified of rain and practiced avoidance. The team members understand that the client is:
- A. Controlling the intensity of the anxiety
- B. Fearful of the internal source of distress
- C. Aware of the basic source of the anxiety
- D. Attempting to undo the source of anxiety

49. A female client continues to exhibit seductive behavior, pressured speech, and psychomotor agitation. Which of the following is the best nursing intervention?
- A. Provide a safe environment.
- B. Indicate that the behavior is not acceptable.
- C. Encourage group activity.
- D. Promote highly competitive activities.

50. The activity therapist is implementing an individualized program for a manic client exhibiting hostility and excessive energy. Which of the following activities would be most appropriate?
- A. Writing short stories
- B. Team sports
- C. Ping-Pong
- D. Walking

51. A scantily dressed client approached the nurse, saying, "I am a striptease dancer and I am ready for visitors." Which action by the nurse would be most appropriate?
- A. Inform the client that all privileges will be suspended indefinitely.
- B. Assure the client that her behavior is appropriate.
- C. Redirect the client to her room and assist her with a change of clothes.
- D. Allow the client to remain as dressed.

52. Which of the following foods would be most appropriate for a client in the manic phase?
- A. Finger sandwiches, orange slices, and a banana
- B. Pasta, meatballs, and a salad
- C. Fried chicken steak with sauce and a salad
- D. Beef stew, mashed potatoes, and a banana

53. A 40-year-old male client discharged from a psychiatric unit 4 days ago presented at the clinic talking loudly, cursing, and crying. Family members stated that they are unable to cope with the behavior and alternative living arrangements must be made. Which living arrangement is most suitable?
- A. Long-term psychiatric hospitalization
- B. Nursing home placement
- C. Group home placement
- D. Independent living

54. The physician orders fluoxetine (Prozac) for a depressed client. Which of the following should the nurse remember about fluoxetine?
- A. Because fluoxetine is a tricyclic antidepressant, it may precipitate a hypertensive crisis.
- B. The therapeutic effect of the drug occurs 2 to 4 weeks after treatment is begun.
- C. Foods such as aged cheese, yogurt, soy sauce, and bananas should not be eaten with this drug.
- D. Fluoxetine may be administered safely in combination with monoamine oxidase (MAO) inhibitors.

55. The nurse is caring for a 38-year-old male client who was in an automobile accident 3 months ago. He complains of neck pain and brags about the pending insurance settlement. The nurse suspects that the client is:
- A. Malingering
- B. Suffering from conversion reaction
- C. Exhibiting somatization disorder
- D. A hypochondriac

56. A 58-year-old female client is admitted to the psychiatric unit. During the nursing assessment, she states, "My mother just walked by the window and I saw her go into the nurses station." This behavior is an example of:
  A. Hallucinations
  B. Fantasies
  C. Delusions
  D. Derealization

57. The client tells the nurse that God is broadcasting messages through his brain, which is acting as a transmitter. What would be the best response by the nurse?
  A. "Describe the messages to me."
  B. "God will punish you for thinking this way."
  C. "Do you really believe that God would send you a message?"
  D. "I do not hear messages being transmitted."

58. In caring for a 39-year-old client who acknowledges noncompliance and demonstrates bizarre behaviors, neologism, and thought insertion, the nurse should:
  A. Convey acceptance of the client.
  B. Spend time focusing on thought insertion.
  C. Ignore the behaviors.
  D. Assist with identification of target symptoms.

59. A 25-year-old female client accused her roommate of stealing her comb and began biting, clawing, and scratching her. Which of the following would be the best nursing intervention?
  A. Provide a safe environment for both clients.
  B. Notify the lawyer advocate.
  C. Isolate the aggressor and place in restraints.
  D. Discuss the angry behavior and available consequences.

60. A 23-year-old client physically attacks another person on the psychiatric unit and accuses the person of stealing. The nurse is aware that his behavior is an example of:
  A. Displacement
  B. Impulsive behavior
  C. Identification
  D. Impulse gratification

61. A 54-year-old female client is admitted to a psychiatric unit in a catatonic state. She is mute and exhibits catalepsy and waxy flexibility. In attempting to communicate with the client, the nurse should give the highest priority to which nursing action?
  A. Acknowledge the client's inability to use the spoken word.
  B. Use clear, concrete statements.
  C. Encourage the client to engage in conversation.
  D. Speak in abstract terms.

62. In a conversation between the nurse and a 50-year-old female client, the client tells the nurse that the hospital staff poisoned her meal and she refuses to eat. The most appropriate nursing intervention is to:
  A. Focus on the delusion.
  B. Focus on the fears and insecurities.
  C. Agree with the client's decision.
  D. Challenge the client's delusional system.

63. The emergency room nurse encounters a 20-year-old female wandering around and exhibiting extreme hyperactivity and bizarre behavior. She laughs, giggles, and is annoying to staff and other clients. Her thoughts are poorly organized. The main focus of nursing care for this client would be to:
  A. Provide a safe environment.
  B. Encourage social interaction.
  C. Discuss the bizarre behavior.
  D. Provide information regarding illness.

64. A 26-year-old was admitted with a diagnosis of schizoaffective disorder. The nurse would assess for:
  A. Mood and thought disturbance
  B. Controlled anger
  C. Uniqueness and individuality
  D. Echopraxia

65. A 34-year-old female client is diagnosed as having bipolar disorder and is acutely psychotic. The client suffers from paranoid delusions. She remarks to the nurse that the FBI and AT&T are plotting against her. In documenting the statement, the nurse may refer to it as a delusion of:
  A. Grandeur
  B. Control
  C. Persecution
  D. Reference

66. A 70-year-old man was admitted to a psychiatric unit because he physically abused his wife. He said to the nurse, "My wife is having an affair with an 18-year-old and I want it investigated." The best response by the nurse is:
  A. "That remark is absolutely ridiculous."
  B. "I understand that you are upset. We will talk about it."
  C. "That seems rather doubtful."
  D. "An 18-year-old is too young. He does not want your wife."

67. A 54-year-old male mental health client is resentful, mistrustful, and rigid in his beliefs. He threatens to kill the physician because of the plots against him. Which action by the nurse represents unsafe nursing practice?
  A. Encourage verbalization of feelings.
  B. Challenge the client's delusional system and implement a referral.
  C. Evaluate the seriousness of the homicidal statement.
  D. Encourage the client to identify fears and suspicions.

68. A 38-year-old male client complains that his legs are misshaped and of a number of other physical defects. Which of the following statements suggest that the client is suffering from a somatic delusion?
    A. "I have a foul odor coming from all over my body."
    B. "My animal has worms coming from the rectum."
    C. "My mother says that my legs are short. I don't think they are."
    D. "I have a problem with my mother. She accuses me of having a body odor."

69. In planning care for a delusional, paranoid person, it is important for the nurse to consider which one of the following characteristics?
    A. Bright affect and extreme suspiciousness
    B. Motor immobility
    C. Regressive and primitive behaviors
    D. Anger and aggressive acts

70. During a mental status examination, a 54-year-old client exhibits rhyming, punning, and perseveration. Which part of the psychiatric assessment is the nurse addressing?
    A. Emotional status
    B. Interpersonal style
    C. Speech and language
    D. Thinking and perception

71. A 48-year-old male client with a diagnosis of schizophrenia experiences confusion over his identity. He frequently exhibits echolalia. The nurse is aware that this is an attempt by the client to:
    A. Identify with the person speaking
    B. Imitate nurse's movements
    C. Alleviate alogia
    D. Alleviate avolition

72. A 28-year-old client, diagnosed as having borderline personality disorder, presented at the mental health clinic and demanded to see a counselor immediately. Which one of the following is the best nursing strategy?
    A. Instruct the client to leave the clinic.
    B. Confront demanding behaviors.
    C. Explain the rules and set limits.
    D. Help the client problem-solve.

73. An 18-year-old male with a diagnosis of antisocial personality disorder was admitted for psychological testing. He reported to the nurse that on two occasions he ran away from his parent's home after he set their house on fire. Which is the best nursing intervention?
    A. Discuss psychological testing.
    B. Discuss alternatives to pyromania.
    C. Limit the client's social interactions.
    D. Coax the client to follow the unit rules.

74. A 15-year-old girl tells the nurse that she wants to talk with her mother. The nurse is aware that the girl's mother does not want any further contact with her daughter. The client asks permission to use the telephone. What is the nurse's best response?
    A. "Why do you want to call your mother?"
    B. "No, not at this time. Tell me more about how you feel toward your mother."
    C. "I don't believe it will be healthy to call her."
    D. "Tell me how you feel, now that your mother has abandoned you."

75. A newly admitted 19-year-old male client who has been diagnosed as having antisocial personality disorder is manipulative, cold, and callous. He is charming and intelligent. What is the most effective nursing intervention for this client?
    A. Allow permissive behavior.
    B. Ignore the behavior.
    C. Set limits on all interactions and behaviors.
    D. Discuss interpersonal relationships.

76. After 3 weeks of treatment, a severely depressed client suddenly begins to feel better and starts interacting appropriately with other clients and staff. The nurse knows that this client has an increased risk for:
    A. Suicide
    B. Exacerbation of depressive systems
    C. Violence toward others
    D. Psychotic behavior

77. In caring for a client diagnosed as having borderline personality disorder, the care plan should include which one of the following?
    A. Punitive actions
    B. Client's control over routine decisions
    C. Strict isolation
    D. Client's freedom to make choices about dependent behavior

78. The nurse in the mental health clinic has been interacting, individually and during group sessions, with a female client for approximately 3 months. The client displays periods of intense anger, impulsiveness, and cooperativeness and frequently expresses feelings of self-devaluation. The nurse interprets this as:
    A. Primitive idealization
    B. Chameleonlike behavior
    C. Omnipotence
    D. Derealization

79. In assessing a client with borderline personality disorder, the nurse should be aware of which one of the following traits?
    A. Predictability
    B. Controlled anger
    C. Primitive dissociation
    D. Stable and friendly relationships

80. A realistic nursing intervention for a client who has problems with negative transference would be to:
    A. Clarify the actual source of hate and bitterness.
    B. Discuss satisfying past relationships.

C. Focus on future relationships.

D. Avoid discussion of the unresolved conflicts.

81. A psychotic client who believes that he is God and rules all the universe is experiencing which type of delusion?

A. Somatic

B. Grandiose

C. Persecutory

D. Nihilistic

82. A long-term goal for the nurse in planning care for a depressed, suicidal client would be to:

A. Provide him with a safe and structured environment.

B. Assist him to develop more effective coping mechanisms.

C. Have him sign a "no-suicide" contract.

D. Isolate him from stressful situations that may precipitate a depressive episode.

83. A client confides to the nurse that he tasted poison in his evening meal. This would be an example of what type of hallucination?

A. Auditory

B. Gustatory

C. Olfactory

D. Visceral

84. A 27-year-old male client is a voluntary admission on a psychiatric unit. He manipulates the staff, brags about his criminal behavior, and exhibits irritability and aggressiveness. He causes disruption on the unit and fear among the other clients. The nurse determines that this behavior is which one of the following disorders?

A. Schizoid personality

B. Passive-aggressive personality

C. Borderline personality

D. Antisocial personality

85. A 21-year-old female client tells the nurse that she finds it necessary to occasionally masturbate and asks for a professional opinion. The best statement by the nurse is:

A. "Only men masturbate to relieve tension."

B. "There is a possibility that masturbation causes voyeurism."

C. "Masturbation causes an orgasmic disorder in both males and females."

D. "Masturbation releases tension that is sexual in nature."

86. An 18-year-old client tells the female mental health worker that she is sexually attracted toward her. The nurse should intervene by:

A. Confronting the mental health worker

B. Encouraging the client to discuss feelings

C. Limiting the interaction

D. Avoiding all behaviors

87. A client diagnosed with a bipolar disorder continues to be hyperactive and to lose weight. Which of the following nutritional interventions would be most therapeutic for him at this time?

A. Small, frequent feedings of foods that can be carried

B. Tube feedings with nutritional supplements

C. Allowing him to eat when and what he wants

D. Giving him a quiet place where he can sit down to eat meals

88. Communication is a transaction that:

A. Influences the past

B. Is limited to a one-way process

C. Has limited dimensions

D. Symbolizes the representational system

89. The physician observes his client sitting calmly and interacting with other clients. The nurse's progress notes state that the client is "angry, hostile, and combative." Which one of the following requests by the physician would be appropriate?

A. "Ask the nurse for clarification of the statement. He is not causing a problem."

B. "Escort my client to the quiet room."

C. "Why did the nurse document that my client is angry, hostile, and combative?"

D. "I demand that the nurse clarify her statement."

90. After reading the nurse's progress note that indicates his client is isolating, the physician requests a statement regarding the meaning of "isolating." Identify the communication technique.

A. Clarification

B. Focusing

C. Voicing doubt

D. Probing

91. A 40-year-old male client jumped from his chair, yelling and cursing at the nurse. What would be the best nursing response?

A. "I don't want you to do that ever again."

B. "I will limit your smoking privileges."

C. "You seem angry. Tell me more about how you feel."

D. "I can see that you need attention; everyone does at times."

92. Which of the following communication techniques would be most effective for the nurse to use during a nurse-client interaction?

A. Facilitative

B. Nonverbal

C. Public

D. Intrapersonal

93. The nurse enters the room of a 50-year-old client, who is lying in a fetal position with his head covered, and says, "How are you feeling this morning?" The client responds, "I'm feeling fine." The behavior exhibited by the client is:

A. Assertive

B. Aggressive

C. Passive

D. Passive-aggressive

94. A 30-year-old male client is admitted to the psychiatric unit with a diagnosis of bipolar disorder. For the last 2 months, his family describes him as being "on the move," sleeping 3 to 4 hours nightly, spending lots of money, and losing approximately 10 lb. During the initial assessment with the client, the nurse would expect him to exhibit which of the following?
    A. Short, polite responses to interview questions
    B. Introspection related to his present situation
    C. Exaggerated self-importance
    D. Feelings of helplessness and hopelessness

95. The nurse must be alert to nonverbal expressions. Because the meaning attached to nonverbal behavior is subjective, it is important for the nurse to:
    A. Validate its meaning.
    B. Increase the client's awareness.
    C. Investigate the connotative meaning.
    D. Validate feelings.

96. The primary goal of a therapeutic relationship between the nurse and the client includes:
    A. Establishing a relationship that promotes growth of the client
    B. Developing the nurse's personal identity
    C. Establishing an intimate purposeful interaction
    D. Developing therapeutic impasses

97. Which statement by the nurse would assist the client with developing feelings of importance?
    A. "I would like to sit and talk with you. What would you like to talk about today?"
    B. "I don't want to talk right now because I don't have time."
    C. "Let me tell you what I did last night."
    D. "Hang in there until things improve."

98. High levels of anxiety are experienced by many mentally ill clients. The condition:
    A. Narrows the perceptual field and decreases attention span
    B. Helps increase communication skills
    C. Greatly increases the thinking process
    D. Helps with problem-solving skills

99. It is important to use which one of the following therapeutic statements when trying to obtain general information?
    A. "Tell me your feelings about your family situation."
    B. "Are you OK today?"
    C. "You seem to be upset. Why do you feel this way?"
    D. "I hope that you are packed and ready to leave."

100. Accurate and complete documentation in a client's record:
    A. Should reflect the nursing process
    B. Should be available to all hospital personnel
    C. Make it an illegal document
    D. Guarantee pertinent and accurate information

101. Which of the following statements might cause a barrier in communication?
    A. "I don't understand. Would you please explain?"
    B. "You are wrong to show hostility for no apparent reason."
    C. "I'm sorry, I'll stay with you for a while."
    D. "Please explain your position in more detail."

102. The nurse wishes to establish a supportive therapeutic relationship with a 22-year-old woman with a diagnosis of schizoid personality disorder. In developing a plan of care, it is most important for the nurse to:
    A. Allow the client's need for distance in a relationship.
    B. Minimize affiliative needs.
    C. Encourage her to participate in intensive group therapy.
    D. Assign different nurses each day until she finds one to whom she can relate.

103. When developing a therapeutic relationship with a client, which one of the following techniques is most essential for the nurse to use?
    A. Genuineness
    B. Confrontation
    C. Catharsis
    D. Giving advice

104. A 24-year-old client walks with a shuffling gait, a bent head, looks distressed, and makes no eye contact. Which of the following behaviors is the nurse most interested in helping the client resolve?
    A. Nonverbal
    B. Verbal
    C. Aggressive
    D. Passive

105. An 18-year-old, newly diagnosed schizophrenic client exhibits withdrawn, regressive, and isolative behaviors. The nurse's initial approach should be to:
    A. Speak in realistic, literal terms.
    B. Use self-disclosure.
    C. Demand information.
    D. Explain in depth the rules and regulations.

106. A 30-year-old client is fearful and refuses to talk. Which one of the following interpersonal techniques is most effective when attempting to engage the client in conversation?
    A. Silence
    B. Introducing historical events
    C. Broad openings
    D. Focusing

107. A 43-year-old client, with a diagnosis of bipolar disorder, has been hospitalized for a number of weeks. She asks the nurse, "Do you think that the doctor is ever going to discharge me?" The best response by the nurse is:
    A. "Ask your doctor."

    B. "Tell me more about your feelings."
    C. "Do you think that you are ready?"
    D. "Let the doctor know your feelings."

108. The nurse is developing a care plan for a client with a paranoid personality disorder. He has been hospitalized after repeatedly yelling and calling the police day and night on his neighbors, who he suspects of plotting to have him removed from his home. The nurse wishes to assist the client to be less socially isolated. Which of the following goals would be most applicable?
    A. Share his belongings with others
    B. Engage in group activities and share his feelings freely
    C. Have as much control as possible over his environment
    D. Participate in solitary activities

109. The nurse observes that a client receiving thioridazine (Mellaril) is restless, agitated, and exhibiting tremors of the upper extremities. Which of the following is the best nursing intervention?
    A. Discuss the symptoms with the physician.
    B. Administer a PRN antiparkinson agent.
    C. Report the incident to the nurse manager.
    D. Ignore the syndrome.

110. The nurse must recognize the side effects of haloperidol (Haldol). These are:
    A. Diarrhea and amenorrhea
    B. Orthostatic hypotension and increased sweating
    C. Decreased sweating and increased sexual activity
    D. Headache and orthostatic hypotension

111. A nursing responsibility is to teach clients about their medications and how to care for self after discharge. A client, who is taking risperidone (Risperdal) frequently requests an antacid. Which instruction is most important?
    A. "You can take antacids anytime."
    B. "Wait 1 hour after each dose of Risperdal before taking an antacid."
    C. "It is OK to take an antacid and Risperdal at the same time, if you have heartburn."
    D. "When you go home, ask the physician about antacids."

112. A 32-year-old client is being discharged on haloperidol (Haldol). Which of the following nursing instructions is most important?
    A. "Do not stop taking Haldol abruptly."
    B. "If you forget to take your morning dose of Haldol, double the dose at bedtime."
    C. "Drink plenty of fluids, and that includes cocktails."
    D. "When you go home, sit outside and enjoy the sunshine."

113. The nursing instructions to a client, who is taking alprazolam (Xanax) three times a day, should include:
    A. The potential for dependence and tolerance
    B. The importance of discontinuing Xanax immediately if addiction is suspected
    C. The importance of increasing the amount of caffeine consumption
    D. Reassurance that Xanax is not habit forming

114. A 23-year-old female client has been admitted to the inpatient psychiatric unit with a diagnosis of catatonic schizophrenia. She appears weak and pale. The nurse would expect to observe which behaviors in this client?
    A. Scratching and catlike motions of the extremities
    B. Exaggerated suspiciousness and excessive food intake
    C. Stuporous withdrawal, hallucinations, and delusions
    D. Sexual preoccupation and word salad

115. Because valproic acid (Depakene) may cause side effects, it is important that the nurse observe for:
    A. Confusion
    B. Drowsiness
    C. Oliguria
    D. Bulimia

116. A 36-year-old person was rushed to the emergency room complaining of restlessness, drooling, and tremors. The daughter informed the nurse that her mother was taking chlorpromazine (Thorazine). The nurse recognized the behaviors as extrapyramidal symptoms (EPS). The drug of choice used to alleviate these symptoms is:
    A. Paroxetine (Paxil)
    B. Carbamazepine (Tegretol)
    C. Benztropine (Cogentin)
    D. Lorazepam (Ativan)

117. A 31-year-old client is receiving an antiparkinson medication. What adverse side effects would the nurse observe, if the client is toxic?
    A. Decrease in psychotic symptoms
    B. Anxiety
    C. Hot, moist skin
    D. Moist mucous membranes

118. The nurse should know that the primary reason for administering lithium carbonate is for which of the following disorders?
    A. Schizoaffective
    B. Obsessive-compulsive
    C. Manic-depressive
    D. Schizophrenia

119. Which one of the following symptoms would the nurse observe if the client's lithium level is 1.8 mEq/L?
    A. Bradycardia
    B. Hypotension
    C. Psychosis
    D. Constipation

120. The nurse includes medication education in the

discharge plans for a client diagnosed as having a bipolar disorder and taking lithium carbonate. The instructions are:
A. Do not skimp on dietary sodium intake.
B. Have serum lithium levels checked monthly.
C. Maintain a low-fat diet.
D. Adjust the dose if you feel out of control.

121. A 20-year-old woman has recently been diagnosed with paranoid schizophrenia. She has been started on haloperidol (Haldol) and seems to be responding less to hallucinations. She has begun to attend an art group for brief periods each day. In planning care to assist the client to be more connected to reality, the nurse should:
A. Reinforce perceptions and thinking that are in touch with reality.
B. Challenge her expressions of distorted thinking.
C. Use peer pressure to discourage delusions.
D. Ignore distorted thinking and bizarre behavior.

122. A 75-year-old client has been taking chlordiazepoxide (Librium) for a year. The nurse should advise the client that:
A. Librium is the drug of choice for long-term relief of anxiety.
B. Smoking will not cause a problem.
C. Librium should be used with caution in the elderly.
D. An afternoon cocktail along with Librium will help reduce anxiety.

123. A 25-year-old male client is preparing for discharge. The physician ordered sertraline (Zoloft) to be taken daily. Which one of the following instructions should the nurse give the client?
A. Take sertraline with food to avoid stomach irritation.
B. If a dose of sertraline is forgotten, double the next dose.
C. Do not mix alcohol or over-the-counter medications with sertraline.
D. Stop the medication abruptly if the side effects are suspected.

124. The physician informed the client that succinylcholine chloride (Anectine) would be administered prior to the electroconvulsive therapy (ECT). The nurse should tell the client that this medication is given:
A. Orally
B. To facilitate prolonged muscular activity
C. To relax skeletal muscles during the ECT procedure
D. To control respirations during ECT

125. Persons who suffer from seizure disorders are often prescribed a combination of medications to control seizures. The nurse should know that these are:
A. Pentobarbital (Nembutal) and phenobarbital (Luminal)

B. Alprazolam (Xanax) and primidone (Myidone)
C. Phenytoin (Dilantin) and phenobarbital (Luminal)
D. Phenytoin (Dilantin) and pentobarbital (Nembutal)

126. A 34-year-old client has a diagnosis of bipolar disorder. The nurse should be aware that the medication of choice for this disorder is:
A. Risperidone (Risperdal)
B. Clozapine (Clozaril)
C. Lorazepam (Ativan)
D. Lithium carbonate (Eskalith)

127. An 60-year-old client is receiving flurazepam (Dalmane) 30 mg at bedtime. Which statement by the client would assure the nurse that medication teaching has been effective?
A. "Nurse, please double the dose, I'm not sleeping."
B. "Will this medication take away the pain?"
C. "I am dizzy and weak in the morning. Please tell the doctor about this."
D. "When the doctor comes, tell him I want to be discharged."

128. A 22-year-old is taking tranylcypromine (Parnate), a monoamine oxidase (MAO) inhibitor. The nurse's discharge teaching about the medication should emphasize which of the following instructions?
A. Stop the medication if side effects occur.
B. Avoid eating chocolate.
C. Use over-the-counter medications for headaches.
D. Eat yogurt to ensure absorption of tranylcypromine.

129. When barbiturates are prescribed to induce sleep for a depressed client, it is important for the nurse to:
A. Check for "cheeking" of the medication.
B. Check the respiratory rate frequently throughout the tour of duty.
C. Explain the differences between absorption and excretion.
D. Check for decreased circulation.

130. A 43-year-old female client has been taking barbiturates for a number of months. She tells the home health nurse that she would like to see her deceased mother. The initial nursing action should be to assess for:
A. Physical and psychological dependence
B. Suicidal ideation
C. Seizure activity
D. Toxicity

131. A 38-year-old male client presents at the emergency room complaining of pain on the right side of the abdomen under the rib cage. He suffers from alcoholism and decreased hepatic function-

ing. The nurse should know that which one of the following is used to treat alcohol withdrawal symptoms?
A. Valproic acid (Depakene)
B. Thiamine
C. Chlordiazepoxide (Librium)
D. Pyridoxine

132. A long-term alcoholic client says to the nurse, "I'm tired of using and I want to stop. The doctor mentioned a medication that can help me maintain sobriety." The nurse is aware that the medication is:
A. Carbamazepine (Tegretol)
B. Clonidine (Catapres)
C. Disulfiram (Antabuse)
D. Folic acid

133. Electroconvulsive therapy (ECT) has been effective in the treatment of severe depression. The nurse should know that the side effects of ECT are:
A. Decreased levels of serotonin
B. Long bone fractures
C. Irreversible brain damage
D. Confusion and temporary memory loss

134. A 36-year-old male client is scheduled for electroconvulsive therapy (ECT). Prior to the client's ECT treatment, it is important for the nurse to explain which of the following:
A. A general anesthesia with the use of a muscle relaxant drug is used during the treatment.
B. The procedure is incapacitating for many persons.
C. ECT has been used since the 1930s. There is absolutely no risk involved.
D. Permanent memory loss is a major side effect.

135. A 56-year-old male client returned to the psychiatric unit from electroconvulsive therapy (ECT). The nurse should know that which of the following is a projected outcome of ECT therapy?
A. The client's anxiety remains high and he has limited understanding of the procedure.
B. The client is reoriented to time, place, and situation.
C. The client is fearful and limits social interaction.
D. The client has increased cyanosis and multiple bruises.

136. A 44-year-old female client, with a history of severe depression, has not responded to antidepressant medications. The nurse caring for the client knows that the treatment of choice would be:
A. Psychotherapy
B. Electroconvulsive therapy (ECT)
C. Insulin coma therapy
D. Pharmacoconvulsive therapy

137. A 45-year-old male client is considering electroconvulsive therapy (ECT). He questions the nurse about the number of necessary treatments. The nurse's best explanation is:

A. "The most common range is usually between 6 and 10 treatments."
B. "One treatment every 3 months until the depression subsides."
C. "The American Psychiatric Association recommends a total of 30 treatments."
D. "There are those who require a maintenance ECT."

138. A 33-year-old female client asks about the length of time it will take to make her feel better after the first ECT treatment. The nurse's best explanation is:
A. Seven days
B. Fifteen days
C. Twenty-eight days
D. Twenty-one days

139. Some persons, after receiving electroconvulsive therapy (ECT), complain of physical discomfort. The nurse should assess for all of the following except:
A. Increased salivation
B. Headache
C. Nausea
D. Muscle soreness

140. After the nurse explains electroconvulsive therapy (ECT) to an outpatient client who is scheduled for the first treatment, the client states, "I'm too scared and can't decide what to do." The best response by the nurse is:
A. "There is no room for concern. You will be all right."
B. "ECT is a safe, effective treatment. There is no degree of risk."
C. "Tell me more about how you feel."
D. "Let your family make the decision for you."

141. The nurse is providing care to a 25-year-old woman experiencing an acute phase of catatonic schizophrenia. One nursing goal is to decrease the client's isolated behavior. Which of the following nursing actions would best contribute to that goal?
A. Provide a colorful environment.
B. Speak in concise, simple terms to prevent sensory overload.
C. Avoid setting limits on her behavior.
D. Encourage participation in group therapy.

142. The nurse's intervention in the management of violent behavior in the psychiatric setting should include which one of the following?
A. Responding in a confrontational, aggressive, or threatening manner
B. Challenging the client's violent behavior
C. Conveying control by using clear, calm statements and a confident physical stance
D. Overidentifying with the client's experience

143. A 33-year-old male client has a history of assaultive behavior. He is hostile, verbally abusive, and demands immediate discharge. The best nursing intervention to manage the behavior would be to:

    A. Limit the physical distance during the verbal intervention.
    B. Control and force stabilization of the situation.
    C. Shift the focus of his hostility.
    D. Quickly establish therapeutic rapport.

144. A 41-year-old physically violent female was transported to the emergency room for a psychiatric assessment. The best approach by the nurse would be to:
    A. Have a sense of humor.
    B. Use brief statements during the assessment.
    C. Provide close contact.
    D. Use open-ended, neutrally posed questions.

145. The best nursing intervention for a client who has a history of assaultive behavior and is labile, combative, and unable to regain control is to:
    A. Apply physical restraints.
    B. Use active listening.
    C. Administer a chemical restraint.
    D. Encourage the use of functional coping skills.

146. When a client is placed in mechanical restraints, it is important for the nurse to:
    A. Obtain a physician's written order at least every 48 hours.
    B. Apply the restraints to maintain limited movement.
    C. Observe the client every 60 minutes and document the information.
    D. Document the type of restraints and the client's response.

147. A 25-year-old suicidal client is preparing for discharge. Which of the following is most important for the nurse to consider?
    A. Knowledge of rehabilitation resources
    B. Denial of suicidal ideation and implementing healthy problem-solving skills
    C. Verbalizes an understanding of the medication regimen
    D. Verbalizes somatic complaints and suicidal ideation

148. During a routine visit to a 38-year-old client, the home health nurse determines that the client has profound feelings of guilt and hopelessness. The client tells the nurse that she has no purpose in life and asks the nurse to keep a secret about her suicidal intention. How should the nurse respond?
    A. Explain that secrets are not entertained.
    B. Discuss steps that will resolve negative lifestyles that increase suicide risk.
    C. Inform the client that preoccupation with self is evident and that she should express hope for the future.
    D. Reassure the client that her secret is sacred because of their long-time friendship.

149. A 50-year-old male client who lost his wife in an automobile accident and is now a paraplegic says to the nurse, "I'm so depressed and in such severe pain, just give me an overdose of morphine." The best response by the nurse is:
    A. "I can see that you are very upset, so I'll increase the amount of morphine."
    B. "I'm unable to alter the prescribed dose."
    C. "I can see that you are very distraught and uncomfortable. I'll give you the prescribed medication."
    D. "You have too much to live for. I don't want to hear that."

150. Which one of the following statements would indicate to the nurse that a client is experiencing suicidal ideation?
    A. "I lost my job and I'm tired of looking for another one."
    B. "I've had enough. I'm just a burden and I have no other choice but to end my life."
    C. "Oh God, I don't know what to do. Please help me."
    D. "If my wife had lived, we would be happy and I would not feel so lonely."

151. Which of the following statements by the nurse would assess for suicidal risk?
    A. "You seem desperate. Do you have a lethal means for suicide?"
    B. "You say that you won't be around much any longer. Tell me what that means."
    C. "Tell me about your lifestyle."
    D. "Have you written any suicide notes?"

152. A 23-year-old female client was admitted to the emergency room for treatment of an overdose of lithium carbonate. She was later transferred to the psychiatric unit. The client said to the nurse, "I will never do that again. My brother died 6 months ago and he still loves me." A possible cause of the suicide attempt is:
    A. A maturational crisis
    B. The inability to express feelings
    C. Psychopathology
    D. Social crisis

153. In planning care for the suicidal client, it is important for the nurse to remember that the attempt may be:
    A. Associated with secondary gain importance
    B. Associated with functional coping skills
    C. From an adequate support group
    D. A direct correlation between feelings and a stable lifestyle

154. Nurses who provide nursing care for the chronic suicidal client often experience:
    A. Countertransference from the client
    B. Assertive behavior from the client
    C. Feelings of despair and jubilation
    D. Feelings of professional inadequacy

155. Cues to suicide are frequently subtle and difficult to interpret. Which one of the following would the nurse assess as a nonverbal cue?

A. Purchasing a new car
B. An increase in psychomotor behavior
C. Purchasing a world trip
D. A decrease in psychomotor activity

156. Anorexia nervosa, or restrictive eating, is characterized by deliberate starvation. The nurse should be aware that one of the features central to the diagnosis is:
A. Obsession with weight gain
B. Body image disturbance
C. Disregard for the feelings of others
D. Healthy relationships

157. A 14-year-old female client was admitted with a diagnosis of anorexia nervosa. During the initial interview, the nurse determined that the client lacked a sense of competence except for weight control. The nurse is aware that this feature is known as:
A. Paralyzing sense of ineffectiveness
B. "Good girl, bad girl" syndrome
C. Disavowing human emotions
D. Internalizing perceptions

158. The primary nursing goal for a client diagnosed as having anorexia nervosa should be aimed at:
A. Promoting improved nutrition
B. Living up to family expectations
C. Preparing food
D. Alleviating depression

159. When caring for a client with self-imposed starvation, which daily nursing assessment should the nurse make?
A. Peripheral edema
B. Hyperthyroid-like state
C. Medication compliance
D. Behavioral change

160. The best approach to establish adequate eating patterns is to assume a positive expectation of the client. Which is the best statement by the nurse?
A. "I'll give you a 1-hour time limit."
B. "I will allow you space to eat in peace."
C. "I will sit quietly with you while you eat."
D. "There are people who would truly appreciate the food that you waste."

161. If an anorectic client is being forced to eat, it is important for the nurse to implement which one of the following interventions?
A. Discuss eating behaviors
B. Provide three large meals daily
C. Observe bathroom behavior
D. Use praise or flattery

162. As the anorectic client's physical condition improves, it is important for the nurse to focus on:
A. Self-determination
B. Dependent behavior
C. Sleep disturbance
D. Rigid daily routine

163. The best nursing approach to mealtime activity for the anorectic client is to provide a:
A. High-calorie dessert
B. Pleasant environment
C. Meal high in fat
D. Low-calorie diet

164. The nurse should understand that clients diagnosed as having anorexia nervosa:
A. Need to control one aspect of their lives
B. Are outgoing and seek support from others
C. Send a message of effective control over their basic needs
D. Exhibit increased internal awareness

165. A 23-year-old female client was admitted to the psychiatric unit. During the assessment interview, the nurse determined that the client was shy, sensitive, stubborn, and extremely underweight. Which of the following statements made by the client would help the nurse determine that she is suffering from an eating disorder?
A. "I eat every morsel of food but I can't gain any weight."
B. "I'm sensitive toward others."
C. "I have not had a menstrual period in 6 months and I'm not pregnant."
D. "My parents are concerned about me."

166. A 19-year-old female college student was admitted to the psychiatric unit because of an eating disorder. During the nursing assessment, the client stated that she was depressed over her social life and weight problems. She mentioned that she has numerous episodes of purging. Which one of the following diagnoses would be most suitable?
A. Compulsive eating disorder
B. Bulimia nervosa
C. Anorexia nervosa
D. Body dysmorphic disorder

167. The nurse, working with a client who has been diagnosed as having bulimia nervosa and who has frequent episodes of bingeing and purging, needs to understand that this disorder is:
A. A symptomatic feature of other psychological conditions
B. A mood disorder
C. An attempt to control the family environment
D. Primary to a psychological disturbance

168. When planning care for a client diagnosed as having bulimia nervosa, the nurse should consider which of the following nursing interventions as a major priority?
A. Providing external limits to help contain the client's anxiety during mealtime
B. Helping the client recognize that the physical symptoms may be life-threatening
C. Intervening when intrafamilial conflicts occur
D. Conveying a judgmental attitude

169. A 23-year-old female client who was admitted with

an eating disorder complains to the nurse in a hostile manner that she wants to be discharged because she has been hospitalized for too long. What is the best response by the nurse?
A. "Ask your social worker about discharge plans."
B. "You need to deal with your hostility."
C. "Tomorrow will be better."
D. "You seem upset. Tell me how you are feeling right now."

170. A 50-year-old female client weighing 450 pounds, confided in the nurse that she was sexually molested as a young child. The nurse should be aware that obesity is thought to represent:
A. Direct self-destruction behavior
B. A defense against intimacy with the opposite sex
C. Financial distress
D. Self-satisfaction

171. A 23-year-old female presents herself at the mental health clinic stating that she is concerned about her bizarre eating behavior. During the nursing assessment, the client states that she has a history of gorging and purging. The nurse observes that the client has dental enamel erosion and calluses on the knuckles. Which one of the following assessments would be most helpful when developing a plan of care?
A. Spiritual cleansing
B. Eating patterns of the family
C. Introverted behavior
D. Hunger prior to bingeing

172. When planning short-term goals for a client diagnosed as having an eating disorder and who expressed emotional conflicts in a destructive manner, the nurse would consider which one of the following?
A. Functional coping skills
B. Motivation for change
C. Excessive involvement in food preparation
D. Alliance building

173. In evaluating the success of care and to determine if the person diagnosed as having an eating disorder is ready for discharge, the nurse would ask which one of the following questions?
A. "Is the person feeling loved and does life matter?"
B. "Is the person willing to discard the use of laxatives?"
C. "Does the person feel powerless and helpless?"
D. "Is success inadequately measured?"

174. An obese 18-year-old is admitted to the psychiatric unit diagnosed as having depression and an eating disorder. The chief complaint is an ugly appearance. She yells at the nurse to do something about it. Which one of the following is the best response by the nurse?
A. "You seem angry, tell me what your feelings are now."

B. "You obviously need to lose some weight."
C. "You are not ugly. Don't worry."
D. "Don't yell. Your feelings may be expressed differently."

175. When establishing a nursing plan of care for an obese client, which one of the following is an outcome criterion?
A. Acknowledging a relationship between food and spiritual needs
B. Achieving and maintaining weight within normal parameters for size and age
C. Achieving psychological testing to determine emotional deficits
D. Gaining an immediate insight into family dynamics

176. The nurse working with clients who are substance-dependent should know that a hallmark of the maladaptive behavior is:
A. Intolerance
B. Withdrawal
C. Irritability
D. Blackouts

177. A 43-year-old mother of three children who is dying of metastasized breast cancer is still able to communicate. A nursing action to promote optimum care would be to:
A. Provide her with opportunities to have some control over her environment.
B. Encourage her to try experimental treatments.
C. Discourage her from making decisions about treatment.
D. Encourage her to verbalize her regrets.

178. A 56-year-old male chronic alcoholic tells the substance abuse clinic nurse that he has not had anything to drink in the past 48 hours. Which of the following is the most serious withdrawal syndrome?
A. Blackout
B. Alcohol withdrawal delirium
C. Hypotension
D. Tissue adaptation

179. A 45-year-old divorced woman tells the nurse at the mental health clinic that she has been self-medicating with cocaine in order to deal with loneliness and depression. The nurse determines that she is:
A. Psychologically dependent
B. Physically dependent
C. In the "postcoke" blues
D. Overly aggressive

180. The nurse working with substance disorder clients should be aware that all of the following factors influence abuse except:
A. Biological factors
B. Amnestic syndrome
C. Ethnic influences
D. Personality factors

181. A 35-year-old chronic alcoholic is suffering from peripheral neuropathy. The nurse informs the client that it is the result of a nutritional deficiency. Which one of the following is the drug of choice for this disorder?
    A. Thiamine
    B. Vitamin K
    C. Vitamin A
    D. Ascorbic acid

182. Frequently, persons with substance abuse problems are very sensitive. It is important for the nurse to:
    A. Be judgmental and objective.
    B. "Rescue" the person.
    C. Criticize recidivism.
    D. Emphasize self-diagnosis.

183. In planning care for the medically unstable alcoholic client, which of the following would be of immediate concern?
    A. Simplifying the environment
    B. Initiating pharmacological therapy
    C. Recommending a therapeutic community
    D. Determining psychosocial needs

184. The nurse should know that maintaining abstinence depends primarily on:
    A. Alcoholics Anonymous
    B. Goal achievement
    C. Family involvement
    D. Psychopharmacological therapy

185. A 50-year-old male client is admitted to the emergency room. His symptoms are incoherent speech, agitation, disorientation, visual hallucinations, and increased blood pressure. The nurse determines that the client is suffering from:
    A. Alcoholic myopathy
    B. Delirium tremens
    C. Korsakoff's syndrome
    D. Gastritis

186. Methadone maintenance programs are available at licensed clinics. The nurse is aware that the expected outcome of methadone maintenance is to:
    A. Augment the addict's craving for narcotics.
    B. Provide a longer-acting narcotic that is a substitute for heroin.
    C. Administer a legally controlled drug.
    D. Improve psychological well-being and family and social functioning.

187. A 50-year-old male client is suffering from alcoholic hallucinosis. He tells the nurse that he sees bugs crawling on the wall. The nurse's best response is:
    A. "I'll remove the bugs from the wall."
    B. "You are confused because of your alcoholism."
    C. "You see shadows from the fan rotating. I'll stay with you until you feel less anxious."
    D. "No, I don't agree."

188. The emergency room nurse assesses a client suffering from chronic alcoholism and observes confabulation. The client reports that she feels nervous, lethargic, and has some memory loss. The nurse would recognize this disorder as:
    A. Korsakoff's psychosis
    B. Vascular dementia
    C. Wernicke's encephalopathy
    D. Esophageal varices

189. A 48-year-old recovering male client who is ready for discharge confides in the nurse that he would like to attend Alcoholics Anonymous (AA) meetings. Which response by the nurse would be most supportive?
    A. "AA groups are not for everyone."
    B. "Members of AA help others to recover from alcoholism."
    C. "Tell me how you will benefit from the program."
    D. "Group members pay a small fee and can receive lifelong support."

190. The nurse is aware that the primary goal of a residential treatment program for substance abusers is to:
    A. Discuss legal problems.
    B. Emphasize morals and values.
    C. Emphasize self-reliance and resocialization.
    D. Discuss the disengagement of family members.

191. The nurse is aware that the medication commonly used for opioid intoxication is:
    A. Benztropine (Congentin)
    B. Methohexital sodium (Brevital)
    C. Nalorphine (Nalline)
    D. Chlordiazepoxide (Librium)

192. A 45-year-old woman has recently been divorced after 25 years of marriage. Her ex-husband is planning to marry the woman with whom he has been having an affair for 5 years. The wife comes to the mental health clinic for help. She has never required psychiatric care in the past. She describes feeling enraged and betrayed. She states, "I just don't know where to turn or what to do." The nurse realizes that the most appropriate treatment approach for her would be:
    A. Intensive psychotherapy
    B. Crisis intervention
    C. Relaxation therapy
    D. Electroconvulsive therapy (ECT)

193. A 6-year-old boy who was recently admitted to the hospital with a diagnosis of autism grabs a toy and hits another child. The most appropriate response to the child's attempts to hurt himself or others is to:
    A. Isolate him for 24 hours.
    B. Encourage him to explain his angry thoughts.
    C. Assume a nonpunitive attitude and stop the attempt to hurt himself or others.
    D. Call his parents to get their input.

194. A 74-year-old exhibits more frequent memory loss

and disorientation to time and place. The family tells the nurse that their loved one has been recently diagnosed with Alzheimer's disease. The nurse should know that the characteristics of this disease are:
A. Slow and insidious with a gradual and progressive loss of cognitive abilities
B. Abrupt onset and runs a variable course
C. Self-limiting
D. Rapid functional decline in multiple cognitive areas

195. A 78-year-old nursing home resident exhibits little emotional control and is often argumentative with other residents and staff. The best nursing approach is to:
A. Confront the argumentative behavior.
B. Redirect attention and set limits on maladaptive abusive behavior.
C. Administer PRN medications to control behavior.
D. Isolate the client until the behavior improves.

196. A 67-year-old female client is in the third stage of Alzheimer's disease. The nurse is aware that which of the following characteristics is indicative of this stage?
A. Memory difficulty with functional attributes
B. Objectively dysfunctional with the inability to adapt to unfamiliar environments
C. Gradually becomes mute and inattentive and requires assistance with basic needs
D. Exhibits neurological signs, contractures, and aspiration of oral intake is noted

197. In planning care for the client in the very last stage of Alzheimer's disease, which of the following nursing goals is inappropriate:
A. Promote quality of life.
B. Determine the living will status.
C. Provide for spiritual needs.
D. Provide for medically assisted suicide.

198. A 55-year-old male tells the nurse at the mental health clinic that he has suffered a great deal of stress, disappointments, and accomplished few successes in life. The nurse should know that the feelings may be expressed in the form of:
A. Shame and doubt
B. Delusional thinking
C. Self-approval
D. Identity confusion

199. A 67-year-old day-program client complains of dizziness, weakness, and forgetfulness. The initial nursing intervention should provide for:
A. Safety needs
B. Palliative treatment
C. Spiritual needs
D. Psychotherapy

200. The nurse working on an Alzheimer's disease unit should be aware that one of the first cognitive changes in a person diagnosed as having the disease would be:
A. Memory disturbance
B. Apraxia
C. Agraphia
D. Agnosia

201. Many confused elderly persons smoke. The most appropriate nursing intervention would be to:
A. Restrict the number of cigarettes.
B. Restrict smoking privileges.
C. Monitor smoking periods.
D. Initiate a smoker's anonymous group.

202. The home health nurse visits a 65-year-old client who is on a homebound status. The nurse determines that the client is fearful and depressed. When revising the care plan, which one of the following is the best intervention?
A. Provide a support system.
B. Initiate a daily schedule.
C. Create a socialization session.
D. Assist with a mobility regimen.

203. The home health nurse determines that the client's condition is grounds for considering the psychiatrically homebound status. Which one of the following criteria should be considered?
A. Requirement for 4-hour supervision
B. Vulnerability in the community
C. Lack of family support
D. Mild anxiety

204. An 83-year-old uncooperative and confused nursing home resident who grew up in another culture has difficulty understanding the nursing staff. The nurse providing care for this client should have a(an):
A. Understanding of cultural relativity
B. Reminiscence group
C. Resocialization group
D. Group discussion about feelings and culture

205. A 66-year-old male diagnosed as having schizophrenia is a nursing home resident. He complains to the nurse that his neck is stiff and he has difficulty swallowing. The best nursing intervention is to assess for:
A. Dysphonia
B. Tardive dyskinesia
C. Akathisia
D. Echolalia

206. A 65-year-old female nursing home resident with a diagnosis of schizophrenia has a number of open wounds that she constantly picks. She ask the nurse for lotion to soothe them. The nurse should evaluate the behavior for:
A. Primary gain
B. Physiological changes
C. Secondary gain
D. Nutritional deficits

207. A crisis is an internal disturbance. The nurse should know it is characterized by:
A. Precipitating events that are perceived as a threat to self
B. Decreased anxiety
C. Cognitive orientation
D. Resolving the perceived threat to self

208. A disheveled looking 35-year-old woman enters the mental health clinic crying and wringing her hands. She says to the nurse, "My life is ruined. I've lost everything and I don't know what to do anymore." Which is the best nursing intervention?
A. Refer to social service.
B. Refer to psychotherapy.
C. Clarify the problem.
D. Discuss antianxiety medication.

209. A client who has frequent appointments at the mental health clinic states that she lost her job, feels out of control, and is unable to cope with her present lifestyle. Which type of event precipitates the crisis state?
A. Dispositional
B. Maturational
C. Adventitious
D. Situational

210. A client was referred to the crisis intervention center. During the assessment, she said to the nurse, "I don't need to be here because all of my problems have been solved." Which defense mechanism is the client using?
A. Denial
B. Displacement
C. Projection
D. Rationalization

211. A 55-year-old widow is unable to cope with the tasks of daily living. A recent hurricane completely destroyed her home. She is unable to identify any available family support. Identify the crisis phase.
A. General reorganization
B. Disorganization
C. Denial
D. Local reorganization

212. Which one of the following is most essential when planning care for a client who is experiencing a crisis?
A. Focus on emotional deficits.
B. Explore underlying personality dynamics.
C. Explore previous coping strategies.
D. Provide financial assistance.

213. During the initial interview with a client in crisis, the mental health professional should first:
A. Evaluate the potential for self-harm.
B. Assess the adequacy of the support system.
C. Determine the level of precrisis functioning.
D. Assess for substance abuse.

214. The most significant goal for a client experiencing a crisis is to:
A. Restore the client to precrisis functioning.
B. Prescribe psychotherapy.
C. Evaluate the effects of early childhood development on the crisis.
D. Provide a list of resources.

215. Which one of the following questions would be most effective when evaluating the outcome of crisis intervention?
A. Has education helped with positive behavioral changes?
B. Has the person developed maladaptive coping strategies?
C. Has the person grown from the experience?
D. Can the person analyze a plan of action for dealing with stressors?

216. You are working with a client who is experiencing a crisis. The client states, "I can no longer function." The nurse directs the client to a quieter environment. The client does not respond to the instruction. After evaluating the situation, the nurse is aware that the client is exhibiting a:
A. Decrease in the perceptual field
B. Level of calmness
C. Strong sense of self
D. Physical disorder

217. A 22-year-old widow tells the nurse that her husband died 3 months ago. She feels alone and vulnerable. Which statement by the widow would indicate that her coping skills are adaptive?
A. "I can't understand why this happened to me."
B. "I will find a support group."
C. "I'm mentally healthy. I can solve my own problems."
D. "What am I to do? God and my husband have abandoned me."

218. When planning crisis intervention for a chronically mentally ill client, it is most essential for the nurse to consider which one of the following:
A. Personal strengths
B. Psychotic episodes
C. Incompetency
D. Family support

219. A 20-year-old male athlete has been recently diagnosed with diabetes. He denies that he has a physical problem. The nurse observes that his speech is monotone, and he states that he is ready to commit suicide. Which one of the following would be an expected outcome of crisis intervention? The client:
A. Expresses optimism and hope for the future
B. Expresses the desire for long-term therapy
C. Demonstrates dysfunctional coping mechanisms
D. Verbalizes feelings of despair

220. The 45-year-old couple have suddenly been faced

with the decision of placing their elderly parents in a nursing home. They call the crisis intervention center and ask for assistance. This type of crisis can often be prevented by:
A. Restitution
B. Anticipatory guidance
C. Appropriate referrals
D. Generic approach

221. A 13-year-old client is admitted to an inpatient adolescent psychiatric unit for treatment of adolescent adjustment reactions. Which of the following characteristics is the nurse likely to see this client exhibit?
A. Verbalizations about a positive body image
B. Acceleration in achieving masculine or feminine social role
C. Aggression, resistance, acting-out behavior
D. Weight loss

222. An 18-year-old client with a serious substance abuse problem during the last year comes to the mental health clinic for treatment. He is restless and pacing. A symptom the nurse should pay attention to would be:
A. Characteristics of his feces
B. His hemoglobin level
C. His level of consciousness
D. The color of his nailbeds

223. An adolescent girl experiencing anxiety reaction is admitted to an inpatient psychiatric unit. As the client begins to adjust to the daily routine on the unit, the nurse would like her to concentrate on completing tasks. Which nursing action would be most appropriate to accomplish this goal?
A. Assess the cause of her anxiety.
B. Administer major tranquilizers.
C. Encourage increased fluid intake.
D. Minimize family contact.

224. A couple whose 3-month-old son just died of sudden infant death syndrome (SIDS) is having difficulties with activities of daily living. However, one important goal of nursing care for them is to:
A. Delay the grieving process.
B. Plan funeral arrangements for their son.
C. Accept that the death could have been prevented.
D. Minimize the discussion of death with others.

225. During the initial interview, the nurse initiates the beginning phases of discharge planning for the client. Which one of the following should the nurse consider?
A. Moral reasoning
B. Sociopolitical topics
C. Sociocultural data
D. Evaluative process

226. An important aspect of nursing care for a mildly retarded 8-year-old would be to:
A. Encourage the parents to concentrate on her rather than the family.

B. Modify her environment to promote independence and impulse control.
C. Delay extensive diagnostic studies until she is older.
D. Provide 1:1 tutorial education and minimize peer interaction.

227. The nurse should be aware that a person who is diagnosed as having a borderline personality disorder displays which of the following characteristics?
A. Global amnesia
B. Intense anger
C. Stable interpersonal relationships
D. Affective stability

228. Which one of the following interventions should the nurse include when planning care for a client diagnosed as having histrionic personality disorder?
A. Accept the client's provocative behavior.
B. Accept the behavior as positive.
C. Set firm limits on attention-seeking behaviors.
D. Emphasize passive-aggressive behavior.

229. A 28-year-old male client who is narcissistic and shows little regard for his peers and the hospital staff is preoccupied with, and has fantasies about, success, power, and intelligence. The best nursing intervention is:
A. Encourage expression of grandiosity.
B. Limit feedback.
C. Criticize the haughty and uncaring attitude.
D. Discuss the unrealistic sense of entitlement.

230. The nursing care plan for a 30-year-old client diagnosed as having obsessive-compulsive personality disorder should include which one of the following interventions?
A. Confront the client about the nonconstructive, compulsive responses during the ritualistic event.
B. Explore activities that are pleasurable.
C. Encourage the client to indirectly express feelings of anger and resentment.
D. Limit decision making.

231. A 41-year-old male client experienced severe depression after the death of his wife. The physician prescribed an antidepressant. Which one of the following nursing instructions is most important?
A. Use sugarless hard candy, chew sugarless gum, and sip water frequently for a dry mouth.
B. Continue with an afternoon cocktail because it is relaxing.
C. Return to your trucker's position.
D. Adjust the amount of the antidepressant when taking over-the-counter medications.

232. Some persons after receiving ECT complain of physical discomfort. The nurse should assess for:
A. Increased salivation
B. Amnesia
C. Abated depression
D. Muscle soreness

233. Prior to the administration of ECT, the nurse instructs the client to:
    A. Drink plenty of fluids.
    B. Remove jewelry and eyeglasses.
    C. Remove a partial plate.
    D. Wear tight-fitting street clothes.

234. A 43-year-old female client diagnosed as having depression is preparing for discharge. To evaluate the effectiveness of therapy during the hospitalization, the nurse should assess the client for:
    A. Ability to control others
    B. Stigmatization of self
    C. Ability to establish realistic goals
    D. Vegetative symptoms

235. Discharge instructions for a 20-year-old female client diagnosed as having a bipolar disorder should include:
    A. Principles of integrity
    B. Emphasis on medication compliance
    C. Emphasis on independence and discourage follow-up care
    D. Medicaid information

236. When planning short-term goals for a 34-year-old hospitalized manic client, the nurse should include:
    A. Protection from self-inflicted harm
    B. Meals in excess of metabolic requirement
    C. Strict participation in unit activities
    D. Enforced medication

237. During hospitalization for a 39-year-old client diagnosed as having dysthymic disorder, the nurse counselor provides instructions on which one of the following?
    A. Psychotic symptoms
    B. Importance of a social support system
    C. Importance of making future goals
    D. Senescence

238. The nurse working with substance use disorder clients should be aware that:
    A. Control is a constant underlying dynamic.
    B. Addiction in men is more open than in women.
    C. Consent of the victim is a vehicle for its development.
    D. Family environment is unaffected by the disorder.

239. A 75-year-old female client suffers from confusion and memory loss and exhibits confabulation. Nursing interventions should include which one of the following?
    A. Promote dependence.
    B. Maintain a stable environment.
    C. Promote afternoon naps.
    D. Confront cognitive errors.

240. In planning care for the client in the late stage of Alzheimer's disease, the nurse should include which one of the following?
    A. Promote quality of life.
    B. Initiate the living will.
    C. Promote reality orientation.
    D. Provide for medically assisted suicide.

241. A client is admitted to the emergency room accompanied by her husband, who reports that she has taken an overdose of amitriptyline (Elavil). He further reports that she has been depressed for 2 years. The highest priority nursing action at this time should be to:
    A. Ask the husband who the client's physician is.
    B. Assess the client's vital signs.
    C. Ask the client if she has drug allergies.
    D. Assess the client's suicide potential.

242. Because of the pharmacological effects of amitriptyline (Elavil) in the body at high doses, the nurse should watch the client for:
    A. Arrhythmias
    B. Nausea and vomiting
    C. Headache
    D. Leg cramps

243. The physician orders that the client with an amitriptyline (Elavil) overdose be admitted to the hospital intensive care unit for 3 days. The most likely reason for this is that:
    A. The client's respirations may drop after the half-life of the drug has passed.
    B. The client may make another suicide attempt.
    C. Blood plasma levels of amitriptyline may need to be monitored closely.
    D. Toxic cardiac effects may not respond to treatment.

244. Which of the following statements is correct concerning personality disorders?
    A. Personality disorders generally emerge after age 45.
    B. Persons with personality disorders usually have insight into their disorder.
    C. Personality disorders are a variant of character traits that go beyond the range found in most people.
    D. Persons with personality disorders demonstrate adaptive ability to perceive and relate to themselves and the environment.

245. A client is admitted to the inpatient unit of a psychiatric hospital with the diagnosis of borderline personality disorder. Initially, on admission, which of the following symptoms would the nurse expect to find during the admission interview?
    A. Rapid mood shifts with isolating behaviors
    B. Intrusiveness with reluctance to discuss personal problems
    C. Compliance with overtones of stable self-image
    D. Affective instability and disrupted self-esteem

246. Three days after admission to the inpatient setting, the borderline client tells the evening weekend nurse, "I'm so glad you're working this

evening. Those day nurses just don't like me. They're mean to me and make me do things that I really don't want to do." The client is demonstrating which ego defense mechanism?
A. Denial
B. Rationalization
C. Splitting
D. Projection

247. The borderline client becomes restless and disruptive during group therapy every afternoon, even attempting to manipulate and undermine the nurse therapist. Which verbal intervention by the nurse therapist would be the most therapeutic at this time?
A. "Please sit down and let the others clients voice their opinion for a while."
B. "If you are unable to sit still, I will have to ask you to leave the therapy room."
C. "Let's see if anyone else in the room has had similar feelings and behavior and how they learned to deal with them."
D. "You may stay in the therapy room if you will show more respect for me and the other clients."

248. The physician has ordered carbamazepine (Tegretol) for the borderline client. The nurse administering the drug knows that the most likely rationale for this drug is to:
A. Improve global functioning
B. Control anger
C. Elevate the mood
D. Diminish anxiety

249. A long-term goal for the borderline personality–disordered client is to:
A. Stay in psychotherapy for a minimum of 2 years.
B. Adjust medications as needed after discharge.
C. Develop insight into maladaptive behaviors.
D. Demonstrate improved coping behaviors.

250. A 25-year-old male is brought to the emergency room by the police in handcuffs. He is dirty and disheveled with incoherent speech. He was picked up by the police after a phone call from his neighbor reporting that he was tearing down the door to his apartment. The neighbor told the police that the man had just used PCP. The nurse should be aware that:
A. The client will most probably calm down with quiet, reassuring words during the initial assessment.
B. She should ask the emergency room physician to order a sedative immediately.
C. The most effective intervention at this time would be to call a family member to stay with the client.
D. Clients experiencing PCP toxicity or psychosis do not respond well to attempts at interaction.

251. The client is placed in a dimly lit room and restrained. As the staff is applying the restraints, the client shouts, "Get those snakes off my body! Get them off now!" The nurse recognizes that the client is:
A. Experiencing visual and tactile hallucinations
B. Having paranoid delusions
C. Morbidly afraid of snakes
D. Disoriented to his whereabouts

252. The physician orders lorazepam (Ativan) 2 mg IM stat for a prisoner. As the nurse enters the room to administer the medication, the client says, "Don't come any closer! I know that you are trying to kill me with that needle!" The most appropriate comment by the nurse would be:
A. "I will leave for now, but I will be back in 15 minutes to give this medication to you."
B. "I know you are frightened right now, but this medication will help you to be less afraid."
C. "Which side would you like your injection in?"
D. "OK, I'll tell the doctor that you don't want the medication."

253. One hour after lorazepam (Ativan) injection, the client begins to calm down. When the nurse enters the room, the client asks, "When can I get out of here? I feel much better than when I first came in." The most therapeutic response by the nurse is:
A. "You can be released when the physician orders it."
B. "None of your family has arrived to take you home."
C. "Let's talk about how you were feeling when you first came in."
D. "OK, I'll release the restraints if you promise not to become violent."

254. The client is released from restraints after a violent episode. He tells the nurse, "I'm embarrassed to go home. My neighbor will probably never want to see me again." Which comment by the nurse is most therapeutic for the client?
A. "If your neighbor is your friend, he will probably just forget about the whole incident."
B. "There's no need to be embarrassed about this. Things like this happen to people all the time."
C. "That's a very real problem. What do you think you could say to your neighbor?"
D. "I don't think you are going home. I think the police are going to take you to jail."

255. A 30-year-old female is admitted to the psychiatric hospital with bizarre thought patterns of short duration. There is no history of substance abuse or trauma. A full psychological workup has been ordered. Which of the following examinations would best determine glucose metabolism in the brain?
A. Computed tomography (CT)
B. Magnetic resonance imaging (MRI)

C. Brain electrical activity mapping (BEAM)
D. Positron emission tomography (PET)

256. Which of the following would be a direct violation of a client hospitalized in a psychiatric facility?
A. A paranoid schizophrenic client is told by the nurse that if he makes a will while in the hospital, it will be valid.
B. A chronically ill but stable client is paid minimum wage for working in the hospital laundry.
C. A member of the treatment team confiscates an outgoing letter to the editor of the local newspaper written by a client.
D. The nurse removes an expensive piece of jewelry from a client's room and informs her that it will be placed in the hospital safe until discharge.

257. A severely depressed and suicidal client is admitted on a physician's emergency certificate (PEC). Which of the following criteria is the most likely justification for this involuntary commitment?
A. Dangerous to self
B. Dangerous to others
C. Gravely disabled
D. Mentally incompetent

258. A nurse is admitted to an inpatient substance abuse treatment facility. Legally, she:
A. Must relinquish her driver's license to the Office of Motor Vehicles.
B. Cannot refuse treatment or refuse to participate in the prescribed therapies.
C. Maintains all of her civil rights.
D. Should notify the state Board of Nursing and relinquish her license to practice.

259. The nurse is admitting a client to the inpatient psychiatry hospital. Which of the following questions would elicit information relative to the client's general fund of knowledge?
A. "On a scale of 1 to 10, how would you rate your mood today?"
B. "What would you do if you found a stamped, self-addressed envelope lying on the ground?"
C. "Do you know today's date?"
D. "Can you name five state capitals?"

260. An admitted client tells the nurse that he is feeling depressed and would be better off dead. Which of the following information, if present, would place the client at highest immediate risk for suicide? The client:
A. Plans to take an overdose but has no medication on hand to do so
B. Wants to kill himself but doesn't have a definite plan
C. Verbalizes that he has a plan and has the means available in his suitcase
D. Plans to jump off the river bridge after discharge

261. A client tells the nurse that he is an angel and has the capacity to become invisible and can go through locked doors. This is an example of a(an):
A. Grandiose delusion
B. Auditory hallucination
C. Paranoid delusion
D. Visual hallucination

262. A client admitted for a complete psychological work-up is about to have the Rorschach test administered. A major benefit of a projective psychological test is that it:
A. Requires no special skills to evaluate the results
B. Bypasses a client's conscious resistance
C. Is fairly simple to administer
D. Assists in establishing rapport with a client

263. A client has been diagnosed with borderline personality disorder. Psychological tests that may help confirm or differentiate this diagnosis are:
A. Weschler Adult Intelligence Scale and Stanford-Binet
B. Stanford-Binet and Minnesota Multiphasic Personality Inventory
C. Minnesota Multiphasic Personality Inventory and Rorschach
D. Rorschach and Weschler Adult Intelligence Scale

264. An elderly client is admitted to the hospital with possible Alzheimer's disease. The most useful psychological test to aid in diagnosis would be:
A. Bender Gestalt
B. Dexamethasone suppression test
C. Thematic apperception test
D. Family kinetic drawings

265. A 50-year-old male is admitted to the psychiatric facility for treatment. His wife reports that he has been treated for schizophrenia several times in his adult life. He takes an oral hypoglycemic agent for control of diabetes mellitus. He has been basically noncompliant with his medications. He is scheduled for some psychological tests. Which of the following, if present, would definitely invalidate the results of psychological tests?
A. Test-taking experience
B. Diabetes mellitus
C. Psychosis
D. Objectivity

266. A client admitted with paranoid schizophrenia approaches the nurse and says, "I'm Jesus Christ and I'm here to forgive your sins." The most therapeutic response to the client at this time would be:
A. "I understand that you think you are Jesus Christ, but I don't believe that you are."
B. "I'm your nurse for the evening shift today. Why don't we sit in the day room and we can talk about why you are here."
C. "You know that you are not Jesus Christ, and if

you continue to say that you are, the other clients may not want to associate with you."

D. "I'll have to report this to your physician. He'll be very interested in hearing about this."

267. The paranoid schizophrenic client is placed on haloperidol (Haldol) 5 mg PO bid. As the nurse prepares to give the medication as ordered, the client tells the nurse, "I'm not taking this medication. I know it's poison, and Jesus Christ doesn't need medication." Which of the following interventions would be most appropriate for this client?
A. Tell the client that he must take his medication or it will be given by injection.
B. Put the medication in the client's food while he's not looking so that he will get the medication without knowing.
C. Wait a few minutes and go back later to offer the medication again to the client.
D. Chart that the client has refused the medication. No other action is necessary.

268. The client has been on haloperidol (Haldol) for 3 days. He tells the nurse that his neck is stiff and his tongue is pulling to one side of his mouth. The nurse assesses that the client is experiencing:
A. Tardive dyskinesia
B. Acute panic level of anxiety
C. Akathisia
D. Acute dystonia

269. Which of the following will give the client the most immediate relief from these unpleasant side effects from neuroleptics?
A. Lorazepam (Ativan) 1 mg PO
B. Diazepam (Valium) 5 mg PO
C. Haloperidol (Haldol) 2 mg IM
D. Benztropine (Cogentin) 1 mg IM

270. The client is to be discharged tomorrow. Which of the following statements reflects that he has learned a more adaptive way to cope with his illness and medication?
A. "From now on, I'm going to take my medication as the doctor has ordered. And if I have any side effects, I will call him."
B. "If I have any problems with my medication, I know now that I should just reduce my Haldol."
C. "When I get to feeling better, I'll be able to stop taking my Haldol."
D. "I'm not really sure why I take this medication anyway. It just causes me to have bad side effects."

271. A 15-year-old female his been admitted to the adolescent unit of the psychiatric hospital for observation, diagnosis, and treatment of possible anorexia nervosa. She is 65 inches tall and weighs 85 pounds. On admission she tells the nurse, "I don't know why my parents admitted me. I'm just trying to lose enough weight to stay on the gymnastic team." The highest priority nursing diagnosis would be:
A. Anxiety
B. Altered growth and development
C. Altered nutrition, less than body requirements
D. Self-esteem disturbance

272. A 15-year-old is admitted to the inpatient psychiatric facility after transfer from the emergency room of the local hospital for treatment of an overdose of acetaminophen (Tylenol). On admission, she is sobbing quietly, sitting in a wheelchair with her hands in her lap, eyes downcast. She offers nothing verbally, but does respond to the nurse's questions in monosyllables and short phrases. The highest priority goal for this client at this time is to:
A. Be introduced to other adolescents on the unit
B. Meet her primary nurse
C. Refrain from self-destructive behavior
D. Speak with her immediate family members

273. Two days after admission, the adolescent client attends insight therapy group. When asked by another adolescent in the group why she had been admitted, she began to cry and asked the therapist if she was required to answer. The most therapeutic response by the therapist would be:
A. "You are not required to answer, but there are others here who may have been through similar circumstances and can identify with your feelings."
B. "If you want to get well and get out of here, you should take every opportunity to participate in your treatment."
C. "Let's ask the other members of the group what they think of your question."
D. "If you don't participate, I'll have to report it to your physician and you may be here a long time."

274. Three days after admission, the adolescent client tells the nurse, "You know, I really did a stupid thing by swallowing those Tylenol." Select the most therapeutic response by the nurse.
A. "Well, it was pretty stupid, but you're OK now, so it doesn't do any good to beat yourself up about it."
B. "There's really no need to dwell on it now. Try to concentrate on getting well and getting back to your life."
C. "Did you do it to get attention from your family?"
D. "How were you feeling right before you decided to take the Tylenol?"

275. The adolescent client is to be discharged in the morning. The primary nurse asks the client what she has learned during hospitalization that will help her after discharge. Which statement by the client reflects that she has learned adaptive behav-

iors that will prevent another suicide attempt in the future?
- A. "I learned that if I ever want to kill myself, I'll have to take something stronger than Tylenol."
- B. "I know that I'm not the only teenager in the world who has ever attempted suicide."
- C. "I probably should have just run away from home like my best friend did."
- D. "If I ever get that depressed again, I'll find someone to talk to before I do anything I'll regret."

276. A 25-year-old college student presents at the health clinic and tells the nurse that he feels overwhelmed and nervous about upcoming exams. He further reports that he hasn't been able to concentrate while reading textbook assignments and has difficulty paying attention in class. Several times in the last week, he has had to get up and leave class because he felt as though he couldn't breathe and his heart was pounding. The most appropriate nursing diagnosis based on this interview assessment is:
- A. Impaired gas exchange
- B. Alteration in sensory experiences
- C. Alteration in thought processes
- D. Moderate anxiety

277. The physician prescribes propranolol (Inderal) for the client. The nurse recognizes the most likely rationale for using this drug in the absence of arrythmias or blood pressure problems is that it is known to:
- A. Block the autonomal arousal associated with anxiety attacks
- B. Activate the chemotrigger receptor zone in the brain
- C. Stimulate production of serotonin as the synapse
- D. Inhibit reuptake of norepinephrine at the synapse

278. A client is being treated with sertraline (Zoloft) for a major depressive episode. One week after medication initiation, the client tells the nurse, "I've only been taking this drug for a week but I'm sleeping better and my appetite has improved." The nurse should know that:
- A. It will take a minimum of 3 to 4 weeks from onset of administration for therapeutic effects to occur.
- B. Sleep disturbances and appetite problems are not affected by Zoloft.
- C. The change in environment and activity is the most likely reason for the client's perceived improvement.
- D. The rapid onset of Zoloft can improve insomnias and appetite disturbances as early as 1 week after initiation.

279. A 40-year-old female is admitted to the hospital for a series of electroconvulsive therapy treatments.

Her diagnosis is major depression and she has been on a variety of antidepressants over a period of 3 years without significant remission. The highest priority intervention at the time of admission would be to:
- A. Ask her to sign a copy of the Patient's Legal Rights.
- B. Call her physician to notify him of the client's admission.
- C. Order the client a dinner tray from the kitchen.
- D. Assess the client for suicidal ideation and potential.

280. A female client has electroconvulsive therapy scheduled for tomorrow. Legally, who should sign the client's consent for this treatment?
- A. The client
- B. The client's husband
- C. A member of the treatment team
- D. Written consent is not necessary

281. The client's husband approaches the nurse as he is leaving the hospital and asks, "Will my wife have any permanent side effects from this electroshock treatment?" The most accurate response by the nurse is:
- A. "Yes, your wife may have permanent memory loss for remote events."
- B. "Yes, your wife may have permanent memory loss for recent events."
- C. "Your wife may have temporary memory loss for remote events."
- D. "Your wife may have temporary memory loss for recent events."

282. A 42-year-old man is admitted to the inpatient unit for treatment of alcohol addiction. On admission, his vital signs are BP 130/88, P 90, R 24, T 97.6°F. He reports that his last drink was 4 hours ago. He has a history of drinking a fifth of whiskey a day for the last 20 years. He has been referred to the treatment center by his employee assistance program at work. The nurse should look for signs of withdrawal:
- A. Within 24 hours of the last drink
- B. 72 hours after the last drink
- C. Three to five days after the last drink
- D. One week after the last drink

283. The client tells the nurse 2 hours after admission for alcohol addiction treatment, "You know, I haven't had any real food for over 3 days." Assessment reveals the following data: BP 170/100, P 110, R 28, and T 97°F. The client's skin is dry with poor turgor; his mucous membranes are dry. The most relevant nursing diagnosis at this time is:
- A. Knowledge deficit
- B. Fluid volume deficit
- C. Altered nutrition: less than body requirements
- D. Ineffective individual coping

284. The alcohol-addicted client complains of feeling tremulous. The BP is now 170/110, P 116, R 30, T 97°F. Which of the following drugs would most likely give the client the most immediate relief from the withdrawal symptoms and effectively reduce the vital signs?
A. Benztropine (Cogentin) 2 mg PO
B. Oxazepam (Serax) 30 mg PO
C. Lorazepam (Ativan) 1 mg IM
D. Meperidine (Demerol) 100 mg IM

285. The alcohol-addicted client safely detoxes and begins to attend 12-step meetings and group therapy to develop insight. Which of the following statements would indicate that the client has insight and is exploring more adaptive ways to cope?
A. "I really get tired of being confronted all the time by the counselor."
B. "I know I probably drink more than the average guy, but when I work all day and come home hot and tired, I deserve a drink if I want one."
C. "I realize now that my drinking hurt my family. After discharge, I'm going to get hooked up with a sponsor and Alcoholics Anonymous."
D. "I know why the employee assistance program referred me to this program. My drinking was affecting the quality of my work."

286. Prior to a client's discharge from the drug treatment program, the client's wife approaches the nurse and says, "I'm so afraid that when my husband leaves here that he will want to go back to drinking. What can I do to prevent that?" The most therapeutic response by the nurse is:
A. "There is a support group for family members and friends of alcoholics called Al-Anon. It's an informal meeting where you can go and talk with other individuals about day-to-day living with spouses after discharge."
B. "You could try going out and having a few beers with him when he gets the urge to drink."
C. "You can't prevent it, but you can make sure that he doesn't drink at home. Just go home before he leaves the hospital and find all of his hidden bottles and empty them."
D. "Tell your husband that if he drinks again that you will leave him."

287. A client is being treated in the inpatient psychiatric setting for cocaine abuse. After initial detoxification, the client participates eagerly in therapy and becomes charming and ingratiating to the primary nurse. The client's primary diagnosis is cocaine dependence; the secondary diagnosis is antisocial personality disorder. The nurse should recognize these behaviors as:
A. Abnormal, indicating that the client has not completed detoxing

B. Unusual at this time, indicating that the client is probably sneaking drugs into the treatment setting
C. Characteristics for clients with the diagnosis of antisocial personality disorder
D. Normal for any client at this stage of treatment of cocaine abuse

288. A frightened young woman calls the emergency room and tearfully tells the nurse, "I've been raped. Please help me!" Before making a recommendation, the nurse would need to know:
A. If the client was injured, in a safe place, and had transportation available
B. If the client knew her assailant, her whereabouts, and if she had notified the police
C. If she had insurance, could get to the hospital on her own, and if pregnancy was possible
D. If she had bathed, douched, or changed clothes

289. The rape victim drives herself to the emergency room and agrees to be examined. The client asks the nurse, "Will I have to notify the police? I'm just so embarrassed." Which response by the nurse is the most appropriate?
A. "You won't have to notify the police. I will do it for you."
B. "No, of course not. You will only need to do so if you intend to press charges if the rapist is located and arrested."
C. "It's not something you have to make a decision about tonight. Why don't you wait a couple of days, then make up your mind?"
D. "Rape is a reportable offense and I will need to call the police. The decision to pursue legal action will be yours."

290. After the rape examination, the nurse prepares to discharge the client from the emergency room. Discharge instructions from the nurse should include:
A. Information concerning bathing, douching, and testing for sexually transmitted diseases and pregnancy
B. The names and phone numbers of local attorneys who defend rape victims
C. When to return to the emergency room for follow-up
D. The phone number of the battered women's shelter and the crisis intervention center

291. As the nurse is making rounds, the client tells the nurse, "The shopatouliens took my shoes out of my room last night." The client's statement is an example of:
A. An auditory hallucination
B. A neologism
C. Word salad
D. Derailment

292. The client tells the nurse that the CIA has put ra-

dio implants in his head to control his thoughts. The nurse should recognize the client's statement as:
A. Magical thinking
B. Paranoid delusions
C. Autistic thinking
D. Somatic delusions

293. A client with schizophrenia tells the nurse, "I could have prevented the earthquake in California in 1980 if I had wanted to." Which disturbance in thinking is the client experiencing?
A. Magical thinking
B. Word salad
C. Derailment
D. Blocking

294. The nurse enters a client's room to help her get prepared for an afternoon walk outside the hospital. The client says, "I'm too depressed and tired. I want to wait until I begin to feel better before I go walking." Which of the following is the most therapeutic response by the nurse?
A. "OK, but tomorrow you will have to go outside with the group."
B. "I'll tell the doctor how depressed you are. Maybe he will want to order a different antidepressant for you."
C. "Walking even if you don't feel like it could help your depression to get better sooner."
D. "No problem. I'll just chart that you refused."

295. A 12-year-old male is referred to a urologist for assessment and treatment of enuresis. The urologist orders imipramine (Tofranil). The most likely reason for this is that:
A. The client is probably clinically depressed and needs an antidepressant.
B. The antidepressant has some anticholinergic effects that may result in urinary continence through the night.
C. One of the major side effects of imipramine is urinary retention.
D. The client is probably just wetting the bed for extra attention from the parents.

296. A 13-year-old female is preoccupied with her appearance and takes pleasure in participating in activities with groups of peers from her school class. She dresses and styles her hair to look like her favorite rock singer. She is in which stage of the life cycle according to Erikson?
A. Stage 3: initiative versus guilt
B. Stage 4: industry versus inferiority
C. Stage 5: identity versus role diffusion
D. Stage 6: intimacy versus isolation

297. A 25-year-old client has just begun to see a nurse therapist in the outpatient clinic. Which of the following tasks is considered high priority and essential for the development of the therapeutic relationship between nurse and client?
A. Client insight
B. Trust and rapport
C. Motivation and mutual needs
D. Client self-awareness

298. The nurse in interviewing a client alone who has the potential for loss of control. Which seating arrangement would pose the least threat for the client and less danger for the nurse?
A. The client is asked to sit on a small couch close to the door; the nurse sits across the room from the door with her back to the wall.
B. The client and the nurse sit side by side on a small sofa with the door to the interview room closed.
C. The client and nurse sit in separate chairs, at least 3 feet apart and the door to the interview room open. The nurse should sit closer to the door than the client.
D. The client chooses to sit in a chair blocking the nurse's exit from the room.

299. The nurse is interviewing a client with a history of violence. Which of the following should be avoided by the nurse?
A. Attempt to calm the client by approaching him directly and telling him the consequences of losing control.
B. Anticipate that loss of control is a distinct possibility with the client's history and plan accordingly.
C. Take heed of verbal threats if any occur and summon help immediately, terminating the interview.
D. Interview the client with another staffperson present.

300. The nurse asks a new client on admission, "Have you ever felt that thoughts were being put into your head by someone or some outside source?" The nurse is trying to determine the presence of which type of thought disruption?
A. Persecutory delusion
B. Auditory hallucination
C. Thought insertion
D. Thought broadcasting

301. The nurse is completing an admission assessment on a psychotic client. He tells the nurse, "Every time I walk into a room and see people laughing, I know they are laughing at me. And when they quit laughing at me, they start talking about me, no matter where I go." The nurse determines that the client is experiencing:
A. Somatic delusions
B. Tactile hallucinations
C. Paranoid delusions
D. Ideas of reference

302. After admission, a psychotic client goes into the dayroom where several other clients are watching a movie (a comedy) on television. The client joins

the other clients and watches the movie without any sign of emotion on his face. His affect could be described as:
- A. Constricted
- B. Flat
- C. Labile
- D. Appropriate

303. The psychotic client tells the nurse, "The ball will fall in the stall. Call me at the mall." The nurse assesses the client's verbalizations as:
- A. Neologisms
- B. Circumstantiality
- C. Slang associations
- D. Auditory hallucinations

304. The nurse is assessing a client's memory. Which assessment question would help the nurse to determine if the client's immediate recall is intact?
- A. "When did you graduate from high school?"
- B. "What did you have for breakfast this morning?"
- C. "What were those three objects that I asked you to remember 5 minutes ago?"
- D. "What important news event happened 6 months ago?"

305. Which of the following statements reflects a client's true emotional insight?
- A. "I don't really have a mental illness, I just have a slight case of the nerves."
- B. "I know I have an illness but I would be okay if everybody would just quit making unreasonable demands of me."
- C. "I know I shouldn't get angry and fly off the handle with my family. I am painfully aware that they are hurt and even sometimes scared of me."
- D. "I'm ashamed of how I've treated my friends and coworkers. When I get back to work, I'm going to see what I can do different so that I won't create problems."

306. A psychotic client tells the nurse on admission that he is hearing voices telling him to kill the president. Which nursing diagnosis is the most appropriate for this client?
- A. Sensory-perceptual alterations
- B. Altered thought processes
- C. Self-care deficit
- D. Spiritual distress

307. A depressed client is accompanied to the hospital for admission by his wife who tells the nurse that her husband no longer seems to enjoy anything, not even his favorite hobbies or interests. The nurse recognizes that the client is experiencing:
- A. Euphoria
- B. Dysphoria
- C. Grief
- D. Anhedonia

308. A manic client tells the nurse, "I keep hearing voices that tell me that I'm rich and very powerful." The client is experiencing:
- A. Mood-incongruent hallucinations
- B. Mood-congruent hallucinations
- C. Mood-incongruent delusions
- D. Mood-congruent delusions

309. A depressed client who has failed to respond to pharmacotherapy is being admitted for electroconvulsive therapy (ECT). Which of the following, if present, would the nurse recognize as an absolute contraindication to ECT?
- A. Suicidal ideation
- B. Hypertension
- C. Ruptured cervical disk
- D. Brain tumor

310. The nurse correctly identifies that a client is experiencing neuroleptic malignant syndrome. The recommended emergency treatment for this condition is to:
- A. Decrease the neuroleptic and monitor the vital signs every 2 hours.
- B. Discontinue the neuroleptic and administer dantrolene sodium (Dantrium).
- C. Administer dantrolene sodium (Dantrium) but continue the neuroleptic.
- D. Discontinue the neuroleptic and monitor the vital signs every 4 hours.

Focus on Psychiatric Drug Dosage Calculation

311. The physician ordered naproxen sodium (Anaprox) 250 mg PO per liquid to a nursing home resident for severe pain. Using a 125 mg/5 ml solution, how many milliliters did the nurse administer?
- A. 5 ml
- B. 10 ml
- C. 15 ml
- D. 20 ml

312. A 28-year-old woman was seen at the local ambulatory care center with a diagnosis of genital herpes. The woman had a history of obsessive-compulsive behavior. The physician ordered acyclovir 200 mg every 4 hours times 5 days. The nurse administered how many 200 mg tablets?
- A. ½ tablet
- B. 1 tablet
- C. 1½ tablets
- D. 2 tablets

313. The physician ordered doxepin 75 mg HS for a nursing home resident with a PEG tube. Using a 10 mg/ml elixir, how many milliliters did the nurse administer?
- A. 5.5 ml

B. 6.5 ml
C. 7.5 ml
D. 8.5 ml

314. A 35-year-old man was being treated for uncomplicated gonorrhea. The physician ordered doxycycline (Vibramycin) 300 mg PO. On hand were 100 mg tablets. The nurse instructed the client to take how many tablets?
A. 1 tablet
B. 2 tablets
C. 3 tablets
D. 4 tablets

315. A 55-year-old was admitted to the local mental health unit with symptoms of chronic alcoholism. The physician ordered disulfiram (Antabuse) 375 mg PO. On hand were 250 mg tablets. How many tablets did the nurse administer?
A. ½ tablet
B. 1 tablet
C. 1½ tablets
D. 2 tablets

316. A 65-year-old nursing home resident began having symptoms of an anxiety attack. The physician ordered alprazolam (Xanax) 0.25 mg bid. On hand were 0.5 mg tablets. How many tablets did the nurse administer?
A. ½ tablet
B. 1 tablet
C. 1½ tablets
D. 2 tablets

317. A 72-year-old was diagnosed with Parkinson's disease. The physician ordered amantadine (Symmetrel) 100 mg bid. Using a 50 mg/5 ml elixir, how many milliliters did the nurse administer?
A. 5 ml
B. 7 ml
C. 9 ml
D. 10 ml

318. The physician ordered amitriptyline (Elavil) 50 mg HS to a 67-year-old nursing home resident for major depression. On hand were 25 mg tablets. The nurse instructed the client to take how many tablets?
A. ½ tablet
B. 1 tablet
C. 1½ tablets
D. 2 tablets

319. A 20-year-old cerebral palsy client was admitted with seizure activity. The physician ordered amobarbital 400 mg IV. Using a 250 mg/1 ml vial, how many milliliters did the nurse administer IV?
A. 1.2 ml
B. 1.4 ml
C. 1.6 ml
D. 1.8 ml

320. A client with manic-depressive disorder was undergoing an exploratory laparotomy. The physician ordered alfentanil (Alfenta) 50 μg/kg IV as the anesthetic for this general surgery. The client weighed 52 kg and would receive 2600 μg IV. Using a 500 μg/1 ml vial, how many milliliters did the client receive?
A. 3.2 ml
B. 4.2 ml
C. 5.2 ml
D. 6.2 ml

321. A 34-year-old was diagnosed with exogenous obesity. The physician ordered amphetamine sulfate 20 mg PO AC. On hand were 10 mg tablets. The nurse instructed the client to take how many tablets?
A. ½ tablet
B. 1 tablet
C. 1½ tablets
D. 2 tablets

322. An 80-year-old was prescribed amoxapine 50 mg tid for depression. On hand were 100 mg tablets. The nurse instructed the client to take how many tablets?
A. ½ tablet
B. 1 tablet
C. 1½ tablets
D. 2 tablets

323. The physician ordered clomipramine (Anafranil) 75 mg HS to a 70-year-old nursing home resident for an obsessive-compulsive disorder. On hand were 50 mg tablets. The nurse administered how many tablets?
A. ½ tablet
B. 1 tablet
C. 1½ tablets
D. 2 tablets

324. A 77-year-old alcoholic was given scopolamine hydrobromide 0.4 mg SC to calm the delirium he was experiencing. Using a 1 mg/ml vial, how many milliliters did the nurse administer SC?
A. 0.2 ml
B. 0.4 ml
C. 0.6 ml
D. 0.8 ml

325. An 18-year-old was admitted for an overdose of diazepam. The physician ordered physostigmine 2 mg IV to reverse the CNS effects of the diazepam. Using a 1 mg/ml vial, how many milliliters did the nurse administer?
A. 1 ml
B. 2 ml
C. 3 ml
D. 4 ml

326. A 34-year-old was receiving lorazepam (Ativan) for anxiety. The client became heavily sedated. The physician ordered flumazenil 0.2 mg to be given IV over 30 seconds to reverse the sedation effects of Ativan. Using a 0.1 mg/ml vial, how many milliliters did the nurse administer?

A. 0.5 ml
B. 1 ml
C. 2 ml
D. 3 ml

327. A 57-year-old client was experiencing depression secondary to chronic myelocytic leukemia. The physician ordered cytarabine 200 mg for 5 days to treat the leukemia. Using a 500 mg/ml vial, how many milliliters did the nurse administer?
A. 0.1 ml
B. 0.2 ml
C. 0.3 ml
D. 0.4 ml

328. A mentally retarded 25-year-old was experiencing drug-induced extrapyramidal symptoms. The physician ordered trihexyphenidyl (Artane) 5 mg PO daily. Using a 2 mg/5 ml elixir, how many milliliters did the nurse administer?
A. 10.5 ml
B. 11.5 ml
C. 12.5 ml
D. 13.5 ml

329. A 68-year-old developed a generalized rash secondary to severe anxiety. The physician ordered hydroxyzine (Atarax) 75 mg tid for the itching. Using a 50 mg/ml vial, how many milliliters did the nurse administer?
A. 0.5 ml
B. 1.0 ml
C. 1.5 ml
D. 2.0 ml

330. A 74-year-old was diagnosed with Hansen's disease. The physician ordered dapsone 100 mg every day. The nurse instructed the client to take how many 25 mg tablets?
A. 1 tablet
B. 2 tablets
C. 3 tablets
D. 4 tablets

331. A 44-year-old was experiencing symptoms of a severe urinary tract infection. The physician ordered trimethoprim-sulfamethoxazole (Bactrim) 160 mg TMP/800 mg SMZ every 12 hours for 10 to 14 days. The pharmacist dispensed 160 mg TMP/800 mg SMZ tablets. The nurse instructed the client to take how many tablets?
A. ½ tablet
B. 1 tablet
C. 1½ tablets
D. 2 tablets

332. A depressed client was found to have type III hyperlipidemia. The physician ordered gemfibrozil (Lopid) 600 mg bid 30 minutes before meals. On hand were 300 mg capsules. The nurse instructed the client to take how many capsules?
A. 1 capsule
B. 2 capsules

C. 3 capsules
D. 4 capsules

333. A 78-year-old man was admitted with Parkinson's symptoms. The physician ordered benztropine mesylate (Cogentin) 1 mg every day IV. Using a 1 mg/ml vial, how many milliliters did the nurse administer?
A. 0.5 ml
B. 1 ml
C. 1.5 ml
D. 2.0 ml

334. A 55-year-old was experiencing extrapyramidal symptoms secondary to neuroleptic drug therapy. The physician ordered biperiden (Akineton) 2 mg tid IV. Using a 5 mg/ml vial, how many milliliters did the nurse administer?
A. 0.1 ml
B. 0.2 ml
C. 0.3 ml
D. 0.4 ml

335. A 55-year-old was being prepared for electroshock therapy. The physician ordered methohexital (Brevital) 100 mg IV given 1 ml/5 seconds as a general anesthesia for the shock therapy. Using a 500 mg/ml vial, how many milliliters did the nurse administer?
A. 0.1 ml
B. 0.2 ml
C. 0.3 ml
D. 0.4 ml

336. The physician ordered bromocriptine (Parlodel) 1.25 mg bid with meals to improve the symptoms of Parkinson's disease in an 87-year-old client. On hand were 2.5 mg tablets. The nurse instructed the client to take how many tablets?
A. ½ tablet
B. 1 tablet
C. 1½ tablets
D. 2 tablets

337. A 22-year-old was being treated with buproprion 150 mg tid PO for depression. On hand were 100 mg tablets. The nurse instructed the client to take how many tablets?
A. ½ tablet
B. 1 tablet
C. 1½ tablets
D. 2 tablets

338. A 76-year-old nursing home resident was complaining about not sleeping at night. The physician ordered chloral hydrate (Noctec) 500 mg ½ hour HS. Using a 250 mg/ml elixir, how many milliliters did the nurse administer?
A. 6 ml
B. 8 ml
C. 10 ml
D. 12 ml

339. A 27-year-old was admitted for mixed seizures. The physician ordered carbamazepine (Tegretol) 400 mg bid. On hand were 200 mg chewable tablets. The nurse instructed the client to chew how many tablets?
A. ½ tablet
B. 1 tablet
C. 1½ tablets
D. 2 tablets

340. A 21-year-old was diagnosed as having bipolar manic-depressive psychosis. The physician ordered lithium carbonate (Carbolith) 300 mg PO. Using a 300 mg/5 ml elixir, how many milliliters did the nurse administer?
A. 2.0 ml
B. 2.5 ml
C. 5.0 ml
D. 5.5 ml

341. A 17-year-old was admitted to the ER hallucinating. The physician ordered loxapine 25 mg IM for this psychotic disorder. Using a 50 mg/ml vial, how many milliliters did the nurse administer?
A. 0.5 ml
B. 1.0 ml
C. 1.5 ml
D. 2.0 ml

342. An obese client was admitted to the ER with hypertension. The physician ordered clonidine (Catapres) 0.8 mg PO. On hand were 0.2 mg tablets. The nurse instructed the client to take how many tablets?
A. 1 tablet
B. 2 tablets
C. 3 tablets
D. 4 tablets

343. A 32-year-old was being treated with prazepam (Centrax) 20 mg HS for anxiety. How many 5 mg capsules must the nurse administer?
A. 1 capsule
B. 2 capsules
B. 3 capsules
D. 4 capsules

344. The physician ordered fluoxetine (Prozac) 20 mg every day to a 38-year-old with major depressive disorder. Each pulvule contains 20 mg. How many pulvules did the nurse administer?
A. 1 pulvule
B. 2 pulvules
C. 3 pulvules
D. 4 pulvules

345. A 17-year-old with cerebral palsy was complaining of painful spasms in both legs. The physician ordered chlorzoxazone (Parafon Forte DSC) 500 mg tid. On stock were 250 mg tablets. The nurse administered how many tablets?
A. ½ tablet
B. 1 tablet

C. 1½ tablets
D. 2 tablets

346. A 35-year-old was experiencing myoclonic seizures secondary to narcotic withdrawal. The physician ordered clonazepam (Klonopin) 0.5 mg tid to be given as a preventive measure to reduce seizure activity. On hand were 1 mg tablets. How many tablets did the nurse administer?
A. ½ tablet
B. 1 tablet
C. 1½ tablets
D. 2 tablets

347. A 44-year-old was diagnosed with schizophrenia. The physician ordered clozapine 300 mg every day after 2 weeks. On hand were 100 mg tablets. How many tablets did the nurse administer?
A. 1 tablet
B. 2 tablets
C. 3 tablets
D. 4 tablets

348. A 67-year-old was complaining of motion sickness while riding in a car. The physician ordered cyclizine (Marezine) 50 mg IM. Using a 50 mg/ml vial, how many milliliters did the nurse administer?
A. 0.5 ml
B. 1.0 ml
C. 1.5 ml
D. 2.0 ml

349. A 60-year-old was complaining of nausea and vomiting. The physician ordered prochlorperazine (Compazine) 10 mg IM. Using a 5 mg/ml vial, how many milliliters did the nurse administer?
A. 0.5 ml
B. 1.0 ml
C. 1.5 ml
D. 2.0 ml

350. A 72-year-old complained of nocturnal leg cramps. The physician ordered cyclandelate (Cyclan) 400 mg bid. On hand were 200 mg tablets. The nurse administered how many tablets?
A. ½ tablet
B. 1 tablet
C. 1½ tablets
D. 2 tablets

351. A 69-year-old was diagnosed with neuroblastoma. The client weighed 45 kg. The physician treated the malignant tumor with cyclophosphamide (Cytoxan) 5 mg/kg (225 mg) IV. Using a 500 mg/ml vial, how many milliliters did the nurse administer?
A. 0.45 ml
B. 1.0 ml
C. 1.45 ml
D. 2.45 ml

352. A 65-year-old experienced severe pruritus secondary to neuroleptic drugs. The physician or-

dered cyproheptadine (Periactin) 4 mg tid. Using a 2 mg/5 ml elixir, how many milliliters did the nurse administer?
A. 4 ml
B. 6 ml
C. 8 ml
D. 10 ml

353. A 26-year-old developed cytomegalovirus retinitis secondary to AIDS. The physician ordered ganciclovir 5 mg/kg (340 mg) to be given over 1 hour IV. The client weighed 68 kg. Using a 500 mg/ml vial, how many milliliters did the nurse administer?
A. 0.48 ml
B. 0.68 ml
C. 0.88 ml
D. 1.00 ml

354. A 75-year-old was complaining of insomnia. The physician ordered flurazepam (Dalmane) 15 mg HS. On hand were 15 mg capsules. How many capsules did the nurse administer?
A. ½ capsule
B. 1 capsule
C. 1½ capsules
D. 2 capsules

355. A physician ordered quazepam 7.5 mg HS for his 84-year-old grandmother who was suffering from insomnia. On hand were 15 mg tablets. How many tablets must the grandmother take?
A. ½ tablet
B. 1 tablet
C. 1½ tablets
D. 2 tablets

356. A schizophrenic client underwent an exploratory laparotomy. The physician ordered meperidine (Demerol) 50 mg IM for severe postoperative pain. Using a 25 mg/ml vial, how many milliliters did the nurse administer?
A. 0.5 ml
B. 1.0 ml
C. 1.5 ml
D. 2.0 ml

357. A 75-year-old nursing home resident was demonstrating signs of depression. The physician ordered desipramine (Norpramin) 25 mg PO. On hand were 10 mg tablets. How many tablets did the nurse administer?
A. 1 tablet
B. 1½ tablets
C. 2 tablets
D. 2½ tablets

358. A 24-year-old was being treated for depression with trazodone (Desyrel) 150 mg HS. On hand were 300 mg tablets. The nurse instructed the client to take how many tablets?
A. ½ tablet
B. 1 tablet

C. 1½ tablets
D. 2 tablets

359. A 28-year-old was diagnosed with exogenous obesity. The physician ordered diethylpropion (Tenuate) 25 mg tid 1 hour before meals. The pharmacist dispensed 25 mg tablets. The nurse instructed the client to take how many tablets?
A. ½ tablet
B. 1 tablet
C. 1½ tablets
D. 2 tablets

360. A 28-year-old was diagnosed with major depression and severe anxiety. The physician ordered doxepin (Sinequan) 50 mg daily. Using a 10 mg/ml vial, how many milliliters did the nurse administer?
A. 2 ml
B. 3 ml
C. 4 ml
D. 5 ml

361. A 19-year-old developed severe cystic acne. The client weighed 68 kg. The physician ordered isotretinoin (Accutane) 0.5 mg/kg (34 mg) bid. The pharmacist dispensed 40 mg tablets. The nurse instructed the client to take how many tablets?
A. ½ tablet
B. 1 tablet
C. 1½ tablets
D. 2 tablets

362. A 65-year-old was complaining of insomnia. The physician ordered ethchlorvynol (Placidyl) 500 mg ½ hour HS. How many 500 mg tablets should the nurse instruct the client to take?
A. ½ tablet
B. 1 tablet
C. 1½ tablets
D. 2 tablets

Answers

1. **(A)** Nursing process phase: planning; client need: safe, effective care environment; content area: psychiatric nursing

Rationale
(A) These clients are at high risk for seizures during the first week after cessation of alcohol intake. (B) Fluid intake should be increased to prevent dehydration. (C) Environmental stimuli should be decreased to prevent precipitation of seizures. (D) Application of restraints may cause the client to increase his or her physical activity and may eventually lead to exhaustion.

2. **(B)** Nursing process phase: analysis; client need: psychosocial integrity; content area: psychiatric nursing

Rationale

(A) The length of hospitalization has decreased due to more effective medication management, milieu therapy, and case management. (B) Many persons who are severely mentally ill use community-based services such as day treatment programs that incorporate rehabilitation philosophy and focus on strengths rather than on pathology. (C) Most family members are supportive of their mentally ill family members and accept them as part of their lifestyle. Family and network support interventions are available to help minimize the burden of care for family members. (D) Deinstitutionalization began when large public mental hospitals were overcrowded and had fallen into disrepair. New therapies raised the hope that effective treatments might be delivered in community settings.

3. **(A)** Nursing process phase: analysis; client need: psychosocial integrity; content area: psychiatric nursing

Rationale

(A) Because of the stigma associated with a mental illness, many clients are fearful of rejection and reprisal. The nurse protects the psychological space of the client through confidentiality. (B) It is impossible for clients to be anonymous during a hospital stay. (C) Insanity defense is a concern for only those mentally ill hospitalized clients diagnosed as criminally insane. (D) The health-care provider, not the mentally ill client, experiences moral distress during an ethical dilemma.

4. **(B)** Nursing process phase: implementation; client need: psychosocial integrity; content area: psychiatric nursing

Rationale

(A) This response is evaluative and nontherapeutic. Feedback should focus on the behavior. (B) The nurse is presenting reality and making it clear that the behavior is not acceptable. (C) This response indicates that there is an external source of power that may cause the client to blame others for his behavior. (D) Advice giving indicates that the nurse knows best and may foster dependent behavior.

5. **(C)** Nursing process phase: implementation; client need: psychosocial integrity; content area: psychiatric nursing

Rationale

(A) Isolation from others may lead to more hostility. (B) Acting out indicates aggressiveness, which is not a healthy behavior. (C) Encourage clients to communicate anger without abridging the rights of others. (D) Improving self-care may increase self-esteem but will not decrease anger.

6. **(B)** Nursing process phase: implementation; client need: psychosocial integrity; content area: psychiatric nursing

Rationale

(A) This response negates the client's thinking. (B) This statement acknowledges the client's thinking and is nonaccusatory. (C) This response is judgmental and may put the client on the defensive. (D) This statement is seeking clarification that is not needed.

7. **(C)** Nursing process phase: analysis; client need: psychosocial integrity; content area: psychiatric nursing

Rationale

(A) A person suffering from psychosis exhibits gross impairment in reality testing, personality disintegration, regressive behavior, disorganized speech, and reduced level of awareness. (B) A character disorder is a personality disorder manifested by a chronic, habitual, maladaptive pattern of reaction that is relatively inflexible and often causes significant personal distress and impaired social functioning. Character traits are typically ego-syntonic. (C) Neurosis is subjective psychological pain that is beyond what is appropriate in the conditions of one's life. (D) This is a group of disorders characterized by physical symptoms that are affected by emotional factors.

8. **(B)** Nursing process phase: analysis; client need: psychosocial integrity; content area: psychiatric nursing

Rationale

(A) Personality disorder patterns of behavior are inflexible and maladaptive, causing significant functional impairment. (B) A person suffering from psychosis may exhibit a disturbance in one or more major areas of functioning. (C) Neurosis is an emotional disturbance of all kinds other than psychosis. (D) This is a group of disorders characterized by physical symptoms that are affected by emotional factors.

9. **(C)** Nursing process phase: assessment; client need: psychosocial integrity; content area: psychiatric nursing

Rationale

(A) Compensation is the process by which a person attempts to make up for real or perceived deficits by strongly emphasizing some other feature that he or she regards as an asset. (B) Identification operates unconsciously and is an attempt to modify behavior and to pattern oneself after another person. (C) Rationalization is used to justify ideas, actions, or feelings with seemingly acceptable reasons or explanations. (D) Projection enables a person to justify his or her own unacceptable feelings and impulses by attributing the behaviors to others.

10. **(B)** Nursing process phase: assessment; client need: psychosocial integrity; content area: psychiatric nursing

Rationale

(A) Projection enables a person to justify his or her own acceptable feelings and impulses by attributing the behaviors to others. (B) Compensation is the process by which a person attempts to make up for real or perceived deficits by strongly emphasizing some other features that he regards as an asset. (C) Reaction formation is the development of attitudes and behaviors that are opposite to what one really feels or would like to do. (D) Rationalization is used to justify ideas, actions, or feelings with seemingly acceptable reasons or explanations.

11. **(D)** Nursing process phase: analysis; client need: psychosocial integrity; content area: psychiatric nursing

Rationale

(A) Rationalization is used to justify ideas, actions, or feelings with seemingly acceptable reasons or explanations. (B) Compensation is the process by which a person attempts to make up for real or perceived deficits. (C) Identification is the process by which a person patterns himself or herself after another person. (D) A fantasy is a daydream that serves to express unconscious wishes and is an attempt to resolve emotional conflict.

12. **(A)** Nursing process phase: assessment; client need: psychosocial integrity; content area: psychiatric nursing

Rationale
(A) Displacement is a shift of emotions from a person or object to another neutral or less-threatening person or object. (B) Projection enables a person to identify his or her own unacceptable feelings and impulses by attributing the behaviors to others. (C) Rationalization is used to justify ideas, actions, or feelings with seemingly acceptable reasons or explanation. (D) Sublimation allows a person to divert unacceptable impulses and motives into personally and socially acceptable channels.

13. **(D)** Nursing process phase: assessment; client need: psychosocial integrity; content area: psychiatric nursing

Rationale
(A) Regression is a retreat to an earlier stage of development. (B) Repression banishes or excludes unacceptable impulses and thoughts from consciousness. (C) Reaction formation allows a person to adopt attitudes and behaviors that are opposite to his or her impulses. (D) The client is using conversion reaction, which is the process of converting emotional stress into impaired physical functions.

14. **(D)** Nursing process phase: analysis; client need: safe, effective care environment; content area: psychiatric nursing

Rationale
(A) Regression is when a person returns to an earlier stage of development. (B) When rationalizing, a person attempts to justify behaviors that are not socially acceptable. (C) This defense mechanism allows the person to divert unacceptable impulses and motives into personally and socially acceptable channels. (D) Denial is a primitive defense mechanism that allows a person to resolve emotional conflict and avoid realities that are disagreeable.

15. **(A)** Nursing process phase: analysis; client need: psychosocial integrity; content area: psychiatric nursing

Rationale
(A) Displacement is when an individual transfers hostile and aggressive feelings from one object to another object or person. (B) Projection enables a person to justify his or her own unacceptable feelings and impulses by attributing the behaviors to another. (C) Reaction formation enables a person to adopt attitudes and behaviors that are opposite to his or her own impulses. (D) Sublimation allows a person to divert unacceptable impulses and motives into personally and socially acceptable channels.

16. **(D)** Nursing process phase: analysis; client need: psychosocial integrity; content area: psychiatric nursing

Rationale
(A) Displacement is when an individual transfers hostile and aggressive feelings from one object to another object or person. (B) Projection enables a person to justify his or her own unacceptable feelings and impulses by attributing the behaviors to another. (C) Reaction formation enables a person to adopt attitudes and behaviors that are opposite to his or her own impulses. (D) With repression, a person forgets or excludes unacceptable impulses and thoughts from consciousness.

17. **(C)** Nursing process phase: assessment; client need: psychosocial integrity; content area: psychiatric nursing

Rationale
(A) When rationalizing, a person attempts to justify behaviors that are not socially acceptable. (B) A fantasy is a daydream that serves to express unconscious wishes. (C) Introjection is when a person incorporates with oneself the attributes of another individual. (D) When compensating, a person attempts to make up for real or perceived deficits.

18. **(A)** Nursing process phase: implementation; client need: psychosocial integrity; content area: psychiatric nursing

Rationale
(A) Forming a therapeutic alliance with the client reduces the threat that the nurse may pose to the client. (B) The goal of therapy is to assist the client to reduce anxiety and learn to delay ritualistic behavior. (C) Clients use compulsive rituals to control anxiety. Rationalizing irrational behaviors is not an appropriate intervention because it may cause the anxiety level to increase. (D) Referring the client is not the most appropriate nursing intervention.

19. **(A)** Nursing process phase: analysis; client need: psychosocial integrity; content area: psychiatric nursing

Rationale
(A) Regression is partial or symbolic return to earlier stages of development. (B) Undoing is used to amend or reverse previous thoughts, feelings, or actions. (C) Repression is an involuntary exclusion of unacceptable feelings or thoughts that are automatically pushed into one's unconscious. (D) Reaction formation enables a person to adopt attitudes and behaviors that are opposite to his or her own impulses.

20. **(A)** Nursing process phase: analysis; client need: psychosocial integrity; content area: psychiatric nursing

Rationale
(A) Sublimation allows a person to divert unacceptable impulses and motives into personally and socially acceptable channels. (B) Reaction formation enables a person to adopt attitudes and behaviors that are opposite to his or her own behaviors. (C) Displacement is when an individual transfers hostile and aggressive feelings from one object to another object or person. (D) Conversion reaction allows a person to convert emotional stress into impaired physical functions.

21. **(D)** Nursing process phase: assessment; client need: psychosocial integrity; content area: psychiatric nursing

Rationale
(A) Projection enables a person to justify his or her own unacceptable feelings and impulses by attributing the behaviors to others. (B) Displacement operates unconsciously and is used by an individual to transfer hostile and aggressive feelings from one object to another object or person. (C) Reaction formation enables a person to adopt attitudes and behaviors that are opposite to his or her own behaviors. (D) Denial is characterized by avoidance of disagreeable realities and unconscious refusal to acknowledge a thought, feeling, need, or desire. The client is denying that he has a substance abuse problem.

22. **(C)** Nursing process phase: assessment; client need: psychosocial integrity; content area: psychiatric nursing

Rationale
(A) Undoing is a mental mechanism and is used to amend or

reverse previous thoughts, feelings, or actions. (B) When rationalizing, a person attempts to justify behaviors that are not socially acceptable. (C) Denial is a primitive defense mechanism that allows a person to resolve emotional conflict and avoid realities that are painful. (D) Sublimation allows a person to divert unacceptable impulses and motives into personally and socially acceptable channels.

23. **(C)** Nursing process phase: analysis; client need: psychosocial integrity; content area: psychiatric nursing

Rationale
(A) Reaction formation enables a person to adopt attitudes and behaviors that are opposite to his or her own impulses. (B) A person diagnosed as having a somatization disorder has multiple physical complaints that can not be explained by any medical condition. (C) Conversion reaction allows a person to convert emotional stress into impaired physical functions. (D) A fantasy is a daydream that serves to express unconscious wishes.

24. **(C)** Nursing process phase: assessment; client need: psychosocial integrity; content area: psychiatric nursing

Rationale
(A) Regression is returning to an earlier stage of development in order to cope with a less than desirable situation. (B) Reaction formation is attempting to make amends for unacceptable feelings. (C) Denial is used to protect the ego from a disturbing reality. (D) Projection is criticizing in others what is disturbing in oneself.

25. **(A)** Nursing process phase: assessment; client need: psychosocial integrity; content area: psychiatric nursing

Rationale
(A) Introjection is an intense type of identification in which the person incorporates the qualities of another person into his or her own ego system. (B) A fantasy is a daydream that serves to express unconscious wishes. (C) When repressing, a person forgets or excludes unacceptable impulses and thoughts from consciousness. (D) Projection enables a person to justify his or her own unacceptable feelings and impulses by attributing the behavior to others.

26. **(B)** Nursing process phase: analysis; client need: safe, effective care environment; content area: psychiatric nursing

Rationale
(A) An intentional tort is a willful act that violates another person's rights. The nurse did not intentionally give Haldol to harm the client. (B) The nursing action was an unreasonable or careless act. The nurse is negligent and liable for the client's death. (C) The amount of Haldol given was within a therapeutic range. (D) An assault is a threatening act that causes another person to fear.

27. **(B)** Nursing process phase: implementation; client need: safe, effective care environment; content area: psychiatric nursing

Rationale
(A) The client has the right to refuse treatment. Restraining and forcing the medication is against the client's constitutional rights and "The Patient Self-Determination Act." (B) The client has a right to self-determination. Accept the client's decision. (C) Pleading is not a therapeutic nursing in-

tervention. Paternalism is operating and may not be beneficial. (D) This response is not a good choice.

28. **(C)** Nursing process phase: implementation; client need: safe, effective care environment; content area: psychiatric nursing

Rationale
(A) Psychiatric clients have the right to leave the hospital if they are not a danger to self or others. (B) The nurse may ask the client to remain hospitalized, but this is not the best response. (C) When clients demand discharge from a psychiatric unit, they are asked to put their intentions in writing. They may be detained against their will for a period of time depending on the laws of the state. (D) This is not the best response. However, a client may discuss discharge with the physician.

29. **(A)** Nursing process phase: implementation; client need: safe, effective care environment; content area: psychiatric nursing

Rationale
(A) A client who is harmful to self may be detained until it has been determined that there are no further indications of self-destructive behavior. (B) A client may sign a legal document to be discharged AMA. However, because of self-destructive behavior, it is important to maintain a safe environment for all clients. (C) This is not the best response. This situation calls for a nursing intervention. (D) Self-destructive behavior is confidential information and not available for public knowledge.

30. **(B)** Nursing process phase: analysis; client need: safe, effective care environment; content area: psychiatric nursing

Rationale
(A) Anonymity is a situation in which the name is not disclosed. (B) Disclosure of information by psychiatric professionals is limited to authorized individuals. (C) It is not a duty to provide information to anyone unless the client has provided authorization. (D) Habeas corpus provides for patients held against their will to be discharged immediately, if judged sane.

31. **(D)** Nursing process phase: implementation; client need: safe, effective care environment; content area: psychiatric nursing

Rationale
(A) The one exception to confidentiality relates to the Tarasoff decision. (B) The client's rights are important but are not a priority in this situation. (C) Never assume anything. (D) It is the responsibility of the clinic to warn the potential victim under protection of the third-party law, which stems from the famous court case *Tarasoff v. Regents of University of California (1976)*.

32. **(B)** Nursing process phase: analysis; client need: safe, effective care environment; content area: psychiatric nursing

Rationale
(A) The client is disclosing information about herself. (B) Privileged communication is the right of all clients to discuss information with their attorney. (C) Information cannot be disclosed without a client's permission. (D) Psychiatric clients have the right to reasonable access to telephones.

33. (B) Nursing process phase: analysis; client need: safe, effective care environment; content area: psychiatric nursing

Rationale

(A, C, & D) Clients under an involuntary status retain all rights unless the state assumes the client is incompetent. (B) An involuntarily admitted client has a right to sign a voluntary admission and agree to receive treatment and abide by hospital rules.

34. (B) Nursing process phase: implementation; client need: safe, effective care environment; content area: psychiatric nursing

Rationale

(A) Clients need outside activity. However, safe practice is essential. (B) To manage effectively, client groups should not be larger than 10. (C) The response supports unsafe care practices. (D) This is an appropriate response. However, the therapist needs to be reminded that health-care practices must be delivered safely.

35. (B) Nursing process phase: implementation; client need: safe, effective care environment; content area: psychiatric nursing

Rationale

(A) Restraints and seclusion are not a form of punishment. (B) It is important to provide safeguards in order to protect clients who are out of control. (C) It is against the law to leave a client in restraints and seclusion for an undetermined length of time. (D) Clients in restraints or seclusion must be checked on a routine basis according to the hospital policy.

36. (C) Nursing process phase: analysis; client need: safe, effective care environment; content area: psychiatric nursing

Rationale

(A) Psychiatric clients have the right to refuse treatment under the U.S. Constitution. (B) Clients have the right to refuse treatment once started. (C) Paternalism is operating when the nurse uses persuasion and manipulation to get the client actively engaged in treatment that is believed best for the client. (D) There is no indication that the client's constitutional rights have been abused.

37. (D) Nursing process phase: analysis; client need: safe, effective care environment; content area: psychiatric nursing

Rationale

(A) Clients have the right to informed consent. (B) Clients have the right to treatment under the U.S. Constitution. (C) Clients have the right to refuse treatment under the U.S. Constitution. (D) Judicial commitment is not one of the eight ethical guidelines.

38. (A) Nursing process phase: analysis; client need: safe, effective care environment; content area: psychiatric nursing

Rationale

(A) The client voluntarily admitted himself for psychiatric care. (B) A state determines judicial commitment. (C) Informal admission resembles an admission to a general hospital. (D) Involuntary admission is characterized by an unwilling and forceful admission.

39. (C) Nursing process phase: assessment; client need: psychosocial integrity; content area: psychiatric nursing

Rationale

(A) Physiological changes are physical symptoms of moderate anxiety. (B) Impairment of psychological functioning may be a response to anxiety. (C) Anxiety is primarily of intrapsychic origin and a response to real or imagined threats to self. (D) It is the uncertainty in a person's life that may cause anxiety.

40. (A) Nursing process phase: implementation; client need: health promotion and maintenance; content area: psychiatric nursing

Rationale

(A) The first priority is to reduce the anxiety to a tolerable level to prevent pathological behavior. (B) Probing the cause of anxiety is recommended only if the client is experiencing mild or well-controlled anxiety. (C) In moderate anxiety, the perceptual field narrows and the person remains alert. Decompensation is unlikely at this level. (D) Anxiety is on a continuum that becomes problematic if there is no appropriate intervention.

41. (D) Nursing process phase: implementation; client need: safe, effective care environment; content area: psychiatric nursing

Rationale

(A) In severe anxiety, the sensory perception is greatly reduced, lessening the capacity to problem-solve. (B) The source of the problem should be probed only if the person is experiencing mild and well-controlled anxiety. (C) An anxiolytic medication may be ordered by the physician, but the initial intervention is to assure the client of safety and provide psychological support. (D) Clients exhibiting severe anxiety require immediate psychological and sometimes physical support.

42. (B) Nursing process phase: implementation; client need: health promotion and maintenance; content area: psychiatric nursing

Rationale

(A) "Why" questions may be perceived as threatening. (B) The use of reflection of feelings signifies understanding, empathy, and respect for the client. (C) This question is limiting and does not focus on the "here and now." (D) Giving advice is nontherapeutic. It shifts responsibility to the nurse and reinforces the client's dependence.

43. (C) Nursing process phase: analysis; client need: psychosocial integrity; content area: psychiatric nursing

Rationale

(A) Antianxiety medications should be used cautiously and sparingly because of the addictive properties. The medications may alleviate the symptoms of anxiety but they interfere with understanding the source of the anxiety. (B) Anxiety that is communicated interpersonally often affects family members. The immediate focus should be on the client. (C) Educating clients is one of the essential nursing responsibilities. (D) Cognitive restructuring is associated with community-based therapy.

44. (B) Nursing process phase: implementation; client need: psychosocial integrity; content area: psychiatric nursing

Rationale

(A) Verbalization of feelings is not the first priority. (B) The number one priority is ruling out a neurological disorder. (C) Physical therapy should not be attempted until organic causes are ruled out. (D) Assistance with future planning is important, but not at this time.

45. **(A)** Nursing process phase: planning; client need: safe, effective care environment; content area: psychiatric nursing

Rationale

(A) Physical symptoms are a defense mechanism that absorbs and neutralizes the anxiety generated by unacceptable, unconscious impulses. (B) The symptoms are not voluntarily controlled. Dependence is not a key issue. (C) Symptoms arise from anxiety and are not used to manipulate others. (D) The symptoms develop from exposure to a specific traumatic event.

46. **(C)** Nursing process phase: planning; client need: safe, effective care environment; content area: psychiatric nursing

Rationale

(A) Psychosis is characterized by gross impairment in reality testing. There is no indication of psychotic behavior. (B) Depression is characterized by dysphoric mood, changes in appetite, insomnia, and slowing of mental processes. (C) Somatization disorder is characterized by multiple physical complaints of several years' duration and is often accompanied by anxiety and depressed mood. (D) The client considers his physical problems real. They are not of delusional intensity.

47. **(D)** Nursing process phase: planning; client need: psychosocial integrity; content area: psychiatric nursing

Rationale

(A) The development of phobic behavior is fear that arises through a process of displacing an unconscious conflict to an external object symbolically related to the conflict. (B) Free-floating anxiety is not tied to a specific stimulus. (C) The client is seeking help for her phobic behavior. (D) Persons suffering from phobic behaviors use avoidance.

48. **(A)** Nursing process phase: analysis; client need: psychosocial integrity; content area: psychiatric nursing

Rationale

(A) The phobic person controls the intensity of the anxiety by avoiding the object with which the anxiety is associated. (B) The phobic person fears a specific external object rather than the internal source of distress. (C) Because phobias are displaced fears and at an unconscious level, the basic source is out of awareness. (D) This is not a good choice because the source of anxiety is an internal conflict at an unconscious level.

49. **(A)** Nursing process phase: implementation; client need: safe, effective care environment; content area: psychiatric nursing

Rationale

(A) Promoting client safety by providing a quiet environment may calm the hyperactive client. (B) This intervention shows little understanding of the disease. (C) Because of the psychomotor agitation, the client may have difficulty remaining in a group activity. Constant disruptions create distractions. (D) Avoid highly competitive activities because they may bring out hostility and aggressive behaviors.

50. **(D)** Nursing process phase: analysis; client need: psychosocial integrity; content area: psychiatric nursing

Rationale

(A) A person with excessive energy is unable to sit and concentrate for any length of time. (B) Team sports will provide a release of excess energy, but may create unnecessary external stimuli. (C) Competition is to be discouraged during the manic phase because it may cause overly aggressive behaviors. (D) Walking is the best choice because it is less competitive and provides an opportunity for the release of energy.

51. **(C)** Nursing process phase: implementation; client need: psychosocial integrity; content area: psychiatric nursing

Rationale

(A) Matter-of-fact intervention, rather than an angry approach, is more effective. (B) Providing false assurances is not an appropriate form of treatment. (C) Keep the client's dignity in mind at all times. (D) The lack of an appropriate intervention is a form of rejection. Inappropriate behaviors may cause future embarrassment.

52. **(A)** Nursing process phase: analysis; client need: physiological integrity; content area: psychiatric nursing

Rationale

(A) Provide preferred nutritious snacks. Making them accessible throughout the day will help replace burned calories. (B) The client is too hyperactive to sit for a meal. (C) This is not a balanced meal. (D) This is a meal that requires the client to sit.

53. **(C)** Nursing process phase: analysis; client need: psychosocial integrity; content area: psychiatric nursing

Rationale

(A) Long-term psychiatric care fosters dependence. The goal of therapy is to promote independence. (B) A nursing home client becomes dependent on the system. (C) A group home will assist the client with structure and help him develop a level of independence. (D) The client requires some form of structure, which is not available with independent living.

54. **(B)** Nursing process phase: implementation; client need: physiological integrity; content area: psychiatric nursing

Rationale

(A) Fluoxetine is not a tricyclic antidepressant. It is an atypical antidepressant. (B) This statement is true. (C) These foods are high in tyramine and should be avoided when the client is taking MAO inhibitors. Fluoxetine is not an MAO inhibitor. (D) Fatal reactions have been reported in clients receiving fluoxetine in combination with MAO inhibitors.

55. **(A)** Nursing process phase: analysis; client need: psychosocial integrity; content area: psychiatric nursing

Rationale

(A) Because the client is complaining of neck pain and bragging about an insurance settlement, the nurse suspects he is feigning pain. (B) Conversion is a defense operating unconsciously. The client clearly states his motive. (C) Somatization disorder applies to clients who have sought medical attention for recurrent and multiple somatic complaints. (D) Hypochondriasis is characterized by constantly worrying about health or fear of having some disease.

56. (A) Nursing process phase: assessment; client need: psychosocial integrity; content area: psychiatric nursing

Rationale

(A) An hallucination is a false sensory perception in the absence of an actual external stimulus. (B) Fantasies are a defense mechanism used in an attempt to resolve an emotional conflict. (C) A delusion is a false belief based on incorrect inference about external reality even with evidence to the contrary. (D) Derealization is a perception that the immediate environment is suddenly strange.

57. (D) Nursing process phase: implementation; client need: psychosocial integrity; content area: psychiatric nursing

Rationale

(A) Focus on the feelings provoked by the delusion rather than on the delusional content. (B) This response may cause more delusional thinking and block communication. (C) This statement challenges the client's belief by focusing on the delusion and may further distance the client from reality. (D) This response represents reality and does not challenge the client's belief system.

58. (A) Nursing process phase: implementation; client need: psychosocial integrity; content area: psychiatric nursing

Rationale

(A) Conveying acceptance shows that the nurse is willing to meet the client's needs. (B) Thought insertion is only one symptom that contributes to the client's behavior. (C) Ignoring the behaviors may create a nontherapeutic relationship because it does not convey acceptance. (D) Before attempting to probe for the target symptoms, the client should show improvement in the disease process.

59. (A) Nursing process phase: implementation; client need: safe, effective care environment; content area: psychiatric nursing

Rationale

(A) Client safety is the nurse's first priority. (B) If a client is dissatisfied with psychiatric or mental health care, the lawyer advocate may be contacted by the client. (C) Restraints dehumanize and interfere with a client's autonomy. It is important to use alternative strategies. (D) Because anger narrows the perceptual field, postpone discussion of anger and consequences until the client is in control.

60. (B) Nursing process phase: analysis; client need: safe, effective care environment; content area: psychiatric nursing

Rationale

(A) Displacement operates on an unconscious level. An emotion, idea, or wish is transferred from the original object to a more acceptable substitute. (B) Poor control of impulsive behavior shows limited insight and poor judgment. (C) Identification is an ego defense mechanism whereby a person tries to become like someone he or she admires. (D) Gratification or a source of satisfaction comes from getting needs met. This client has poor impulse control.

61. (B) Nursing process phase: planning; client need: psychosocial integrity; content area: psychiatric nursing

Rationale

(A) Acknowledging the client's inability to speak without encouraging alternative methods to convey messages will decrease trust and hinder the total communication process. (B) The use of simple concrete terms will help the client understand the meaning of the spoken word. (C) An attempt to encourage a conversation at this time may increase anxiety and psychotic behaviors. (D) Persons with schizophrenia think concretely. Abstract terms may be misinterpreted.

62. (B) Nursing process phase: implementation; client need: psychosocial integrity; content area: psychiatric nursing

Rationale

(A) Focusing on the delusional content may increase anxiety. (B) Focusing on the fears and insecurities promotes the client's trust and willingness to be helped. (C) Agreeing with the client may reinforce the delusion. (D) Challenging the client's delusional system is not appropriate because it may increase tension and force the client to defend it.

63. (A) Nursing process phase: planning; client need: psychosocial integrity; content area: psychiatric nursing

Rationale

(A) The client is unable to control her mental state of health. Providing a safe environment with reduced external stimuli will provide feelings of security and safety. (B) Social interaction should not be encouraged until after the mood has been stabilized. (C) Discussion of the bizarre behavior may increase anxiety and cause anger and a defensive attitude. (D) The main focus of nursing care is to provide a safe environment that will protect the client. With disorganized thoughts, the client may not be capable of processing the information.

64. (A) Nursing process phase: assessment; client need: psychosocial integrity; content area: psychiatric nursing

Rationale

(A) Schizoaffective disorder is manifested by schizophrenic behaviors, along with symptoms of mood disorders, either manic or depression. (B) Persons with thought disorders have difficulty controlling anger. (C) Persons with schizophrenia lack feelings of uniqueness and individuality because of extremely weak ego boundaries. (D) Echopraxia is that behavior in a person suffering from schizophrenia characterized by purposeless imitation of movement by others.

65. (C) Nursing process phase: analysis; client need: psychosocial integrity; content area: psychiatric nursing

Rationale

(A) Delusion of grandeur is when the person has an exaggerated feeling of importance. (B) Delusion of control is a belief that one's feelings, impulses, thoughts, or actions are not one's own but have been imposed by some external force. (C) Delusion of persecution is the feeling of being threatened and belief that others intend harm or persecution toward him or her. (D) Delusion of reference is the conviction that events or actions of others in the immediate environment have a particular and unusual significance.

66. (B) Nursing process phase: implementation; client need: psychosocial integrity; content area: psychiatric nursing

Rationale
(A) This response criticizes the client and may cause unnecessary anger and conflict. (B) This response gives recognition and acknowledgment of feelings. (C) Denying the belief serves no purpose, because delusional ideas are not eliminated by this approach. (D) This response rejects the client's belief and may cause the client to limit further interaction.

67. **(B)** Nursing process phase: analysis; client need: psychosocial integrity; content area: psychiatric nursing

Rationale
(A) Do not agree or disagree with the beliefs. When the client feels that he and his beliefs are accepted, trust begins to develop. (B) Persons suffering from delusions of persecutory type think they are being treated malevolently. Delusional ideas are not eliminated by challenging. Reinforce and focus on reality. Warn the physician about the behavior. Breach of client-nurse confidentiality should be considered but should not pose an ethical or legal dilemma. (C) For the protection of society, homicidal statements must be taken seriously and thoroughly assessed. (D) After trust is established, the client will begin to discuss and identify fears and suspicions.

68. **(A)** Nursing process phase: analysis; client need: psychosocial integrity; content area: psychiatric nursing

Rationale
(A) Somatic delusions focus on the body and may include the false belief that all or part of the body is distorted. (B) The client is not focusing on self. (C) The client's statement is not a delusion. He is focusing on the mother's thinking. (D) This statement does not indicate a delusion. The client is having a problem with his mother.

69. **(D)** Nursing process phase: analysis; client need: psychosocial integrity; content area: psychiatric nursing

Rationale
(A) Paranoid clients exhibit a flat, dull affect and suspicious behaviors. (B) Abnormalities in motor behavior are characteristics of catatonic schizophrenia. (C) Regressive and primitive features are present is disorganized schizophrenia. (D) The paranoid client is often angry, aggressive, and guarded.

70. **(C)** Nursing process phase: assessment; client need: psychosocial integrity; content area: psychiatric nursing

Rationale
(A) Emotional status is the overall mood state or affective reaction. (B) Interpersonal style assesses eye contact, involvement or withdrawal, receptivity or negativity, and independence or dependence. (C) Speech characteristics include clarity, articulation, organization, and appropriateness of word choice. (D) This is the ability to understand and express meaning in an appropriate manner.

71. **(A)** Nursing process phase: analysis; client need: psychosocial integrity; content area: psychiatric nursing

Rationale
(A) Echolalia is a parrotlike repetition of overheard words or fragments of speech. It is an attempt to identify with the person speaking. (B) The term used for imitating a person's movement is echopraxia. (C) Alogia is a brief, empty verbal response. (D) Avolition is a lack of initiative and goal-directed activities.

72. **(C)** Nursing process phase: implementation; client need: safe, effective care environment; content area: psychiatric nursing

Rationale
(A) Instructing the client to leave without an explanation may cause anger and alienation. (B) Confrontation in an open setting may be perceived as punitive. (C) Clear boundaries and set limits will provide firm structure necessary for clients diagnosed with a personality disorder. (D) One of the health teachings of a person diagnosed with borderline personality disorder is problem-solving, which is a long-term issue.

73. **(B)** Nursing process phase: implementation; client need: psychosocial integrity; content area: psychiatric nursing

Rationale
(A) A discussion related to the psychological testing is not a nursing priority. (B) The intervention must focus on denial, self-gratification, and the need for changing behaviors. (C) Antisocial personalities see themselves as victims. Limiting social interactions may reinforce this thinking. (D) The word "coax" leaves room for misinterpretation. Explanations must be concise, concrete, and clearly stated.

74. **(B)** Nursing process phase: implementation; client need: psychosocial integrity; content area: psychiatric nursing

Rationale
(A) Asking the client a "why" question can be intimidating and implies that the client must defend the request. (B) This response is direct and explores the relationship between mother and daughter that may provide relevant information. (C) This response is judgmental and opposes the client's request. (D) Probing for information that is difficult to answer may place the client on the defensive.

75. **(C)** Nursing process phase: implementation; client need: psychosocial integrity; content area: psychiatric nursing

Rationale
(A) Because of the client's impulsive and manipulative behavior, allowing permissive behavior will destroy the milieu. The staff must set and maintain consistent rules and regulations for these clients because it is critical to developing and maintaining a therapeutic alliance. (B) Ignoring the behavior allows the client to gain power and control over the milieu. (C) Setting strict limits conveys external control. (D) Discussing interpersonal relationships with an antisocial personality is futile. It is impossible for the person to have a satisfying interpersonal relationship because he or she has learned to place trust only in self.

76. **(A)** Nursing process phase: assessment; client need: safe, effective care environment; content area: psychiatric nursing

Rationale
(A) When the severely depressed client suddenly begins to feel better, it often indicates that the client has made the decision to kill himself or herself and has developed a plan to do so. (B) Improvement in behavior is not indicative of an exacerbation of depressive symptoms. (C) The depressed client has a tendency for self-violence, not violence toward others. (D) Depressive behavior is not always accompanied by psychotic behavior.

77. **(B)** Nursing process phase: planning; client need: health promotion and maintenance; content area: psychiatric nursing

Rationale

(A) Do not threaten with punitive actions. Ultimatums increase confrontation, which may result in a power struggle. (B) Independence fosters feelings of control. (C) Clients with this disorder have little tolerance for being alone. Strict isolation may increase their fear of abandonment. (D) This intervention is counterproductive because these persons exhibit helplessness, dependence, and regressive behavior.

78. **(B)** Nursing process phase: analysis; client need: health promotion and maintenance; content area: psychiatric nursing

Rationale

(A) Primitive idealization is the assignment of unrealistic powers to an individual on whom one is dependent. (B) The client's behavior is inconstant. (C) Omnipotence is a fantasy of unlimited power or greatness. (D) Derealization is a feeling of disconnectedness from the environment.

79. **(C)** Nursing process phase: analysis; client need: psychosocial integrity; content area: psychiatric nursing

Rationale

(A) These clients are unpredictable due to impulsiveness and lack of responsibility. (B) These persons demonstrate poorly controlled anger. (C) Clients diagnosed as having a borderline personality disorder use the defense mechanism of splitting. (D) One criterion for the borderline personality disorder is a pattern of unstable and intense interpersonal relationships.

80. **(A)** Nursing process phase: planning; client need: psychosocial integrity; content area: psychiatric nursing

Rationale

(A) Clarifying the actual source of hate and bitterness may heighten self-awareness of these feelings to assist with resolution. (B) A discussion of satisfying past relationships deals with positive transference rather than negative transference. (C) Focus on helping the client bring an unconscious event into consciousness, to examine its cause and meaning. Future relationships are not part of the problem. (D) Transference is a form of resistance and further avoidance may sabotage the treatment.

81. **(B)** Nursing process phase: assessment; client need: psychosocial integrity; content area: psychiatric nursing

Rationale

(A) These delusions are related to the belief that an individual has an incurable illness. (B) These delusions are related to feelings of self-importance and uniqueness. (C) These delusions are related to feelings of being conspired against. (D) These delusions are related to denial of self-existence.

82. **(B)** Nursing process phase: planning; client need: psychosocial integrity; content area: psychiatric nursing

Rationale

(A) This statement represents a short-term goal. (B) Long-term therapy should be directed toward assisting the client to cope effectively with stress. (C) Suicide contracts represent short-term interventions. (D) This statement represents an unrealistic goal. Stressful situations cannot be avoided in reality.

83. **(B)** Nursing process phase: assessment; client need: safe, effective care environment; content area: psychiatric nursing

Rationale

(A) Auditory hallucinations involve sensory perceptions of hearing. (B) Gustatory hallucinations involve sensory perceptions of taste. (C) Olfactory hallucinations involve sensory perceptions of smell. (D) Visceral hallucinations involve sensory perceptions of sensation.

84. **(D)** Nursing process phase: assessment; client need: psychosocial integrity; content area: psychiatric nursing

Rationale

(A) A hallmark of the schizoid personality is a marked withdrawal from social contact. (B) Characteristics of this disorder are procrastination, postponement of routine tasks, irritability, and argumentativeness. (C) Borderline personality characteristics include instability of interpersonal relationships, poor self-image, and lack of control over impulses. (D) Persons with antisocial personality disorders lack empathy and remorse, and are callously unconcerned for the feelings of others. These persons use manipulation to control others.

85. **(D)** Nursing process phase: implementation; client need: psychosocial integrity; content area: psychiatric nursing

Rationale

(A) Masturbation is a common practice among both sexes. (B) There is no research that indicates masturbation causes voyeurism. (C) There is no evidence that masturbation causes an orgasmic disorder. (D) Masturbation is used to release tension and frustration. Both sexes obtain sexual satisfaction.

86. **(B)** Nursing process phase: implementation; client need: psychosocial integrity; content area: psychiatric nursing

Rationale

(A) Confronting the mental health worker is a distraction from the main issue. (B) Encouraging the discussion of feelings may prevent unconditional acceptance of the client and help the client with her sexual identity. (C) Limiting the interaction will deny the client therapeutic nursing care. (D) A behavior that interferes with the rights of others requires an intervention.

87. **(A)** Nursing process phase: implementation; client need: health promotion and maintenance; content area: psychiatric nursing

Rationale

(A) The manic client is unable to sit still long enough to eat an adequate meal. Small, frequent feedings with finger foods allow him to eat during periods of activity. (B) This type of therapy should be implemented when other methods have been exhausted. (C) The manic client should not be in control of his treatment plan. This type of client may forget to eat. (D) The manic client is unable to sit down to eat full meals.

88. **(D)** Nursing process phase: implementation; client need: psychosocial integrity; content area: psychiatric nursing

Rationale

(A) Communication may be influenced by past experiences. It does not influence the past. (B) Communication is not a one-way process. It is a circular process. (C) The process of communication is dynamic and has multiple dimensions. (D) During an interaction, persons use a variety of symbols that may identify the representational system.

89. **(A)** Nursing process phase: assessment; client need: safe, effective care environment; content area: psychiatric nursing

Rationale
(A) The physician is requesting additional information to help clarify information that does not seem relevant. (B) There is no indication that the client should be removed from the milieu. (C) "Why" questions may be perceived as threatening and cause barriers to communication. (D) Demands are barriers to open communication. Avoiding communication barriers will facilitate constructive communication.

90. **(A)** Nursing process phase: assessment; client need: safe, effective care environment; content area: psychiatric nursing

Rationale
(A) Clarifying unclear communication increases understanding and will assist with misperceptions. (B) "Focusing" is not therapeutic. It concentrates on a single point of the communication. This technique is used with clients who move very quickly from one thought to another. (C) "Voicing doubt" expresses uncertainty. (D) "Probing" involves persistent questioning.

91. **(C)** Nursing process phase: implementation; client need: psychosocial integrity; content area: psychiatric nursing

Rationale
(A) This is a form of rejection and may interfere with any further interaction. (B) Denying privileges sends a signal that the nurse conditionally accepts the client. (C) Making observations and encouraging the client to verbalize feelings will help the client recognize specific behaviors. (D) The nurse acknowledges the problem but conveys a lack of empathy and understanding.

92. **(A)** Nursing process phase: implementation; client need: psychosocial integrity; content area: psychiatric nursing

Rationale
(A) Facilitative communication moves beyond social chitchat and into an interpersonal relationship. Interpersonal communication plays a major role in psychiatric nursing. (B) Nonverbal communication does not include the spoken word. However, it may influence the outcome of the interaction. (C) Public communication occurs when speaking to a group. (D) Intrapersonal communication occurs when persons communicate between themselves.

93. **(C)** Nursing process phase: analysis; psychosocial integrity; content area: psychiatric nursing

Rationale
(A) Assertive behavior is an accurate statement about feelings, beliefs, and opinions. It is stated in a manner than promotes self-respect and respects others. (B) Aggressive behavior is inconsiderate, offensive, and violates the basic rights of others. (C) Passive behavior is a response that discounts one's own rights in order to avoid conflict. (D) Passive-aggressive behavior is expressed through sarcasm, resistance, manipulation, procrastination, and the use of covert aggression instead of words.

94. **(C)** Nursing process phase: assessment; client need: safe, effective care environment; content area: psychiatric nursing

Rationale
(A) During the manic phase of bipolar disorder, clients have short attention spans and may be abusive toward authority figures. (B) Introspection requires focusing and concentration; clients with mania experience flight of ideas, which prevents concentration. (C) Grandiosity and an inflated sense of self-worth are characteristic of this disorder. (D) Feelings of helplessness and hopelessness are symptoms of the depressive stage of bipolar disorder.

95. **(A)** Nursing process phase: analysis; client need: psychosocial integrity; content area: psychiatric nursing

Rationale
(A) The nurse should always validate the meaning and significance of a specific behavior. (B) The nurse is unable to increase the client's awareness until validation of the meaning is obtained. (C) Nonverbal behaviors may have several meanings. However, it is important to validate the meaning prior to any investigation. (D) Feelings encompass a wide range of expressions and may be part of the meaning of the nonverbal behavior.

96. **(A)** Nursing process phase: implementation; client need: psychosocial integrity; content area: psychiatric nursing

Rationale
(A) A therapeutic interaction helps bring about insight and behavioral change that is directed toward growth. (B) The primary concern during the development of a nurse-client relationship is the client. (C) The nurse must maintain professionalism and discourage intimate interactions. (D) Therapeutic impasses are elements of a complex therapeutic nurse-client relationship but not the primary goal.

97. **(A)** Nursing process phase: implementation; client need: psychosocial integrity; content area: psychiatric nursing

Rationale
(A) This statement acknowledges the importance of the client's role. (B) This statement indicates that the nurse does not value the client. (C) This statement tells the client that the nurse is more interested in talking about her personal life. (D) This statement is meaningless in a nurse-client relationship.

98. **(A)** Nursing process phase: assessment; client need: safe, effective care environment; content area: psychiatric nursing

Rationale
(A) Sensory perception is greatly reduced, making concentration difficult, and there may be a decompensation of ego functions. (B) High levels of anxiety decrease communication skills because of the cognitive interruption. (C) High levels of anxiety decrease the thought processes and the ability to stay focused. (D) High levels of anxiety limit cognitive functioning, thus hindering insight and problem-solving abilities.

99. (A) Nursing process phase: implementation; client need: psychosocial integrity; content area: psychiatric nursing

Rationale
(A) The nurse's statement allows the client to take the initiative and share any pertinent or nonessential information. (B) This statement is nontherapeutic and limits the response to "yes" or "no." (C) "Why" questions can be intimidating and may be perceived as threatening. (D) This statement focuses on discharge and may be misinterpreted.

100. (A) Nursing process phase: implementation; client need: safe, effective care environment; content area: psychiatric nursing

Rationale
(A) Documentation related to delivery of care must reflect the use of the nursing process. (B) Information in a client's record is confidential and available to authorized personnel only. (C) The client's record is a legal document. (D) There is no guarantee that documentation is pertinent or accurate.

101. (B) Nursing process phase: assessment; client need: psychosocial integrity; content area: psychiatric nursing

Rationale
(A) This statement seeks clarification. (B) This statement is one of disagreement and may provoke defensiveness. (C) This statement offers self. (D) This statement explores the situation.

102. (A) Nursing process phase: planning; client need: psychosocial integrity; content area: psychiatric nursing

Rationale
(A) The nurse must recognize the client's need for distance in a relationship. Trying to become too close or friendly will cause the client to feel threatened and withdraw. (B) The client's affiliation needs should be considered and planned for in an individualized manner. (C) Intensive group therapy would be too threatening to this client and contribute to further withdrawal from social interactions. (D) Consistent interactions by a few nurses would be more therapeutic for this client.

103. (A) Nursing process phase: assessment; client need: psychosocial integrity; content area: psychiatric nursing

Rationale
(A) Genuineness implies honesty, sincerity, and active involvement in the development of a therapeutic relationship. (B) Confrontation should not be used until after a therapeutic relationship and a level of trust has developed. (C) It is important to develop a therapeutic relationship prior to encouraging catharsis. The nurse will be ready to support the client and protect the vulnerable state. (D) Advice giving is not therapeutic. It encourages dependence.

104. (A) Nursing process phase: assessment; client need: psychosocial integrity; content area: psychiatric nursing

Rationale
(A) The behavior presented is nonverbal and may indicate decreased self-esteem. Assisting with negative self-esteem and self-worth may increase the optimal level of functioning. (B) There is no indication of verbal communication. (C) The client does not exhibit aggressive behavior. (D) Passive behavior is expressed through both verbal and nonverbal patterns.

105. (A) Nursing process phase: implementation; client need: psychosocial integrity; content area: psychiatric nursing

Rationale
(A) When addressing a client with a schizophrenic disorder, use realistic and concrete terms. (B) The use of self-disclosure is inappropriate if the client can not benefit from it. (C) Demanding information is a barrier to communication. (D) It is important to keep the conversation simple until the client has a better understanding of his disease process.

106. (C) Nursing process phase: implementation; client need: psychosocial integrity; content area: psychiatric nursing

Rationale
(A) When the nurse remains silent, it only fosters silence in the patient. (B) A conversation about history may cause intimidation, increased fear, and an uncomfortable feeling. (C) Broad openings allow the client to take the initiative. (D) Focusing on specifics is not therapeutic.

107. (B) Nursing process phase: implementation; client need: psychosocial integrity; content area: psychiatric nursing

Rationale
(A) This response leaves the client's question unanswered. (B) This response explores the client's feelings about the length of stay and allows the client to self-pace the information. (C) This response may be a challenge to the client and may cause an unnecessary scene. (D) This response is inappropriate because it does not provide the opportunity for the client to discuss feelings with the nurse.

108. (C) Nursing process phase: planning; client need: safe, effective care environment; content area: psychiatric nursing

Rationale
(A) Sharing his belongings with others may be a long-term goal but may never be achieved in this client, who constantly feels vulnerable to exploitation by others. (B) Engaging in group activities and freely sharing his feelings may also be a long-term goal that may never be achieved. (C) Feelings of helplessness and lack of control can reinforce this client's suspicions and pattern of social isolation. The client and nurse must work jointly toward the goal of ensuring that the client has as much control as possible. (D) The client should not be encouraged to engage in solitary activities because such activities promote social isolation.

109. (B) Nursing process phase: implementation; client need: safe, effective care environment; content area: psychiatric nursing

Rationale
(A) The nurse must be cognizant of any side effects that the client exhibits from a neuroleptic agent. If the signs and symptoms are frequent, it is important to notify the physician. (B) The side effects from a neuroleptic medication are treatable with an antiparkinson agent. (C) Reporting the incident to a nurse manager is not a priority issue. (D) Ignoring the syndrome does not provide the quality of care that the client needs.

110. (D) Nursing process phase: assessment; client need: safe, effective care environment; content area: psychiatric nursing

Rationale

(A) There is no indication that diarrhea or amenorrhea is a side effect of Haldol. (B) Orthostatic hypotension is a side effect, but increased sweating is not. (C) Decreased sweating is a side effect, but persons complain of impotence. (D) Headache and orthostatic hypotension are side effects of Haldol.

111. (B) Nursing process phase: implementation; client need: health promotion and maintenance; content area: psychiatric nursing

Rationale

(A) The client should be told that antacids may decrease the absorption of Risperdal and the full effectiveness of the medication is not obtained. (B) Waiting 1 hour before taking an antacid may allow less interference with absorption of the medication. (C) It is not "OK" to take antacids with Risperdal because antacids decrease the effectiveness of the medication. (D) A nursing responsibility is to instruct the client about medications. It may help the client with independence and decrease recidivism.

112. (A) Nursing process phase: implementation; client need: health promotion and maintenance; content area: psychiatric nursing

Rationale

(A) Abrupt withdrawal may precipitate nausea, vomiting, tremors, and lower the seizure threshold. (B) "Doubling" the dose of Haldol may cause an overdose. (C) Do not mix Haldol and alcohol because they potentiate each other's effect. (D) Photosensitivity is a major side effect of Haldol. You must advise the client to use plenty of sunscreen and wear protective clothing.

113. (A) Nursing process phase: implementation; client need: health promotion and maintenance; content area: psychiatric nursing

Rationale

(A) Benzodiazepines are addictive. It is the responsibility of the nurse to teach the client about dependence, tolerance, and more effective coping skills. (B) Abrupt withdrawal could produce panic, paranoia, tremors, and lowering of the seizure threshold. (C) Caffeine should be discouraged because it interferes with the effectiveness of the drug. (D) Xanax is addictive and should not be prescribed for an indefinite period of time.

114. (C) Nursing process phase: assessment; client need: psychosocial integrity; content area: psychiatric nursing

Rationale

(A) This is not a characteristic of catatonic schizophrenia. (B) This is not a characteristic of paranoid schizophrenia that is not generally seen in catatonic schizophrenia. The symptoms can result in an unwillingness or inability to eat. (C) Stuporous withdrawal, hallucinations, and delusions are characteristics of catatonic schizophrenia. (D) Sexual preoccupation is more a characteristic of sexual disorders and the manic phase of bipolar disorder. Word salad is a speech pattern in which words do not make sense and is not characteristic of catatonic schizophrenia.

115. (B) Nursing process phase: assessment; client need: safe, effective care environment; content area: psychiatric nursing

Rationale

(A) Confusion is not reported as a side effect of Depakene. (B) Drowsiness is a side effect of Depakene. Persons who have been prescribed Depakene should be instructed on the dangers of operating heavy machinery and driving a car. (C) There are no data that support genitourinary problems. (D) Anorexia is a side effect of Depakene, but there are no data that support bulimia.

116. (C) Nursing process phase: analysis; client need: health promotion and maintenance; content area: psychiatric nursing

Rationale

(A) Paxil is a third-generation antidepressant medication. (B) Tegretol is an anticonvulsant medication and is also used as a mood stabilizer. (C) Cogentin is the drug of choice to treat extrapyramidal symptoms associated with antipsychotic drugs. (D) Ativan is an antianxiety agent. It is not prescribed for EPS.

117. (B) Nursing process phase: assessment; client need: safe, effective care environment; content area: psychiatric nursing

Rationale

(A) Antiparkinson medication may cause an intensification of psychotic symptoms. (B) A side effect of an antiparkinson medication is anxiety. (C) A side effect is hot, dry, flushed skin. (D) An antiparkinson medication may cause dry mucous membranes.

118. (C) Nursing process phase: analysis; client need: safe, effective care environment; content area: psychiatric nursing

Rationale

(A) Lithium carbonate is not the drug of choice prescribed for schizoaffective disorder. (B) Lithium carbonate is not the drug of choice for obsessive-compulsive disorders. (C) Lithium carbonate is the drug of choice for controlling manic episodes in persons with manic-depressive illness. (D) Neuroleptic medications are the drug of choice for schizophrenia.

119. (C) Nursing process phase: assessment; client need: safe, effective care environment; content area: psychiatric nursing

Rationale

(A) Bradycardia is not a symptom of lithium carbonate overdose. (B) Hypertension is a common symptom with clients whose lithium carbonate serum level is above the therapeutic range. (C) When the serum level of lithium is greater than the therapeutic range, psychotic behaviors range from mild to severe. (D) When the lithium serum level is determined to be toxic, severe diarrhea may be a problem.

120. (A) Nursing process phase: implementation; client need: health promotion and maintenance; content area: psychiatric nursing

Rationale

(A) It is important for the client to consume sufficient sodium in the diet because sodium depletion will decrease renal excretion of lithium and cause the drug to accumulate. (B) Serum lithium levels should be checked every 1 to 2 months to determine the blood serum level and prevent toxicity. (C)

The client is advised to choose foods from the four food groups and avoid "junk foods." (D) Leaving the adjustment to the client is irresponsible.

121. **(A)** Nursing process phase: planning; client need: safe, effective care environment; content area: psychiatric nursing

Rationale
(A) The plan should focus on reinforcing perceptions and thinking that is in touch with reality. (B) Challenging the client's hallucinations and delusions is not effective and can impede the development of a trusting therapeutic relationship. (C) Using peer pressure to discourage distorted thinking and bizarre behavior is not therapeutic. (D) Ignoring distorted thinking and bizarre behavior is not therapeutic in assisting this client to become more connected to reality.

122. **(C)** Nursing process phase: implementation; client need: health promotion and maintenance; content area: psychiatric nursing

Rationale
(A) Librium is used for the temporary relief of anxiety, not as a long-term medication. (B) Nicotine decreases the effects of Librium and should be avoided. (C) Librium should be used cautiously in the elderly and in persons with a history of drug addiction. (D) Central nervous system depressants (including alcohol) should be avoided.

123. **(C)** Nursing process phase: implementation; client need: health promotion and maintenance; content area: psychiatric nursing

Rationale
(A) There is no indication that sertraline causes stomach irritation. If sertraline is taken with food, it decreases the time it takes to reach peak plasma concentration. (B) The medication should be taken exactly as prescribed. Do not double-dose. (C) Taking other medications with sertraline could "precipitate" a life-threatening situation. (D) Abrupt stopping of the medication may cause withdrawal symptoms.

124. **(C)** Nursing process phase: implementation; client need: safe, effective care environment; content area: psychiatric nursing

Rationale
(A) Succinylcholine chloride is not given orally due to poor absorption from the gastrointestinal tract. (B) Succinylcholine is rapidly destroyed in the body, thus making the onset rapid and the action brief. (C) Succinylcholine chloride is the medication of choice used to relax the skeletal muscles prior to ECT to prevent bone fractures. (D) Succinylcholine is not administered to control respirations.

125. **(C)** Nursing process phase: analysis; client need: safe, effective care environment; content area: psychiatric nursing

Rationale
(A) Pentobarbital is a sedative-hypnotic medication, not for the control of seizures. Phenobarbital is used to control seizure activity. (B) Alprazolam is an antianxiety agent. Primidone is an anticonvulsant medication. (C) Phenytoin is an anticonvulsant, has only minor side effects, and is used in conjunction with phenobarbital to control seizure activity with less sedating side effects. (D) Phenytoin is used to control

seizures. Pentobarbital is a sedative-hypnotic. These medications are not prescribed in combination for seizure disorders.

126. **(D)** Nursing process phase: analysis; client need: safe, effective care environment; content area: psychiatric nursing

Rationale
(A) Risperidone is an antipsychotic agent prescribed for schizophrenia and related psychosis. (B) Clozapine is an antipsychotic used in the management of severely ill persons with schizophrenia. (C) Lorazepam is indicated for anxiety disorders. (D) Lithium carbonate is the drug of choice for maintenance therapy in clients diagnosed as having a bipolar disorder. It reduces the hyperactivity that is characteristic of the disorder.

127. **(C)** Nursing process phase: analysis; client need: health promotion and maintenance; content area: psychiatric nursing

Rationale
(A) The dosage of flurazepam is 15 to 30 mg at bedtime. Doubling that amount may "precipitate" a life-threatening situation. (B) Flurazepam is a sedative-hypnotic used primarily for insomnia, not pain. (C) The client verbalizes an understanding of the side effects and wants relief. (D) The request for discharge is not relevant to information about the medication.

128. **(B)** Nursing process phase: implementation; client need: health promotion and maintenance; content area: psychiatric nursing

Rationale
(A) Stopping the medication abruptly may produce a headache, depression, and hallucinations. (B) Chocolate contains enough tyramine or other related pressor amine materials to cause dangerous hypertensive episodes. (C) Do not use over-the-counter medications because many of these medications could "precipitate" a hypertensive episode. (D) Yogurt is a food to be avoided because it contains high levels of vasopressors.

129. **(A)** Nursing process phase: implementation; client need: safe, effective care environment; content area: psychiatric nursing

Rationale
(A) It is important for the nurse to check for "checking" of the medication to prevent a possible suicide attempt. (B) Sleep induced by hypnotic doses of barbiturates involves no more depression of the respiratory system than occurs in normal sleep. (C) This option is not a priority and is of least importance. (D) Circulation is not significantly affected by sedative or hypnotic doses of barbiturates.

130. **(B)** Nursing process phase: assessment; client need: safe, effective care environment; content area: psychiatric nursing

Rationale
(A) It is possible that the client is addicted to barbiturates but the addiction is not a priority. (B) The first priority is to assess for suicidal ideation. The client tells the nurse that she would like to see her deceased mother. (C) Barbiturate withdrawal is a possibility and requires assessment after suicidal ideation is determined. (D) Assessing for toxicity is not the initial action.

131. **(C)** Nursing process phase: assessment; client need: safe, effective care environment; content area: psychiatric nursing

Rationale
(A) Valproic acid is used for management of seizures and should be used cautiously in clients who suffer from hepatic disease. It is not the drug of choice for alcohol withdrawal. (B) Because alcoholics suffer from a marked dietary and vitamin deficiency, thiamine is given to prevent polyneuritis. (C) Librium is used for treating the withdrawal symptoms of alcohol. It is rapidly absorbed in the intestines and does not depress the brain center. (D) Pyridoxine is a B vitamin necessary for the prevention of neuritis that frequently occurs in persons suffering from alcoholism.

132. **(C)** Nursing process phase: implementation; client need: safe, effective care environment; content area: psychiatric nursing

Rationale
(A) Carbamazepine is an anticonvulsant medication. (B) Clonidine is an antihypertensive medication. (C) Disulfiram is sometimes used during the rehabilitation phase of alcohol abuse and acts as a deterrent to alcohol consumption. (D) This medication is used in treating macrocytic anemia due to folic acid deficiency.

133. **(D)** Nursing process phase: analysis; client need: safe, effective care environment; content area: psychiatric nursing

Rationale
(A) It is not clear how ECT effects a therapeutic response. It is believed that there is a significant increase in the circulating levels of several neurotransmitters. (B) Clients are administered a skeletal muscle relaxant to prevent injuries during the seizure activity. (C) There are no research data that support irreversible brain damage or changes in brain functioning caused by ECT. (D) During a course of ECT, clients have some short-term memory deficit and confusion.

134. **(A)** Nursing process phase: implementation; client need: safe, effective care environment; content area: psychiatric nursing

Rationale
(A) According to the American Psychiatric Association standards, ECT should be given under general anesthesia with the use of a muscle relaxant drug. (B) The procedure is not incapacitating. Clients resume normal activity soon after the treatment is completed. (C) ECT has been in use since the 1930s. However, there is a degree of risk with any procedure requiring a general anesthesia. (D) There are no research data that support permanent memory loss caused by ECT therapy.

135. **(B)** Nursing process phase: evaluation; client need: safe, effective care environment; content area: psychiatric nursing

Rationale
(A) The nurse caring for the client should explain the procedure prior to therapy and answer questions to decrease anxiety. (B) A projected outcome of ECT therapy is reorientation to time, place, and situation. (C) Most clients are confused immediately after ECT therapy. If the nurse orients the client, fear is reduced. (D) This is not an outcome of ECT therapy.

136. **(B)** Nursing process phase: planning; client need: safe, effective care environment; content area: psychiatric nursing

Rationale
(A) Psychotherapy and pharmacotherapy are continued to aid against the return of symptoms. (B) Most severely depressed clients who fail to respond to other forms of therapy respond to ECT. (C) Insulin coma therapy has been discontinued as a treatment for mental illness. (D) Pharmacoconvulsive therapy is no longer a treatment for mental illness.

137. **(A)** Nursing process phase: implementation; client need: safe, effective care environment; content area: psychiatric nursing

Rationale
(A) For severe depression, a series of 6 to 10 treatments over a duration of 2 to 4 weeks is recommended. (B) Persons may require one treatment a month as "maintenance" therapy. (C) The American Psychiatric Association does not recommend a specific number of treatments. (D) There are those who may be prescribed "maintenance ECT." After the series of treatments, a reduced schedule is recommended.

138. **(A)** Nursing process phase: evaluation; client need: health promotion and maintenance; content area: psychiatric nursing

Rationale
(A) Treatments are given three times a week for approximately 2 to 4 weeks. After three treatments, the client should begin to see beneficial effects. (B) The client should see improvement in less than 15 days. (C) ECT treatments are normally completed in 4 weeks. The client's condition should begin to improve after three treatments. (D) Beneficial effects should be evident during the first week of treatment, if the client has received at least three ECT treatments.

139. **(A)** Nursing process phase: assessment; client need: safe, effective care environment; content area: psychiatric nursing

Rationale
(A) Methscopolamine or atropine sulfate is given prior to ECT to decrease secretions. Persons usually complain of a dry mouth. (B) Most patients have a headache ranging from mild to severe. (C) Occasionally, persons complain of nausea. (D) Muscle and joint soreness are common physical complaints.

140. **(C)** Nursing process phase: implementation; client need: psychosocial integrity; content area: psychiatric nursing

Rationale
(A) This statement does not respect the client's concern and is belittling. (B) ECT is relatively safe. When anesthesia is used, there is a degree of risk. (C) This response explores further into the client's feelings about fears related to the treatment. (D) A family member can be supportive and may help the person with decision making. It is possible that a family member may be asked to give consent. However, it is a difficult decision to make for someone else and the client should be encouraged to make the decision.

141. **(B)** Nursing process phase: planning; client need: safe, effective care environment; content area: psychiatric nursing

Rationale
(A) The client with catatonic schizophrenia has a diminished ability to deal with external stimulation. (B) As part of the plan to decrease the catatonic client's withdrawn behavior, the nurse should speak in simple, concise terms to avoid sensory overload of the client. (C) These clients need to have limits set on their behavior to promote safety. (D) In the acute phase of catatonic schizophrenia, clients are unable to participate in group therapy.

142. **(C)** Nursing process phase: implementation; client need: safe, effective care environment; content area: psychiatric nursing

Rationale
(A) This intervention may actually precipitate a violent reaction. (B) This intervention may make the nurse the target of violence. (C) A key to managing violent behavior is to respond in a calm, controlled, nonthreatening, and caring manner. A confident physical stance communicates control and may de-escalate violence. (D) This intervention is nontherapeutic and may lead to increased aggression.

143. **(D)** Nursing process phase: implementation; client need: psychosocial integrity; content area: psychiatric nursing

Rationale
(A) Physical distance is important during a verbal intervention. A large personal space is necessary with clients who are anxious and assaultive. (B) If attempts to establish a therapeutic relationship fail, then force is needed to control the situation. (C) Shifting the focus of hostility may be accomplished only after a therapeutic rapport is established. (D) Quickly establishing rapport through verbal restraints should be attempted prior to any extreme form of control.

144. **(B)** Nursing process phase: implementation; client need: psychosocial integrity; content area: psychiatric nursing

Rationale
(A) Humor is not therapeutic for clients who exhibit violence. (B) The nurse needs to determine that the environment is safe to assess the client and then use a structured interview and brief statements to acquire the necessary information. (C) Clients exhibiting violent behavior need a larger personal space than those clients who are nonviolent. (D) Many violent persons have difficulty expressing anger and rage in a nonverbal manner. Open-ended questions may increase the client's agitated state because of the verbal deficit.

145. **(A)** Nursing process phase: implementation; client need: safe, effective care environment; content area: psychiatric nursing

Rationale
(A) A safe environment for all clients and staff must be maintained. Combative and violent behavior causes anxiety. Therefore, the out-of-control client should be immobilized until the behavior is under control. (B) Because active listening is one of the early interventions, it is unlikely that it will be effective once the client has lost control. (C) A chemical restraint is useful in decreasing the risk of violent behavior. After the physical restraints have been applied, a chemical restraint may be administered if there is a standing or PRN order. (D) This intervention is appropriate but not until after the client is nonviolent and ready to consider more effective coping behaviors.

146. **(D)** Nursing process phase: implementation; client need: safe, effective care environment; content area: psychiatric nursing

Rationale
(A) The use of mechanical restraints requires a physician's order at least every 24 hours. (B) Restraints that are applied too tightly may interfere with circulation, causing damage to the extremities. (C) Clients in mechanical restraints are observed every 15 minutes and the information is documented. (D) The type of restraints and the client's response are documented in the progress notes.

147. **(B)** Nursing process phase: evaluation; client need: health promotion and maintenance; content area: psychiatric nursing

Rationale
(A) Knowledge of rehabilitation resources may set stage for vocational training that will foster self-esteem. (B) A discharge outcome is denial of suicidal ideation and implementating functional coping skills. (C) Understanding the medication regimen is no indication that the client is free from self-mutilation and suicide ideation. (D) Discussing somatic complaints and suicide ideation is an indication that the client is depressed and not ready for discharge.

148. **(A)** Nursing process phase: implementation; client need: safe, effective care environment; content area: psychiatric nursing

Rationale
(A) The nurse has an ethical and legal responsibility for providing safety, preserving life, and notifying others about the client's intention. (B) This intervention is a long-term goal. (C) The client is preoccupied with destroying self. The nurse immediately intervenes regarding the client's ambivalent behavior and helps the client express hope for the future. (D) Most cultures consider suicide an immoral act. Social sanctions and the code of ethics help the nurse respond with appropriate nursing interventions and do not allow for the nurse to keep secrets about suicide intentions.

149. **(C)** Nursing process phase: implementation; client need: safe, effective care environment; content area: psychiatric nursing

Rationale
(A) The amount of morphine cannot be altered unless it is ordered by the person prescribing the medication. (B) Although the nurse does not respond to the medication request, she does not take the opportunity to address the depressed state. (C) The nurse is acknowledging the depressed state and pain, and expressed concern and empathy. (D) This statement does not address the client's concern and feelings and shows contempt. It does not provide therapeutic support.

150. **(B)** Nursing process phase: analysis; client need: safe, effective care environment; content area: psychiatric nursing

Rationale
(A) The client indicates that the loss of employment has caused emotional stress and loss of energy, but not suicide. (B) The client clearly states that there are no alternatives to suicide. (C) This is the bargaining stage of the grieving process. (D) The client is reflecting on his life and attempting to put it in perspective.

151. (A) Nursing process phase: assessment; client need: safe, effective care environment; content area: psychiatric nursing

Rationale

(A) The nurse asked the client a direct question about the intent and lethality. This will provide concrete information and assist the nurse with formulating an appropriate nursing intervention. (B) This nurse is indirectly seeking clarification. (C) Knowing the lifestyle of the client may assist the nurse with interventions. (D) Many persons write suicide notes. Determining the content may be helpful during the planning of care.

152. (C) Nursing process phase: assessment; client need: safe, effective care environment; content area: psychiatric nursing

Rationale

(A) Maturational crises are periods requiring role changes. This client is in the adult stage of life and may or may not be confronted with a role change. (B) The client exhibited the ability to express feelings during the admission period. (C) Clients with depressive and manic-depressive illness are more likely to attempt suicide than any other risk group. (D) Social crises involve multiple losses with environmental changes.

153. (A) Nursing process phase: planning; client need: health promotion and maintenance; content area: psychiatric nursing

Rationale

(A) A secondary gain may be avoidance on conflict. (B) A client would be more likely to attempt suicide if the coping skills were dysfunctional. (C) An adequate support group should meet the client's needs. (D) An unstable lifestyle is more likely to cause a person to attempt suicide.

154. (D) Nursing process phase: evaluation; client need: safe, effective care environment; content area: psychiatric nursing

Rationale

(A) It is the nurse or therapist who exhibits emotional reaction to the client. (B) Clients who are suicidal tend to be nonassertive. They have little respect for self. (C) Nurses may exhibit despair. An emotionally healthy nurse should not be jubilant. (D) The client's psychological symptoms may be so overwhelming that the nurse feels inadequate.

155. (B) Nursing process phase: assessment; client need: safe, effective care environment; content area: psychiatric nursing

Rationale

(A) Purchasing a new car indicates that the client is not in despair and willing to enjoy life. (B) An increase in psychomotor activity is an indication that the vegetative state has been lifted and the client is at risk for suicide. (C) A world tour may provide joy and happiness—not gloom and despair. (D) A depressed client who has a decrease in psychomotor activity lacks the energy to act on suicidal thoughts.

156. (B) Nursing process phase: assessment; client need: physiological integrity; content area: psychiatric nursing

Rationale

(A) These persons are obsessed with losing weight. (B) Persons diagnosed with anorexia nervosa exhibit an intense fear of gaining weight. They deny being thin even when grossly un-

derweight and will refer to self as being too "fat." (C) Anorectics show empathy, concern, and attend to the needs of others. (D) Relationships are impaired.

157. (A) Nursing process phase: analysis; client need: physiological integrity; content area: psychiatric nursing

Rationale

(A) A lack of a sense of competence in any area outside of weight control is known as a "paralyzing sense of ineffectiveness." (B) Anorectic clients have been compliant and are known as "good little girls." (C) Anorectic clients speak about having an internal void or emptiness. They lack a sense of responsibility. (D) Anorectic persons lack the capacity to identify internal perceptions.

158. (A) Nursing process phase: implementation; client need: physiological integrity; content area: psychiatric nursing

Rationale

(A) Because there is a concern for physiological complications, restoration of adequate nutrition is a primary goal. (B) Living up to family expectations has been an ordeal for the anorectic person. (C) Anorectics are preoccupied with thoughts and preparation of food. (D) Depression is a psychological dysfunction that must be treated after the fear of physical complications has been abated.

159. (A) Nursing process phase: assessment; client need: physiological integrity; content area: psychiatric nursing

Rationale

(A) It is important for the nurse to assess for peripheral edema, which may be evident in the advanced stage of anorexia nervosa. (B) Hypothyroid-like state is a physical symptom of anorexia nervosa, not a hyperthyroid-like state. (C) Pharmacological therapy may or may not be used because there are no medications specifically indicated for eating disorders. (D) Change takes place over a long period of time. Most anorectic clients are extremely resistant to change.

160. (C) Nursing process phase: implementation; client need: psychosocial integrity; content area: psychiatric nursing

Rationale

(A) This statement allows too much time for eating. It is important to set limits to forestall mealtime. (B) Vigilance is necessary during mealtime, because there is no guarantee that the client is eating. (C) This response is nonjudgmental and indicates a caring behavior. Because anorectic persons are manipulative, close observation during mealtimes is necessary. (D) Attempting to instill guilt is an inappropriate nursing intervention.

161. (C) Nursing process phase: implementation; client need: psychosocial integrity; content area: psychiatric nursing

Rationale

(A) Food discussions reinforce maladaptive behaviors by allowing the person to avoid dealing with the hidden issues. (B) Frequent small meals are more tolerable than large meals. (C) Observing bathroom behavior may be necessary if the nurse suspects that the client is discarding food or purging. (D) Avoid praise and flattery because the anorectic person has a sense of mistrust.

162. (A) Nursing process phase: implementation; client need: psychosocial integrity; content area: psychiatric nursing

Rationale
(A) Focusing on self-determination fosters adaptive coping skills that may be carried over to daily life after discharge. (B) Foster trust and encourage independence. (C) Sleep disturbance may be a problem but is not an important issue. (D) As the condition improves, a flexible routine may increase a sense of responsibility.

163. (B) Nursing process phase: implementation; client need: physiological integrity; content area: psychiatric nursing

Rationale
(A) The client may equate eating dessert with a loss of control. (B) Providing a pleasant environment is critical to the nursing care. (C) Anorectic clients need food high in protein—not high in fat. (D) A high-calorie diet of 1200 to 1500 calories per day is required to meet the weight-restoration goal.

164. (A) Nursing process phase: analysis; client need: psychosocial integrity; content area: psychiatric nursing

Rationale
(A) Anorectic persons thrive on self-control through their weight and diet. (B) Anorectic persons rarely identify the need for support and eventually withdraw from others. (C) Anorectic persons lack insight and have a sense of ineffectiveness that leads to weight control. (D) Anorectic persons have decreased emotional awareness and recognition of body sensations.

165. (C) Nursing process phase: assessment; client need: physiological integrity; content area: psychiatric nursing

Rationale
(A) The client is rationalizing about her eating habits and weight. (B) A characteristic of anorexia nervosa is a sensitive feeling toward others. However, many persons have that particular trait. (C) A diagnostic criterion for anorexia nervosa is amenorrhea of at least three consecutive menstrual cycles. (D) The client is making a matter-of-fact statement about her parents.

166. (B) Nursing process phase: analysis; client need: safe, effective care environment; content area: psychiatric nursing

Rationale
(A) Compulsive overeaters are not physically hungry but choose food as a method of nurturing themselves. (B) Persons with bulimia nervosa frequently eat large amounts of food and then purge themselves. Purging is one criterion for bulimia nervosa. (C) Self-starvation and excessive weight loss are characteristics of anorexia nervosa. (D) Body dysmorphic disorder is a preoccupation with an imagined defect in body shape and size.

167. (A) Nursing process phase: analysis; client need: safe, effective care environment; content area: psychiatric nursing

Rationale
(A) Research indicates that bulimina nervosa is a symptomatic feature of other psychological conditions and not a disorder itself. (B) Persons who suffer from bingeing and purging have mood changes. These behaviors are by-products of star-vation rather than psychopathology. (C) Bulimia nervosa is a morbid fear of obesity. (D) Anorexia nervosa is an illness occurring secondarily to a psychological disturbance.

168. (A) Nursing process phase: planning; client need: safe, effective care environment; content area: psychiatric nursing

Rationale
(A) Establishing expectations and providing limitations will help decrease the client's anxiety at mealtime. (B) Helping the client recognize indirect self-destructive behavior must be included as part of therapy. (C) Immediate attention is on bingeing and purging. Family involvement is important as the client's condition improves. (D) The nurse needs to convey a caring and sensitive attitude to establish trust, not a judgmental attitude.

169. (D) Nursing process phase: implementation; client need: psychosocial integrity; content area: psychiatric nursing

Rationale
(A) The nurse directs the client to social service rather than using a nursing judgment. (B) This statement is nontherapeutic because it is a demand. (C) The nurse is giving false assurances. (D) The nurse is offering self and acknowledges the client's feelings.

170. (B) Nursing process phase: assessment; client need: psychosocial integrity; content area: psychiatric nursing

Rationale
(A) Excessive overweight is categorized as indirect self-destructive behavior. (B) Obesity is a response to an emotional need. "Fat and ugly" is a protection from the danger of intimacy and getting emotionally hurt. (C) Financial distress may play a role in obesity, but obese persons eat to escape from emotional stress and pain. (D) Obese persons exhibit dissatisfaction with self. Characteristics include dependency traits, greed, and impatience.

171. (B) Nursing process phase: assessment; client need: psychosocial integrity; content area: psychiatric nursing

Rationale
(A) Research has shown that some bulimic persons purge to rid themselves of the "evil" that lurks within. (B) The environment within the family structure is often marked by chaos and conflict, which triggers inner conflicts and self-defeating behaviors. (C) The bulimic person tends to be an extrovert rather than an introvert. (D) Hunger before bingeing is not considered an important factor relative to other factors.

172. (A) Nursing process phase: planning; client need: safe, effective care environment; content area: psychiatric nursing

Rationale
(A) After the client's strengths and functional coping skills have been identified, short-term goals can be established. (B) Many persons with an eating disorder are resistant to change and lack the motivation to sincerely get involved in treatment. (C) Excessive involvement in food preparation is a dysfunctional coping skill. Building on the client's strengths is more important than exposing the deficits. (D) Persons with an eating disorder have difficulty accepting nurturing and therefore have difficulty forming a therapeutic alliance.

173. **(A)** Nursing process phase: evaluation; client need: health promotion and maintenance; content area: psychiatric nursing

Rationale

(A) Fitting into family and society and perception of self are issues that the person with an eating disorder struggles with because they value other people's opinions more than their own. (B) Laxative abuse leads to metabolic complications and should be addressed during the early intervention period. The person needs to be made aware of the self-destructive behavior. (C) If the person continues to feel powerless and helpless, the interventions were unsuccessful and goals need to be modified. (D) Continually evaluating goals encourages the nurse to adequately measure the client's success.

174. **(A)** Nursing process phase: implementation; client need: psychosocial integrity; content area: psychiatric nursing

Rationale

(A) This response verbalizes the perceived and allows the client to express feelings. (B) Telling the client what to do implies that the nurse knows best and may nurture dependent behavior. (C) This indicates that the nurse is devaluing the client's feelings. (D) The nurse is giving advice and negating the client's feelings.

175. **(B)** Nursing process phase: planning; client need: safe, effective care environment; content area: psychiatric nursing

Rationale

(A) Some persons may have a relationship between food and spiritual needs. This is not identified as an outcome. (B) Achieving and maintaining weight within normal parameters for size and age is an identified expected outcome. (C) Psychological testing is not determined as an essential outcome. (D) Gaining insight into family dynamics is accomplished over a long period of time.

176. **(B)** Nursing process phase: analysis; client need: psychosocial integrity; content area: psychiatric nursing

Rationale

(A) A hallmark is tolerance. Tolerance is the need for increased amounts of a substance to get the desired effect. (B) Withdrawal is the physiological and cognitive behavioral changes that take place after a person disengages in heavy use of the substance. (C) Irritability is a psychological symptom. It is not a hallmark of the maladaptive behavior. (D) A blackout is a physical symptom.

177. **(A)** Nursing process phase: planning; client need: psychosocial integrity; content area: psychiatric nursing

Rationale

(A) In planning to assist the dying client to have an optimum quality of life during her remaining time, the nurse should provide the client with opportunities to have some control over her environment. This would decrease feelings of helplessness and dependence, which could contribute to the development of depression. (B) The client should be provided with information about available treatments, but the decision should be the client's. (C) The client should be encouraged to make decisions about treatment. (D) The client should be encouraged to express her thoughts and feelings. The nurse should not direct the expression to particular topics but be open to listening if they come up.

178. **(B)** Nursing process phase: assessment; client need: psychosocial integrity; content area: psychiatric nursing

Rationale

(A) The person appears to function effectively while drinking, but has a loss of short-term memory. (B) Delirium tremens, or alcohol withdrawal delirium, is the most serious form of the withdrawal syndrome. (C) Involvement of the autonomic nervous system causes the blood pressure and pulse to increase. (D) Tissue adaptation is not a withdrawal syndrome.

179. **(A)** Nursing process phase: assessment; client need: safe, effective care environment; content area: psychiatric nursing

Rationale

(A) Persons who are chronic abusers of cocaine are psychologically dependent. (B) Cocaine is not determined to cause physical dependence. (C) The "postcoke" blues is known as the cocaine crash that occurs after a brief postuse euphoria. (D) The client states that she is depressed. There is no evidence of aggression.

180. **(B)** Nursing process phase: analysis; client need: physiological integrity; content area: psychiatric nursing

Rationale

(A) Research has shown that there is a hereditary factor involved in the development of substance abuse. (B) Amnestic syndrome is organic brain changes related to the chronic use of alcohol. (C) There is a high incidence of alcohol use in many ethnic groups. (D) Certain personality traits may play a role in the development and maintenance of substance abuse.

181. **(A)** Nursing process phase: implementation; client need: physiological integrity; content area: psychiatric nursing

Rationale

(A) Vitamin B increases metabolic functions. It is essential for the metabolism of carbohydrates and fats. (B) Vitamin K is necessary for clotting blood. (C) Vitamin A is necessary for visual adaptation. (D) Ascorbic acid is used for persons suffering from scurvy.

182. **(D)** Nursing process phase: implementation; client need: psychosocial integrity; content area: psychiatric nursing

Rationale

(A) Professionals often get frustrated and angry at the chemically dependent person but must be nonjudgmental and objective. (B) It is important for the nurse to be aware of feelings and allow the client to work through the dependency behavior. (C) The nurse working with chemically dependent persons see many failures. The nurse should accept the client and develop an attitude of hope. (D) Persons who self-diagnose are usually motivated to change. Self-diagnosis forms the cornerstone of treatment.

183. **(B)** Nursing process phase: planning; client need: safe, effective care environment; content area: psychiatric nursing

Rationale

(A) Simplying the client's environment is accomplished after the client's immediate life-threatening needs are under control. (B) Benzodiazepines are administered to prevent the more severe forms of withdrawal. Vitamin B replaces the thiamine deficiency, and multivitamins replace the vitamins lost because of an inadequate diet. (C) Residential treatment is recommended after the life-threatening needs are under control. (D) A full psychosocial assessment is deferred until the client is stabilized medically.

184. **(B)** Nursing process phase: analysis; client need: health promotion and maintenance; content area: psychiatric nursing

Rationale
(A) Alcoholics Anonymous is a program of recovery for alcoholics as an outpatient group. (B) The client needs to accept ownership of his problem and motivation to change behaviors. (C) Involvement of the family is an important contribution, but maintaining abstinence depends on the person affected. (D) Medications are part of a comprehensive treatment program. The person must be committed to the program.

185. **(B)** Nursing process phase: assessment; client need: physiological integrity; content area: psychiatric nursing

Rationale
(A) The person experiences pain, tenderness, and edema in the skeletal muscles. (B) The symptoms describe withdrawal delirium tremens. (C) Wernicke-Korsakoff syndrome is an organic disorder marked by dementia. (D) Gastritis is inflammation of the stomach. There is no indication that it is part of his symptoms.

186. **(D)** Nursing process phase: evaluation; client need: health promotion and maintenance; content area: psychiatric nursing

Rationale
(A) Methadone alleviates the addict's craving for narcotics. (B) This is a rationale for administering methadone. It is not an outcome of treatment. (C) Methadone is prescribed and legally controlled, but this is not an expected outcome. (D) An expected outcome of methadone maintenance is to improve the psychological well-being and family and social functioning of the addict.

187. **(C)** Nursing process phase: implementation; client need: safe, effective care environment; content area: psychiatric nursing

Rationale
(A) By participating in this activity, the nurse reinforces the reality of the hallucination. The client needs to be reassured that insects are not in his room. (B) This response presents reality but does not address visual hallucinations. (C) This reinforces reality and may help decrease the client's anxiety. (D) This response presents a harsh reality and provokes the need for defensive behavior.

188. **(A)** Nursing process phase: assessment; client need: physiological integrity; content area: psychiatric nursing

Rationale
(A) The symptoms described are those associated with Korsakoff's psychosis, which is caused by a deficiency in thiamine. (B) Vascular dementia is characterized by sudden cognitive and functional losses. (C) Symptoms of Wernicke's encephalopathy are paralysis of ocular muscles, diplopia, somnolence, and stupor. (D) The symptoms presented do not reflect esophageal varices.

189. **(B)** Nursing process phase: implementation; client need: health promotion and maintenance; content area: psychiatric nursing

Rationale
(A) This statement is nontherapeutic and is not supportive of the client's desires. (B) AA groups share their experiences and strengths. The sponsorship program avails itself as an informal network of support. (C) This statement is pushing for answers and may place the client on the defensive. (D) There is no fee for attending AA meetings. However, if needed, members can receive lifelong support.

190. **(C)** Nursing process phase: analysis; client need: psychosocial integrity; content area: psychiatric nursing

Rationale
(A) Legal problems may be an issue, but they are not a primary goal. (B) A person does not directly benefit from such a discussion. Moral and value topics cause arguments and disagreements. (C) Residential treatment programs help the client with self-esteem, responsibility for drug abuse, and working toward recovery. (D) Many family members disengage themselves from the addicted person. The primary goal is to work closely with the client in the therapeutic community center.

191. **(C)** Nursing process phase: analysis; client need: physiological integrity; content area: psychiatric nursing

Rationale
(A) Benztropine is used for all forms of parkinsonism. (B) Methohexital is a short-acting anesthetic. (C) Nalorphine is a narcotic antagonist used for opioid intoxication. (D) Chlordiazepoxide is used for the temporary relief of anxiety.

192. **(B)** Nursing process phase: planning; client need: psychosocial integrity; content area: psychiatric nursing

Rationale
(A) The client is experiencing difficulty coping with a severe crisis after coping effectively previously. Intensive psychotherapy is not indicated. (B) Crisis intervention is the most appropriate treatment approach. The client's coping mechanisms are overwhelmed by the stressor, and she needs assistance to identify resources and work through the problem-solving process. (C) Relaxation therapy may be used in conjunction with crisis intervention to assist her in coping with anxiety. (D) ECT is used to treat major depression when psychopharmacological treatment is ineffective. It is not indicated in this situation.

193. **(C)** Nursing process phase: implementation; client need: psychosocial integrity; content area: psychiatric nursing

Rationale
(A) Isolating the child would only increase his withdrawal. (B) The autistic child has minimal verbal skills and could not be expected to be able to explain his angry thoughts or feelings. (C) The nurse must intervene to protect the child physically while assuming a nonpunitive approach. The autistic child cannot be expected to limit his own behavior. (D) Getting parental input could be helpful from a preventative standpoint but is not an appropriate intervention at the time when the behavior is occurring.

194. **(A)** Nursing process phase: assessment; client need: psychosocial integrity; content area: psychiatric nursing

Rationale
(A) The disease is characterized by a slow and insidious onset with progressive loss of cognitive abilities. (B) Multi-infarct dementia has an abrupt onset and progresses in steps. (C) Alzheimer's disease is not self-limiting. It is slow and progressive. (D) Alzheimer's disease is a chronic progressive disorder that ravages the mind.

195. **(B)** Nursing process phase: implementation; client need: safe, effective care environment; content area: psychiatric nursing

Rationale
(A) Confrontation may be interpreted as a threat and may increase the agitated state. (B) Setting limits provides a sense of security and stability. (C) Administer PRN medications after other nursing interventions have failed. Extreme caution should be used when giving medication because of impaired circulation. (D) Isolating the client takes away some of her dignity and self-esteem.

196. **(C)** Nursing process phase: analysis; client need: safe, effective care environment; content area: psychiatric nursing

Rationale
(A) Memory difficulty with functional attributes is the forgetful phase or first stage. (B) Objectively dysfunctional with the inability to adapt to unfamiliar environments is the confusional phase or second stage. (C) The characteristics of the dementia phase, or stage three, are those addressed in this answer. (D) These characteristics are evident during the latest stages of the disease.

197. **(D)** Nursing process phase: planning; client need: safe, effective care environment; content area: psychiatric nursing

Rationale
(A) Quality-of-life issues are particularly important during the late stages of Alzheimer's disease. (B) A living will describes a client's wishes and should be initiated early in the disease process. (C) For many clients, spiritual needs are important and can be provided. (D) There are situations when suicide is accepted. However, medically assisted suicides are not legal in most states and are not supported by the ANA.

198. **(A)** Nursing process phase: assessment; client need: psychosocial integrity; content area: psychiatric nursing

Rationale
(A) The person expresses shame about the lack of accomplishments and unfulfillment. There may be doubt about the purpose or sense of direction in life. (B) There is no evidence of delusional thinking. (C) There is no indication that the person exhibits self-approval. (D) There are no statements from the client concerning identity confusion.

199. **(A)** Nursing process phase: implementation; client need: safe, effective care environment; content area: psychiatric nursing

Rationale
(A) Maintaining a safe environment for all clients is a primary priority. (B) Palliative treatment alleviates the signs and symptoms without curing. This intervention is necessary but not during the initial intervention. (C) Spirituality may be an integral part of the day program, but is not the primary issue. (D) Psychotherapy is not the initial treatment of choice.

200. **(A)** Nursing process phase: analysis; client need: psychosocial integrity; content area: psychiatric nursing

Rationale
(A) Initially the person has difficulty remembering recent events. (B) Apraxia is the inability to carry out simple activities. This occurs during the second phase of the disease. (C) Agraphia is the inability to read or write and is part of the late stages of the disease. (D) Agnosia is the loss of sensory ability to recognize objects. This deficit is evident during phase three.

201. **(C)** Nursing process phase: implementation; client need: safe, effective care environment; content area: psychiatric nursing

Rationale
(A) Restricting the number of cigarettes will not help eliminate the hazard of burns or possible fire. (B) Restricting privileges may be implemented. However, this intervention does not consider safety measures. (C) Monitoring smoking times will help assure safety. (D) The objective in dealing with a confused person is to prevent a hazardous situation. A smoker's anonymous group will not accomplish the goal.

202. **(A)** Nursing process phase: planning; client need: psychosocial integrity; content area: psychiatric nursing

Rationale
(A) Providing a support system for the client will establish a caring environment and assist with psychosocial needs. (B) Many clients have difficulty with a daily schedule. A member of the support team may provide assistance. (C) Creating socializing sessions may be included as part of the support system activity. (D) Assisting the client with mobility may not alleviate fear and depression.

203. **(B)** Nursing process phase: assessment; client need: psychosocial integrity; content area: psychiatric nursing

Rationale
(A) Requirement for 24-hour supervision is a criterion—not a 4-hour period. (B) Vulnerability in the community is grounds for considering a person psychiatrically homebound. (C) Lack of family support may be grounds for resident care in a guest home rather than homebound status. (D) Mild anxiety is not a consideration for homebound care.

204. **(A)** Nursing process phase: implementation; client need: psychosocial integrity; content area: psychiatric nursing

Rationale
(A) Caregivers must have an understanding of the norms of other cultures in order to accept the client and provide professional care. (B) Persons in the early stages of cognitive disorders benefit from reminiscence groups, if they are not disruptive and understand the language. (C) Resocialization groups benefit those persons with cognitive disorders and those who are cooperative because little cognitive processing is required. (D) Discussing feelings and culture would be successful in the presence of an interpreter and would not be beneficial to all of the residents.

205. **(B)** Nursing process phase: implementation; client need: safe, effective care environment; content area: psychiatric nursing

Rationale
(A) Dysphonia is a speech disorder caused by a dysfunction of the vocal cords. (B) Tardive dyskinesia is involuntary movement of the tongue, stiff neck, and difficulty in swallowing. (C) Akathisia is exhibited by rocking from foot to foot, pacing, and the inability to sit still. (D) Echolalia is the parrotlike repetition of overheard words.

206. (C) Nursing process phase: evaluation; client need: psychosocial integrity; content area: psychiatric nursing

Rationale
(A) Primary gain is the relief from emotional conflict. (B) Physiological changes occur with aging and should not be overlooked. (C) Secondary gain may be derived from personal attention of others that fulfills certain psychological needs. (D) Older persons are at risk for nutritional deficits and need to have their meals monitored to ensure an adequate intake of food.

207. (A) Nursing process phase: assessment; client need: safe, effective care environment; content area: psychiatric nursing

Rationale
(A) Persons in crisis perceive the event as a personal threat to self, and it usually involves a loss or sense of loss. (B) Levels of anxiety may increase to the point of acute personality disorganization unless intervention is swift and goal-directed. (C) One characteristic of a crisis state is cognitive rigidity. (D) Resolution of the perceived threat is not a characteristic. Resolution is the result of working through the crisis state.

208. (C) Nursing process phase: implementation; client need: safe, effective care environment; content area: psychiatric nursing

Rationale
(A) A nursing intervention must assess decompensation and help restore functioning prior to any referral. (B) Crisis therapy is intense and short-term. Lengthy psychotherapy is not appropriate for crisis intervention. (C) Focus should be on the immediate problem and on returning the client to the precrisis state of functioning. (D) An antianxiety medication may be prescribed after crisis therapy if it is determined that the client is unable to find relief from anxiety.

209. (D) Nursing process phase: assessment; client need: health promotion and maintenance; content area: psychiatric nursing

Rationale
(A) A dispositional crisis is an acute response to an external situational stressor. (B) Maturational crises are identifiable in relation to transitional stages of human development. (C) An adventitious crisis is caused by a natural disaster and affects many people at the same time. (D) A situational crisis represents an external event perceived as harmful.

210. (A) Nursing process phase: assessment; client need: safe, effective care environment; content area: psychiatric nursing

Rationale
(A) The client denies the reality of the situation and rejects the available support resources. (B) Displacement is a shift of emotions from one person or object to another. There is no evidence of displacement. (C) Projection attributes one's

own thoughts or impulses that are unacceptable to oneself to another. (D) Rationalization offers logical reasons to justify unacceptable feelings.

211. (B) Nursing process phase: assessment; client need: safe, effective care environment; content area: psychiatric nursing

Rationale
(A) General reorganization takes place when the person is able to integrate new patterns of behavior and coping into personality and family. (B) Disorganization occurs when the person ceases to function effectively. The person is preoccupied with the event and flooded with high levels of anxiety. (C) The client is past the denial stage. She is exhibiting maladaptive behavior. (D) Local reorganization is the ability to resume normal activities of daily living.

212. (C) Nursing process phase: planning; client need: safe, effective care environment; content area: psychiatric nursing

Rationale
(A) Focusing on emotional deficits undermines the crisis intervention process. (B) Exploring underlying personality dyamics is useful only if it relates to the crisis problem. (C) Enquiring about previous coping strategies will provide insight as to the relationship to the current crisis situation. (D) The client may have a financial problem, but providing financial assistance is not one of the interventions.

213. (A) Nursing process phase: assessment; client need: psychosocial integrity; content area: psychiatric nursing

Rationale
(A) An essential component of the initial interview is to assess the lethality potential. (B) Determining the adequacy of the client's support system is important. However, it is not the first priority. (C) An important intervention in a crisis situation is to help the client return to a precrisis level of functioning. The primary concern is the potential for suicide. (D) During the initial interaction, a complete enquiry into the nature of the crisis is essential. This should include substance abuse.

214. (A) Nursing process phase: planning; client need: psychosocial integrity; content area: psychiatric nursing

Rationale
(A) The primary goal in crisis intervention is to determine the precipitating event and return the client to a precrisis level of functioning. (B) Crisis intervention is a form of preventive psychiatry. The therapy is short-term and goal-directed. Psychotherapy is long-term. (C) In a crisis situation, time is limited. Evaluating the effects of early childhood development should be left for any follow-up therapy. (D) Providing a list of resources may establish a link between crisis therapy and future need.

215. (C) Nursing process phase: analysis; client need: safe, effective care environment; content area: psychiatric nursing

Rationale
(A) Education is not used during crisis intervention. Positive changes are accomplished through tense, goal-directed, short-term therapy. (B) Crisis therapy helps the client develop adaptive coping strategies. Maladaptive coping provides a roadblock to resolving the crisis. (C) Through adaptive changes, a crisis is

resolved and psychological growth is experienced. (D) It is important for the person to describe rather than analyze a plan of action for dealing with stressors that precipitated the crisis.

216. **(A)** Nursing process phase: analysis; client need: psychosocial integrity; content area: psychiatric nursing

Rationale

(A) Anxiety increases during a crisis state, causing a decrease in the perceptual field. (B) Typically, clients in crisis are scared, confused, and anxious. (C) The client in crisis feels helpless and vulnerable. (D) A physical disorder cannot be ruled out and must be included in the triage assessment. However, because tension is so intolerable, it takes over the emotional rather than the physical aspect of the client.

217. **(B)** Nursing process phase: assessment; client need: psychosocial integrity; content area: psychiatric nursing

Rationale

(A) The client is still in the phase of shock and denial. (B) The client understands the importance of a support group, and she is willing to accept the help. (C) This statement indicates that the client is angry, and she is depending solely on self. (D) This statement indicates pain, abandonment, and anger.

218. **(A)** Nursing process phase: planning; client need: safe, effective care environment; content area: psychiatric nursing

Rationale

(A) Each person has strengths as well as weaknesses. Building on the strengths reinforces the positive elements. (B) There is a possibility that the client may become psychotic. However, in order to assist the client to return to a precrisis level of functioning, the nurse must work with the healthy aspects of the client. (C) The client may be incompetent to care for self. The health-care team must fill the void. (D) An external support system, including a supportive family that will help prevent further chaos and decrease the risk of another crisis situation, is a necessary strategy.

219. **(A)** Nursing process phase: planning; client need: safe, effective care environment; content area: psychiatric nursing

Rationale

(A) The suicidal client views life as hopeless. Discussing suicidal feelings and conveying a message to the client that he is a worthwhile person will provide a sense of security and optimism. (B) After crisis intervention is complete, long-term therapy may be initiated to help the client learn improved interpersonal skills and a sense of belonging. (C) New and functional coping skills should be an outcome of crisis intervention. (D) If the client verbalizes feelings of despair, then crisis intervention has been less than successful.

220. **(B)** Nursing process phase: implementation; client need: safe, effective care environment; content area: psychiatric nursing

Rationale

(A) Restitution completes the grief work. It is not part of the crisis prevention strategy. (B) Anticipatory guidance is an educational process that helps persons and families distinguish between normal and unusual experiences. It helps persons foresee future events that may become problematic. (C) Referral to other agencies may take place after crisis intervention therapy.

(D) The generic approach is designed to reach large numbers of high-risk persons who have experienced loss and disruption.

221. **(C)** Nursing process phase: assessment; client need: psychosocial integrity; content area: psychiatric nursing

Rationale

(A) The client usually has a poor self-concept. (B & D) This is not a characteristic of adolescent adjustment reaction. (C) These are characteristics of clients who are experiencing adolescent adjustment reactions.

222. **(C)** Nursing process phase: assessment; client need: physiological integrity; content area: psychiatric nursing

Rationale

(A, B, & D) Characteristics of feces, hemoglobin level, and color of nailbeds are not markedly affected by drug use. (C) Consciousness level is an important nursing assessment of a client suspected of substance abuse, because many drugs affect the consciousness level. Both the client's behavior and verbalizations and the nurse's objective and subjective assessment would yield these data.

223. **(A)** Nursing process phase: planning; client need: safe, effective care environment; content area: psychiatric nursing

Rationale

(A) Assessing the cause of the client's anxiety is an important part of the nursing plan. Both the client and the nurse need to work together to establish a plan. (B) Major tranquilizers would only mask the anxiety. (C) Increased fluid intake is not related to completing tasks. (D) Decreasing family contact is not a major factor in completing tasks.

224. **(B)** Nursing process phase: assessment; client need: psychosocial integrity; content area: psychiatric nursing

Rationale

(A) Delaying the grieving process would not be helpful. (B) Planning funeral arrangements is an important part of the grieving process for the parents. This task helps validate the reality of the infant's death. (C) This is not correct because the infant's death could not have been prevented. (D) Minimizing discussion would not be helpful. Usually, talking about the loss facilitates the grief process.

225. **(C)** Nursing process phase: planning; client need: health promotion and maintenance; content area: psychiatric nursing

Rationale

(A) Moral reasoning is highly individualistic and is part of the universal principles of justice and ethical reasoning. It does not benefit the client. (B) Sociopolitical topics are highly explosive and serve no purpose. (C) Sociocultural data are relevant for successful discharge planning because they may help the nurse understand the client's living arrangement, support system, and economic status. (D) The evaluative process helps determine successes and/or failures of the discharge plan after implementation of the interventions.

226. **(B)** Nursing process phase: planning; client need: psychosocial integrity; content area: psychiatric nursing

Rationale

(A) The parents should focus on the welfare of the total family and not just the affected child. (B) A major nursing goal is to modify the child's environment to promote independence and impulse control. The child's strengths should be accentuated because there are varying levels of disability due to retardation. (C) The sooner diagnostic studies are done, the sooner appropriate treatment can begin. (D) Increased peer interaction is important for assisting a retarded child to learn socialization skills.

227. (B) Nursing process phase: analysis; client need: psychosocial integrity; content area: psychiatric nursing

Rationale
(A) Global amnesia is loss of a whole lifetime of experience. This is not a characteristic of the borderline personality disorder. (B) Because borderline personality disorder persons are unable to tolerate their own "bad" image, they project it on others. The anger tends to be directed at those persons who remind them of a nurturing or frustrating parent. (C) One essential feature of the borderline personality disorder is a pervasive pattern of intense, unstable, and chaotic relationships. (D) These persons exhibit intense fluctuation of mood, including depression and hypomanic episodes.

228. (C) Nursing process phase: planning; client need: health promotion and maintenance; content area: psychiatric nursing

Rationale
(A) One characteristic of the histrionic personality disorder is the inappropriate, sexually provocative behavior that is not acceptable. (B) Acceptance of the behaviors will not provide the client with guidelines that promote alternatives. (C) These persons need to be the center of attention. Setting and enforcing limits is essential in promoting adaptive behaviors. (D) Emphasizing passive-aggressive behavior will not help the client meet his or her needs and may show disrespect for others.

229. (D) Nursing process phase: implementation; client need: psychosocial integrity; content area: psychiatric nursing

Rationale
(A) Expression of grandiosity is an inflated self-concept and may be compensation for feelings of diminished self-worth. Nursing intervention is geared toward heightened self-esteem. (B) Do not limit feedback. Feedback that focuses on the behavior may help the client consider modification of his behavior. (C) Do not criticize the haughty, uncaring attitude. Acknowledge and accept the client as a person. (D) One diagnostic criterion for the narcissistic personality disorder is a sense of entitlement. These clients show an arrogant attitude based on feelings of entitlement and envy. Discussion of the behavior may help the client work through feelings of reasonable expectations of especially favorable treatment.

230. (B) Nursing process phase: implementation; client need: psychosocial integrity; content area: psychiatric nursing

Rationale
(A) Confrontation during the ritualistic response increases the client's anxiety level. The client needs time to complete the ritual. It is best to confront after the ritual because the client's anxiety level is lowered by performing the ritual. (B) For persons diagnosed as having obsessive-compulsive disorder, work organizes their lives at the exclusion of pleasure. (C) The client must feel free to express feelings of anger and

resentment directly rather than indirectly. (D) Limiting decision making will reduce autonomy and increase the struggle for power. Provisions for progressive opportunities for effective decision making will help reduce power struggles.

231. (A) Nursing process phase: implementation; client need: health promotion and maintenance; content area: psychiatric nursing

Rationale
(A) Antidepressants cause dry mouth, which can be relieved by frequent sips of water, sucking on sugarless hard candy, or chewing sugarless gum. (B) Alcohol enhances the depressant effects that the antidepressant was prescribed to relieve. (C) Antidepressants affect the central nervous system and may cause dizziness and drowsiness. (D) Advise the client not to adjust his antidepressant and not to consume other medications because it could precipitate a life-threatening situation.

232. (D) Nursing process phase: assessment; client need: safe, effective care environment; content area: psychiatric nursing

Rationale
(A) Methscopolamine (atropine sulfate) is given prior to ECT to decrease secretions. Persons usually complain of dry mouth. (B) Temporary memory loss—not amnesia—is a side effect of ECT. Research indicates that memory deficits do not persist beyond 3 months. (C) Depression is an emotional discomfort, not a physical discomfort. (D) Muscle and joint soreness is a common physical complaint.

233. (B) Nursing process phase: implementation; client need: safe, effective care environment; content area: psychiatric nursing

Rationale
(A) The client is given nothing by mouth (NPO) for 4 to 8 hours prior to treatment. (B) These items should be removed because of breakage and possible misplacement. (C) Partial plates should be left in the mouth to provide even pressure on the teeth and jaw during the tonic phase of seizures. (D) Loose-fitting, comfortable clothing is recommended.

234. (C) Nursing process phase: evaluation; client need: psychosocial integrity; content area: psychiatric nursing

Rationale
(A) Persons have control or lack of control over self, but not of others. (B) Persons who suffer from mood disorders are very often stigmatized by others because of the emotional disability. (C) An expected outcome of therapy during hospitalization is for the client to establish realistic plans for the future. (D) Vegetative symptoms are changes in physiological functioning that may be predominant during the early phases of the depressed state.

235. (B) Nursing process phase: implementation; client need: health promotion and maintenance; content area: psychiatric nursing

Rationale
(A) Integrity involves values and honesty. Providing information about integrity is individualistic and serves no purpose. (B) Clients need information about the importance of compliance with medications even when feeling well or if feeling that the medication is not working. (C) Referral or follow-up care will provide a support system and continuity of care and

should not be discouraged. Independence should be encouraged. (D) The goal of nursing is to prevent undue dependence. Encouragement of government resources may promote learned helplessness.

236. (A) Nursing process phase: planning; client need: safe, effective care environment; content area: psychiatric nursing

Rationale

(A) Persons suffering from mania experience a disturbance in suicidal behavior. (B) A goal for this client should be to eat enough to maintain energy needs, not to gain weight. (C) Manic clients exhibit hyperactivity and irritability. They are unable to engage in strict participation. (D) Clients have the rights and may refuse medications.

237. (B) Nursing process phase: implementation; client need: psychosocial integrity; content area: psychiatric nursing

Rationale

(A) There is no evidence of psychotic symptoms with a person suffering from a dysthymic disorder. (B) Persons with mood disorders frequently experience disruptions in relationships. A supportive social network will enhance social skills, promote self-esteem, and facilitate positive relationships. (C) Persons in a depressed mood and who have possibly lost interest in life should take one day at a time. Planning for the future requires decision making and may be anxiety provoking. (D) Senescence is a chronological period and does not apply to a 39-year-old person.

238. (A) Nursing process phase: analysis; client need: psychosocial integrity; content area: psychiatric nursing

Rationale

(A) The substance abuser lacks control over the psychoactive substance and the family attempts to control the use of the agent. (B) Addiction in women is hidden because it carries a greater stigma than for men. (C) The disorder is self-inflicted and develops without the consent of its victims. (D) Substance abuse disorder directly affects the person and can have equally devastating effects on family members.

239. (B) Nursing process phase: implementation; client need: safe, effective care environment; content area: psychiatric nursing

Rationale

(A) Promoting independent functioning is a desirable caregiving goal for all clients. (B) Stability in the environment reduces anxiety and provides a sense of security that may reduce confusion. (C) Elimination of daytime naps may help a normal nighttime sleep pattern. (D) Making an issue of the client's confusion and confabulation is not supportive and is rarely useful.

240. (A) Nursing process phase: planning; client need: safe, effective care environment; content area: psychiatric nursing

Rationale

(A) Quality-of-life issues are particularly important during the late stages of Alzheimer's disease. (B) A living will describes a client's wishes and should be initiated early in the disease process when the client is still aware of decision making. (C) Reality orientation serves no purpose because of global memory loss. (D) There are situations when suicide is accepted. However, medically assisted suicide is not legal in most states.

241. (B) Nursing process phase: analysis; client need: safe, effective care environment; content area: psychiatric nursing

Rationale

(A) Although the name of the physician is important, it is of low priority on admission to the emergency room. (B) Assessment of the client's vital signs is the highest priority intervention because the status must be determined. (C) History of drug allergies is an important part of the client's history, but low priority at the time of admission. (D) Because of the reported suicide attempt, the client is obviously at high risk for suicide and assessing suicide risk is of lower priority than assessing the current status by taking the vital signs.

242. (A) Nursing process phase: assessment; client need: physiological integrity; content area: psychiatric nursing

Rationale

(A) In high doses, this drug becomes arrhythmogenic. (B) Nausea and vomiting are not common side effects nor toxic effects of tricyclics. (C) Headache is not an effect in the presence of sedation. (D) Although this drug has a central nervous system-depressing effect, it has no effect on the skeletal muscle.

243. (D) Nursing process phase: analysis; client need: physiological integrity; content area: psychiatric nursing

Rationale

(A) The client's respirations are more likely to be depressed before the drug has peaked. (B) Clients admitted to the intensive care unit after a suicide attempt are always on close observation. (C) Monitoring blood plasma levels of a drug is not a criterion for admission to an intensive care unit. (D) Toxic cardiac effects may not appear for 3 days after the overdose.

244. (C) Nursing process phase: assessment; client need: health promotion and maintenance; content area: psychiatric nursing

Rationale

(A) The onset of personality disorders is before age 30. (B) Persons with personality disorders are usually in a state of denial regarding their maladaptive patterns of behavior. (C) Personality and character traits are stable and predictable following early adolescence but become exaggerated to the point that they cause significant functional impairment and subjective distress when a personality disorder emerges. (D) Persons with personality disorders are ego-syntonic and feel no anxiety or remorse for their maladaptive behavior. They do not recognize their own behavior as maladaptive.

245. (D) Nursing process phase: assessment; client need: health promotion and maintenance; content area: psychiatric nursing

Rationale

(A) Rapid mood shifts are common in person with borderline personality disorders but they cannot tolerate being alone for fear of abandonment. (B) Persons with borderline personality disorders demonstrate intrusiveness due to their need for attention and will openly discuss personal problems although their perception of the nature of the problem may be very different from how others may view it. (C) Initially, most borderline personality-disordered persons are compliant but demonstrate evidence of alteration of self-image, which fluctuates with mood swings. (D) Persons with borderline personality disorders show marked affective lability and verbalize feelings of worthlessness.

246. (C) Nursing process phase: analysis; client need: psychosocial integrity; content area: psychiatric nursing

Rationale
(A) Denial is the ego's way of defending itself against attack when threatened by a confrontation too painful to face. The client initiated the comment and has not been confronted. (B) The client is not attempting to justify behavior. (C) Clients with this disorder polarize and place people in all-good and all-bad categories. This is called splitting. (D) Projection is when clients attribute their own thoughts or feelings to another person. In this situation, the client has clearly attributed her own thoughts to self.

247. (C) Nursing process phase: implementation; client need: psychosocial integrity; content area: psychiatric nursing

Rationale
(A) The nurse therapist is placing limits but not validating what the client is experiencing. (B) This statement is maladaptively reinforcing the undesirable behavior and offering punitive consequences. In fact, the client may be manipulating the therapist to allow her to leave therapy and avoid appropriate confrontation. A power struggle could ensue. (C) This response places necessary limits without threatening the client but redirects the flow of conversation to include other clients. It also validates what the client may be experiencing. (D) The nurse therapist is demonstrating feelings of countertransference and is, at this point, nontherapeutic.

248. (A) Nursing process phase: implementation; client need: physiological integrity; content area: psychiatric nursing

Rationale
(A) Carbamazepine inhibits nerve impulses by limiting influx of sodium ions across the cell membrane in the motor cortex, thereby improving overall functioning. (B & D) Drugs used to control anger or diminish anxiety are generally of the anxiolytic class or in some way depress the central nervous system. Carbamazepine is not of this class. (C) Drugs that elevate or stabilize the mood are either some form of lithium or an antidepressant. Carbamazepine is classed as an anticonvulsant.

249. (D) Nursing process phase: planning; client need: health promotion and maintenance; content area: psychiatric nursing

Rationale
(A) Most psychoanalytical theorists recommend a minimum of 7 years of therapy to reconstruct the personality. (B) Clients should never adjust their own medications after discharge without the physician's direction to do so. (C) Although a client should develop insight into maladaptive behaviors in order to recognize which should be changed, just having insight will not effectively assist the client to live a more adaptive life. (D) Demonstrating more-adaptive coping behaviors after developing insight will have a longer-lasting positive effect on the client.

250. (D) Nursing process phase: analysis; client need: safe, effective care environment; content area: psychiatric nursing

Rationale
(A) A client experiencing PCP-induced toxicity or psychosis is likely to become violent at another person's attempt to calm him. (B) The physician will most likely need an assessment of the client before ordering medication. (C) Although calling a family member to be with the client may have a calming effect, the client may not respond favorably to any degree of questioning at this time. (D) This is the correct choice because clients under the influence of PCP are known to strike out in response to unfamiliar stimuli.

251. (A) Nursing process phase: assessment; client need: safe, effective care environment; content area: psychiatric nursing

Rationale
(A) The client is experiencing visual and tactile hallucinations: He actually sees snakes and feels them on his skin. (B) The client's comments are not a fixed, false belief. He is perceiving sensory stimulation, but there are no snakes in the room. (C) He may be morbidly afraid of snakes, but his statements indicate that he is actually seeing and feeling snakes on his skin. (D) His comments do not indicate that he is unaware of his whereabouts.

252. (B) Nursing process phase: implementation; client need: psychosocial integrity; content area: psychiatric nursing

Rationale
(A) The nurse has failed to address the real issue here and is delaying a stat order unnecessarily. (B) The nurse is correctly addressing the client's real feelings and is intervening to promote comfort. (C) The nurse is ignoring the client's concerns and fears. (D) Although the client has the right to refuse medication, he is in protective custody and the nurse has a responsibility to give the stat medication as ordered.

253. (C) Nursing process phase: implementation; client need: psychosocial integrity; content area: psychiatric nursing

Rationale
(A) The nurse is not taking primary responsibility for assessing the client for potential for continued violence. (B) There is no indication that the family has been notified, nor has the nurse completed an assessment to determine readiness for restraint release. (C) This is therapeutic because the nurse is encouraging the client to review the events immediately prior to the violent episode. This in turn could allow the client to connect cause and effect related to his violence. (D) Release from restraint is not done simply at the client's request. Also, no therapeutic alliance has been formed.

254. (C) Nursing process phase: implementation; client need: psychosocial integrity; content area: psychiatric nursing

Rationale
(A) This comment fails to address the client's emotional distress. (B) This statement tells the client that he shouldn't feel the way he does and makes light of the gravity of the situation. (C) This response validates the client's perception of the situation and his emotional response to it. Also, asking the client

to think about his options promotes his problem-solving ability. (D) The nurse is ignoring the client's emotional need and overlooking the opportunity to assist the client with insight and options.

255. **(D)** Nursing process phase: analysis; client need: safe, effective care environment; content area: psychiatric nursing

Rationale

(A) The CT is a series of computer-constructed x-rays that stacks "slices" of the brain, giving a three-dimensional view of brain structure. (B) The MRI demonstrates pictorially radio waves emitted by the brain, induced by a magnetic field. Primarily, MRI is used to view brain structure although newer MRI techniques show brain activity. (C) The BEAM uses computed tomography techniques to display electroencephalographic readings. It shows structure and some brain activity, but the display of the graphic readings obscures the structures underlying the cerebrum. (D) The PET uses tomography and injection of a radioactive substance, which is taken up by certain areas of the brain. The injected substances are taken up in different amounts, depending on the level of activity in the brain and the type of tissue being viewed.

256. **(C)** Nursing process phase: analysis; client need: safe, effective care environment; content area: psychiatric nursing

Rationale

(A) Hospitalized clients maintain all civil rights, including making a will. (B) Clients admitted to psychiatric hospitals have the right to be employed if jobs exist that they can effectively manage while treatment continues. Hospitals are not required to supply job opportunities. (C) Clients maintain the right to privacy and communication, which includes the right to write letters and expect them to mailed as requested. Staff members who open a client's mail or deliberately fail to mail it as requested are violating both the client's rights and federal law concerning the United States Postal Service. (D) Hospitals are not responsible for valuables that clients choose to keep in their possession or inadvertently fail to place in the hospital safe. The nurse's action is legal and appropriate.

257. **(A)** Nursing process phase: assessment; client need: health promotion and maintenance; content area: psychiatric nursing

Rationale

(A) The fact that the client is known to be suicidal justifies commitment because she is a danger to herself. (B) There is no supportive data that the client is homicidal. No verbal threats have been made. (C) There is no supportive data that the client is psychotic or out of touch with reality. (D) Mental incompetence is a legal term, not a medical term, therefore it is not included as a criterion for commitment.

258. **(C)** Nursing process phase: analysis; client need: health promotion and maintenance; content area: psychiatric nursing

Rationale

(A) All clients maintain the right to retain licenses, privileges, or permits that have been established by law, including driver's licenses. (B) Clients have the civil right to refuse treatment and medications in most states, even if voluntarily committed. (C) Although some variations occur from state to state, currently, psychiatric clients basically maintain all of

their civil rights. (D) Because the license to practice nursing is establishing by law, the client does not need to relinquish it because of admission. Some states have impaired nurse programs, which require that the state Board of Nursing be notified when a nurse enters treatment.

259. **(D)** Nursing process phase: assessment; client need: safe, effective care environment; content area: psychiatric nursing

Rationale

(A) This question is asking the client to subjectively evaluate his mood. (B) This question is to determine the client's judgment. (C) This is an orientation question. (D) This question requires that the client recall learned information that is part of his general fund of knowledge.

260. **(C)** Nursing process phase: assessment; client need: physiological integrity; content area: psychiatric nursing

Rationale

(A) A client who has a definite plan is at high risk, but without the means to complete the plan, the risk is lower. (B) Verbalizing suicidal ideation is high risk, but not having a definite plan reduces the risk. (C) This client is at high immediate risk. He has a definite plan and admits to having the means on hand. Immediate attention should be directed to the suitcase. (D) Jumping off the river bridge is a definite plan, but the means are not immediately available because the client is in the hospital and discharge is not imminent.

261. **(A)** Nursing process phase: assessment; client need: safe, effective care environment; content area: psychiatric nursing

Rationale

(A) This is a fixed false belief that is greater than the client's actual ability. (B) The client's statement does not reflect that he is having a sensory experience without external stimuli. (C) The client is reflecting a fixed false belief but it is not paranoid in nature. (D) The client's statement does not reflect that he is having a sensory experience without external stimuli.

262. **(B)** Nursing process phase: analysis; client need: safe, effective care environment; content area: psychiatric nursing

Rationale

(A) Only clinical psychologists are educationally prepared to evaluate the results of the Rorschach. (B) Because there are no direct questions administered to the client, all responses are spontaneous and largely subconscious thematically. (C) Although the Rorschach requires only the cards, paper, and a pencil, that is not a major benefit. (D) Establishing rapport with the client is not a major benefit, but establishing some level of trust is necessary to elicit the client's cooperation and to put him at ease.

263. **(C)** Nursing process phase: assessment; client need: safe, effective care environment; content area: psychiatric nursing

Rationale

(A) Both of these tests are designed to determine intelligence and intellectual functioning ability. (B) The Stanford-Binet is an intelligence test but the Minnesota Multiphasic Personality inventory would be very beneficial in identifying specific traits and attitudes regarding relationships. (C) The Minnesota Multiphasic Personality Inventory would be an effective tool to confirm or differentiate the personality diagnosis and the Rorschach, being a projective test, would identify themes and attitudes that might not be reflected on the Minnesota Multiphasic Personality Inventory. (D) As above, the Rorschach would be beneficial, but the Weschler Adult Intelligence Scale would not.

264. (A) Nursing process phase: assessment; client need: safe, effective care environment; content area: psychiatric nursing

Rationale
(A) The Bender Gestalt is a visual motor examination that is used to screen for organic dysfunction versus a primary psychological problem. (B) The dexamethasone suppression test is used to determine the presence of excessive cortisol levels in the blood often found in endogenous depression. (C) The thematic apperception test is a projective test, not a visual motor test. (D) The family kinetic drawings are also projective, not visual motor.

265. (C) Nursing process phase: analysis; client need: safe, effective care environment; content area: psychiatric nursing

Rationale
(A) Test-taking experience would not invalidate the results of tests; in fact, it could assist the client to complete some of the objective tests because of previous experience taking tests. (B) Diabetes could but would not necessarily invalidate the results of the psychological tests. If his diabetes is not in control, it might impact on his concentration and endurance. (C) The presence of psychosis would definitely invalidate the results because the client's thinking may be bizarre and too much out of touch with reality to follow instructions and stay on task to completion. (D) A client's objectivity would not invalidate the results.

266. (B) Nursing process phase: implementation; client need: safe, effective care environment; content area: psychiatric nursing

Rationale
(A) Casting doubt on the client's beliefs is appropriate after the nurse-client relationship is established and the client has developed some level of trust with the nurse. This client is paranoid and there is no evidence that trust has been developed yet. (B) This is the most therapeutic response because the nurse redirects the client to a reality-based subject. Also, making an opportunity to spend time with the client gives the nurse an opportunity to do a more thorough assessment. (C) Confronting the client with the fact that his belief is false will only reinforce his belief that it is true and factual. Also because the client is paranoid, the nurse has probably destroyed the possibility that trust can be built at this time. (D) The nurse is missing the opportunity to be therapeutic with this client. Passing the client on to the physician indicates that she is not able to be therapeutic with the client.

267. (C) Nursing process phase: implementation; client need: safe, effective care environment; content area: psychiatric nursing

Rationale
(A) It is neither appropriate nor therapeutic to threaten the client with an injection in order to get him to take it. Further,

he is paranoid and he will suspect the nurse even more. (B) It is never appropriate to hide medication in a client's food. It is especially nontherapeutic with the paranoid client. (C) This is the most therapeutic response because there is no power struggle, no reinforcement of the delusional material, plus, the client, even though paranoid, has the right to refuse medication. (D) Simply charting that the client refused the medication is not enough. He needs the medication. If the nurse cannot therapeutically intervene with the client, she should consult other members of the treatment staff for assistance or further instructions.

268. (D) Nursing process phase: assessment; client need: physiological integrity; content area: psychiatric nursing

Rationale
(A) Tardive dyskinesia occurs when prolonged blockade of dopamine has occurred, which is not the case with this client. Also, the cardinal symptoms of tongue protrusion, lip smacking, chewing, and choreiform movements are absent. (B) The client is not exhibiting signs of panic level anxiety. (C) The signs and symptoms of akathisia include restlessness and inner agitation. The client has not complained of these subjective symptoms. (D) The client is exhibiting classic signs of acute dystonia: sudden spasms of the neck and the tongue pulling to one side.

269. (D) Nursing process phase: implementation; client need: safe, effective care environment; content area: psychiatric nursing

Rationale
(A) Ativan will probably act to give the client some relief by relaxing the muscles by depressing the central nervous system, but it is not the drug of choice in this situation. Also the oral route of administration is slower to act and will not give the client quick relief. (B) Valium will act as Ativan, but the oral route will not give the client relief fast enough. (C) Haldol is the drug that is causing the side effects. To give more would only increase the intensity of his symptoms. (D) Cogentin parenterally is the drug of choice for this client. It is the first-line choice of drugs for extrapyramidal symptoms associated with the use of neuroleptics.

270. (A) Nursing process phase: evaluation; client need: psychosocial integrity; content area: psychiatric nursing

Rationale
(A) This statement reflects that the client has gained knowledge and insight into the nature of his illness and the need for medication compliance. (B) Clients should never adjust their medication without the instruction of the physician to do so. (C) This statement reflects no insight into his illness or desire for compliance with medications. (D) This statement shows no insight into the nature or chronicity of his illness.

271. (C) Nursing process phase: analysis; client need: safe, effective care environment; content area: psychiatric nursing

Rationale
(A) Although the client may be experiencing some level of anxiety, it is not the highest priority nursing diagnosis. (B) From the client's statement, there is no indication that there is a growth and development alteration. (C) The client's weight-to-height ratio indicates more than 25 percent weight loss, which validates the nursing diagnosis of altered nutrition, less than body requirements. (D) The client probably

does have a self-esteem disturbance, but there are no data to support this in the assessment information.

272. **(C)** Nursing process phase: planning; client need: safe, effective care environment; content area: psychiatric nursing

Rationale

(A) Although it will be important for this client to meet her peers on the unit, it is not the highest priority. (B) She will eventually meet with her primary nurse to develop a master treatment plan, but that can only take place after she has been assessed by the multidisciplinary treatment team. (C) The highest priority goal must always be safety and maintenance of the therapeutic environment. (D) The client may or may not desire to speak to her family members at the time of admission but care should be taken to ensure that her parents or legal guardians are kept informed of her status.

273. **(A)** Nursing process phase: implementation; client need: psychosocial integrity; content area: psychiatric nursing

Rationale

(A) This response offers the client a choice about whether to self-disclose or not initially, and also offers reassurance that there is mutual support in the group. (B) The client has probably not bonded with anyone on the unit yet and may feel reluctant to self-disclose. Also, at this stage of the therapeutic relationship, the therapist should refrain from telling the client what she should do. (C) What the other clients in the group may think about her question is not relevant, nor is it therapeutic. (D) This response sounds like a threat and will do little to enhance the trust necessary to build a therapeutic relationship.

274. **(D)** Nursing process phase: implementation; client need: psychosocial integrity; content area: psychiatric nursing

Rationale

(A) This response by the nurse is demeaning and fails to validate the client's feelings. (B) The nurse dismisses the importance of the suicide attempt and misses an opportunity to interact therapeutically with the client. (C) This response is too blunt for this stage of the relationship. Also, most adolescents can't accurately relate "why" they took an overdose, but they can talk about feelings and events immediately preceding the overdose. (D) This is therapeutic because it encourages the client to identify circumstances leading up to the suicide attempt and to explore more adaptive alternatives.

275. **(D)** Nursing process phase: evaluation; client need: health promotion and maintenance; content area: psychiatric nursing

Rationale

(A) The client has not learned a more adaptive alternative to suicide, but has learned that a more lethal method of suicide will be necessary if she feels that suicide is her only choice. (B) Although this response reflects universality, it does not identify a learned adaptive behavior. (C) This response does not reflect a more adaptive way to cope with suicidal thoughts. (D) This is the correct response because it is a safe and adaptive alternative to suicide.

276. **(D)** Nursing process phase: analysis; client need: physiological integrity; content area: psychiatric nursing

Rationale

(A) There is no history or physical evidence that the client has actually experienced pathological or obstructed breathing patterns. (B) The client has reported no alterations in visual, auditory, gustatory, olfactory, or tactile senses. (C) The client has reported nothing to the nurse that reflects disruption in thought patterns or thought processes. (D) The client has reported classic symptoms of a moderate level of anxiety: impaired concentration, inability to maintain attention, difficulty breathing, and rapid pulse.

277. **(A)** Nursing process phase: analysis; client need: physiological integrity; content area: psychiatric nursing

Rationale

(A) Although this drug has not been officially approved for psychiatric indications, effectiveness in blocking the autonomal arousal during an anxiety attack has been well documented. (B) Activation of the chemotrigger receptor zone in the brain would result in nausea and vomiting. Inderal is a beta adrenergic receptor antagonist, therefore, it acts in a different part of the brain. (C & D) Inderal has no direct action in the synapse.

278. **(D)** Nursing process phase: evaluation; client need: safe, effective care environment; content area: psychiatric nursing

Rationale

(A) The onset of action for Zoloft is 1 to 3 weeks. (B) Sleep disturbances and appetite problems are two of the symptoms targeted within the first week of administration. (C) Change in environment will have a positive impact on the client but will not likely be sufficient to improve sleep patterns or appetite. It is also unlikely that the client's activity level has changed such that it would improve the condition of the mood. (D) Zoloft is known to improve middle and terminal insomnia, appetite disturbances, and anxiety as early as 1 week after drug initiation.

279. **(D)** Nursing process phase: implementation; client need: safe, effective care environment; content area: psychiatric nursing

Rationale

(A) Although the client will be asked to read and/or sign a copy of the Patient's Legal Rights, it is not the highest priority intervention. (B) The physician will need to be notified of the client's admission, but he will also need to know at that time if the client is having suicidal thoughts. The nurse will be prepared to report this in a timely way if she completes the assessment for suicidal potential first. (C) If the client has not had dinner, it would be appropriate after admission to get her a tray from the kitchen, but nutritional needs never take priority over safety needs. (D) The highest priority intervention should always be the client's safety and, in this instance, that would mean assessing the client for the presence of suicidal ideation and potential.

280. **(A)** Nursing process phase: implementation; client need: safe, effective care environment; content area: psychiatric nursing

Rationale

(A) Unless the client is unconscious, sedated, or has been declared incompetent in a court of law, she should sign her own consent. (B) The husband is designated as the next of kin who may sign a client's consent only in the event she is unable to do so. (C) A treatment team member is not allowed to sign a consent for a client unless that person has been legally given the power of attorney for the client. Even if that were the case, it would be unethical for the team member to sign the consent because of a conflict of interest. (D) A signed and witnessed informed consent is required before this therapy is done.

281. (D) Nursing process phase: implementation; client need: health promotion and maintenance; content area: psychiatric nursing

Rationale
(A) Electroconvulsive therapy has no known permanent effect on remote memory. (B) Electroconvulsive therapy has no known permanent effect on recent memory. (C) Electroconvulsive therapy has no known temporary effect on remote events. (D) Electroconvulsive therapy is known to cause temporary memory loss for recent events.

282. (A) Nursing process phase: analysis; client need: safe, effective care environment; content area: psychiatric nursing

Rationale
(A) The nurse should anticipate withdrawal within the first 24 hours after the last drink. (B) The client will most likely be in acute but subsiding withdrawal by 72 hours after the last drink. (C) The client should be reaching some degree of stabilization between 3 and 5 days after the last drink. (D) The client should be nearing the end of withdrawal or completely and safely withdrawn at the end of 1 week.

283. (B) Nursing process phase: analysis; client need: physiological integrity; content area: psychiatric nursing

Rationale
(A) Although the client probably has some degree of knowledge deficit, it is not the most relevant nursing diagnosis because physiological integrity is always higher priority than cognitive integrity. (B) The client is obviously exhibiting signs of acute dehydration, dry skin membranes with poor skin turgor. (C) By history, he admits to nutritional deficits, but the fluid deficit takes priority over nutritional deficits. (D) There is evidence that the client has coped ineffectively, but that is not the most relevant nursing diagnosis.

284. (C) Nursing process phase: analysis; client need: physiological integrity; content area: psychiatric nursing

Rationale
(A) Cogentin is an anticholinergic that is used to reverse the extrapyramidal symptoms associated with the use of neuroleptics. (B) Serax is frequently used to treat the symptoms of alcohol withdrawal but the onset of action with the oral route of administration is 30 to 60 minutes. (C) Ativan would give the client the quickest relief because of the parenteral route of administration. It is a benzodiazepine but has a longer half-life than Serax, therefore, it would be more effective because it will be in the body longer than Serax. (D) Demerol is a schedule II narcotic and synthetic opioid. This drug is not indicated for alcohol withdrawal.

285. (C) Nursing process phase: evaluation; client need: safe, effective care environment; content area: psychiatric nursing

Rationale
(A) This statement reflects neither insight nor more adaptive

ways to cope. (B) This statement reflects minimal insight and a lot of rationalization. There is no evidence of more adaptive coping. (C) The client is verbalizing that he recognizes the consequences of alcohol abuse, and realizes that a sponsor and a support group will enhance his chances of recovery and sobriety and that alcohol will not. (D) This statement reflects insight but no improved methods of coping.

286. (A) Nursing process phase: implementation; client need: health promotion and maintenance; content area: psychiatric nursing

Rationale
(A) This is the most therapeutic response because it will guide the client's wife to a support group where she can confidentially discuss concerns about her spouse and address her own issues of codependence. It is also where a lot of teaching and mutual support takes place. (B) Having a "few beers" with the husband will not prevent him from drinking, rather it will encourage it. (C) Although it is true that the wife will not be able to prevent the spouse from drinking, emptying bottles at home is a codependent behavior. (D) Threatening the recovering alcoholic will neither cause nor prevent the client's drinking, but it could result in arguments or power struggles that could be detrimental to the relationship.

287. (C) Nursing process phase: analysis; client need: safe, effective care environment; content area: psychiatric nursing

Rationale
(A) There is not a specific withdrawal for cocaine abuse except to assess and treat target symptoms as they occur. The client's behavior has nothing to do with cocaine withdrawal; he is predominantly demonstrating personality traits. (B) There are no data given to support the suspicion that the client is sneaking drugs into the facility. These behaviors are typical of the client with antisocial personality disorder. (C) This response is correct because charming and ingratiating behaviors are characteristic traits of the antisocial personality-disordered individual. (D) The client' behavior is unrelated to his cocaine abuse or treatment.

288. (A) Nursing process phase: assessment; client need: safe, effective care environment; content area: psychiatric nursing

Rationale
(A) If the client is in a safe place, she will be able to talk openly. If she is injured, she may need an ambulance. If no other injuries are evident and the client has transportation, the nurse could then offer the client options about examination, treatment, and notification of the authorities. (B) It is not relevant for the nurse to know if the client knows her assailant. (C) Whether the client has insurance has no relevance to the care that she may need following a rape. It would be important to determine if the client could be pregnant, but not during initial telephone contact with the client. (D) If the client makes the decision to be examined, she should be instructed not to bathe, douche, or change clothes, because the victim holds the burden of proof in a court of law in the event that she presses charges. It is not the high priority question on initial contact.

289. (D) Nursing process phase: implementation; client need: psychosocial integrity; content area: psychiatric nursing

Rationale

(A) The nurse will need to notify the police if the client has not already done so. Further, it will be the responsibility of the nurse to make sure the police have been notified even if the client states that she called the police before she left home. (B) The nurse is in error. The police will need to be notified whether the client intends to pursue legal recourse or not. (C) After the client reaches the emergency room, it is the nurse's responsibility to notify the police. The client has the option of waiting to pursue legal counsel if she plans to go to court, provided the rapist is arrested and the district attorney determines if enough evidence is present to obtain a conviction. (D) This is the correct answer because the nurse is legally obligated to report the offense; the client is not obligated to pursue legal action even if the district attorney recommends legal action.

290. **(A)** Nursing process phase: implementation; client need: health promotion and maintenance; content area: psychiatric nursing

Rationale

(A) Bathing and douching are important hygienic needs after the rape examination. Also, the client will need to know how, when, and where she should obtain these further examinations. (B) It would be inappropriate to give out or recommend a specific attorney related to the client's emergency room visit. (C) Any follow-up that becomes necessary should be done at a rape crisis center, primary physician's office, or the health clinic. (D) The client is not battered, she has been raped. She will not need the phone number of the battered women's shelter, but it would be appropriate to refer her to the crisis intervention center.

291. **(B)** Nursing process phase: assessment; client need: safe, effective care environment; content area: psychiatric nursing

Rationale

(A) There is no evidence that the client is experiencing a false sensory perception with lack of external stimuli. (B) The client has created a new word by combining syllables of other words for an idiosyncratic reason. This is a neologism. (C) Word salad is an incoherent mixture of phrases and words that are illogical. There is only one illogical word in the client's statement. (D) This is not a psychiatric term.

292. **(A)** Nursing process phase: assessment; client need: safe, effective care environment; content area: psychiatric nursing

Rationale

(A) In magical thinking, the client believes that thoughts, words, or actions can assume power or cause or prevent events. (B) The client's statement reflects a false belief and is not paranoid in nature. (C) Autistic thinking is characterized by a preoccupation with one's inner and private world. There are no data to support this in the client's statement. (D) The client's statement is a false belief, but does not indicate that there is a problem with the bodily functions.

293. **(A)** Nursing process phase: assessment; client need: safe, effective care environment; content area: psychiatric nursing

Rationale

(A) Magical thinking is when thoughts, words, or actions are assumed by the client to have power, such as causing or pre-

venting events. (B) Word salad is a incoherent mixture of phrases and words that are illogical and have no meaning to the listener. (C) Derailment is a deviation in the client's thought without thought blocking. (D) Thought blocking is the interruption in the client's flow of speech because the idea cannot be recalled.

294. **(C)** Nursing process phase: analysis; client need: psychosocial integrity; content area: psychiatric nursing

Rationale

(A) Allowing the client to remain inside without further explanation is not therapeutic. Also, telling the client that she must go out tomorrow is a violation of her right to refuse treatment. (B) Telling the physician how depressed and tired the client is, is not a sound rationale for changing the client's antidepressant. (C) Walking will enhance and release the client's endorphins and enkephalins, which could contribute to improvement in mood. (D) The nurse is not recognizing that the client is experiencing a lack of motivation along with the depression.

295. **(C)** Nursing process phase: analysis; client need: physiological integrity; content area: psychiatric nursing

Rationale

(A) If the client was depressed, he would most likely be referred to a psychiatrist for medication, not a urologist. (B) Some antidepressants do have a side effect that is similar to anticholinergic effects, such as dry mouth and drowsiness, but it does not usually result in urinary retention. (C) One of the common side effects of imipramine is urinary retention. This is not a recommended use, but it has been well documented that it has been effective in treating enuresis. (D) Although the client may be attention-seeking, enuresis is not a conscious effort to achieve that end.

296. **(C)** Nursing process phase: analysis; client need: safe, effective care environment; content area: psychiatric nursing

Rationale

(A) Stage 3 is usually between ages 3 and 5 years, and characterized by the desire and motivation to complete tasks for the sake of doing them, guilt from the desire to be aggressive, and wanting to mimic adults. (B) Stage 4 is usually between the ages 6 and 11, and characterized by creating, building, and accomplishing. During this stage the child becomes socially decisive and may experience feelings of inferiority and inadequacy. (C) The client is in stage 5. She is in the correct age range (11 through the end of adolescence), and is attempting to develop ego identity. She is further interested in her appearance, enjoys her peer group, and is demonstrating hero worship. (D) Stage 6 is usually between ages 21 and 40. It is characterized by tasks related to work and love, intense relationships, and lifelong attachments.

297. **(B)** Nursing process phase: assessment; client need: health promotion and maintenance; content area: psychiatric nursing

Rationale

(A) It is not a high priority or even essential that the client begin therapy with insight. Insight usually occurs in the working phase of the therapeutic relationship. (B) Ideally, rapport and some degree of trust should be established in the initial interview with the client if possible. (C) Motivation on the part of the client is desirable, but mutual needs are not therapeutic. (D) It is desirable for the nurse therapist to have a high level of self-awareness, but not so for the client.

298. **(C)** Nursing process phase: planning; client need: safe, effective care environment; content area: psychiatric nursing

Rationale
(A) The nurse should always have a clear exit from the room. (B) A small sofa will probably place the nurse in the client's personal space, which the client could interpret as a threat. (C) Sitting in two separate seats is preferable to both sitting on a small sofa in each other's personal space. The nurse should always sit nearer the door than the client and always have a clear exit. (D) It is unsafe for the client to deliberately block the nurse's exit from the room.

299. **(A)** Nursing process phase: analysis; client need: safe, effective care environment; content area: psychiatric nursing

Rationale
(A) The client should not be approached quickly or touched. Most of all, the client should not be given an ultimatum. (B) If the history of violence is known, then the nurse can take measures to ensure her safety and the safety of the client. (C) If the client threatens the nurse verbally, the interview should come to an immediate end and appropriate help summoned. (D) It is very appropriate to ask another staffperson to interview the client with the nurse if the nurse feels afraid or assesses that the client cannot maintain control during the interview.

300. **(C)** Nursing process phase: assessment; client need: safe, effective care environment; content area: psychiatric nursing

Rationale
(A) The nurse has not asked if the client thinks others are trying to hurt him or take his belongings. (B) The client has not been asked if he is hearing voices. (C) The client is being asked directly if he thinks someone is inserting thoughts into his head. (D) The nurse has not asked the client if he hears his thoughts out loud or if he thinks others could hear his thoughts.

301. **(D)** Nursing process phase: assessment; client need: safe, effective care environment; content area: psychiatric nursing

Rationale
(A) There are no data indicating that the client believes that his body is diseased, changed, or in any way abnormal. (B) The client is not complaining of feeling anything on his skin that is not actually there. (C) There are no data to indicate that he believes that people are against him or plotting to harm him. (D) The client is experiencing ideas of reference because his statement reflects that he believes other people's words and behavior refer to him when there is no validation to support that.

302. **(B)** Nursing process phase: assessment; client need: safe, effective care environment; content area: psychiatric nursing

Rationale
(A) Constricted affect is one in which there is a clear reduction (not absence) in the range and intensity. (B) The client is demonstrating virtually no signs of affective expression. (C) The client's affect is not rapidly shifting from one extreme to another. (D) The client's affect is incongruent with the content of the movie, therefore, it is inappropriate.

303. **(C)** Nursing process phase: assessment; client need: safe, effective care environment; content area: psychiatric nursing

Rationale
(A) The client is not using words known only to him. (B) The client is not being circumstantial because there is no logic to his conversation. (C) The client is verbalizing slang associations. He has put them together in a sentence in which many of the words rhyme. (D) The client is not hearing voices.

304. **(C)** Nursing process phase: assessment; client need: safe, effective care environment; content area: psychiatric nursing

Rationale
(A) This question will elicit remote memory. (B) This question will elicit recent memory. (C) This question will elicit immediate recall. (D) This question will elicit recent past memory.

305. **(D)** Nursing process phase: assessment; client need: safe, effective care environment; content area: psychiatric nursing

Rationale
(A) The client may have some slight awareness of having an illness but has a degree of denial at this same time. (B) The client has awareness of the illness but is blaming it on others. (C) The client is demonstrating intellectual insight only. There is no indication from his statement that this knowledge will be applied to future experiences. (D) The client is verbalizing emotional awareness of the effect of his behavior on others and is planning to change his behavior.

306. **(A)** Nursing process phase: analysis; client need: safe, effective care environment; content area: psychiatric nursing

Rationale
(A) The client is experiencing a sensory experience without external stimuli validating the nursing diagnosis. (B) The client's statement does not reflect that he is experiencing fixed, false beliefs. (C) Many psychotic clients do experience self-care deficits, but there is no evidence in the client's statement to validate this. (D) There is no evidence in the client's statement that there is spiritual distress.

307. **(D)** Nursing process phase: assessment; client need: safe, effective care environment; content area: psychiatric nursing

Rationale
(A) The client is not experiencing intense elation with feelings of grandeur according to the wife's report. (B) The client's mood goes beyond an unpleasant mood, which is usually transient. (C) There are no data indicating that a major loss has occurred. (D) The client has lost interest in, and withdrawn from, all regular and pleasurable activities.

308. **(B)** Nursing process phase: assessment; client need: safe, effective care environment; content area: psychiatric nursing

Rationale
(A) The client is having hallucinations, but they are not mood-incongruent. (B) The client is having hallucinations that are congruent with his manic and elevated mood. His hallucinations are reinforcing his mood. (C & D) The client is not experiencing delusions.

309. **(D)** Nursing process phase: analysis; client need: safe, effective care environment; content area: psychiatric nursing

Rationale
(A) Suicidal ideation in the presence of pharmacotherapy is an indication for treatment. (B) Hypertension can be medicated and monitored during and after ECT. (C) Clients who receive ECT are given a centrally acting muscle paralyzer that prevents muscle contractions which could complicate cervical disk disease. (D) Brain tumor is one of the few absolute contraindications for ECT, because ECT will further increase intracranial pressure.

310. **(B)** Nursing process phase: implementation; client need: safe, effective care environment; content area: psychiatric nursing

Rationale
(A) A neuroleptic is the offending agent and should be discontinued. The vital signs should be monitored every 15 minutes. (B) This is the recommended emergency treatment for this condition. Dantrolene, which is centrally acting, will reverse the severe muscle rigidity associated with neuroleptic malignant syndrome. (C) The neuroleptic should be discontinued and dantrolene administered. (D) Discontinuing the neuroleptic is correct, but the vital signs should be monitored every 15 minutes after dantrolene is administered.

Focus on Psychiatric Drug Dosages

311. **(B)** Nursing process phase: implementation; client need: safe, effective care environment; content area: psychiatric nursing—dosage calculation

Rationale
125 mg : 5 ml = 250 mg : x = 10 ml
Math calculation explains incorrect answers.

312. **(B)** Nursing process phase: implementation; client need: safe, effective care environment; content area: psychiatric nursing—dosage calculation

Rationale
200 mg : 1 tablet = 200 mg : x = 1 tablet
Math calculation explains incorrect answers.

313. **(C)** Nursing process phase: implementation; client need: safe, effective care environment; content area: psychiatric nursing—dosage calculation

Rationale
10 mg : 1 ml = 75 mg : x = 7.5 ml
Math calculation explains incorrect answers.

314. **(C)** Nursing process phase: implementation; client need: safe, effective care environment; content area: psychiatric nursing—dosage calculation

Rationale
100 mg : 1 tablet = 300 mg : x = 3 tablets
Math calculation explains incorrect answers.

315. **(C)** Nursing process phase: implementation; client need: safe, effective care environment; content area: psychiatric nursing—dosage calculation

Rationale
375 mg divided by 250 mg × 1 tablet = 1½ tablets
Math calculation explains incorrect answers.

316. **(A)** Nursing process phase: implementation; client need: safe, effective care environment; content area: psychiatric nursing—dosage calculation

Rationale
0.25 mg divided by 0.5 mg × 1 tablet = ½ tablet
Math calculation explains incorrect answers.

317. **(D)** Nursing process phase: implementation; client need: safe, effective care environment; content area: psychiatric nursing—dosage calculation

Rationale
50 mg : 5 ml = 100 mg : x = 10 ml
Math calculation explains incorrect answers.

318. **(D)** Nursing process phase: implementation; client need: safe, effective care environment; content area: psychiatric nursing—dosage calculation

Rationale
25 mg : 1 tablet = 50 mg : x = 2 tablets
Math calculation explains incorrect answers.

319. **(C)** Nursing process phase: implementation; client need: safe, effective care environment; content area: psychiatric nursing—dosage calculation

Rationale
250 mg : 1 ml = 400 mg : x = 1.6 ml
Math calculation explains incorrect answers.

320. **(C)** Nursing process phase: implementation; client need: safe, effective care environment; content area: psychiatric nursing—dosage calculation

Rationale
500 μg : 1 ml = 2600 μg : x = 5.2 ml
Math calculation explains incorrect answers.

321. **(D)** Nursing process phase: implementation; client need: safe, effective care environment; content area: psychiatric nursing—dosage calculation

Rationale
10 mg : 1 tablet = 20 mg : x = 2 tablets
Math calculation explains incorrect answers.

322. **(A)** Nursing process phase: implementation; client need: safe, effective care environment; content area: psychiatric nursing—dosage calculation

Rationale
100 mg : 1 tablet = 50 mg : x = ½ tablet
Math calculation explains incorrect answers.

323. (C) Nursing process phase: implementation; client need: safe, effective care environment; content area: psychiatric nursing—dosage calculation

Rationale

50 mg : 1 tablet = 75 mg : x = 1.5 tablets
Math calculation explains incorrect answers.

324. (B) Nursing process phase: implementation; client need: safe, effective care environment; content area: psychiatric nursing—dosage calculation

Rationale

1 mg : 1 ml = 0.4 mg : x = 0.4 ml
Math calculation explains incorrect answers.

325. (B) Nursing process phase: implementation; client need: safe, effective care environment; content area: psychiatric nursing—dosage calculation

Rationale

1 mg : 1 ml = 2 mg : x = 2 ml
Math calculation explains incorrect answers.

326. (C) Nursing process phase: implementation; client need: safe, effective care environment; content area: psychiatric nursing—dosage calculation

Rationale

0.1 mg : 1 ml = 0.2 mg : x = 2 ml
Math calculation explains incorrect answers.

327. (D) Nursing process phase: implementation; client need: safe, effective care environment; content area: psychiatric nursing—dosage calculation

Rationale

500 mg : 1 ml = 200 mg : x = 0.4 ml
Math calculation explains incorrect answers.

328. (C) Nursing process phase: implementation; client need: safe, effective care environment; content area: psychiatric nursing—dosage calculation

Rationale

2 mg : 5 ml = 5 mg : x = 12.5 ml
Math calculation explains incorrect answers.

329. (C) Nursing process phase: implementation; client need: safe, effective care environment; content area: psychiatric nursing—dosage calculation

Rationale

50 mg : 1 ml = 75 mg : x = 1.5 ml
Math calculation explains incorrect answers.

330. (D) Nursing process phase: implementation; client need: safe, effective care environment; content area: psychiatric nursing—dosage calculation

Rationale

25 mg : 1 tablet = 100 mg : x = 4 tablets
Math calculation explains incorrect answers.

331. (B) Nursing process phase: implementation; client need: safe, effective care environment; content area: psychiatric nursing—dosage calculation

Rationale

160 mg / 800 mg : 1 tablet = 160 mg / 800 mg : x = 1 tablet
Math calculation explains incorrect answers.

332. (B) Nursing process phase: implementation; client need: safe, effective care environment; content area: psychiatric nursing—dosage calculation

Rationale

300 mg : 1 capsule = 600 mg : x = 2 capsules
Math calculation explains incorrect answers.

333. (B) Nursing process phase: implementation; client need: safe, effective care environment; content area: psychiatric nursing—dosage calculation

Rationale

1 mg : 1 ml = 1 mg : x = 1 ml
Math calculation explains incorrect answers.

334. (D) Nursing process phase: implementation; client need: safe, effective care environment; content area: psychiatric nursing—dosage calculation

Rationale

5 mg : 1 ml = 2 mg : x = 0.4 ml
Math calculation explains incorrect answers.

335. (B) Nursing process phase: implementation; client need: safe, effective care environment; content area: psychiatric nursing—dosage calculation

Rationale

500 mg : 1 ml = 100 mg : x = 0.2 ml
Math calculation explains incorrect answers.

336. (A) Nursing process phase: implementation; client need: safe, effective care environment; content area: psychiatric nursing—dosage calculation

Rationale

2.5 mg : 1 tablet = 1.25 mg : x = ½ tablet
Math calculation explains incorrect answers.

337. (C) Nursing process phase: implementation; client need: safe, effective care environment; content area: psychiatric nursing—dosage calculation

Rationale

100 mg : 1 tablet = 150 mg : x = 1½ tablets
Math calculation explains incorrect answers.

338. (C) Nursing process phase: implementation; client need: safe, effective care environment; content area: psychiatric nursing—dosage calculation

Rationale

250 mg : 5 ml = 500 mg : x = 10 ml
Math calculation explains incorrect answers.

339. (D) Nursing process phase: implementation; client need: safe, effective care environment; content area: psychiatric nursing—dosage calculation

Rationale

200 mg : 1 tablet = 400 mg : x = 2 tablets
Math calculation explains incorrect answers.

340. (C) Nursing process phase: implementation; client

need: safe, effective care environment; content area: psychiatric nursing—dosage calculation

Rationale

$$300 \text{ mg} : 5 \text{ ml} = 300 \text{ mg} : x = 5 \text{ ml}$$

Math calculation explains incorrect answers.

341. (A) Nursing process phase: implementation; client need: safe, effective care environment; content area: psychiatric nursing—dosage calculation

Rationale

$$50 \text{ mg} : 1 \text{ ml} = 25 \text{ mg} : x = 0.5 \text{ ml}$$

Math calculation explains incorrect answers.

342. (D) Nursing process phase: implementation; client need: safe, effective care environment; content area: psychiatric nursing—dosage calculation

Rationale

$$0.2 \text{ mg} : 1 \text{ tablet} = 0.8 \text{ mg} : x = 4 \text{ tablets}$$

Math calculation explains incorrect answers.

343. (D) Nursing process phase: implementation; client need: safe, effective care environment; content area: psychiatric nursing—dosage calculation

Rationale

$$5 \text{ mg} : 1 \text{ capsule} = 20 \text{ mg} : x = 4 \text{ capsules}$$

Math calculation explains incorrect answers.

344. (A) Nursing process phase: implementation; client need: safe, effective care environment; content area: psychiatric nursing—dosage calculation

Rationale

$$20 \text{ mg} : 1 \text{ pulvule} = 20 \text{ mg} : x = 1 \text{ pulvule}$$

Math calculation explains incorrect answers.

345. (D) Nursing process phase: implementation; client need: safe, effective care environment; content area: psychiatric nursing—dosage calculation

Rationale

$$250 \text{ mg} : 1 \text{ tablet} = 500 \text{ mg} : x = 2 \text{ tablets}$$

Math calculation explains incorrect answers.

346. (A) Nursing process phase: implementation; client need: safe, effective care environment; content area: psychiatric nursing—dosage calculation

Rationale

$$1 \text{ mg} : 1 \text{ tablet} = 0.5 \text{ mg} : x = \tfrac{1}{2} \text{ tablet}$$

Math calculation explains incorrect answers.

347. (C) Nursing process phase: implementation; client need: safe, effective care environment; content area: psychiatric nursing—dosage calculation

Rationale

$$100 \text{ mg} : 1 \text{ tablet} = 300 \text{ mg} : x = 3 \text{ tablets}$$

Math calculation explains incorrect answers.

348. (B) Nursing process phase: implementation; client need: safe, effective care environment; content area: psychiatric nursing—dosage calculation

Rationale

$$50 \text{ mg} : 1 \text{ ml} = 50 \text{ mg} : x = 1 \text{ ml}$$

Math calculation explains incorrect answers.

349. (D) Nursing process phase: implementation; client need: safe, effective care environment; content area: psychiatric nursing—dosage calculation

Rationale

$$5 \text{ mg} : 1 \text{ ml} = 10 \text{ mg} : x = 2 \text{ ml}$$

Math calculation explains incorrect answers.

350. (D) Nursing process phase: implementation; client need: safe, effective care environment; content area: psychiatric nursing—dosage calculation

Rationale

$$200 \text{ mg} : 1 \text{ tablet} = 400 \text{ mg} : x = 2 \text{ tablets}$$

Math calculation explains incorrect answers.

351. (A) Nursing process phase: implementation; client need: safe, effective care environment; content area: psychiatric nursing—dosage calculation

Rationale

$$500 \text{ mg} : 1 \text{ ml} = 225 \text{ mg} : x = 0.45 \text{ ml}$$

Math calculation explains incorrect answers.

352. (D) Nursing process phase: implementation; client need: safe, effective care environment; content area: psychiatric nursing—dosage calculation

Rationale

$$2 \text{ mg} : 5 \text{ ml} = 4 \text{ mg} : x = 10 \text{ ml}$$

Math calculation explains incorrect answers.

353. (B) Nursing process phase: implementation; client need: safe, effective care environment; content area: psychiatric nursing—dosage calculation

Rationale

$$500 \text{ mg} : 1 \text{ ml} = 340 \text{ mg} : x = 0.68 \text{ ml}$$

Math calculation explains incorrect answers.

354. (B) Nursing process phase: implementation; client need: safe, effective care environment; content area: psychiatric nursing—dosage calculation

Rationale

$$15 \text{ mg} : 1 \text{ capsule} = 15 \text{ mg} : x = 1 \text{ capsule}$$

Math calculation explains incorrect answers.

355. (A) Nursing process phase: implementation; client need: safe, effective care environment; content area: psychiatric nursing—dosage calculation

Rationale

$$15 \text{ mg} : 1 \text{ tablet} = 7.5 \text{ mg} : x = \tfrac{1}{2} \text{ tablet}$$

Math calculation explains incorrect answers.

356. (D) Nursing process phase: implementation; client need: safe, effective care environment; content area: psychiatric nursing—dosage calculation

Rationale

$$25 \text{ mg} : 1 \text{ ml} = 50 \text{ mg} : x = 2 \text{ ml}$$

Math calculation explains incorrect answers.

357. (D) Nursing process phase: implementation; client need: safe, effective care environment; content area: psychiatric nursing—dosage calculation

Rationale

$$10 \text{ mg} : 1 \text{ tablet} = 25 \text{ mg} : x = 2\tfrac{1}{2} \text{ tablets}$$

Math calculation explains incorrect answers.

358. (A) Nursing process phase: implementation; client need: safe, effective care environment; content area: psychiatric nursing—dosage calculation

Rationale
      300 mg : 1 tablet = 150 mg : x = ½ tablet
Math calculation explains incorrect answers.

359. (B) Nursing process phase: implementation; client need: safe, effective care environment; content area: psychiatric nursing—dosage calculation

Rationale
      25 mg : 1 tablet = 25 mg : x = 1 tablet
Math calculation explains incorrect answers.

360. (D) Nursing process phase: implementation; client need: safe, effective care environment; content area: psychiatric nursing—dosage calculation

Rationale
      10 mg : 1 ml = 50 mg : x = 5 ml
Math calculation explains incorrect answers.

361. (B) Nursing process phase: implementation; client need: safe, effective care environment; content area: psychiatric nursing—dosage calculation

Rationale
      40 mg : 1 tablet = 34 mg : x = 0.85 tablet, round off to 1 tablet
Math calculation explains incorrect answers.

362. (B) Nursing process phase: implementation; client need: safe, effective care environment; content area: psychiatric nursing—dosage calculation

Rationale
      500 mg : 1 tablet = 500 mg : x = 1 tablet
Math calculation explains incorrect answers.

unit**three**

INTEGRATED
PRACTICE TESTS

test 1

1. A client with pregnancy-induced hypertension (PIH) at 34 weeks' gestation has been admitted to the obstetric unit for observation. Which of the following laboratory results indicate that her condition is worsening?
   A. Elevated liver function tests (LFTs)
   B. Proteinuria of 3+
   C. Increased platelets
   D. Elevated erythrocyte sedimentation rate

2. Scoliosis is defined as a lateral curvature of the spine. The best rationale for the compensatory curve that often develops in the spine is to:
   A. Maintain body alignment.
   B. Distribute weight evenly.
   C. Straighten the spine.
   D. Allow for chest expansion.

3. A client is to receive 30 units of NPH insulin and 4 units of regular insulin at 8 A.M. The nurse would:
   A. Inject air into the regular insulin first.
   B. Draw up the insulins in separate syringes.
   C. Inject air into the NPH insulin first.
   D. Ask the pharmacy for the desired mixture.

4. The physician ordered norethindrone (Norlutin) 7.5 mg PO for a young woman experiencing breakthrough bleeding. The pharmacist dispensed 5 mg tablets and instructed the client to take____tablets.

   A. 0.5 tablet
   B. 1.0 tablet
   C. 1.5 tablets
   D. 2.0 tablets

5. The nurse is doing a physical assessment on a 6-month-old infant. The baby is sitting quietly on the mother's lap. Which of the following parts of the assessment should the nurse do first?
   A. Auscultate heart and lungs.
   B. Examine eyes, ears, and mouth.
   C. Examine head and move toward the feet.
   D. Palpate peripheral pulses.

6. The 74-year-old client is being discharged by the nurse. The primary source of long-term care for older adults with acquired immune deficiency syndrome (AIDS) is:
   A. Nursing home care
   B. Home health care
   C. Hospital nursing care
   D. Community AIDS clinics

7. The client who has been in mechanical restraints asked the nurse when they can be removed. Which one of the following is the best response by the nurse?
   A. "Please tell me why you were physically violent."
   B. "When apologies are made for creating such a disturbance."
   C. "When your behavior is under control and you are no longer a danger to yourself or others."
   D. "When the medication has calmed your violent behavior."

8. After the spontaneous vaginal delivery of a term newborn with clear amniotic fluid, the nurse attempts to clear the airway using bulb suctioning. Proper technique with bulb suction includes which nursing action?
   A. Suction the nose first, with the bulb compressed before insertion.
   B. Suction the pharynx first, with the bulb compressed before insertion.
   C. Suction the nose first with a Dee Lee mucus trap.
   D. Suction the pharynx only after insertion of an oral-gastric tube.

9. A 53-year-old male is admitted with uncontrolled hypertension. He suddenly develops double vision,

slurring of speech, left-sided weakness, and dizziness. These symptoms resolve within 12 hours. The client is scheduled for a carotid endarterectomy. Which of the following symptoms should the nurse closely monitor for with this client?
A. Sudden rise in blood pressure and bounding pulse
B. Increased respirations and increased pulse
C. Increased temperature and increased respirations
D. Sudden decrease in pulse and tachycardia

10. During a routine pelvic examination, a client, 6 months' pregnant, states that she feels hot, sweaty, and that her heart is racing. Which of the following nursing interventions is best?
A. Get her an ice pack for her forehead.
B. Administer nasal oxygen at 7 L/min.
C. Place the client in Trendelenburg's position.
D. Assist her to a left lateral position.

11. A 40-year-old male is admitted following an accident in which he suffered blunt trauma to the chest. He has a fracture of the right fifth and sixth ribs. Which of the following complications of lower or middle rib fracture would the nurse monitor for?
A. Laceration of the pericardium
B. Laceration of the trachea
C. Laceration of the spine
D. Laceration of the sternum

12. The nursing diagnosis of highest priority for a client who has experienced a postpartum hemorrhage is:
A. Alteration in comfort
B. Anxiety
C. Altered tissue perfusion
D. High risk for infection

13. A 12-year-old male was admitted to the pediatric unit for evaluation brought about by a flare-up of polyarticular arthritis. He was diagnosed 5 years ago and at that time had a positive rheumatoid factor. Which of the following information is the most important when planning care?
A. Limited joint movement is probably caused by ankylosis of the joint.
B. Joint inflammation restricts muscle-strengthening exercise in the area of involved joint.
C. Iridocyclitis is more likely to occur in males than females.
D. Positive latex fixation test.

14. Your client has called to check on the score on the biophysical profile she had done. She has a score of 10, which you would interpret as:
A. Reassuring, with repeat testing in approximately 1 week
B. Equivocal, with repeat testing within 24 hours
C. Worrisome, with a need for speedy delivery
D. Abnormal, with immediate retesting to confirm results

15. The nurse administers lorazepam (Ativan) to the client for the first time. The client asks, "Why are you giving me this drug? I usually take Xanax." Which of the following nursing diagnoses would be the most appropriate at this time?
A. Ineffective individual coping
B. Spiritual distress
C. Knowledge deficit
D. Impaired adjustment

16. The nurse evaluates the outcome of thyroid hormone replacement therapy. Initially, the expected response is:
A. A decreased pulse rate
B. Improved wound healing
C. Diuresis and weight loss
D. Increased serum potassium

17. The nurse, in caring for a 4-year-old child postoperatively from a tonsillectomy and adenoidectomy, monitors for signs and symptoms of hemorrhage. Which of the following would be an early indication of hemorrhage?
A. Swallowing infrequently
B. Dark brown emesis of approximately 25 ml
C. Pulse rate of 95 beats per minute
D. Drooling of bright red secretions.

18. When the client's IV infusion infiltrates, which action should the nurse initially take?
A. Apply cool compresses to relieve edema.
B. Gently massage the site to relieve pain.
C. Apply moist heat to the venipuncture site.
D. Discontinue the infusion and restart elsewhere.

19. A pregnant client is started on an iron supplement. What information can the nurse give the client to aid in absorption of the supplement?
A. "Take your iron with milk."
B. "Take your supplement with your prenatal vitamins."
C. "Take your iron with orange juice."
D. "Take your iron in the morning with breakfast."

20. A 68-year-old male is admitted after a car accident with multiple contusions to his right chest, arms, and legs. He has chest tubes placed to the right chest wall. After several hours the client becomes very anxious, short of breath, and has noticeable jugular venous distension (JVD). His heart sounds are muffled, his BP is 62/28, and there is slight serosanguineous drainage from the chest tubes. Which of the following conditions would the nurse suspect from the client's signs and symptoms?
A. Pneumothorax
B. Hemothorax
C. Myocardial infarction
D. Cardiac tamponade

21. During an otoscopic examination on a 9-month-

old infant, the nurse pulls the pinna in what direction?

A. Down and back
B. Down and forward
C. Up and back
D. Up and forward

22. A 15-year-old male client who had been incarcerated for stealing was admitted to the adolescent psychiatric unit. His roommate accused him of name calling and stealing cigarettes. What is the best nursing intervention?

A. Ignore the behavior because the client has not had time to adjust.
B. Explore the meaning of the client's behavior.
C. Demand that the client return the cigarettes to the owner.
D. Explore with the client his self-serving attitude.

23. A 7-year-old had developed a nonproductive cough. The child weighed 23 kg. The physician ordered benzonatate 8 mg/ kg (184 mg) in three to six divided doses. How many 100 mg tablets would the nurse instruct the mother to give?

A. ½ tablet
B. 1 tablet
C. 1½ tablets
D. 2 tablets

24. Which lunch menu should the nurse recommend for the child with celiac disease?

A. Hot dog, french fries, milk, and cake
B. Spaghetti, garlic bread, salad, and pudding
C. Pizza, cookies, and malt
D. Baked fish, corn on the cob, and apple

25. A 42-year-old male is receiving peritoneal dialysis. The nurse knows that which of the following is a complication of peritoneal dialysis?

A. Hypoglycemia
B. Hypertension
C. Hypovolemia
D. Hypervolemia

26. After reviewing danger signs of pregnancy, which of the following should the client report immediately?

A. Intermittent vomiting
B. Vaginal bleeding
C. Leukorrhea
D. Urinary frequency

27. As the nurse, you are teaching a 27-year-old, first-time mother of a healthy term girl. Which of the following statements by the newborn's mother indicates a need for further teaching?

A. "I need to place my daughter on her side to sleep."
B. "I need to place my daughter on her back to sleep."
C. "I need to place my daughter on her abdomen to sleep."
D. "I need to place my daughter upright to burp her before I put her to sleep after her bottle."

28. Joseph, age 8, has been diagnosed as having Legg-Calvé-Perthes disease. The right femur is involved. The major emphasis in planning nursing care for Joseph while he is undergoing therapy is to:

A. Prevent flexion of the right hip.
B. Control pain that is especially acute at night.
C. Prevent weight bearing on the head of the right femur.
D. Encourage Joseph to walk despite discomfort at the right hip.

29. The nurse, in planning program activities for clients in a day treatment setting, should:

A. Facilitate diversional activities for the lower functioning clients.
B. Focus on pathology.
C. Provide for meaningful social interaction.
D. Provide for the multifaceted needs.

30. A 56-year-old female is admitted with weakness, nausea, vomiting, anorexia, weight loss, diarrhea, and numbness and tingling to her extremities. Her tongue is beefy red and smooth. The sclera are slightly jaundiced. She has systolic murmur, and percussion reveals an enlarged liver and spleen. She has positive Babinski's and Romberg's signs. Her Schilling's test results are also positive. The nurse realizes that all of these indicators are signs of which of the following conditions?

A. AIDS
B. Pernicious anemia
C. Adult respiratory distress syndrome (ARDS)
D. Parkinson's disease

31. Your client arrives in your clinic for her first pre-natal visit. She states that her last menstrual period was May 12 to 16. using Naegele's rule, determine her expected date of confinement (EDC).

A. February 23
B. August 15
C. February 19
D. March 3

32. A 52-year-old male is admitted with a diagnosis of pernicious anemia. Which of the following nursing interventions would be appropriate for this client?

A. Administer vitamin B_6 injections as ordered.
B. Promote independence and encourage the client to pursue any chosen activities.
C. Ensure accurate collection of Harvard's test for pernicious anemia.
D. Provide frequent oral care and oral anesthetics.

33. A 13-year-old female diagnosed with systemic lupus erythematosus (SLE) is in the rheumatology clinic for a check-up. She has been on hydroxychloroquine (Plaquenil) for 2 years. Which of the following is most important for planning care for this adolescent?

A. Physical assessment identifies a malar rash.
B. Subjective data reveal she walks home from school with friends in the afternoon.

C. The mother reports her last eye examination was 1 year ago.

D. Client had a weight gain of 4 lb over the last 6 months.

34. Which of the following statements indicates the best understanding to the nurse about placenta functioning?
    A. "The placenta filters out harmful substances."
    B. "The placenta is where my blood circulates through my baby."
    C. "The umbilical cord has one vein and one artery."
    D. "The placenta gives my baby oxygen and nutrients."

35. A 58-year-old male is admitted from ICU with a pneumonectomy of the left lung 3 days ago. The nurse realizes that pneumonectomy clients must be monitored closely for the development of which of the following conditions?
    A. Pleural effusion
    B. Hypoglycemia
    C. Hemothorax
    D. Congestive heart failure

36. Which nursing action is not appropriate for the infant or child with acute and severe GI bleeding?
    A. Assess the degree of blood loss and hemodynamic status.
    B. Note the child's vital signs, capillary refill, skin color, and LOC.
    C. Start rapid IV fluids of normal saline or lactated Ringer's solution.
    D. Test all stools for blood.

37. You are providing care for a primigravida who at 34 weeks' gestation has been diagnosed with HELLP syndrome. Her level of anxiety is very high. The most therapeutic comment you can make to help decrease her anxiety is:
    A. "You don't have a thing to worry about. You have lots of people here who will take good care of you and your baby."
    B. "You are only making things worse for you and your baby by being so upset. If you will calm down, we can do a better job of helping you."
    C. "We see this kind of thing all the time. You should just rest and not worry about a thing."
    D. "I know when things like this happen so quickly it can be very upsetting for you."

38. A 58-year-old male is 4 days' postoperative for a coronary bypass graft surgery. The nurse encourages him to cough and deep-breathe to clear the thick secretions out of his lungs. The client states it hurts too much to breath. Which of the following nursing actions would be appropriate to help this client minimize the pain from his chest incision?
    A. Administer morphine sulfate as ordered.
    B. Use incentive spirometer every hour.

C. Use a pillow to splint the chest.
D. Teach diaphragmatic breathing to the client.

39. Which of the following laboratory results is consistent with a diagnosis of diabetic ketoacidosis in a child?
    A. Blood pH of 7.36 and a bicarbonate of 15 mEq/L
    B. Bicarbonate level of 24 mEq/L
    C. Serum glucose of 350 mg/dl and ketonuria
    D. Blood glucose level of 30 mg/dl

40. A diabetic client experiences hyperglycemic rebound following a period of hypoglycemia. The nurse explains that this phenomenon is called:
    A. Dawn phenomenon
    B. Insulin resistance
    C. Insulin sensitivity reaction
    D. Somogyi effect

41. A female client asks the nurse why women are more susceptible to cystitis than men. The nurse replies, "Women are more likely than men to develop cystisis because of":
    A. Wearing pantyhose.
    B. Poor hygiene practices.
    C. Inadequate fluid intake.
    D. The length of the male urethra.

42. A 33-year-old was experiencing sever irritability secondary to acute alcohol withdrawal. The physician ordered lorazepam (Ativan) 4 mg IV tid. Using a 4 mg/ml vial, how many milliliters did the nurse administer?
    A. 0.5 ml
    B. 1.0 ml
    C. 1.5 ml
    D. 2.0 ml

43. A 38-year-old female is admitted with fever and dyspnea and is intubated and placed on a ventilator for her respiratory distress. After the endotracheal tube has been placed in the client, the nurse would immediately do which of the following?
    A. Check for bilateral breath sounds.
    B. Call for a chest x-ray.
    C. Obtain stat arterial blood gases.
    D. Check the client's vital signs.

44. A client is 9 weeks' pregnant. She confides to the nurse that cocaine is her drug of choice. Which of the following is an effect of cocaine on the maternal-fetal unit?
    A. Cocaine decreases norepinephrine levels, increasing maternal risk for HELLP syndrome.
    B. Cocaine increases norepinephrine, causing vasoconstriction and decreased placental perfusion.
    C. Cocaine accelerates fetal growth and development by increasing the fetal metabolic rate.
    D. Placental villi increase in number to offset the insult.

45. A 49-year-old male is admitted with signs and symptoms of pulmonary embolism. The nurse is aware that which of the following are risk factors associated with pulmonary embolism?
   A. Hypervolemia
   B. Arthritis
   C. Long bone fracture
   D. Osteoporosis

46. A child with neutropenia was just admitted to the pediatric unit. Which of the following actions by the nurse would take highest priority?
   A. Encourage eating raw vegetables and fruits for the vitamin C content.
   B. Prohibit any activity and maintain strict bedrest.
   C. Report immediately any temperature elevation.
   D. Screen visitors.

47. The best nursing approach to a client who refuses to participate in unit activities is to:
   A. Initiate a form of punishment for lack of attendance.
   B. Enforce the attendance rule and discuss feelings.
   C. Explore with the client his or her feelings related to the unit activities.
   D. Continue to observe the client's noncompliance.

48. A 35-year-old female has two chest tubes connected to a pleurovac to wall suction at 20 cm. The nurse would use which of the interventions to facilitate drainage from the client's chest?
   A. Hang the chest tubes off the bed.
   B. Encourage deep breathing.
   C. Keep the client flat in the bed.
   D. Milk the chest tubes every hour.

49. The nurse is explaining sleep behaviors to a class of parents. Which of the following statements is more indicative of a sleep terror as opposed to a nightmare?
   A. The child is aware of and reassured by another's presence.
   B. The child may be able to describe the dream.
   C. The child may be delayed in the return to sleep.
   D. The nightmare usually occurs 1 to 4 hours after falling asleep.

50. Danger signs of pregnancy that a woman should immediately report to her health-care provider are:
   A. Constipation and urinary frequency
   B. Nocturia and linea nigra
   C. Abdominal pain and hematuria
   D. Leg cramps and pyrosis

51. A 46-year-old female is 3 days' postoperative from a craniotomy. The client develops diabetes insipidus. The nurse realizes that which of the following cause diabetes insipidus?
   A. Increased antidiuretic hormone (ADH) production
   B. Decreased ADH production
   C. Hypovolemia
   D. Renal failure

52. A 70-year-old female has been diagnosed with terminal breast cancer. She is receiving radiation and chemotherapy treatments, and the physician has consulted the hospital hospice program to review her case for home care. What is the most important action the nurse can do for a dying client?
   A. Explain progress of the disease process to the client.
   B. Provide pain medications as needed for the client.
   C. Listen to the needs and fears of the client.
   D. Teach the family about home care of the client.

53. A 44-year-old with arthritis was high risk for drug-induced gastric ulcers from taking nonsteroidal anti-inflammatory drugs. The physician ordered misoprostol (Cytotec) 100 μg qid with food. The nurse instructed the client to take how many 200 μg tablets?
   A. ½ tablet
   B. 1 tablet
   C. 1½ tablets
   D. 2 tablets

54. A 12-year-old male with sickle-cell anemia has been admitted to the pediatric unit for treatment. This client was diagnosed with sickle-cell disease at 8 months old. This year he has been admitted to the hospital three times for sickle-cell crisis. The physician ordered 2 units of packed red blood cells. Because of the client's history, which of the following nursing assessments is the most important during the blood transfusions?
   A. Assessment for neurological impairments caused by the crisis.
   B. Assessment for a reduction in pain because hydration has begun.
   C. Assessment for signs and symptoms of cardiac failure related to hydration.
   D. Assessment for a bacterial infection that possibly triggered the crisis.

55. A 78-year-old male is admitted for shortness for breath on exertion and extreme fatigue. Some time after lunch, the client asks the nurse if there are any large print magazines in the hospital for him to read. He tells the nurse that it is the only type of print he can read from. The nurse would identify which of the following conditions as the reason for the client's visual problem:
   A. Cataracts
   B. Presbyopia
   C. Xerostomia
   D. Arcus senilis

56. A 46-year-old female is admitted after a severe concussion following a fall. She is diagnosed with syndrome of inappropriate antidiuretic hormone secretion (SIADH). The nurse would observe for which of the following symptoms associated with this disorder?
    A. Polyuria
    B. Hematuria
    C. Hypoglycemia
    D. Abdominal cramping

57. Which of the following statements by a 23 weeks' pregnant client indicates to the nurse the need for further instruction on improving circulation?
    A. "I should avoid crossing my legs while sitting."
    B. "I should put on my support panty hose after I have walked to the bathroom."
    C. "I should elevate my legs whenever I sit at work."
    D. "I should dorsiflex my feet if I have been standing for a long period of time."

58. A 30-year-old male is admitted with a diagnosis of Addison's disease. The nurse realizes that a client with Addison's disease develops which of the following signs and symptoms?
    A. Hypertension and hypokalemia — hypotension
    B. Bronze skin color and fatigue
    C. Chronic thirst and pica
    D. Constipation and bloody stools

59. What is the single most effective mechanism to prevent and control the spread of hepatitis A in any setting?
    A. Education
    B. Hand washing
    C. Avoidance of illicit drug use
    D. Immunization to prevent HBV infection

60. The second stage of labor is complete when:
    A. The cervix is completely dilated.
    B. The client begins the pushing process.
    C. The infant is delivered.
    D. The placenta has been delivered.

61. A 28-year-old female is admitted with Cushing's syndrome. Which of the following physical changes would the nurse expect to observe in a client with this disorder?
    A. Bronzing of the skin, weight loss, and alopecia
    B. Hyperactivity, acne, and ecchymosis
    C. Moon face, hirsutism, and thin extremities
    D. Buffalo hump, thin extremities, and girdle obesity

62. A 16-year-old client with severe PIH is being treated with IV magnesium sulfate. The occurrence of which of the following client conditions would warrant stopping the infusion of the magnesium sulfate?
    A. Nausea, vomiting, and diarrhea
    B. The presence of facial edema
    C. Complaints of dizziness and lightheadedness
    D. The absence of deep-tendon reflexes (DTR)

63. A 22-year-old male client who is diagnosed as having antisocial personality disorder is sexually aggressive toward a young female client. What is the best nursing intervention?
    A. Explore feelings related to the inappropriate behavior.
    B. Encourage nurturing rather than seductive behavior.
    C. Set limits on the interaction and the behavior.
    D. Teach morally correct behavior.

64. A 25-year-old client who has just looked at her client record asks the nurse the meaning of the following letters and numbers: G5T2P1A1L3. Which of the following explanations by the nurse would be most accurate?
    A. This means you have been scheduled for five prenatal visits, you have been on time for two, canceled one, missed one, and were late for three.
    B. This means you have five children, two were born when they were due, one was early, and two were overdue.
    C. This means you have had five pregnancies, two babies were born when they were due, you had one baby born before 36 weeks, one abortion, and three living children.
    D. This means you have five children, two were born early, three were born at term, and you miscarried one time.

65. Which of the following information is most important in teaching parents about the hygiene of a preschooler?
    A. The parent should assist with or supervise all of his or her hygiene needs, especially bathtime, until age 5.
    B. The preschooler is fearful of being pulled down the drain because of the inability to judge size.
    C. The child cannot dress himself or herself completely until age 4.
    D. Specific instructions and directions with no options are best to ensure proper bathing and dressing.

66. The nurse recognizes that the most common cause of the mild normocytic normochromic anemia noted with hypothyroidism is:
    A. Decreased oxygen demand by the tissues
    B. Increased production of erythropoietin
    C. Deficient iron absorption in the diet
    D. Significant blood loss from menorrhagia

67. The 73-year-old was admitted from the nursing home with a urinary tract infection. The physician ordered cefazolin (Ancef) 750 mg IM every 8 hours. The 1-gm vial of powdered cefazolin was supplied with directions on the right side of the label as follows: "Add 2.5 ml sterile water . . . provides an approximate volume of 3.0 ml (330 mg/ml). How much does the nurse draw up?

A. 1.5 ml
B. 2.0 ml
C. 2.3 ml
D. 2.5 ml

68. A 9-year-old had orthopedic surgery because of multiple fractures to the right femur yesterday. The nurse brings a pain injection in after the mother requests the medicine. The nurse observes facial grimacing and a stiff body in the child. Which of the following behaviors is the most characteristic response of a school-age child receiving pain management?
   A. Expresses fear vocally.
   B. Physical resistance.
   C. Stalling behavior.
   D. Uncooperative.

69. The physician ordered estropipate (Ogen) 0.625 mg PO to prevent osteoporosis. The nurse instructed the client to take how many 1.5 mg tablets?
   A. 0.5 tablet
   B. 1.0 tablet
   C. 1.5 tablets
   D. 2.0 tablets

70. A 67-year-old female has a pressure ulcer on her sacrum; the area of broken epidermis is approximately 2 inches in diameter. The nurse would chart an estimate of the size and label the pressure area as a decubitus ulcer:
   A. Stage I
   B. Stage II
   C. Stage III
   D. Stage IV

71. A 16-year-old client from an influential family comes in for her first prenatal visit at 10 weeks' gestation. She is of average weight, denies use of alcohol but admits to smoking two to three cigarettes a day. Her initial laboratory shows that she is anemic. The nurse understands the factors that increase this client's nutritional risk factors include:
   A. Age and smoking
   B. Age and anemia
   C. Smoking and weight
   D. Socioeconomic status and age

72. A primipara in the eighth week of pregnancy attended a prenatal class on self-care in the first trimester of pregnancy. In conversing with the nurse in charge of education, the client reviews activities she should avoid at this stage of pregnancy. Which of the following statements would indicate that the client needs further instruction?
   A. "Someone else at home should clean out the cat litter box."
   B. "I should call my health-care provider before I take any kind of medicine."
   C. "I should eat five small meals a day."
   D. "I can relax in my hot tub at the end of the day."

73. A client is 4 days' postdelivery for a cesarean birth. Which of the following is true regarding uterine involution after a cesarean section?
   A. The uterus involutes 1 cm/day.
   B. Lochia increases about day 5.
   C. Lochia decreases about day 5.
   D. There is less risk for endometritis.

74. Administering blood transfusions under pressure places children at risk for developing a particular complication. The nurse identifies which complication as being associated with this practice?
   A. Air emboli
   B. Hemolytic reaction
   C. Allergic reaction
   D. Hypothermia

75. A 35-year-old female is treated for iron-deficiency anemia. The nurse reinforces dietary teaching to promote the client's recovery. Which foods does the nurse recommend as the best sources of dietary iron?
   A. Fried oysters, stewed tomatoes, salad, and juice
   B. Liver and onions, carrot and raisin salad, and milk
   C. Kidney beans and rice, spinach, orange sections, and tea
   D. Hamburger on whole wheat toast, sliced tomatoes, and corn

76. A prenatal examination at 38 weeks' gestation would require further investigation with these findings:
   A. Nocutria and epistaxis
   B. Lower-limb edema and leg cramps
   C. Moderate leukorrhea and urinary frequency
   D. Periorbital edema and proteinuria

77. A 44-year-old male is recovering from a myocardial infarction. The nurse explains that the Valsalva maneuver should be avoided because this maneuver will initially:
   A. Increase afterload
   B. Decrease afterload
   C. Decrease preload
   D. Increase preload

78. A 25-year-old female client was admitted to the psychiatric unit with panic disorder. Her symptoms are irritability, palpitations, tachycardia and sweating. She is fearful that she is suffering from a myocardial infarction. The initial nursing intervention should be to:
   A. Discuss the symptom complex.
   B. Provide safety and reduce the anxiety to a more tolerable level.
   C. Discuss the incapacitating disorder.
   D. Provide an anxiolytic medication.

79. A 6-year-old boy has asthma. His mother asks the nurse if he can participate in any sports. The nurse would recommend which of the following?
   A. Basketball

    B. Long-distance running
    C. Swimming
    D. Soccer

80. An 18-year-old woman was diagnosed with hypogonadism. She was treated with human chorionic gonadotropin (Pregynl) 500 units three times a week for 3 weeks. Once reconstituted, the vial will contain 1000 U/ml. How many milliliters will the nurse administer?
    A. 0.5 ml
    B. 1.0 ml
    C. 1.5 ml
    D. 2.0 ml

81. A mother has her 12-year-old daughter in the arthritis clinic. The physician prescribes naproxen (Naprosyn)—first dose 500 mg, then 250 mg every 8 hours—for signs and complaints of inflamed joints and pain. The mother asks how long it will take for the naproxen to be effective. Which of the following is the most accurate response by the nurse?
    A. "It is a long-acting drug and will take several months for therapeutic effect."
    B. Therapeutic effects may not be noticed for 3 to 4 weeks."
    C. "The medicine works rapidly, so she will be moving her joints better in 24 hours."
    D. "She will have relief of pain after the first dose, but the inflammation will not decrease for several days."

82. A client gave birth 10 minutes ago. The placenta has still not delivered. The nurse should:
    A. Inform the primary health-care provider.
    B. Apply traction to the umbilical cord.
    C. Prepare the client for surgery.
    D. Reassure the client that this is normal.

83. The nurse is caring for a 4-year-old child admitted with a history of spontaneous pneumothorax. The child has a closed-chest drainage system. The purpose of the water in the closed-chest drainage chamber is to:
    A. Decrease the danger of sudden change in pressure in the tube.
    B. Prevent entrance of air into the pleural cavity.
    C. Provide faster removal of chest secretions by capillary.
    D. Facilitate emptying bloody drainage from the chest.

84. The physician ordered chloral hydrate 750 mg PO for a 69-year-old nursing-home client with insomnia. Using a 500 mg/5 ml elixir, how many milliliters did the nurse administer?
    A. 5.5 ml
    B. 6.5 ml
    C. 7.5 ml
    D. 8.5 ml

85. A 54-year-old paraplegic is being discharged; the client will be cared for in the home. The nurse teaches the client and the caregiver interventions to prevent pressure ulcers. Such interventions include:
    A. Proper hand-washing technique
    B. Taking frequent rest periods
    C. Allowing family to provide self-care needs
    D. Maintaining a diet high in protein and vitamins C and E

86. A physical finding in a term newborn that would need further evaluation by the health-care team is:
    A. Cyanotic hands and feet with a respiratory rate of 54 per minute
    B. Dark blue marks over the buttocks and overriding cranial sutures
    C. Tufts of hair at the base of the spine
    D. Periobital edema and nevus flammeus over the forehead

87. A diabetic client has an area of broken skin in the groin. Pus and serous drainage are oozing from the area, and red streaks are noted radiating from the groin. The vital signs are within normal limits. The home health nurse would want the following laboratory tests run:
    A. Blood cultures and electrolyte panel
    B. CBC and wound culture
    C. BUN, creatinine, and liver function panel
    D. Prothrombin time and partial thromboplastin time

88. A client at 20 weeks' gestation reports to you that she is craving cornstarch and has been eating small amounts on a daily basis. The nurse knows the medical term for this condition is:
    A. Pytalism
    B. Couvade
    C. Pyrosis
    D. Pica

89. A 45-year-old female performs the repetitive act of checking the front door of her house to make certain that it is locked. She feels out of control and requests admission to the hospital. During the initial interview, the nurse observes that the client is restless and has difficulty focusing on the topic. The nurse is aware that the client's behavior represents an effort to:
    A. Relieve tension
    B. Control her thoughts
    C. Seek attention
    D. Control a phobia

90. A 6-month-old male infant was diagnosed at the clinic with mild phimosis. Which of these nursing interventions is important for an infant with mild phimosis?
    A. Teaching the parents foods high in potassium
    B. Teaching the parents proper cleansing technique
    C. Monitoring urinary output
    D. Monitoring abdominal girth

91. Discharge instructions for a client recovering from severe iron-deficiency anemia should emphasize the need for:
    A. Planned rest periods
    B. Fluid intake of 3000 cc daily
    C. A diet high in vitamin B_{12}
    D. A diet high in folic acid

92. A 2-year-old has been diagnosed with a urinary tract infection. While teaching the mother, the nurse identifies the following factor that has predisposed her daughter to a urinary tract infection:
    A. Increased fluid intake
    B. Frequent emptying of the bladder
    C. Ingestion of highly acidic juices
    D. Short urethra in young females

93. A couple is using breathing techniques to manage their labor. The prime reason for utilizing paced breathing patterns in labor is to:
    A. Maintain adequate oxygenation of the mother and the fetus.
    B. Provide a means of attention focusing.
    C. Eliminate need for analgesics.
    D. Increase mental relaxation.

94. A 33-year-old woman is placed on warfarin (Coumadin) therapy following replacement of the mitral valve. The nurse gives the client a list of foods that should be consumed in moderation. These foods are high in:
    A. Vitamin C
    B. Protein
    C. Calcium
    D. Vitamin K

95. A 9-year-old client has been treated for rhinitis over the last 2 months. The nurse correctly identifies which of the following as the most significant in producing symptoms of allergic rhinnitis?
    A. Antigen
    B. B lymphocytes
    C. Histamine
    D. Leukotrienes

96. For many women, one of the first signs of pregnancy is a fullness or tingling of the breasts. These changes are a result of:
    A. The presence of breast milk
    B. An enhanced sexual drive
    C. A decreased blood supply
    D. Hormonal changes

97. An 8-year-old boy was admitted to the hospital with an acute illness. During his admission assessment, the nurse notes the child's religious affiliation as Mormon. What beliefs about diet and food practices are common to this religion?
    A. May not have blood transfusions
    B. May eat meat from animals that are vegetable eaters, are cloven hoofed, and chew their cud

C. Avoidance of tea, coffee, chocolate, or products containing caffeine
    D. Fast for 6 hours before receiving Holy Communion

98. A client who has tried unsuccessfully to become pregnant for 2 years has been scheduled for a hysterosalpingography. The nurse identifies the purpose of this test as:
    A. It is an immunological test to determine sperm and cervical mucus compatibility and interaction.
    B. It is an examination of the lining of the uterus to detect secretory changes and how receptive it is to implantation of a fertilized egg.
    C. Examination of pelvic structures by inserting a small telescope through a small incision in the abdomen.
    D. Examination of the uterine cavity and tubes using a contrast material inserted through the cervix.

99. A 2-kg premature infant was experiencing respiratory distress syndrome. The physician ordered beractant 4 ml/kg. How many milliliters did the nurse administer?
    A. 2 ml
    B. 4 ml
    C. 6 ml
    D. 8 ml

100. A 15-year-old female is seen at the clinic and is diagnosed with a urinary tract infection. In preparing to teach her, the nurse would include which of the following in the plan of care?
    A. Informing her that the cause of such infection in adolescents is usually sexual activity.
    B. Drinking large amounts of carbonated beverages would help to dilute the urine.
    C. Douching would help to rid the vagina of bacteria.
    D. It is best to take showers because baths may contribute to bacterial growth that may predispose a female to a urinary tract infection.

101. During a group therapy session, the clinical nurse specialist supports the client as she discusses her ritualistic behavior. Which response by the nurse is most therapeutic?
    A. "I know that the ritual is troubling and difficult to control."
    B. "You have control over your behavior and you can change."
    C. "These thoughts began when you were a teenager."
    D. "I know that you can avoid the ritualistic thoughts if you try."

102. A cold-stressed infant was warmed to 99°F (core temperature) over a period of 4 hours. The infants' temperature has ranged from 98.4°F to 99.6°F for the last 24 hours. The infant has been

ingesting formula, 1 oz every 3 to 4 hours. The nurse should monitor which of the following laboratory results?
A. Serum calcium
B. Serum glucose
C. Serum sodium
D. Serum bilirubin

103. A 44-year-old client with chronic renal failure is being discharged. The nurse teaches the following home-care intervention to manage pruritus:
A. Keep the home warm and dry.
B. Clothing made of polyester will promote comfort.
C. Use a good laundry detergent to be sure clothes are clean.
D. Inspect the skin for redness, heat, swelling, and pain.

104. When comparing a child with PKU with an unaffected sibling, the child with PKU typically has:
A. A shorter stature
B. A larger abdomen
C. A larger head circumference
D. Lighter skin pigmentation

105. A 4-year-old male is admitted to the children's surgical unit for first stage repair of hypospadias. In considering the level of development of the preschool-age child, which of the following statements accurately describes this stage of development?
A. He is experiencing the electra complex.
B. He is beginning to question his sexuality.
C. He is anxious over penile size.
D. He is afraid of mutilation.

106. The nurse is caring for a client who has just received an epidural anesthetic. The nurse's first action should be:
A. Assess the client's blood pressure.
B. Document the client's tolerance of the procedure.
C. Assess the pain perception in the lower extremities.
D. Raise the client's head 45 degrees.

107. An alcoholic client is being discharged from the inpatient treatment setting on disulfiram (Antabuse). The nurse should instruct the client to avoid the use of:
A. Vinegar-based dressings, cough elixirs, and cologne
B. Cough elixirs, cologne, and acetaminophen
C. Cologne, acetaminophen, and penicillin
D. Acetaminophen, penicillin, and vinegar-based dressings

Contain alcohol

108. A 20-year-old client has third-degree burns on 9 percent of the body. The nurse explains to the family that one leg has been burned and that third degree means that:

A. Subcutaneous tissues and possibly underlying tissues are involved
B. Destruction of epidermis and dermis has occurred
C. Only the epidermis has been lost
D. The leg is covered by erythema and blisters

109. A 15-year-old female has been coming to the allergy clinic for immunotherapy weekly for the last 2 months. What is the minimal amount of time a nurse should observe the client for a systemic reaction after the immunotherapy?
A. 10 minutes
B. 20 minutes
C. 30 minutes
D. 60 minutes

110. Because of the client's history of a difficult vaginal delivery (shoulder dystocia), which of the following nursing measures is important in her neonatal care?
A. Avoid eliciting Moro's reflex.
B. Avoid pulling the infant up from under her arms.
C. Assess the symmetry of the scarf sign.
D. Prepare for a casting procedure to prevent movement.

111. A nurse is teaching a 65-year-old client about closed-angle glaucoma. Which of the following statements indicates a clear understanding of closed-angle glaucoma?
A. "I should never take over-the-counter medications without consulting my doctor."
B. "If I forget to take my eye drops, I just wait for the next dose."
C. "I can stop taking my eye drops when my vision improves."
D. "I will return to my eye doctor for a check-up every 2 years."

112. A 17-year-old female suspects she is 10 days' pregnant. Because she cannot come to the clinic this week, the client tells the nurse that she will use a home pregnancy test. The nurse should reinforce:
A. Consumer tests have a higher rate of false-positives
B. Consumer tests are easy to use
C. Repeating negative results in a week if amenorrhea continues
D. Keeping her results private

113. When planning care for a client with pheochromocytoma, which nursing diagnosis is most appropriate to include in the plan of care?
A. Activity intolerance
B. Ineffective airway clearance
C. Potential fluid volume excess
D. Altered elimination: constipation

114. The nurse is caring for a 38-year-old client with an obsessive-compulsive disorder who is ready to focus on strategies that will reduce anxiety. Which

one of the following nursing interventions would be most appropriate?
- A. Allow the client to complete the ritualistic act.
- B. Offer protection from injury.
- C. Provide simple exercises.
- D. Assist the client to gain control over the compulsive act.

115. A 24-year-old client at term who is 5 cm dilated, fully effaced, and at 0 station is no longer able to cope effectively with her uterine contractions. She has requested that an epidural block be administered. Immediately after an epidural block has been administered, the nurse would observe the client for?
- A. Increased frequency and intensity of uterine contractions
- B. Increased variability in the fetal heart tracing
- C. Increased maternal palpitations
- D. Decreased maternal blood pressure

116. On assessment, the nurse might find that the client with acromegaly will often have:
- A. Vitiligo
- B. Dry skin
- C. Joint pain
- D. Sparse hair growth

117. The nurse is assessing a young child for strabismus. She explains to the child's mother the importance for detecting strabismus by which of the following statements?
- A. "Corneal light reflexes may fall symmetrically within each pupil."
- B. "Epicanthal folds may develop in the affected eye."
- C. "Amblyopia may result."
- D. "Color-blindness may result."

118. One hour after delivery, a client has a temperature of 99°F. This is a likely first indication of
- A. Thrombophlebitis
- B. Breast engorgement
- C. Dehydration
- D. Hypovolemic shock

119. Which of the following statements by the psychiatric client would indicate that a dose of benztropine (Cogentin) has been effective?
- A. "I'm beginning to feel sleepy since you gave me that shot."
- B. "I should be able to think more clearly now."
- C. "My neck isn't as stiff as it was this morning."
- D. "My mouth is very dry now that you've given me the Cogentin."

120. During a nonstress test, what is the nurse assessing for to assure fetal well-being?
- A. Contractions
- B. Decelerations
- C. Accelerations
- D. Fetal movement

121. When reading an EKG, the nurse correctly identifies the QRS complex on an EKG as representing what phase of electrical activity within the heart?
- A. Atrial depolarization
- B. Ventricular depolarization
- C. Electrical recovery from ventricular contraction
- D. Impulse conduction from the SA node to the AV node

122. Which of the following indicates expected behavior from a 4-year-old?
- A. The child may tell "tall tales" and may have imaginary playmates.
- B. Extra demands for attention because of fear of loss of love are common.
- C. The child still clings to the security blanket.
- D. The child will be more tranquil than at 3 years old.

123. A 24-year-old was experiencing postpartal depression. The physician ordered nortriptyline (Aventyl) 100 mg PO HS. The nurse instructed the client to take how many 50 mg tablets?
- A. ½ tablet
- B. 1 tablet
- C. 1½ tablets
- D. 2 tablets

124. An 8-year-old child is admitted to the pediatric unit with a diagnosis of acute glomerulonephritis (AGN). A nursing care plan would include which of the following?
- A. Forcing fluids on him
- B. Increasing the sodium in his diet
- C. Weighing him daily
- D. Taking his vital signs once per shift

125. A 16-year-old girl developed macrocytic anemia secondary to pregnancy. The physician ordered 1 mg of folic acid IM for 4 to 5 days. Using a 5 mg/ml vial, the nurse administered how many milliliters?
- A. 0.1 ml
- B. 0.2 ml
- C. 0.3 ml
- D. 1.0 ml

126. A 2-day-old term male is receiving his discharge physical by the nurse. Which of the following physical examination findings could indicate congenital cataracts?
- A. Absence of the red reflex
- B. Edematous eyelids
- C. Absence of tears
- D. Strabismus

127. A 23-year-old female is 7 months' pregnant. She has not received prenatal health care, and she has a folic acid deficiency. The nurse reinforces dietary teaching. Which best provides folic acid for this client?
- A. Lentil soup, sliced applies, bagel, and coffee

B. Scrambled eggs, bacon, whole wheat toast, and milk

C. Broiled chicken, corn, whole wheat toast, and tea

D. White beans and rice, spinach, cornbread, and milk

128. A 38-year-old female entered the mental health clinic complaining that she has an irrational fear of spiders. She said to the nurse, "I can't even tolerate looking at a picture of a spider without having a severe anxiety attack." The best nursing action is to:
A. Acknowledge the client's feelings and concerns.
B. Discuss the desensitization procedure.
C. Explain the relationship between phobia and fear.
D. Suggest the client resume normal life activities.

129. The upper portion of the female uterus that can easily be palpated in the postpartum woman is the:
A. Cervix
B. Fundus
C. Body
D. Crest

130. Ivan, a 12-year old hemophiliac patient, is admitted to the hospital for a bleed following a fall at school. Which of the following is characteristic of hemophilia and therefore would most likely be observed when initially assessing Ivan?
A. Petechiae
B. Dehydration
C. Hemarthrosis
D. Neutropenia

131. A client with non–insulin-dependent diabetes mellitus (NIDDM) is found in a coma; the skin is warm, dry, and flushed. The nurse would expect the physician to order:
A. Epinephrine
B. Fluid
C. Prednisone
D. Bicarbonate

132. A 6-year-old returned to the pediatric unit 8 hours ago after having an open reduction to repair a fractured radius. The nurse is assessing the child's neurovascular status. Which of the following would require immediate attention?
A. Coolness to the affected fingers with a palpable radial pulse
B. Coolness to the affected fingers with a capillary refill of 5 seconds
C. Edema and bruised appearance to the affected fingers
D. Edema to the fingers and a capillary refill of 2 seconds to the affected arm

133. A client at term has just delivered a term infant. Which of the following actions by the nurse should have first priority?

A. Suction the nose and mouth of the infant.
B. Check the heart rate of the infant.
C. Place identification bands on the infant.
D. Dry the infant.

134. The nurse asks the psychiatric client on admission, "Do you think you have a mental illness?" What area of the mental status is the nurse assessing?
A. Mood
B. Thought processes
C. General fund of knowledge
D. Insight

135. A client with acute leukemia is started on allopurinol (Zyloprim). Which nursing intervention should be implemented while the client takes allopurinol?
A. Restrict sodium intake.
B. Encourage a bland diet.
C. Encourage fluid intake.
D. Discourage carbonated fluids.

136. Which finding indicates that a client who takes nitroglycerine (NTG) needs further teaching to prevent complications?
A. Took six NTG before notifying the physician.
B. Places the tablet under the tongue until dissolved.
C. Stores the medication in an airtight, dark bottle.
D. Reports that he premedicates prior to sexual intercourse.

137. When the client's membranes spontaneously rupture, the nurse's first action is to:
A. Change the client's linen.
B. Notify the primary health-care provider.
C. Assess fetal heart tones.
D. Document the client's response to the event.

138. The clinical manifestation of sickle-cell disease is the result of:
A. Hypertension
B. Hypotension
C. Intravascular clotting
D. Edema

139. The best nursing intervention for a client with a social phobia is to:
A. Recommend psychoanalysis.
B. Provide reassurance and support.
C. Encourage public speaking.
D. Explain the dysfunctional behavior.

140. A term infant who is classified as macrosomic is likely the product of a mother who has:
A. Pregnancy-induced hypertension
B. Lupus
C. Gestational diabetes
D. HIV

141. A diabetic client had 30 units of NPH insulin SC at 8 A.M. The nurse might plan for this client to have a snack between:
A. 10 A.M. and 2 P.M.
B. 12 noon and 4 P.M.

C. 2 P.M. and 8 P.M.
D. 4 P.M. and 7 P.M.

142. The nurse identifies that the best way to determine the effectiveness of nasotracheal suctioning is:
A. Check chest rays before and after suctioning.
B. Ask the client if she can breathe more easily.
C. Observe the rate and rhythm of respirations.
D. Auscultate the chest before and after suctioning.

143. A client delivered her firstborn via cesarean section 8 hours ago. She is eager to breastfeed her baby and she is requesting pain medication. The nurse should advise her that:
A. If she receives an analgesic, she will be too drowsy to nurse her baby.
B. The analgesic will be given just after breastfeeding.
C. The pain medication will inhibit her milk production.
D. She should pump her breast to avoid contamination of her milk.

144. When assessing the client with aplastic anemia, the nurse identifies pancytopenia associated with aplastic anemia, which will be reflected in the client's laboratory work as:
A. RBCs 900,000; WBCs 1000; and platelets 25,000
B. RBCs 3 million; WBCs 6000; and platelets 85,000
C. Hct 36 and Hgb 12
D. Hct 42 and Hgb 14

145. A 28-year-old nullipara, 32 weeks' gestation, is admitted to the labor unit with abdominal pain and intermittent, mild vaginal bleeding. She is physically exhausted and disoriented. She states she has a cold. There is evidence of nasal inflammation. This client states she free-based cocaine 1 hour ago. The nurse recognizes that the client is at greatest risk for:
A. Abruptio placenta
B. Malnutrition
C. Congenital malformation
D. Pulmonary embolism

146. A client receives an injection of NPH Humulin insulin 20 units subcutaneously at 6:30 A.M. The nurse should monitor the client most closely for evidence of hypoglycemia around:
A. 8:30 A.M. to 9:30 A.M.
B. 9 A.M. to 11 A.M.
C. 12:30 P.M. to 2:30 P.M.
D. 10 P.M. to 12 A.M.

147. A 47-year-old was treated with isoniazid 5 mg/kg PO every day for tuberculosis. The client weighed 57 kg and required 285 mg per dose. Using a 50 mg/5 ml elixir, how many milliliters did the nurse administer?
A. 25.5 ml

B. 26.5 ml
C. 27.5 ml
D. 28.5 ml

148. Which of the following nursing diagnoses of a psychiatric client should be the highest priority when developing a plan of care?
A. Knowledge deficit related to psychiatric medications
B. Impaired mobility related to lack of motivation
C. Self-esteem related to depression
D. High risk for self-harm related to ineffective coping skills

149. The descent of the fetal head into the pelvis prior to delivery is called:
A. Quickening
B. Effacement
C. Lightening
D. Station

150. An 11-year-old was admitted with hypertension. The child weighed 52 kg. The physician ordered verapamil 0.3 mg/kg (15.6 mg) over 2 minutes IV bolus. Using a 2.5 mg/ml vial, how many milliliters did the nurse administer IV?
A. 6.24 ml
B. 7.24 ml
C. 8.24 ml
D. 9.24 ml

151. A child is admitted to the hospital with asthma. His current peak expiratory flow rate is in the red zone. The nurse would interpret this information as:
A. A medical alert since the child is below 50 percent of his personal best
B. A signal that he is clear since he is 80 to 100 percent of his personal best
C. A signal of caution since he is 50 to 80 percent of his personal best
D. A signal of caution since he is 80 percent of his personal best

152. A 74-year-old male client reports difficulty with urination. He reports symptoms of frequency, urgency, nocturia, and urge incontinence. Based on the symptoms expressed by the client, the initial action by the nurse is to:
A. Obtain a urine sample for creatinine clearance function.
B. Obtain a computerized axial tomography (CAT) scan.
C. Perform a mental status examination for cognitive function.
D. Perform a physical examination for prostate enlargement.

153. A client gave birth to her first infant (a boy) 15 minutes ago over a second-degree midline episiotomy. Vital signs are temperature 99.8°F, BP 110/68, pulse 102, respirations 22. Pitocin 10 mg was added to the IV fluids after delivery of the pla-

centa and is infusing at 125 cc/hr. The fundus is firm at the umbilicus, and lochia is moderate rubra with one quarter sized clot noted. The infant is being held by the new father while the new mother states, "We really wanted a little girl, but a boy is fine." Which of the following nursing diagnoses are most appropriate for this stage of labor?
A. High risk for injury related to uterine atony and hemorrhage
B. Altered family processes, potential for growth
C. Potential for infection related to altered skin integrity
D. Anxiety related to a new parenting role

154. Patrick has leukemia. Patient-family education would appropriately include that the side effects of cancer chemotherapy are usually:
A. Impossible to relieve
B. Temporary and reversible
C. Caused by effects on the cancer cells
D. Mostly psychological

155. A 37-year-old client dances toward her room, examines the door, turns around three times, and then backs into the door, pushing it open. This ritualistic behavior is performed several times a day. The best nursing action is to:
A. Approach the client in a calm, direct, nonauthoritative manner.
B. Interrupt the ritualistic behavior.
C. Avoid discussing the behavior.
D. Explain that the ritual is part of the anxiety behavior.

156. The most common internal congenital abnormality associated with a single umbilical artery in a newborn is:
A. Imperforate anus
B. Hepatosplenomegaly
C. Renal anomalies
D. Cardiac malformations

157. The client asks the nurse how to tell the difference between true and false labor. She is frustrated because she has been having irregular contractions and a backache for several days. What is the nurse's best response?
A. "When you are really in labor, you'll know it."
B. "When your cervix begins to soften and your contractions vary in frequency, you need to go to the hospital."
C. "The baby will get more active and you'll notice a clear vaginal discharge."
D. "Your health-care provider will have to check for cervical change to determine when you are really in labor."

158. A client has been in seclusion and restraints for 4 hours because of an outburst of angry behavior in which he injured another client on the unit. What criterion will the nurse use to determine if the client should be released from restraints?

A. The client apologizes to the injured client and offers to pay for the necessary treatment.
B. The physician must see the client in restraints and make the determination about whether he should be released or not.
C. The minimum amount of time spent in seclusion and restraints for violent behavior resulting in injury to self or others is 6 hours.
D. The violent behavior has subsided and a therapeutic alliance between nurse and client has occurred.

159. Which of the following approaches by the nurse is best when administering an IM injection of an antibiotic to a 2-year-old?
A. Tell the child it will not hurt, secure the child, and administer the antibiotic IM.
B. Tell the child there will be a little stick in the arm and explain that it will hurt a little.
C. Allow the child to assist in drawing up the medication beforehand.
D. Enter the room with medication prepared, briefly state you are giving him a shot, administer it, and comfort the child.

160. The home health nurse has recommended biofeedback for the client who is experiencing incontinence. The following information is most important in evaluating the client for biofeedback as a treatment modality:
A. Medical factors and motivation
B. Medical factors and family support
C. Mental status and family support
D. Mental status and motivation

161. A 28-year-old multigravida expresses concern about the darkened blotches on her face and neck. Which of the following responses by the nurse is most appropriate?
A. "That is your body's announcement to the world that you are pregnant."
B. "Let's review your diet for the past 24 hours. This hyperpigmentation is diet related."
C. "These skin changes are normal and often fade after the baby is born."
D. "Have you considered using pigment-lightening cream?"

162. A nurse is caring for a client with end-stage renal disease (ESRD). The physician recommends continuous ambulatory peritoneal dialysis (CAPD) for this client. The most important reason for the physician's recommendation is:
A. CAPD is more rapid and effective in renal clearance.
B. CAPD increases the client's socialization during treatment.
C. CAPD increases the client's feelings of self-control.
D. CAPD requires scheduled interaction with dialysis personnel.

163. A nurse working with the health department is preparing a health promotion program for a group of older adults that will focus on normal aging changes. The nurse identifies that the most significant physiological changes that occur with normal aging are:
   A. Loss of skin turgor, increase in lean body mass, and decreased immune function
   B. Loss of skin turgor, increase in bone density, and loss of visual acuity
   C. Loss of lean body mass, decrease in bone density, and depressed immune function
   D. Loss of lean body mass, loss of visual acuity, and increase in bone density

164. A common assessment used to evaluate fetal presentation, position, and engagement is called:
   A. Leopold's maneuver
   B. Babinski's assessment
   C. Walker's maneuver
   D. Lamaze technique

165. It is important for the nurse to understand that repetitive ritualistic behavior aims to:
   A. Control the environment.
   B. Send love messages.
   C. Prevent or reduce distress.
   D. Seek attention.

166. In order to assess a child's capillary filling time, the nurse would do which of the following?
   A. Palpate the carotid artery.
   B. Inspect the bucal membranes.
   C. Ascultate the heart.
   D. Palpate the skin to produce a slight blanching.

167. The nurse is instructing a 70-year-old client scheduled for discharge. The client is beginning continuous ambulatory peritoneal dialysis (CAPD). The most important information the nurse gives this client is:
   A. Information about performing sterile technique.
   B. Information about follow-up appointments.
   C. Information about a low-sodium diet.
   D. Information about prescribed diuretics.

168. An expectant mother is in her third trimester and has low-back discomfort. Which exercise should the nurse suggest to alleviate her low-back pain?
   A. Deep knee bends
   B. Pelvic floor exercises
   C. Double leg lifts
   D. Pelvic tilts

169. An older adult is being treated for a gynecologic malignancy. The head nurse indicates to the staff that a conference is necessary to discuss the sexual function of this client. The rationale for the request made by the head nurse is:
   A. Sex is not particularly important to women over 70.
   B. Gynecologic malignancy hinders all sexual relationships.
   C. Sexual counseling is based on the needs of each individual.
   D. Women don't engage in sexual relations because of the lack of a partner.

170. The physician ordered the nurse to give 30 units of Novolin N NPH insulin and 10 units of Novolin R regular insulin for the client with unstable type I diabetic. How would the nurse draw up the insulin order?
   A. Draw up the NPH insulin first, then the regular insulin.
   B. Draw up the regular insulin first, then the NPH insulin.
   C. Draw up the insulins in two separate syringes.
   D. Withdraw NPH insulin and then inject air into the regular insulin vial.

171. When planning nursing care for a 5-year-old child, which nursing action is most appropriate for the child placed under an oxygen mist tent?
   A. Encourage the child to keep stuffed animals in bed with him or her.
   B. Encourage the use of a battery-operated tape player for music.
   C. Use only synthetic blankets under the tent.
   D. Use a plastic or vinyl doll for play.

172. A 28-year-old was having severe anxiety from acute alcohol withdrawal. The physician ordered chlordiazepoxide (Librium) 25 mg tid IM. Using a 100 mg/ml vial, how many milliliters did the nurse administer?
   A. 0.25 ml
   B. 0.50 ml
   C. 0.75 ml
   D. 1.0 ml

173. A home health nurse is caring for a client who has had a head injury. The client is started on a bowel management program. Which statement made by the family would indicate to the nurse that the instruction has been understood?
   A. "The program should be done during the week but not on weekends."
   B. "The program should be initiated before breakfast every third day."
   C. "The program requires being placed on the toilet 1 hour after initiation."
   D. "The program will cause diarrhea, and good skin care is necessary."

174. A nurse on a geriatric unit is admitting an 80-year-old. Family members report that the client has lost 16 lb recently. Laboratory values for this client include: serum albumin 2 gm/dl, serum transferrin 100 mg/dl, and lymphocytes 750 cells/mm. The nurse correctly identifies that this client is experiencing:
   A. Dementia

B. Diarrhea
C. Malnutrition
D. Depression

175. An 18-year-old client who is visiting the clinic for a yearly physical tells the nurse that her menses are 2 weeks late. She asks the nurse how to know for sure if she is pregnant. Which of the following explanations by the nurse would be most accurate?
A. A positive pregnancy test is the best indicator of pregnancy.
B. The best way to know if you are pregnant is through an ultrasound.
C. If the examination reveals a bluish coloration and softness of the cervix, you are pregnant.
D. If you don't have a period for 2 months, you are pregnant.

176. The family of a 78-year-old client express concern that they think their family member is dehydrated. Which symptoms, if experienced by the client, would the nurse expect to see in making a diagnosis?
A. Mental confusion, dry mouth, and hypertension
B. Constipation, elevated temperature, and hypertension
C. Sunken eyeballs, diarrhea, and hypotension
D. Mental confusion, hypotension, and weak pulse

177. Early clinical signs of polycythemia in a newborn are:
A. Jaundice
B. Plethoric and cyanotic look
C. Hepatosplenomegaly
D. Elevated temperature

178. The nurse is caring for a client receiving docusate sodium (Colace). Which action by the nurse is essential when caring for clients receiving this medication?
A. Close monitoring of serum electrolyte values
B. Reducing the amount of dietary fiber
C. Encouraging 2500 ml of fluids daily
D. Testing monthly for blood in the feces

179. The nurse is presenting a program on cataracts at a senior citizen center. The nurse reports that the cardinal symptom in the detection of cataracts is:
A. A continuous dull ache behind the eye
B. A sharp pain that radiates through the eye
C. A slowly progressive, painless loss of vision
D. A small node growing on the inner lens

180. The parents of a terminally ill girl who has been hospitalized many times tell a nurse that they think they will lose their daughter during the present hospitalization. The nurse should:
A. Reply quietly, "She does seem to be quite sick this time."
B. Ask the doctor to order a sedative for the parents.
C. Introduce another topic of conversation.
D. Say soothingly, "You shouldn't have waited so long to bring her here."

181. Your client who has been breastfeeding her newborn for 2 weeks reports that she has an area in her left breast that is warm to the touch and painful. She has been experiencing an elevated temperature and chills. The most likely diagnosis for this client is:
A. An upper respiratory infection
B. Mastitis
C. Blocked lactiferous duct
D. Cystitis

182. A 74-year-old client is admitted to the hospital with symptoms of right upper quadrant pain and a 4-lb weight loss in the last month. Laboratory results indicate an elevated serum alkaline phosphatase and decreased albumin. The physician orders a CT scan and an abdominal ultrasound to confirm the diagnosis. The client asks the nurse why the physician would order both these tests. The nurse correctly identifies the reason for this order is:
A. The physician is afraid of a malpractice suit if he makes an error in diagnosis.
B. The CT scan would find a lesion, and ultrasound would indicate abdominal function.
C. CT scans may help document lesions but may miss lesions that are tumorous.
D. These symptoms are rare and need both visual and auditory equipment to diagnose.

183. A newly diagnosed diabetic is being discharged; the client is to give himself insulin when he goes home. Prior to discharging the client, the nurse sees that he:
A. Explains all of the details about how to give the insulin
B. Administers the injection into an orange
C. Administers the injection to a significant other
D. Administers the insulin to himself

184. A client asks for a list of foods that are rich in iron. Which of the following foods would the nurse recommend?
A. Milk, nuts, and poultry
B. Citrus fruits, tomatoes, and broccoli
C. Potatoes, bananas, and yogurt
D. Eggs, green leafy vegetables, and liver

185. A psychotic client has been taking chlorpromazine (Thorazine) 25 mg tid for 2 years. He approaches the nurse and tells her, "My tongue seems to want to stick out of my mouth, and I'm afraid that people will think that I'm sticking my tongue out at them. What should I do?" The nurse's next action should be to:
A. Report these symptoms to the physician.
B. Assess for signs of tardive dyskinesia by using the abnormal inventory movement scale (AIMS).
C. Call the physician and obtain an order for benztropine (Cogentin).
D. Chart the client's complaint in the record and pass the word along to the oncoming shift.

186. The nurse knows that HIV causes which of the following abnormal T-cell ratios?
    A. Increase in helper T cells and decrease in suppressor T cells
    B. Decrease in cytotoxic cells and increase in helper T cells
    C. Increase in cytotoxic cells and decrease in memory cells
    D. Decrease in helper T cells and increase in suppressor T cells

187. Your client has given birth to her first baby by cesarean section. Which assessment data would cause you to suspect a pulmonary embolism?
    A. Dyspnea and complaints of a sharp, stabbing pain in her chest
    B. Hypertension with cool, moist skin
    C. Decreased hematocrit and tachycardia
    D. Palpitations and vasoconstriction

188. A 6-month-old infant is being discharged on a liquid iron preparation. The nurse would need to teach which of the following to the mother concerning the administration of the iron preparation?
    A. An adequate dosage will turn the infant's stools a tarry green color.
    B. Mix the iron preparation with the infant's formula.
    C. Bathe the infant's teeth with the iron preparation.
    D. Notify the physician of constipation.

189. The nurse caring for a client with rheumatoid arthritis (RA) recognizes that as RA evolves, pannus formation is identified when:
    A. Synovium thickens, becomes hyperemic, and fluid accumulates in joint space.
    B. Inflammatory granulation tissue develops over the popliteal bursae.
    C. Granulation tissue is invaded with fibrous tissue.
    D. Fibrous tissue calcifies, causing a firm, bony union.

190. The nurse is caring for an infant who is receiving gavage feedings. To determine the length of tube needed to reach the stomach, the nurse should:
    A. Advance the tube until resistance is met.
    B. Advance the tube as far as necessary to aspirate gastric contents.
    C. Measure the distance from the nose to the earlobe to the epigastric area of the abdomen.
    D. Measure from the mouth to the umbilicus and add half the distance.

191. A 43-year-old client who shares a hospital room with another person is constantly rearranging the furniture and the linens. The roommate complains to the charge nurse. The best nursing intervention is to:
    A. Separate the roommates.
    B. Confront the behavior.
    C. Limit the behavior in a supportive manner.

    D. Increase the medication.

192. The nurse admits a 13-year-old in labor. The client is a G4 P0 AB3, 40 weeks' gestation. On assessment, the nurse notes that the fundal height is 40 cm, cervix is 100 percent effaced, 3 cm dilated, and at −4 station. Based on these findings, what is the priority area of concern that should be considered?
    A. Because the client has already had three babies, she will be at risk for hemorrhage.
    B. The client will be emotionally upset because she has "lost" three other babies.
    C. Because she is so young, her pelvis may be underdeveloped and not adequate for the fetus to pass through.
    D. The fetus may be too small to survive the delivery.

193. The nurse recognizes that which one of the following clients would be of most concern to develop pneumonia?
    A. A 45-year-old after thyroidectomy
    B. A 32-year-old with history of HIV infection
    C. An 87-year-old after colon resection
    D. A 5-year-old after tonsillectomy

194. The nurse recognizes that the principal hormones secreted by the anterior pituitary (adenohypophysis) include:
    A. Thyroid-stimulating hormone (TSH), adrenocorticotropic hormone (ACTH), and calcitonin
    B. Adrenocorticotropic hormone (ACTH), thyroid-stimulating hormone (TSH), and growth hormone (GH)
    C. Thyroid-stimulating hormone (TSH), follicle-stimulating hormone (FSH), and antidiuretic hormone (ADH)
    D. Adrenocorticotropic hormone (ACTH), oxytocin, and aldosterone

195. A client calls the clinic to report sore nipples after 3 days of breastfeeding. The nurse should:
    A. Instruct her to use nipple shields while nursing.
    B. Encourage her to nurse less frequently, but for longer time periods.
    C. Encourage her to continue nursing the baby through the discomfort.
    D. Observe and assess the infant's position on the breast.

196. A 27-year-old developed a respiratory infection secondary to a tuberculin lung. The physician ordered streptomycin 1 gm every day IM to be given along with antituberculin drugs. Using a 1 gm/ml vial, how many milliliters did the nurse administer IM?
    A. 0.5 ml
    B. 1.0 ml
    C. 1.5 ml
    D. 2.0 ml

197. A 6-year-old child has been diagnosed with iron-

deficiency anemia. Which of the following foods should the nurse recommend to increase the amount of iron in the diet?
A. Milk
B. Orange or yellow vegetables
C. Meat
D. Citrus fruits

198. A manic client is being admitted for assessment, diagnosis, and stabilization. On admission, the client paces and is intrusive and loquacious. The nurse is able to redirect the focus of the client, but with difficulty, because he continues to dominate the conversation and stays wide of the point when asked a question. The client's speech could best be described as:
A. Pressured and tangential
B. Tangential and loud
C. Loud and illogical
D. Illogical and pressured

199. A client confides in the nurse that she has been taking megadoses of vitamin A because someone told her it would help the baby's vision. The nurse's response should be based on the knowledge that vitamin A:
A. Does accelerate retinal development and will increase the chance of the baby having good vision
B. Has teratogenic effects on the fetus when taken in large doses
C. Is one of the vitamins that is frequently deficient in the body, and extra doses will be beneficial
D. Is a water-soluble vitamin that requires frequent doses to maintain the appropriate level in the body

200. The nurse is assessing a client who recently received third-degree burns on 22 percent of the body. When no bowel sounds are detected, the nurse suspects that:
A. A stress ulcer has developed.
B. Hypovolemia has caused decreased blood supply to the intestines.
C. Ileus has occurred.
D. The gastrointestinal tract is empty.

201. A 35-year-old client is being seen in the clinic today for possible systemic lupus erythematosus (SLE). When performing the assessment, the nurse knows that the most significant sign or symptom present in SLE is:
A. Recurrent petechiae on the abdomen
B. Recurrent low-grade afternoon fever
C. Recurrent multiple ecchymoses over entire body
D. Recurrent butterfly rash over cheeks and nose

202. A 24-year-old G1 now P1 with O negative blood type has just delivered the placenta. She plans to bottle feed. Ten units of oxytocin (Pitocin) is added to IV fluids of 1000 cc normal saline and hung. What is the purpose of giving the client Pitocin?
A. To prevent the breast milk from coming in
B. To promote the formation of clotting factors
C. To prevent the formation of anti-Rh antibodies
D. To stimulate uterine contractions and prevent hemorrhage

203. A 32-year-old post-appendectomy client's incision has become infected and now requires wound care every 8 hours. When packing the incision with a saline-soaked 4 × 4 bandage, the nurse accidentally drops the dressing on the client's chest. The most appropriate intervention by the nurse would be to:
A. Use that bandage because the client just had a bed bath.
B. Resoak this bandage in sterile normal saline for 5 minutes and place it in the incision.
C. Use this bandage last and place it on top of the other sterile bandages used to dress the wound.
D. Discard this bandage and prepare a new one.

204. On afternoon rounds, the nurse sees the parent of a terminal cancer client weeping silently. What would be the most appropriate nursing intervention?
A. Tell her you understand how she feels.
B. Tell her she mustn't cry. Everything is going to be all right.
C. Go immediately to her bedside and ask her what she is crying about.
D. Sit in the chair beside her. Put your hand on her hand and wait for her to speak.

205. An 85-year-old client in a skilled-care facility has an infected leg ulcer. Hot, moist packs are ordered. The nurse knows to use extreme caution in applying these packs, based on the knowledge that many elderly clients have:
A. Reduced sensation to temperature stimuli
B. No sensitivity to pain
C. Increased sensation to nerve pathways
D. Thickened integumentary areas

206. A newly admitted 63-year-old male client is agitated and crying. He asks the nurse just prior to bedtime to talk with him about his emotional state. The nurse's best response should be:
A. "No, you control your actions."
B. "It is time for bed, we will talk in the morning."
C. "I can see that you are upset. I'm here when you want to talk."
D. "I don't have time; I'll find someone to talk with you."

207. An infant born at 33 weeks' gestation weighing 1250 gms and falling below the 10th percentile would be classified as:
A. Post-term AGA
B. Preterm LGA
C. Preterm SGA
D. Term SGA

208. Which of the following is an accurate descriptor of Hirschsprung's disease?
  A. Protrusion of a portion of bowel through a weakness in the abdominal wall, resulting in intestinal obstruction
  B. Twisting of the intestines, resulting in a lack of peristalsis
  C. One portion of intestine invaginates into another, resulting in intestinal obstruction
  D. Absence of nerve cells in an intestinal segment, resulting in a lack of peristalsis

209. The nurse is caring for an older adult with a diagnosis of AIDS. The client complains of pain in the oral cavity. The nurse notes a lesion on the mucosa of the mouth that resembles cottage cheese. The nurse correctly identifies this lesion as:
  A. Oral squamous-cell carcinoma
  B. Oral candidiasis
  C. Oral Kaposi's sarcoma
  D. Oral herpes simplex

210. A client is detoxing from a large ingestion of lysergic acid (LSD). He tells the nurse that every time someone enters his room, he sees continuous, slow blurring images following behind the person. He is afraid he has permanently damaged his vision. The nurse should recognize the client's symptoms as:
  A. Detached retina
  B. Trailing phenomenon
  C. Visual hallucinations
  D. Illusions

211. A 24-year-old pregestational diabetic client attending a class on breastfeeding indicated to the nurse that she was interested in breastfeeding. However, she stated, "My mother told me the baby would get too much sugar and be too fat if I breastfed because my milk would have too much sugar in it." Which of the following explanations regarding breastfeeding and diabetes would be most accurate?
  A. "She's right, you shouldn't breastfeed. Your milk will pick up the sugar from your blood."
  B. "You should definitely breastfeed. It has advantages for you and your baby."
  C. "You can breastfeed. The insulin you take will counteract the high sugar levels in your milk."
  D. "You would have to add 500 extra calories to your diet if you breastfed. That is too may calories for a diabetic woman."

212. An accurate nursing assessment of a 46-year-old client for early signs and symptoms of tuberculosis would include:
  A. Elevated white blood cell (WBC) count, diaphoresis, hypertension, and anorexia
  B. Fatigue, low-grade afternoon fever, weight loss, and cough
  C. Chest pain, enlarged cervical lymph nodes, joint pain, and chills
  D. Bradycardia, weight gain, subnormal temperature, and elevated sedimentation rate

213. You are the nurse caring for a 55-year-old client who was in a motor vehicle accident and had extensive abdominal trauma requiring liver repair, an exploratory laparotomy, and a splenectomy. It is the second day postoperatively and he begins to cough forcefully. On assessment you notice several abdominal sutures are broken, the incision is open, and part of the intestine is protruding. You would recognize that which of the following interventions would be least beneficial to the client?
  A. Gently push the intestine back into the abdominal cavity, then cover the area with a sterile dressing.
  B. Cover the entire area with sterile dressings and apply enough sterile saline solution to keep the dressing moist.
  C. Prepare the client for surgery.
  D. Place the client in a low Fowler's position with knees flexed.

214. A client had one male child born at 40 weeks' gestation. Her second pregnancy ended at 11 weeks. Which of the following is an accurate description?
  A. Gravida II para I ab I
  B. Gravida II para I ab 0
  C. Gravida II para II ab I
  D. Gravida I para I ab I

215. Which one of the following nursing interventions would be most beneficial to do when caring for a client in a coma?
  A. Effective communication to client and family
  B. Range-of-motion exercises every hour
  C. Begin discharge planning as early as possible
  D. Maintaining skin integrity by frequent turning

216. A 69-year-old client has been diagnosed with a nosocomial infection. The nurse recognizes that the term nosocomial infection means:
  A. Infection acquired at home
  B. Communicable diseases
  C. Health facility acquired infections
  D. Sexually transmitted

217. A client who is 26 weeks' pregnant asks what she can do to relieve her constipation. The best nursing response would be:
  A. "Perform an enema until the fluid returned is clear."
  B. "Try eating a cereal high in fiber each morning, have a high-fiber snack, and increase your intake of fluids."
  C. "Take a laxative now, and every third day until delivery."
  D. "Constipation is normal in pregnancy and nothing to worry about."

218. A 45-year-old farmer is admitted to the emergency department with complaints of itching and blistering of the hands and face. He tells you that he was spraying a vegetable garden yesterday with

chemicals. The emergency department nurse suspects that this client has:
A. Contact dermatitis
B. Erythema nodosum
C. Erysipelas
D. Seborrhea

219. The appropriate techniques the nurse uses to assess a client with complaints of itching and blistering of the hands and face after exposure to a chemical aerosol are:
A. Patch test and observation
B. Neurological checks and observation
C. History and inspection
D. History and vital signs

220. The most concerning problem associated with fetal alcohol syndrome (FAS) is:
A. Central nervous system deficits
B. Facial malformations
C. Hypoplastic nails
D. Eye malformations

221. In compliance with routine universal precautions, the nurse would wear which of the following when giving an IM injection?
A. No protective barrier necessary
B. Mask, gloves, gown
C. Gloves and gown only
D. Gloves only

222. The client was 2 days' postoperative for an above-the-knee amputation of his right leg. The physician ordered meperidine 50 mg and hydroxyzine (Vistaril) 25 mg IM for pain. The meperidine was in a 100 mg/2 ml vial and the hydroxyzine 25 mg/ml. How many milliliters did the nurse draw up to give this pain medication?
A. 1 ml
B. 1.5 ml
C. 2 ml
D. 2.5 ml

223. A quick way to determine the size of an endotracheal airway for a child is by using:
A. Clark's rule
B. Body surface area
C. Pinky rule
D. Hopkin's rule

224. A 22-year-old client returns to the hospital room following a cardiac catheterization of the left side of the heart. The catheter was inserted into the femoral artery through the left groin. The nurse assesses the following frequently:
A. Neurovascular signs in the right foot
B. Neurovascular signs in the left foot
C. Level of consciousness
D. Heart sounds

225. The physician ordered clorazepate (Tranxene) 7.5 mg PO as an adjunct therapy with seizure disorders to a 37-year-old having narcotic withdrawal.

On hand were 3.75 mg tablets. How many tablets did the nurse administer?
A. ½ tablet
B. 1 tablet
C. 1½ tablets
D. 2 tablets

226. A client, 28 weeks' gestation, presents to the clinic for her routine prenatal visit. When obtaining her weight, the nurse notes that the client has gained 12 lb since her last prenatal visit. The nurse's response will be based on the knowledge that:
A. This is an excessive weight gain for this gestational age.
B. This is an average weight gain for this gestional age.
C. This weight gain is inadequate to meet the needs of the pregnancy.
D. The weight gain puts the client at risk for eclampsia.

227. The nurse recognizes that which of the following best describes the prodromal phase of the acute infectious disease process:
A. Multiplying of the organism at the site and is the time between earliest symptoms and appearance of rash or fever
B. Invasion of the infectious agent into the host and established itself
C. Decline in symptoms
D. Interaction between host and infectious organisms causes symptoms of acute illness

228. Which of the following classifications of drugs is useful in diminishing the signs and symptoms of psychotic behavior?
A. Anticholinergics
B. Anxiolytics
C. Beta blockers
D. Neuroleptics

229. A 75-year-old home health client complained of constipation. The physician ordered lactulose (Chronulac) 15 ml every day. Using a 3.33 gm/5 ml elixir, how many grams did the client receive?
A. 5 gm
B. 7 gm
C. 9 gm
D. 10 gm

230. A pregnant client in the 30th week of gestation complains of swelling of her ankles and fingers. Edema of the hands can be a sign of pregnancy-induced hypertension (PIH). Which of the following symptoms would indicate to the nurse the development of PIH?
A. A blood pressure of 160 over 90. Her blood pressure was 142/112 four weeks ago.
B. Proteinuria of 2+
C. Frequent headaches
D. Heartburn

231. A 60-year-old female attending a local hospital

health screening is found by the nurse to have a blood pressure of 180/100 mm Hg. Which of the following approaches by the nurse is best?
A. Teach information about a low-salt diet.
B. Check the blood pressure again.
C. Instruct the client to see her physician.
D. Send the client to the emergency department.

232. A 40-year-old female client has been admitted to the hospital with thrombophlebitis. Which of the following symptoms would the nurse expect to find?
A. Tenderness in the calf
B. Both ankles swollen
C. Large thrombosed veins
D. Contracted feet

233. The client was admitted with a severe asthmatic reaction to a bee sting. The physician ordered epinephrine 1 mg subcutaneously stat. The ampule was labeled 1:1000. How much should the nurse give?
A. 0.2 ml
B. 0.3 ml
C. 0.5 ml
D. 1.0 ml

234. An expectant mother and her partner attended prepared childbirth classes. In labor, they expressed a desire to not have continuous fetal monitoring to permit maternal mobility. The nurse should do which of the following?
A. Determine if the couple understands the risks and benefits of continuous fetal monitoring.
B. Reassure them that continuous fetal monitoring will prevent a poor outcome.
C. Carefully explain that their request will put their infant at risk.
D. Offer to transfer them to a birthing center that can support their request.

235. While evaluating a client's technique for self-administration of insulin, the nurse checks to see whether:
A. The site is rubbed following the injection.
B. NPH insulin is vigorously shaken to mix it.
C. The site is prepared with a sterile 2 × 2 gauze.
D. A mixture is administered immediately after preparation.

236. The term parity refers to the number of:
A. Times the client has been pregnant
B. Deliveries the client has had regardless of gestation
C. Pregnancies carried 20 weeks or more
D. Live births the client has had

237. A client who has undergone drug treatment for infertility for 5 years without success asks the nurse what is involved in gamete intrafallopian tube transfer (GIFT). Which of the following explanations by the nurse would be most accurate?
A. The GIFT procedure involves stimulation of the ovaries to produce eggs, extraction of the eggs through laparoscopy, mixing the eggs with sperm obtained from the partner, and injecting the sperm-egg mix into the woman's fallopian tubes.
B. The GIFT procedure involves mixing eggs obtained from the woman with sperm from her partner in a petri dish. After the eggs have become fertilized and embryos are developing, the healthiest three or four embryos are then implanted into the woman's uterus.
C. The GIFT procedure involves stimulation of ovulation through fertility drugs, and then proceeding with artificial insemination using either the partner's sperm (if the sperm count is high enough) or sperm from a donor.
D. The GIFT procedure involves taking eggs from the ovaries of a client, mixing them with sperm obtained from the client's partner in a petri dish, and then implanting any resulting embryos into the uterus of a donor woman.

238. A 6-year-old was admitted with herpes simplex encephalitis. The child weighed 23 kg. The physician ordered vidarabine (Vira-A) 15 mg/kg (345 mg) times 10 days. Using a 200 mg/ml vial, how many milliliters would the nurse administer?
A. 1.5 ml
B. 1.6 ml
C. 1.7 ml
D. 1.8 ml

239. To prevent thrombophlebitis, the physician ordered heparin 8000 units subcutaneously every 8 hours. On hand is a 4 ml vial of heparin sodium injection 10,000 units/ml. How many milliliters will the nurse draw up to deliver 8000 units?
A. 0.8 ml
B. 1 ml
C. 1.5 ml
D. 2 ml

240. The clinical manifestations of respiratory distress syndrome (RDS) in a 28-week AGA infant would be:
A. Jitteriness and elevated temperature
B. Acrocyanosis and abdominal breathing
C. Expiratory grunting and cyanosis
D. Paleness and decreased respiratory rate

241. A 58-year-old male arrives for his clinic appointment. On review of his chart, you notice the nurse's notes indicate pedal pulses are slightly impaired. According to the pulse scale, his pedal pulses should be described as:
A. 1+
B. 2+
C. 3+
D. 4+

242. A client reports to the nurse that she is hearing voices telling her to stay out of group therapy.

Which of the following responses by the nurse is the most therapeutic?
A. "Well, you should respond to the voices by telling them that you will go to group therapy anyway."
B. "Are the voices male or female?"
C. "I understand that you hear the voices, but I do not."
D. "Just keep on taking your medication and the voices will go away."

243. A 71-year-old male client in an acute-care facility is taking digoxin. Which of the following neurological symptoms would indicate digoxin toxicity?
A. Decreased heart rate and arrhythmias
B. Headache, blurred vision, and confusion
C. Loss of appetite with nausea and vomiting
D. Hallucinations, weakness, and depression

244. A 3-year-old male is admitted to the hospital with a suspected diagnosis of Wilms' tumor. The child's mother describes that he has no energy and has just about stopped eating. On assessment, the nurse could expect to find which of the following additional symptoms?
A. Anemia
B. Hypotension
C. Weight gain
D. Hypothermia

245. A 70-year-old nursing home client was diagnosed with gastric ulcer. The physician ordered cimetidine 300 mg qid with meals. Using a 300 mg/2 ml elixir, how many milliliters did the nurse administer?
A. 0.5 ml
B. 1.0 ml
C. 1.5 ml
D. 2.0 ml

246. A 32-year-old client at 32 weeks' gestation with gestational diabetes has been on a 2000-kcal ADA diet for 4 weeks. Which of the following laboratory reports would indicate that the physician will most likely order insulin therapy?
A. A fasting blood glucose level of 90
B. A HbA1c level of 5 percent
C. A 2-hr postprandial blood glucose level of 130
D. A before-lunch blood glucose level of 105

247. A 56-year-old male is scheduled for a resting thallium myocardial scan. In preparing to teach the client about his test, the nurse would include which of the following?
A. The test requires no venipuncture.
B. The test detects areas of perfusion in the myocardium.
C. The test measures coronary artery insufficiency during treadmill walking.
D. The test is used instead of cardiac catheterization.

248. A public health nurse is asked to present an AIDS prevention program to a group of older adults in the community. The nurse reports to the administrator of this program that she will present this program to the Ladies Garden Club. The most probable reason the nurse chose a woman's group was:
A. Women comprise the fastest growing at-risk population for HIV infections.
B. Women are more apt to come in contact with sexual body fluids than men.
C. Women live longer than men and are more likely to seek sexual activity later in life.
D. Women experience greater changes in the immune system as they get older.

249. The nurse teaches the diabetic client about symptoms that might occur. Symptoms of severe hyperglycemia include:
A. Tremulousness, hunger, and diaphoresis
B. Kussmaul respirations and dry skin
C. Nausea, diaphoresis, and clammy skin
D. Abdominal pain and diaphoresis

250. A client arrives at the clinic for her first prenatal visit. Her baseline weight is 200 lb and she is 5 ft 1 inch. What information should the nurse provide the client in regard to weight gain in pregnancy?
A. "Because you are so obese, you need to avoid any weight gain during this pregnancy."
B. "Because you are overweight, you need to follow a strict diet during your pregnancy."
C. "Based on your weight, you will need to gain 15 to 25 lb during your pregnancy."
D. "The expected weight gain in pregnancy for all women is 25 to 35 lb."

251. The nurse confirms with the laboratory findings that the client is experiencing dehydration and makes plans to intervene. The most appropriate nursing intervention for the client with dehydration is:
A. Rehydrate using IV fluids and weigh daily.
B. Rehydrate orally with water and monitor urinary output.
C. Rehydrate orally with juice, tea, and coffee and weigh daily.
D. Rehydrate using IV fluids and monitor urinary output.

252. A young woman was experiencing severe pain postoperatively from a tubal ligation. The physician ordered fentanyl 0.1 mg every 1 to 2 hours PRN pain IV. Using a 0.05 mg/ml vial, how many milliliters did the nurse administer?
A. 0.5 ml
B. 1.0 ml
C. 1.5 ml
D. 2.0 ml

253. The nurse asks the client on admission to serially subtract the number 7 from 100. The nurse is assessing the client's:

A. Remote memory
B. Mood
C. Ability to calculate
D. Orientation

254. A 15-year-old client who is being seen in the obstetric-gynecologic clinic because her periods had stopped asked the nurse what caused this condition. A serum hCG was negative. Which of the following explanations by the nurse would be most accurate?
    A. It could be caused by endometrial tissue outside the uterus that causes scar tissue.
    B. It could be caused by strenuous exercise that results in a weight loss of 10 or more pounds.
    C. It could be caused by monthly hormonal changes that also cause headaches, irritability, and depression.
    D. It could be caused by a bacterial infection that has spread throughout the pelvic organs.

255. A 22-year-old client was found to have trichomoniasis during her annual pap smear. The physician ordered 2 gm metronidazole (Flagyl) IV to be administered as outpatient. Using a 1500 mg/5 ml vial, the nurse withdrew how many milliliters to be mixed with 500 cc dextrose in water?
    A. 5 ml
    B. 5.5 ml
    C. 6 ml
    D. 6.7 ml

256. A 1-day-old male infant has just been fed 1 ounce of formula and burped. He is placed in the crib by the nurse. To prevent aspiration, in which position should the nurse place the infant?
    A. Place the infant on his right side with the crib flat
    B. Place the infant on his left with the crib flat
    C. Place the infant on his abdomen with the crib flat
    D. Place the infant on his abdomen with the foot of the crib elevated

257. A 15-year-old was admitted with rheumatoid arthritis. The physician ordered phenylbutazone (Butazolidin) 200 mg PO. The nurse instructed the teen to take how many 100 mg tablets?
    A. ½ tablet
    B. 1 tablet
    C. 1½ tablets
    D. 2 tablets

258. A 63-year-old has been prescribed hydrochlorothiazide during his hospital stay. Which of the following laboratory reports should the nurse review?
    A. Serum sodium levels
    B. Serum potassium levels
    C. Cholesterol levels
    D. Thyroid panel

259. The nurse is involved in developing antenatal services. Which of the following is an example of fostering family attachment in the prenatal period?
    A. Large, frequent, culturally diverse education classes
    B. Weekday clinic appointments during routine business hours
    C. Preconception classes held on the weekend
    D. "Expectant Mothers" classes to discuss routine hospital interventions

260. The client was admitted with the right toe partially severed from a lawnmower accident. The physician was preparing to suture the toe and asked the nurse to prepare the syringe with 30 mg of 2% lidocaine. A 2000 mg/100 ml vial was on hand. How much should the nurse draw up?
    A. 0.5 ml
    B. 1.5 ml
    C. 2.0 ml
    D. 2.5 ml

261. The physician ordered potassium chloride 30 mEq added to each 1000 ml IV fluids. On hand on the unit was a 30 ml multiple-dose vial of potassium chloride 2 mEq/ml. How many milliliters are needed to deliver 30 mEq of potassium chloride?
    A. 5 ml
    B. 10 ml
    C. 15 ml
    D. 20 ml

262. The nurse suspects a 9-year-old child is having a hemolytic transfusion reaction. Which of the following is the first action the nurse should take?
    A. Take the child's vital signs and compare them to the baseline set.
    B. Notify the physician of the child's physical status.
    C. Dilute the blood with an equal amount of normal saline.
    D. Stop the blood transfusion and maintain a patent IV with normal saline and new tubing.

263. Which serum laboratory value indicates to the nurse that the client is experiencing hypoglycemia?
    A. 50 mg/dl
    B. 110 mg/dl
    C. 130 mg/dl
    D. 155 mg/dl

264. A 78-year-old woman is admitted to the hospital for assessment and diagnosis of possible Alzheimer's disease. It would be essential for the nurse to ask the family:
    A. "Has her mood changed recently?"
    B. "Have you noticed any major appetite changes lately?"
    C. "Are her bowel habits about the same?"
    D. "Has she grown more forgetful over the last 6 months?"

265. A 28-year-old gravida I, now para I, is ready to be discharged home with her 2-day-old daughter. She tells

the nurse, "I'm so worried about SIDS. Is there anything I can do to help prevent this from happening to my baby?" Which of the following explanations by the nurse would be most accurate?

A. The best thing you can do is place your baby on her stomach on a firm surface when you lay her down. This will prevent choking.

B. Keep your baby on her right side. That way the stomach contents will empty better into the small intestine, and she won't spit up and choke.

C. You can place the infant on her back when you lay her down, and avoid soft surfaces like bean-bags and pillows.

D. Lay your baby down on one side or the other. You can also put a small pillow under her head.

Answers

1. **(A)** Nursing process phase: evaluation; client need: physiological integrity; content area: maternity nursing

Rationale

(A) Increased liver function tests are characteristic of HELLP (hemolysis, elevated liver enzymes, low platelets) syndrome. HELLP syndrome develops as PIH worsens. (B) Proteinuria of 3+ is one of the signs and symptoms that are diagnostic for PIH. It does not indicate worsening of the condition. (C) Platelets decrease as PIH worsens. (D) The erythrocyte sedimentation rate normally increases in the second and third trimesters of pregnancy. It is not an indicator of PIH.

2. **(A)** Nursing process phase: analysis; client need: physiological integrity; content area: pediatric nursing

Rationale

(A) The spine develops a compensatory curve in the opposite direction to maintain body alignment. (B) The compensatory curve does not develop to distribute body weight evenly. (C) The compensatory curve adds another curve to the spine, rather than straightens it. (D) The compensatory curve does not develop to allow for chest expansion. If both curves continue to develop, chest expansion will be severely limited.

3. **(C)** Nursing process phase: implementation; client need: safe, effective care environment; content area: medical/surgical nursing

Rationale

(A) If NPH is drawn up first, this intermediate-acting insulin could be mixed with regular insulin. (B) The client would receive two injections, and this is not necessary. (C) After air is injected into the NPH, the regular insulin is drawn into the syringe first. If some regular insulin should get into the vial of NPH, the action of the NPH would not be greatly affected. (D) The nurse can mix the two insulins without the assistance of the pharmacy.

4. **(C)** Nursing process phase: implementation; client need: safe, effective care environment; content area: maternity nursing—dosage calculation

Rationale

5 mg : 1 tablet = 7.5 : x = 1.5 tablets

Math calculation explains incorrect answers.

5. **(A)** Nursing process phase: analysis and planning; client need: health promotion and maintenance; content area: pediatric nursing

Rationale

(A) If an infant is quiet, begin with auscultating the heart, lungs, and abdomen. This is difficult to do if the child is fussing. (B) Traumatic assessments such as eyes, ears, and mouth should be completed last or while the infant is crying. (C) The head-to-toe assessment should be altered to meet the developmental needs of the infant. (D) Percussion and palpation of areas should follow auscultation.

6. **(B)** Nursing process phase: analysis; client need: safe, effective care environment; content area: medical/surgical—gerontological nursing

Rationale

(A) Although the problems associated with AIDS make treatment and care a major challenge, long-term care facilities such as nursing homes have been reluctant to accept older adults with the disease because of the fear that the other residents and their families would react negatively and the lack of trained staff to care for the client. (B) Most persons with AIDS, including older adults, are cared for in their homes. As the disease progresses, functional assistance is needed by the family and home health care is instituted. (C) The hospital nurse may care for an older adult with AIDS during the initial phase of diagnosis and during admission for acute health problems. But hospital nursing care is not available for long-term care of AIDS. (D) Community AIDS clinics are rare. Researchers and other health-care providers have identified that the major issues common to older persons with AIDS are the need for accessible and affordable health care, community-based respite and hospice programs, and support groups.

7. **(C)** Nursing process phase: analysis; client need: safe, effective care environment; content area: psychiatric nursing

Rationale

(A) "Why" questions may put the client on the defensive and increase the agitated state. (B) Apologies are no assurance that the client has the ability to control his behavior. (C) The decision to release the client from mechanical restraints is based on assessment data that indicate the client's ability to control his violent behavior. (D) Current medication practice involves a combination of neuroleptics and antianxiety medications. However, there is no assurance that the medication will calm the violent behavior.

8. **(B)** Nursing process phase: implementation; client need: safe, effective care environment; content area: pediatric nursing

Rationale

(A) Suctioning the nose first could lead to aspiration. (B) In order to prevent aspiration, the pharynx is suctioned first. (C) Suctioning the nose first could lead to aspiration. Intubation and suctioning or a Dee Lee trap may be used with meconium fluid. (D) An oral-gastric tube may be inserted to decrease abdominal distention, but it is not indicated *before* suctioning may occur.

9. **(A)** Nursing process phase: analysis; client need: safe, effective care environment; content area: medical/surgical nursing

Rationale

(A) A sudden increase in blood pressure and a bounding pulse are indicative of a cerebral vascular accident (CVA). Because the client suffered an incident of transient ischemic attacks (TIA) the previous day, the client would be at high risk for a CVA. (B) Increased respirations and increased pulse can be related to the client's increased anxiety over his upcoming surgery or could be indicative of pain. (C) An increased temperature and increased respirations would alert the nurse to a possible infection. (D) A sudden decrease in blood pressure and tachycardia indicate hypovolemia or shock, late indicators that there is a serious problem.

10. **(D)** Nursing process phase: implementation; client need: physiological integrity; content area: maternity nursing

Rationale

(A) The clamminess is related to vena cava syndrome and is a result of low blood pressure. (B) Nasal oxygen is not needed; simply assisting the mother to a lateral Sims' position will improve her blood pressure. (C) This position is indicated for a client in shock. This client needs to be positioned on her side to alleviate symptoms. (D) Changing to a left lateral position alleviates vena cava compression from the gravid uterus.

11. **(A)** Nursing process phase: analysis; client need: safe, effective care environment; content area: medical/surgical nursing

Rationale

(A) Laceration of the pericardium is a possible complication resulting from this type of rib fracture. The nurse would need to monitor for chest pain, increasing aspiration, tachycardia, and falling blood pressure. (B) A laceration of the trachea would be difficult. The trachea is protected by bone and is not considered a complication of this type of fracture. (C) Laceration of the spine would be difficult for a floating rib and is not a complication of this type of fracture. (D) Laceration of the sternum would not be a complication because it a very thick bone.

12. **(C)** Nursing process phase: implementation; client need: safe, effective care environment; content area: maternity nursing

Rationale

(A) Though clients may experience postpartum pain, this is not usually associated with hemorrhage. (B) Clients may be anxious; however, the priority focus in this situation should be adequate organ perfusion. (C) Altered tissue perfusion results with hemorrhage and should be the nurse's highest priority to maintain the client's physiological well-being. (D) Though postpartum patients are at an increased risk for infection, this diagnosis is not related to hemorrhage.

13. **(A)** Nursing process phase: assessment; client need: physiological integrity; content area: pediatric nursing

Rationale

(A) After establishment of the disease process, limited movement in joints is a result of ankylosis or soft-tissue contractures. This characteristic is important in planning care because it identifies limitations to joint movement. Early in the disease process, limited joint movement is caused by inflammation and muscle spasms. Inflammation and muscle spasms will decrease, making joint movement easier, whereas ankylosis is a fixation in the joint. (B) When joints are inflamed, isometric and tensing exercises can be done to assist maintaining muscle strength. (C) Pauciarticular and polyarticular arthritis are more prevalent in females. Iridocyclitis is more prevalent in pauciarticular arthritis and, therefore, more common in females. (D) The latex fixation test measures rheumatoid factor. It is positive at onset; therefore, this information is already known. Rheumatoid factor is associated with severe disease process.

14. **(A)** Nursing process phase: analysis; client need: safe, effective care environment; content area: maternity nursing

Rationale

(A) A biophysical profile score was developed to identify the fetus in danger of death. It consists of five parameters, which receive a score of 0 to 2. A reassuring score of 10 indicates that at the time of the test, the fetus is well prepared to withstand the stress of labor. (B) Scores of 5 to 6 are equivocal and should be repeated within 24 hours. (C) Scores of 4 or less are considered worrisome. A fetus with this low a score will seldom increase the score with repeat testing, therefore, a speedy delivery would be the best choice. (D) Scores that are worrisome or abnormal usually do not improve with retesting.

15. **(C)** Nursing process phase: analysis; client need: safe, effective care environment; content area: psychiatric nursing

Rationale

(A) This nursing diagnosis refers to a state in which the individual is at high risk for demonstrating an inability to manage stressors because of a lack of adequate resources. There are no data available to support this. (B) Spiritual distress describes when a client experiences a disturbance in the belief or value system that provides strength, hope, and life meaning. (C & D) A knowledge deficit exists when the client experiences a deficiency in the level of cognitive knowledge concerning the condition or treatment. Impaired adjustment exists when the client is unwilling to modify the lifestyle or behavior that would contribute to an improved health status. This client is asking for information so that an adjustment can be made.

16. **(C)** Nursing process phase: evaluation; client need: physiological integrity; content area: medical/surgical nursing

Rationale

(A) After the initial response to therapy, an increased pulse rate will be noted. (B) This is not an initial response to hormone replacement therapy. (C) Diuresis, decreased edema, and weight loss will often be the initial response to hormone replacement therapy. (D) This sign is not a positive initial response to therapy.

17. **(D)** Nursing process phase: assessment; client need: safe, effective care environment; content area: pediatric nursing

Rationale

(A) Swallowing frequently, not infrequently, would be a sign or symptom of hemorrhage. (B) Dark-brown emesis is old blood and is usually present in the emesis after tonsillectomy and adenoidectomy. (C) A pulse rate of 95 beats per minute is a normal pulse rate for a 4-year-old child. (D) Drooling of bright-red secretions may be an early indication of hemorrhage after tonsillectomy and adenoidectomy.

18. **(D)** Nursing process phase: implementation; client need: safe, effective care environment; content area: medical/surgical nursing

Rationale
(A) Warm compresses are applied to promote absorption of fluid. (B) This action is inappropriate; it will not relieve pain. (C) Moist heat should be applied to the site after the IV has been discontinued. (D) As soon as infiltration is noted, the infusion should be stopped and the IV cannula removed. The infusion should then be started elsewhere.

19. **(C)** Nursing process phase: implementation; client need: health promotion and maintenance; content area: maternity nursing

Rationale
(A & B) Milk and calcium supplements decrease absorption of iron. (C) Research has shown that iron is absorbed best if taken at bedtime with citrus juice. (D) Iron is absorbed best at bedtime and on an essentially empty stomach.

20. **(D)** Nursing process phase: analysis; client need: physiological integrity; content area: medical/surgical nursing

Rationale
(A) A pneumothorax would not be a possibility with this client because there is patency from the chest tube, indicating that the tube is operational. Heart sounds would not be muffled and there would be no breath sounds to one side. (B) A hemothorax would not be a possibility because the chest tube is patent and draining fluid. This indicates that there is no accumulation of fluid in the chest wall. The breath sound would also be decreased or absent to one side. (C) A myocardial infarction would present with pain radiating or none radiating. The heart sounds would not be muffled, and the client may also exhibit nausea, vomiting, and diaphoresis. (D) Cardiac tamponade usually follows blunt trauma to the chest wall. Muffled heart sounds are an indicator to the nurse that fluid is accumulating inside the pericardial sac. JVD, decreasing BP, and weak rapid pulses are indicators of this condition.

21. **(A)** Nursing process phase: assessment; client need: health promotion and maintenance; content area: pediatric nursing

Rationale
(A) To straighten the ear canal in an infant, the pinna is pulled down and back. (B & D) The pinna is not pulled forward to straighten the ear canal. (C) With older children, usually over the age of 3, the pinna is pulled up and back to allow visualization of the tympanic membrane.

22. **(B)** Nursing process phase: implementation; client need: psychosocial integrity; content area: psychiatric nursing

Rationale
(A) It is important for the nurse to intervene early and to set limits that may help prevent recurrence of the behavior. (B) Information that gives details about the client's behavior can be used to modify the behavior. (C) Making demands may escalate the client's anger and frustration, thus displacing the aggressive behavior toward others. (D) Exploring attitudes rather than behaviors may indicate that the nurse is being judgmental.

23. **(D)** Nursing process phase: implementation; client need: safe, effective care environment; content area: pediatric nursing—dosage calculation.

Rationale
$$100 \text{ mg} : 1 \text{ tablet} = 184 \text{ mg} : x = 2 \text{ tablets}$$
Math calculations explains incorrect answers.

24. **(D)** Nursing process phase: implementation; client need: health promotion and maintenance; content area: pediatric nursing

Rationale
(A) Hot dogs, bread, and cake contain gluten. This child needs a gluten-free diet. (B & C) All these foods contain gluten. (D) These foods are gluten-free and should be recommended for this child's diet.

25. **(C)** Nursing process phase: analysis; client need: safe, effective care environment; content area: medical/surgical nursing

Rationale
(A) Hyperglycemia, not hypoglycemia, is a complication of peritoneal dialysis. (B) Hypotension, not hypertension, caused by excessive fluid removal is a complication of peritoneal dialysis. (C) This is correct. Hypovolemia caused by excessive fluid removal is a complication in most dialysis treatments. (D) Hypovolemia, not hypervolemia, is the correct complication seen in peritoneal dialysis caused by excessive fluid removal from the client's intravascular space.

26. **(B)** Nursing process phase: evaluation; client need: physiological integrity; content area: maternity nursing

Rationale
(A) Intermittent vomiting is not a danger sign; continuous vomiting is. (B) Vaginal bleeding is the number one danger sign to be reported because of the high risk of injury to the mother and the fetus. The client should seek health care. (C) Leukorrhea, vaginal discharge, is not a threat to the mother's life or her fetus. Vaginal discharge is a common occurrence during pregnancy. (D) Urinary frequency is a common discomfort of pregnancy because of the increased pressure on the maternal bladder.

27. **(C)** Nursing process phase: evaluation; client need: health promotion and maintenance; content area: pediatric nursing

Rationale
(A) The mother is correct to place the infant on the side as recommended by the American Academy of Pediatrics (AAP). (B) The mother is correct to place the infant in a supine position to sleep as recommended by the AAP. (C) The mother needs further teaching because the abdomen is no longer recommended as a sleep position for healthy newborns. Only infants with breathing problems or excessive vomiting should sleep prone. (D) The upright position is appropriate for burping, which is indicated after feedings.

28. **(C)** Nursing process phase: implementation; client need: physiological integrity; content area: pediatric nursing

Rationale

(A) A major goal of therapy is to keep the head of the femur in the acetabulum, which will be accomplished by abduction. (B) While pain is present, it most often occurs after prolonged weight bearing and activity. Major emphasis on treatment is to keep the spherical shape of the femur head through rest and non–weight-bearing. (C) Correct. The ultimate outcome of this aseptic necrosis of the femoral head depends on early and efficient treatment. Children are on bedrest with non–weight-bearing traction, cast, brace, or harness sling. (D) Joseph will be on bedrest and not allowed to bear weight on the right femur.

29. (C) Nursing process phase: planning; client need: psychosocial integrity; content area: psychiatric nursing

Rationale

(A) Diversional activity for the lower functioning client may precipitate anxiety and regression. (B) Program activities should focus on strengths rather than pathology. This may help the client relinquish the sick role and demonstrate more adaptive behavior. (C) Day treatment centers provide social interaction, recreational and learning activities for those persons who might otherwise be isolated. (D) Day treatment centers provide for social skills training, opportunities for socialization, structure, and support for the client. The remaining needs are provided by significant others.

30. (B) Nursing process phase: analysis; client need: safe, effective care environment; content area: medical/surgical nursing

Rationale

(A) AIDS is an immune disorder that would present with signs of a depressed immune system with decreased resistance to infectious diseases. (B) This is correct. Pernicious anemia is characterized by decreased gastric production of hydrochloric acid and vitamin B_{12} deficiency. A beefy red tongue is a hallmark sign for this disorder. (C) The client did not present with any signs of respiratory distress that might indicate ARDS. (D) The client is not presenting with a neurological disorder such as Parkinson's disease. Signs of this disease would include extrapyramidal disorders.

31. (C) Nursing process phase: analysis; client need: health promotion and maintenance; content area: maternity nursing

Rationale

(A, B & D) The correct answer is C. (C) Naegele's rule, the most common method of determining a delivery date, is obtained by subtracting 3 months from the first day of the last menstrual period and then adding 1 year and 7 days to that date. The correct answer is determined by: May minus 3 months is February. Adding 1 year and 7 days to the 12th results in an EDC of February 19.

32. (D) Nursing process phase: implementation; client need: safe, effective care environment; content area: medical/surgical nursing

Rationale

(A) The client is given vitamin B_{12} injections for pernicious anemia and not vitamin B_6 injections, since this is a disorder characterized by vitamin B_{12} deficiency. (B) The client should be assisted with daily activities, and safety precautions should be established since this client tends to be weak. (C) The Schilling's test—not the Harvard's test—is the definitive test for pernicious anemia. (D) This is correct. Frequent oral care because of a red, swollen tongue and painful oral mucosa is important to this client, and a nurse familiar with the discomforts of this disorder would provide appropriate care.

33. (C) Nursing process phase: assessment; client need: physiological integrity; content area: pediatric nursing

Rationale

(A) Dermatologic reactions can occur with antimalarial drugs, but malar rash is a symptom and result of the disease process. (B) Fatigue is to be avoided; however, exercise in moderation and involvement with friends are encouraged. (C) Frequent eye examinations are encouraged because of the possible side effects of retinal damage from hydroxychloroquine. (D) Weight gain can be a problem in clients with SLE and should be watched closely. The usual weight gain for a female during the adolescent period (12 to 18 years old) is 15 to 55 lb. Four pounds in 6 months does not mean there is a problem.

34. (D) Nursing process phase: evaluation; client need: health promotion and maintenance; content area: maternity nursing

Rationale

(A) The placenta does not filter out harmful substances. Whatever the mother takes in, the fetus eventually gets. (B) The maternal blood and fetal blood do not directly mix. Maternal nutrients and fetal wastes permeate the capillary walls of the placental villi. (C) The umbilical cord has two arteries and one vein. (D) The placenta is the connection between maternal nutrition and fetal waste.

35. (D) Nursing process phase: analysis; client need: safe, effective care environment; content area: medical/surgical nursing

Rationale

(A) A pleural effusion can result from congestive heart failure from fluid build up in the pleural spaces. A pneumonectomy can lead to congestive heart failure—not a pleural effusion. (B) Hypoglycemia, or low blood sugar, cannot develop as the result of a pneumonectomy. (C) A hemothorax is blood entering the pleural cavity as a result of chest trauma. In a pneumonectomy, the lung has been removed; the only possibility here is third spacing of fluid and the client would have chest tubes inserted to avoid this complication. (D) This is correct. Congestive heart failure can develop from a pneumonectomy because of the fact that the client has lost 50 percent of the functional lung surface. This increases the work load of the other lung and can cause fluid accumulation around the heart.

36. (D) Nursing process phase: implementation; client need: physiological integrity; content area: pediatric nursing

Rationale

(A) This assessment will give the nurse an indication of the amount of blood loss and hemodynamic stability. (B) Altered vital signs, delayed capillary refill, cyanosis, and diminished LOC are expected with acute and severe GI bleeding. (C) Intravenous fluids are needed to enhance hemodynamic status. (D) Hematesting stools can be done after the child is stabilized.

37. (D) Nursing process phase: implementation; client

need: psychosocial integrity; content area: maternity nursing

Rationale

(A) Telling a client with something as serious as HELLP syndrome that they should not worry is not therapeutic. You have no way of knowing that everything will be OK. (B) Blaming the client for any part of the event is not therapeutic. It is not necessary to scold or admonish her. This can cause further guilt if there is not a good outcome. (C) Downplaying the serious nature of the event is not being honest with a client. This is not a therapeutic comment. (D) Validating the feelings of your client is very important. Letting her know that you recognize her anxiety and are there for her is the most therapeutic comment in this situation.

38. **(D)** Nursing process phase: implementation; client need: safe, effective care environment; content area: medical/surgical nursing

Rationale

(A) This would not help the client clear the thick secretions from his lungs. Morphine sulfate can decrease deep breathing and increase the client's chance of developing pneumonia. (B) An incentive spirometer is used to help the client improve his tidal volume and improve deep breathing. It does not help alleviate pain and is uncomfortable with a fresh chest incision. (C) Using a pillow as a splint helps the client cough following abdominal or thoracic surgery. It does not alleviate pain with breathing. (D) This is correct. The client can benefit from diaphragmatic breathing by using accessory muscles. He can deep breath without placing pressure on his incision.

39. **(C)** Nursing process phase: analysis; client need: health promotion and maintenance; content area: pediatric nursing

Rationale

(A) While the bicarbonate value will fall in diabetic ketoacidosis, this is a slightly alkalotic pH value. Diabetic ketoacidosis will produce a pH of less than 7.25. (B) This is within normal limits. (C) Correct. The child in diabetic ketoacidosis has insufficient insulin to use glucose. These values represent hyperglycemia and ketones being excreted in the urine. Both of these values represent the changes occurring with diabetic ketoacidosis. (D) A glucose of 30 mg/dl is hypoglycemia, a condition not found in diabetic ketoacidosis.

40. **(D)** Nursing process phase: analysis; client need: safe, effective care environment; content area: medical/surgical nursing

Rationale

(A) The "Dawn phenomenon" is not preceded by hypoglycemia. (B) The data are not sufficient to justify insulin resistance. (C) The data do not support insulin sensitivity. (D) The data support the Somogyi effect.

41. **(D)** Nursing process phase: implementation; client need: health promotion and maintenance; content area: medical/surgical nursing

Rationale

(A) This is not accurate. (B) While cystitis may occur because of poor hygiene practices, it is not the reason why men are less prone to cystisis than women. (C) While low fluid intake is a factor in the development of cystitis, it is not the reason why males are less prone to cystitis than women. (D) The length

of the male urethra makes the development of cystitis less likely in men than among females.

42. **(B)** Nursing process phase: implementation; client need: safe, effective care environment; content area: psychiatric nursing—dosage calculation

Rationale

$$4 \text{ mg} : 1 \text{ ml} = 4 \text{ mg} : x = 1 \text{ ml}$$

Math calculation explains incorrect answers.

43. **(A)** Nursing process phase: implementation; client need: safe, effective care environment; content area: medical/surgical nursing

Rationale

(A) The very first action a nurse should do after the placement of an endotracheal tube is to check the breath sounds of the client to make sure that the tube is in the correct place and that there is bilateral expansion of the lungs. (B) This would be done after you have assessed your client and after the physician has written the order. (C) This is a respiratory therapist's function and also needs a physician's orders. However the nurse is responsible for making sure the physician's orders have been carried out. (D) You would check the client's vital signs only after you have assessed the breath sounds and tube placement.

44. **(B)** Nursing process phase: assessment; client need: physiological integrity; content area: maternity nursing

Rationale

(A) Cocaine quickly raises norepinephrine and serotonin blood levels and then suddenly lowers them. (B) Cocaine increases the amount of norepinephrine in the maternal circulation, causing vasoconstriction of the maternal vessels; thus decreased oxygen perfuses the placenta. (C) Cocaine impacts the fetus by leading to small-for-gestational-age infants. (D) The response of the placenta to cocaine is related to the acute spasm of uterine blood vessels, resulting in abruption.

45. **(C)** Nursing process phase: analysis; client need: safe, effective care environment; content area: medical/surgical nursing

Rationale

(A) Hypovolemia—not hypervolemia—can predispose an individual to pulmonary embolus and can produce hypercoagulability of the blood. (B) Arthritis is an inflammation of the joints and would not predispose a client to pulmonary embolus. (C) A long-bone fracture can predispose a client to pulmonary embolus by causing trauma and a change in the peripheral blood flow. (D) Osteoporosis is the thinning of the density of the bone and does not predispose a client to pulmonary embolus.

46. **(C)** Nursing process phase: implementation; client need: safe, effective care environment; content area: pediatric nursing

Rationale

(A) Raw vegetables, fruit, and fish should be prohibited because they can introduce bacteria. (B) Total restriction of activity is not necessary. Games or toys that can be disinfected and watching TV are appropriate activities. (C) Any temperature elevation is significant, and temperature elevations of 100.5°F or greater are reported to the physician. (D) Visitors with colds, sore throats, or infections should be prohibited from visiting.

47. **(C)** Nursing process phase: implementation; client need: psychosocial integrity; content area: psychiatric nursing

Rationale

(A) One of the least constructive interventions is to threaten the patient with punishment. (B) It is almost always detrimental to force the client to do anything. (C) This intervention does not put the client on the defensive and shows that the nurse is willing to understand the reason for the uncooperative behavior. (D) This intervention limits the client's progression in his treatment.

48. **(B)** Nursing process phase: implementation; client need: safe, effective care environment; content area: medical/surgical nursing

Rationale

(A) The chest tubes should be coiled on the bed to prevent dependent loops that impede drainage. (B) This is correct. Deep breathing helps to push pleural air out into the tube and aid drainage. (C) The client needs to be turned from side to side every 2 hours to increase the air flow and blood from the chest. (D) Milk the chest tubes only when a blockage is suspected. Milking too frequently will defeat the purpose of the suction and decrease the ability of the chest tubes to function properly.

49. **(D)** Nursing process phase: analysis and planning; client need: health promotion and maintenance; content area: pediatric nursing

Rationale

(A) The child is not very aware of another's presence and may push that person away in the midst of a night terror. (B) The child has no memory of the night terror dream or the yelling and screaming that he did. (C) The child is hard to keep awake after a night terror; they fall back asleep rapidly. (D) Night terrors usually occur in 1 to 4 hours past falling asleep. A nightmare or dream usually occurs in the second part of the night.

50. **(C)** Nursing process phase: assessment; client need: health promotion and maintenance; content area: maternity nursing

Rationale

(A) Constipation is a common complaint during pregnancy because of the decreased motility. Urinary frequency is common in the first few weeks of pregnancy as the growing uterus begins to put pressure on the urinary bladder. It is again common in the third trimester when lightening has occurs. These are not emergency situations. (B) Nocturia, urination during the hours of sleep, is a result of the increased renal flow that occurs at night when the pregnant woman is lying down. This may act to reduce lower-extremity edema; however, it is somewhat of a problem because it causes interruption of sleep. Linea nigra is the darkening of the linea alba, the line between the symphysis and the umbilicus. This darkening is a result of the increased pigmentation that normally occurs during pregnancy as a result of hormonal changes. Neither of these is an emergency situation. (C) Abdominal pain may indicate infection or preterm labor, and hematuria would be concerning because it may indicate a UTI. The nurse would need to educate the client concerning the danger and warning signs of complications of pregnancy. (D) Leg cramps are quite common, especially in the third trimester. The physiological reason has never been supported in research; however,

some explanations are calcium-phosphorus metabolism or pressure from the enlarging uterus on the pelvic blood vessels. Pyrosis, or heartburn, is a common complaint at various stages during pregnancy. This common complaint is explained by the fact that the hormonal effects on the smooth muscles cause the cardiac valve between the esophagus and stomach to work less efficiently, allowing acidic stomach secretions to reflux into the esophagus. Teaching safe relief measures for these common complications is necessary.

51. **(B)** Nursing process phase: analysis; client need: physiological integrity; content area: medical/surgical nursing

Rationale

(A) An increase in the production of ADH would cause fluid retention, leading to syndrome of inappropriate antidiuretic hormone (SIADH) and not diabetes insipidus which is marked by dehydration. (B) This is correct. There is a decrease in the amount of ADH produced by the pituitary. The syndrome is marked by excessive urination, dehydration, and fluid and electrolyte imbalances. (C) Hypovolemia would be a result of diabetes insipidus and not a cause for this disorder. (D) Renal failure would not be a cause of diabetes insipidus.

52. **(C)** Nursing process phase: implementation; client need: psychosocial integrity; content area: medical/surgical nursing

Rationale

(A) The client may not be ready or may not want to know about the course of her terminal condition. This is not a necessary action unless the client asks about it. (B) Pain medication is important for terminal cancer clients; however, when a client is dying, psychosocial skills and therapeutic communication are more important to prepare the client for the journey ahead. (C) This is correct. The most important action that you can do for any terminal client is to listen. They want to talk about their fears and concerns. You have to be able to mentally handle this difficult part of nursing. You will be of no assistance to your client unless you are comfortable with discussing death and dying. (D) This is not appropriate unless the client's family asks for this assistance. This is usually done by nurses who work in a hospice program; however, you could prepare the client's family by teaching them some simple care tasks. Never teach until they are ready. During this stage following confirmation of a terminal diagnosis, the family may be too upset or stressed to comprehend any instructions.

53. **(A)** Nursing process phase: implementation; client need: safe, effective care environment; content area: medical/surgical nursing—dosage calculation

Rationale

200 μg : 1 tablet = 100 μg : x = ½ tablet
Math calculation explains incorrect answers.

54. **(C)** Nursing process phase: assessment; client need: physiological integrity; content area: pediatric nursing

Rationale

(A) Neurological impairment can be indicative of a stroke. By giving the blood products, the viscosity of the blood will be decreased. (B) Increasing hydration does decrease sickling and reduces pain. This is the desired effect—not the adverse effect. (C) When administering fluid or blood products, clients should be watched carefully for cardiac failure caused by an increased workload on the heart. (D) An infection can trigger a crisis, so the client should be watched for an infection. The immediate concern would be cardiac functioning.

55. **(B)** Nursing process phase: assessment; client need: safe, effective care environment; content area: medical/surgical nursing

Rationale

(A) Cataracts cause an opacity of the lens and lead to a gradual loss of vision. Images are usually hazy and the client is bothered by glare. (B) This is correct. This condition is marked by the inability to read objects up close and is caused by the loss of elasticity of the lens of the eye. This is a common result of the aging of the eye lens. (C) Xerostomia is a condition seen in the elderly where they suffer from frequent dry mouth. (D) Arcus senilis is the deposition of lipids in the iris of the eye. It is usually seen as a slight yellow ring around the iris and is associated with aging.

56. **(D)** Nursing process phase: assessment; client need: physiological integrity; content area: medical/surgical nursing

Rationale

(A) Polyuria is seen in head injuries that result in diabetes insipidus. This syndrome is marked by a decrease in antidiuretic hormone. (B) Hematuria can be related to a number of causes associated with trauma to the kidneys, ureters, or bladder. However, it is not associated with SIADH. (C) Hypoglycemia is not associated with the water intoxication seen in SIADH. Electrolyte imbalances are more common in SIADH. (D) This is correct. SIADH causes nausea, abdominal cramps, vomiting, anorexia, and excessive weight gain in clients.

57. **(B)** Nursing process phase: implementation; client need: health promotion and maintenance; content area: maternity nursing

Rationale

(A) Dependent edema of the lower extremities may occur because of poor venous return related to crossing the legs. (B) To prevent dependent edema, support panty hose should be put on in the morning prior to putting the lower extremities in a dependent position, that is, walking. (C) Sitting with feet elevated facilitates venous return. (D) Dorsiflexion improves circulation and prevents venous stasis.

58. **(B)** Nursing process phase: assessment; client need: physiological integrity; content area: medical/surgical nursing

Rationale

(A) Hypertension and hypokalemia are not found in this disorder. Addison's disease is caused by adrenal hypofunction and decreased glucocorticoid and androgen secretion. (B) This is correct. Bronze skin discoloration is a hallmark sign of Addison's disease. The client may also suffer from extreme fatigue, weight loss, and lightheadedness. (C) Chronic thirst is usually seen in diabetes insipidus. Pica can belong to a variety of physiological and psychological disorders. (D) Constipation and bloody stools can be indicative of lower gastrointestinal disorders. Any condition from cancer to bleeding ulcers can be indicated by theses findings; however, they are not usually associated with Addison's disease.

59. **(B)** Nursing process phase: implementation; client need: physiological integrity; content area: pediatric nursing

Rationale

(A) Education of children and parents is important, but action is needed to prevent and control hepatitis. (B) The single most effective method of prevention is the use of hand washing. (C) Illicit drug use places individuals at risk for the development of hepatitis B. (D) The current vaccine is only effective against the hepatitis B organism.

60. **(C)** Nursing process phase: assessment; client need: physiological integrity; content area: maternity nursing

Rationale

(A) Stage 1 is completed when the cervix is completely dilated. (B) Pushing occurs at the end of stage 1 and beginning of stage 2. (C) Stage 2 begins when the client is fully dilated and is complete on delivery of the infant. (D) From the time the infant delivers until delivery of the placenta is stage 3. The delivery of the placenta is the beginning of the recovery stage, stage 4.

61. **(C)** Nursing process phase: assessment; client need: safe, effective care environment; content area: medical/surgical nursing

Rationale

(A) These are physical changes associated with Addison's disease, which is caused by a decrease in glucocorticoid production. (B) Acne and ecchymosis are physical changes seen in Cushing's syndrome; however, hyperactivity is not associated with this disorder. (C) This is correct. Cushing's syndrome is a disease where there is an excessive amount of glucocorticoid and hyperplasia of the adrenal cortex. Other physical symptoms associated with this disease include purplish striae, delayed wound healing, and a buffalo hump noted in the upper back. (D) These are normal physical changes associated with aging.

62. **(D)** Nursing process phase: evaluation; client need: physiological integrity; content area: maternity nursing

Rationale

(A) Nausea, vomiting, and diarrhea are not adverse reactions to magnesium sulfate. (B) Facial edema is characteristic of severe PIH and not an adverse reaction to the medication. (C) Dizziness and lightheadedness are characteristic adverse reactions to terbutaline, a tocolytic. These symptoms are generally not seen with magnesium sulfate. (D) The absence of deep-tendon reflexes is an early indication of magnesium toxicity. The infusion should be stopped.

63. **(C)** Nursing process phase: implementation; client need: safe, effective care environment; content area: psychiatric nursing

Rationale

(A) Antisocial people lack concern for others and have a disregard for social norms. The client would not see the behavior as inappropriate. (B) Because antisocial persons lack the ability to trust and look for immediate gratification, encouraging nurturing behavior would be futile. (C) Setting limits conveys external control (D) The antisocial personality disorder person does not see self realistically and sees no merit in the values and morals of society.

64. **(C)** Nursing process phase: implementation; client need: health promotion and maintenance; content area: maternity nursing

Rationale

(A, B, & D) GTPAL stands for *g*ravida (number of times pregnant), *t*erm (number of babies delivered after 36 weeks' gestation), *p*reterm (number of babies born before 36 weeks' gestation), *a*borta (number of pregnancies miscarried or therapeutically aborted), and *l*iving (number of children now living). (C) The client has had five pregnancies (including this one): two were term, one preterm, one abortion or miscarriage, and three living children.

65. **(A)** Nursing process phase: assessment; client need: health promotion and maintenance; content area: pediatric nursing

Rationale

(A) The parent should supervise or assist with hygiene, especially baths, until the age of 5 to prevent injury or drowning and ensure proper technique. (B) The preschooler is fearful about the drain, but physiological safety takes priority over psychological safety. (C) Usually the 3-year-old can dress himself or herself except for back buttons and should be allowed to do such. (D) Options can be allowed if they exist. The option to bathe and dress should not be allowed.

66. **(A)** Nursing process phase: analysis; client need: physiological integrity; content area: medical/surgical nursing

Rationale

(A) A mild normocytic, normochromic anemia frequently accompanies hypothyroidism caused by reduced oxygen demand by the tissues. (B) A mild normocytic, normochromic anemia frequently accompanies hypothyroidism, caused by reduced—not increased—production of erythropoietin by the kidney. (C) Deficient iron absorption is seen in macrocytic, microcytic, and hypochromic anemia and not normocytic, normochromic anemia. (D) Microcytic and hypochromic—not normocytic, normochromic—anemia can develop in a client with significant blood loss from the relatively common menorrhagia.

67. **(C)** Nursing process phase: implementation; client need: safe, effective care environment; content area: medical/surgical nursing—dosage calculation

Rationale

750 mg divided by 330 mg × 1 ml = 2.3 ml
Math calculation explains incorrect answers.

68. **(C)** Nursing process phase: analysis; client need: safe, effective care environment; content area: pediatric nursing

Rationale

(A) Adolescents are very vocal about the pain they feel, but will not protest pain measures. (B) An older infant, toddler, and preschool-age child will push stimulus away and show physical resistance. (C) School-aged children will attempt to put off the pain medication and make excuses delaying the procedure. (D) Toddlers will be uncooperative and may need physical restraint.

69. **(A)** Nursing process phase: implementation; client need: safe, effective care environment; content area: maternity nursing—dosage calculation

Rationale

1.5 mg : 1 tablet = 0.625 mg : x = 0.5 tablet
Math calculation explains incorrect answers.

70. **(B)** Nursing process phase: analysis; client need: safe, effective care environment; content area: medical/surgical nursing

Rationale

(A) A stage I pressure area is characterized by no break in the skin. (B) A stage II pressure area is characterized by loss of skin, frequently into the dermis. (C) A stage III area exposes or involves subcutaneous tissue. (D) A stage IV area extends beyond subcutaneous tissue.

71. **(B)** Nursing process phase: analysis; client need: health promotion and maintenance; content area: maternity nursing

Rationale

(A) Adolescents are at increased risk for nutritional problems, but research has shown that smoking less than one-half pack of cigarettes per day has little effect on the pregnancy. (B) Adolescents have increased nutritional needs because their bodies are still growing and they frequently have poor food habits. Anemia early in pregnancy is often difficult to resolve because of constantly increasing demands from the fetus and pregnancy. (C) Research has shown that smoking less than one-half pack of cigarettes per day has little effect on the pregnancy. The fact that the client is of average weight is a positive factor. (D) The fact that this client is in a higher socioeconomic group is favorable. As noted above, age is a factor.

72. **(D)** Nursing process phase: evaluation; client need: health promotion and maintenance; content area: maternity nursing

Rationale

(A) Cats can carry the organism *Toxoplasma*, which can cause fetal anomalies. The organism is found in the stool of many cats. (B) Many medications, including over-the-counter (OTC) medicines, cross the placenta to the fetus. The greatest danger of causing developmental defects in the fetus from drugs exists during the first 12 weeks. (C) Gastrointestinal motility is decreased in pregnancy because of the influences of the hormone estrogen. The hormone hCG may also have an influence on morning sickness. Pregnant women should avoid empty and/or overloaded stomachs. Five to six small meals a day accomplishes this goal. (D) Any activity or condition that raises the body temperature over 102°F for more than 10 minutes can cause fetal central nervous system damage. Heat stress is to be avoided by pregnant women.

73. **(B)** Nursing process phase: assessment; client need: physiological integrity; content area: maternity nursing

Rationale

(A) After a cesarean birth, there is about a 5-day delay in involution. (B) Lochia will increase when the uterus begins to involute, around day 5. (C) Lochia is scant the first few days, then as involution occurs, the lochia increases. (D) Because of delayed involution, there is an increased risk of an infection, endometritis.

74. **(A)** Nursing process phase: implementation; client need: safe, effective care environment; content area: pediatric nursing

Rationale

(A) Air emboli may occur when blood is transfused under pressure. (B) These reactions are associated with blood incompatibility rather than pressure. (C) The client reacts to allergens in the donor's blood. The reaction itself is not associated with pressure. (D) This reaction occurs when blood is not allowed to warm to room temperature or not prewarmed with a mechanical blood warmer.

75. (B) Nursing process phase: implementation; client need: health promotion and maintenance; content area: medical/surgical nursing

Rationale
(A) While oysters are a fairly good source of iron, they are not the best source. (B) Organ meats such as liver are very high in iron. Raisins are also a good source of iron. (C) While dried beans and spinach are good sources of iron, liver is the better choice. (D) Organ meats are a better source of iron than hamburger.

76. (D) Nursing process phase: evaluation; client need: safe, effective care environment; content area: maternity nursing

Rationale
(A) Urinary frequency and epistaxis (nosebleeds) are common discomforts that occur during pregnancy. Increased estrogen levels can cause edema of the mucous membranes of the nasal cavity, causing nasal stuffiness and epistaxis. Following lightening, which frequently occurs by 38 weeks, urinary frequency is common. (B) Lower-limb edema is common during the third trimester because of the impaired venous return that occurs as a result of the weight of the gravid uterus. The cause of leg cramps is not well explained in research literature. (C) Leukorrhea is a common finding in pregnancy because of the hormonal influence on the vaginal walls. This would be concerning only if the discharge became odorous, discolored, or caused itching or pain. Good perineal care is important for the client. Urinary frequency is also common at term if lightening has taken place and the gravid uterus is placing increased pressure on the urinary bladder. (D) Periorbital edema and proteinuria are worrisome because they are two of the signs of pre-eclampsia. These symptoms would need further evaluation.

77. (C) Nursing process phase: implementation; client need: physiological integrity; content area: medical/surgical nursing

Rationale
(A) The Valsalva maneuver should be avoided because of its effect on preload. (B) The rationale is explained under A. (C) Preload will be decreased initially because of the increased pressure inside the thoracic cavity caused by the Valsalva maneuver. (D) Following a decrease in preload, the heart will be flooded with blood to be pumped. However, D is not the correct answer because an increase in preload is not the initial effect of the Valsalva maneuver.

78. (B) Nursing process phase: implementation; client need: safe, effective care environment; content area: psychiatric nursing

Rationale
(A) The symptom complex expressed by the client mimics myocardial infarction and is called cardiac neurosis. During acute panic attacks, problem solving is disrupted. (B) The first priority is to provide safety and reduce the client's immediate anxiety to a moderate level. (C) Panic disorder can be severe, although it is rarely incapacitating. (D) A careful history must be developed to determine the use of other drugs.

Anxiolytic medication may be prescribed after the client has been assessed.

79. (C) Nursing process phase: implementation; client need: health promotion and maintenance; content area: pediatric nursing

Rationale
(A, B, & D) Exercise-induced asthma is common to all persons with asthma. This is rare in activities that require only short bursts of energy (i.e., baseball, gymnastics, skiing) compared with those that involve endurance exercise such as soccer, basketball, and distance running. (C) Swimming, even long-distance swimming, is recommended because the child breathes air saturated with moisture, and exhaling under water prolongs expiration and increases end-expiratory pressure.

80. (A) Nursing process phase: implementation; client need: safe, effective care environment; content area: maternity nursing—dosage calculation

Rationale
$$1000 \text{ U} : 1 \text{ ml} = 500 \text{ U} : x = 0.5$$
Math calculation explains incorrect answers.

81. (B) Nursing process phase: implementation; client need: safe, effective care environment; content area: pediatric nursing

Rationale
(A) The therapeutic effects may not be seen immediately, but are apparent in 2 to 4 weeks. (B) The normal time for the effects to be apparent is anywhere from 2 to 4 weeks. (C) The naproxen does not work that quickly for the inflammatory response from arthritis. (D) Beneficial effects for arthritis will be longer than for other conditions such as menstrual cramps.

82. (D) Nursing process phase: implementation; client need: safe, effective care environment; content area: maternity nursing

Rationale
(A) The primary health-care provider should be present until after the delivery of the placenta. If the physician or midwife is not there at this time, this is a normal finding and would not be an indication to call them. (B) The primary health-care provider may sometimes apply tension to the cord to facilitate delivery of the placenta. This is not the role of the nurse, and traction on the cord will increase the risk of complication such as uterine inversion. (C) Fifteen minutes is still within the acceptable time frame for the third stage of labor. If the client does not deliver the placenta within 30 minutes, the physician will explore the uterus and may determine that the client has a placenta accreta, which would require surgical intervention. (D) The normal time frame for delivery of the placenta is 5 to 30 minutes. Most placentas deliver within 5 minutes, but 15 minutes is certainly within the expected time frame for this stage.

83. (C) Nursing process phase: analysis; client need: safe, effective care environment; content area: pediatric nursing

Rationale
(A) The purpose of the water in the closed drainage system is to prevent entrance of air into the pleural cavity. It is not to decrease the danger of sudden change in pressure in the tube. (B) The purpose of the water in the closed drainage system is

to prevent entrance of air into the pleural cavity. (C) The purpose of the water in the closed drainage system is to prevent entrance of air into the pleural cavity. It is not to foster removal of chest secretion by capillary. (D) The purpose of the water in the closed drainage system is to prevent entrance of air into the pleural cavity. It is not to facilitate emptying bloody drainage from the chest.

84. **(C)** Nursing process phase: implementation; client need: safe, effective care environment; content area: psychiatric nursing—dosage calculation

Rationale
$$500 \text{ mg} : 5 \text{ ml} = 750 \text{ mg} : x = 7.5 \text{ ml}$$
Math calculation explains incorrect answers.

85. **(D)** Nursing process phase: implementation; client need: health promotion and maintenance; content area: medical/surgical nursing

Rationale
(A) Proper hand washing would not help prevent pressure ulcers. (B) The client needs to remain as active as possible to promote circulation in order to prevent pressure ulcers. (C) The client should remain as independent as possible. (D) A diet high in proteins and vitamins C and E promotes healthy skin and tissues to resist forces tending to cause pressure ulcers.

86. **(C)** Nursing process phase: assessment; client need: physiological integrity; content area: maternity nursing

Rationale
(A) Cyanotic hands and feet, acrocyanosis, is a common finding in the newborn. A respiratory rate of 54 falls within the normal range. (B) Dark blue marks over the buttocks, mongolian spots, and overriding cranial sutures are common findings in the newborn. (C) Tufts of hair at the base of the spine would need further evaluation. This infant may have a spinal abnormality known as spina bifida. (D) Vertex deliveries often produce an infant with periorbital edema. Nevus flammeus, reddened areas over the brow or base of the neck, are common findings in a newborn.

87. **(B)** Nursing process phase: analysis; client need: safe, effective care environment; content area: medical/surgical nursing

Rationale
(A) The data do not indicate a need for blood cultures or an electrolyte panel at this time. (B) The data indicate that the client has cellulitis; therefore, a WBC and wound culture would be most appropriate at this time. (C) The data do not indicate a need to check kidney or liver function. (D) The data do not indicate a need to check blood coagulation.

88. **(D)** Nursing process phase: assessment; client need: safe, effective care environment; content area: maternity nursing

Rationale
(A) Pytalism is the disorder that occurs in pregnancy characterized by excessive salivation. (B) Couvade is the condition in which the male partner suffers many of the common symptoms of pregnancy. (C) Pyrosis is acid indigestion and is characterized by burping and acidic taste in the mouth (D) Pica is a persistent compulsion to ingest nonfood items that contain little or no nutritional value.

89. **(A)** Nursing process phase: analysis; client need: psychosocial integrity; content area: psychiatric nursing

Rationale
(A) Compulsions are attempts to relieve tension. (B) Obsessions are recurring thoughts that cannot be dismissed from the consciousness. (C) Compulsive behavior is a defense against anxiety. It is not an attention-seeking behavior. (D) The client is suffering from a compulsive disorder—not a phobia.

90. **(B)** Nursing process phase: analysis; client need: physiological integrity; content area: pediatric nursing

Rationale
(A) Teaching the parents foods high in potassium is not an appropriate intervention for phimosis. (B) Teaching the parents proper cleansing is an important intervention for phimosis, which is a narrowing or stenosis of the preputial opening of the foreskin that prevents retraction of the foreskin over the glans penis. (C) Monitoring urinary output is not an appropriate nursing intervention for mild phimosis. However, occasionally if the narrowing obstructs the flow of urine, this may result in a dribbling stream of urine or cause ballooning of the foreskin with accumulated urine during voiding. (D) There is no reason to measure abdominal girth for a child with mild phimosis.

91. **(A)** Nursing process phase: implementation; client need: health promotion and maintenance; content area: medical/surgical nursing

Rationale
(A) The client may feel weak and fatigue easily because of tissue hypoxia caused by diminished RBCs with oxygen-carrying capacity. Rest is indicated. (B) A high fluid intake is desirable, but is not the priority intervention for a client recovering from iron deficiency. (C) A diet rich in vitamin B_{12} will not necessarily prevent iron deficiency anemia. (D) A diet high in folic acid is indicated for anemia caused by folate deficiency, not iron deficiency anemia.

92. **(D)** Nursing process phase: implementation; client need: health promotion and maintenance; content area: pediatric nursing

Rationale
(A) Increased fluid intake leads to diuresis. Diuresis enhances the antibacterial properties of the renal medulla. (B) The single most important factor influencing the occurrence of UTI is urinary stasis. The act of frequently emptying the bladder flushes away organisms preventing UTI. (C) Concentrated and alkaline urine predisposes a client to UTI. Ingestion of highly acidic juices, such as cranberry, acidify the urine. (D) The short urethra, which measures 3/4 inch in young girls, provides a ready pathway for the invasion of organisms.

93. **(A)** Nursing process phase: analysis and planning; client need: physiological integrity; content area: maternity nursing

Rationale
(A) During labor, a natural response to contractions is to hold one's breath or to breathe more rapidly. Paced breathing alters that negative response by ensuring an adequate oxygen supply to both the mother and the fetus. (B) Paced breathing does provide a focus. However, the physiological need of oxygenation is the priority. (C) The breathing patterns are used

to modify the mother's response to the contraction, to change a typically negative response to a positive one. There may be less need for analgesics. (D) Mental relaxation is an outcome of the breathing patterns. It is secondary to adequate oxygenation.

94. (D) Nursing process phase: implementation; client need: health promotion and maintenance; content area: medical/surgical nursing

Rationale
(A) Vitamin C does not affect the actions of warfarin. (B) A diet high in protein will be needed for healing and will not affect the actions of warfarin. (C) Calcium will not affect the actions of warfarin. (D) Vitamin K is the antidote for warfarin, and altering the amount of vitamin K in the diet will cause prothrombin times, the test used to monitor the effects of warfarin, to fluctuate.

95. (C) Nursing process phase: assessment; client need: physiological integrity; content area: pediatric nursing

Rationale
(A) An antigen is the external stimulus that activates the immune response. (B) B lymphocytes stimulate the production of antibodies that work to destroy antigen. (C) Histamine is the mediator responsible for acting on local receptors producing inflammation. Histamines cause vasodilitation, which results in mucus production and sneezing, which are common symptoms in allergic rhinnitis. (D) Leukotrienes are secondary mediators that increase vascular permeability that aid the inflammatory response.

96. (D) Nursing process phase: analysis; client need: physiological integrity; content area: maternity nursing

Rationale
(A) Breast milk does not develop in the breast early in pregnancy. (B) Though some women do experience an increase in sexual drive early in pregnancy, the changes in the breast are not a result of this. (C) The tender breasts that occur with early pregnancy result from an increased blood supply. (D) The hormones of pregnancy, particularly estrogen and progesterone, prepare the body for breastfeeding. Estrogen has an influence on the development of the ducts, and progesterone causes alveolar and lobule development. Blood vessels enlarge and become prominent, and the darkening and enlargement of the tubercles of Montgomery are related to the action of estrogen.

97. (C) Nursing process phase: assessment; client need: psychosocial integrity; content area: pediatric nursing

Rationale
(A) This is a belief of the Jehovah Witness faith. (B) Particular types of meat are not forbidden. (C) The Mormon faith encourages the avoidance of such stimulants as tea, coffee, chocolate, and products containing caffeine. (D) Mormons may fast for 24 hours on the first Sunday each month.

98. (D) Nursing process phase: analysis and planning; client need: safe, effective care environment; content area: maternity nursing

Rationale
(A) This is the Sperm Immobilization Antigen-Antibody Test (B) This is a description of an endometrial biopsy. (C) A laparoscopy involves inserting a small telescope through an ab-

dominal incision to visualize abdominal or pelvic structures. (D) Radiopaque dye is inserted through a cannula into the uterus and tubes, and visualized on a radiographic screen taken to observe the structures.

99. (D) Nursing process phase: implementation; client need: safe, effective care environment; content area: pediatric nursing—dosage calculation

Rationale
$$4 \text{ ml} / \text{kg} \times 2 \text{ kg} = 8 \text{ ml}$$
Math calculation explains incorrect answers.

100. (D) Nursing process phase: planning; client need: health promotion and maintenance; content area: pediatric nursing

Rationale
(A) Sexual intercourse may produce transient bacteriuria in females and is associated with increased risk of UTI, but it would not be appropriate to teach that it is usually the cause of UTI in adolescents. (B) Drinking large amounts of carbonated beverages would be contraindicated with a UTI because this may be a contributing factor to UTI. (C) Douching may contribute to bacteriuria in females and is not recommended. (D) UTIs have been related to the use of hot tub or whirlpool baths, and thus if one is predisposed to UTIs it is best to avoid tub baths.

101. (A) Nursing process phase: implementation; client need: psychosocial integrity; content area: psychiatric nursing

Rationale
(A) The client is aware that the thoughts and behaviors are irrational and out of his control. (B) During certain periods the client is able to control troubling and unwanted thoughts. Change is gradual and characterized by an uneven course. (C) The client is aware of the time frame and does not need a reminder. (D) Trying to avoid the ritualistic thoughts creates anxiety. It is difficult to control the irrational thoughts until the client recognizes the stimuli that trigger the anxiety.

102. (D) Nursing process phase: assessment; client need: health promotion and maintenance; content area: maternity nursing

Rationale
(A) Hypocalcemia is strongly associated with newborns of diabetic mothers, perinatal asphyxia, trauma, and low-birth-weight and preterm birth. (B) Glucose levels normally fall in the newborn over the first few hours of life. Infants with risk factors (large or small for gestational age, low birth weight, cold stress, or neonatal asphyxia) may require frequent glucose monitoring for the first few hours of life. Hypoglycemia is treated by feeding the infant. (C) Water intoxication results in hyponatremia and is associated with excessive feeding of water to infants. Diluting formula with water is one cause of water intoxication. (D) Cold stress of the newborn may result in acidosis and raise the level of free fatty acids. In the presence of acidosis, albumin binding of bilirubin is weakened and bilirubin is freed, resulting in hyperbilirubinemia.

103. (D) Nursing process phase: implementation; client need: safe, effective care environment; content area: medical/surgical nursing

Rationale
(A) Heat and dryness make pruritus worse. (B) Polyester clothing does not allow for ventilation and would make pruritus worse. (C) Strong detergents might produce increased irritation and discomfort. (D) The skin should be inspected for the cardinal signs of inflammation; infection could be the cause of the inflammation or could follow the pruritus.

104. **(D)** Nursing process phase: assessment; client need: health promotion and maintenance; content area: pediatric nursing

Rationale
(A) This is not characteristic of children with PKU. (B) This feature is not characteristic of children with PKU. (C) A large head is not characteristic of children with PKU. (D) True. Children with PKU have decreased melanin and are characteristically fair skinned with blue eyes and blonde hair.

105. **(D)** Nursing process phase: analysis; client need: health promotion and maintenance; content area: pediatric nursing

Rationale
(A) The Electra complex is a phenomenon of female development in which the girl wishes to marry her father and kill her mother. (B) Adolescence, not the preschool-age child, is a period during which individuals commonly question their own sexual orientation. (C) Penile size is not a concern of a 4-year-old male. (D) Mutilation and castration anxiety are normal development in reference to Freud's oedipal or phallic stage for the preschool child.

106. **(A)** Nursing process phase: implementation; client need: safe, effective care environment; content area: maternity nursing

Rationale
(A) The most common side effect of epidural anesthesia is a drop in maternal blood pressure, which also decreases perfusion to the fetus and can result in fetal distress. (B) The nurse cannot determine how well the client tolerated the procedure until a blood pressure is evaluated. It is standard practice to assess the client prior to documentation. (C) The epidural will take approximately 15 minutes to affect the lower extremities. The client and the fetus could suffer serious side effects if BP is not evaluated prior to that time. (D) Raising the head of the bed will most likely drop the client's blood pressure and cause the epidural to settle below the intended level of anesthesia. The client is kept nearly flat for the first hours, then may raise the head of the bed, depending on tolerance and the effect on the anesthesia.

107. **(A)** Nursing process phase: implementation; client need: health promotion and maintenance; content area: psychiatric nursing

Rationale
(A) Vinegar-based salad dressing, cough elixirs, and cologne all contain alcohol and could cause a severe reaction in the presence of Antabuse. (B) Cough elixirs and cologne contain alcohol; acetaminophen does not. (C) Cologne contains alcohol; acetaminophen and penicillin do not. (D) Acetaminophen and pencillin do not contain alcohol; vinegar-based salad dressing does.

108. **(A)** Nursing process phase: analysis; client need: safe, effective care environment; content area: medical/surgical nursing

Rationale
(A) Third-degree burns may extend into subcutaneous tissue, muscle, and nerves. (B) Loss of dermis and epidermis are characteristic of second-degree burns. (C) Loss of only the epidermis would mean that the burns were first-degree. (D) Blisters and erythema are seen in second-degree burns.

109. **(C)** Nursing process phase: evaluation; client need: safe, effective care environment; content area: pediatric nursing

Rationale
(A) A systemic reaction is an immediate hypersensitivity that begins within minutes of an exposure to an antigen. However, 10 minutes may not be long enough for the major organs to respond with symptoms. (B) Within 20 minutes, symptoms can be present, but symptoms in some organs may not be apparent for 30 minutes. (C) Systemic reactions that produce severe symptoms occur within 30 minutes in the cardiovascular, respiratory, gastrointestinal, and integumentary systems; therefore, a minimal waiting period should be 30 minutes. (D) System reactions begin within minutes of exposure to an antigen, and a delayed reaction may occur up to 24 hours. Major organ response will produce symptoms within 30 minutes.

110. **(B)** Nursing process phase: analysis and planning; client need: safe, effective care environment; content area: pediatric nursing

Rationale
(A) The Moro reflex may be asymmetrical in a newborn with a fractured clavicle. Fractured clavicles are most often associated with difficult vaginal deliveries of greater-than-average-gestational-age newborns. It is not contraindicated to be elicited. (B) The client should be supported at the upper and lower back to be lifted up to prevent pain or further trauma. (C) The scarf sign assessment is contraindicated in a client with suspected or confirmed clavicle fractures. (D) A cast is usually not indicated. A sling or Ace-type dressing may be applied for immobilization if any treatment at all is indicated.

111. **(A)** Nursing process phase: implementation; client need: safe, effective care environment; content area: medical/surgical nursing

Rationale
(A) Medications that dilate the pupil could further increase intraocular pressure by blocking drainage from the eye through the canal of Schlemm. (B) Doses of eye drops should not be missed. (C) Eye drops will probably be given over the client's lifetime. (D) Clients with glaucoma should see their ophthalmologist at least yearly.

112. **(C)** Nursing process phase: implementation; client need: health promotion and maintenance; content area: maternity nursing

Rationale
(A) Consumer tests actually have higher rates of false-negatives. This is related to the test being performed too soon after a missed period. (B) There are many variables that must be controlled for, such as specimen contamination, timing, or movement of sample. The ease of testing is relative. (C) Because there is an increased chance of false-negative, it is important to determine pregnancy at the earliest time to provide

prenatal care and minimize fetal risk. (D) Home testing does ensure privacy, so the client is the only one who will know the results.

113. (A) Nursing process phase: planning; client need: physiological integrity; content area: medical/surgical nursing

Rationale

(A) Fatigue is a common complaint with pheochromocytoma because of basal metabolic rate. (B) A poor cough reflex and constipation are not usually noted with pheochromocytoma. (C) Mild dehydration and hemoconcentration are usually present in pheochromocytoma. (D) A poor cough reflex and constipation are not usually noted with pheochromocytoma.

114. (C) Nursing process phase: implementation; client need: psychosocial integrity; content area: psychiatric nursing

Rationale

(A) The client at this stage is unable to engage in activities that will interrupt obsessive themes. (B) Protection from injury is an intervention used when the client is overwhelmed with anxiety. (C) Providing simple activities may reduce anxiety and interrupt obsessive themes and ritualistic behaviors. (D) It is important for the client to have some control over his behavior before engaging in simple activities.

115. (D) Nursing process phase: assessment; client need: safe, effective care environment; content area: maternity nursing

Rationale

(A) An epidural block does not affect uterine contractions. Administration of IV Pitocin would increase the frequency and intensity of uterine contractions. (B) Fetal heart rate variability is not affected by an epidural block. Any fetal heart tracing changes seen would likely be either tachycardia, bradycardia, or a pattern of late decelerations, which are associated with a decrease in placental perfusion. (C) An epidural block does not cause palpations and tremors. The tocolytic terbutaline is most commonly associated with these side effects. (D) Hypotension in the woman is the most common side effect of epidural block.

116. (C) Nursing process phase: assessment; client need: physiological integrity; content area: medical/surgical nursing

Rationale

(A) Increased skin pigmentation is usually noted, not vitiligo. (B) Increased oil and sweat production of the skin is usually noted in acromegaly. (C) Joint pain resulting from skeletal changes and arthritis is common in acromegaly. (D) Hair growth may increase in acromegaly.

117. (C) Nursing process phase: implementation; client need: health promotion and maintenance; content area: pediatric nursing

Rationale

(A) The corneal light reflex test is used to detect strabismus. If the eyes are normal orthophoric, twin red reflexes fall symmetrically within each pupil. (B) Epicanthal folds may give a false impression of malalignment of the eyes; however, they do not develop as a result of strabismus. (C) If strabismus is not corrected by age 4 to 6 years, amblyopia, a type of blindness, will develop. Amblyopia is blindness resulting from the

brain suppressing the image produced by the affected eye. (D) Strabismus does not result in color perception deficit.

118. (C) Nursing process phase: assessment; client need: physiological integrity; content area: maternity nursing

Rationale

(A) Thrombophlebitis signs and symptoms include calf pain, redness, and warmth. (B) Breast engorgement can occur in 48 hours. (C) An immediate low-grade elevation in temperature is related to dehydration in labor and delivery. (D) Some of the hypovolemic shock symptoms include excessive or bright-red bleeding, a boggy fundus, and a high temperature.

119. (C) Nursing process phase: evaluation; client need: physiological integrity; content area: psychiatric nursing

Rationale

(A) Drowsiness is a side effect of benztropine, not the therapeutic effect. (B) The anticholinergic effect of benztropine does not enhance thought processes. (C) Benztropine reverses the extrapyramidal effects caused by the administration of a neuroleptic. (D) Dryness of the mouth is a side effect of benztropine, not the therapeutic effect.

120. (C) Nursing process phase: assessment; client need: safe, effective care environment; content area: maternity nursing

Rationale

(A) The purpose of the test is to evaluate the presence of accelerations in response to fetal movements. Contractions are not indicators of fetal well-being. (B) Decelerations seen in response to fetal movement are indicative of a poor fetal outcome. (C) The purpose of the test is to evaluate the presence of accelerations in response to fetal movements. The test is said to be reactive when there are at least two fetal heart rate accelerations in response to fetal movement in 20 minutes, each increasing at least 15 beats and lasting at least 15 seconds. (D) Fetal movement is an important part of the nonstress test, but the purpose of the test is to evaluate fetal response to fetal movement.

121. (B) Nursing process phase: analysis; client need: safe, effective care environment; content area: medical/surgical nursing

Rationale

(A) The P wave on an EKG represents atrial depolarization. (B) Depolarization of ventricular cells produces the QRS complex. (C) The T wave on the EKG represents electrical recovery or restored electronegativity. (D) This action describes atrial depolarization.

122. (A) Nursing process phase: assessment; client need: health promotion and maintenance; content area: pediatric nursing

Rationale

(A) Tall tales and imaginary playmates are normal for the 4-year-old. (B & C) The 3-year-old is more likely to have a security blanket or other object and to fear loss of love. (D) The 4-year-old is typically more aggressive than the 3-year-old and will become more tranquil at 5 years old.

123. (D) Nursing process phase: implementation; client need: safe, effective care environment; content area: psychiatric nursing—dosage calculation

Rationale
$$50 \text{ mg} : 1 \text{ tablet} = 100 \text{ mg} : x = 2 \text{ tablets}$$
Math calculation explains incorrect answers.

124. **(C)** Nursing process phase: planning; client need: physiological integrity; content area: pediatric nursing

Rationale
(A) Fluid restriction is seldom necessary in the treatment of AGN. Forcing fluids would be contraindicated because of the edema associated with AGN. (B) Sodium may be restricted during the edematous phase. Increasing sodium in the diet would be contraindicated. (C) A record of daily weight is the most useful means to assess fluid balance in a child with AGN. (D) Regular measurements of vital signs, not once a shift, are essential to identify the acute hypertension associated with AGN.

125. **(B)** Nursing process phase: implementation; client need: safe, effective care environment; content area: maternity nursing—dosage calculation

Rationale
$$5 \text{ mg} : 1 \text{ ml} = 1 \text{ mg} : x = 0.2 \text{ ml}$$
Math calculation explains incorrect answers.

126. **(A)** Nursing process phase: assessment; client need: health promotion and maintenance; content area: pediatric nursing

Rationale
(A) The absence of the red reflex could indicate congenital cataracts or a hemorrhage of the retina. (B) Edema of the eyelids is normal for up to 2 days after delivery. (C) Tears may be present or absent in the newborn. Purulent drainage is abnormal and should be reported. (D) Strabismus is normal because of the lack of binocularity.

127. **(D)** Nursing process phase: implementation; client need: health promotion and maintenance; content area: medical/surgical nursing

Rationale
(A) While lentils are a good source of folic acid, the other foods are not. (B) Eggs, milk, and most meats are not good sources of folic acid. (C) Most meats are not good folate sources. Dark-green leafy vegetables are a better folic acid source than corn. (D) Dried beans and spinach are two foods that contain high levels of folate.

128. **(A)** Nursing process phase: implementation; client need: psychosocial integrity; content area: psychiatric nursing

Rationale
(A) Acknowledgment of the client's feelings and concerns about the phobic behavior demonstrates understanding. (B) Desensitization is a technique that may be appropriate when the client shows a willingness to be exposed to a series of increasingly anxiety-provoking situations. (C) If the client's perceptual field is narrow or disrupted, the client will be unable to assimilate the information about phobias and fear. (D) The client was not seeking advice when she entered the clinic.

129. **(B)** Nursing process phase: assessment; client need: physiological integrity; content area: maternity nursing

Rationale
(A) The cervix is the neck of the uterus. (B) The fundus is the upper portion of the uterus, which can be palpated abdominally in the postpartum woman. (C) The body of the uterus refers to the entire upper portion of the uterus. (D) This is not an appropriate term for the top portion of the uterus.

130. **(C)** Nursing process phase: assessment; client need: physiological integrity; pediatric nursing

Rationale
(A) Bleeding will be most pronounced and localized at the point(s) of injury. You would expect to see bleeding in joints and tissue surrounding the areas injured in his fall. (B) Dehydration is not a typical sign observed with hemophilia after a fall. (C) True. Bleeding in the joint at the point of injury is typical and may be severe. (D) Neutropenia is not a symptom associated with hemophilia.

131. **(B)** Nursing process phase: planning; client need: physiological integrity; content area: medical/surgical nursing

Rationale
(A) Epinephrine is contraindicated because it causes a further elevation of serum glucose. (B) The medical diagnosis and the condition of the skin indicate that the client is in hyperglycemic, hyperosmolar, nonketotic coma. One of the highest priorities for such clients is fluid replacement because of losses from osmotic diuresis. The need for insulin is not as great as in ketosis because the pancreas is producing some insulin. (C) Prednisone would also cause can even greater elevation of the serum glucose. (D) The client does not need bicarbonate if acidosis is not present.

132. **(B)** Nursing process phase: assessment; client need: safe, effective care environment; content area: pediatric nursing

Rationale
(A) Coolness to the extremity should be watched for progression and diminishing pulse. A palpable radial pulse indicates circulation to the area. (B) Coolness to the fingers and a slow capillary refill indicate decreased circulation to the extremity. This would require immediate attention to prevent nerve and/or tissue damage. (C) Edema and discoloration are a concern, but each could be used as a baseline for the child. An increase in either from the baseline could indicate decreasing circulation to the area. (D) Edema to the extremity should be watched for any increase. A capillary refill of 2 to 3 seconds is considered normal.

133. **(D)** Nursing process phase: implementation; client need: physiological integrity; content area: maternity nursing

Rationale
(A) The oropharynx of the infant should be suctioned by the physician while the head is on the perineum. Immediate suctioning after delivery can stimulate the vagus nerve and lower the heart rate of the infant. (B) The heart rate should be checked at 1 minute after birth, and after the infant is dried and warmed. (C) Placement of the identification bands can be done anytime after the infant is stabilized. (D) Cold stress is extremely dangerous to the newborn. It increases oxygen demands and can cause hypoxia. Drying the infant has first priority.

134. (D) Nursing process phase: assessment; client need: safe, effective care environment; content area: psychiatric nursing

Rationale

(A) The nurse would have asked the client to rate his mood on a scale of 1 to 10 if she had been assessing the mood. (B) Although the nurse has asked the client what he thinks about a subject, neither the content nor the process has been specifically addressed. (C) The nurse has not requested that the client answer questions specific to previously learned material. (D) The nurse is assessing insight. If the client responds by saying "Yes," then the nurse should explore to what degree.

135. (C) Nursing process phase: implementation; client need: safe, effective care environment; content area: medical/surgical nursing

Rationale

(A) Sodium restriction is not necessary unless the client is taking allopurinol for treatment of recurrent calcium oxalate stones. (B) A bland diet is unnecessary. (C) When a client is taking allopurinol, a daily urine output of 2 L/day is desirable to flush uric acid from the body. (D) Carbonated beverages, in moderation, are not contraindicated.

136. (A) Nursing process phase: evaluation; client need: safe, effective care environment; content area: medical/surgical nursing

Rationale

(A) This behavior would indicate a need for further teaching. The client should notify the physician if original pain is unrelieved by three doses of NTG. (B) This action should be taken by the client receiving NTG. It does not indicate a need for further teaching. (C) This action should be taken by the client receiving NTG. It does not indicate a need for further teaching. (D) This action should be taken by the client receiving NTG. It does not indicate a need for further teaching.

137. (C) Nursing process phase: implementation; client need: safe, effective care environment; content area: maternity nursing

Rationale

(A) Because of the risk of cord prolapse with the rupture of membranes, the nurse must first assure fetal well-being before performing comfort measures. (B) Because of the risk of cord prolapse with the rupture of membranes, the nurse must first assure fetal well-being before notifying the physician or midwife. (C) The nurse should first evaluate fetal well-being by assessing the fetal heart tones. There is a high risk of cord prolapse with the rupture of the amniotic membranes. (D) Because of the risk of cord prolapse with the rupture of membranes, the nurse must first assure fetal well-being before documenting the client response.

138. (C) Nursing process phase: analysis; client need: health promotion and maintenance; content area: pediatric nursing

Rationale

(A) Hypertension is not a manifestation of sickle-cell disease. (B) Hypotension is not a manifestation of sickle-cell disease. (C) True. The primary manifestation of sickle-cell disease is intravascular clotting with clumping of sickled red blood cells. (D) Slight edema may be present at sites of injury; however, it is not a primary manifestation of the disease.

139. (B) Nursing process phase: implementation; client need: safe, effective care environment; content area: psychiatric nursing

Rationale

(A) Psychoanalysis is a long-term therapy, which may be a choice after the anxiety has been reduced to a manageable level. (B) The best intervention is to provide support and reassurance in order to decrease the anxiety level and increase the client's feelings of self-worth. (C) Encouraging public speaking will further increase the level of anxiety and may cause an intense, disorganizing flood of panic. (D) Most persons with phobic reactions are aware of them and recognize them as excessive or unreasonable.

140. (C) Nursing process phase: assessment; client need: physiological integrity; content area: maternity nursing

Rationale

(A) Infants whose mothers have experienced pregnancy-induced hypertension usually are small for gestational age. (B) Lupus erythematosus is an autoimmune disease. Pregnancy does not appear to worsen this disease. If a woman already has renal damage and hypertension, placental damage can lead to a spontaneous abortion. The presence of this disease during pregnancy does not produce a macrosomic infant. (C) Gestational diabetes frequently produces a macrosomic infant. Alterations in glucose metabolism in the diabetic mother affect the fetus and the newborn. The newborn appears plump, plethoric, and puffy. Occasionally, infants of diabetic mothers may be small because of placental insufficiency in utero. (D) Macrosomia is not seen in infants born of HIV-positive mothers.

141. (C) Nursing process phase: planning; client need: safe, effective care environment; content area: medical/surgical nursing

Rationale

(A) NPH SC peaks in 6 to 12 hours. (B–D) The rationale is the same.

142. (D) Nursing process phase: evaluation; client need: safe, effective care environment; content area: medical/surgical nursing

Rationale

(A) This is not routinely done and will not show immediate improvement in ventilation after suctioning. (B) Although this action may be done, it is not the best way to evaluate effectiveness of suctioning. (C) Although this action may be done, it is not the best way to evaluate effectiveness of suctioning. (D) Before and after auscultation of the chest is the best way to determine effectiveness of suctioning.

143. (B) Nursing process phase: implementation; client need: physiological integrity; content area: maternity nursing

Rationale

(A) Increasing postcesarean birth comfort should not prevent a mother from initiating breastfeeding. A low dose may be given just after breastfeeding to prevent a peak drug level in the beast milk and to prevent drowsiness. (B) The analgesic will peak within 15 to 30 minutes after administration to avoid interference with the breastfeeding process. (C) There is no evidence that analgesics inhibit milk production. They may permit sufficient relaxation to provide for the milk letdown reflex. (D) Taking an analgesic is not equivalent to milk contamination.

144. (A) Nursing process phase: assessment; client need: physiological integrity; content area: medical/surgical nursing

Rationale
(A) With pancytopenia, all hematologic values will be greatly diminished. (B) While these laboratory values are low, they do not indicate pancytopenia. (C & D) These laboratory values are within normal limits.

145. (A) Nursing process phase: assessment; client need: physiological integrity; content area: maternity nursing

Rationale
(A) Abruptio placenta is associated with acute cocaine-induced hypertension and usually occurs within 1 hour of use. (B) Because the client is pregnant, she has increased nutritional requirements, which are not likely to be met because of the substance abuse. However, this is not her greatest risk factor at this time. (C) Fetal vasoconstriction is related to the increased incidence of congenital malformations in the first trimester. This client is 32 weeks' gestation. (D) Pulmonary emboli are most often associated with thromboembolic disease.

146. (C) Nursing process phase: implementation; client need: physiological integrity; content area: medical/surgical nursing

Rationale
(A, B, & D) The time ranges specified do not identify the peak action time for Humulin NPH insulin given at 6:30 A.M. (C) Humulin NPH insulin exerts its maximum effect about 4 to 10 hours after administration. Beef or porcine NPH insulin peaks about 6 to 12 hours after administration.

147. (D) Nursing process phase: implementation; client need: safe, effective care environment; content area: medical/surgical nursing

Rationale
285 mg divided by 50 mg/5 ml = 28.5 ml
Math calculation explains incorrect answers.

148. (D) Nursing process phase: analysis; client need: physiological integrity; content area: psychiatric nursing

Rationale
(A) This nursing diagnosis is lower priority than those concerning safety and physiological integrity because it has a teaching-learning focus. (B) While there are some physiological hazards that can occur with impaired mobility, it is unlikely when it is related to lack of motivation that a physical impairment is present. This would make it a lower priority. (C) This nursing diagnosis addresses the integrity of the ego. When it is related to a depressed mood, suicidal ideation should be assessed. There are no data to indicate that the client with this diagnosis is suicidal, although the potential is always present. (D) This nursing diagnosis should receive the highest priority on the plan of care, and the client should be assessed regularly for suicidal intent, plan, and available means.

149. (C) Nursing process phase: assessment; client need: physiological integrity; content area: maternity nursing

Rationale
(A) Quickening refers to the first movements of the growing fetus that are felt by the mother. (B) Effacement refers to the shortening and thinning of the cervix that occurs prior to delivery. (C) Lightening refers to the tilting or dropping of the fetal head forward and downward into the true pelvis. This usually occurs 2 to 3 weeks before labor in the primigravida but frequently does not occur until the beginning of labor in many multigravidas. (D) Station is defined as the location of the presenting part of the fetus in relation to the ischial spines of the birth canal.

150. (A) Nursing process phase: implementation; client need: safe, effective care environment; content area: pediatric nursing—dosage calculation

Rationale
2.5 mg : 1 ml = 15.6 mg : x = 6.24 ml
Math calculation explains incorrect answers.

151. (A) Nursing process phase: assessment; client need: physiological integrity; content area: pediatric nursing

Rationale
(A) Red means medical alert since the child is below 50 percent of her personal best. Red equals below 50 percent of personal best and signals medical alert, possible severe airway narrowing, take bronchodilator immediately, call practitioner if child does not return to yellow or green zone immediately. (B) The green zone indicates 80 percent to 100 percent of his personal best and symptom-free. Green equals 80 to 100 percent of personal best, all clear, no symptoms present, follow routine treatment plan. (C) The yellow zone indicates 50 to 80 percent of his personal best and thus a caution signal. Yellow equals 50 to 80 percent of personal best, caution signal, acute exacerbation may be present, may need increase in maintenance therapy, call practitioner if remains in this color zone. (D) Eighty percent of his personal best still indicates caution since the child is in the yellow zone. Yellow equals 50 to 80 percent of personal best, caution signal, acute exacerbation may be present, may need an increase in maintenance therapy, call practitioner if remains in this color zone.

152. (D) Nursing process phase: assessment; client need: physiological integrity; content area: medical/surgical—gerontological nursing

Rationale
(A) Creatinine clearance is a 24-hour test and is used to measure renal functioning. This client does not present with symptoms of difficulty with renal function. (B) Computerized axial tomography (CAT scan) is an expensive procedure used to detect tumors or other masses. This assessment would not be the initial assessment of the nurse but might be required if other assessment data are negative. (C) The nurse might perform a complete mental status examination to determine cognitive function, but there is no evidence to suggest that this client is experiencing cognitive impairment. (D) Benign prostatic hypertrophy (BPH) is the most common cause of urinary obstruction in males, occurring in about 50 percent by the age of 60 and increasing with age.

153. (B) Nursing process phase: analysis; client need: psychosocial integrity; content area: maternity nursing

Rationale
(A) The postpartum assessment revealed that the client had a firm fundus at the appropriate fundal height. In addition, the

lochial flow was appropriate for a newly delivered client. One clot is not of serious concern when it is smaller than a silver dollar. Actual problems have priority over those at risk. (B) This family has entered a new phase of development. The nurse needs to plan and implement measures to promote attachment and bonding so that the parents can assume their roles. This is an actual problem. (C) There is a potential for infection. However, actual problems have priority over potential problems. (D) There is no evidence of anxiety at this time. Altered family would be a more appropriate nursing diagnosis.

154. (B) Nursing process phase: implementation; client need: physiological integrity; content area: pediatric nursing

Rationale

(A) This is incorrect. We can relieve many of the side effects of chemotherapy. (B) True. Most of the side effects of cancer chemotherapy are temporary and reversible once the chemotherapy is eliminated from the body. (C) The side effects of chemotherapy are often caused by the effects on the normal cells in the body. (D) Most of the side effects of chemotherapy are physical in nature, not psychological.

155. (A) Nursing process phase: implementation; client need: psychosocial integrity; content area: psychiatric nursing

Rationale

(A) A calm, direct, and nonauthoritative manner decreases anxiety, allows the client to regain some control, and decreases powerlessness and agitation. (B) When the client is interrupted during the ritualistic behavior, anxiety escalates. (C) Ignoring the behavior is nontherapeutic. However, the less focus placed on the ritual, the less anxiety will occur. (D) Explaining the rationale will be helpful, if the client is receptive to learning.

156. (C) Nursing process phase: assessment; client need: physiological integrity; content area: maternity nursing

Rationale

(A) A single umbilical artery is not associated with an imperforate anus. (B) Hepatosplenomegaly, enlargement of the spleen and liver, has many causes. A single umbilical artery is not related to hepatosplenomegaly. (C) Because of the time frame of the development of the renal system in conjunction with the development of the umbilical arteries, renal anomalies are frequently seen in infants with a single umbilical artery. This finding would warrant further evaluation. (D) Cardiac malformations are not generally associated with a single umbilical artery.

157. (D) Nursing process phase: implementation; client need: health promotion and maintenance; content area: maternity nursing

Rationale

(A) This statement does not give information that increases the client's knowledge or that decreases her frustration. (B) Softening of the cervix may occur weeks before the onset of labor and is an objective sign the client will not be aware of. True labor is characterized by contractions increasing in frequency and regularity. (C) Typically, the fetus will decrease in activity as it settles into the pelvis in preparation for labor. The clear vaginal discharge could be interpreted as ruptured membranes, but the statement does not have adequate infor-

mation for the client to understand rupture of membranes. (D) Many signs and symptoms can occur as labor approaches, but the defining characteristic of labor is cervical effacement and dilatation.

158. (D) Nursing process phase: planning; client need: health promotion and maintenance; content area: psychiatric nursing

Rationale

(A) The client may recognize the need to apologize and make some kind of restitution, but neither is a criterion for restraint release. (B) In most hospitals, the physician does make the determination about whether the client is ready to be released from restraints, but does so only after the nurse's assessment. (C) There is not a minimum amount of time that must be spent in seclusion and restraint before release can be considered. (D) When the violent behavior has subsided and the client and nurse have formed a therapeutic alliance, then release from restraints can be considered.

159. (D) Nursing process phase: implementation; client need: psychological integrity; content area: pediatric nursing

Rationale

(A) Honesty is preferred. An IM antibiotic will probably hurt. (B) Children take things literally and will assume you are putting a real stick in the arm. (C) Although seeing and holding supplies may be beneficial in some instances, the child is not able to properly prepare an IM. (D) Brief explanations presented positively and immediately before a procedure are best.

160. (D) Nursing process phase: evaluation; client need: safe, effective care environment; content area: medical/surgical—gerontological nursing

Rationale

(A–C) While medical and mental factors as well as family support are important in the assessment for incontinence, biofeedback requires that the client be cognitively intact and motivated to learn bladder inhibition and sphincter contraction. (D) Biofeedback requires that the client be cognitively intact and motivated to learn bladder inhibition and sphincter contraction.

161. (C) Nursing process phase: implementation; client need: psychosocial integrity; content area: maternity nursing

Rationale

(A) Although the increased pigmentation cannot be presently changed, this response does not therapeutically address her concerns. (B) This hyperpigmentation is not diet-related or associated with an increased intake of iron. (C) Changes during pregnancy in skin pigmentation are common. These changes are associated with elevated levels of melanocyte-stimulating hormone stimulated by increased hormone levels. (D) It is not advisable to suggest using a product that could potentially impact fetal development.

162. (C) Nursing process phase: planning; client need: psychosocial integrity; content area: medical/surgical—gerontological nursing

Rationale

(A) Hemodialysis allows more rapid renal clearance and removal of excess body fluid than does CAPD. (B) Hemodialysis provides a social environment for interaction, and some hemodialysis centers offer clients the opportunity to engage in art and music therapy. (C) Because CAPD is done at home, the client develops an increased feeling of self-control, which is important to the independent client. (D) Hemodialysis, not CAPD, provides the client with three well-defined dialysis days per week in which they will interact with the dialysis personnel.

163. **(C)** Nursing process phase: analysis; client need: safe, effective care environment; content area: medical/surgical—gerontological nursing

Rationale
(A) There are changes in the skin turgor of the older adult that are a result of the aging process; however, there is a decrease in lean body mass, and the immune function is depressed, not decreased. (B) There are changes in the skin turgor of the older adult and loss of visual acuity that are a result of the aging process; however, there is a decrease in bone density, not an increase. (C) The most significant normal physiological aging changes in older adults include the loss of lean body mass, decrease in bone density, and depressed immune function. These make the older adult vulnerable to fractures and to infections, particularly respiratory infections. (D) As a result of the aging process, there is a loss of lean body mass and of visual acuity in the older adult; however there is a decrease in bone density, not an increase.

164. **(A)** Nursing process phase: assessment; client need: health promotion and maintenance; content area: maternity nursing

Rationale
(A) This palpation of the fetal outline through the abdomen of the mother allows the examiner to feel for parts of the fetus and then to identify the fetal position or lie. (B) Babinski's reflex is a reflex response of the newborn. (C) This is not a correct response. Walker's maneuver is not a term used in this context. (D) The Lamaze technique describes a type of psychoprophylaxis for childbirth in which the mother is instructed in breathing techniques that permit her to facilitate delivery by relaxation.

165. **(C)** Nursing process phase: analysis; client need: psychosocial integrity; content area: psychiatric nursing

Rationale
(A) It is not a conscious effort to control the environment, but the environment may have accommodated the ritualistic behavior. (B) Ritualistic behavior is not associated with love messages. (C) Ritualistic behavior is employed to relieve anxiety caused by unconscious impulses that are frightening. (D) Ritualistic behavior is an attempt to find relief from anxiety, not to seek attention.

166. **(D)** Nursing process phase: assessment; client need: physiological integrity; content area: pediatric nursing

Rationale
(A) Palpating the carotid artery provides information concerning the pulse. (B) Inspecting the bucal membranes provides assessment data related to cyanosis. (C) Auscultating the heart provides assessment data concerning heart sound. (D) Press the skin lightly on a central site, such as the forehead or the top of the hand, to produce a slight blanching.

The time it takes for the blanched area to return to its original color is the capillary refill time.

167. **(A)** Nursing process phase: implementation; client need: physiological integrity; content area: medical/surgical—gerontological nursing

Rationale
(A) A major limiting factor of CAPD is peritonitis resulting from breaks in sterile technique or contamination of the system. There is also a greater risk of infection at the catheter insertion site that is placed in the abdominal cavity. (B) Information about follow-up appointments is necessary, but is not crucial to the health of this client. (C) Weight gain may occur in CAPD clients as a result of carbohydrate absorption, which occurs because of the glucose concentration in the dialysate. This can be controlled by physical activity levels and dietary consciousness, but a sodium restriction is not necessary. (D) Clients having CAPD are not prescribed diuretics. The dialysate solution is the vehicle for the removal of excess fluids and harmful toxins.

168. **(D)** Nursing process phase: implementation; client need: health promotion and maintenance; content area: maternity nursing

Rationale
(A) Deep knee bends put increased stress on the lower part of the already unstable lower body. (B) Pelvic floor exercises increase support for the gravid uterus during pregnancy. (C) Double leg lifts cause the back to arch and strain, increasing low back discomfort. (D) Pelvic tilting works the abdominal muscles in the front and buttocks, thus rolling back the pelvis and flattening the arch in the lumbar spine. This action increases comfort in the lower back.

169. **(C)** Nursing process phase: planning; client need: safe, effective care environment; content area: medical/surgical—gerontological nursing

Rationale
(A) The most important determinant of frequency of sexual activity for a woman is the presence of a healthy and interested sexual partner. (B) Some medical therapies and surgical interventions may improve function. There is no evidence to suggest that this malignancy cannot be treated with one of these therapies. (C) Counseling clients about their sexual function as a result of treatment is important because some medical therapies and surgical interventions may improve function and this information needs to be shared with the client. (D) The most important determinant of frequency of sexual activity for a woman is the presence of a healthy and interested sexual partner; however, there is no evidence to suggest that this client does not have a partner.

170. **(B)** Nursing process phase: implementation; client need: safe, effective care environment; content area: medical/surgical nursing

Rationale
(A & D) Regular insulin is drawn up first, then NPH insulin. (B) This is correct. (C) Regular insulin can be mixed with NPH insulin in the same syringe.

171. **(D)** Nursing process phase: implementation; client need: safe, effective care environment; content area: pediatric nursing

Rationale
(A) Not suitable toys since moisture will dampen the toys and make it difficult to keep them dry. (B) The toy may be a source of sparks and a potential fire hazard. (C) Synthetic blankets can initiate sparks, which may cause a fire. (D) Vinyl or plastic items do not absorb moisture and can be easily wiped dry.

172. **(A)** Nursing process phase: implementation; client need: safe, effective care environment; content area: psychiatric nursing—dosage calculation

Rationale

$$100 \text{ mg} : 1 \text{ ml} = 25 \text{ mg} : x = 0.25 \text{ ml}$$

Math calculation explains incorrect answers.

173. **(B)** Nursing process phase: evaluation; client need: physiological integrity; content area: medical/surgical—gerontological nursing

Rationale
(A) A bowel management program continues on a regular basis, even on weekends. (B) Breakfast is best as the triggering meal because the gastrocolic and duodenocolic reflexes are strongest on an empty stomach. The program is implemented on a regular schedule, either every day or every third day. (C) Toileting is begun 15 minutes after the triggering of the rectal reflex, not 1 hour. (D) The goal of bowel management is to produce a soft, well-formed stool, not diarrhea.

174. **(C)** Nursing process phase: assessment; client need: safe, effective care environment; content area: medical/surgical—gerontological nursing

Rationale
(A) There is no information given in this situation that would lead the nurse to believe that this client is experiencing dementia. (B) While the client may be experiencing diarrhea, the symptoms noted are indicative of severe malnutrition. (C) Signs of severe malnutrition include weight loss of over 10 percent of usual body weight, serum albumin less than 2.1 gm/dl, serum transferrin less than 100 mg/dl, and lymphocytes less than 800 cells per millimeter. (D) While depression may be the reason that this client is malnourished, there is no information that would indicate depression in this client.

175. **(B)** Nursing process phase: implementation; client need: health promotion and maintenance; content area: maternity nursing

Rationale
(A) A positive pregnancy test is a presumptive sign of pregnancy. Certain medications, premature menopause, blood in urine, or malignant tumors that produce hCG may result in false-positive findings. (B) There are only three signs that are accepted as positive confirmation of pregnancy. They are (1) auscultation of fetal heart sounds, (2) fetal movement felt by an examiner, and (3) visualization of the fetus by ultrasound. (C) A bluish coloration of the cervix is known as Chadwick's sign. Softening of the cervix is known as Goodell's sign. Cervical changes are probable signs of pregnancy. Other probable causes are a cervical infection or hormonal imbalances. (D) Amenorrhea is a presumptive sign of pregnancy. It can be caused by emotional stress, strenuous physical exercise, endocrine problems, chronic disease, or early menopause.

176. **(D)** Nursing process phase: assessment; client need: physiological integrity; content area: medical/surgical—gerontological nursing

Rationale
(A) Mental confusion and dry mouth are symptoms of dehydration, but the client will have hypotension, not hypertension. (B) None of these symptoms are indicative of dehydration, but elevated temperature may indicate an infectious process. (C) While diarrhea may lead to dehydration, this is not a symptom of dehydration, and a facial appearance in which the eyes appear sunken may be a normal aging change. (D) Mental confusion, a weak rapid pulse, and orthostatic hypotension are indicators of dehydration.

177. **(B)** Nursing process phase: assessment; client need: physiological integrity; content area: maternity nursing

Rationale
(A) Jaundice may be a result of polycythemia after a period of time as the breakdown of the increased RBCs takes place. (B) Infants with polycythemia have a ruddy or plethoric look. There is also usually a cyanotic tinge to the skin. (C) Hepatosplenomegaly refers to an enlargement of the liver and spleen. (D) Polycythemia does not cause an elevated temperature.

178. **(C)** Nursing process phase: implementation; client need: safe, effective care environment; content area: medical/surgical—gerontological nursing

Rationale
(A) Close monitoring of serum electrolyte values is not necessary with docusate sodium, but including a diet of adequate bulk and 2500 to 3000 ml of fluids is essential for this drug to act effectively. (B) Reducing the amount of dietary fiber is not appropriate with this drug. A diet containing adequate bulk and 2500 to 3000 ml of fluids is essential for this drug to act effectively. (C) Docusate acts like a detergent by permitting water and fatty substances to penetrate and be well mixed with the fecal material. A diet containing adequate bulk and 2500 to 3000 ml of fluids is essential for this drug to act effectively. (D) Testing monthly for blood in the feces is not indicated in the use of docusate sodium.

179. **(C)** Nursing process phase: assessment; client need: safe, effective care environment; content area: medical/surgical—gerontological nursing

Rationale
(A, C, & D) Symptoms of cataracts include blurred vision, sensitivity to bright light and glare, and a slowly progressive loss of vision. (B) A sharp pain that radiates through the eye should be assessed immediately because most visual impairments are not manifested by pain.

180. **(A)** Nursing process phase: implementation; client need: psychosocial integrity, content area: pediatric nursing

Rationale
(A) Correct. This is a therapeutic statement that validates the parents' observations. (B) This action does not address the parents' concerns, and sedation would be very nontherapeutic for parents and child! (C) To change the subject gives the parents the message that you do not want to address their concerns and does not assist in their coping. (D) This is a very judgmental, accusatory statement that will induce guilt and may further complicate the parents' abilities to cope.

181. **(B)** Nursing process phase: analysis; client need: safe, effective care environment; content area: maternity nursing

Rationale
(A) An upper respiratory infection will not include a reddened, painful area on the breast. (B) Mastitis is an inflammation of the breast tissue that is caused by a bacterial infection. *Staphyloccus aureus* is generally the causative agent. The bacteria usually enters the breast through a cracked nipple and multiplies in the breast milk. (C) Although a blocked duct may occur in breastfeeding mothers, this is not the primary cause of mastitis. (D) Cystitis is an inflammation of the bladder.

182. **(C)** Nursing process phase: analysis; client need: safe, effective care environment; content area: medical/surgical—gerontological nursing

Rationale
(A) There is no evidence to suggest that using both of these tests would prevent malpractice litigation. CT scan may help document lesions but may miss 10 percent of tumors. (B) A CT scan may help document lesions but may miss 10 percent of tumors. Ultrasound does not indicate abdominal function but is a radiologic technique used to examine abdominal and other organs that contain air. (C) A CT scan may help document lesions but may miss 10 percent of tumors. Diagnosis of disorders with symptoms experienced by this client are often made by using a combination of abdominal ultrasound, CT scan, angiography, and biopsy. (D) These symptoms are typical of hepatic tumors, the most common form of metastatic carcinoma.

183. **(D)** Nursing process phase: evaluation; client need: health promotion and maintenance; content area: medical/surgical nursing

Rationale
(A) Knowledge of a psychomotor skill is evaluated best by demonstration. (B) The nurse must see a demonstration of the procedure as it will be done in the home. (C) The client should show that fear of sticking one's self with a needle can be overcome. (D) This is the exact procedure that will be carried out at home.

184. **(D)** Nursing process phase: implementation; client need: health promotion and maintenance; content area: maternity nursing

Rationale
(A) This list of foods is highest in phosphorus, calcium, and protein (B) This list of foods is highest in vitamin C (C) This list of foods is highest in vitamin B$_1$, calcium, and potassium (D) This list of foods is highest in iron. Other sources of iron include dried beans and peas, enriched breads and cereals, and red meats.

185. **(B)** Nursing process phase: assessment; client need: physiological integrity; content area: psychiatric nursing

Rationale
(A) The symptoms should be reported to the physician, but an assessment should be completed before calling. (B) The AIMS should be completed before the physician is notified because he will, no doubt, ask for the results. (C) The addition of a drug such as benztropine in the presence of a low-potency drug like chlorpromazine will sometimes make the symptoms

of tardive dyskinesia worse. (D) Although the client's complaint should be recorded in the chart and passed on to the next shift, the client needs some immediate relief.

186. **(D)** Nursing process phase: analysis; client need: physiological integrity; content area: medical/surgical nursing

Rationale
(A) HIV causes a decreased ratio of helper to suppression T cells. (B) HIV causes a decrease in helper T cells. (C) HIV causes a decreased ratio of helper to suppression T cells. (D) HIV causes a decreased ratio of helper to suppressor T cells.

187. **(A)** Nursing process phase: analysis; client need: safe, effective care environment; content area: maternity nursing

Rationale
(A) A pulmonary embolism is a rare complication of deep-vein thrombosis. Signs and symptoms of pulmonary embolism may include a sharp chest pain or chest discomfort, tachypnea, dyspnea, and anxiety. (B) Hypertension and cool, moist skin are not indicative of a pulmonary embolism. (C) Tachycardia may be present with a pulmonary embolism; however, a decreased hematocrit is not related. (D) A gallop rhythm of the heart may be heard when a large emboli is present. Vasoconstriction is not related.

188. **(A)** Nursing process phase: implementation; client need: health promotion and maintenance; content area: pediatric nursing

Rationale
(A) When an adequate dosage of iron is reached, the stools will turn a tarry green color. The nurse should enquire about its occurrence on follow-up visits. (B) Iron supplements should be administered between meals and feedings when the presence of free hydrochloric acid is greatest. Gastric alkalinity impairs absorption of iron. (C) Liquid preparations of iron supplements may stain the teeth; therefore, the medication is given through a syringe or dropper placed at the back of the mouth. (D) Constipation is an infrequent side effect, especially in infants. The physician should be notified if diarrhea develops.

189. **(A)** Nursing process phase: analysis; client need: physiological integrity; content area: medical/surgical nursing

Rationale
(A) This process describes pannus formation in RA. (B) RA involves inflammatory granulation tissue that develops over the synovial membrane and articular cartilage, not popliteal bursae. (C & D) This process does not describe or identify pannus formation in RA.

190. **(C)** Nursing process phase: implementation; client need: safe, effective care environment; content area: pediatric nursing

Rationale
(A) The procedure for measuring the length of the nasogastric tube is to measure the distance from the nose to the earlobe to the epigastric area of the abdomen. While advancing the tube, if you meet resistance prior to complete insertion, you would pull back on the tube and attempt to insert it again. (B) The procedure for measuring the length of the epigastric tube is to measure the distance from the nose to the earlobe to the epigastric area of the abdomen. You advance the tube only this length. You do not advance until you get gastric con-

tents. (C) This is the correct procedure for measuring the length of the nasogastric tube for gavage feedings. (D) The procedure for measuring the length of the epigastric tube is to measure from the nose to the earlobe to the epigastric area of the abdomen. It would be both incorrect and unsafe to measure from the mouth to the umbilicus and add half the distance.

191. **(C)** Nursing process phase: implementation; client need: psychosocial integrity; content area: psychiatric nursing

Rationale

(A) This option will have no effect on the client's ritualistic behavior. (B) Confrontation without support may increase the anxiety and associated behaviors. (C) Limiting the behavior with kindness and support sets the external controls. (D) Increasing the medication is not the best intervention.

192. **(C)** Nursing process phase: evaluation; client need: safe, effective care environment; content area: maternity nursing

Rationale

(A) The client has had three abortions, and statistically this will not increase her risk of hemorrhage. (B) The nurse might assume that the client will be emotionally upset for this reason. There is not enough information to determine either whether the abortions were elective or the client's state of mind. (C) In most females, the pelvis does not fully mature until the age of 15. The assessment of a fundal height of 40 cm at 40 weeks' gestation and the −4 station indicates that the fetus has not dropped into the pelvis and engaged. The client is in labor, as indicated by the changes in the cervix. These findings indicate that the fetus is too large for the pelvis size. (D) There is no information given that indicates that the fetus is small.

193. **(C)** Nursing process phase: assessment; client need: safe, effective care environment; content area: medical/surgical nursing

Rationale

(A) All postoperative clients are of some concern for developing infection, but this client is not of most concern to develop pneumonia. (B) Clients with active HIV can predispose pneumonia, but this client reports a history of this and there is no evidence that it is an active state. (C) The elderly population, especially postoperatively, are at the greatest risk to develop pneumonia because of fragile immune responses, which often lead to increased susceptibility to infections. (D) This age group and surgery type can be monitored for other complications postoperatively, but is not a concern for developing pneumonia.

194. **(B)** Nursing process phase: analysis; client need: physiological integrity; content area: medical/surgical nursing

Rationale

(A) Calcitonin is not secreted by the anterior pituitary, but by the thyroid gland. (B) All of these hormones are secreted by the anterior pituitary gland. (C) Antidiuretic hormone (ADH) is not secreted by the anterior, but by the posterior pituitary. (C) Oxytocin is secreted by the posterior pituitary, and aldosterone is secreted by the adrenal cortex.

195. **(D)** Nursing process phase: implementation; client

need: physiological integrity; content area: maternity nursing

Rationale

(A) Taking the infant on and off the nipple will increase soreness, especially before the milk lets down. (B) Nursing on the sorer nipple exposes that nipple to the vigorous sucking at the beginning of the feeding. Start with the other nipple. (C) The breastfeeding style or pattern will continue, so additional trauma and discomfort is likely to occur. (D) Sore nipples are usually caused by improper positioning of the infant on the areola.

196. **(B)** Nursing process phase: implementation; client need: safe, effective care environment; content area: medical/surgical nursing—dosage calculation

Rationale

$$1 \text{ gm} : 1 \text{ ml} = 1 \text{ g} : x = 1 \text{ ml}$$

Math calculation explains incorrect answers.

197. **(C)** Nursing process phase: implementation; client need: health promotion and maintenance; content area: pediatric nursing

Rationale

(A) Milk is a source of protein, calcium, and vitamin D. (B) Green, leafy vegetables contain iron, not the orange and yellow vegetables. (C) Meat is a good source of iron. (D) Citrus fruits are a source of vitamin C.

198. **(A)** Nursing process phase: assessment; client need: safe, effective care environment; content area: psychiatric nursing

Rationale

(A) The client's speech is rapid, increased in amount, and difficult to interrupt. It also remains wide of the point, making it pressured and tangential. (B) The client's speech is tangential, but no data are given to support that it is also loud. (C) No data are given to indicate that the client's speech is illogical or loud. (C) The client's speech is not illogical, but it is pressured.

199. **(B)** Nursing process phase: implementation; client need: health promotion and maintenance; content area: maternity nursing

Rationale

(A) It helps form and maintain skin and membrane tissue and is important in the mineralization of the fetal skeleton. Excessive doses have not been shown to accelerate retinal development or increase vision in the fetus. (B) Vitamin A is a fat-soluble vitamin and is stored in the body. Large doses can be harmful to the client and the fetus. (C) The body is seldom deficient in this vitamin since it is stored in the body. (D) Vitamin A is a fat-soluble vitamin.

200. **(C)** Nursing process phase: analysis; client need: safe, effective care environment; content area: medical/surgical nursing

Rationale

(A) An indication of a stress ulcer would likely be bleeding through the nasogastric tube. (B) The data do not indicate that hypovolemia has occurred. (C) Ileus is a possible complication of burns and is indicated by the lack of bowel sounds. (D) An empty gastrointestinal tract does not cause the absence of bowel sounds.

201. (D) Nursing process phase: client need: health promotion and maintenance; content area: medical/surgical nursing

Rationale

(A) Petechiae on the abdomen are not clinical findings of SLE. (B) Low-grade afternoon fever is not a clinical finding of SLE. (C) Multiple ecchymoses of the body are not clinical findings in clients with SLE. (D) A recurrent butterfly rash on the face is a distinct clinical finding of clients with SLE.

202. (D) Nursing process phase: analysis; client need: safe, effective care environment; content area: maternity nursing

Rationale

(A) There are currently no approved drugs for lactation suppression. (B) An injection of vitamin K_1 is given to the newborn to stimulate the formation of factors II, VII, IX, and X by the liver for clotting. In addition, pregnant and postpartum clients have no need for vitamin K_1 since their blood is already in a hypercoagulability state. (C) Rh_o(D) immune globulin (RhoGAM) is given to prevent the formation of anti-Rh antibodies in the Rh-negative woman who delivers an Rh-positive infant. It is administered within 72 hours of delivery. (D) Pitocin is an oxytocin that promotes firm contraction of the uterus after birth to control postpartum bleeding.

203. (D) Nursing process phase: implementation; client need: safe, effective care environment; content area: medical/surgical nursing

Rationale

(A) The prepared bandage is contaminated and should be discarded. (B) The prepared bandage is contaminated and should not be resoaked and reused. (C) The bandage is contaminated and should not be reused on this dressing. (D) The bandage is contaminated and should be discarded. A new one should be prepared to ensure aseptic technique and prevent introduction of infection.

204. (D) Nursing process phase: implementation; client need: psychosocial integrity; content area: pediatric nursing

Rationale

(A) Telling her you understand how she feels is not an appropriate response. It is a closed statement and does not invite a response. (B) Telling her not to cry, that everything is going to be all right is not an appropriate response. It is a nontherapeutic statement. (C) Going immediately to her bedside and asking her what is she crying about does invite a response; however, it is not as therapeutic as being attentive and letting her know you care by your touch and waiting for her to speak. (D) Sitting in the chair beside her and letting her feel your presence and waiting for her to speak is a therapeutic response.

205. (A) Nursing process phase: implementation; client need: health promotion and maintenance; content area: medical/surgical nursing

Rationale

(A) Elderly clients have reduced sensation to hot and cold, especially in the lower extremities. This is because of vascular, nervous system, and circulatory changes that occur progressively with the aging process. (B) Elderly clients have some reduced sensation to temperature stimuli, but it is not absent altogether, unless other problems are present. (C) Elderly clients have decreased CNS sensation, not increased. (D) Elderly clients have thinning of the skin because of the aging process, which leads to loss of tone and elasticity.

206. (C) Nursing process phase: implementation; client need: psychosocial integrity; content area: psychiatric nursing

Rationale

(A) The client is seeking help to gain control over his agitated emotional state. This response rejects it. (B) The nurse is not acknowledging the client's emotional state, which may increase his agitation. (C) This response acknowledges the client's feelings and indicates that the nurse is supportive. (D) The nurse is willing to refer to another person but is not willing to provide assistance. The client may perceive this as rejection.

207. (C) Nursing process phase: analysis; client need: health promotion and maintenance; content area: maternity nursing

Rationale

(A) Postterm infants are born at 42 weeks' or more after the due date. Average for gestational age (AGA) indicates the infant's weight is normal for a particular gestation, falling between the 10th and 90th percentile. (B) Infants born prior to the 38th week of gestation are considered preterm. Large for gestational age (LGA) indicates the infant is above the 90th percentile in size. (C) An infant born prior to the 38th week of gestation is preterm. Small for gestational age (SGA) indicates the infant falls below the 10th percentile in size. (D) A term infant is born between 38 and 42 weeks' gestation. Small for gestational age indicates the infant falls below the 10th percentile in size.

208. (D) Nursing process phase: analysis; client need: physiological integrity; content area: pediatric nursing

Rationale

(A) This is a description of a gastroschisis or omphalocele. (B) This is a description of torsion or obstruction of the bowel, and this is not a classic feature of Hirschsprung's. (C) This is a description of intussusception. (D) Correct. Hirschsprung's disease is also known as congenital aganglionic megacolon, a disease that results in mechanical obstruction from inadequate motility of part of the intestine, caused by the absence of nerve ganglion cells.

209. (B) Nursing process phase: assessment; client need: physiological integrity; content area: medical/surgical—gerontological nursing

Rationale

(A) Squamous-cell carcinoma may appear in the oral cavity of the client with AIDS. This lesion will appear as a firm keratotic nodule with an indurated base. (B) Oral candidiasis is a common lesion seen in AIDS clients. Its appearance resembles that of cottage cheese, and it may adhere to the mucosa of the mouth or esophagus. (C) Kaposi's sarcoma is a lesion involving the skin, mucous membranes, gastrointestinal tract, or other organs. This skin lesion begins as a bruise-type appearance and develops into firm, purplish nodules. (D) Oral herpes simplex is a viral disorder, which appears initially as a sensation of burning or itching, followed by vesicles that appear on an erythematous base at the mucocutaneous junction of the lips or nose.

210. (B) Nursing process phase: analysis; client need: safe, effective care environment; content area: psychiatric nursing

Rationale

(A) Retinal detachment is characterized by floaters, flashing lights, and/or an increasing shadow or curtain over the field of vision. There are no data to support this. (B) The trailing phenomenon is a perceptual abnormality associated with the use of hallucinogenic drugs. The client sees objects as a series of discontinuous yet discrete images. (C) Visual hallucinations are visual images seen by the client when there are no actual visual stimuli. What the client is describing is a deviation in real visual stimuli. (D) Illusions are misperceptions or misinterpretations of real external stimuli. This client is not misinterpreting or misperceiving. This is an effect of a large dose of lysergic acid.

211. (B) Nursing process phase: implementation; client need: health promotion and maintenance; content area: maternity nursing

Rationale

(A) Blood glucose levels do not affect the amount of lactose in breast milk. (B) Breastfeeding is encouraged in diabetic mothers because it decreases the insulin requirements for insulin-dependent women. In addition, breastfed infants have a decreased risk of developing juvenile diabetes than if they were formula fed. (C) Neither blood glucose nor insulin enter breast milk from the bloodstream of the lactating mother. (D) Adding calories for breastfeeding will not affect dietary control for the diabetic woman. The caloric demands of breastfeeding require adding 500 kcal per day to the diet. However, the energy demands of breastfeeding easily use up these calories.

212. (B) Nursing process phase: assessment; client need: safe, effective care environment; content area: medical/surgical nursing

Rationale

(A) All of these symptoms and diagnostic findings occur in the advanced stage of TB, except anorexia, which is an early symptom. (B) All of these symptoms can occur in the early stage of TB. (C) None of these symptoms occurs in the early stage of TB. (D) None of these findings is evident in the early stage of TB, but appears in the advanced stage. Elevated sedimentation rate is insignificant with TB.

213. (A) Nursing process phase: implementation; client need: physiological integrity; content area: medical/surgical nursing

Rationale

(A) This would be least beneficial to the client because it would increase injury and infection. Nursing actions would never include pushing the intestine or other organs back into the abdominal cavity. (B) The nurse would cover the area and keep it moist. This action would reduce the risk of injury or potential infection. (C) This action would benefit the client because the problem is serious and needs an immediate surgical intervention. (D) A low Fowler's position with knees flexed would benefit the client because it would reduce stress on the abdominal muscles and therefore prevent further injury.

214. (A) Nursing process phase: assessment; client need: physiological integrity; content area: maternity nursing

Rationale

(A–D) Gravida is any pregnancy, regardless of length; para is any delivery after 20 weeks, whether live or dead; ab(abortion) is any delivery occurring prior to the end of 20 weeks' gestation. The client had two pregnancies: gravida II. The client has had one delivery after 20 weeks: para I. The client has had one pregnancy end before 20 weeks: ab I.

215. (D) Nursing process phase: implementation; client need: physiological integrity; content area: medical/surgical nursing

Rationale

(A) Effective communication is always necessary and important when caring for a client in a coma, but it is not the most beneficial nursing intervention listed here. (B) Range-of-motion exercises are beneficial to a client in a coma, but are done every 2 to 4 hours, not every 1 hour. Also, this is not the most beneficial nursing intervention of these listed. (C) Discharge planning begins when the client's prognosis is determined and plan of care is developed. This is not the most beneficial nursing intervention of these listed. (D) Promoting good skin integrity and preventing breakdown by frequent turning is the most beneficial nursing intervention of these listed.

216. (C) Nursing process phase: analysis; client need: physiological integrity; content area: medical/surgical nursing

Rationale

(A) An infection acquired at home is not referred to as nosocomial. (B) Communicable diseases are not referred to as nosocomial. (C) Nosocomial infection is acquired in a health-care facility. A common example is a urinary tract infection (UTI) from an indwelling catheter. (D) Sexually transmitted diseases are not referred to as nosocomial infections.

217. (B) Nursing process phase: implementation; client need: health promotion and maintenance; content area: maternity nursing

Rationale

(A) An aggressive enema during pregnancy is not recommended. This procedure may cause an electrolyte imbalance and can stimulate labor; both would be detrimental for a 26-week-gestation client. (B) High-fiber food and increased fluid intake are the best recommendations for relieving constipation of pregnancy. The client may also increase activity if her physician approves. (C) Laxatives are not recommended in pregnancy. They can be habit-forming and cause electrolyte imbalances if used in excess. (D) This statement is true, but does not help the client resolve her problem.

218. (A) Nursing process phase: analysis; client need: physiological integrity; content area: medical/surgical nursing

Rationale

(A) This describes a temporary localized skin irritation, which often results from chemicals and subsides when the source of irritation is removed. (B) This term refers to red and painful nodules on the legs, associated with rheumatism, certain drugs, and food poisoning. (C) This term describes an acute febrile disease with localized inflammation and redness of skin and subcutaneous tissue accompanied by systemic disturbance. It is caused by *Streptococcus pyogenes*. (D) This describes the term for dry, flaking scalp, trunk, or face—also known as dandruff. It is caused by hypersecretion and altered quality of the sebaceous glands.

219. **(C)** Nursing process phase: assessment; client need: safe, effective care environment; content area: medical/surgical nursing

Rationale
(A) These are not the appropriate techniques used to assess a client with a local skin irritation. The more specific form is inspection, rather than observation. (B) These techniques are not appropriate to assess signs of a localized skin irritation. (C) The appropriate techniques for assessing a client with localized skin irritation include a client history of what happened and inspecting the area(s) of concern. (D) History can be beneficial in the assessment of a local skin irritation, but vital signs are not appropriate unless the client exhibits signs and symptoms of an anaphylactic reaction.

220. **(A)** Nursing process phase: assessment; client need: physiological integrity; content area: maternity nursing

Rationale
(A) Fetal alcohol syndrome (FAS) is characterized by central nervous system deficits. These infants may have microcephaly and mild to moderate mental retardation. (B) Although facial malformations may occur with FAS, these are not the most concerning problem. Facial characteristics of these infants include hirsutism, short palpebral fissure, epicanthal folds, hypertelorism, short nose with long philtrum, thin upper lip and a depressed, broadened nasal bridge. (C) Hypoplastic nails may also occur but are not the most concerning problem of FAS. (D) Eye malformations such as epicanthal folds may occur, though this is not the major concern of FAS.

221. **(D)** Nursing process phase: implementation; client need: safe, effective care environment; content area: medical/surgical nursing

Rationale
(A) Universal precautions and Centers for Disease Control (CDC) guidelines recommend the use of clean gloves when giving direct care to the client, such as administering an IM injection. (B) It is not necessary to wear a gown and mask when performing routine universal precautions, such as administering an IM injection. The use of additional protective barriers depends on the client's illness and needs. (C) It is not necessary to wear a gown when performing routine universal precautions, such as administering an IM injection. Gloves only are necessary according to CDC guidelines. (D) According to CDC guidelines, gloves are used when administering an IM injection as a routine universal precaution procedure.

222. **(C)** Nursing process phase: implementation; client need: safe, effective care environment; content area: medical/surgical nursing—dosage calculation

Rationale
  50 mg divided by 100 mg × 2 ml = 1 ml of meperidine
  25 mg divided by 25 mg × 1 ml = 1 ml of hydroxyzine
  Total = 2 ml
Math calculation explains incorrect answers.

223. **(C)** Nursing process phase: assessment; client need: physiological integrity; content area: pediatric nursing

Rationale
(A) Clark's rule is used in the solving of drug problems. (B)

Body surface area is useful when solving drug problems, but not in determining endotracheal tube size. (C) The diameter of a child's pinky is approximately the size of the trachea. (D) No such rule exists.

224. **(B)** Nursing process phase: assessment; client need: physiological integrity; content area: medical/surgical nursing

Rationale
(A) Neurovascular signs in the right foot would be needed only for comparison with the left foot. (B) Monitoring for normal circulation in an extremity is essential following an invasive procedure into the major artery supplying that extremity. (C) Clients are usually sufficiently awake during the procedure to participate. (D) Heart sounds are not routinely monitored following cardiac catheterization.

225. **(D)** Nursing process phase: implementation; client need: safe, effective care environment; content area: psychiatric nursing—dosage calculation

Rationale
  3.75 mg : 1 tablet = 7.5 mg : x = 2 tablets
Math calculation explains incorrect answers.

226. **(A)** Nursing process phase: implementation; client need: health promotion and maintenance; content area: maternity nursing

Rationale
(A) A weight gain of more than 2 lb/week in the second and third trimesters is considered excessive. (B) An average weight gain is 1 lb/week. This client gained an average of 3 lb/week. (C) The weight gain is excessive, not inadequate. (D) An excessive weight gain in 1 month does not place the client at risk for eclampsia, but weight gain is a warning sign of pre-eclampsia.

227. **(A)** Nursing process phase: analysis; client need: physiological integrity; content area: medical/surgical nursing

Rationale
(A) This statement describes the prodromal phase of the acute infectious disease process, where the organism disseminates itself throughout the body or multiplies at a localized site. (B) This statement describes the incubation stage of an acute infectious disease process. (C) This statement describes the recovery phase of an acute infectious disease process. (D) This statement describes the acute phase of an infectious disease process, which occurs immediately after the organism disseminates in the body. This is the stage of infection where all symptoms and clinical findings are present, it follows the prodromal phase.

228. **(D)** Nursing process phase: analysis; client need: health promotion and maintenance; content area: psychiatric nursing

Rationale
(A) Anticholinergics are sometimes used in the psychiatric setting to reverse or diminish extrapyramidal symptoms associated with the use of antipsychotics. (B) Anxiolytics are primarily prescribed to treat anxiety disorders or for short-term treatment of anxiety. (C) Some beta blockers are used in the psychiatric setting to block the autonomic arousal associated with panic levels of anxiety, but this is an unlabeled use. (D) Neuroleptics, which are also called antipsychotics, are the

drugs of choice for targeting the signs of symptoms of psychoses.

229. (D) Nursing process phase: implementation; client need: safe, effective care environment; content area: medical/surgical nursing—dosage calculation

Rationale
3.33 gm : 5 ml = x : 15 ml = 9.99 gm, round off to 10 gm
Math calculation explains incorrect answers.

230. (A) Nursing process phase: assessment; client need: health promotion and maintenance; content area: maternity nursing

Rationale
(A) A systolic blood pressure of 160 or a diastolic blood pressure of 110 on two occasions at least 6 hours apart is indicative of PIH. (B) Pregnant women normally have 1+ to 2+ proteinuria. Proteinuria of greater than 3+ is indicative of PIH. (C) The increased vascular flow to the head typically causes headaches in pregnant women. If the headache is severe or unrelenting, PIH is suspected. (D) Pregnant women frequently experience heartburn because of the decreased peristalsis and crowding of the stomach and intestines as pregnancy advances. In contrast, right upper quadrant (epigastric) pain is indicative of PIH.

231. (C) Nursing process phase: implementation; client need: health promotion and maintenance; content area: medical/surgical nursing

Rationale
(A) Teaching a low-salt diet would be appropriate when the client is diagnosed as hypertensive. (B) Checking the blood pressure again after the first reading may cause anxiety and not be accurate. (C) The best response would be to refer the client to her physician for further evaluation. (D) A referral to the emergency department would not be needed if the client is stable.

232. (A) Nursing process phase: assessment; client need: safe, effective care environment; content area: medical/surgical nursing

Rationale
(A) Decreased blood flow causes inflammation. (B) Ankle edema bilaterally would occur if thrombophlebitis affects both legs. (C) Venous insufficiency causes large thrombosed veins. (D) Contracted feet can be neurological.

233. (D) Nursing process phase: implementation; client need: safe, effective care environment; content area: medical/surgical nursing—dosage calculation

Rationale
1:1000 means 1 gm in 1000 ml, resulting in 1 mg/ml
Math calculation explains incorrect answers.

234. (A) Nursing process phase: safe, effecting care environment; client need: physiological integrity; content area: maternity nursing

Rationale
(A) The couple is entitled to factual, objective information to make informed choices. (B) This response is promoting a false sense of security. (C) This response utilizes fear and guilt. (D) This response implies that their request is unrealistic and impossible.

235. (D) Nursing process phase: evaluation; client need: safe, effective care environment; content area: medical/surgical nursing

Rationale
(A) Rubbing hastens absorption and can cause irritation. (B) Insulin is destroyed by vigorous shaking. (C) The site is cleaned with an antiseptic or soap and water to prevent infection. (D) Insulin must be given immediately after mixing because absorption and/or action profiles could be altered.

236. (C) Nursing process phase: assessment; client need: health promotion and maintenance; content area: maternity nursing

Rationale
(A) This is the definition of the term gravida. (B) This definition would include abortions as well as fetuses beyond 20 weeks' gestation, and is not an accurate definition of parity. (C) Parity refers to the number of pregnancies carried 20 weeks or longer, regardless of whether the infant is born alive or stillborn. Less than 20 weeks' gestation is an abortion. (D) This is an incomplete definition of parity

237. (A) Nursing process phase: implementation; client need: health promotion and maintenance; content area: maternity nursing

Rationale
(A) This procedure describes the GIFT procedure. (B) In vitro fertilization is the procedure described in this answer. (C) This procedure describes therapeutic intrauterine insemination. (D) This procedure describes a surrogate mother.

238. (C) Nursing process phase: implementation; client need: safe, effective care environment; content area: pediatric nursing—dosage calculation

Rationale
200 mg : 1 ml = 345 mg : x = 1.7 ml

Math calculation explains incorrect answers.

239. (A) Nursing process phase: implementation; client need: safe, effective care environment; content area: medical/surgical nursing—dosage calculation

Rationale
8000 units divided by 10,000 units × 1 ml = 0.8 ml
Math calculation explains incorrect answers.

240. (C) Nursing process phase: analysis; client need: physiological integrity; content area: maternity nursing

Rationale
(A) Jitteriness might indicate metabolic alterations or CNS abnormalities. Elevated temperatures in the newborn usually reflect maternal temperature or result from overheating by caregivers. (B) Acrocyanosis, mild cyanosis of the hands and feet, is normal in a newborn. Abdominal movement with respirations in a newborn is normal. (C) Expiratory grunting and central cyanosis indicate respiratory distress in an infant. A 28-week-gestation infant would most likely have undeveloped lungs and an inadequate supply of surfactant, leading to respiratory distress. (D) Paleness and decreased respiratory rate would not be typical of RDS. The common clinical manifestation is an infant who is dyspneic with rapid breathing, expiratory grunting, cyanotic, and limp.

241. (C) Nursing process phase: assessment; client need: health promotion and maintenance; content area: medical/surgical nursing

Rationale
(A) A 1+ pedal pulse would indicate markedly impaired. (B) A 2+ pedal pulse would indicate markedly impaired. (C) A 3+ pedal pulse would indicate slightly impaired. (D) A 4+ pedal pulse would indicate normal pulse.

242. (C) Nursing process phase: implementation; client need: psychosocial integrity; content area: psychiatric nursing

Rationale
(A) Instructing the client to create a dialogue with the voices only reinforces the client's ability to test reality accurately. (B) It may be appropriate to determine at some point if the voices are male or female, but this response is not therapeutic. (C) This response is therapeutic because it validates what the client is experiencing and it presents reality. (D) Medication may make the voices go away, but it will not happen immediately. The client needs to know that what she is experiencing is an alteration in her perception of the world around her.

243. (B) Nursing process phase: assessment; client need: safe, effective care environment; content area: medical/surgical nursing

Rationale
(A) Decreased heart rate and arrhythmia are not neurological signs, but common cardiac symptoms caused by digoxin toxicity. (B) Headache, blurred vision, and confusion are neurological symptoms of digoxin toxicity. (C) Loss of appetite with nausea and vomiting are common GI symptoms and may not be caused by digoxin toxicity. (D) Hallucinations, weakness, and depression are neurological symptoms and may not be caused by digoxin toxicity.

244. (A) Nursing process phase: assessment; client need: physiological integrity; content area: pediatric nursing

Rationale
(A) The most common presenting sign of Wilms' tumor is swelling of the mass within the abdomen. Other symptoms are the result of compression from the tumor mass, metabolic alterations secondary to the tumor, or metastasis. Anemia, which is secondary to hemorrhage within the tumor, results in pallor, anorexia, and lethargy. (B) Hypertension, not hypotension, is a symptom that occurs occasionally with Wilms' tumor and is probably caused by the excretion of excess amounts of renin by the tumor. (C) Weight loss, not weight gain, is another common symptom of malignancy in general. (D) Hyperthermia, not hypothermia, is another common symptom of malignancy in general.

245. (D) Nursing process phase: implementation; client need: safe, effective care environment; content area: medical/surgical nursing—dosage calculation

Rationale
$$300 \text{ mg} : 2 \text{ ml} = 300 \text{ mg} : x = 2 \text{ ml}$$
Math calculation explains incorrect answers.

246. (C) Nursing process phase: analysis; client need: psychosocial integrity; content area: maternity nursing

Rationale
(A) The desired target range for a fasting blood glucose level in a pregnant woman is 60 to 90. (B) Good glycemic control in a pregnant woman is indicated by HbA1c values of 2.5 to 6 percent. (C) Pregnant diabetic clients are kept under strict glycemic control. The desired target range for a 2-hr postprandial blood glucose level in the pregnant woman is 60 to 120. (D) The target range for before lunch, dinner, and bedtime blood glucose levels in pregnant women is 60 to 105.

247. (B) Nursing process phase: analysis; client need: safe, effective care environment; content area: medical/surgical nursing

Rationale
(A) The test is invasive and requires an IV access for thallium infusion. (B) Radioactive thallium enters cardiac tissue with good perfusion and does not enter areas with poor blood flow or damage. (C) Thallium scanning during exercise would not be resting, and the test does not determine coronary artery function. (D) Cardiac catherization is used in diagnosing cardiac disease and may be required in addition to thallium scanning to evaluate the extent of coronary artery disease.

248. (A) Nursing process phase: analysis; client need: health promotion and maintenance; content area: medical/surgical—gerontological nursing

Rationale
(A) In comparison to younger clients with AIDS, a higher proportion of older clients with AIDS are caucasians and women. Women comprise the fastest growing at-risk population for HIV infection and for AIDS in the United States and around the world. (B) Women are no more likely to come in contact with sexual body fluids than are men. (C) While women do live longer than men, women report a lower incidence of sexual activity in later life than do men. (D) Changes in the immune system are normal aging processes. There is no evidence to support that women experience greater changes in the immune system as they get older.

249. (B) Nursing process phase: assessment; client need: physiological integrity; content area: medical/surgical nursing

Rationale
(A) These are symptoms of hypoglycemia. (B) Without treatment, clients with severe hyperglycemia will be dehydrated and have dry skin. Kussmaul respirations may also be present. (C) Nausea is a sign of hyperglycemia, but diaphoresis and clammy skin will be evident with hypoglycemia. (D) Abdominal pain is present with hyperglycemia; diaphoresis is present in hypoglycemia.

250. (C) Nursing process phase: implementation; client need: health promotion and maintenance; content area: maternity nursing

Rationale
(A & B) These are not correct because dieting or avoiding weight gain in pregnancy can result in poor pregnancy outcomes. The glucose and nutrients needed for fetal growth are not readily available from maternal stores and must be acquired through daily nutrition. (C) This is the recommended weight gain for the moderately to severely obese client for optimal perinatal outcomes. (D) Weight gain is based on pre-pregnancy weight. The underweight client will be encouraged

to gain 35 to 45 lb, the average-weight client 25 to 35 lb, and the overweight client 15 to 25 lb.

251. **(B)** Nursing process phase: implementation; client need: safe, effective care environment; content area: medical/surgical—gerontological nursing

Rationale
(A & D) The oral route for fluids is preferred whenever possible. Because of the normal aging changes, renal function is decreased, leading to diminished ability to filter, to concentrate, and to dilute urine in response to water, salt, or excess or diminished fluids. (B) The oral route for fluids is preferred whenever possible. Careful monitoring of intake and output is an important part of the treatment regimen. (C) The oral route for fluids is preferred whenever possible; however, tea and coffee are diuretics in nature and should be avoided.

252. **(D)** Nursing process phase: implementation; client need: safe, effective care environment; content area: maternity nursing—dosage calculation

Rationale
$$0.05 \text{ mg} : 1 \text{ ml} = 0.1 : x = 2 \text{ ml}$$
Math calculation explains incorrect answers.

253. **(C)** Nursing process phase: assessment; client need: safe, effective care environment; content area: psychiatric nursing

Rationale
(A) Recall of events of the far past is not being assessed. (B) Mood is assessed by asking the client to subjectively evaluate his own emotional state. (C) By asking the client to serially subtract 7's, the nurse is assessing the client's ability to calculate. (D) The client has not been asked to give data concerning person, place date, time, or situation.

254. **(B)** Nursing process phase: implementation; client need: health promotion and maintenance; content area: maternity nursing

Rationale
(A) The endometrium is the lining of the uterus that prepares for a pregnancy each month. When pregnancy does not occur, the endometrium is shed. Sometimes endometrial tissue is found on pelvic organs outside the uterine cavity. This tissue also bleeds at time of the menses. This bleeding leads to pain and scarring of the pelvic organs that can lead to infertility. The name of this condition is endometriosis. Endometriosis does not cause menstrual periods to cease. (B) Menstrual regularity requires the maintenance of weight and body fat above a certain level. A woman who weighs less than 115 lb, or who has lost 10 or more pounds through strenuous exercise, often experiences cessation of menses. This condition is known as hypogonadotropic amenorrhea. (C) These are the symptoms of premenstrual syndrome (PMS), which include edema, emotional instability, panic attacks, irritability, impaired ability to concentrate, headache, fatigue, and backache. The cause of PMS is unknown. There is no cessation of the menstrual period. (D) A generalized infection of the female pelvic organs (or PID) is a significant cause of infertility. It is most frequently caused by sexually transmitted organisms. It causes severe lower abdominal pain and tenderness. Cessation of menses is not a symptom of PID.

255. **(D)** Nursing process phase: implementation; client need: safe, effective care environment; content area: maternity nursing—dosage calculation

Rationale
$$1500 \text{ mg} : 5 \text{ ml} = 2000 \text{ mg} : x = 6.7 \text{ ml}$$
Math calculation explains incorrect answers.

256. **(A)** Nursing process phase: implementation; client need: safe, effective care environment; content area: maternity nursing

Rationale
(A) Turning the infant to the right side promotes emptying of the stomach contents into the small intestine. A side-lying position also facilitates drainage from the oropharynx. (B) The infant should be turned from one side to the other in order to help develop even contours of the head and to ease pressure on other parts of the body. However, after a feeding, the infant should be positioned on the right side. (C) The prone position has been associated with an increased incidence of sudden infant death syndrome (SIDS). (D) The prone position has been associated with SIDS. Elevating the foot of the crib increases the risk of aspiration.

257. **(D)** Nursing process phase: implementation; client need: safe, effective care environment; content area: pediatric nursing—dosage calculation

Rationale
$$100 \text{ mg} : 1 \text{ tablet} = 200 \text{ mg} : x = 2 \text{ tablets}$$
Math calculation explains incorrect answers.

258. **(B)** Nursing process phase: evaluation; client need: physiological integrity; content area: medical/surgical nursing

Rationale
(A) Sodium levels would be important, but an adverse effect of hydrochlorothiazide would be a manifestation of low potassium. (B) Potassium would be the first laboratory parameter to review. (C) Cholesterol levels would not be affected by hydrochlorothiazide. (D) Thyroid levels would not be affected by hydrochlorothiazide.

259. **(C)** Nursing process phase: implementation; client need: health promotion and maintenance; content area: maternity nursing

Rationale
(A) Family attachment would be better facilitated in smaller, culturally unique classes. (B) Having appointments during routine business hours often eliminates support persons from accompanying the expectant mother for her health care. (C) Weekend classes expand the participation to the expectant family and their designates. (D) Expectant mothers would exclude her support systems from participating in class.

260. **(B)** Nursing process phase: implementation; client need: safe, effective care environment; content area: medical/surgical nursing—dosage calculation

Rationale
$$30 \text{ mg divided by } 2000 \text{ mg} \times 100 \text{ ml} = 1.5 \text{ ml}$$
Math calculation explains incorrect answers.

261. **(C)** Nursing process phase: implementation; client need: safe, effective care environment; content area: medical/surgical nursing—dosage calculation

Rationale
       30 mEq divided by 2 mEq $\times$ 1 ml = 15 ml
Math calculation explains incorrect answers.

262. (D) Nursing process phase: evaluation; client need: physiological integrity; content area: pediatric nursing

Rationale
(A) Assessing and monitoring for shock is necessary and should occur following stopping the transfusion, which is the cause of the reaction. (B) After stopping the transfusion and assessing the child's physiological status, the physician would be notified of the client's status. (C) Diluting the blood with normal saline is inappropriate and should never occur. (D) The incompatibility of the blood product being given with the client's blood is causing the hemolytic reaction. Therefore, the first action is to remove the cause by stopping the blood transfusion but maintaining a patent IV for possible medication administration.

263. (A) Nursing process phase: analysis; client need: physiological integrity; content area: medical/surgical nursing

Rationale
(A) A serum glucose level of 50 mg/dl is below the normal range of 60 to 120 mg/dl. (B) This serum glucose level is WNL. (C & D) This value is above the normal range and represents hyperglycemia.

264. (D) Nursing process phase: assessment; client need: safe, effective care environment; content area: psychiatric nursing

Rationale
(A) Mood changes are not early indicators of Alzheimer's disease. (B) Changes in eating habits are more common in Alzheimer's disease than changes in appetite because the client may forget when she last ate. (C) Assessing for changes in bowel habits on admission is important but is not essential in assessing for the symptoms associated with Alzheimer's disease. (D) Progressive memory loss is a cardinal sign of Alzheimer's disease. It would be important to particularly find out if recent or remote memory is involved.

265. (C) Nursing process phase: implementation; client need: health promotion and maintenance; content area: maternity nursing

Rationale
(A) The prone position is associated with the occurrence of SIDS. A firm surface is appropriate. (B) Lying an infant on the right side after feedings promotes gastric emptying. However, an infant should not be restricted to lying on one side (C) It is recommended that healthy infants be placed on their backs or sides because of the association between the prone position and SIDS. (D) A side-lying position is appropriate for infant positioning. However, placing a small pillow under the head of the infant will cause flexion of the neck and can occlude the airway.

test 2

1. When assessing a 46-year-old female client for a possible thyroid malfunction, the nurse recognizes which clinical finding that is present in most clients with hypothyroidism?
   A. Weakness
   B. Diarrhea
   C. Tachycardia
   D. Restlessness

2. A 55-year-old woman was 1 day postoperative after undergoing a hysterectomy. She was complaining of severe pain. The physician ordered meperidine (Demerol) 50 mg IM every 3 to 4 hours for pain. Using a 75 mg/ml vial, the nurse withdrew how many milliliters?
   A. 0.5
   B. 0.6
   C. 0.7
   D. 0.8

3. Which nursing measures are appropriate to decrease pain in children with acute otitis media and draining exudate from a ruptured eardrum?
   A. Local application of heat to the affected ear
   B. Local application of heat to both ears
   C. Insertion of sterile earplugs
   D. Ice compress to the affected ear while the child is sitting up playing

4. A 40-year-old woman is admitted from the postpartum unit with a diagnosis of intrarenal failure, oliguric phase. The nurse would check which of the following for the best clinical indicator of how well the nephrons in the kidney are functioning?
   A. Serum creatinine
   B. Blood urea nitrogen
   C. Creatinine clearance
   D. Urine output

5. An 84-year-old woman has had cataract surgery on her left eye. When preparing her for discharge, the nurse teaches her to:
   A. Lie on her left side at night.
   B. Take tub baths.
   C. Clean drainage from the eye with a sterile cotton ball and water.
   D. Take aspirin as needed for pain.

6. A 24-year-old client has just received a mastoidectomy. The nurse knows that the caregiver has understood instructions for postoperative care when he or she hears:
   A. "He must lie on the unoperated side for 4 hours after surgery."
   B. "He will be able to fly to California in 3 days on his business trip."
   C. "Vertigo or dizziness is to be expected and does not need to be reported."
   D. "I will need to learn how to change the dressing."

7. The nurse explains to a client who has many allergies the reason why the following type of insulin has been prescribed for him:
   A. Pork
   B. Beef
   C. Humulin
   D. Ultralente

8. A 35-year-old female client who experienced recurrent panic attacks developed signs of agoraphobia. Which one of the following is not a symptom of the disease?
   A. Fear of crowds
   B. Fear and avoidance of being alone
   C. Intrusive thoughts about incapacitating physical health
   D. Psychosis

9. In providing nutritional counseling to the parents of a preschooler, it is most important for the nurse to stress which explanation?

A. Quality is more important than quantity.

B. Strict table manners should be enforced.

C. A preschooler consumes three-quarters of an adult portion.

D. Food dislikes are only stubbornness and must be overcome now.

10. A client with severe PIH at 28 weeks' gestation complains of epigastric pain. Which action by the nurse would be most appropriate?

A. Check the chart to see when the client last received an antacid.

B. Pad the siderails of the bed and position the client on her left side.

C. Start an IV line stat.

D. Check the fetal heart rate.

11. A 12-year-old boy received an allergy shot during his clinic visit. What symptom would the nurse identify as an early sign of an anaphylactic response?

A. A blood pressure reading of 95/60

B. Complaints of abdominal cramping

C. A heart rate of 90

D. A sense of impending doom

12. A client is scheduled for keratoplasty. When preparing this client for surgery, the nurse explains that he should:

A. Remain on bedrest until the sutures are removed.

B. Be out of bed the evening of surgery.

C. Begin caring for himself as soon as possible.

D. Start progressive ambulation following the first dressing change.

13. While discussing the advantages of breastfeeding with expectant parents, it is important for the nurse to reinforce which of the following?

A. It is a safe, natural, highly effective form of contraception.

B. Breastfeeding promotes uterine involution.

C. Breastfed babies do not develop colic.

D. Breastfeeding mothers need to supplement their diet with about 1000 extra calories per day.

14. A 10-year-old was brought to the emergency room after a bicycle accident. X-rays confirm a simple fracture to the right humerus. The nurse cleaned the abrasions on the right arm, then covered them with sterile 4 by 4s prior to casting. When teaching the parents cast care at home, which of the following would be indicative of an infection?

A. Increased pain to the extremity

B. Temperature of 100°F orally

C. Hot areas felt on the cast

D. Blood-tinged drainage on the cast

15. A 34-year-old male client has been diagnosed with acquired immune deficiency syndrome (AIDS) and pneumonia. The nurse will perform the following assessment every 8 hours:

A. Inspection of the IV site

B. Vital signs, especially respiratory status

C. Nonverbal signs of pain

D. Inspection of oral mucous membranes

16. A 36-year-old man with a history of severe anxiety is admitted with hyperventilation syndrome. The nurse needs to monitor the client for which of the following conditions?

A. Respiratory alkalosis

B. Respiratory acidosis

C. Metabolic alkalosis

D. Metabolic acidosis

17. Parents are often confused regarding the best disciplinary strategy for young children. Which disciplinary strategy should a nurse recommend for young children?

A. Time-out

B. Spanking

C. Scolding

D. Reasoning

18. A 24-year-old woman is admitted with a diagnosis of pneumonia. She is having difficulty breathing and her chest x-ray reveals moderate pulmonary edema. When checking the client's laboratory values, the nurse would be alert for which of the following?

A. Platelet count less than 300,000 μl

B. Hemoglobin 9.0 gms/dl

C. White blood cell count 12,500 μl

D. Potassium 4.0 mEq/l

19. A 76-year-old client with lung cancer has the field of radiation outlined with purple ink. The nurse cares for the skin within the purple markings by:

A. Putting nothing on the area

B. Washing the area with mild soap and water

C. Applying lotion to prevent drying

D. Cleaning it with half-strength hydrogen peroxide

20. An expectant mother is in her third trimester. Which of the following developmental tasks is specific to this client?

A. Anticipation of fetal movements

B. Readjustment of her life as a careerperson

C. Developing inner strength

D. Visualizing the infant with a distinct personality

21. To facilitate client and family acceptance of a colostomy in a schoolage child, the nurse should:

A. Teach the client and family to remove the appliance from the skin each time the bag needs emptying.

B. Encourage the child to wear clothing over the colostomy in the presence of family.

C. Encourage the child and family to participate in changing or emptying the appliance.

D. Inform the family that the stoma will be pale white in appearance.

22. A 40-year-old man is admitted following a fall with a fracture at the C2 to C3 of the spine. Which of the following problems would the nurse be alert for if this client has sustained damage to the spinal cord?
    A. Facial nerve paralysis
    B. Decreased respiratory function
    C. Bowel and urine incontinence
    D. Urine retention, intact anal wink

23. A 66-year-old woman has been admitted to the unit following a total abdominal hysterectomy. She has been receiving hydromorphone (Dilaudid) for pain every 4 hours. When the nurse goes into the room, the client is on the floor and one of the siderails has been left down on the bed. The client is complaining of severe neck pain and pain in her right knee. What should the nurse do to assist this client?
    A. Get the client more pain medication, even if it is not a scheduled dose.
    B. Ask the client to roll onto her unaffected side to inspect her back and spine.
    C. Instruct the client to move her arms and legs one by one in order to assess range of motion.
    D. Immobilize the client with pillows and towels on the floor and instruct her not to move.

24. The nurse correctly identifies which of the following as the psychosocial stage identified by Erikson that is met by the mother when promptly attending to her infant's cries of hunger?
    A. The "oral sensory"
    B. "Trust vs. mistrust"
    C. "Sensorimotor"
    D. "Maternal person–radius significant relationship"

25. A 61-year-old woman complains of occasional periods of tinnitus and vertigo. When she asks a nurse what she should do about these occasional "spells," the nurse replies:
    A. "It's part of the aging process; don't worry about it."
    B. "You should have a medical evaluation to prevent hearing loss."
    C. "A few drops of half-strength peroxide may be instilled in the ears to remove cerumen."
    D. "Just take special precautions to protect the ears from loud noises."

26. The nurse is preparing a child for allergy skin testing. The mother tells the nurse she hasn't given the child corticosteroids in 2 days. Which of the following actions taken by the nurse would be the most appropriate?
    A. Apply a positive control solution to see if the skin reacts.
    B. Continue with the skin testing.
    C. Discontinue preparation and reschedule skin testing in 1 week.
    D. Notify the physician for further instructions.

27. A client received 10 units of regular insulin at 12 noon. At what time would the nurse assess for signs of hypoglycemia?
    A. 1 to 2 P.M.
    B. 3 to 4 P.M.
    C. 5 to 6 P.M.
    D. 8 to 9 P.M.

28. The nurse should teach the mother of an infant with recurrent seborrheic dermatitis (cradle cap) that prevention may include which of the following?
    A. Adequate scalp hygiene and shampooing
    B. Allergy shot or treatments
    C. Avoidance of any soap products on the scalp
    D. Delaying the introduction of cow's milk until after the first year

29. Which of the following clients should be viewed as having a high potential for experiencing urinary retention as a side effect of an antipsychotic?
    A. Children under 10 years of age
    B. Postmenopausal women
    C. Young women on birth control pills
    D. Elderly men with enlarged prostates

30. A 54-year-old client is being prepared for discharge following a laryngectomy for cancer of the larynx. In helping this client make a successful psychosocial adaptation to his illness, the nurse will recommend support groups in the community and:
    A. Participating in community activities
    B. Joining a variety of organizations
    C. Withdrawing from social interaction until he is stronger
    D. Maintaining open communication with supportive others

31. A 39-year-old female client is being evaluated in the emergency department for a possible thyroid malfunction complication. The nurse recognizes that the most significant clinical finding often noted in a client with thyrotoxic crisis is:
    A. Body temperature of 99°F
    B. Fatigue
    C. Tachycardia
    D. Cool, dry skin

32. A 63-year-old man is brought to the emergency room having developed chest pain while shoveling snow in his driveway. The nurse recognizes that he has most likely had a myocardial infarction (MI) upon viewing positive results to the following test:
    A. CK enzymes
    B. CK-MB fraction
    C. Myoglobin
    D. AST (SGOT)

33. A 60-lb child was admitted with glomerulonephritis. The physician ordered penicillin G benzathine (Bicillin) 1.2 million units IM. How many milliliters will the nurse administer from a 600,000 unit/ml vial?

A. ½ ml
B. 1 ml
C. 1½ ml
D. 2 ml

34. A client in the third trimester of her pregnancy attends a prenatal class on breastfeeding. She tells the lactation consultant that she would like to breastfeed, but has inverted nipples. She asks if there is anything that she can do to make the nipples more erect. Which of the following explanations by the nurse regarding preparing inverted nipples for breastfeeding would be most accurate?
A. There is nothing you can do before the baby is born. Once the baby starts nursing, the nipples will soon pop out.
B. You should roll the nipples between your thumb and forefinger, and toughen them by rubbing them with a washcloth.
C. Breast shells are made for inverted nipples. If you start wearing them now, the nipple will be erect enough for the baby to grasp by your due date.
D. You should be wearing a breast shield under your bra to help break down the tissue that is causing your nipples to go in instead of out.

35. The home health nurse visits a 52-year-old female client who exhibits religious delusions. The most appropriate intervention for the nurse to take is to:
A. Promote the client's return to a reality-based orientation.
B. Argue to disprove the delusion.
C. Discuss the delusion.
D. Agree with the patient until the prescribed medication is effective, then discuss reality.

36. A 50-year-old man is admitted with complaints of extreme weakness and fatigue. His laboratory work reveals a potassium level of 5.8 mEq/L. The nurse needs to be aware that which of the following conditions can cause an increased potassium level?
A. Syndrome of inappropriate antidiuretic hormone (SIADH)
B. Addison's disease
C. Cushing's syndrome
D. Diabetes insipidus

37. An important nursing intervention when caring for an infant with diarrhea would be:
A. Monitoring for signs of alkalosis
B. Monitoring hydration status
C. Placing the infant on reverse isolation
D. Positioning the infant in an infant seat

38. When planning health-promotion classes for mothers with children, the nurse identifies the type of injury a child is most susceptible to at a given age as most closely dependent on which of the following characteristics?

A. Physical health
B. Developmental level
C. Gender
D. Educational level

39. A 48-year-old man is admitted after a car accident. He has fractured his left clavicle and left radius, and has bruising to his left chest wall. He has two chest tubes connected to a one-unit disposable suction system. The nurse would clamp the chest tubes when which of the following occurs?
A. Transporting to another unit
B. To check for an air leak
C. To change the dressing around the tube insertions site
D. To obtain a drainage specimen from the collection device

40. A 4-month-old infant is to receive the second immunization of DPT in the series. Prior to administration, the nurse would ask the mother if the child had any adverse reactions following the previous injection. The nurse would also investigate which of the following?
A. If the child had persistent, inconsolable crying lasting longer than 3 hours
B. If any member of the household has HIV
C. If the infant is allergic to eggs
D. If a family history of seizures exists

41. Which symptom will be noted on nursing assessment of the client with acute hypoparathyroidism?
A. Hypercalcemia
B. Hypernatremia
C. Positive Chvostek's sign
D. Negative Trousseau's sign

42. Which nursing intervention will be most effective in preventing renal calculi formation caused by hypercalcemia?
A. Restrict fluids to 1000 cc/24 hr.
B. Administer phosphate binders as ordered.
C. Administer vitamin D supplements as prescribed.
D. Force fluids up to 3 L/day unless contraindicated.

43. When assessing the toddler, the nurse should know which type of play is characteristic?
A. Cooperative
B. Associative
C. Parallel
D. Onlooker

44. The physician has ordered loxapine hydrochloride (Loxitane C) 100 mg PO qid for a client. The nurse should:
A. Question the order.
B. Give the medication as ordered.
C. Give half doses only.
D. Ask another nurse to give the medication.

45. When planning care, which nursing diagnosis is

the most pertinent for a client with diabetes insipidus?
A. Fluid volume excess
B. Fluid volume deficit
C. Altered cardiac output
D. Altered nutrition: less than body requirements

46. An infusion of 1000 cc D$_5$W every 8 hr is ordered. The nurse initiates the venipuncture. Intravenous cannulation is successful when:
A. The IV cannula threads easily
B. The client has veins that can be easily visualized
C. Backflow of blood is noted in the hub of IV cannula
D. The IV drips freely after the cannula and tubing are connected

47. To prevent urinary tract infections in young girls, the nurse would teach which of the following?
A. Wear cotton panties.
B. Cleanse the perineum with soap and water after voiding.
C. Void infrequently.
D. Decrease fluids.

48. Antacids such as aluminum hydroxide (Amphojel) are routinely administered to clients in chronic renal failure (CRF) to:
A. Bind phosphate.
B. Neutralize stomach acid.
C. Decrease gastric acid production.
D. Bind histamine at H$_2$ receptor sites.

49. A 22-year-old client with a history of mitral stenosis is having an annual checkup. The nurse recognizes the following as being an abnormal finding in his or her other assessment of the cardiovascular system:
A. Visible pulsation at the point of maximum intensity (PMI)—fifth intercostal space (ICS) at midclavicular line (MCL)
B. Capillary refill of 2 seconds
C. Inability to percuss right-sided heart border
D. No jugular venous distention (JVD) with patient at 45-degree angle

50. A 38-year-old female client presented herself at the mental health clinic complaining of insomnia, hopelessness, and irritability. She told the nurse that she feels like hurting herself. The best response by the nurse is:
A. "Do you like yourself?"
B. "Are other family members depressed?"
C. "The mental health specialist will see you tomorrow."
D. "Tell me how you feel about your life now."

51. During a routine well-child visit, the nurse notes a 6-month-old has a closed posterior fontanelle with an open anterior fontanelle. What nursing action is most appropriate considering this finding?

A. Continue with the child's physical examination because this finding is normal.
B. Notify the physician immediately because this occurrence is usually part of a pathological condition.
C. Question the mother regarding the head growth and intelligence of her other children.
D. Request routine skull x-rays to rule out any underlying physical problem.

52. A client is experiencing breast engorgement. Which of the following statements indicates to the nurse a need for additional teaching?
A. "I should wear a supportive bra 24 hours a day."
B. "Nursing my baby every 2 hours will help empty the ducts."
C. "Ice packs will help the milk to flow more freely."
D. "Expressing a small amount of milk will help my baby to latch on."

53. In providing information to the parents of a 15-month-old, which of the following explanations by the nurse provides the most accurate growth and development information?
A. The growth rate slows between 12 and 18 months.
B. The growth rate increases between 12 and 18 months.
C. The growth rate remains unchanged between 12 and 18 months.
D. The growth rate halts completely between 12 and 18 months.

54. A diabetic client has just had surgery. The nurse knows that diabetics are especially prone to the following complication of surgery:
A. Urinary retention
B. Hemorrhage
C. Thrombophlebitis
D. Hypostatic pneumonia

55. A pregnant client at 24 weeks' gestation was admitted to the labor unit for induction of labor 24 hours after fetal demise. The nurse identifies which of the following statements made by the client as characteristic of the shock and numbness dimension of mourning?
A. "If only I had stayed off my feet last week. We moved into a new house. I shouldn't have been lifting anything. That is what caused this to happen!"
B. "The doctor said he couldn't hear the heartbeat of my baby. Would you hook up the monitor? Maybe the baby just moved. This is like a bad dream'"
C. "This is hard to deal with. I guess I will just have to go on with my life, but I will always remember this baby and what he meant to me and my husband."
D. "I feel so tired, and as though I just can't con-

centrate on anything. Even the simplest things seem too difficult. I just don't care about anything since the doctor told me my baby died."

56. A 35-year-old man was admitted with pneumocystic carnii pneumonia. He weighed 82 kg. The physician ordered AZT 2 mg/kg (164 mg) to be given IV. Using a 100 mg/ml vial, how many milliliters did the nurse administer?
    A. 1.24
    B. 1.44
    C. 1.64
    D. 1.84

57. When administering $MgSO_4$ for treatment of PIH, which of the following findings are of concern?
    A. Respirations of 16 per minute
    B. Reflexes of 2+
    C. Irritability and nervousness
    D. Urinary output less than 20 ml/hr

58. A 19-year-old client is found at the site of a motorcycle accident. Blood is spurting from the calf of the right leg. A nurse, who stops to help the victim, would apply:
    A. Pressure in the right groin
    B. Pressure in the right popliteal area
    C. A tourniquet to the right thigh
    D. Direct pressure to the spurting artery

59. Cefazolin (Ancef Gm T) is to be administered in a 50 cc IV piggyback (PB) over 30 minutes. The tubing delivers 10 gtt/cc. At how many cubic centimeters per hour should the IV controller be regulated?
    A. 50 cc/hr
    B. 100 cc/hr
    C. 17 gtt/min
    D. 8 gtt/min

60. A 13-month-old has Down syndrome and the parents are being interviewed by the nurse. Which interview technique is most appropriate for encouraging the parents to talk?
    A. "Does your child sleep well during the night?"
    B. "Did you expect to have a Down syndrome child?"
    C. "Does your child ever have any difficulty with her feedings?"
    D. "Can you tell me about your usual day with your child?"

61. A non-breastfeeding mother is experiencing breast engorgement. Which of the following comfort measures would be most appropriate for this client?
    A. Hand-expressing after the infant nurses
    B. Having the client stand under a warm shower
    C. Increasing the infant feedings
    D. Applying ice packs to both breasts

62. A client who is receiving haloperidol (Haldol) approaches the nurse and says, "I feel like my insides are crawling and I can't stand still." The nurse should recognize the client's subjective symptoms are:
    A. Akinesia
    B. Akathisia
    C. Tardive dyskinesia
    D. Dystonia

63. Which of the following statements by the nurse is most accurate when teaching a child client's mother about the purpose of the DDST II?
    A. The DDST II measures development in children from birth to 6 years old.
    B. The DDST II measures IQ in children from birth to 6 years old.
    C. The DDST II is diagnostic of mental retardation in children from birth to 6 years old.
    D. The DDST II measures stress levels in children from birth to 6 years old.

64. Baby Smith is 3 hours old. The nurse knows that infants pass through phases of instability during the transition period. Which of the following assessments requires the nurse's immediate attention?
    A. Periods of deep sleep between the two reactivity periods
    B. Periodic breathing with brief periods of tachycardia
    C. Heart rate between 100 to 120 during sleep periods
    D. Nasal flaring and intercostal retractions

65. Which of the following approaches to management would not be appropriate for the child with type I diabetes mellitus? The child('s):
    A. Will need to eat a morning, afternoon, and bedtime snack.
    B. Will need extra food when extra activity is planned.
    C. Appetite should be a guide for the amount of calories needed.
    D. Daily exercise regimen should be planned.

66. A newborn infant has a myelomeningocele. The nurse providing care for this infant does a thorough assessment to determine if the most frequently associated anomaly with myelomeningocele is present. Which of the following is that anomaly?
    A. Complete paralysis of lower extremities
    B. Hyperreflexia
    C. Hydrocephalus
    D. Vesicostomy

67. A 72-year-old man is admitted with acute exacerbation of chronic obstructive pulmonary disease (COPD). The nurse notes some abnormal findings during the assessment of this client. Which of the following would represent an abnormal assessment finding seen in a COPD client?
    A. Using abdominal muscles for breathing when at rest

B. A costal angle of less than 90 degrees

C. A costal angle greater than 90 degrees

D. Using thoraic muscles for breathing when at rest

68. A client who is a devout Catholic can only use the calendar method of birth control. She tells the nurse that she understands she must abstain from intercourse on the 14th to the 17th day of her menstrual cycle because pregnancy can only occur within 2 days of ovulation. The nurse's response should be based on the knowledge that:

A. Ovulation occurs on the 14th day of the menstrual cycle.

B. Day of ovulation can vary for the individual, making this method totally unreliable.

C. If abstinence is observed from days 4 to 17 of the menstrual cycle, the method can be fairly reliable.

D. The ovum can survive up to 5 days after ovulation, so the client could get pregnant from the 14th to the 19th day of her menstrual cycle.

69. A 75-year-old home health client developed acute gouty arthritis. The physician ordered phenylbutazone (Butazolidin) 400 mg PO every 8 hours. The home health nurse instructed the client to take how many 100 mg tablets?

A. 2

B. 4

C. 6

D. 8

70. A 4-year-old child has had respiratory infections three times in the last 12 months. The parents are smokers and refuse to quit smoking. What would be the next action for the nurse to take?

A. Assist parents to establish home rules to restrict smoking in certain areas.

B. Consult the social services department to set up counseling.

C. Have the physician prescribe medication to help parents to stop smoking.

D. Notify the office of Child Protection.

71. A 54-year-old female client tells the nurse that she lost her job and husband 3 months ago. She says that she no longer has a bedroom of her own because her daughter and family have moved in with her. During the initial interview, the nurse asks several questions. Which one of the following questions would determine cognitive changes?

A. "How many hours of sleep do you get each night?"

B. "What feelings have you had during the past 3 months?"

C. "Do you feel that you have control over your present situation?"

D. "You lost your husband. Did that interfere with your social life?"

72. Judy H. has just delivered a full-term newborn boy

and the nurse is preparing to give the infant his vitamin K injection. Judy asks the nurse to explain the reason her baby already needs a shot. The nurse's explanation includes that babies:

A. Cannot get enough fat in their diet and need vitamin K to better utilize what they do get

B. Lack a clotting factor and must have vitamin K to decrease their chance of bleeding

C. Are born with a sterile gut and are not able to produce vitamin K on their own initially

D. Are born with hypovitaminemia and must have vitamin K for clotting purposes

73. Which factors predispose an infant to fluid imbalances?

A. A decreased surface area

B. A lower metabolic rate

C. A decreased daily exchange of extracellular fluid

D. Immature kidney function

74. Fluid replacement using isotonic IV fluids is ordered. Which fluid is isotonic?

A. $D_{20}W$

B. .45 NS (normal saline)

C. D_5 .45 NS

D. D_5W

75. Which of the following should the nurse observe for in a client with mastitis?

A. Symptoms include sudden onset of flulike symptoms and a tender, reddened area on the breast.

B. The greater the involvement in the breast, the more likely the elevation in body temperature.

C. The onset is usually between 6 and 10 weeks postpartum.

D. Mastitis improves when breastfeeding is terminated.

76. A 38-year-old male client has been transferred to the unit after being admitted with a diagnosis of Addison's disease. In planning the care of this client, the nurse should include which of the following?

A. Teach the client relaxation techniques.

B. Provide potassium-rich snacks as tolerated.

C. Provide a low-sodium diet.

D. Encourage activity and independence with self-care.

77. A client has been on lorazepan (Ativan) for the treatment of a generalized anxiety disorder. Unknown to the client's physician, the client has increased his own dosage of lorazepam to 1 mg four times a day. The physician is preparing to discontinue the pharmacological therapy by slowly tapering the dosage. The client would be expected to experience early withdrawal symptoms of:

A. Anxiety, irritability, insomnia, and fatigue

B. Irritability, insomnia, fatigue, and increased appetite

C. Insomnia, fatigue, increased appetite, and diaphoresis

D. Fatigue, increased appetite, diaphoresis, and anxiety

78. A 27-year-old client had twin infants born at 37 weeks' gestation 5 years ago. Twelve months ago, she spontaneously aborted an 8-week fetus. She has now missed one menstrual period and is experiencing breast tenderness and nausea in the morning. She states, "I know I am pregnant because of my symptoms." Which of the following responses by the nurse would be most accurate?

A. "Amenorrhea, breast changes, and morning sickness are positive signs of pregnancy."

B. "Missing a period, breast tenderness and enlargement, and nausea in the morning are probable signs of pregnancy."

C. "Missing a period, breast tenderness, and nausea are presumptive signs of pregnancy."

D. "Amenorrhea, morning sickness, and a positive pregnancy test are the only positive signs of pregnancy."

79. A 35-year-old was diagnosed with multiple sclerosis. The physician ordered Betaseron 0.25 mg (8 IU) IM every other day. Using a 0.3 mg/ ml vial, how many milliliters did the nurse administer?

A. 0.5 ml

B. 0.6 ml

C. 0.7 ml

D. 0.8 ml

80. Baby Jane, 11 months old, is admitted with suspected respiratory syncytial virus (RSV). What type of isolation should the nurse place in effect?

A. Contact isolation

B. Universal isolation

C. Respiratory isolation

D. Generalized isolation

81. To prevent a client who is withdrawing from a benzodiazepine from experiencing rebound or recurrence of symptoms, the nurse anticipates that the physician will order the drug to be:

A. Administered every other day

B. Reduced by 25 percent weekly

C. Changed to another drug of the same classification instead of the drug originally prescribed

D. Changed to a barbiturate with a long half-life

82. A 48-year-old woman is admitted with respiratory distress. During auscultation of the client's lungs, the nurse hears a noise occurring on inspiration and expiration and producing a squeaking or grating sound. Which of these abnormal breath sounds did the nurse hear?

A. Bronchial

B. Pleural friction rub

C. Rhonchi

D. Resonance

83. The nurse recognizes that the most common clinical finding noted in a client who is experiencing "thyroid storm" is:

A. Hypothermia

B. Tachycardia

C. Lethargy

D. Hypotension

84. Which nursing intervention is a priority preoperatively for a client with a pheochromocytoma?

A. Restrict liquids to prevent fluid overload.

B. Encourage adherence to a low-calorie diet.

C. Administer sedatives as ordered to decrease anxiety.

D. Monitor BP every 4 hours and administer antihypertensives as ordered.

85. Baby Wilson is born with a spinal cord defect. The physician asks the nurse to help evaluate whether this is a meningocele or a myelomeningocele. An observation that the nurse should make to determine this is:

A. Quality of sucking

B. Movement of lower extremities

C. Head circumference

D. Skin covering the defect

86. A 79-year-old man is admitted with digoxin toxicity. He is confused and has severe headaches and nausea. During the chart review, the nurse notes that the client has been on the same dose of digoxin for 13 years. The nurse realizes that the client's dosage of the medication should be reevaluated. Which physiological change associated with aging is most likely to affect drug absorption?

A. Increased appetite

B. Decreased activity

C. Decreased total-body water

D. Increased body weight

87. A 41-year-old female client tells the mental health nurse that she has lost 25 lb in the last month and does not know why. In planning care for the client, what should be the initial intervention?

A. Force adequately nutritious meals.

B. Sit with the client as she eats.

C. Teach the client about the need for adequate nutrition.

D. Monitor skin turgor and muscle tone.

88. Sarah R. has stated that her friend told her she should be allowed to put her newborn to breast as soon as he is born. However, she does not really understand why. Her nurse is supportive of this procedure and explains:

A. "Early feedings stimulate earlier passage of meconium, reducing the chances of bilirubin elevations and also lessening the chance of hypoglycemia."

B. "Early feedings ensure that the infant does not become dehydrated. It is important to ensure that babies are fed during the first 2 hours be-

cause newborns don't have enough reserve to go much beyond that."
C. "Feeding your baby in the delivery room is very important since he will go to the newborn nursery very quickly while you will go to the recovery room. Since you are breastfeeding, they will not feed him again until you are moved up to postpartum."
D. "It is important to stimulate the root, suck, and swallow reflexes right away. Babies should go to breast very soon after birth so that these reflexes can be examined to ensure an intact neurological system."

89. A mother brings her 6-month-old infant in for a well-baby check-up. The mother asks the nurse if her baby can have solid food. What would the nurse teach the mother about introducing solid foods into her baby's diet?
A. "Begin with a single cereal and see how your baby tolerates it."
B. "Begin with fruit juices that have been diluted by half with water."
C. "Begin with a single strained fruit, omitting citrus fruit."
D. "Begin with a single cereal mixed with fruit juice."

90. During the postpartum period, the uterus on palpation should be:
A. Firm and midline
B. Soft and below the umbilicus
C. Above the umbilicus and to the right of midline
D. At the umbilicus and boggy

91. A nurse is preparing to discharge 17-year-old Lucy T. 18 hours following the birth of her first child. The nurse would like her to understand about hyperbilirubinemia. The teaching plan should include:
A. Demonstrating for Lucy how to assess her baby's skin color for the presence of jaundice by using the blanch test.
B. Explaining to Lucy how bilirubin moves through the GI tract.
C. Showing Lucy how to correctly apply phototherapy.
D. Explaining to Lucy how to assess her baby for signs of kernicterus.

92. The nurse expects to find the functional murmurs most frequently located at which auscultation site in the small child?
A. Aortic area
B. Pulmonic area
C. Erb's point
D. Apical area

93. A nurse working in a public health department is asked by a pregnant client what factors could indicate a potentially complicated pregnancy. Which

of the following explanations by the nurse would be most accurate?
A. Black women younger than age 35 are at a higher risk for complications of their pregnancy.
B. Women aged 20 or less, pregnant for the second time with the same partner, have more complicated pregnancies.
C. Nondiabetic, nonisoimmunized, pregnant women with hydramnios are more likely to have a complicated pregnancy.
D. Women with a pregnancy in which placental size is increased have a higher risk of complications.

94. Carbamazepine (Tegretol) is prescribed for the client withdrawing from benzodiazepine. The nurse should understand that the most likely rationale for this is that:
A. Carbamazepine acts as a central nervous system depressant.
B. Carbamazepine diminishes impulsiveness.
C. Blood pressure, pulse, and respirations will be less affected by the withdrawal of the benzodiazepine.
D. It permits a more rapid and better tolerated withdrawal than does a gradual taper of the benzodiazepine alone.

95. A client was experiencing a severe exacerbation of shortness of breath resulting from chronic obstructive pulmonary disease. The physician ordered theophylline oral solution 160 mg PO every 6 hours. The pharmacy sent theophylline oral solution 80 mg per 15 ml. How many milliliters are required to deliver the prescribed order?
A. 15
B. 20
C. 25
D. 30

96. A nurse is caring for a client who is 2 hours' postpartum. The offgoing nurse reports that the client has third-degree lacerations. Care for this client should be based on the knowledge that a third-degree laceration involves:
A. The skin and mucous membranes of the posterior fourchette and proximal vagina only
B. The skin and mucous membranes as well as the muscle and fascia up to the anal sphincter
C. Skin and mucous membranes, muscle, and fascia through the anal sphincter
D. Tissue around the urethra as well as the skin and mucous membranes of the proximal vagina

97. Braces are often ordered for the treatment of scoliosis in a child when the curve is less than 40 degrees. Satisfactory results of this treatment are dependent on:
A. Fit and appearance of the brace

B. Teaching and counseling by the nursing personnel
C. Reinforcement by the parents
D. Compliance and cooperation of the client

98. A client at 6 weeks' gestation called the obstetrical clinic and reported a small amount of painless spotting when she got up to go to the bathroom this morning. She also stated that she had intercourse last night and there had been no further bleeding. She also asked what could be causing the bleeding. Which of the following explanations by the nurse would be most accurate?
   A. "You are probably having a miscarriage. You need to go to the emergency room right away."
   B. "What you are experiencing is the bleeding caused by implantation of the embryo. It is nothing to be concerned about."
   C. "Some women continue to have a small period each month. Just go to bed during that time so you don't lose the baby."
   D. "The penetration of the penis during intercourse can cause slight bleeding. Don't worry about it, but do call back if the bleeding continues or you start cramping."

99. A client who is 5 days' postpartum is unable to get more than an hour of rest at a time. Her baby girl was born via emergency cesarean section. She states that motherhood is not what she thought it would be. The client is most likely to be experiencing:
   A. Postpartum psychosis
   B. Postpartum blues
   C. Depression
   D. Homeostasis

100. The nurse should be aware that the client with anorexia nervosa thrives on:
   A. Acceptance of self
   B. Self-control
   C. Attending to the needs of self
   D. Socially competent feelings

101. A 20-month-old boy with a tracheostomy is transferred from the pediatric intensive care unit to the pediatric floor. The mother comes to the desk and requests suction catheters because her child needs suctioning. Which of the following suction catheter sizes would be most appropriate for this child?
   A. 6 Fr.
   B. 8 or 10 Fr.
   C. 10 or 12 Fr.
   D. 12 Fr.

102. A 72-year-old man is admitted with aspiration pneumonia after being discharged home 1 week ago. He had a stroke 2 months ago and has visible right-sided weakness. Which of the following factors may have contributed to the client's condition?
   A. Decreased gag reflex
   B. Decreased self-care ability

C. Facial paralysis and weakness
D. Decreased ventilatory effort

103. A nurse has assessed Patty J., a 3-hour-old term neonate. The findings include vital signs (VS): respiration (R) 45, heart rate (HR) 163, T 37.4°C, BP 67/41. Patty has a cephalohematoma and molding. Her glucose is 53. In the assessment findings, the one item that places Patty most at risk is her:
   A. Glucose level
   B. Temperature
   C. Respiratory rate
   D. Cephalohematoma

104. The newborn's Apgar score will be assessed by the nurse: The score reflects:
   A. Newborn behavior
   B. Physiological integrity at 1 and 5 minutes of life
   C. Gestational age
   D. Fetal distress

105. A 65-year-old postmenopausal woman was discharged with advanced breast cancer. The physician ordered testolactone (Teslac) 250 mg qid PO. She had 50 mg tablets on hand. The nurse instructed her to take how many tablets?
   A. 2
   B. 3
   C. 4
   D. 5

106. As part of the discharge teaching for the school-age child with asthma, the nurse should encourage exercise. Which rationale would guide the nurse's decision to recommend forms of exercise in the discharge teaching plan?
   A. Both moderate and strenuous exercise have been found to be advantageous for children with asthma.
   B. Only mild forms of exercise can be tolerated by children with asthma since exercise may trigger an episode.
   C. Only a minority of these children can participate in sports with little difficulty.
   D. Children with exercise-induced asthma are often restricted to certain exercise activities.

107. The normal interaction between the parasympathetic and sympathetic nervous systems causes the fetal heart rate to increase and decrease. This is reflected on the monitor strip as:
   A. Long-term and short-term variability
   B. Sinusoidal heart rate pattern
   C. Periodic changes in heart rate
   D. Nonreassuring changes in heart rate

108. A client is receiving clozapine (Clozaril). The nurse should assess the client carefully for the serious adverse side effect of:
   A. Parkinsonian-like symptoms
   B. Anemia

C. Agranulocytosis

D. Hypertension

109. Dede O. asks the nurse how long it will be before her baby's cord dries up and falls off. The nurse's best response is:

A. "Keep it clean around the base, and it should fall off on its own in about a week to 10 days."

B. "If you put alcohol on it with every diaper change, it should dry up and you can pull it off in about a week."

C. "Just leave it alone, and it will take about 2 to 3 weeks for all of it to completely fall off."

D. "When your change her diaper, be sure that the diaper doesn't cover the cord and it should fall off on its own in about 3 days."

110. Which of the following statements is most accurate when the nurse describes the treatment of pain in children?

A. Infants do not feel pain.

B. Children tolerate pain better than adults.

C. Narcotics are more dangerous to use in children.

D. Children may deny having pain to avoid painful injections.

111. Ida L. is a 15-year-old gravida I who is talking with the school nurse about her pregnancy. Which statement most indicates that Ida needs further nutritional instruction?

A. "I heard that gaining a lot of weight during my pregnancy is bad for me and the baby, so I'm going to eat a lot of fruit and vegetables and cut out the meat."

B. "I don't want my baby to be sick or me to be fat. Guess I'll have to stop eating so many burgers and fries."

C. "I hope my baby doesn't make me look like a blimp. Oh well, I guess I can lose whatever weight I gain, just so my baby comes out OK."

D. "I'm really worried about all this weight they say you gain when you're pregnant. Maybe if I eat really good food I won't gain too much."

112. A 70-year-old woman is admitted with a fractured right hip and right radius. The client is placed on bedrest and receives pain medication every 6 hours. The nurse would need to monitor this client for development of which metabolic disorder?

A. Hypoglycemia

B. Negative nitrogen balance

C. Hypercalcemia

D. Hyperkalemia

113. An 18-year-old client was seen in the local ambulatory care center suffering moderate pain from a football injury. The physician ordered buprenorphine (Buprenex) 0.5 mg every 6 hr PRN for pain. Using a 0.3 mg/ml elixir, how many milliliters did the nurse instruct the client to take?

A. 1.4

B. 1.5

C. 1.6

D. 1.7

114. Mary G. asks how long it will be before she can give her newborn baby a tub bath. Her nurse's best response would be:

A. "You can bathe the baby any time after you have been discharged. Just remember to keep him warm."

B. "Newborns don't really need tub baths since they don't get dirty. Sponge baths are really best."

C. "You should wait until the baby's cord has dried up and fallen off. After that a tub bath is fine."

D. "Tub baths are fine as long as you don't bathe the baby right after he has eaten. It is easy to cause him to spit up since you move him around so much during a bath."

115. The nurse is planning the care of a client in the acute manic phase of bipolar disorder. A nursing goal is for the client to meet her nutritional needs. The most appropriate nursing action to meet this goal would be to:

A. Engage the client in frequent conversations at meal times.

B. Encourage the client to eat small, frequent meals.

C. Have the client keep detailed records of intake and output.

D. Provide the client with literature on the four food groups.

116. A newborn delivered by a diabetic mother is admitted to the nursery. The mother's diabetes was frequently unregulated. This newborn is at risk for:

A. Hypoglycemia

B. Hyperglycemia

C. Hypercalcemia

D. Being small for gestational age

117. A 32-year-old client being seen in the obstetric clinic at 18 weeks' gestation had a blood pressure of 140/90 at her 12-week visit and 148/92 at this visit. The nurse identifies that which of the following procedures will give the most important information regarding pregnancy risks for this client?

A. Vaginal examinations

B. Fundal heights

C. Vital signs

D. Fetal heart tones

118. You are caring for a gravida I, 26 weeks' gestation client in preterm labor. She is 2 cm dilated with intact membranes. Which electronic fetal monitoring equipment would be recommended for this client?

A. Internal fetal scalp electrode

B. External Doppler

C. Intrauterine pressure catheter (IUPC)

D. Electronic fetal monitoring (EFM) is not recommended at this gestational age

119. A 36-year-old female is admitted with severe weight loss, dry skin, and muscle wasting. The client states she has had continuous diarrhea for 2 weeks and has fainted twice at work. The nurse recognizes this type of nutritional disorder to be called which of the following?
A. Kwashiorkor
B. Marasmus
C. Anorexia
D. Pellagra

120. A 29-year-old primipara in the 26th week of gestation is admitted to the labor unit with uterine contractions every 6 to 8 minutes for the past 3 hours that are not affected by ambulation or position change, an increase in vaginal discharge, and a vaginal examination with the following results: membranes intact, presenting part at −1 station, cervix 80 percent effaced, cervix closed. Because of these findings, which of the following measures are important in her care?
A. Initiate IV fluid therapy, place on complete bedrest, NPO except for ice chips, and do continuous fetal and uterine contraction monitoring.
B. Monitor the client for 2 hours, offer emotional support, teach her the difference between false and true labor, and send her home.
C. Place the client in Trendelenburg's position, call for staff assistance stat, and initiate IV fluid therapy ASAP.
D. Initiate IV therapy, and notify the nursery and pediatrics to prepare for the delivery of a preterm infant.

121. Hand washing is crucial in preventing the spread of infection. The nurse recognizes that this practice is aimed at breaking the "chain of infection" during which phase of the cycle?
A. Portal of entry to host
B. Reservoir
C. Method of transmission
D. Portal of exit from source

122. Baby R., a 6-hour-old newborn who was just received into the NICU by ambulance after an unexpected home birth, was admitted with an axillary temperature of 95.8°F. You know that the best way to warm a hypothermic neonate is to:
A. Warm him quickly to decrease the length of cold stress.
B. Place him on an open warmer with an additional heat lamp.
C. Warm him slowly to avoid possible apneic episodes.
D. Place him in a closed isolette with blankets from a warmer.

123. The nurse recognizes that the clinical manifestation of multisystem organ failure is present in a client with:
A. A nosocomial infection

B. Bacteremia
C. Septic shock (hyperdynamic stage)
D. Septic shock (hypodynamic stage)

124. A 16-year-old client developed a severe asthmatic condition. The physician ordered methylprednisolone (Solu-Medrol) 100 mg IV every 6 hr. On hand was Solu-Medrol 80 mg/ ml. How many milliliters are needed to deliver 100 mg/ml?
A. 0.5
B. 0.7
C. 1.0
D. 1.3

125. At her monthly prenatal visit, Kaye R., who is 18 weeks pregnant, asks the nurse if having intercourse with her husband will hurt the baby. The nurse's best reply would be:
A. "Yes, it would be best for the baby if you and your husband waited until after the baby is a few weeks old to continue your sexual relationship."
B. "No, there is no reason why you should have to stop having intercourse. It will be fine to continue as long as you like."
C. "It can hurt the baby later in your pregnancy, but not right now. It is OK to continue until you are in your third trimester."
D. "As long as you are not having complications with your pregnancy, it is OK to continue to have intercourse. You may find that you need to change your sexual position later in pregnancy as your abdomen enlarges."

126. Lithium is prescribed for a client with bipolar disorder. His serum lithium level after 1 week is 0.4 mEq/L. The nurse should:
A. Notify the physician; this is not a therapeutic level.
B. Place the laboratory report in the client's chart.
C. Give an additional dose of 300 mg a day.
D. Call the physician; this is a toxic level.

127. The nurse would expect the normal appearance of a third-postoperative-day surgical wound to:
A. Have slight erythema at the distal portion and slight sanguineous drainage
B. Have minimal or an absence of redness or swelling, with edges well approximated
C. Have minimal-to-moderate swelling and slight purulent discharge
D. Have slight scar tissue and minimal serous drainage

128. Betty R. is worried that her newborn will not sleep once she takes him home because they live so close to a railroad track. As her nurse, you explain to her that newborns can decrease their response to annoying stimuli after repeated exposure. This response is known as:
A. Level of comfort

B. Habituation
C. Responsibility
D. Consolability

129. A nursing intervention for a client with nephro-lithiasis includes encouragement of oral fluids of 2500 ml/day unless contraindicated by other health problems. The most important rationale for increased oral intake (2500 ml/day) would be:
   A. Increased fluids are encouraged to facilitate passage of the stone and help prevent infection.
   B. To prevent hemorrhage in the ureter by stone irritation.
   C. A client having nephrolithiasis is on a clear liquid diet, so large amounts of water are encouraged.
   D. Fluids are encouraged so the stone will expand and show up better on x-ray.

130. A gestational diabetic mother expresses a desire to breastfeed her newborn. The nurse should advise her to:
   A. Resume her pre-pregnancy diet and insulin dose.
   B. Formula feed, because diabetes is a contra-indication for breastfeeding.
   C. Supplement her diet with an additional 500 to 600 calories per day.
   D. Formula feed so that she does not predispose the infant to diabetes.

131. A diabetic is found in a coma. The body is drenched with perspiration, and the pulse rate is 110. The nurse should have the following ready:
   A. Orange juice
   B. An IV insulin drip
   C. Glucagon
   D. IV glucose

132. The most important nursing consideration when providing discharge planning for a 3-year-old with sickle-cell anemia is which of the following?
   A. Teach parents and child how to prevent sickling.
   B. Have the child receive genetic counseling.
   C. Facilitate the adjustment of the family to a short-term disease.
   D. Identify the complications of multiple blood transfusions.

133. An 18-year-old client with a prenatal history of PIH has just arrived on the postpartum floor after delivery of an 8-lb female infant. The nurse knows that because of the client's history, which of the following medications should be avoided in her care?
   A. Oxytocin (Pitocin)
   B. Bromocriptine (Parlodel)
   C. Ferrous sulfate
   D. Propoxyphene and acetaminophen (Darvocet)

134. A 72-year-old client is being interviewed by a nurse in a community nursing center. The client reports feeling "tired all the time" and is having difficulty remembering things. The nurse notes a weight loss of 20 lb since the last visit. In addition to physical and mental status examinations, the nurse completes a sexual history on this client. The rationale for this action by the nurse is:
   A. The number of clients with AIDS over age 60 has risen steadily in the past decade.
   B. Older adults may masturbate because of a lack of a sexual partner and have guilt feelings that are manifested in physical symptoms.
   C. The number of clients reporting diminished sexual desire increases steadily over age 60 and reaches a peak at age 80.
   D. AIDS is the fifth leading cause of death in persons over the age of 65.

135. The nurse therapist is working with a client diagnosed with borderline personality disorder. Two hours before the therapist is to leave the city for vacation, the client telephones to say that she is having suicidal thoughts. The most therapeutic intervention by the nurse therapist would be to:
   A. Cancel her vacation and see the client immediately.
   B. Postpone her flight until she can make arrangements to see the client.
   C. Tell the client to telephone the hotline at the crisis intervention center.
   D. Refer the client to the therapist on call for her after completing a suicide assessment.

136. When giving instructions to a client with a urinary tract infection (UTI), the nurse emphasizes to the client to avoid which one of the following foods because it will increase the urine pH and can lead to a recurrent UTI?
   A. Meat
   B. Citrus fruits
   C. Cranberry juice
   D. Eggs

137. The purpose of the false pelvis is:
   A. To provide support for the uterus
   B. To act as the birth passage for the fetus
   C. To provide protection for the fetus during the birth process
   D. To give the health-care provider a way to determine the size of the pelvis before labor

138. After a client's IV fluids have been infusing for a period of time, the flow is interrupted. Which one of the following would be the nurse's initial intervention?
   A. Move the client's arm to a new position.
   B. Lower the receptacle below the level of the needle.
   C. Flush cannula or needle with sterile saline.
   D. Check for swelling at the needle site.

139. A client asks why iron is so important to her diet when she is pregnant. The nurse's response should be based on the understanding that iron:
A. Helps maintain the acid-base balance in tissues and is important in DNA and RNA synthesis
B. Is needed for the formation of hemoglobin in both the mother and the fetus
C. Is needed to facilitate mineralization of the fetal skeleton and deciduous teeth
D. Aids in protein metabolism, including RNA and DNA synthesis

140. A 10-year-old has ascites secondary to nephrotic syndrome. The child weighs 36 kg. The physician orders bumetanide (Bumex) 0.1 mg/kg (3.6 mg). Using a 0.25 mg/ml vial, how many milliliters should the nurse administer IV?
A. 14.0
B. 14.5
C. 15.0
D. 15.5

141. The home health nurse visits Laura G. 2 weeks' postpartum. When she calculates the calories Laura is providing for her newborn, she discovers that he is receiving 684 calories per day. The infant's weight is 9 lb 6 oz. The best nursing diagnosis for this infant is:
A. Knowledge deficit related to infant nutritional requirements
B. Altered nutrition, less than body requirements
C. Altered nutrition, more than body requirements
D. Fluid volume excess

142. A primary goal in developing a plan of care for a client with an organic brain syndrome is:
A. The client will maintain social skills.
B. The client will complete all ADL independently.
C. The client will be safe from injury.
D. The client will maintain nutritional status.

143. A client at term gestation is admitted to the labor unit with a diagnosis of ruptured membranes times 20 hours. An external fetal and contraction monitor is applied. The monitor shows a fetal heart rate of 160 with good variability. No contraction pattern is noted. The nurse should monitor the results of which of the following laboratory tests?
A. Amniocentesis
B. Cervical cultures
C. Urinalysis
D. CBC with differential

144. To increase the weekly weight gain of a client's breastfeeding, 2-week-old newborn, the nurse should inform the client to:
A. Supplement with formula.
B. Nurse him more often during the night.

C. Decrease his feedings and increase the length to 10 minutes.
D. Keep him nursing at the breast for more than 10 minutes.

145. A 67-year-old client receiving IV fluids at 150 cc/hr begins experiencing headache, flushed skin, rapid pulse, increased blood pressure, increased respirations, coughing, and shortness of breath. The nurse recognizes that these symptoms may indicate possible:
A. Circulatory overload
B. Drug overload
C. Superficial thrombophlebitis
D. Air embolism

146. Using Leopold maneuvers, the nurse determines that the baby's back is facing the maternal left side. The baby's head is in the pelvis with the cephalic prominence on the right. The nurse should listen for the heart tones over the mother's abdominal:
A. Upper left quadrant
B. Lower left quadrant
C. Upper right quadrant
D. Lower right quadrant

147. A physical assessment is done by the nurse on a client who is 12 hours' postpartum. Assessment findings are as follows: Breasts soft, nipples clean, dry, and intact; bowel sounds slightly hypoactive, no BM, positive flatus; firm fundus at two fingerbreadths above the umbilicus; lochia moderate rubra without clots; Second-degree midline episiotomy without edema or redness and edges well approximated; Homan's sign negative. Which of the following actions by the nurse is best?
A. These are expected findings. No action is warranted.
B. Notify the physician of the decreased bowel sounds.
C. Assist the client up to the bathroom to void.
D. Discourage ambulation secondary to the possibility of thrombophlebitis.

148. A client admitted and treated for depression is to be discharged tomorrow. The nurse knows that the client has made previous suicide attempts. Which response by the nurse would be the most therapeutic to determine if the client has learned more adaptive coping?
A. "You know, making a suicide attempt is really silly. You have so much to be grateful for."
B. "Be sure to take your medications after you leave here tomorrow. Call someone if you get down again."
C. "Don't think of sad things after you go home. Try to think happy thoughts."
D. "If you begin to think of suicide after you get home, what will you do instead of hurting yourself?"

149. Julia G. is 26 weeks' pregnant and works as a computer programmer. She spends most of her day working at a desk. She tells the nurse that she has a comfortable chair and can't understand why her feet continue to swell. The nurse should advise Julia to:
    A. Quit her desk job since women should not work beyond their second trimester.
    B. Be sure to take her coffee breaks so that she can prop up her feet.
    C. Take several breaks throughout the day to walk around.
    D. Decrease her salt intake in order to prevent fluid retention.

150. A client with nephrotic syndrome is receiving prednisone daily. Which of the following nursing actions would be most helpful in monitoring fluid retention?
    A. Assessing urine specific gravity
    B. Measuring abdominal girth
    C. Measuring urinary output
    D. Obtaining a daily weight

151. The nurse who is caring for a 31-year-old client with suspected tuberculosis is aware of the importance of proper isolation care. Therefore, which one of the following isolation methods is specifically used to prevent the transmission of pulmonary tuberculosis in clients with positive sputum or chest x-ray reports?
    A. Respiratory
    B. Tubercle bacilli
    C. Contact
    D. Acid-fast bacilli

152. Constipation during pregnancy is usually caused by:
    A. Decreased activity caused by the growing uterus
    B. Decreased motility caused by the relaxation of the smooth muscle
    C. Decreased levels of progesterone
    D. Increased levels of human chorionic gonadotropin

153. A 24-year-old client has a diagnosis of bronchial asthma. The nurse knows that which one of these medications would be of least benefit to the client during an asthma attack?
    A. Epinephrine
    B. Terbutaline sulfate
    C. Cromolyn sodium
    D. Theophylline

154. Betty B. is a type II diabetic who has a cardiac complication. She asks you to recommend a contraceptive technique that would be appropriate for her. You know the best choice for Betty would be:
    A. Oral contraceptives
    B. Sterilization
    C. An intrauterine device
    D. A barrier device

155. Which of the following analgesic orders should the nurse question in an adolescent allergic to aspirin?
    A. Lortab liquid
    B. Tylox
    C. Percodan
    D. Vicodin

156. A client at 37 weeks' gestation should be advised to see her primary health-care provider immediately if she has the following symptoms:
    A. Increased vaginal mucus that requires the use of a vaginal pad
    B. Constipation with increased discomfort with hemorrhoids
    C. Shortness of breath while climbing several flights of stairs
    D. Bloated feeling and blurred vision

157. An appropriate nursing intervention when caring for a 3-year-old client with upper respiratory infection would be which of the following?
    A. Give tepid water baths to reduce fever.
    B. Encourage increasing cereal consumption to increase caloric intake.
    C. Have the child wear heavy clothing to prevent chilling.
    D. Give small amounts of favorite fluids frequently to prevent dehydration.

158. You are caring for a client who is 36 weeks' gestation. She is complaining of nasal congestion, red palms, and a flushed appearance. The information you give the client is based on the knowledge that:
    A. These signs indicate PIH.
    B. This is an unusual complaint in pregnancy and requires follow-up.
    C. These symptoms result from increased peripheral blood flow.
    D. These are symptoms of melasma, which is an acute disease of pregnancy.

159. The nurse is doing postoperative teaching to a client having cataract surgery. The nurse correctly instructs the client to:
    A. Avoid bending at the waist or lifting heavy objects.
    B. Avoid sleeping on the back or the affected side.
    C. Avoid instilling the eye drops in the eye until healed.
    D. Avoid foods high in caffeine and nicotine.

160. A 28-year-old breastfeeding client who is 48 hours' postpartum has complained of sore nipples. On assessment, the nurse notes that the nipples are reddened bilaterally, but without cracking or blistering. The nurse should teach the client which of the following techniques to reduce nipple soreness?
    A. Limit nursing time to 5 minutes on each breast.

Then increase nursing time by 1 minute at each feeding.
B. Dry the nipples with a soft cloth, and then rub them with A&D ointment after each feeding.
C. When the infant latches on, make sure the nipple and most of the areola is taken into the mouth.
D. Breastfeed the baby only every other feeding. Use a breast pump to maintain the client's milk supply.

161. An obsessive-compulsive client with a type A personality was being treated with dipyridamole 50 mg tid IV for long-term therapy of chronic angina pectoris. Using a 75 mg/ml vial, how many milliliters did the nurse administer?
A. 0.57
B. 0.67
C. 0.77
D. 0.87

162. In preparing the Alzheimer's client for inpatient care, which elements of the nursing care plan should be considered highest priority?
A. Safety and the client's ability to perform self-care
B. The client's ability to perform self-care and drug allergies
C. Drug allergies and dietary preferences
D. Dietary preferences and safety

163. A 26-year-old client has second-degree burns covering the face and anterior chest. The nurse places highest priority on the following outcome in planning for this client's care:
A. Airway will remain open, with free exchange of air.
B. Fluid loss will be balanced with fluid intake.
C. Electrolytes will remain within normal limits.
D. Peripheral pulses will remain palpable.

164. A nurse is visiting the home of a client newly diagnosed with diabetic retinopathy. The client seems quiet and does not initiate conversation. The most appropriate response by the nurse at this time is:
A. "Some people with retinopathy fear going blind, what about you?"
B. "You will get used to your poor vision in time and will be just fine."
C. "Other people have experienced retinopathy; it's not that bad."
D. "I can't help you with your problems unless you talk to me."

165. The purpose of genetic counseling is to:
A. Assist couples in reproductive decision making without unduly influencing their decision.
B. Remove the burden of reproductive decision making from couples.
C. Provide information to couples so that they are able to terminate their pregnancy without guilt.

D. Make reproductive decisions for couples who are at high risk.

166. Evaline S. has experienced a spontaneous abortion at 14 weeks. The nurse who is caring for her should monitor for which of the following complications:
A. Hyperglycemia and hypotension
B. Leukorrhea and depression
C. Hemorrhage and infection
D. Fluid and electrolyte imbalance

167. A 60-year-old male presents at the mental health clinic because he is miserable, lonely, and feels hopeless. The nurse counselor formulates outcome criteria for this client. Which one is unrealistic?
A. Displays a consistent, optimistic attitude
B. Identifies helpful resources and support systems
C. Initiates social interactions
D. Demonstrates external locus of control

168. When assessing the client, the nurse correctly identifies which of the following as a positive Chvostek's sign?
A. The facial muscles on one side of the face contract when that side is tapped.
B. The facial muscles on both sides of the face contract when one side is tapped.
C. The client experiences pain in the abdomen after deep palpation occurs.
D. Application of cuff pressure just above systolic pressure produces carpopedal spasm.

169. A 16-year-old client just delivered a term female infant. Which of the following actions by the nurse would best facilitate the attachment process?
A. Once the Apgar scores are obtained, the nurse wraps the baby in a blanket and gives her to the mother to hold.
B. Immediately after delivery of the infant, she is placed on the mother's chest with a blanket over her.
C. After the infant is stabilized in the nursery and given a bath, she is dressed and taken out to her mother.
D. After the infant has been taken to the nursery, the nurse encourages the mother to look at her through the nursery window.

170. Tracheoesophageal (TE) fistula is best described as an abnormal connection between the:
A. Stomach and esophagus
B. Trachea and esophagus
C. Esophagus and diaphragm
D. Trachea and mainstream bronchus

171. A nurse enters the nursing station and tells another nurse on duty, "That client really angers me. She is so manipulative and never appreciates anything you do for her." The nurse is experiencing:
A. Burnout

B. Countertransference
C. Transference
D. Denial

172. Hemodilution of pregnancy leads to the following signs in the woman:
A. A slight elevation of BP in response to overload
B. A decrease in hematocrit level by the second trimester
C. Supine hypotension in later pregnancy
D. Reduction in pulse rate and increase in cardiac output

173. A 90-year-old client is admitted to the nursing home. The psychosocial history obtained by the nurse indicates the client is a widower of 5 years, he retired 10 years ago as a certified public accountant, he is Jewish and attends Beth Israel Synagogue, and he has no children. The most important information for the nurse to share in interdisciplinary team conference is:
A. His lack of family support
B. His educational status
C. His religious affiliation
D. His financial status

174. A young adult female had iron-deficiency anemia. Which laboratory value indicates recovery from this condition?
A. Hemoglobin of 14 gm/dl
B. Hemoglobin of 10.1 gm/dl
C. Hematocrit of 28 percent
D. Hematocrit of 31 percent

175. The nurse is administering IV fluids to an adolescent without an IV pump. He is to receive 1000 cc IV fluid over 12 hours. The drop factor is 60 gtt/ml. The nurse should regulate the flow so that the number of drops per minute is approximately:
A. 63 gtt/min
B. 73 gtt/min
C. 83 gtt/min
D. 93 gtt/min

176. A multipara was 6 cm 30 minutes ago. Now she is vomiting. The nurse should first:
A. Administer an ordered antinausea plus analgesic medication IM.
B. Turn her on her left side and place a cool cloth on her throat.
C. Perform a vaginal examination.
D. Withhold all liquids by mouth except ice chips.

177. A 75-year-old client complains of anorexia and fatigue. The nurse notes that the client has dry skin with some scaling and is wearing a heavy sweater even though the room is a pleasant temperature. The most appropriate nursing action based on these observations is:
A. Obtain laboratory work to test thyroid function.
B. Obtain laboratory work to test for metastatic carcinoma.

C. Do nothing because these are normal findings in older adults.
D. Teach the client to use less soap when bathing.

178. The nurse is performing a history and physical on a young child with hepatitis. The nurse knows that many young children obtain hepatitis A infection from:
A. An infected mother
B. A parenteral route
C. Contaminated water
D. Diapered children in day-care centers

179. The nurse is caring for a client who has been admitted for routine surgery. The client's history of alcoholism was not known, and he experienced abrupt withdrawal from alcohol after chronic consumption. The serious physiological symptom that resulted was:
A. Blackouts
B. Delirium tremens
C. Hypocalcemia
D. Constricted pupils

180. A 65-year-old client is admitted to the hospital with complaints of dull pains in the head which occasionally progress to severe. The blood chemistry indicates a serum glutamic oxaloacetic transaminase (SGOT) of 44 units/L, alkaline phosphatase of 147 units/L, acid phosphatase 1.1 units/L, potassium 5.1 mmol/L, and fasting blood sugar of 108 ml. The nurse recognizes that these laboratory findings suggest:
A. The client may have myocardial infarction.
B. The client may have hyperkalemia.
C. The client may have Paget's disease.
D. The client may have diabetes.

181. A client who delivered a male infant 24 hours ago had her 2-year-old daughter in the room. The newborn was brought into the room for sibling visitation. The 2-year-old turned her head away and stated, "I hate that baby. Send him back." The client then asked the nurse to take the baby back to the nursery. Which of the following nursing diagnoses would be most appropriate?
A. Altered parenting related to postpartum depression
B. Altered role performance related to postpartum psychosis
C. Low self-esteem related to lack of confidence in ability to provide care for two children
D. Altered family processes related to sibling rivalry

182. Which of the following foods should be omitted from the diet of a child with PKU?
A. Squash
B. Fruit juices
C. Cheese
D. Bananas

183. A 17-year-old client with a newly diagnosed preg-

nancy tells the nurse, "My grandmother told me, 'For every child a tooth.' Is this true? I want to keep my teeth. " Which of the following explanations by the nurse is most accurate?

A. "If you take good care of them, you shouldn't lose any teeth."

B. "Yes, it's true. The baby takes the calcium it needs from your teeth."

C. "Yes, the baby takes the calcium from your teeth if you don't drink enough milk."

D. "You won't lose any teeth if you take calcium supplements."

184. The bedridden client is placed on dactinomycin (actinomycin). The initial nursing action prior to administration of actinomycin is:

A. Inspect the skin for discoloration.

B. Inspect the oral cavity for lesions.

C. Obtain baseline vital signs.

D. Obtain signed consent from family.

185. A 32-year-old was diagnosed with macrocytic anemia. The physician ordered leucovorin 5 mg IM. Using a 3 mg/ml vial, how many milliliters did the nurse administer?

A. 0.67

B. 1.67

C. 2.67

D. 3.67

186. A laboring client is completely dilated, +3, and pushing. She has not had anesthesia. In the labor room, she utilized an upright position to bear down. Now she is in the lithotomy position. She says she cannot feel the urge to push. The nurse should:

A. Apply fundal pressure.

B. Assist her in breath holding for more than 5 seconds.

C. Assess fetal descent.

D. Reposition her and encourage her to push when the urge presents itself.

187. A 8-year-old female was admitted to the pediatric unit with a history of pauciarticular juvenile rheumatoid arthritis. Presently, the child is in a flare-up, and the rheumatologist has prescribed corticosteroids. The mother voices her concern that the corticosteroids will impede her daughter's growth. The best response from the nurse is:

A. The corticosteroids will affect the growth less than the inflammation caused by the disease process.

B. The corticosteroids will only interrupt growth when taken over a long period of time.

C. The corticosteroids will be given by alternating high and low doses between days to minimize disturbances to growth.

D. The corticosteroids will produce weight gain rather than interrupt growth.

188. You are an RN working in a prenatal clinic. Your client, who is 32 weeks' gestation, asks if she can continue her current exercise regimen. What guidelines should you share with this client?

A. She can continue her normal routine as long as she does not add any new activities without consulting her physician.

B. She needs to be sure that her heart rate does not exceed 140 beats per minute, and strenuous activities should not exceed 15 minutes in duration.

C. She should stop exercising at this time in her pregnancy because of the increased risk of preterm labor.

D. She can continue exercising as long as her caloric intake does not decrease.

189. A 3-year-old male is admitted to the pediatric clinic with an admitting diagnosis of rule-out Wilms' tumor. Which of the following examining techniques should the nurse be careful to avoid when performing the physical examination?

A. Illiciting his reflex activity

B. Illiciting the function of his cranial nerves

C. Palpating his pulses

D. Palpating his abdomen

190. A client is placed on levothyroxine (Synthroid) 0.025 mg PO daily. Before administering this medication to the client, the nurse should check the medical history to determine:

A. If the client is being administered an anticoagulant medication

B. If the client is being administered an antibiotic medication

C. If the client has a history of liver disease

D. If the client has a history of kidney disease

191. A psychiatric client was raped as a young woman, but she has no memory of the event, although police records support the complaint and her family reports that it happened. The client is using the ego defense mechanism of:

A. Repression

B. Regression

C. Projection

D. Blocking

192. A client is bearing down during second stage. Her blood pressure is continuing to rise as the fetal heart rate drops. The nurse knows that this necessitates:

A. Fundal pressure

B. Forceps or vacuum extraction

C. A change in breathing pattern

D. An emergency cesarean section

193. Nursing care of the child receiving a blood transfusion involves multiple precautions and responsibilities. Which nursing action should the nurse avoid?

A. Vital signs with blood pressure should be taken

before the infusion and then every 15 minutes for 1 hour during the infusion.

B. The first 50 ml of blood or one-third volume of blood (whichever is less) should be administered slowly, while the nurse remains at the bedside.

C. Administer the transfusion using a blood filter.

D. The blood transfusion should begin within 1 hour of receiving the blood from the blood bank or stored in the unit refrigerator.

194. A 65-year-old client is admitted to a psychiatric unit for depression. His vital signs on admission were: blood pressure 180/98, pulse 88, respirations 22, and temperature 98°F. The physician orders include: theophylline 450 mg PO bid, furosemide (Lasix) 40 mg PO every morning, and trazodone 100 mg PO bid. The nurse is monitoring the client's laboratory values. Which laboratory value noted by the nurse would indicate a potential adverse reaction to furosemide?
A. Chemistry indicates increased blood sugar.
B. Chemistry indicates decreased blood urea nitrogen.
C. Urinalysis indicates a trace of protein.
D. Urinalysis indicates a trace of blood.

195. Which hormone is secreted by the placenta after the 12th week of gestation and is primarily responsible for maintenance of the pregnancy?
A. Estrogen
B. Prolactin
C. Progesterone
D. Human chorionic gonadotropin

196. A nurse is evaluating the teaching of a diabetic client. The client gives evidence that the teaching for diabetes has been understood with which of the following statements?
A. "I can decrease the risk of complications by keeping my blood sugar as close to normal as possible."
B. "I should have a thorough eye examination at least every 2 years."
C. "I should not take my insulin if I have fever, the flu, a respiratory infection, or other illness."
D. "I should soak my feet in hot water once a day and more often as needed."

197. Baby girl Bishop was born with cystic fibrosis. The statement that most clearly defines this disorder is a:
A. Recessive disorder in which abnormal secretions occur from exocrine glands
B. Dominant disorder in which secretions produced in the lungs lead to respiratory infections
C. Recessive disorder in which structural changes occur in the hemoglobin molecule
D. Dominant disorder in which an enzyme deficiency leads to fatty deposits in the brain

198. The nurse identifies that the correct procedure for nasotracheal suctioning is to apply suction:
A. To the mouth first and then the trachea
B. For at least 30 seconds each time
C. When inserting the catheter
D. When withdrawing the catheter

199. The client is scheduled to have cataract surgery. The client asks the nurse how long she should expect to be hospitalized. The most appropriate nursing response is:
A. "You need to discuss your hospital stay with your physician."
B. "Most cataract surgery is performed as outclient surgery."
C. "Hospital stay usually depends on the ability of the client."
D. "There is no way of knowing how long you will be hospitalized."

200. A client is receiving lithium carbonate for the medical diagnosis of bipolar disorder. Which of the following symptoms would indicate that the client was toxic?
A. Headache
B. Lethargy
C. Fatigue
D. Coarse hand tremors

201. A 3-year-old child is admitted to the hospital to receive chemotherapy for a diagnosis of neuroblastoma. Which of the following effects would most likely occur after the chemotherapy begins?
A. Painful lesions in the mouth
B. Brittle ridging of the nails
C. Increase in the leukocyte count
D. Swelling in the joints of the hands and feet

202. The nurse assesses a client's venipuncture site. Which statement concerning phlebitis is accurate?
A. The vein feels soft when palpated.
B. The venipuncture site appears inflamed.
C. No blood return is noted with aspiration.
D. The site appears edematous and is cool to touch.

203. A client has been admitted to an inpatient substance abuse clinic with alcoholism. He is a professional man who is in danger of losing his job of 30 years because of his drinking. He states, "Look, I know I've had a little trouble lately, but this is a mistake. I can quit anytime I want. I don't belong here. I don't need this kind of help." The best nursing response would be:
A. "You probably could do this as an outpatient. I'll call your family to discuss it."
B. "Why do you think you are here?"
C. "You're an alcoholic, and it's time to admit it."
D. "You are here because your drinking is jeopardizing your job."

204. A pregnant client may complain of indigestion at the end of her first trimester secondary to:

A. An increase in gastric acids
B. A decrease in gastric acids
C. Pressure from the growing fetus
D. Relaxation of the smooth muscle

205. A 4-year-old is diagnosed with a severe asthma episode. The medication the nurse would be prepared to administer in the emergency treatment of this episode would be which of the following?
A. Epinephrine
B. Corticosteroids
C. Cough syrup with codeine
D. Antibiotics

206. A primigravida is being induced with 10 units of oxytocin added to lactated Ringers'. She is 42 weeks' gestation and is alone in labor. Currently her blood pressure is 150/90, pulse 100, respirations 20, dilation 4 cm, 80 percent effaced, and at −2 station. She complains of nausea as she changes from right to left lateral position every 30 minutes. The client received an epidural at 3 cm. Fetus is in a posterior position. Which of the following is the highest priority nursing diagnosis?
A. Ineffective individual coping related to inadequate support systems
B. Risk for fetal injury related to fetal malpresentation
C. Risk for maternal injury related to alteration in contractile pattern
D. Risk for fluid volume deficit related to vomiting and mild diuresis with oxytocin administration.

207. A 16-year-old female diagnosed with systemic lupus erythematosus was admitted to the hospital for a "pulse" method for administering corticosteroids. During assessment rounds, the nurse observes the teenager crying, and she tells the nurse she is afraid all of her hair will fall out. Assessment of the hair and scalp reveals thinning of hair on top of her head. Which of the following information is most accurate on which to base an appropriate response?
A. Alopecia is an unavoidable symptom of system lupus erythematosus.
B. Hair regrows when the disease activity is in remission.
C. Hair regrowth can occur with the use of a topical medication specifically for hair growth.
D. When alopecia occurs, it is permanent.

208. A client complains to the nurse that she thinks she has a thyroid disorder, particularly hypothyroidism, and asks what tests she should have performed to determine this diagnosis. The nurse correctly informs the client that the best test to determine hypothyroid disorder is:
A. Serum T_3
B. Serum T_4
C. Thyroid releasing hormone (TRH)
D. Thyroid directed antibodies (TDA)

209. A 15-year-old adolescent male refuses to attend group with the other clients. When confronted, he begins cursing and shoving the furniture around in the day room of the adolescent unit. The client is primarily demonstrating the defense mechanism of:
A. Reaction formation
B. Sublimation
C. Acting out
D. Splitting

210. A client is admitted to the hospital with a thyroid nodule. In discussion, the client expresses the fear that the nodule is cancerous and states, "I know I will die soon." The most appropriate response by the nurse is:
A. "I know you are frightened, but thyroid nodules are usually benign."
B. "I know you are frightened, but your doctor can do surgery."
C. "I know that the nodule is not cancerous and will not cause death."
D. "I know that the nodule is bothersome but try to get your mind off it."

211. A 14-year-old large, obese adolescent is being assessed by the nurse on admission to the clinic. The nurse suspects that the client may have a slipped femoral capital epiphysis. Which of the following symptoms would indicate a slipped femoral capital epiphysis?
A. Limp and complaint of hip pain
B. Limp and complaint of ankle pain
C. Curvature of the thoracic spine
D. Curvature of the lumbar spine

212. A 72-year-old was diagnosed with Bell's palsy. The physician ordered phenytoin (Dilantin) 200 mg PO. Using a 125 mg/5 ml elixir, how many milliliters did the nurse administer?
A. 2
B. 4
C. 6
D. 8

213. A 65-year-old female client is admitted to the hospital. On the admissions procedure, the nurse documents an absent dorsalis pedis pulse. The location of this pulse would be where?
A. The back of the knee area
B. Below the medial malleolus of the ankle
C. Below the inguinal ligament
D. Dorsum of the foot lateral to great toe

214. The nurse is assessing a child with croup. Examining the child's throat using a tongue depressor may precipitate which of the following?
A. Bleeding
B. Expiratory crackles
C. Complete obstruction
D. Throat abscess

215. Pytalism is caused by:

A. Increased blood flow to the mouth
B. A decrease in saliva production
C. An increased progesterone level
D. A decrease in the pH of the secretions

216. A 44-year-old male client is undergoing discharge planning from his physician and is sent to the interdisciplinary team for his chronic hypertension. The nurse identifies which of the following approaches as most important?
    A. Keeping doctors' appointments
    B. Attending a hypertension support group
    C. Recommending a smoking cessation program and providing support
    D. Enforcing adherence to the prescribed medication regimen

217. The client was recovering from shingles on his left shoulder. The physician ordered vitamin B_{12} 1 mg IM every day. The stock vial of liquid was labeled 1000 µg/ml. How many milliliters should the nurse draw up?
    A. 0.5 ml
    B. 1 ml
    C. 1.5 ml
    D. 2 ml

218. A 50-year-old woman has come to the clinic for her routine appointment. She is on a diet and exercise program to reduce her weight. Which of the following would be the greatest cardiac risk factor?
    A. All maternal and paternal relatives are obese.
    B. The patient has smoked for a short period of time in the past.
    C. The patient has a job which requires walking.
    D. The patient has an intense job, but is not stressed.

219. A 43-year-old client, diagnosed as having schizophrenia, is admitted to the psychiatric unit. The client is unkempt and exhibits persecutory psychosis. During the initial interview, the nurse determines that the client is suicidal. Which one of the following is the best nursing intervention?
    A. Consult the clinical nurse specialist regarding suicide precautions.
    B. Implement suicide precautions promptly.
    C. Identify and empathize with the client's suicide behavior.
    D. Avoid the client's depersonalizing behavior.

220. A 10-year-old client was diagnosed with uncomplicated urinary tract infection. The preteen weighed 45 kg. The physician ordered 4 mg/kg (180 mg) every 12 hours. Using a 100 mg/5 ml liquid, how many milliliters did the child receive?
    A. 6 ml
    B. 7 ml
    C. 8 ml
    D. 9 ml

221. The nursing assessment of a laboring client reveals: dilation, 5 cm; effacement, 80 percent; station, 0; presentation, vertex; membranes, ruptured; contractions, 3 to 5 minutes apart, 60 seconds long. The client is uncomfortable during her contractions but relaxing well in between. She wants to walk to the nursery to see the newborns. The nurse's best response is:
    A. "Walking will stimulate the uterus to contract and a change of scenery will help."
    B. "Because your membranes are ruptured, you cannot walk around because of the risk of cord prolapse."
    C. "I know you are getting tired, why don't you get in the whirlpool?"
    D. "Would you like me to call for your epidural now before it is too late?"

222. In assessing a child postoperatively with a diagnosis of Wilms' tumor, the nurse is aware that which one of the following symptoms is most likely to occur if the child is developing a complication of intestinal obstruction?
    A. Increase in bowel sounds
    B. Increase in abdominal distention
    C. Increase in blood pressure
    D. Increase in urinary output

223. The primary reason AIDS in the older adult is often missed as a diagnosis by health-care providers is:
    A. The elderly do not often engage in IV drug use.
    B. The symptoms are similar to other common chronic illnesses.
    C. The older adult rarely engages in sexual activity.
    D. The older adult rarely engages in homosexual activity.

224. A pregnant diabetic client at term comes into the obstetrical unit in active labor. In initiation of IV therapy, the nurse would include which of the following in her plan of care?
    A. Hang an IV solution of normal saline to prevent hyperglycemia.
    B. Hang an IV solution of $D_{10}W$ to prevent hypoglycemia.
    C. Hang lactated Ringer's solution mixed with the prescribed amount of insulin and flush the IV tubing.
    D. First flush the IV line with 250 ml of lactated Ringer's mixed with either a protein solution or 10 units of insulin.

225. Iron is best absorbed when given with orange juice or on an empty stomach. A 19-year-old female is treated with ferrous gluconate (Fergon), an oral iron preparation, but refuses to take the medicine because it upsets her stomach. In order to decrease the likelihood of gastric irritation, the nurse should give the medication:
    A. With milk
    B. Undiluted

C. With food

D. At bedtime

226. A 42-year-old female with a history of brain cancer is admitted to the unit 2 days following a craniotomy for the removal of a temporal lobe tumor. The client develops polyuria of an abrupt onset. She is diagnosed with diabetes insipidus. The nurse taking care of the client would realize that the client has developed which type of diabetes insipidus?

A. Primary

B. Secondary

C. Transient

D. Surgical

227. During the mental status examination, the nurse should assess for risk for violence. Which is the best question by the nurse?

A. "Have you had aggressive behaviors in the past?"

B. "Do you feel like hurting yourself or anyone else?"

C. "Do you have trouble with impulse control?"

D. "Tell me how your family engages in violent behavior."

228. Clinical symptoms associated with acute hypocalcemia that the nurse should assess for include:

A. Nausea and vomiting

B. Paresthesia and tetany

C. Polydipsia and polyuria

D. Anorexia and vomiting

229. A 29-year-old female is being seen in the clinic today for a possible urinary tract infection (UTI). She is not vegetarian and was not NPO before a urine specimen was collected. The nurse recognizes that which one of the following urinalysis findings is abnormal?

A. pH 5.5 and low hyaline casts

B. Specific gravity 1.010 and 2 to 3 RBC

C. 20 to 25 WBC and pH 8.5

D. Crystals and specific gravity 1.025

230. A client gave birth to a male infant who died shortly after birth. The infant was anencephalic. The client and her husband are asked if they would like to see their baby. They ask the nurse what they should do. Which of the following answers by the nurse is best?

A. "It would be best to remember your baby as you imagined him. Some things are best left unseen."

B. "This is a hard decision, but some parents have told us that they were glad they saw and held their baby."

C. "You shouldn't rush into a decision. We don't want to add to any guilt you must already be feeling."

D. "It would be best to view the baby at the funeral home. They can 'fix him up' so you have good memories."

231. A 70-year-old client at a free health screening was found to have a thyroid disorder. A nursing student assisting with the screening asks the instructor why the client had not sought medical attention for this disorder sooner. The instructor correctly informs the student:

A. Older adults do not seek medical care because they fear nursing home placement.

B. Older adults do not seek medical care because of limited financial resources.

C. Older adults do not seek medical care because they fear loss of independence.

D. Older adults do not seek medical care because they exhibit few symptoms.

232. A 10-year-old female has been treated for allergic rhinitis in the allergy clinic for the last 2 months. She is scheduled for skin testing today. What measure by the nurse would promote the accuracy of the results?

A. Assessing the child's lungs to make sure there is no wheezing

B. Making sure the child has not taken an antihistamine in the last 4 days

C. Skin testing for allergens that were positive on her radioallergosorbent test (RAST)

D. Using the child's upper back instead of the upper forearm for skin testing

233. A head nurse in team conference indicates to the staff that the 79-year-old client recently admitted needs close observation of the "geriatric triad" during hospitalization. The geriatric triad refers to three conditions requiring special attention, including:

A. Falls, incontinence, and family support

B. Falls, cognitive change, and social isolation

C. Falls, incontinence, and sensory deprivation

D. Falls, cognitive change, and incontinence

234. A young woman was experiencing gastric acidity during the first trimester of pregnancy. The physician ordered aluminum hydroxide gel (Amphojel) 10 ml 1 hour after meals. How many milligrams will the client receive from a 600 mg/5 ml suspension?

A. 600

B. 900

C. 1000

D. 1200

235. In providing anticipatory guidance for the parents of a 4-month-old, the nurse discusses the development of motor skills. The nurse should explain that at around 7 months of age, the infant will most likely be able to:

A. Walk with support

B. Stand holding onto furniture

C. Feed herself successfully with a spoon

D. Sit alone using her hands for support

236. An 18-year-old primigravida at 9 weeks' gestation is admitted to the obstetrical unit for severe nausea and vomiting. This is her fourth admission for this diagnosis in the last 5 weeks. IV fluids are started and IV push promethazine (Phenergan) given. What is the purpose of giving the client promethazine?
   A. Hyperemesis is associated with maternal neurosis. Promethazine decreases anxiety.
   B. Hyperemesis is caused by maternal exhaustion. Promethazine is a sleep aid.
   C. Hyperemesis results in fluid and electrolyte imbalance. Promethazine is an electrolyte replacement.
   D. Hyperemesis is uncontrolled vomiting. Promethazine is an antiemetic.

237. When teaching the client with diabetes, the nurse identifies that the onset of action for regular insulin given subcutaneously is about:
   A. ½ to 1 hour
   B. 2 to 4 hours
   C. 4 to 6 hours
   D. 5 to 7 hours

238. The primary goal in planning nursing care for the suicidal client is to:
   A. Administer an antidepressant agent.
   B. Determine appropriate follow-up care treatment.
   C. Teach the client to challenge irrational thoughts.
   D. Understand the issues motivating the client's behavior.

239. Normal urinary frequency in the first trimester occurs because of:
   A. Stasis of the urine because of obstruction of the ureters
   B. The enlarging uterus applying pressure on the bladder
   C. Bacterial growth in the bladder resulting in urinary tract infection
   D. The enlargement of the uterus, causing it to rise out of the pelvic cavity

240. A 55-year-old female client is scheduled for cardiac catheterization tomorrow. The nurse is preparing the preoperative checklist. Which of the following laboratory tests would the nurse make sure is completed prior to surgery?
   A. Creatinine clearance
   B. Coagulation studies
   C. Urine protein
   D. Uric acid level

241. A 2-year-old was diagnosed with hypoparathyroidism. The physician ordered calcitriol 0.25 µg every day. On hand are 0.5 µg tablets. How many tablets should the mother give the child?
   A. ½ tablet
   B. 1 tablet

   C. 1½ tablets
   D. 2 tablets

242. A 25-year-old male client is in the hospital with AIDS and is put on blood and body fluid precautions. The nurse has noticed that he has had no questions about his isolation precautions. Which of the following explanations would best describe the isolation?
   A. No visitors
   B. Precautions when handling blood and body fluids
   C. Negative air flow required
   D. Semiprivate room recommended

243. A client is prescribed ferrous sulfate tablets twice daily. She is a 40-year-old with iron-deficiency anemia. The nurse should teach the client which of the following?
   A. It will discolor her teeth.
   B. It will give her urine an odor.
   C. It will give her bad breath.
   D. It will darken her stools.

244. A 30-year-old client has to be urged daily to attend all prescribed activities. She reluctantly attends, but refuses to actively participate. When questioned, she states, "I'm here because I need a rest and to have my medications regulated. I've been through all that before and I don't need it now." The client is demonstrating:
   A. Resistance to treatment
   B. Secondary gain
   C. Free association
   D. A phobia to therapy

245. The nurse teaches the mother of a 2-month-old infant that approximately 12 to 24 hours after the administration of diphtheria, pertussis, and tetanus (DPT) vaccine, a normal reaction that the infant may experience is:
   A. Lethargy
   B. Mild fever
   C. Diarrhea
   D. Nasal congestion

246. A 45-year-old client is recovering from thrombophlebitis and has completed heparin therapy in the hospital. She asks the nurse to review the particulars on the proper use of her TED hose. Which of the following statements by the nurse is most accurate when teaching the client about TED hose?
   A. Apply them upon arising.
   B. Do not remove them to sleep.
   C. Cutting the top would be appropriate, if they feel tight.
   D. Wear the same pair always.

247. The client was seen in the emergency room for a puncture wound to the bottom of his left foot. The wound happened within 24 hours and was showing signs of inflammation with red streaking around the wound. The physician ordered cef-

tazidime 200 mg IM as the initial dose. The stock vial of powder was labeled 500 mg when reconstituted with 1.5 ml of sterile water. The total volume once reconstituted is 1.8 ml. How many milliliters are need to deliver 200 mg?
A. 0.5
B. 0.6
C. 0.7
D. 0.8

248. When the nurse is coordinating the therapeutic plan with the interdisciplinary team, the nurse correctly identifies that the primary goal of physiological care for the child with nephrosis is which of the following?
A. Reduce hematuria
B. Reduce excretion of urine protein
C. Increase the ability of tissues to retain fluid
D. Increase blood pressure

249. For which of the following conditions, if present, would the nurse be administering lorazepam (Ativan)?
A. Euphoria
B. Anxiety
C. Depressed mood
D. Psychosis

250. Which laboratory values would the nurse use to confirm the diagnosis of dehydration in the client?
A. Elevated sodium (Na), elevated hematocrit (Hct), and elevated blood urea nitrogen (BUN)
B. Decreased sodium (Na), decreased potassium (K+), and elevated blood urea nitrogen (BUN)
C. Decreased sodium (Na), elevated potassium (K+), and elevated blood urea nitrogen (BUN)
D. Elevated sodium (Na), elevated hematocrit (Hct), and decreased blood urea nitrogen (BUN)

251. A diagnosis of Wilms' tumor for a 3-year-old is confirmed within a few hours after admission to the hospital. In planning preoperative care, which of the following nursing actions should the nurse plan to include?
A. Teaching the side effects of chemotherapy
B. Taking once-a-shift vital signs
C. Supporting the family
D. Forcing fluids every 2 hours

252. When caring for a 33-year-old client with a UTI, the nurse knows that which of the following would be of least benefit in the care and treatment of UTI?
A. Antibiotics usually used for UTI are Bactrim (trimethoprim-sulfamethoxazole), nitrofurantoin, ampicillin, and cephalosporin.
B. Obtain a urine for culture and sensitivity before and after treatment with antibiotics.
C. Increase fluid intake, empty bladder frequently, and teach importance of follow-up culture.
D. Antibiotic therapy would be prescribed for a 3 to 5-day duration.

253. When prednisone is given orally in the treatment of a child with cancer, it is important to remember that it:
A. Increases the rate of wound healing
B. Stimulates secretions of the adrenal gland
C. Obscures the inflammatory symptoms of infection
D. Increases antibody production in the body

254. An expectant mother, 28 weeks' gestation, expresses concern about the birth of her baby. She tells the nurse at the prenatal clinic that she and her partner have herpes simplex, type 2. The nurse should:
A. Advise her that she will not be able to deliver vaginally.
B. Advise her that her pregnancy will lessen the severity of the disease if it reoccurs.
C. Reassure the client that avoiding public restrooms will prevent disease transmission.
D. Reassure her that a vaginal delivery is possible if the herpes is inactive.

255. The nurse recognizes that an increase in growth hormone after bony epiphyseal closure will cause the development of:
A. Acromegaly
B. Dwarfism
C. Sheehan's syndrome
D. Midgetism

256. The nurse is preparing a pain medication for a client diagnosed with AIDS who is experiencing pain. The nurse recognizes that as the client progresses from the transition phase to the AIDS phase, the usual form of pain management for an older adult with this diagnosis is:
A. Aspirin (ASA)
B. Acetaminophen (Tylenol)
C. Nonsteroidal anti-inflammatory drugs (NSAIDS)
D. Narcotic analgesics

257. A 75-year-old male is admitted with shortness of breath and chest pain. His arterial blood gas on room air has a PaO_2 of 65 mm Hg. What does this PaO_2 reading indicate to the nurse?
A. Pulmonary embolus
B. Hypoxia
C. Normal oxygenation
D. Respiratory acidosis

258. A client asks what the term "lightening" means. The nurse's best response would be:
A. "This is when the pregnant woman first feels fetal movement."
B. "These are the sensations the pregnant woman feels as the cervix begins to dilate."
C. "This is when the presenting part descends into the pelvis."
D. "This is the chronic nasal stuffiness that many pregnant women experience."

259. A 38-year-old truck driver was admitted to the psychiatric unit with severe apathy. The physician ordered caffeine 500 mg IM as a mild CNS stimulant. Using a 250 mg/ml vial, how many milliliters did the nurse administer?
A. 0.5
B. 1.0
C. 1.5
D. 2.0

260. A 72-year-old was discharged to home health services with the diagnosis of osteomyelitis. The physician ordered ciprofloxacin (Cipro) 750 mg every 12 hours. The home health nurse instructed the family member to give how many 500 mg tablets?
A. ½ tablet
B. 1 tablet
C. 1½ tablets
D. 2 tablets

261. A 21-year-old client is being treated in the emergency department today for asthma. The nurse knows that asthma is an obstructive lung disease characterized by which one of the following clinical findings?
A. Gradual onset of bradycardia
B. Facial flushing with warm dry skin
C. Hypoinflation of lung capacity
D. Sudden onset of dyspnea

262. When assessing the client with hypoparathyroidism, the nurse correctly identifies which of the following as a positive Trousseau's sign?
A. The facial muscles on one side of the face contract when that side is tapped.
B. The facial muscles on both sides of the face contract when one side is tapped.
C. The client experiences pain in the abdomen after deep palpation occurs.
D. Application of cuff pressure just above systolic pressure produces carpopedal spasm.

263. Magnesium sulfate is used in the treatment of preeclampsia to:
A. Prevent seizures.
B. Decrease BP.
C. Increase urine output.
D. Decrease edema.

264. The nurse should be aware that the expected outcome for a suicidal client is to:
A. Display a consistently optimistic, hopeful attitude.
B. Demonstrate voluntary medication compliance.
C. Discuss previous suicide attempts.
D. Verbalize anger.

265. Which of the following analgesic medications to be used for a hemophiliac, if mentioned by the mother, would indicate the need for further teaching?
A. Aspirin
B. Meperidine
C. Acetaminophen
D. Codeine

Answers

1. (A) Nursing process phase: assessment; client need: physiological integrity; content area: medical/surgical nursing

Rationale
(A) Complaints of weakness are present in most clients with hypothyroidism. This may be caused by changes in muscle function, anemia, or numerous other factors. (B) Clients with hypothyroidism experience constipation, not diarrhea. (C) Client with hypothyroidism exhibit bradycardia, not tachycardia. (D) Clients with hypothyroidism exhibit lethargy and apathy, not restlessness.

2. (C) Nursing process phase: implementation; client need: safe, effective care environment; content area: maternity nursing

Rationale
$$75 \text{ mg} : 1 \text{ ml} = 50 \text{ mg} : x = 0.7 \text{ ml}$$
Math calculation explains incorrect answers.

3. (A) Nursing process phase: implementation; client need: physiological integrity; content area: pediatric nursing

Rationale
(A) The application of heat generally relieves discomfort in children with otitis media. If the child lies on the affected side, drainage of exudate will be facilitated and comfort enhanced. (B) It is not necessary to apply this measure to both ears, and it is difficult for the child to comply with this measure. (C) Sterile earplugs will not assist with pain relief. (D) Ice compresses may provide comfort by decreasing edema, but positioning on the affected side is necessary to facilitate drainage.

4. (C) Nursing process phase: assessment; client need: physiological integrity; content area: medical/surgical nursing

Rationale
(A) Serum creatinine is used to assess glomerular filtration rate and does not screen for nephron damage. (B) Blood urea nitrogen (BUN) evaluates renal function and is used as an assessment for hydration. (C) Creatinine clearance is a urine study to assess renal function and to monitor progress of renal insufficiency. It determines the efficiency of the kidney to clear creatinine from the bloodstream. The test becomes abnormal when 50 percent of the total nephron units have been damaged. (D) Urine output measures only quantity of volume and not the functional ability of the kidney nephrons.

5. (C) Nursing process phase: implementation; client need: health promotion and maintenance; content area: medical/surgical nursing

Rationale
(A) The client should not be on her left side because the pull of gravity on circulation could increase pressure in the opera-

tive site. (B) Tub baths are not usually recommended after cataract surgery because getting in and out of the tub could increase pressure in the eyes. (C) This is the recommended method for cleaning drainage from the eye following cataract surgery. (D) Aspirin decreases the aggregation of platelets and could promote bleeding in the eye.

6. **(A)** Nursing process phase: implementation; client need: safe, effective care environment; content area: medical/surgical nursing

Rationale

(A) Lying on the unoperated side prevents pressure increases in the operative site. (B) Flying should be avoided for at least a week. (C) Vertigo or dizziness should be reported. (D) The client will return to the physician's office to have the dressing removed.

7. **(C)** Nursing process phase: implementation; client need: physiological integrity; content area: medical/surgical nursing

Rationale

(A) Pork insulin differs by one amino acid from human insulin; this amino acid could act as an antigen. (B) Beef insulin has three amino acids that could act as antigens. (C) Humulin insulin is human insulin produced by recombinant DNA. (D) Ultralente is a type of insulin classified by action, not source.

8. **(C)** Nursing process phase: assessment; client need: safe, effective care environment; content area: psychiatric nursing

Rationale

(A) Fear of being in a crowd is a symptom of agoraphobia. (B) Fear of being alone or being in open places from which escape might be difficult is another symptom of agoraphobia. (C) Persons with agoraphobia do not exhibit intrusive thoughts about incapacitating physical health. (D) Psychosis is not a symptom of agoraphobia. However, during times of acute panic, persons may experience impaired concentration and disorganized thought processes.

9. **(A)** Nursing process phase: assessment; client need: health promotion and maintenance; content area: pediatric nursing

Rationale

(A) The overall quality is most important. The child may eat more or less during each meal to balance out the day's or week's intake. (B) Until age 5, the child is not completely ready for the social side of eating. A 3- to 4-year-old cannot sit through long meals. (C) The child, on average, consumes one-half of an adult portion. (D) Food likes and dislikes may be related to genetic sensitivity. As long as the overall nutritional requirements are met, no specific food has to be a part of the diet.

10. **(B)** Nursing process phase: implementation; client need: safe, effective care environment; content area: maternity nursing

Rationale

(A) Epigastric pain is located in the right upper quadrant of the abdominal area, as opposed to "heartburn," or acid reflux, which is a burning sensation located just below the xiphoid process. (B) Epigastric pain is caused by hepatic edema and hemorrhage in clients with severe PIH. This right upper quad-

rant pain is a sign of impending seizures. (C) It is unlikely that there will be time to start an IV before the onset of seizures. The client needs to be protected from injury first. (D) Although fetal well-being is a concern, the priority is to ensure the safety of the mother. Fetal heart tones can be obtained after the seizures have ceased. However, it is likely that the fetus will be delivered during the seizures.

11. **(D)** Nursing process phase: analysis; client need: physiological integrity; content area: pediatric nursing

Rationale

(A) This is an acceptable BP. A BP of 95/60 falls between the 5th and 50th percentile for 12-year-old boys. However, hypotension is a sign of an anaphylactic reaction. (B) Abdominal pain is considered a symptom of anaphylaxis, but not an early one. (C) A heart rate of 90 falls within an acceptable range of 55 to 90 for a 12-year-old client who is awake in a resting state. Tachycardia is a sign of anaphylactic reaction. (D) This complaint by the client is an early symptom of anaphylactic reaction.

12. **(D)** Nursing process phase: implementation; client need: health promotion and maintenance; content area: medical/surgical nursing

Rationale

(A) Sutures will probably not be removed for 6 months. (B) This surgery requires more time for healing so that the surgery will not be disrupted. (C) The surgery requires time for healing to occur so that the surgery will not be disrupted. (D) Progressive ambulation following the first dressing change is standard procedure for this surgery.

13. **(B)** Nursing process phase: implementation; client need: health promotion and maintenance; content area: maternity nursing

Rationale

(A) Although breastfeeding suppresses ovulation after childbirth, it is an ineffective method of birth control. Predicting ovulation is difficult when menstruation has not resumed. (B) Oxytocin is released by the brain with successful latch-on. Oxytocin stimulates the uterus to contract and involution occurs. (C) Both bottle-fed and breastfed infants may develop colic. Colic may be related to reduced gastric acidity in the newborn. (D) Nutritional recommendations for lactating mothers include the addition of 300 to 500 calories per day above the nonpregnant level.

14. **(C)** Nursing process phase: assessment; client need: physiological integrity; content area: pediatric nursing

Rationale

(A) Increased pain can be related to infection, but without other symptoms this would not be conclusive. (B) The temperature should be watched for further elevation. A low-grade temperature can be the result of the inflammatory process. (C) Infected areas are hot to touch, and the heat can radiate through the cast. (D) Bloody drainage on the cast does not mean infection, but drainage can be a medium for infection.

15. **(D)** Nursing process phase: assessment; client need: safe, effective care environment; content area: medical/surgical nursing

Rationale

(A) The IV site should be inspected more frequently. (B) The vital signs should be taken more frequently. (C) Nonverbal signs of pain should be assessed more frequently. (D) The oral mucous membranes should be assessed every 8 hours for signs of an opportunistic infection.

16. **(A)** Nursing process phase: analysis; client need: physiological integrity; content area: medical/surgical nursing

Rationale
(A) Respiratory alkalosis results from alveolar hyperventilation. In the acute stage it is also called hyperventilation syndrome. (B) Respiratory acidosis is an increase in $PaCO_2$ in the bloodstream (greater than 45 mm Hg) caused by decreased oxygen. (C) Metabolic alkalosis is a condition marked by increased amounts of base and decreased amounts of acid in the blood. It is usually secondary to an underlying cause. (D) Metabolic acidosis is a physiological state of excess acid and deficient amount of base in the blood. It is usually produced by an underlying disorder.

17. **(A)** Nursing process phase: implementation; client need: psychosocial integrity; content area: pediatric nursing

Rationale
(A) Time-out is a great disciplinary strategy for young children. By isolating the child, the reinforcer for misbehavior is eliminated and the child becomes bored. The child then agrees to behave appropriately to reenter the family or group. (B) Spanking can result in severe physical or emotional injury and thus is not recommended. (C) Verbal scolding criticizes the child and often creates feelings of shame. The form of discipline is not recommended. (D) Reasoning is more appropriate for older children. Reasoning involves an explanation of why the behavior is wrong and of negative consequences.

18. **(B)** Nursing process phase: analysis; client need: physiological integrity; content area: medica/surgical nursing

Rationale
(A) A platelet count of this nature is normal and would would not affect the client's ability to oxygenate her tissues. (B) This is a very low hemoglobin and, because hemoglobin carries oxygen, this could affect the client's tissue oxygenation. (C) This is an elevated WBC, which would be expected in a client with a diagnosis of pneumonia. (D) This is a normal potassium level and would not affect the client's respiratory status.

19. **(A)** Nursing process phase: implementation; client need: safe, effective care environment; content area: medical/surgical nursing

Rationale
(A) Nothing (not even water) should be put on the site. (B) Soap and water might be irritating to the skin. (C) Lotion is contraindicated. (D) Nothing should be put on intact skin.

20. **(D)** Nursing process phase: assessment; client need: psychosocial integrity; content area: maternity nursing

Rationale
(A) Anticipating fetal movement is an example of incorporation of the idea of being pregnant, associated with the first trimester. (B) Social-role adjustment is associated with the first trimester. (C) Developing inner strength, becoming more introspective, is evidenced in the second trimester. (D) Seeing the infant separate from the mother is a task associated with the third trimester.

21. **(C)** Nursing process phase: implementation; client need: psychosocial integrity; content area: pediatric nursing

Rationale
(A) The appliance is not changed unless it comes loose from the skin and begins leaking. (B) This is not a therapeutic intervention to promote acceptance. (C) The child and family should participate and learn care of the stoma and appliance to gain acceptance. (D) A pale, white stoma would indicate insufficient blood flow, which could cause tissue necrosis.

22. **(B)** Nursing process phase: assessment; client need; safe, effective care environment; content area: medical/surgical nursing

Rationale
(A) Facial nerve paralysis is indicative of a condition known as Bell's palsy and can affect one side of the face. It is usually attributed to trauma to the facial nerve, a tumor next to the nerve, or possibly an unknown infection. (B) The client with spinal cord damage to the C2 to C3 area would have difficulty breathing or respiratory depression. The nurse needs to monitor the client closely for any changes in case mechanical ventilation needs to be initiated. (C) Bowel and urinary incontinence can be seen with lower lumbar fractures as well as cervical fractures. However, there is a more important problem that the nurse needs to monitor for in this client. (D) Damage to a small section of the spinal cord can cause this type of injury in lower spinal cord injuries. This would not be seen if there was damage to the spinal cord at the cervical section of the spine.

23. **(D)** Nursing process phase: implementation; client need: safe, effective care environment; content area: medical/surgical nursing

Rationale
(A) The nurse would not leave the client's side to get more pain medication. The client is injured, and the nurse must protect the client from further injury. (B) No one should move any client complaining of neck pain. If the client has any type of cervical fracture, you could do permanent damage to the spinal cord by asking the client to move around. (C) The nurse would not ask the client to move her extremities. If the client has injured her neck, she needs to be kept still in order to avoid further injury to the spinal cord if a cervical fracture has occurred. (D) The nurse would immobilize the client, call for assistance, and not leave the client. The nurse would want to avoid possible further injury to the neck in case there has been cervical fracture.

24. **(B)** Nursing process phase: assessment; client need: psychological integrity; content area: pediatric nursing

Rationale
(A) The "oral sensory" is the psychosexual stage identified by Freud to be present from birth to 1 year. (B) "Trust versus mistrust" is the psychosocial stage identified by Erikson and met by attention to basic needs. (C) "Sensorimotor" is the cognitive stage identified by Piaget to depict the period of birth to 2 years old. (D) Sullivan described the "radius of significant relationships."

25. **(B)** Nursing process phase: implementation; client need: promotion and maintenance; content area: medical/surgical nursing

Rationale
(A) The client has minor symptoms of Ménière's disease and may need medical attention to prevent hearing loss. (B) The rationale has been given under A. (C) Cerumen is not the problem. (D) Medical attention may be needed to prevent hearing loss.

26. (A) Nursing process phase: implementation; client need: safe, effective care environment; content area: pediatric nursing

Rationale
(A) A positive control solution consists of a solution that will produce a positive skin reaction. The positive control test will detect skin-reaction suppression. (B) False-negative results can occur if medication suppression is present. (C) Rescheduling for 1 week would ensure an appropriate time lapse between corticosteroid administration and testing. The usual waiting period between corticosteroid administration and testing is 48 to 96 hours. (D) Notifying the physician for directions is acceptable, but the only way to determine medicine suppression is to apply a negative control solution.

27. (B) Nursing process phase: planning; client need: safe, effective care environment; content area: medical/surgical nursing

Rationale
(A–D) The action of regular insulin peaks in 3 to 4 hours.

28. (A) Nursing process phase: implementation; client need: safe, effective care environment; content area: pediatric nursing

Rationale
(A) Adequate shampooing, often with a sulfur and salicylic acid compound, may treat cradle cap. Adequate scalp hygiene may prevent the condition. (B) Atopic dermatitis (AD) is associated with allergies, but seborrheic dermatitis is not allergic in nature. (C) Avoidance of shampooing because of a "fear of hurting soft spots" may contribute to the condition. (D) The delaying of cow's milk may decrease the risk of AD, which is allergy based, but does not affect seborrhea.

29. (D) Nursing process phase: analysis; client need: physiological integrity; content area: psychiatric nursing

Rationale
(A) No available studies indicate that urinary retention is a problem for young children. (B) Studies done with postmenopausal women on antipsychotics have not identified urinary retention as a side effect. (C) There are no data to indicate that this age group has a problem with urinary retention. (D) Literature significantly support the findings that elderly men with enlarged prostate glands experience urinary retention, dribbling, urinary hesitation, and increased urinary tract infections while taking antipsychotics because of the anticholinergic activity.

30. (D) Nursing process phase: implementation; client need: psychosocial integrity; content area: medical/surgical nursing

Rationale
(A & B) Immediately following discharge, the client might encounter negative reactions to his disfigurement. He needs to be ready to deal with such reactions prior to participating in community activities. (C & D) The client needs open communication with supportive others until he has developed the psychosocial strengths to cope with his disfigurement.

31. (C) Nursing process phase: assessment; client need: physiological integrity; content area: medical/surgical nursing

Rationale
(A) Clients in a thyrotoxic crisis exhibit a very high (102 to 106°F) body temperature. 99°F is considered within a normal range for adults. (B) Clients in thyrotoxic crisis exhibit restlessness and then manic behavior until comatose. They do not exhibit fatigue. (C) Clients in thyrotoxic crisis exhibit severe tachycardia (resting pulse greater than 90 beats per minute). (D) Clients in thyrotoxic crisis exhibit diaphoresis and not dryness of skin. Because of an elevated body temperature, the skin is usually warm to the touch rather than cool.

32. (C) Nursing process phase: analysis; client need: safe, effective care environment; content area: medical/surgical nursing

Rationale
(A) These enzymes are not specific for heart muscle and take 4 to 6 hours to become elevated. (B) A positive CK-MB fraction is highly indicative of MI. (C) A positive myoglobin is most sensitive for MI and should be positive 1 hour following an MI. (D) AST is not specific for heart muscle and will not show up as positive for approximately 6 hours following an MI.

33. (D) Nursing process phase: implementation; client need: safe, effective care environment; content area: pediatric nursing

Rationale
600,000 U : 1 ml = 1,200,000 U : x = 2 ml
Math calculation explains incorrect answers.

34. (C) Nursing process phase: implementation; client need: physiological integrity; content area: maternity nursing

Rationale
(A) The statement that there is nothing that can be done is false. However, the infant is capable of drawing out an inverted nipple. (B) Rolling and toughening of nipples has been associated with an increased incidence of preterm labor. This statement is incorrect. (C) Nipple inversion is caused by adhesions that pull the nipple into the breast tissue. Breast shells provide a gentle suction that pulls out flat or inverted nipples. (D) Breast shields have been used to protect sore or cracked nipples once breastfeeding has been initiated. They are not used prenatally.

35. (A) Nursing process phase: implementation; client need: psychosocial integrity; content area: psychiatric nursing

Rationale
(A) Delusions are false beliefs. To promote health, take the first opportunity to engage the patient in reality-oriented conversation. (B) Argument is inappropriate and useless because patients will defend and hold on to their delusions. (C) As little reference as possible should be made to the delusional concerns to prevent increasing entrenchment of the delusions. (D) Agreeing with the delusional thinking reinforces the delusions.

36. **(B)** Nursing process phase: assessment; client need: safe, effective care environment; content area: medical/surgical nursing

Rationale

(A) SIADH causes electrolyte imbalances, such as hyponatremia and low serum osmolality. It does not cause hyperkalemia. (B) Addison's disease is marked by hyponatremia, hyperkalemia, and hypocalcemia. (C) Cushing's syndrome produces hypernatremia and water retention caused by glucocorticoid excess. (D) Diabetes insipidus leads to hypovolemia with reduced serum osmolality and hyponatremia. This is a result of increased fluid volume intake and excessive polyuria caused by a deficiency of vasopressin (antidiuretic hormone).

37. **(B)** Nursing process phase: implementation; client need: physiological integrity; content area: pediatric nursing

Rationale

(A) Infants with diarrhea would be subject to acidosis. (B) Infants with diarrhea can lose a large volume of fluid in a short amount of time and can quickly experience shock from dehydration. (C) Reverse isolation is not indicated with diarrhea. (D) Infants are positioned in infant seats primarily to ease respiratory effort or minimize gastric reflux. This positioning would not be a key nursing intervention for an infant with diarrhea.

38. **(B)** Nursing process phase: assessment; client need: health promotion and maintenance; content area: pediatric nursing

Rationale

(A) Physical health does not correlate to the type of injury. (B) The curiosity related to a developmental stage impels the child to investigate activities and mimic behaviors of others. This predisposes the child to numerous hazards in childhood. (C) Gender does not determine the type of injury a child may be susceptible to at a given age. However, a preponderance of boys tend to be involved in injuries because of behavioral characteristics, especially aggression. (D) Educational level does not correlate to the type of injury. Cognitive characteristics predispose children to injury.

39. **(B)** Nursing process phase: analysis; client need: safe, effective care environment; content area: medical/surgical nursing

Rationale

(A) You do not clamp chest tubes to transport the client to another unit; however, you would clamp the tubes if you had to change the collection system. (B) You would clamp the chest tubes to check for an air leak or any time the chest tube system has been inadvertently interrupted. (C) You would not need to clamp the tubes to change the dressings unless you were going to interrupt the suction to the system. (D) You do not need to clamp the chest tubes when obtaining a sample of the drainage. The disposable systems have self-sealing sampling ports. This allows obtaining specimens without interrupting the flow.

40. **(A)** Nursing process phase: assessment; client need: physiological integrity; content area: pediatric nursing

Rationale

(A) An inconsolable cry lasting longer than 3 hours within 48

hours of receiving should be carefully reviewed prior to further administration. (B) Oral polio is contraindicated if a member of the household has HIV. (C) Administration of MMR would be carefully reviewed if the infant were allergic to eggs. (D) DPT is not contraindicated in infants with a family history of seizures.

41. **(C)** Nursing process phase: assessment; client need: physiological integrity; content area: medical/surgical nursing

Rationale

(A) Clients with hypoparathyroidism are hypocalcemic. (B) Hyponatremia is not routinely noted in acute hyperparathyroidism. (C) Clients with acute hyperparathyroidism are hypocalcemic and exhibit a positive Chvostek's sign. (D) Clients with acute hyperparathyroidism are hypocalcemic and also exhibit a positive Trousseau's sign.

42. **(D)** Nursing process phase: implementation; client need: health promotion and maintenance; content area: medical/surgical nursing

Rationale

(A) Fluids should be encouraged, not restricted. (B) Although phosphate binders may be given to decrease calculi formation, it is not a nursing intervention; a high fluid intake will be more effective. (C) Vitamin D is restricted for those clients with hypercalcemia. (D) Fluids up to 3 L/day should be encouraged to dilute the urine.

43. **(C)** Nursing process phase: assessment; client need: psychosocial integrity; content area: pediatric nursing

Rationale

(A) In cooperative play, children use the play activity to achieve a desired goal. Children must organize their group and play with others. This type of play is too high-level for the toddler. (B) Children easily lend and share toys when playing together in the same or similar activity. The group has no real organization. Toddlers have difficulty in lending and sharing toys and playing with others. (C) During this characteristic play of toddlers, children play beside each other, but not with each other. (D) This is the characteristic play of infants because their primary interest is watching other children playing.

44. **(A)** Nursing process phase: implementation; client need: safe, effective care environment; content area: psychiatric nursing

Rationale

(A) The nurse should question the order because the maximum safe dose is 250 mg/day. (B) If the nurse gives the medication as ordered, he or she will overdose the client. (C) The nurse should never make the independent decision to change the dosage of a medication. That function is the responsibility of the physician. (D) Asking another nurse to administer the medication could still result in an overdose for the client if he or she fails to question the order.

45. **(B)** Nursing process phase: planning; client need: physiological integrity; content area: medical/surgical nursing

Rationale

(A, C, & D) This nursing diagnosis is not usually associated with diabetes insipidus. (B) Absent or diminished vasopressin secretion causes increased water loss in the urine and increased plasma osmolality and sodium levels. Severe dehydration and hypernatremia may develop if thirst is diminished or water is not available.

46. **(D)** Nursing process phase: evaluation; client need: safe, effective care environment; content area: medical/surgical nursing

Rationale
(A) Although venous cannulation is necessary for IV therapy, it is not the final step. (B) This is one of the initial steps to successful IV cannulation. (C) This is one of the steps to initiating successful IV cannulation. (D) After venipuncture, the IV tubing must be connected. Once the IV fluid drips freely, IV therapy is under way.

47. **(A)** Nursing process phase: implementation; client need: health promotion and maintenance; content area: pediatric nursing

Rationale
(A) Cotton panties, not nylon panties, should be worn because of their absorbency, which keeps uropathogens away from the urethra. (B) Perineal hygiene should consist of wiping from front to back. It is not necessary to wash the perineum with soap and water after each voiding. (C) Children should be encouraged to void frequently to prevent urinary stasis, which would provide a medium for bacterial growth. (D) Generous fluid intake should be encouraged to promote urinary transport and lower the concentration of pathogens in the urine.

48. **(A)** Nursing process phase: analysis; client need: safe, effective care environment; content area: medical/surgical nursing

Rationale
(A) Phosphate levels are typically elevated in CRF. This medication will bind phosphate, allowing it to be passed through the intestines. (B) Although this is one action of Amphojel, it is not the rationale for administering it in CRF. (C) Antacids neutralize gastric acids; they do not decrease production. This is not the rationale for administering Amphojel in CRF. (D) This is the action of antiulcer drugs such as ranitidine (Zantac) and cimetidine (Tagamet).

49. **(A)** Nursing process phase: analysis; client need: physiological integrity; content area: medical/surgical nursing

Rationale
(A) A visible PMI is abnormal. (B & D) The finding is normal. (C) The right border of the normal heart should not be detected by percussion.

50. **(D)** Nursing process phase: implementation; client need: safe, effective care environment; content area: psychiatric nursing

Rationale
(A) This question focuses on self-esteem and may elicit a "yes" or "no" answer. (B) This question focuses only on the family, not on the client. (C) The nurse is legally responsible for accurately assessing and immediately implementing suicide precautions. (D) This question focuses on feelings, indicates concern, and establishes the foundation for suicide assessment and intervention.

51. **(A)** Nursing process phase: implementation; client need: physiological integrity; content area: pediatric nursing

Rationale
(A) The posterior fontanelle usually closes by 2 months of age, while the anterior fontanelle closes between 12 and 18 months of age. (B) This finding is normal and thus does not warrant an immediate notification of the physician. (C) This line of questioning is totally inappropriate and would serve only to alarm the mother. (D) The nurse would not request skull x-rays unless ordered by the physician.

52. **(C)** Nursing process phase: evaluation; client need: health promotion and maintenance; content area: maternity nursing

Rationale
(A) Wearing a well-fitting, supportive bra 24 hours a day will provide comfort because it will immobilize the breasts. (B) Frequent nursing helps to empty the ducts and relieves intraductal pressure. (C) Ice packs may alleviate the discomfort, but they will inhibit milk flow. (D) Expressing small amounts of milk softens the areola and makes it easier for the infant to latch on.

53. **(A)** Nursing process phase: implementation; client need: health promotion and maintenance; content area: pediatric nursing

Rationale
(A–C) The growth rate slows between 12 and 18 months, with a decrease in kilocalories per kilogram from 108 during infancy to 102 and in fluid needs from 140 ml/kg to 115 ml/kg. By 30 months, the birth weight has quadrupled, whereas the weight had tripled by 12 months. (D) Toddlers do require slightly more vitamins and minerals to meet the demands of muscle tissue and other growth. Growth is not halted.

54. **(A)** Nursing process phase: assessment; client need: physiological integrity; content area: medical/surgical nursing

Rationale
(A) A neurogenic bladder would make urinary retention a more likely complication. Urinary retention could lead to a urinary tract infection. (B) The diabetic is not at greater risk for hemorrhage. (C) The diabetic is not at greater risk for thrombophlebitis. (D) The diabetic is at greater risk for any infection, but urinary retention is a better answer for the reasons given under rationale A.

55. **(B)** Nursing process phase: evaluation; client need: psychosocial integrity; content area: maternity nursing

Rationale
(A) This dimension of mourning is that of searching and yearning. It is characterized by feelings of restlessness, anger, guilt, and ambiguity. It is yearning for the baby and searching for the answer for why the loss occurred. (B) The dimension of shock and numbness is expressed by parents through feelings of stunned disbelief, panic, distress, or anger. Parents have said that they feel as though it is all a bad dream and they yearn to wake up. (C) This is the phase of reorganization. Reorganization is characterized by the ability of the parents to place the loss in perspective. Families have said that they will never forget the baby who died, but that they have moved on with their lives. (D) This is the dimension of disorganization.

Disorganization is characterized by feelings of depression, difficulty concentrating, and generally feeling physically and emotionally ill. Many parents feel they will never get over their loss.

56. **(C)** Nursing process phase: implementation; client need: safe, effective care environment; content area: psychiatric nursing

Rationale
$$100 \text{ mg} : 1 \text{ ml} = 164 \text{ mg} : x = 1.64 \text{ ml}$$
Math calculation explains incorrect answers.

57. **(D)** Nursing process phase: assessment; client need: safe, effective care environment; content area: maternity nursing

Rationale
(A) This is a normal respiratory rate. (B) 2+ reflexes are expected with PIH. (C) $MgSO_4$ more typically results in mild sedation because of the CNS effects. (D) A urinary output of less than 30 ml/hr is considered an abnormal amount. Toxicity may result when the kidney function is decreased as a result of reabsorption of the drug. Decreased urine output is a common side effect of $MgSO_4$ toxicity.

58. **(D)** Nursing process phase: implementation; client need: physiological integrity; content area: medical/surgical nursing

Rationale
(A, B, & D) The most effective method to stop bleeding has been found to be direct pressure to the area. Applying pressure to the femoral artery would be using a pressure point. (C) Tourniquets can cause damage if not properly used.

59. **(B)** Nursing process phase: analysis; client need: safe, effective care environment; content area: medical/surgical nursing

Rationale
$$\frac{50 \text{ cc}}{30 \text{ min}} = \frac{x}{60 \text{ min}}$$
$$30x = 3000 \text{ cc}$$
$$\frac{3x}{3} = \frac{300}{3}$$
$$x = 100 \text{ cc}$$
Math calculation explains incorrect answers.

60. **(D)** Nursing process phase: assessment; client need: physiological integrity; content area: pediatric nursing

Rationale
(A) This closed-ended question requires only a "yes" or "no" response and offers little information. (B) This closed-ended question will not elicit feelings and problem areas for discussion. (C) This question may imply a lack of parental skill and encourage defensiveness. (D) This open-ended question allows the parent to respond with detail information during the interview.

61. **(D)** Nursing process phase: implementation; safe, effective care environment; content area: maternity nursing

Rationale
(A) If the client does not plan to breastfeed, having the infant

nurse will only increase her engorgement by increasing milk flow. Also, after nursing, one should not be able to express milk. (B) A warm shower will further stimulate milk production. (C) Because the infant is bottle-feeding, increasing the feedings will have no effect on the engorgement. (D) Applying ice packs to the breasts will constrict the vessels and prevent further engorgement; this is also a comfort measure. Applying a binder to the chest may also help.

62. **(B)** Nursing process phase: assessment; client need: safe, effective care environment; content area: psychiatric nursing

Rationale
(A) Akinesia is described as a decrease in spontaneous facial expressions, gestures, speech, or body movements. These symptoms, if present, would be objective, not subjective. (B) Akathisia is characterized as subjective feelings of restlessness or the objective signs of restlessness or both. (C) Tardive dyskinesia is characterized by involuntary or rhythmic movements of the tongue, jaw, or extremities after at least 6 months on a neuroleptic. (D) Dystonia is described as abnormal positioning or spasm of the muscles of the head, neck, limbs, or trunk, which develops within a few days after initiation of an antipsychotic medication.

63. **(A)** Nursing process phase: assessment; client need: health promotion and maintenance; content area: pediatric nursing

Rationale
(A) The DDST II measures development in the areas of personal-social, fine-motor, language, and gross-motor skills in children from birth to 6 years. (B) The DDST II does not measure IQ. (C) The DDST II does not diagnose mental retardation, though developmental delays may be identified. (D) The DDST II does not measure stress or anxiety.

64. **(D)** Nursing process phase: evaluation; client need: safe, effective care environment; content area: maternity nursing

Rationale
(A) Infants go into such a deep sleep between the periods of reactivity that they are virtually unresponsive. This is normal behavior. (B) Periodic breathing is a normal breathing pattern for a newborn. Periods of apnea lasting more than 20 seconds are worrisome. Brief periods of tachycardia up to 180 beats per minute are also normal with activity. (C) This is a normal heart rate for a term newborn during periods of sleep. (D) Nasal flaring and retractions indicate respiratory distress. Further evaluation is necessary.

65. **(C)** Nursing process phase: planning; client need: health promotion and maintenance; content area: pediatric nursing

Rationale
(A) This is true. Children with type I diabetes mellitus require snacks to prevent hypoglycemia during the time of peak insulin levels. (B) This is true. Children will need extra food during times of decreased activity. (C) This is incorrect. Appetite should not be a guide for the amount of calories needed. Children with type I diabetes mellitus require adequate calories with their insulin, despite their appetite. (D) This is true. It is important to have a regular exercise regimen.

66. **(C)** Nursing process phase: analysis and planning;

client need: physiological integrity; content area: pediatric nursing

Rationale

(A) Varying degrees of paralysis may be present, depending on the location and severity of the defect. Therefore complete paralysis is not the most common anomaly because of the widely varying manifestation of paralysis. (B) Reflexes will be altered. The neurological assessment will determine the neurosegmental level of the lesion and may result in findings from hyperreflexia to diminished or absent reflexes, dependent on the nerves involved. (C) Ninety to 95 percent of children with myelomeningocele have hydrocephalus, which is the most frequently associated anomaly. (D) A vesicostomy is not an anomaly. It is a procedure in which the anterior wall of the bladder is brought to the abdominal wall, creating a stoma for urinary drainage.

67. **(C)** Nursing process phase: assessment; client need: physiological integrity; content area: medical/surgical nursing

Rationale

(A) This is a normal breathing pattern for an adult man when at rest or sleeping. (B) This is a normal finding in a client with no history of respiratory problems. The costal angle is the angle between the ribs and sternum above the xiphoid process. (C) The costal angle widens if the client's chest wall is expanded chronically as seen in COPD. (D) The diaphragm, not the thoracic muscles, would be used for breathing at rest. Thoracic muscles would be used in instances of extreme physical exertion.

68. **(C)** Nursing process phase: analysis; client need: health promotion and maintenance; content area: maternity nursing

Rationale

(A) Ovulation occurs on the 14th day of the cycle plus or minus 2 days before the onset of the next menses. (B) Ovulation does vary somewhat, but with accurate charting of the menstrual cycle, the method can be fairly reliable. (C) Days 4 to 17 of the menstrual cycle are considered the fertile period, and if intercourse is avoided during that time, this method can be fairly reliable. (D) The ovum can only survive 1 to 2 days following ovulation.

69. **(B)** Nursing process phase: implementation; client need: safe, effective care environment; content area: medical/surgical—gerontological nursing

Rationale

100 mg : 1 tablet = 400 mg : x = 4 tablets
Math calculation explains incorrect answers.

70. **(A)** Nursing process phase: implementation; client need: health promotion and maintenance; content area: pediatric nursing

Rationale

(A) Limiting smoking to specific rooms can reduce smoke in the child's environment. (B) Parents must show a need and willingness to be counseled. If parents do not want to quit smoking, then restricting areas is the next step to see if the child's allergy response improves. (C) Certain medications help people to stop smoking, but the person must want to stop smoking. (D) This is not a reportable problem. The child's condition must be worse for it to be reportable, and the par-

ents can be worked with to restrict smoking to specific area so that the child's exposure can be reduced.

71. **(C)** Nursing process phase: assessment; client need: safe, effective care environment; content area: psychiatric nursing

Rationale

(A) This question assesses physical changes. (B) The nurse is assessing for changes in mood. (C) The question focuses on the client's cognitive changes. (D) The question focuses on behavioral changes.

72. **(C)** Nursing process phase: implementation; client need: health promotion and maintenance; content area: maternity nursing

Rationale

(A) Infants should receive about 15 percent of their calories from fat. They can easily do this if fed commercial formula or breast milk. This has nothing to do with their vitamin K intake. (B) Infants are not normally missing clotting factors at birth. (C) This is a true statement. Normal intestinal flora help synthesize vitamin K, folic acid, and biotin. Because the gut is sterile at birth, production of vitamin K is delayed. (D) Full-term infants whose mothers have maintained a good diet during their pregnancy should not be born with vitamin deficiencies.

73. **(D)** Nursing process phase: analysis; client need: health promotion and maintenance; content area: pediatric nursing

Rationale

(A) Infants have increased surface areas for their body weight. (B) Infants have increased metabolic rates. (C) Infants have an increased daily exchange of extracellular fluid. (D) Immature kidney function in young infants predisposes them to fluid imbalances.

74. **(D)** Nursing process phase: analysis; client need: safe, effective care environment; content area: medical/surgical nursing

Rationale

(A) This fluid is hypertonic. (B & C) This solution is hypotonic. (D) D_5W and NS (0.9 percent) are isotonic fluids.

75. **(A)** Nursing process phase: assessment; client need: physiological integrity; content area: maternity nursing

Rationale

(A) High temperature, malaise, and a warm, lumpy, tender area on the affected breast are indicators of mastitis. (B) Because of the body's ability to wall off the infection, the less systemic response there is. (C) The onset of mastitis is 2 to 4 weeks postpartum. (D) Most mothers benefit from continuing to breastfeed because it helps the affected breast to empty the ducts.

76. **(A)** Nursing process phase: implementation; client need: safe, effective care environment; content area: medical/surgical nursing

Rationale

(A) This is correct. The nurse must teach the client relaxation exercises to help reduce stress. Increased stress can exacerbate symptoms in Addison's disease. (B) Clients with Addison's disease have increased potassium levels and should be given a potassium-sparing diet. You would want to encourage small, frequent meals as tolerated by the client. Client's with Addison's disease tend to suffer from anorexia and weight loss. (C) The client with Addison's disease has low sodium levels and needs a diet with sodium supplementation. (D) The client with Addison's disease needs frequent rest intervals and a safe environment. The client may need assistance with activities of daily living and rest should be encouraged.

77. **(A)** Nursing process phase: assessment; client need: safe, effective care environment; content area: psychiatric nursing

Rationale
(A) Anxiety, irritability, insomnia, and fatigue are early symptoms of benzodiazepine withdrawal. (B) Irritability, insomnia, and fatigue are symptoms of withdrawal; increased appetite is not. (C) Insomnia, fatigue, and diaphoresis are signs of withdrawal; increased appetite is not. (D) Fatigue, diaphoresis, and anxiety are signs of withdrawal; increased appetite is not.

78. **(C)** Nursing process phase: implementation; client need: health promotion and maintenance; content area: maternity nursing

Rationale
(A) Only three signs are accepted as positive confirmation of pregnancy. They are auscultation of the fetal heartbeat, fetal movement felt by the health-care provider, and visualization of the fetus on ultrasound. (B) Probable signs of pregnancy include abdominal enlargement, cervical changes, ballottement, Braxton-Hicks contractions, and a positive pregnancy test. (C) These symptoms are the presumptive signs of pregnancy, which include amenorrhea, breast enlargement and tenderness, nausea and vomiting, emotional lability, and fatigue. (D) Amenorrhea and morning sickness are presumptive signs of pregnancy. A positive pregnancy test is a probable indicator of pregnancy.

79. **(D)** Nursing process phase: implementation; client need: safe, effective care environment; content area: medical/surgical nursing

Rationale
$$0.3 \text{ mg} : 1 \text{ ml} = 0.25 \text{ mg} : x = 0.8 \text{ ml}$$
Math calculation explains incorrect answers.

80. **(A)** Nursing process phase: implementation; client need: safe, effective care environment; content area: pediatric nursing

Rationale
(A–D) Contact isolation is recommended because RSV is mainly transmitted through direct contact with respiratory secretions (inoculation from hand to eye, nose, or mucous membranes). Direct inoculation may occur from large-particle aerosols or self-inoculation from fomites.

81. **(B)** Nursing process phase: analysis; client need: physiological integrity; content area: psychiatric nursing

Rationale
(A) Administering the drug every other day constitutes reducing the daily dosage by 50 percent. The client will most likely experience some withdrawal symptoms at this dosage. (B) Reducing the daily dosage by 25 percent is recommended to prevent the client from experiencing withdrawal symptoms. (C) Cross-tolerance among the benzodiazepines is well documented. This would not be appropriate. (D) The use of barbiturates for benzodiazepine withdrawal is not recommended.

82. **(B)** Nursing process phase: assessment; client need: physiological integrity; content area: medical/surgical nursing

Rationale
(A) Bronchial sounds are normal breath sounds heard over the bronchial or tracheal tree. (B) A pleural friction rub, which produces a grating or high-pitched squeaking noise, can be heard in the lateral lung fields during inspiration and expiration. (C) Rhonchi are abnormal breath sounds, also called wheezes, caused by moving air colliding with secretions in the airway. They are usually heard on inspiration. (D) Resonance is not heard during auscultation, but is a normal sound heard during percussion at the interspaces of the chest wall.

83. **(B)** Nursing process phase: assessment; client need: physiological integrity; content area: medical/surgical nursing

Rationale
(A) A clinical finding noted in thyroid storm is fever, not hypothermia. (B) Tachycardia is commonly noted in clients with thyroid storm. (C) Common clinical findings noted in clients with thyroid storm are restlessness and anxiety, not lethargy. (D) A clinical finding noted in clients with thyroid storm is hypertension, not hypotension.

84. **(D)** Nursing process phase: implementation; client need: physiological integrity; content area: medical/surgical nursing

Rationale
(A) A fluid intake of 3 L/day is encouraged because mild dehydration and hemoconcentration are usually present because of epinephrine and release of renin by the kidneys. (B) A low-calorie diet is not indicated because the basal metabolic rate is increased. (C) Sedatives should not be administered routinely preoperatively; they can mask changes in the client's neurological status. (D) Treatment of pheochromocytoma focuses on controlling hypertension and the paroxysmal attacks. Monitoring and controlling blood pressure is a priority.

85. **(B)** Nursing process phase: assessment; client need: physiological integrity; content area: pediatric nursing

Rationale
(A) Quality of sucking would be a reflection of overall cerebral functioning. This is not an accurate method of differentiating between meningocele and myelomeningocele. (B) Meningoceles are sacks that contain meninges and spinal fluid, but no neural elements; therefore the lower extremities should not be affected. Myelomeningoceles contain meninges, spinal fluid, and nerves, which cause neurological deficits in the lower extremities. (C) Head circumference is not an accurate observation to distinguish between these two defects. (D) Neither defect is covered with skin.

86. **(C)** Nursing process phase: assessment; client need: physiological integrity; content area: medical/surgical nursing

Rationale

(A) Elderly people are likely to have a decrease in appetite, not an increase, because of decreased taste sensation and decreased gastric motility. (B) Decreased activity would not have an effect on drug absorption in elderly people. (C) This is correct. The decrease in total body water associated with aging can affect drug absorption in the system. A smaller amount of medication may be required. (D) In elderly people approaching 80, there is usually an increase in adipose tissue of the trunk area and a decrease in fat of the extremities. Weight usually decreases with advancing age, which can affect drug absorption. This client has probably had a weight change over 13 years.

87. **(B)** Nursing process phase: planning; client need: physiological integrity; content area: psychiatric nursing

Rationale

(A) Avoid a power struggle. The focus on food diverts attention from the underlying dynamics. (B) This provides support and encourages the client to eat adequate amounts of nutritious foods. (C) Depressed clients very often suffer from nutritional changes. Teaching is a necessary part of discharge planning but not the initial intervention. (D) Monitoring the physical changes is part of the holistic nursing care.

88. **(A)** Nursing process phase: implementation; client need: health promotion and maintenance; content area: maternity nursing

Rationale

(A) This is a true statement. Early passage of meconium reduces the enterohepatic circulation and therefore influences later bilirubin levels. In addition, feeding stimulates glucagon secretion and therefore glycolysis, decreasing the chance of hypoglycemia. (B) Infants do not dehydrate this quickly. They are born with additional water weight and will actually lose weight in the first couple of days. (C) In some facilities, babies go to the newborn nursery while the mother is in the recovery room. However, more and more institutions are allowing the infant to remain with the mother if she is well. This is a good time for bonding. However, if the infant must go to the nursery, not being fed right away in the delivery room will not be problematic. If the mother is too ill to feed the infant, he will be fed in the nursery. (D) These reflexes are normally present and will remain so even if the infant does not go to breast right away. Evaluating these reflexes does give an indication of an intact neurological system; however, this can be evaluated at a later time.

89. **(A)** Nursing process phase: implementation; client need: health promotion and maintenance; content area: pediatric nursing

Rationale

(A) Rice cereal is usually the first solid food because of its increased iron content, its easy digestion, and its low allergic quality. (B) After 6 months, fruit juices can be introduced, but rice cereal is recommended because it is easily digested and has a low allergy response. (C) Fruit juice should be introduced in small amounts to prevent abdominal cramps and diarrhea. (D) Introduce only one new food at a time to determine tolerance. Juices mixed with cereals will enhance iron absorption.

90. **(A)** Nursing process phase: assessment; client need: safe, effective care environment; content area: maternity nursing

Rationale

(A) The uterus changes locations as involution occurs, but it should remain firm and midline at all times. (B) The uterus should not be soft. This indicates that the uterus is not contracting as it should and increases the client's risk of hemorrhage. (C) The uterus should be midline at all times. This position is indicative of a full bladder, which pushes the uterus up and over to the right. (D) The uterus should not be boggy. This indicates that the uterus is not contracting as it should and the client is at risk for hemorrhage.

91. **(A)** Nursing process phase: implementation; client need: health promotion and maintenance; content area: maternity nursing

Rationale

(A) With earlier postpartal discharges taking place, mothers need to be taught how to adequately assess their infants for jaundice and be instructed on when they should contact their health-care provider. (B) Though this might be interesting information for Lucy, it is not necessary for her to completely understand the pathophysiology of hyperbilirubinemia in order to provide good care for her newborn once she is discharged. (C) Lucy would need to have her infant evaluated by a health-care provider and have an order for phototherapy prior to its use. She would receive instructions at that time. (D) Kernicterus, the deposit of unconjugated bilirubin in brain cells, results in death or impaired intellectual, perceptive, or motor function. Lucy would need to have her baby evaluated long before the jaundice reached this stage.

92. **(C)** Nursing process phase: assessment; client need: physiological integrity; content area: pediatric nursing

Rationale

(A) S_2 is louder than S_1 at the aortic area. (B) The splitting of S_2 is best heard in the pulmonic area. (C) Functional murmurs are most often heard at this second to third (LIS) sternal border area (Erb's point). (D) S_1 is heard longest at the apical area. If an S_3 or S_4 is present, it is usually best heard here.

93. **(D)** Nursing process phase: implementation; client need: health promotion and maintenance; content area: maternity nursing

Rationale

(A) Race is not a significant risk factor in women between the ages of 20 and 35. (B) Women who are young and pregnant for at least the second time, but with a different partner, are at a higher risk of developing PIH. (C) Hydramnios unaccompanied by fetal hydrops or diabetes is not a risk factor. (D) Pregnancies in which placental size is increased, such as multiple fetuses, diabetes, syphilis, isoimmunized pregnancies, or hydatidiform moles, are at higher risk because the placenta plays an important role in pathophysiological processes.

94. **(D)** Nursing process phase: analysis; client need: physiological integrity; content area: psychiatric nursing

Rationale

(A) Carbamazepine does not act as a central nervous system depressant. (B) It has been well documented that carbamazepine diminishes impulsiveness in some psychiatric disorders, but withdrawal from a benzodiazepine is not one of those conditions. (C) Carbamazepine has little effect on blood pressure, pulse, and respirations. (D) Studies indicate that benzodiazepine withdrawal is enhanced and hastened by the concurrent use of carbamazepine.

95. **(D)** Nursing process phase: implementation; client need: safe, effective care environment; content area: medical/surgical nursing

Rationale

160 mg divided by 80 mg $\times$ 15 ml = 30 ml

Math calculation explains incorrect answers.

96. **(C)** Nursing process phase: planning; client need: physiological integrity; content area: maternity nursing

Rationale

(A) This is the definition of a first-degree laceration. (B) This is the definition of a second-degree laceration. (C) This is the definition of a third-degree laceration. (D) This describes a periurethral tear and a cervical tear.

97. **(D)** Nursing process phase: evaluation; client need: health promotion and maintenance; content area: pediatric nursing

Rationale

(A) While fit and appearance of the brace are important, therapy will not be successful if the brace is not worn for the amount of time required. (B) Teaching and counseling by the nurse is very important, but the ultimate success of the treatment depends on the client's compliance and cooperation. (C) Parents should be active in the treatment regimen; however, ultimate success is up to the client. (D) Correct. These braces often must be worn for 18 to 23 hours a day for many months or years. Compliance and cooperation by the client are difficult but crucial to successful reduction of the curvature.

98. **(D)** Nursing process phase: implementation; client need: physiological integrity; content area: maternity nursing

Rationale

(A) Signs of a miscarriage are bleeding with cramps, severe pain with or without vaginal bleeding, vaginal bleeding as heavy as a menstrual period, or light staining that continues for more than 3 days. (B) Implantation occurs from 7 to 10 days after conception. (C) Slight bleeding at the time when a period would have been expected is common. No special precautions are indicated. (D) The cervix becomes very vascular and soft during pregnancy. Deep penetration of the penis during intercourse may cause bleeding if the cervix is bumped.

99. **(B)** Nursing process phase: assessment; client need: psychosocial integrity; content area: maternity nursing

Rationale

(A) Postpartum psychosis is associated with a previous history of mental illness. (B) Postpartum blues is associated with a sudden onset and is often related to an unanticipated birth event, such as cesarean section. Mothers often express feelings of being overwhelmed. (C) Characteristics of depression include alterations in weight, sleep, and eating patterns. It is a disorder that affects mood and is related to loss. (D) In homeostasis, an effort is made to maintain balance.

100. **(B)** Nursing process phase: analysis; client need: psychosocial integrity; content area: psychiatric nursing

Rationale

(A) Clients diagnosed as having anorexia nervosa are never satisfied with their body image. (B) Limiting food intake is a means of controlling the client's inner world. (C) Many persons with anorexia nervosa have spent their lives attending to the needs of others. (D) These persons have feelings of social incompetence.

101. **(B)** Nursing process phase: implementation; client need: safe, effective care environment; content area: pediatric nursing

Rationale

(A) Size 6 Fr would be usual size for a newborn to 18 months. This would be too small to suction out secretions. (B) Catheters in an 8 Fr or 10 Fr would be the appropriate size for an 18- to 24-month old. (C) The 10 Fr would be appropriate in some cases, but 12 Fr would be too large. Ten to twelve Fr would be appropriate for ages 2 to 4 years. (D) A 12 Fr is too large and is appropriate for a client 7 years old or older.

102. **(A)** Nursing process phase: assessment; client need: physiological integrity; content area: medical/surgical—gerontological nursing

Rationale

(A) This is correct. A decreased gag reflex makes the client more susceptible to aspiration of food or liquids. (B) A decreased self-care ability would not contribute to this client's aspiration pneumonia. However, if the client is not receiving proper care at home, this could increase the client's risks for malnutrition or starvation because of his inability to prepare food. (C) Facial paralysis or weakness would not contribute to this client's condition. The client can pocket food in the affected side of the mouth during meals and would need to be monitored; however, this would not affect the client's ability to swallow. (D) A decreased ventilatory effort is an age-related change seen in the elderly, which would not affect the client's ability to swallow foods or liquids.

103. **(D)** Nursing process phase: evaluation; client need: safe, effective care environment; content area: maternity nursing

Rationale

(A) This is a normal glucose level for a newborn. Levels fall after birth and stabilize at about 50 to 60 mg/dl in the first 4 to 6 hours. (B) This is a normal axillary temperature for a newborn. It should average between 97.6 and 98.6°F (36.5 to 37°C) with a range from 97 to 99°F (36.1 to 37.2°C). (C) Patty's respiratory rate is within normal limits. Rate varies with level of alertness and ranges between 30 to 60 beats per minute. With crying, rates may go slightly above 60 beats per minute. (D) The cephalohematoma, a collection of blood between a skull bone and the periosteum, places Patty at risk for hyperbilirubinemia. As the hematoma resolves, the breakdown of the RBCs may lead to hyperbilirubinemia.

104. **(B)** Nursing process phase: assessment; client need: physiological integrity; content area: maternity nursing

Rationale

(A) Newborn behavior is assessed by using Brazelton's neonatal assessment tool. (B) The Apgar score reflects the newborn's physical condition at 1 and 5 minutes. (C) Gestational age estimation is determined by using a standardized tool to assess external physical characteristics and/or neuromotor development. (D) Fetal distress may be evaluated by fetal scalp blood sampling. The test measures the CO_2 and the O_2 levels in the fetal blood.

105. **(D)** Nursing process phase: implementation; client need: safe, effective care environment; content area: maternity nursing

Rationale

$$50 \text{ mg} : 1 \text{ tablet} = 250 \text{ mg} : x = 5 \text{ tablets}$$

Math calculation explains incorrect answers.

106. **(A)** Nursing process phase: implementation; client need: health promotion and maintenance; content area: pediatric nursing

Rationale

(A) Swimming is a superb exercise for children with asthma. The air that they breathe is saturated with moisture. Perhaps even more important is the fact that underwater exhalation is prolonged, which increases the end-expiratory pressure in the lungs. (B) Children are encouraged to participate in all forms of exercise as long as their asthma is controlled. (C) Most of these children can participate in sports. (D) Children who experience exercise-induced asthma can still participate in all forms of exercise when appropriately monitored and evaluated.

107. **(A)** Nursing process phase: evaluation; client need: physiological integrity; content area: maternity nursing

Rationale

(A) The interaction between the parasympathetic and sympathetic nervous systems causes the fetal heart rate to increase and decrease. This is reflected in short-term or beat-to-beat changes, or in long-term changes—changes in the baseline over a 1-minute time frame. (B) A sinusoidal pattern is seen when severe fetal brain damage has occurred. There is no longer control by the sympathetic or parasympathetic system. (C) Periodic changes include accelerations and decelerations and are related to several factors, including uterine activity and level of oxygenation of the fetus. (D) Nonreassuring also reflects abnormal. These changes are related to hypoxia of the fetus or other signs of fetal distress.

108. **(C)** Nursing process phase: assessment; client need: safe, effective care environment; content area: psychiatric nursing

Rationale

(A) Clozapine is associated with significantly fewer parkinsonianlike side effects than the conventional antipsychotics. (B) Studies have not reported the incidence of anemia as a specific side effect of clozapine. (C) Clozapine is associated with the occurrence of agranulocytosis in 1 to 2 percent of all clients receiving it. (D) Hypotension, not hypertension, is associated with clozapine treatment.

109. **(A)** Nursing process phase: client need: health promotion and maintenance; content area: maternity nursing

Rationale

(A) This is a correct response. The mother should also be told to notify her health-care provider if she notices any odor, discharge, or skin inflammation around the cord. (B) Alcohol is sometimes used to cleanse the cord several times a day. Mothers should be cautioned not to pull on the cord or attempt to remove it. This can cause bleeding or other injury. (C) It should not take this long for the cord to separate. If it is kept

dry, it will dry and fall off in about 7 to 10 days. (D) The instruction to keep the diaper away from the cord is appropriate; however, the cord will not dry enough to fall off in 3 days.

110. **(D)** Nursing process phase: assessment; client need: safe, effective care environment; content area: pediatric nursing

Rationale

(A) Infants and even fetuses (after 20 weeks) are capable of feeling pain. (B) Pain tolerance increases with age. (C) Narcotics are not more dangerous to young children than to older people. It is uncommon for a child appropriately treated with an opiate to develop respiratory depression or addiction. (D) Children do not always tell the truth about pain if they fear an injection or do not realize the severity of the pain.

111. **(A)** Nursing process phase: assessment; client need: safe, effective care environment; content area: maternity nursing

Rationale

(A) This statement indicates that Ida needs a review of the basic food groups and the need to include foods from each group to maintain a balanced diet. She would need further instruction. (B) Ida seems to understand that her health and the health of her baby depend a great deal on her diet. She realizes that fast foods are not the best choices. (C) Body image is a prime factor for adolescents. Although Ida seems to be concerned about her weight gain, she is showing good judgment regarding her baby's health. (D) Although Ida is concerned about her weight gain, she seems to understand the importance of a good diet.

112. **(B)** Nursing process phase: analysis; client need: safe, effective care environment; content area: medical/surgical nursing

Rationale

(A) This client would not be at risk for developing hypoglycemia. The client has no history of glucose disorders. (B) This is correct. A negative nitrogen balance can result from a lack of adequate protein in the diet, or from the breakdown of tissue as a result of extreme stress, injury, altered mobility, or disease. (C) Hypocalcemia—not hypercalcemia—would be a concern for this client. Extra calcium would be needed by the client to help bone formation. (D) This client would not be at risk for developing hyperkalemia.

113. **(D)** Nursing process phase: implementation; client need: safe, effective care environment; content area: medical/surgical nursing

Rationale

$$0.3 \text{ mg} : 1 \text{ ml} = 0.5 \text{ mg} : x = 1.7 \text{ ml}$$

Math calculation explains incorrect answers.

114. **(C)** Nursing process phase: implementation; client need: health promotion and maintenance; content area: maternity nursing

Rationale

(A) Caregivers need to ensure the warmth of a newborn during a bath. However, tub baths are not recommended right away and at least not until the cord has fallen off. (B) Recommendations for skin care during the early newborn period have changed. In the past, newborns were washed only as necessary to preserve the vernix caseosa. However, with the possible presence of HIV, it is now recommended that neonates be washed soon after birth. Sponge baths are used thereafter until the cord falls off. (C) Once the cord has dried and fallen off, neonates may be immersed in water for bathing. Ensuring warmth is very important. (D) Late evening, before bedtime, seems to be a good time for many infants to receive their baths. Prior to feeding is best to avoid spitting up; however, tub baths are not recommended until after the cord has dried and fallen off.

115. (B) Nursing process phase: planning; client need: physiological integrity; content area: psychiatric nursing

Rationale

(A) Conversations at mealtime would be too stimulating for a client in the acute manic phase. She is too easily distracted. (B) Encouraging small, frequent meals would be the most therapeutic nursing action for a client who has difficulty sitting still long enough for regular meals. (C) Having a manic client keep detailed records is unrealistic. (D) Expecting a manic client to read literature in a meaningful way is unrealistic.

116. (A) Nursing process phase: analysis; client need: physiological integrity; content area: maternity nursing

Rationale

(A & B) Hypoglycemia in the newborn is a result of hyperplasia of the pancreatic beta cells, which leads to increased insulin production. The increased insulin causes a rapid drop in circulating glucose, causing hypoglycemia. (C) Hypocalcemia is a frequent finding because diabetic mothers tend to have higher calcium levels at term. This high level of calcium may cause secondary hypoparathyroidism in the newborn. (D) Infants born to mothers who are diabetic are large for gestational age because of fetal hyperinsulinemia.

117. (B) Nursing process phase: assessment; client need: physiological integrity; content area: maternity nursing

Rationale

(A) A vaginal examination is routinely performed at the first prenatal visit and then not until the last 2 to 4 weeks of pregnancy, unless there is a reason for a cervical check at more frequent intervals. Such reasons include preterm labor and incompetent cervix. Elevated blood pressures are not an indicator for a vaginal examination. (B) The diagnosis of chronic hypertension is that of pressure readings of 140/90 mg Hg or higher on at least two occasions before the 20th week of pregnancy. Mild or moderate hypertension increases the risk of intrauterine growth retardation. Measurement of the fundal height at each prenatal visit is a good indicator of fetal growth in the absence of polyhydramnios or oligohydramnios. (C) The probability of chronic hypertension in this client may result in scheduling more frequent prenatal visits. Monitoring vital signs is important, but holds less significance than fundal heights. (D) Chronic hypertension has little effect on the fetal heart rate.

118. (B) Nursing process phase: planning; client need: safe, effective care environment; content area: maternity nursing

Rationale

(A & C) Internal monitoring is not recommended in this case. The cervix should be at least 3 cm dilated with membranes ruptured for attachment. In most cases, stopping labor for this gestational age is recommended. (B) This is the recom-

mended method for monitoring preterm clients, especially with intact membranes and a less than 3 cm dilated cervix. (D) There is no known contraindication for external electronic fetal monitoring based on gestational age.

119. (B) Nursing process phase: assessment; client need: safe, effective care environment; content area: medical/surgical nursing

Rationale

(A) Kwashiorkor is a disease of depleted protein and is marked by normal body weight and abnormal protein studies. This client has had marked weight loss and would not be considered for this condition. (B) This is correct. The client with marasmus is extremely emaciated and malnourished and is characterized by wasting of subcutaneous fat and muscle. It is usually seen in children, but can be seen in adults with severe intestinal dysfunction. (C) The client did not complain of anorexia, which is the lack of appetite. The client is having a problem with absorption of nutrients from the intestinal tract. (D) Pellagra is a condition resulting from a deficiency in niacin. This is not a consideration for this client.

120. (A) Nursing process phase: implementation; client need: safe, effective care environment; content area: maternity nursing

Rationale

(A) True labor includes regular contractions that do not decrease with position change or ambulation, an increase in vaginal discharge, and cervical changes. The cervix at this gestational age should be long (about 2 cm), thick, and closed. (B) False labor is characterized by a decrease or stop of uterine contractions with position changes or ambulation, no change in vaginal discharge, and no cervical changes. This client is in true labor. (C) Trendelenburg's or knee-chest positioning is indicated when fetal membranes rupture and there is evidence of a prolapsed core (identified by visualization or palpation of the cord on vaginal exam). The fetal membranes are intact on this client. (D) This client is in early labor as evidenced by the lack of cervical dilation and the fetal station. It has not progressed to the point that would warrant preparing for imminent delivery of a preterm infant.

121. (C) Nursing process phase: implementation; client need: safe, effective care environment; content area: medical/surgical nursing

Rationale

(A) "Portal of entry to host" is a source of acquiring an infection, and not a practice to break the "chain of infection." (B) "Reservoir" is a host for infection and not a method to transfer infection from one source to another, and therefore, not a practice to break the "chain of infection." (C) "Method of transmission" of infection is the phase in which hand washing before and after various tasks can break the "chain of infection" and lead to safe, effective client care. (D) "Portal of exit from host" refers to blood, wound drainage, feces, and urine, which can transmit disease because of improper handling and improper hand-washing technique.

122. (C) Nursing process phase: implementation; client need: safe, effective care environment; content area: maternity nursing

Rationale

(A) Infants who are warmed too quickly will experience periods of apnea. (B) Again, this will provide a warming process that will move too quickly. It is not controlled. (C) Hypothermic infants should be warmed slowly to avoid apneic episodes. The infant should be placed in an isolette with a servocontrol mechanism that is set 2 degrees higher than the infant's present temperature. A skin probe is applied to the infant, and the thermostat is increased by 2 degrees at a time as the infant reaches the set temp. The process should occur over 2 to 4 hours until temperature reaches 97.7 to 98.6°F. (D) Warmed blankets placed on the infant in an isolette would interfere with receiving an accurate reading on the isolette thermostat.

123. **(D)** Nursing process phase: analysis; client need: physiological integrity; content area: medical/surgical nursing

Rationale
(A) Nosocomial infections, such as a urinary tract infection, do not present the clinical manifestations of multisystem organ failure, unless untreated for a long time. (B) Bacteremia is the presence of bacteria in the blood and can lead to various problems, but not the initial clinical manifestation of multisystem organ failure. (C) The hyperdynamic stage (warm) of septic shock results in system changes, that is, tachycardia, hypotension, and increased cardiac output, but does not manifest multisystem organ failure. (D) The hypodynamic stage (cool) of septic shock is the advanced stage and causes profound hypotension, decreased cardiac output, changes in level of consciousness, and multisystem organ failure.

124. **(D)** Nursing process phase: implementation; client need: safe, effective care environment; content area: medical/surgical nursing

Rationale
100 mg divided by 80 mg × 1 ml = 1.3 ml
Math calculation explains incorrect answers.

125. **(D)** Nursing process phase: implementation; client need: health promotion and maintenance; content area: maternity nursing

Rationale
(A) Sexual intercourse is not contraindicated for uncomplicated pregnancies. (B) There generally is no reason to discontinue sexual intercourse. However, complications such as ruptured membranes, preterm labor, or infections would place the mother and fetus at high risk. (C) As long as the woman is not having complications in her pregnancy, sexual relations may be continued throughout her pregnancy. (D) Changes in sexual positions may be necessary after the 30th week of pregnancy; however, barring complications, sexual intercourse is not contraindicated.

126. **(A)** Nursing process phase: analysis; client need: safe, effective care environment; content area: psychiatric nursing

Rationale
(A) The client's serum level is below the therapeutic level of 0.6 to 1.2 mEq/L. The nurse should notify the physician. (B) The nurse should place the laboratory report in the chart after notifying the physician. (C) An additional dose of 300 mg will bring the client's serum level up by 0.2 mEq/L, but the nurse cannot give this additional dose without an order from the physician. (D) Toxic level is about 1.2 mEq/L.

127. **(B)** Nursing process phase: assessment; client need: physiological integrity; content area: medical/surgical nursing

Rationale
(A) Erythema may be absent or present along the suture line and not at a specific area. Sanguineous drainage is not present on the third postoperative day unless there is a bleeding problem. (B) A surgical wound heals by primary intention. Therefore, wound edges would be well approximated with minimal erythema and/or edema, and with scant to moderate sanguineous drainage by the third postoperative day. (C) These findings are abnormal and suggest an early infectious process. (D) Scar tissue would not occur until days or weeks after healing has taken place.

128. **(B)** Nursing process phase: implementation; client need: health promotion and maintenance; content area: maternity nursing

Rationale
(A) This is an incorrect response. The level of comfort of the infant may have some influence on the length of sleep; however, this phrase does not describe the infant's response. (B) Habituation refers to an infant's ability to decrease responses to repeated environmental stimuli. (C) This is not a correct description of the newborn's response. (D) Consolability refers to the infant's ability to bring himself or herself or to be brought by others to a lower state.

129. **(A)** Nursing process phase: implementation; client need: physiological integrity; content area: medical/surgical nursing

Rationale
(A) The initial treatment is aimed toward passage of the stone so that infection and the need for a surgical intervention will not develop. (B) Stone irritation may cause hemorrhage in the ureter, regardless of increased fluids. The fluids specifically help facilitate passage of the stone. (C) The client with renal stones is not on a clear liquid diet; this is not necessary. The diet is either NPO (because of other complications) or regular diet. Large amounts of fluids are encouraged, unless contraindicated, to help facilitate passage of the stone. (D) Fluids are encouraged, but not for the purpose of x-ray procedures. Fluids are encouraged to help facilitate passage of the stone.

130. **(C)** Nursing process phase: analysis; client need: physiological integrity; content area: maternity nursing

Rationale
(A) Resuming the prepregnant diet and insulin dosage are recommended for nonnursing mothers with diabetes mellitus. (B) Diabetes mellitus is not a contraindication for breastfeeding. (C) After a vaginal delivery, the majority of gestational diabetes will not need additional diet or medication control. (D) Breastfeeding the baby will not give the newborn diabetes.

131. **(D)** Nursing process phase: analysis; client need: physiological integrity; content area: medical/surgical nursing

Rationale
(A) Orange juice should not be given to a comatose client. (B) The data indicate that the client is in hypoglycemia. (C) Glucagon can be given only subcutaneously or intramuscularly; faster action would be required because the client is comatose. (D) IV glucose is the best answer because it would correct the hypoglycemia most rapidly.

132. (A) Nursing process phase: implementation; client need: health promotion and maintenance; content area: pediatric nursing

Rationale
(A) The aims of therapy are to prevent the sickling and treat the medical emergency of sickle-cell crisis. (B) Genetic counseling for a 5-year-old would be inappropriate. (C) Sickle-cell anemia is a chronic illness with a potentially terminal outcome. (D) Complications of multiple blood transfusions should be discussed prior to the transfusion, not at the time of discharge.

133. (B) Nursing process phase: analysis; client need: safe, effective care environment; content area: maternity nursing

Rationale
(A) Oxytocin (Pitocin) is used to control vaginal bleeding by causing uterine contraction. It does not affect maternal blood pressure. (B) Parlodel is a drug used to suppress lactation. It has been associated with seizures, strokes, and myocardial infarctions in postpartum women. It is contraindicated for use in women with a history of chronic hypertension or PIH. (C) Ferrous sulfate is an iron preparation routinely given to all postpartum women. It has no effect on blood pressure. (D) Darvocet is a category three analgesic used to relieve pain caused by involution of the uterus. It does not increase the maternal blood pressure.

134. (A) Nursing process phase: analysis; client need: physiological integrity; content area: geriatric nursing

Rationale
(A) There were 1400 cases of AIDS reported in 1991; representing a steady rise over the past decade. The number is expected to increase from 3 to 10 percent over the next decade. (B) There is no evidence to suggest that masturbation is brought on by the lack of a sexual partner or that older adults have guilt feelings related to masturbation. (C) Although it is commonly believed that sexual desire diminishes with age, research indicates that older adults continue to enjoy sexual relationships throughout each decade of life. (D) According to the 1992 U.S. Bureau of Census, the five leading causes of death in older adults are heart disease, cancer, stroke, COPD, and pneumonia-influenza.

135. (D) Nursing process phase: assessment; client need: safe, effective care environment; content area: psychiatric nursing

Rationale
(A) The therapist should not cancel her vacation because this is most likely a manipulative attempt by the client for attention. (B) Postponing her flight may be necessary to make arrangements for someone else to see and/or assess the client in person if those arrangements have not already been made prior to the therapist's departure. (C) Instructing the client to call the hotline may be viewed by the client as rejection and may be the deciding factor in making a serious attempt on her life. (D) The therapist should complete a suicide assessment on the phone, obtain a verbal "no suicide" contract, and refer the client to the therapist on call as planned.

136. (B) Nursing process phase: planning; client need: health promotion and maintenance; content area: medical/surgical nursing

Rationale
(A) Meat contributes much of the acid metabolic waste and is considered a food in an acid ash diet that lowers the urine pH. (B) Citrus fruits contribute to an alkaline urine in which the pH is high. This can promote UTI. (C) Cranberry juice increases the acidity of urine and decreases the pH. (D) Eggs contribute much of the acid metabolic waste and are considered a food in an acid ash diet that lowers the urine pH.

137. (A) Nursing process phase: assessment; client need: physiological integrity; content area: maternity nursing

Rationale
(A) The false pelvis is a basin-type structure at the top of the true pelvis. The uterus "rests" on the false pelvis during pregnancy. (B) The true pelvis is the passage the fetus must pass through to deliver vaginally. (C) During the birth process, the fetus progresses through the true pelvis; the false pelvis provides little if any protection at this time. (D) Pelvic measurements are obtained by measurement of the diagonal conjugate, the distance from the sacral promontory and the symphysis pubis, both part of the true pelvis.

138. (D) Nursing process phase: assessment; client need: safe, effective care environment; content area: medical/surgical nursing

Rationale
(A) This is appropriate because the client may have moved his arm, which may have caused the level of the needle to lie against the side of the vein, thereby obstructing the flow of solution, but it is not the initial intervention by the nurse. (B) This may be appropriate because patency of the tubing may be assessed by observation of a return of blood from the client into the IV tubing when the receptacle is lowered, but it is not the initial intervention. (C) The IV may be flushed with normal saline after other aspects related to IV infiltration are assessed. The nurse would never attempt to flush the cannula if resistance is met because such action may force a blood clot into circulation. (D) This is most appropriate and the best initial action because swelling may demonstrate the presence of edema, suggesting infiltration.

139. (B) Nursing process phase: implementation; client need: health promotion and maintenance; content area: maternity nursing

Rationale
(A) Zinc is the mineral that helps maintain the acid-base balance in tissues and is important in DNA and RNA synthesis (B) Iron is needed for the formation of hemoglobin, which carries oxygen to the cells and fetus. During pregnancy, there is an additional demand because of the increase in maternal blood volume, fetal blood formation, fetal iron stores, and blood loss during delivery. (C) Calcium is the mineral that facilitates mineralization of the fetal skeleton and deciduous teeth. (D) Vitamin B_{12} aids in protein metabolism, including RNA and DNA synthesis.

140. (B) Nursing process phase: implementation; client need: safe, effective care environment; content area: pediatric nursing

Rationale
$$0.25 \text{ mg} : 1 \text{ ml} = 3.6 \text{ mg} : x = 14.5 \text{ ml}$$
Math calculation explains incorrect answers.

141. (C) Nursing process phase: planning; client need: safe, effective care environment; content area: maternity nursing

Rationale

(A) It is true that this mother is not knowledgeable of infant nutritional needs; however, this is not the diagnosis of the highest priority that is infant-focused. (B) This is not appropriate since the infant is receiving more than the recommended number of calories. (C) This is the best nursing diagnosis for this infant. The recommended number of calories per day for the first 6 months of an infant's life is 49 kcal/lb/day. The infant is receiving more than 76 kcal/lb. (D) This may be true. However, it depends on how the mother is providing the calories. You are not given enough information to determine this. Perhaps Laura is simply not diluting the formula appropriately; in which case the volume would not be the priority problem.

142. (C) Nursing process phase: planning; client need: physiological integrity; content area: psychiatric nursing

Rationale

(A) The nurse would want to promote social interaction, but it is not the priority goal for this client. (B) A more appropriate goal would be that client accomplishes ADL to the best of his or her ability. (C) The priority nursing goal for clients with organic brain syndrome is the maintenance of client safety. Clients with this disorder have impaired cognitive and psychomotor functioning that puts them at risk for injury. (D) Maintaining nutritional status is important for this client, but not the priority nursing goal.

143. (D) Nursing process phase: assessment; client need: physiological integrity; content area: maternity nursing

Rationale

(A) Amniocentesis is analysis of amniotic fluid to determine the presence of fetal chromosomal anomalies, or in the case of preterm labor, to determine fetal lung maturity. The fetal membranes are ruptured and the infant is at term. Amniocentesis is neither possible nor indicated. (B) Cervical cultures are done to determine the presence of a bacterial infection. It is contraindicated when the membranes are ruptured because of the probability of introducing infectious organisms into the uterine cavity and to the fetus. (C) A urinalysis is performed to detect the presence of glucose, protein, white blood cells, or bacteria in the urine. A urinary tract infection is associated with an increased incidence of preterm contractions, not premature rupture of the membranes. (D) Rupture of the membranes for more than 24 hours before delivery is associated with an increased incidence of endometritis, or infection of the uterine endometrium. An elevated white blood count with a shift to the left in the bands and segmented neurophiles indicates endometritis.

144. (D) Nursing process phase: evaluation; client need: health promotion and maintenance; content area: maternity nursing

Rationale

(A) Supplementing with formula will interfere with the establishment of breastfeeding. At 2 weeks the process is just beginning. (B) Nursing the newborn more often at night will encourage more feeding at night versus daytime feeding. The mother's rest is likely to be compromised and breast milk supply limited. (C) Decreasing the interval will limit the number of feeding opportunities and weight gain. (D) Permitting the newborn to nurse at the breast for a minimum of 10 minutes encourages the intake of the hind milk. The hind milk is rich in nutrients and fat, which will assist the newborn in adding weight.

145. (A) Nursing process phase: assessment; client need: physiological integrity; content area: medical/surgical nursing

Rationale

(A) In addition to the aforementioned symptoms, a client experiencing circulatory overload will exhibit venous distention, syncope, shock, dyspnea, and cyanosis resulting from pulmonary edema. (B) Drug overload may occur from receiving an excessive amount of fluid containing drugs; and symptoms may include dizziness, fainting leading to shock, and symptoms specific to the offending drug. (C) Superficial thrombophlebitis may produce tenderness at first with subsequent pain along the direction of the vein, edema and redness at the injection site, and excessive warmth in the affected arm as compared with the other arm. These signs are characteristic of inflammation. (D) An air embolism results when air gets into the circulatory system. Symptoms may include hypotension, cyanosis, tachycardia, increased venous pressure, and loss of consciousness.

146. (B) Nursing process phase: client need: physiological integrity; content area: maternity nursing

Rationale

(A) The upper left quadrant would be used when the baby is positioned left sacrum anterior (LSA). (B) The baby's head is vertex. The fetal heart tones will be below the umbilicus. The fetal heart tones will be loudest over the baby's back. Positions are in relation to the mother's pelvis. In left occiput transverse (LOT), it would be found in the lower left quadrant. (C) The upper right quadrant would be designated if the baby were in right sacrum anterior (RSA). (D) The lower right quadrant is an area of maximum intensity for right occiput anterior (ROA).

147. (A) Nursing process phase: implementation; client need: physiological integrity; content area: maternity nursing

Rationale

(A) These are normal findings. For the first few hours after birth, the fundus is at the umbilicus. At 12 hours' postpartum, the fundus rises to one to two finger breadths above the umbilicus. Lochia is expected to be moderate and with few or no small clots. The increase in progesterone causes decreased gastrointestinal peristalsis during pregnancy. The GI tract remains hypoactive for the first few days postpartum. A bowel movement is generally not expected until the third postpartum day. (B) Bowel sounds are normally hypoactive. A bowel movement is not yet expected. Because there is positive flatus, this client is not at risk for an ileus. (C) Signs of a full bladder are a firm fundus that is high and deviated to one side. A full bladder may also be palpated or visualized. (D) Homan's sign is the presence of a sharp pain or forced dorsiflexion of the client's foot. A positive Homan's sign indicates the possibility of thrombophlebitis.

148. (D) Nursing process phase: implementation; client need: psychosocial integrity; content area: psychiatric nursing

Rationale

(A) The nurse is making light of the client's experience of depression and suicide attempts. (B) Although the client should take medications as ordered after discharge, the nurse should be more specific about who the client may be able to call if she should have suicidal ideation again. (C) This is nontherapeutic and offers false reassurance. (D) This is the most therapeutic response because the alternative to suicide must come from the client.

149. (C) Nursing process phase: implementation; client need: health promotion and maintenance; content area: maternity nursing

Rationale
(A) Women can successfully work up until the day of delivery if they are not at high risk in their pregnancy. (B) Propping up the feet does increase venous return; however, a couple of times a day for 10 minutes will not be enough to make a major difference in Julia's swelling. (C) Walking is an excellent form of exercise to promote good circulation. Frequent position changes promote good arterial as well as venous circulation. (D) Sodium restriction is not recommended for normal pregnancies.

150. (D) Nursing process phase: implementation; client need: physiological integrity; content area: pediatric nursing

Rationale
(A) Assessing urine specific gravity is one measure of monitoring urine that is important in the care of a child with nephrotic syndrome. However, measuring urine output is more essential. (B) Measuring abdominal girth is one means of monitoring fluid retention in a child with nephrotic syndrome. However, measuring urine output is more essential. (C) Continuous monitoring of fluid retention or excretion is an important nursing function. Measuring urine output is essential to obtain an accurate measurement of output. (D) Daily weight is one means of monitoring fluid retention or excretion in a child with nephrotic syndrome. However, measuring urine output is more essential.

151. (D) Nursing process phase: implementation; client need: safe, effective care environment; content area: medical/surgical nursing

Rationale
(A) Respiratory isolation is indicated to prevent the transmission of infections by direct contact, indirect contact, or airborne (droplet) routes. Examples of infections requiring this isolation are: measles, meningitis, meningococcal pneumonia, mumps, and pertussis. (B) This term describes a type of bacteria and not an isolation method. (C) This type of isolation is indicated to prevent the transmission of highly contagious infections that do not necessitate strict isolation. These examples include draining wounds, influenza, herpes simplex, impetigo, and scabies. (D) This type of isolation is indicated to prevent the transmission of pulmonary tuberculosis (TBC) in clients who have a positive sputum smear or positive chest x-ray for TBC.

152. (B) Nursing process phase: analysis; client need: health promotion and maintenance; content area: maternity nursing

Rationale
(A) Though some activity change may occur with pregnancy, and the result may increase the occurrence of constipation, this is not the primary reason for this discomfort of pregnancy. (B)

Constipation in pregnancy is a result of some relaxation of the intestinal smooth muscles, resulting in slower motility and consequently removal of more water from the lower bowel. Later in pregnancy, the enlarging uterus may displace the bowel, intensifying the problem. (C) Changes in the level of progesterone during pregnancy do not cause constipation. (D) Increased levels of hCG in pregnancy do not cause constipation.

153. (C) Nursing process phase: planning; client need: safe, effective care environment; content area: medical/surgical nursing

Rationale
(A) Epinephrine is a bronchodilator and acts to relieve bronchospasm during asthma attacks. (B) Terbutaline sulfate is a bronchodilator and therefore relieves bronchospasm during asthma attacks. (C) Cromolyn sodium has no bronchodilator, anti-inflammatory, or antihistamine action. Cromolyn is not effective for acute bronchial asthmatic attacks. Cromolyn inhibits the allergic reaction if inhaled before the challenge by an antigen. (D) Theophylline is a bronchodilator and therefore relieves bronchospasm during asthma attacks.

154. (D) Nursing process phase: implementation; client need: health promotion and maintenance; content area: maternity nursing

Rationale
(A) Oral contraceptives are not recommended for diabetics because of the increased risk of thromboembolic and vascular complications and their effect on carbohydrate metabolism. (B) Prior to the discovery and use of insulin, diabetic women were encouraged not to become pregnant. Current medical management has made it possible for these women to conceive and carry a child to term. This remains a high-risk pregnancy but with good management can produce a healthy mother and child. (C) IUDs are associated with an increased risk for infection in these patients. (D) Barrier methods for contraception are usually recommended for diabetics. These methods pose the least risk for complications. Diaphragms, condoms with spermicides, and cervical caps are examples of barrier contraceptives.

155. (C) Nursing process phase: evaluation; client need: safe, effective care environment; content area: pediatric nursing

Rationale
(A) Lortab is an acetaminophen-hydrocodone combination. (B) Tylox is a oxycodone-acetaminophen combination. (C) Percodan contains aspirin and oxycodone. (D) Vicodin contains acetaminophen and oxycodone.

156. (D) Nursing process phase: implementation; client need: safe, effective care environment; content area: maternity nursing

Rationale
(A) An increase in vaginal mucus is typically seen when labor is approaching, and is not a reason for concern in the term client. (B) Constipation and hemorrhoids are common in pregnancy because of the increased absorption of water from the GI tract. The client may need to seek advice, but this is not an emergency. (C) Because of the additional burden of pregnancy, it would not be unusual for the client to be short of breath after extreme exertion such as this. (D) These are both significant signs of PIH related to increasing edema of the retinal vessels and liver engorgement.

157. (D) Nursing process phase: implementation; client need: physiological integrity; content area: pediatric nursing

Rationale

(A) Tepid baths are ineffective in treating febrile children. Antipyretic medications are the most effective for treating fever. (B) Loss of appetite is characteristic, and in most cases children can determine their own need for food. Urging food on anorexic children may precipitate nausea and vomiting. (C) The child should be dressed for comfort, neither wearing heavy clothing nor exposure to the environment is necessary. (D) Adequate fluid intake should be encouraged by offering small amounts of favorite fluids.

158. (C) Nursing process phase: analysis; client need: physiological integrity; content area: maternity nursing

Rationale

(A) Signs of pregnancy-induced hypertension include edema, elevated BP, and proteinuria. (B) This is a very common complaint in pregnant women and is no reason for concern. (C) Increased blood volume and increased blood flow to the face and hands cause nasal congestion and a flushed appearance. (D) Melasma is a common occurrence in pregnancy, characterized by a splotchy, brownish change in pigmentation on the face.

159. (A) Nursing process phase: implementation; client need: physiological integrity, content area: medical/surgical—gerontological nursing

Rationale

(A) The client should be instructed to avoid bending at the waist or lifting heavy objects for at least a month following surgery. (B) The client should be instructed to sleep on the back or unaffected side for 3 to 4 weeks. (C) The client will most likely be prescribed eye drops and should be instructed in their proper installation and in hand-washing techniques. (D) There are no dietary restrictions related to cataract surgery. Caffeine and nicotine may be avoided, however, for other health reasons.

160. (C) Nursing process phase: implementation; client need: physiological integrity; content area: maternity nursing

Rationale

(A) Limiting time at the breast does not prevent sore nipples. (B) Any technique that involves friction will increase nipple soreness. Nipples should be air-dried. If used, A&D ointment must be removed before breastfeeding. (C) The nipple and as much of the areola as possible should be in the infant's mouth. When the infant is positioned properly at the breast, there shouldn't be any pain or tissue damage. (D) Limiting breastfeeding to every other feeding will not alleviate sore nipples. In addition, the mechanical action of the breast pump will increase nipple soreness because of friction.

161. (B) Nursing process phase: implementation; client need: safe, effective care environment; content area: psychiatric nursing

Rationale

75 mg : 1 ml = 50 mg : x = 0.67 ml
Math calculation explains incorrect answers.

162. (A) Nursing process phase: planning; client need: safe, effective care environment; content area: psychiatric nursing

Rationale

(A) The client's safety and ability to perform activities of daily living are high priority. (B) It will be necessary to determine the client's drug allergies, but safety is higher priority at this stage of planning. (C) Dietary preferences and drug allergies are important, but not higher priority over the client's safety. (D) Safety is a high priority but dietary preferences are not.

163. (A) Nursing process phase: planning; client need: physiological integrity; content area: medical/surgical nursing

Rationale

(A) Alveolar and capillary membranes involved in the exchange of gases could have been damaged by the fire. An open airway for exchange of oxygen and carbon dioxide always takes the highest priority in the medical and nursing management of clients. (B) The threat of hypovolemia is secondary to gas exchange, as established by research on cardiopulmonary resuscitation. (C) Gas exchange takes the highest priority. (D) Gas exchange should receive a higher priority than tissue perfusion.

164. (A) Nursing process phase: implementation; client need: psychosocial integrity; content area: medical/surgical—gerontological nursing

Rationale

(A) Anxiety related to fear of blindness is a common experience of persons with retinopathy. This response by the nurse provides the client with information that the feelings are normal and encourages conversation. (B) The goal for clients with retinopathy is to learn to cope with chronic, gradual vision loss, but this statement is false reassurance for a newly diagnosed client at this time. (C) In times of crisis, clients are not concerned with what other people have experienced. This statement minimizes the client's feelings. (D) This statement by the nurse belittles the client and does little to open communications.

165. (A) Nursing process phase: planning; client need: health promotion and maintenance; content area: maternity nursing

Rationale

(A) Genetic counselors should be well informed about the risks of genetic disease and the status of environmental teratogens. They should provide information to couples seeking counseling in order that the couple can make the most informed decision. (B) Couples should ultimately have the final decision in their reproductive health. A counselor should not remove the decision from the couple because they may come to feel that the counselor talked them into a particular decision, leading them to blame the outcome on the counselor. (C) The outcome decision of genetic counseling is not always to terminate the pregnancy. (D) Reproductive decisions should be made by the well-informed couple who are at high risk, not the counselor.

166. (C) Nursing process phase: assessment; client need: safe, effective care environment; content area: maternity nursing

Rationale

(A) There would not be a reason for concern of hyperglycemia following a spontaneous abortion. Hypotension might be a concern if Evaline had experienced a large blood loss. (B) Leukorrhea is a common occurrence during pregnancy but not a concern following a spontaneous abortion. Depression and grief would be a common finding in a woman experiencing a perinatal loss. The nurse would provide appropriate nursing interventions for these symptoms. (C) Hemorrhage and infection are complications following a spontaneous abortion. Retained placental fragments or uterine atony may lead to hemorrhage. Infection is a concern because of the possible instrumentation needed following a spontaneous abortion. (D) There would be a possibility of a fluid imbalance if Evaline had experienced a large blood loss. The information you are given does not indicate this to be true. Also, there is no indicated reason for her to experience an electrolyte imbalance.

167. (D) Nursing process phase: evaluation; client need: psychosocial integrity; content area: psychiatric nursing

Rationale
(A) The goal of therapy is to discourage and interrupt hopelessness and alienation. (B) Positive strokes from members of a support system help increase the client's self-worth and esteem. (C) Clients will experience success when social interactions are pursued. (D) The client must demonstrate internal locus of control and identify factors that contribute to the loss of control.

168. (A) Nursing process phase: analysis; client need: physiological integrity; content area: medical/surgical nursing

Rationale
(A) This response describes a positive Chvostek's sign. (B & C) This response does not describe a positive Chvostek's sign. (D) This response describes a positive Trousseau's sign.

169. (B) Nursing process phase: implementation; client need: psychosocial integrity; content area: maternity nursing

Rationale
(A) Touch is used extensively by parents to become acquainted with the newborn. Wrapping the infant in a blanket blocks the tactile sense. (B) Research indicates that early physical contact favorably affects maternal attachment behaviors. Mother's especially love the feel of the infant's body against theirs. Skin-to-skin contact enhances the tactile senses. (C) The first hours after birth may be a sensitive time for parent-infant interaction. However, the normal nursery routine is to keep the infant under a warmer for approximately 4 hours. A bath is then given, and the infant placed back under the warmer for another hour. Separation of the mother and infant for this period of time is not conducive to attachment. (D) Attachment is strengthened through the use of sensual responses by both the mother and infant. The mother needs to see, touch, smell, and talk to her infant in order for attachment to take place. Viewing an infant through a window blocks sensory feedback.

170. (B) Nursing process phase: assessment; client need: physiological integrity; content area: maternity nursing

Rationale
(A) TE fistula does not involve a connection between the stomach and esophagus. (B) TE fistula is a gastrointestinal defect that can be life-threatening. There is an abnormal connection between the trachea and esophagus. The esophagus may be patent or end in a blind sac. TE fistula may be complicated by rectal atresia or imperforate anus. Surgical

repair is required. (C) The diaphragm is not involved in TE fistula. (D) The mainstream bronchus is not involved in TE fistula.

171. (B) Nursing process phase: analysis; client need: safe, effective care environment; content area: psychiatric nursing

Rationale
(A) Burnout most often occurs when the caregiver becomes uninterested and irritable most often with terminally ill clients or those so chronically ill that progress is minimal or absent. There are no data to support burnout. (B) Countertransference is the unconscious reaction of the nurse to the client's behavior and feelings. (C) Transference is the unconscious reaction of the client toward the caregiver. (D) Denial is defined as the avoidance of awareness of some reality issue by negating incoming sensory data. There are no data to support denial.

172. (B) Nursing process phase: analysis; client need: physiological integrity; content area: maternity nursing

Rationale
(A) Hemodilution is a normal occurrence in pregnancy and does not cause an increase in blood pressure. (B) There is a greater increase in fluid volume in proportion to the increase in red blood cells, causing a drop in the hematocrit. (C) Supine hypotension is caused by pressure of the fetus on the vena cava, decreasing blood flow to the mother's brain. (D) There is an increase in both pulse and cardiac output as pregnancy progresses related to the increased blood volume. Hemodilution is inconsequential.

173. (C) Nursing process phase: planning; client need: psychosocial integrity; content area: medical/surgical—gerontological nursing

Rationale
(A) While the client is a widower and has no children, there is nothing to indicate the lack of family support. While this might be important, this would not be as important in the interdisciplinary team conference, where all disciplines need to plan for the client's care. (B) While this might be important, it is not the most important thing that needs to be known to all disciplines in providing care. (C) The religious and cultural beliefs of a client would need to be known and taken into account with all disciplines in planning care for this client. (D) There is nothing to suggest that financial concerns would need to be known in planning care for the client.

174. (A) Nursing process phase: evaluation; client need: physiological integrity; content area: medical/surgical nursing

Rationale
(A) A hemoglobin of 14 gm/dl is WNL. (B) The hemoglobin value is too low. (C & D) The hematocrit value is too low; it indicates anemia.

175. (C) Nursing process phase: implementation; client need: safe, effective care environment; content area: pediatric nursing

Rationale
Using the formula for calculating flow rate:

$$\frac{\text{What the set delivers}}{60} \times \text{hourly volume} = \text{gtt/min}$$

$$\frac{60}{60} \times 83.3 = 83.3 = 83 \text{ gtt/min}$$

Math calculation explains incorrect answers.

176. **(C)** Nursing process phase: implementation; client need: physiological integrity; content area: maternity nursing

Rationale
(A) Examine the client first to determine if delivery is imminent. Narcotics have a depressant effect on the fetus and should not be administered within 1 hour of delivery. (B) Although this measure will temporarily increase her comfort, it will not determine the cause of the problem. (C) Multiparas can progress rapidly in labor. Vomiting is an indication of the onset of second stage. (D) The fluids by mouth are not contributing to her nausea, her labor progression is.

177. **(A)** Nursing process phase: assessment; client need: physiological integrity; content area: geriatric nursing

Rationale
(A) Common symptoms of thyroid disorders are anorexia, constipation, lack of energy, mental clouding, cold intolerance, fatigue, and skin drying and scaling. (B) Anorexia and fatigue may be experienced with metastatic carcinoma, but dry skin scaling and cold intolerance are not typical characteristics of this disease. (C) Older adults may have dry skin and scaling, but cold intolerance and fatigue are not normal aging changes. (D) This action only deals with the dry skin and scaling and does nothing to assess for the cause of the other symptoms being displayed.

178. **(D)** Nursing process phase: implementation; client need: safe, effective care environment; content area: pediatric nursing

Rationale
(A) Most children acquire hepatitis B perinatally. (B) Hepatitis C transmission is mainly parenteral. (C) Hepatitis E transmission may be acquired through the fecal-oral route or through contaminated water. (D) Children with hepatitis A generally have very mild symptoms, allowing the disease to spread unnoticed. The disease is transmitted orally or through fecal matter.

179. **(B)** Nursing process phase: analysis; client need: physiological integrity; content area: psychiatric nursing

Rationale
(A) Blackouts occur with drinking in clients who are alcoholic. (B) Delirium tremens is a serious sequela to abrupt withdrawal from alcohol. It includes disorientation; confusion; visual and tactile hallucinations that are very disturbing to the client; agitation; tachycardia; tremor; diaphoresis; and fever. Prevention involves obtaining a nursing history of alcohol use on admission, observing for early symptoms of withdrawal, and administering benzodiazepines as ordered. (C) Hypocalcemia is not a symptom of severe alcohol withdrawal. (D) Constricted pupils are not a serious symptom of withdrawal.

180. **(C)** Nursing process phase: analysis; client need: safe, effective care environment; content area: medical/surgical—gerontological nursing

Rationale
(A) The serum glutamic oxaloacetic transaminase (SGOT), which indicates myocardial infarction, is within normal limits. (B) The serum potassium level, which indicates hyperkalemia, is within normal limits. (C) Both alkaline phosphatase and acid phosphatase levels are increased. These parameters indicate liver and bone disorders, particularly Paget's disease. (D) The fasting blood sugar is within normal limits.

181. **(D)** Nursing process phase: analysis; client need: psychosocial integrity; content area: maternity nursing

Rationale
(A) Postpartum depression is characterized by the woman showing less interest in her surroundings and a loss of the usual emotional responses toward her family. She is unable to feel pleasure in her new baby and often has strong feelings of guilt and shame. She feels fatigued and has difficulty concentrating. These feelings are disabling to the women experiencing them. (B) Postpartum psychosis is characterized by tearfulness, guilt feelings, sleep and appetite disturbances, and thoughts of harming the infant or self. (C) There is no evidence that this client has low self-esteem or is feeling unable to care for both her children. (D) Sibling rivalry is characterized by the older child experiencing feelings of jealousy and fear that he or she will be replaced in the parent's affections for the newcomer. Parental reassurance of their love, and time spent alone with the older child can help him or her cope with these feelings.

182. **(C)** Nursing process phase: implementation; client need: health promotion and maintenance; content area: pediatric nursing

Rationale
(A) Squash does not contain high levels of phenylalanine and does not have to be eliminated from the diet. (B) Fruit juices do not contain high levels of phenylalanine. (C) Dairy products contain high levels of phenylalanine and may have to be eliminated or severely restricted in the diet of children with PKU. (D) Bananas do not contain high levels of phenylalanine.

183. **(A)** Nursing process phase: implementation; client need: health promotion and maintenance; content area: maternity nursing

Rationale
(A) Nausea and vomiting in pregnancy may contribute to poor oral hygiene, which can result in caries and tooth loss. Regular brushing and flossing will prevent tooth decay and loss. (B) The calcium in teeth is stable and not affected by pregnancy. (C) An adequate intake of calcium will prevent calcium stores in the bone from being used by the pregnancy. Calcium in the teeth is not affected by fetal needs. (D) Calcium in teeth is stable and not affected by fetal needs. In addition, supplements are a poor replacement for milk and other calcium-rich foods.

184. **(B)** Nursing process phase: implementation; client need: safe, effective care environment; content area: medical/surgical—gerontological nursing

Rationale
(A) This is an important nursing action but is not crucial to the administration of actinomycin. (B) One of the common adverse reactions with actinomycin is ulcerative stomatitis and

pharyngitis, and sores often occur under the tongue. The nurse must inspect the oral cavity for any lesions prior to administration. (C) Darkening of the skin is bothersome and may occur if the client has received previous radiation therapy, but is not critical to administration. (D) There is nothing in this situation to indicate the need for a signed consent for this medication.

185. **(B)** Nursing process phase: implementation; client need: safe, effective care environment; content area: medical/surgical nursing

Rationale

$$3 \text{ mg} : 1 \text{ ml} = 5 \text{ mg} : x = 1.67 \text{ ml}$$

Math calculation explains incorrect answers.

186. **(D)** Nursing process phase: implementation; client need: physiological integrity; content area: maternity nursing

Rationale

(A) Fundal pressure may be needed in the anesthetized mother or for shoulder dystocia. (B) Prolonged breath holding may initiate Valsalva's maneuver. (C) Fetal station is +3, the baby is past the narrowest part of the pelvis. (D) Using an upright position yields a stronger sensation to bear down as the presenting part comes in contact with the pelvic floor. To push with the maximum effort of the uterus, the mother should determine when the urge to bear down is the greatest.

187. **(C)** Nursing process phase: analysis; client need: health promotion and maintenance; content area: pediatric nursing

Rationale

(A) Both the corticosteroids and inflammation will affect the growth. High doses of steroids will stunt growth. Inflammation will cause damage to joints, and deformities develop that interfere with normal growth. (B) Short periods of taking the corticosteroids and low doses will not interrupt growth as with high doses over long periods of time. (C) By alternating the high and low doses between days, the child's growth is less affected. (D) A side effect of corticosteroids is weight gain. They stimulate the appetite as well as cause fluid retention.

188. **(B)** Nursing process phase: implementation; client need: safe, effective care environment; content area: maternity nursing

Rationale

(A) The nurse needs to discuss with the client what her regular routine is and discuss the American College of Gynecologists' (ACOG) recommendations to assure safety for the client and her pregnancy. (B) These are recommendations made by ACOG to assure safe exercise in pregnancy. (C) Gestational age alone does not place a client at risk for preterm labor. Most clients can continue an exercise routine as long as safety guidelines are followed. (D) A pregnant client's caloric intake must increase to meet the extra demands of exercise.

189. **(D)** Nursing process phase: assessment; client need: safe, effective care environment; content area: pediatric nursing

Rationale

(A) The assessment of reflex activity would not be contraindicated in a child with possible Wilms' tumor. (B) The assessment of cranial nerves would not be contraindicated. How-

ever, the extent examined would of course depend on the client's overall health status. (C) The assessment of pulses would not be contraindicated in a child with possible Wilms' tumor. (D) Palpating the abdomen of a child with a possible Wilms' tumor would be contraindicated because manipulation increases the danger of metastasis of the tumor.

190. **(A)** Nursing process phase: analysis; client need: safe, effective care environment; content area: medical/surgical—gerontological nursing

Rationale

(A) Levothyroxine (Synthroid) may alter the effects of oral anticoagulants and may necessitate a decrease in anticoagulation therapy. (B) There is no indication that levothyroxine affects antibiotic medications. (C & D) Levothyroxine is deiodinated in peripheral tissue and only a small amount is metabolized by the liver.

191. **(A)** Nursing process phase: assessment; client need: safe, effective care environment; content area: psychiatric nursing

Rationale

(A) The client has expelled or withheld the rape event from her consciousness. (B) Regression is when the client attempts to return to a previous level of function or development to avoid anxiety or conflict associated with the event. (C) Projection occurs when the client controls unacceptable impulses by acting as though they were outside oneself or attempts to attribute them to someone else. (D) Blocking is a temporary or transient inhibition of thinking. The client is not experiencing blocking.

192. **(C)** Nursing process phase: evaluation; client need: physiological integrity; content area: maternity nursing

Rationale

(A) Fundal pressure is performed by the nurse to shorten the second stage in the anesthetized mother or in the presence of shoulder dystocia. (B) Forceps or vacuum extraction is used when the baby must be born right away, when there is fetal distress, or when the mother is not pushing effectively. (C) Prolonged breath holding during the second stage may precipitate increased blood pressure in the mother and produce an imbalance in the oxygen and carbon dioxide levels in the baby's blood. Gentle pushing, sustaining the push with breath holding of no more than 5 seconds, will alleviate the situation. (D) During pushing, there is an increased amount of pressure on the baby that normally results in a drop in fetal heart rate. This heart rate should recover, not necessitating a cesarean section.

193. **(D)** Nursing process phase: implementation; client need: physiological integrity; content area: pediatric nursing

Rationale

(A) These data will establish a baseline for the comparison of vital signs during and after the infusion. (B) A small volume is given initially to note any immediate reaction. (C) Only blood filters are recommended for use. Regular IV filters should not be used to administer blood. (D) The blood must be transfused within 30 minutes or returned to the blood bank.

194. **(D)** Nursing process phase: evaluation; client need:

physiological integrity; content area: medical/surgical—gerontological nursing

Rationale

(A) Blood glucose concentrations may be increased when furosemide (Lasix) is administered. (B) Furosemide may cause a slight increase in blood urea nitrogen. (C) Proteinuria may occur in older adults, but this may indicate urinary tract infection or kidney disease. (D) Blood in the urine and gastrointestinal bleeding are indicators of potential side effects of furosemide.

195. **(C)** Nursing process phase: assessment; client need: physiological integrity; content area: maternity nursing

Rationale

(A) Estrogen causes growth of the uterus. (B) Prolactin's primary purpose is in the promotion of milk production. (C) Progesterone is secreted by the placenta and inhibits uterine motility. (D) Human chorionic gonadotropin is secreted by the trophoblastic layer of the blastocyst. It maintains the corpus luteum until the placenta tissue produces adequate amounts of pregnancy hormones to take over.

196. **(A)** Nursing process phase: evaluation; client need: health promotion and maintenance; content area: medical/surgical nursing

Rationale

(A) Research has shown that the risk of chronic complications is reduced by maintaining a blood sugar as close to normal as possible. It is logical that the acute complications would be minimized. (B) Following baseline eye examinations, a diabetic should have the eyes examined at least once a year. (C) Insulin should be taken on sick days; more may be needed to cover the illness. (C) Soaking dries the feet, and hot water could injure the feet because of a decrease in sensation.

197. **(A)** Nursing process phase: assessment; client need: physiological integrity; content area: maternity nursing

Rationale

(A) This is a true statement. Cystic fibrosis is a recessive disorder in which abnormal secretions are produced by the exocrine glands. Viscid secretions are produced in the liver, small intestine, pancreas, duodenum, and lungs. Complications such as respiratory distress and meconium ileus often occur in the newborn. (B) Cystic fibrosis is a recessive disorder. (B) Cystic fibrosis does not involve the hemoglobin molecule. (D) Many of the inborn errors of metabolism lead to enzyme deficiencies. Tay-Sachs disease causes fatty deposits in the brain.

198. **(D)** Nursing process phase: implementation; client need: safe, effective care environment; content area: medical/surgical nursing

Rationale

(A) "Sterile" cavities such as the trachea are suctioned first, followed by suction to "dirty" areas such as the mouth. (B) Ten to 15 seconds is the maximum aspiration time for each suction. (C) Suction is not applied when inserting the catheter; this could damage the mucosa. (D) Intermittent suction is applied as the catheter is withdrawn.

199. **(B)** Nursing process phase: analysis; client need: safe, effective care environment; content area: medical/surgical—gerontological nursing

Rationale

(A–D) Most cataract surgery is performed as outclient surgery with the administration of a local anesthetic.

200. **(D)** Nursing process phase: assessment; client need: physiological integrity; content area: psychiatric nursing

Rationale

(A) Headache is a common side effect of lithium. (B) Lethargy is a common side effect of lithium. (C) Fatigue is a common side effect of lithium. (D) Coarse hand tremors is a sign of toxicity.

201. **(A)** Nursing process phase: analysis; client need: physiological integrity; content area: pediatric nursing

Rationale

(A) Stomatitis (painful lesions in the mouth) is a common side effect of chemotherapy. (B) Brittle ridging of the nails does occur with some types of chemotherapy [such as cyclophosphamide (Cytoxan)]; however, this side effect is less common than stomatitis. (C) An increase in the leukocyte count is present with the initial diagnosis. Chemotherapy depresses the bone marrow, which would reduce the leukocyte count. (D) Swelling of the hands and feet is not a usual side effect of chemotherapy.

202. **(B)** Nursing process phase: assessment; client need: physiological integrity; content area: medical/surgical nursing

Rationale

(A) Phlebitis is characterized by swelling, warmth, and redness. (B) Phlebitis is characterized by swelling, warmth, and redness around the insertion site or along the path of the vein. (C) This describes an IV infusion that has become clotted. (D) This describes an infiltrated IV.

203. **(D)** Nursing process phase: implementation; client need: psychosocial integrity; content area: psychiatric nursing

Rationale

(A) This response would reinforce the client's denial about the seriousness of his alcoholism. (B) This response is an example of a nontherapeutic communication called "requesting an explanation." Asking "Why" can be intimidating and encourages the client to become defensive. (C) This response does not assist the client to connect his behavior with his illness or separate the behavior from the client. It sounds judgmental. (D) This response is therapeutic because it assists the client to connect his personal problems with his drinking. A nursing goal for a client with alcoholism is to assist the client to acknowledge the association between his drinking and his personal problems.

204. **(D)** Nursing process phase: analysis; client need: physiological integrity; content area: maternity nursing

Rationale

(A) The normal amount of gastric secretions is somewhat lower in the first and second trimesters of pregnancy; then a dramatic increase occurs in the third trimester. (B) While a slight decrease in gastric acids does occur in the first and second trimesters of pregnancy, this is not a precipitating cause of indigestion in pregnancy. (C) In the first trimester, the fetus is not large enough to apply significant pressure to cause GI symptoms. (D) Progesterone causes relaxation of the smooth muscle, causing decreased motility and relaxation of the cardiac sphincter, which results in indigestion.

205. (A) Nursing process phase: analysis; client need: physiological integrity; content area: pediatric nursing

Rationale
(A) Epinephrine is a B_1 and B_2 agonist, causing increased levels of cyclic AMP producing bronchodilation. It may be given subcutaneously, parenterally, or through inhalation, depending on the severity of the acute episode. (B) Corticosteroids are effective anti-inflammatory drugs that are highly effective in controlling symptoms and reducing hyperreactivity in chronic asthma, but are not the drugs of choice in an acute emergency. (C) Cough syrup with codeine would be contraindicated. Codeine can cause respiratory depression. (D) Antibiotics are used to treat respiratory infections, which may trigger an asthma episode; however, they are not effective during an acute attack of asthma.

206. (C) Nursing process phase: analysis; client need: physiological integrity; content area: maternity nursing

Rationale
(A) Physiological and safety needs come before psychological needs. (B) The fetus is in a posterior position. This can be alleviated (about 70 percent of the time) by changing the mother's position to a lateral Sims' position. The client is already alternating positions. (C) The client is being induced. She also received her epidural early in labor, which may result in a prolonged labor. (D) She is receiving IV fluids. She is not vomiting. Her fluid volume is stable at present.

207. (B) Nursing process phase: assessment; client need: psychosocial integrity; content area: pediatric nursing

Rationale
(A) Alopecia occurs in some clients who are diagnosed with lupus, but not all. (B) Alopecia is experienced during disease exacerbations. During periods of remission, the hair usually regrows. (C) There are topical medications available to treat alopecia. Clients diagnosed with lupus experience regrowth of hair with cessation of disease activity. A dermatologist should be consulted for the benefits of this type of medication with lupus. (D) Alopecia in some conditions is permanent; however, with lupus it is temporary and occurs during the disease process.

208. (B) Nursing process phase: assessment; client need: safe, effective care environment; content area: medical/surgical—gerontological nursing

Rationale
(A) The serum T_3 is of little value since one-third of clients with hypothyroidism have serum T_3 concentrations within normal limits. (B) The diagnosis of hypothyroidism is based on precise and reliable assays of TSH and T_4 serum levels. (C) There is no test known as thyroid releasing hormone (TRH). The TSH is useful in the diagnosis of hypothyroidism. (D) Thyroid-directed antibodies are found in the serum of clients with Hashimoto's disease, an autoimmune inflammatory process of the thyroid gland.

209. (C) Nursing process phase: analysis; client need: safe, effective care environment; content area: psychiatric nursing

Rationale
(A) Reaction formation is an unacceptable impulse that is

transformed into its opposite. The client is not exhibiting this defense mechanism. (B) Sublimation is when an impulse is channeled into a socially acceptable behavior. (C) Acting out is when the client gives in to an impulse to avoid anxiety that would result from the postponement of expression. (D) Splitting is a defense mechanism in which a person views himself as all good or all bad and is unable to integrate positive and negative qualities into a cohesive image.

210. (A) Nursing process phase: implementation; client need: psychosocial integrity; content area: medical/surgical—gerontological nursing

Rationale
(A) This response relates the fear the client is experiencing and at the same time correctly shares with the client knowledge that is true. The 5-year survival rate for all clients even with thyroid cancers is 93 percent. (B) In deciding whether to treat thyroid nodules surgically, the higher risk of surgical morbidity in older adults must be taken into account. (C) This is false reassurance and does little to respond to the client's fears or concerns. (D) This response ignores the client's feelings altogether.

211. (A) Nursing process phase: assessment; client need: physiological integrity; content area: pediatric nursing

Rationale
(A) Slipped femoral capital epiphysis is suspected when an adolescent or preadolescent youngster, who is obese or tall and lanky, begins to limp and complains of pain in the hip continuously or intermittently. The pain is frequently referred to the groin, the knee, or the anteromedial aspect of the thigh. (B) Complaints of a limp and ankle pain would usually be associated with an ankle injury. (C) Curvature of the thoracic spine characterizes the spinal deformity of kyphosis. (D) Curvature of the cervical or lumbar spine beyond physiological limits characterizes the spinal deformity of lordosis.

212. (D) Nursing process phase: implementation; client need: safe, effective care environment; content area: psychiatric nursing

Rationale
$$125 \text{ mg} : 5 \text{ ml} = 200 \text{ mg} : x = 8 \text{ ml}$$
Math calculation explains incorrect answers.

213. (D) Nursing process phase: assessment; client need: physiological integrity; content area: medical/surgical nursing

Rationale
(A) The back of the knee is the popliteal pulse. (B) Below the medial malleolus of the ankle is the tibial pulse. (B) Below the inguinal ligament is the femoral pulse. (D) The dorsum of the foot lateral to the great toe is the dorsalis pedis pulse.

214. (C) Nursing process phase: analysis; client need: physiological integrity; content area: pediatric nursing

Rationale
(A) Croup results from swelling or obstruction in the region of the larynx. No bleeding exists from the inflammation process. (B) Expected pulmonary sounds include a "barky" cough and varying degrees of inspiratory stridor from the laryngeal inflammation, not expiratory crackles. (C) Examination with a tongue depressor is contraindicated because it may

precipitate further or complete obstruction. (D) A throat abscess does not result from an examination with a tongue depressor.

215. **(A)** Nursing process phase: assessment; client need: physiological integrity; content area: maternity nursing

Rationale
(A) There is increased circulation to the tissue, causing an increase in secretion of saliva. (B) Pytalism is the increase of saliva. (C) Increased progesterone does have a relaxant effect on the GI system in pregnancy, but has not been shown to contribute to increased saliva production. (D) The pH of saliva is typically unchanged in pregnancy.

216. **(D)** Nursing process phase: implementation; client need: health promotion and maintenance; content area: medical/surgical nursing

Rationale
(A) Keeping doctors' appointments would not be the highest priority. (B) Attending a support group would be helpful with coping with the disease, but is not the most important. (C) Smoking cessation would be a high priority, but not above medication compliance. (D) Medication compliance would be the highest priority to control chronic hypertension.

217. **(B)** Nursing process phase: implementation; client need: safe, effective care environment; content area: medical/surgical nursing

Rationale
1 mg divided by 1000 µg × 1 ml = 1 ml
Math calculation explains incorrect answers.

218. **(A)** Nursing process phase: assessment; client need: health promotion and maintenance; content area: medical/surgical nursing

Rationale
(A) Obesity is a high risk factor with strong family history. (B) Past smoking would not be a current risk factor. (C) A nonsedentary lifestyle would not be a risk factor. (D) An intense job that does not produce stress would not be a risk factor.

219. **(B)** Nursing process phase: implementation; client need: safe, effective care environment; content area: psychiatric nursing

Rationale
(A) Psychiatric units have suicide guidelines that must be implemented prior to any consultation requests. (B) Immediate implementation of suicide precautions communicates caring and enables the psychiatric staff to monitor and provide protection. (C) Identification can cause the nurse to doubt his or her own coping abilities. By showing empathy, the nurse enables the client to identify the source of distress. (D) Because suicidal behavior arouses feelings of anxiety in the nurse, coping measures include avoiding the client's depersonalizing behavior.

220. **(D)** Nursing process phase: implementation; client need: safe, effective care environment; content area: pediatric nursing

Rationale
100 mg : 5 ml = 180 mg : x = 9 ml
Math calculation explains incorrect answers.

221. **(A)** Nursing process phase: implementation; client need: content area: maternity nursing

Rationale
(A) No single position is best for all of labor. Walking uses gravity and provides an outlet for anxious energy. (B) The client's fetus is vertex and the head is engaged at 0 station. She is not at risk for cord prolapse. She should be permitted to walk if she desires. (C) Bathing is contraindicated with ruptured membranes because of the risk of contamination since the barrier of protection is absent. (D) The client is coping and relaxing well between contractions. An epidural is not indicated at this time.

222. **(B)** Nursing process phase: assessment; client need: physiological integrity; content area: pediatric nursing

Rationale
(A) The bowel sounds with intestinal obstruction are decreased or absent—not increased. (B) Increased abdominal distention, vomiting, absence of stool, and pain are also symptoms of intestinal obstruction. (C) Late signs of intestinal obstruction include tachycardia, fever, hypotension, or shock. (D) Urinary output is not a significant observation unless dehydration is present, and if present, urinary output would be decreased.

223. **(B)** Nursing process phase: health promotion and maintenance; client need: physiological integrity; content area: medical/surgical—gerontological nursing

Rationale
(A) Older adults may not engage in IV drug use as often as the general population, but this is not the primary reason that it is missed as a diagnosis by health-care providers. (B) Older adults in the early stages of human immunodeficiency virus (HIV) infection often present with vague symptoms that can be confused with other disease processes, making an accurate diagnosis difficult. (C) Although it is commonly believed that sexual desire and activity diminish with age, sexual patterns persist throughout the life span. Almost half of all males over the age of 70 report being sexually active. (D) Homosexual activity accounts for about 20 percent of AIDS cases in clients over the age of 70.

224. **(D)** Nursing process phase: implementation; client need: safe, effective care environment; content area: maternity nursing

Rationale
(A) The IV maintenance fluid recommended for pregnant diabetics is either lactated Ringer's or 5% dextrose with lactated Ringer's. The work of labor requires calories provided by the glucose in the IV solution. (B) Laboring women use large amounts of energy to accomplish the work of labor and birth. However, the glucose load in $D_{10}W$ can precipitate hyperglycemia in the mother, which can cause hypoglycemia in the newborn. (C) Insulin is chemically attracted to the plastic in IV tubing. Insulin in the prescribed solution will adhere to the lining of the tubing. This results in varying concentrations of insulin in the solution. (D) Flushing the IV line with 250 to 500 ml of lactated Ringer's or normal saline mixed with 10 units of insulin, or with a protein, will completely coat the IV tubing so that the prescribed solution of insulin will remain stable.

225. **(C)** Nursing process phase: intervention; client need: safe, effective care environment; content area: medical/surgical nursing

Rationale
(A) Iron preparations should not be given with milk or antacids. (B) Iron preparations should be diluted to decrease gastric irritation. (C) While between-meal dosing may increase absorption, gastric distress can be decreased by giving oral iron with food. (D) Gastric irritants should not be given at bedtime when the client will be fasting throughout the night.

226. (B) Nursing process phase: analysis; client need: physiological integrity; content area: medical/surgical nursing

Rationale
(A) Primary diabetes insipidus affects about 50 percent of clients with this disorder. Its origin is idiopathic. It is seen primarily in neonates as a result of congenital malformation of the central nervous system, infection, trauma, or tumor. (B) Secondary diabetes insipidus results from intracranial neoplastic or metastatic lesions or any type of neurosurgery, skull fracture, or head trauma. (C) Transient diabetes insipidus occurs during pregnancy, usually after the fifth or sixth month, and reverses spontaneously after delivery. (D) There is no such thing as surgical diabetes insipidus.

227. (B) Nursing process phase: implementation; client need: safe, effective care environment; content area: psychiatric nursing

Rationale
(A) Keep the focus on the here and now. This question does not directly address suicidal or homicidal behavior. (B) By asking a direct question, it helps the client verbalize feelings instead of acting out the behavior. (C) This question does not deal directly with suicidal or homicidal behavior. (D) This question focuses on the family rather than on the client.

228. (B) Nursing process phase: assessment; client need: physiological integrity; content area: medical/surgical nursing

Rationale
(A & D) These gastrointestinal complaints do not generally accompany hypocalcemia. (B) When acute hypocalcemia occurs, clients should be monitored for paresthesia and tetany. (C) These symptoms are not associated with hypocalcemia; they are present in uncontrolled diabetes.

229. (C) Nursing process phase: evaluation; client need: health promotion and maintenance; content area: medical/surgical nursing

Rationale
(A, B, & D) These findings are normal in a routine urinalysis. (C) Normal findings in a routine urinalysis include a few WBC (4 to 5) and a pH of 4.3 to 8 with an average of 6 in adults. Therefore, these findings of 20 to 25 WBC and pH of 8.5 indicate a UTI.

230. (B) Nursing process phase: implementation; client need: psychosocial integrity; content area: maternity nursing

Rationale
(A) Parents should not feel pressured to make a decision the health-care provider feels is best for them. There is evidence that indicates what the parents imagine is far worse than the reality. (B) A statement that gives the parents permission to do what may seem morbid or distasteful is desirable. Communicating with parents that options are their right, not their obligation, is essential. (C) This statement implies that the parents contributed in some way to the anomalies and death of their baby. Being sensitive to the needs of the parents of actualizing their loss is necessary for their healing. (D) Seeing and/or holding the baby should be one of the first options discussed with the parents. These moments are the only ones they will have alone with their child. It is essential to remember that parents see their infant with very different eyes than health-care professionals. In addition, there are many things a nurse can do to help make the infant more attractive, such as having a perfect hand or foot showing when the infant is brought into the room, putting lotion and powder on the baby to make him smell sweet, wrapping him in a pretty blanket, are all ways to prepare the baby for his parents.

231. (D) Nursing process phase: analysis; client need: health promotion and maintenance; content area: medical/surgical—gerontological nursing

Rationale
(A) While older adults may fear nursing home placement, the reason they do not seek medical care for thyroid disorders is because they exhibit few of the classic symptoms of the disease. (B) While older adults may have limited financial resources, the reason they do not seek medical care for thyroid disorders is because they exhibit few of the classic symptoms of the disease. (C) While older adults may fear loss of independence, the reason they do not seek medical care for thyroid disorders is because they exhibit few of the classic symptoms of the disease. (D) The reason they do not seek medical care for thyroid disorders is because they exhibit few of the classic symptoms of the disease.

232. (B) Nursing process phase: analysis; client need: safe, effective care environment; content area: pediatric nursing

Rationale
(A) If wheezing or bronchospasms are present, allergens used for skin testing could enhance symptoms. Assessment of lungs is a precautionary measure. (B) Antihistamines suppress skin test reactivity and therefore should be withheld for 48 to 96 hours prior to testing. (C) The RAST is done as a supplement test to validate skin testing results. The RAST is not a screening tool. (D) Choosing a site that promotes accuracy depends on location, dermatographism, eczema, and cooperation of the child. Both the upper forearm and the upper back are appropriate sites.

233. (D) Nursing process phase: analysis; client need: health promotion and maintenance; content area: medical/surgical—gerontological nursing

Rationale
(A) While family support is important in providing care to older adults, falls, incontinence, and cognitive changes are the three conditions that are high risk to hospitalized older adults. (B) While the older adult may be high risk for social isolation while hospitalized, falls, incontinence, and cognitive changes are the three conditions that are high risk for hospitalized older adults. (C) While the older adult may be high risk for sensory deprivation while hospitalized, falls, incontinence, and cognitive changes are the three conditions that are high risk to hospitalized older adults. (D) Falls, incontinence, and cognitive changes are the three conditions that are high risk to hospitalized older adults.

234. (D) Nursing process phase: implementation; client need: safe, effective care environment; content area: maternity nursing

$$600 \text{ mg} : 5 \text{ ml} = x : 10 \text{ ml} = 1200 \text{ mg}$$

Math calculation explains incorrect answers.

235. (D) Nursing process phase: implementation; client need: health promotion and maintenance; content area: pediatric nursing

Rationale

(A) At or around 11 months, an infant is able to walk with both hands held, and by age 1 year may be able to walk with one hand held. (B) At or around 9 months, an infant can stand while holding onto furniture and can pull himself or herself to a standing position. (C) At or around 14 months, a child can feed himself or herself successfully with a spoon. (D) At or around 7 months of age, an infant can sit alone leaning onto hands for support.

236. (D) Nursing process phase: analysis; client need: physiological integrity; content area: maternity nursing

Rationale

(A) Promethazine can decrease anxiety; however, it is no longer believed that women experiencing hyperemesis are attempting to "throw up" the pregnancy. (B) Promethazine can have the side effect of causing sleepiness; however, hyperemesis is not associated with maternal exhaustion. (C) Hyperemesis can cause fluid and electrolyte imbalance; however, promethazine is not an electrolyte solution. (D) Promethazine is used as an antiemetic in pregnancies where nausea and vomiting are uncontrolled by other means.

237. (A) Nursing process phase: analysis; client need: physiological integrity; content area: medical/surgical nursing

Rationale

(A) Regular insulin begins working quickly. (B & C) Given subcutaneously, regular insulin peaks in 2 to 4 hours. (D) The duration of regular insulin given subcutaneously is about 5 to 7 hours.

238. (D) Nursing process phase: planning; client need: safe, effective care environment; content area: psychiatric nursing

Rationale

(A) Administering medications is a collaborative intervention and not the primary goal. Other forms of therapy may provide protection for the suicide client prior to the pharmacological treatment. (B) Determining follow-up care is not considered a primary goal. (C) Teaching the client to have a more realistic view of self is an important nursing goal for a suicidal client but is not the primary goal. (D) Collaborating with the client about the issues that motivate the behavior will help the nurse understand and deal with the problems more effectively.

239. (B) Nursing process phase: assessment; client need: physiological integrity; content area: maternity nursing

Rationale

(A) Urine stasis does occur, but this does not cause frequency except in the case of resulting UTI. (B) Pressure of the enlarging uterus on the bladder stimulates the sensation of needing to void even when the bladder is not full. (C)

Though this is a common occurrence in pregnancy, it is not a cause of normal urinary frequency, but can result in frequency from a UTI. (D) As the uterus rises out of the pelvis, urinary frequency should decrease. This occurs in the second trimester.

240. (B) Nursing process phase: assessment; client need: safe, effective care environment; content area: medical/surgical nursing

Rationale

(A) Creatinine clearance would be a parameter of kidney function. (B) Coagulation studies would be required to prevent bleeding complications. (C) Urine protein would be another parameter of kidney function. (D) Uric acid levels would be used to evaluate for gout.

241. (A) Nursing process phase: implementation; client need: safe, effective care environment; content area: pediatric nursing

Rationale

$$0.5 \text{ μg} : 1 \text{ tablet} = 0.25 \text{ μg} : x = \tfrac{1}{2} \text{ tablet}$$

Math calculation explains incorrect answers.

242. (B) Nursing process phase: implementation; client need: safe, effective care environment; content area: medical/surgical nursing

Rationale

(A) "No visitors" is not required with this type of isolation. (B) Universal precautions are followed when handling blood and body fluids. (C) Negative air flow is not required with blood and body fluid isolation. (D) A private room would be preferred.

243. (D) Nursing process phase: implementation; client need: health promotion and maintenance; content area: medical/surgical nursing

Rationale

(A) Ferrous sulfate tablets would not stain teeth. (B) Urine would not be affected—the iron is absorbed in the intestines. (C) Breath would not be affected. (D) Stools would turn black or green because only 50 percent of the iron is absorbed and the rest is excreted in the stool.

244. (A) Nursing process phase: assessment; client need: safe, effective care environment; content area: psychiatric nursing

Rationale

(A) Resistance is the unconscious opposition to treatment or therapy goals. (B) Secondary gain is when the client attempts to gain advantages for the external world by provoking sympathy and attention from others. Because the client did not seek out the nurse to gain attention in order to get out of participating in activities, then she is not trying to obtain secondary gain. (C) The client is not free associating, that is, she is not saying whatever comes to mind. (D) The client is not demonstrating an unnatural fear of therapy or a fear out of proportion to the real degree of threat.

245. (B) Nursing process phase: implementation; client need: health promotion and maintenance; content area: pediatric nursing

Rationale

(A) An infant tends to be restless because of fever, rather than lethargic, after immunization with DPT. (B) It is a common occurrence for an infant who receives the DPT vaccine to have mild fever between 12 and 24 hours after the administration of the vaccine. The mother should be taught to administer acetaminophen (Tylenol) for the fever. Fever over 102°F (30°C) should be reported to the physician or nurse practitioner. (D) Diarrhea has no association with the administration of the DPT vaccine. (D) Nasal congestion has no association with the administration of the DPT vaccine.

246. **(A)** Nursing process phase: implementation; client need: safe, effective care environment; content area: medical/surgical nursing

Rationale
(A) Upon arising would be correct, when no swelling has occurred. (B) Most TEDs are removed for sleep and daily hygiene. (C) Cutting would cause the elasticity to be lost. (D) More than one pair of stockings should be obtained for availability while being washed.

247. **(C)** Nursing process phase: implementation; client need: safe, effective care environment; content area: medical/surgical nursing

Rationale
200 mg divided by 500 mg × 1.8 ml = 0.7 ml
Math calculation explains incorrect answers.

248. **(B)** Nursing process phase: analysis; client need: safe, effective care environment; content area: pediatric nursing

Rationale
(A) Hematuria is not present in a child with nephrosis. (B) The primary objective is to reduce the excretion of urinary protein and maintain a protein-free urine. (C) An objective of therapeutic management is to control edema, not to increase fluid in the tissues. (D) The blood pressure of a child with nephrosis is usually within the normal range. There is no need to elevate it.

249. **(B)** Nursing process phase: analysis; client need: safe, effective care environment; content area: psychiatric nursing

Rationale
(A) Lorazepam is not indicated for use related to elevation of mood. (B) The major indications for the use of lorazepam are for anxiety disorders and short-term relief of symptoms of anxiety. (C) Anxiolytics act to depress the central nervous system and therefore would not be used to treat or reverse a depressed mood. (D) Neuroleptics (antipsychotics) are the drugs of choice for treating psychoses.

250. **(A)** Nursing process phase: assessment; client need: safe, effective care environment; content area: medical/surgical—gerontological nursing

Rationale
(A) Elevated sodium (Na), elevated hematocrit (Hct), and elevated blood urea nitrogen (BUN) should be monitored by the nurse if dehydration is suspected. (B & C) The nurse would expect an elevation—not a drop in sodium values, and potassium would not be a laboratory value used in monitoring for dehydration. (D) The nurse would not recognize a decrease in blood urea nitrogen (BUN) as an indicator of dehydration.

251. **(C)** Nursing process phase: planning; client need: psychosocial integrity; content area: pediatric nursing

Rationale
(A) Teaching the side effects of chemotherapy would be overwhelming, and it is usually best to wait until after surgery to teach the family about chemotherapy. (B) In addition to the usual preoperative observations, vital signs, especially the blood pressure, are monitored frequently. (C) As with all cancers, the diagnosis of Wilms' tumor is a shock to the family. The parents may express guilt about not finding the mass sooner, and with the swiftness of the diagnosis, they will need the support of the nurse. (D) Forcing fluids every 2 hours would not be necessary preoperatively with a diagnosis of Wilms' tumor.

252. **(D)** Nursing process phase: planning; client need: health promotion and maintenance; content area: medica/surgical nursing

Rationale
(A) The antibiotics listed here are the drugs of choice and are most commonly used to treat a UTI. (B) Testing a urine sample for culture and sensitivity is performed before and after treatment of a UTI and therefore is used in the treatment. (C) Increasing fluids, emptying the bladder frequently, and follow-up teaching are included in the care and treatment of a UTI. These interventions will reduce the risk of a recurrent infection. (D) Treatment for a UTI would include antibiotics for a 10-day duration. If it is stopped before that, there is an increased chance of reoccurrence of the UTI, which could lead to renal damage.

253. **(C)** Nursing process phase: analysis; client need: physiological integrity; content area: pediatric nursing

Rationale
(A) Prednisone does not increase the rate of wound healing. (B) Prednisone does not stimulate secretions of the adrenal gland. (C) Correct. Prednisone, like most steroid preparations, will obscure the inflammatory symptoms of infections. It is important to monitor for other signs of infection in these clients. (D) Steroids will not increase antibody production.

254. **(D)** Nursing process phase: implementation; client need: health promotion and maintenance; content area: maternity nursing

Rationale
(A) Vaginal delivery is only contraindicated with two consecutive positive HSV-II cultures close to the time of delivery. (B) Herpes infections seem to be more severe in pregnant women. (C) Herpes transmission occurs by having close contact with another infected person. (D) The route of transmission is from mother to infant via an actively infected birth canal. If the cultures are not active, she should deliver vaginally.

255. **(A)** Nursing process phase: analysis; client need: physiological integrity; content area: medical/surgical nursing

Rationale
(A) This is the correct term to describe this process that produces increased skeletal thickness, hypertrophy of the skin, and enlargement of visceral organs. (B) Dwarfism is a result of growth hormone deficiency. (C) Sheehan's syndrome is the term for pituitary infarction caused mostly by postpartum

hemorrhage. (D) Midgetism is a result of growth hormone deficiency.

256. (D) Nursing process phase: analysis; client need: physiological integrity; content area: medical/surgical—gerontological nursing

Rationale

(A & B) During the hidden phase of AIDS, the client may experience vague symptoms of fatigue, headache, malaise, and swollen lymph nodes. Aspirin and acetaminophen (Tylenol) may help to alleviate these symptoms. (C) Nonsteroidal anti-inflammatory drugs (NSAIDS) are used in the early AIDS phase in only about 19 percent of clients with AIDS; the most usual form of pain management is narcotic analgesics with the opiates. (D) As the client progresses from the transition phase to the AIDS phase, narcotic analgesics, namely the opiate family, are required to maintain a level of comfort.

257. (C) Nursing process phase: analysis; client need: safe, effective care environment; content area: medical/surgical nursing

Rationale

(A) A pulmonary embolus is not a consideration for this client. A PaO_2 of less than 40 mm Hg would indicate an acute respiratory problem. (B) Hypoxia is not a consideration for this client. His PaO_2 would be below 40 mm Hg to indicate an acute respiratory problem. (C) This is correct. This PaO_2 represents normal oxygenation for a client of this age. The normal level for clients over the age of 65 decreases with age as changes occur in the aging lung. Subtract 1 mm Hg for every year the client is over the age of 60 years from 80 mm Hg. (D) Respiratory acidosis cannot be assessed based only on the PaO_2 given here. You need the entire arterial blood gas analysis in order to determine this condition.

258. (C) Nursing process phase: implementation; client need: health promotion and maintenance; content area: maternity nursing

Rationale

(A) This is the definition for quickening. (B) Those sensations are pain-related and do not have a medical term to describe them. (C) Lightening is the term used when the fetus descends into the pelvis in preparation for birth. Common symptoms that accompany this include urinary frequency, increased backache, and an ability to breathe more easily. (D) There is no formal term for this, but it is thought to be related to an increase in estrogen levels in pregnancy.

259. (D) Nursing process phase: implementation; client need: safe, effective care environment; content area: psychiatric nursing

Rationale

250 mg : 1 ml = 500 mg : x = 2 ml
Math calculation explains incorrect answers.

260. (C) Nursing process phase: implementation; client need: safe, effective care environment; content area: medical/surgical—gerontological nursing

Rationale

500 mg : 1 tablet = 750 mg : x = 1½ tablets

Math calculation explains incorrect answers.

261. (D) Nursing process phase: analysis; client need: physiological integrity; content area: medical/surgical nursing

Rationale

(A) Clinical findings of asthma include tachycardia—not bradycardia. (B) Clinical findings of asthma include profuse diaphoresis—not warm, dry skin or facial flushing. (C) In asthma the lungs become overinflated from retained air caused by the difficulty in moving air in and out of the lungs. (D) Clinical findings of an asthma attack include sudden onset of dyspnea. This is caused by the narrowed bronchial lumina and difficulty of expiring air through the narrowed and mucus-clogged airways.

262. (D) Nursing process phase: assessment; client need: physiological integrity; content area: medical/surgical nursing

Rationale

(A–C) The behavior described is not a positive Trousseau's sign. (D) This reaction describes a positive Trousseau's sign.

263. (A) Nursing process phase: implementation; client need: safe, effective care environment; content area: maternity nursing

Rationale

(A) $MgSO_4$ prevent seizures by blocking neuromuscular transmission. (B) With the administration of $MgSO_4$, a slight drop in BP may be seen as a result of the relaxation of smooth muscles. However, $MgSO_4$ is not an antihypertensive drug. (C) $MgSO_4$ treatment does not result in an increase urine output, but may with toxicity actually cause a decrease. (D) Decreasing edema as a result of diuresis caused by the increased perfusion of the kidney is a positive sign. However, decreasing edema is not the primary purpose of $MgSO_4$ administration.

264. (A) Nursing process phase: evaluation; client need: safe, effective care environment; content area: psychiatric nursing

Rationale

(A) Displaying a hopeful attitude indicates that the client feels some sense of self-worth and there is a meaning for living. (B) There is no indication in this answer that the client expresses hope and optimism for living. (C) During the assessment phase, the nurse questions the client about previous suicide behavior. This answer is not an expected outcome. (D) Verbalizing anger is a healthy step, but there remains a danger that the client does not see self as valuable and moves toward self-destructive behavior.

265. (A) Nursing process phase: planning; client need: health promotion and maintenance; content area: pediatric nursing

Rationale

(A) Aspirin is an anticoagulant and is contraindicated in clients with hemophilia. (B) Meperidine (Demerol) can be prescribed for hemophiliacs. (C) Acetaminophen (Tylenol) can be given to children with hemophilia. (D) Codeine can be prescribed for children with hemophilia.

appendix A
State Boards of Nursing

Alabama Board of Nursing
P.O. Box 303900
Montgomery, AL 36130
(334) 242-4060

Alaska Board of Nursing
Department of Commerce &
    Economic Development
3601 C St., Suite 722
Anchorage, AK 99503
(907) 269-8161

American Samoa Health Services
Regulatory Board
LBJ Tropical Medical Center
Pago Pago, American Samoa 96799
(684) 633-1222, Ext. 206

Arizona Board of Nursing
1651 E. Morten Ave., Suite 150
Phoenix, AZ 85020
(602) 255-5092

Arkansas Board of Nursing
University Towers Bldg
Suite 800
1123 S. University
Little Rock, AR 72204
(501) 686-2700

California Board of
RN Nursing
P.O. Box 944210
Sacramento, CA 94244
(916) 322-3350

Colorado Board of Nursing
1560 Broadway, Suite 670
Denver, CO 80202
(303) 894-2430

Connecticut Board of Examiners
for Nursing
410 Capitol Ave., MS# 12 HSR
Hartford, CT 06134
(860) 509-7624

Delaware Board of Nursing
Cannon Bldg., Suite 203
P.O. Box 1401
Dover, DE 19903
(302) 739-4522

District of Columbia Board of
Nursing
614 H St. NW
Washington, DC 20001
(202) 727-7468

Florida Board of Nursing
4080 Woodcock Dr., Suite 202
Jacksonville, FL 32207
(904) 858-6940

Georgia Board of Nursing
166 Pryor St. SW
Atlanta, GA 30303
(404) 656-3943 RN (3921 PN)

Guam Board of Nurse
Examiners
P.O. Box 2816
Agana, Guam 96910
011 (671) 475-0251

Hawaii Board of Nursing
P.O. Box 3469
Honolulu, HI 96801
(808) 586-2695

Idaho Board of Nursing
P.O. Box 83720
Boise, ID 83720-0061
(208) 334-3110

Illinois Department of Profes-
sional Regulation
320 W. Washington St., 3rd Fl.
Springfield, IL 62786
(217) 785-9465/0800
    or
100 W. Randolph, #9-300
Chicago, IL 60601
(312) 814-2715

Indiana State Board
402 W. Washington St., #041
Indianapolis, IN 46204
(317) 232-2960

Iowa Board of Nursing
State Capitol Complex
1223 East Court Avenue
Des Moines, IA 50319
(515) 281-3255

Kansas Board of Nursing
Landon State Office
900 S.W. Jackson St., #551-S
Topeka, KS 66612
(913) 296-4929

Kentucky Board of Nursing
312 Wittington Parkway
Suite 300
Louisville, KY 40222-5172
(502) 329-7006

Louisiana State Board of
Nursing
3510 N. Causeway Blvd., Suite 501
Metairie, LA 70002
(504) 838-5332

Maine State Board of Nursing
158 State House Station
Augusta, ME 04333
(207) 287-1149

...nd Board of Nursing
...40 Patterson Ave.
Baltimore, MD 21215-2254
(410) 764-5124

Massachusetts Board of Registration in Nursing
Leverett Saltonstall Bldg.
100 Cambridge St., Rm. 1519
Boston, MA 02202
(617) 727-9961

State of Michigan CIS/Office of Health Services
Ottawa Towers North
611 W. Ottawa, 4th floor
Lansing, MI 48933
(517) 373-9102

Minnesota Board of Nursing
2829 University Avenue SE, #500
St Paul, MN 55414
(612) 617-2270

Mississippi Board of Nursing
239 N. Lamar St., #401
Jackson, MS 39201
(610) 359-6170

Missouri State Board of Nursing
P.O. Box 656
Jefferson City, MO 65102
(314) 751-0681

Montana Board of Nursing
111 N. Jackson
Helena, MT 59620-0407
(406) 444-2071

Nebraska Board of Nursing
P.O. Box 94986
Lincoln, NE 68509
(402) 471-4376

Nevada Board of Nursing
1755 E. Plumb Lane
Suite 260
Reno, NV 89502
(702) 786-2778

New Hampshire Board of Nursing
Health & Welfare Bldg
6 Hazen Drive
Concord, NH 03301
(603) 271-2323

New Jersey Board of Nursing
P.O. Box 45010
Newark, NJ 07101
(201) 504-6586

New Mexico Board of Nursing
4206 Louisiana Blvd. N.E.
Suite A
Albuquerque, NM 87109-1807
(505) 841-8340

New York Board of Nursing
Cultural Education Center
Room 3023
Albany, NY 12230
(518) 474-3843/3845

Northern Mariana Islands
Public Health Center
P.O. Box 1458
Saipan, MP 96950
011 (670) 234-8950/8954

North Carolina Board of Nursing
3724 National Drive
Raleigh, NC 27602
(919) 782-3211

North Dakota Board of Nursing
919 S. 7th St., Suite 504
Bismarck, ND 58504-5881
(701) 328-9777

Ohio Board of Nursing
77 S. High St., 17th Fl.
Columbus, OH 43215
(614) 466-3947

Oklahoma Board of Nursing
2915 N. Classen Blvd, Suite 524
Oklahoma City, OK 73106
(405) 525-2076

Oregon Board of Nursing
800 N.E. Oregon St., #25, Suite 465
Portland, OR 97232
(503) 731-4745

Pennsylvania Board of Nursing
P.O. Box 2649
Harrisburg, PA 17105
(717) 783-7142

Commonwealth of Puerto Rico Board of Nursing
Call Box 10200
Santurce, PR 00908
(809) 725-8161/7904

Rhode Island Board of Nursing
Cannon Health Bldg.
Three Capitol Hill, Rm. 104
Providence, RI 02908-5097
(401) 277-2827

South Carolina Board of Nursing
110 Centerview Drive
Suite 202
Columbia, SC 29210
(803) 896-4550

South Dakota Board of Nursing
3307 S. Lincoln Ave
Sioux Falls, SD 57105
(605) 367-5940

Tennessee Board of Nursing
426 5th Ave. North
1st fl—Cordell Hull Bldg.
Nashville, TN 37247
(615) 532-5166

Texas Board of Nurse Examiners
P.O. Box 430
Austin, TX 78767
(512) 305-7400

Utah Board of Nursing
160 E. 300 South
P.O. Box 45802
Salt Lake City, UT 84111
(801) 530-6628

Vermont Board of Nursing
109 State St.
Montpelier, VT 05609
(802) 828-2396

Virgin Islands Board of Nursing
Veterans Drive Station
St. Thomas, VI 00803
(340) 776-7397

Virginia Board of Nursing
6606 W. Board St., 4th Fl.
Richmond, VA 23230
(804) 662-9909

Washington State Board of Nursing
P.O. Box 47864
Olympia, WA 98504
(206) 753-2686

West Virginia Board of Examiners for Registered Professional Nurses
101 Dee Drive
Charleston, WV 25311
(304) 558-3596

Wisconsin Board of Nursing
1400 E. Washington Ave.
Madison, WI 53708
(608) 266-2112

Wyoming Board of Nursing
2020 Carey Ave., Suite 100
Cheyenne, WY 82002
(307) 777-7601